Primary Care
of Women

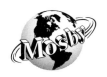

Visit our website at **www.mosby.com**

Primary Care of Women

Editors

KAREN J. CARLSON, MD

Director, Women's Health Associates
Massachusetts General Hospital
Assistant Professor of Medicine
Harvard Medical School
Massachusetts General Hospital
Boston, Massachusetts

STEPHANIE A. EISENSTAT, MD

Physician, Women's Health Associates
Department of Medicine, General Medical Unit
Massachusetts General Hospital
Assistant Professor of Medicine
Harvard Medical School
Boston, Massachusetts

Associate Editors

FREDRIC D. FRIGOLETTO, Jr, MD

Chief, Division of Obstetrics and General Gynecology
Massachusetts General Hospital
Charles Montraville Green and Robert Montraville Green
Professor of Obstetrics and Gynecology
Harvard Medical School
Boston, Massachusetts

ISAAC SCHIFF, MD

Chief, Vincent Obstetrics and Gynecology Service
Massachusetts General Hospital
Joe Vincent Meigs Professor of Gynecology
Harvard Medical School
Boston, Massachusetts

Second Edition

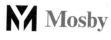 Mosby

An Affiliate of Elsevier

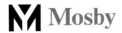

An Affiliate of Elsevier Science

Editor: Liz Fathman
Developmental Editor: Kristen Mandava
Publishing Services Manager: Patricia Tannian
Project Manager: Melissa Mraz Lastarria
Book Design Manager: Gail Morey Hudson
Cover Design: Teresa Breckwoldt

SECOND EDITION

Notice

Pharmacology is an ever-changing field. Standard safety precautions must be followed, but as new research and clinical experience broaden our knowledge, changes in treatment and drug therapy may become necessary or appropriate. Readers are advised to check the most current product information provided by the manufacturer of each drug to be administered to verify the recommended dose, the method and duration of administration, and contraindications. It is the responsibility of the licensed prescriber, relying on experience and knowledge of the patient, to determine dosages and the best treatment for each individual patient. Neither the publisher nor the editor assumes any liability for any injury and/or damage to persons or property arising from this publication.

Mosby, Inc.
An Affiliate of Elsevier
11830 Westline Industrial Drive
St. Louis, Missouri 63146

Printed in United States of America

Library of Congress Cataloging in Publication Data

Primary care of women / editors, Karen J. Carlson, Stephanie A. Eisenstat; associate editors, Fredric D. Frigoletto, Jr., Isaac Schiff. —2nd ed.
    p. ; cm.
   Includes bibliographical references and index.
   ISBN 0-323-01065-2
    1. Women—Medical care. 2. Women—Diseases. I. Carlson, Karen J. II. Eisenstat, Stephanie A.
  [DNLM: 1. Women's Health. 2. Primary Health Care. WA 309 P652 2002]
  RC48.6 .P752 2002
  616'.0082—dc21
                            2001052183

03   04   05 CL/MV 9 8 7 6 5 4 3 2

Contributors

RONALD J. ANDERSON, MD
Associate Professor of Medicine, Department of Medicine, Division of Rheumatology, Allergy and Immunology, Harvard Medical School; Director of Clinical Training Programs, Department of Medicine, Division of Rheumatology, Allergy and Immunology, Brigham and Women's Hospital; Boston, Massachusetts

MEREDITH AUGUST, DMD, MD
Assistant Professor, Department of Oral and Maxillofacial Surgery, Harvard School of Dental Medicine; Assistant Oral and Maxillofacial Surgeon, Massachusetts General Hospital; Boston, Massachusetts

JOHNNY T. AWWAD, MD
Assistant Professor, Department of Obstetrics and Gynecology, American University of Beirut Medical Center; Beirut, Lebanon

MARGARET H. BARON, MD, PhD
Irene and Dr. Arthur M. Fishberg Professor of Medicine, Department of Medicine-Hematology Division, Mount Sinai School of Medicine of New York University; Associate Professor, Department of Biochemistry and Molecular Biology, Ruttenberg Cancer Center and Institute for Gene Therapy and Molecular Medicine; New York, New York

JOSHUA A. BECKMAN, MD
Instructor of Medicine, Department of Medicine, Cardiovascular Division, Harvard Medical School; Associate Attending Physician, Department of Medicine, Brigham and Women's Hospital; Boston, Massachusetts

SUSAN E. BENNETT, MD
Assistant Professor of Medicine, Harvard Medical School; Associate in Medicine, Lown Cardiovascular Center, Brigham and Women's Hospital; Assistant Physician, Massachusetts General Hospital; Boston, Massachusetts

BONNIE L. BERMAS, MD
Instructor in Medicine, Department of Medicine, Harvard University; Associate Director of Clinical Affairs for Women's Health, Division of Women's Health and Rheumatology, Brigham and Women's Hospital; Boston, Massachusetts

KAREN J. CARLSON, MD
Assistant Professor of Medicine, Harvard Medical School; Director, Women's Health Associates, Massachusetts General Hospital; Boston, Massachusetts

DAVID L. CARR-LOCKE, MD, FRCP
Associate Professor, Harvard Medical School; Director, Endoscopy, Brigham and Women's Hospital; Boston, Massachusetts

GRACE CHANG, MD, MPH
Associate Professor, Department of Psychiatry, Harvard Medical School; Associate Physician, Department of Psychiatry, Brigham and Women's Hospital; Boston, Massachusetts

TANUJA CHITNIS, MD
Fellow in Neurology, Department of Neurology, Harvard Medical School; Clinical Fellow in Neurology, Centre for Neurologic Diseases, Brigham and Women's Hospital; Boston, Massachusetts

BUM-CHAE CHOI, MD
Associate Clinical Professor, Department of Obstetrics and Gynecology, Sungkyunkwan University School of Medicine; Seoul, Korea; Director, Department of Obstetrics and Gynecology Center for Recurrent Miscarriage and Infertility, Creation and Love Women's Hospital; Gwang-Jv, Korea

BARBARA ANN COCKRILL, MD
Assistant Professor of Medicine, Harvard Medical School; Assistant Physician, Pulmonary Critical Care Unit, Massachusetts General Hospital; Boston, Massachusetts

KAREN H. COSTENBADER, MD
Fellow, Harvard Medical School; Rheumatology Fellow, Department of Medicine, Division of Rheumatology, Massachusetts General Hospital; Boston, Massachusetts

M. CORNELIA CREMENS, MD
Instructor in Psychiatry and Medicine, Department of Psychiatry and Medicine, Harvard Medical School; Assistant in Psychiatry and Medicine, Massachusetts General Hospital; Boston, Massachusetts

SUSAN M. CUMMINGS, MS, RD
Clinical Programs Coordinator, Massachusetts General Hospital Weight Center, Massachusetts General Hospital; Boston, Massachusetts

COREY STEPHEN CUTLER, MD
Fellow in Hematology-Oncology, Department of Oncology, Dana-Farber Cancer Institute; Boston, Massachusetts

MICHELE G. CYR, MD
Associate Professor of Medicine, Department of Medicine, Brown University School of Medicine; Chief, Division of General Internal Medicine, Department of Medicine, Rhode Island Hospital; Providence, Rhode Island

DAVID M. DAWSON, MD
Professor, Department of Neurology, Harvard Medical School; Brigham and Women's Hospital; Boston, Massachusetts

SHEILA ANN DUGAN, MD, PT
Instructor, Physical Medicine and Rehabilitation, Harvard Medical School; Director of Musculoskeletal Rehabilitation, Department of Physical Medicine and Rehabilitation, Spaulding Rehabilitation Hospital; Clinical Associate, Department of Physical Medicine and Rehabilitation, Massachusetts General Hospital; Associate Physician, Department of Rheumatology and Medicine, Brigham and Women's Hospital; Boston, Massachusetts

LINDA R. DUSKA, MD
Assistant Professor, Harvard Medical School; Assistant in Gynecology and Obstetrics, Vincent Gynecology Service, Division of Gynecologic Oncology, Massachusetts General Hospital; Boston, Massachusetts

BARBARA A. DWORETZKY, MD
Assistant Professor of Neurology, Department of Neurology, Boston Veterans Administration Medical Center; Director, Division of Behavioral Neurology, Department of Neurology, Boston Veterans Administration Medical Center; Boston, Massachusetts

STEPHANIE A. EISENSTAT, MD
Assistant Professor of Medicine, Harvard Medical School; Physician, Women's Health Associates, General Medicine Unit, Department of Medicine, Massachusetts General Hospital; Boston, Massachusetts

DONNA FELSENSTEIN, MD
Assistant Professor of Medicine, Harvard School of Medicine; Physician in Medicine, Department of Infectious Disease, Massachusetts General Hospital; Director of the Sexually Transmitted Disease Unit; Boston, Massachusetts

PATRICIA A. FRASER, MD, MPH, MS
Assistant Professor of Medicine, Harvard Medical School; Associate Physician, Director of Pediatric Rheumatology, Department of Medicine, Brigham and Women's Hospital; Boston, Massachusetts

LAWRENCE S. FRIEDMAN, MD
Associate Professor of Medicine, Harvard Medical School; Physician, Gastrointestinal Unit and Chief, Walter Bauer Firm (Medical Services), Massachusetts General Hospital; Boston, Massachusetts

MARIE GERHARD-HERMAN, MD, RUT, FACC
Assistant Professor of Medicine, Harvard Medical School; Medical Director, Vascular Diagnostic Laboratory, Brigham and Women's Hospital; Boston, Massachusetts

SOHEYLA DANA GHARIB, MD
Assistant Professor, Department of Medicine, Harvard Medical School; Medical Director, Divisions of General Medicine and Women's Health; Boston, Massachusetts

ELIZABETH S. GINSBURG, MD
Assistant Professor of Obstetrics, Gynecology, and Reproductive Biology, Harvard Medical School, Brigham and Women's Hospital; Medical Director of IUE, Department of Obstetrics and Gynecology; Boston, Massachusetts

JULIE GLOWACKI, PhD
Associate Professor, Department of Orthopedic Surgery, Harvard Medical School; Director, Skeletal Biology Laboratories, Department of Orthopedic Surgery, Brigham and Women's Hospital; Associate Professor, Department of Oral and Maxillofacial Surgery, Harvard School of Dental Medicine; Boston, Massachusetts

SAMUEL Z. GOLDHABER, MD
Associate Professor of Medicine, Cardiovascular Division, Harvard Medical School; Director, Venous Thromboembolism Research Group, Director, Cardiac Center's Anticoagulation Service, Department of Cardiology, Brigham and Women's Hospital; Boston, Massachusetts

MICHAEL F. GREENE, MD
Associate Professor of Obstetrics, Gynecology, and Reproductive Biology, Department of Obstetrics and Gynecology, Harvard Medical School; Director of Maternal-Fetal Medicine, Vincent Memorial Obstetrics Division, Massachusetts General Hospital; Boston, Massachusetts

JOSEPH A. GROCELA, MD
Instructor in Surgery, Harvard Medical School; Urology Service, Department of Urology, Massachusetts General Hospital; Boston, Massachusetts

JANET ELIZABETH HALL, MD
Associate Professor of Medicine, Harvard Medical School; Department of Medicine, Reproductive Endocrine Unit, Massachusetts General Hospital; Boston, Massachusetts

LINDA J. HEFFNER, MD, PhD
Associate Professor, Department of Obstetrics and Gynecology, Harvard Medical School; Director of Maternal-Fetal Medicine, Department of Obstetrics and Gynecology, Brigham and Women's Hospital; Boston, Massachusetts

SUSAN E. HERZ, JD, MPH
Adjunct Faculty Member, Massachusetts College of Pharmacy, Northeastern University, Suffolk University, Boston, Massachusetts; Senior Research Associate, Center for Applied Ethics on Professional Practice, Education Development Center, Inc; Newton, Massachusetts

JOSEPH A. HILL, MD
Associate Professor of Obstetrics, Gynecology, and Reproductive Biology, Harvard Medical School; Director, Reproductive Medicine, Department of Obstetrics, Gynecology, and Reproductive Biology, Brigham and Women's Hospital; Boston, Massachusetts

JENNIFER HO, MD
Medical Student, Harvard Medical School;
Boston, Massachusetts

KEITH B. ISAACSON, MD
Associate Professor, Harvard Medical School, Department of
Obstetrics and Gynecology, Massachusetts General Hospital;
Boston, Massachusetts

LINDA S. JAFFE, MD
Instructor in Medicine, Department of Medicine, Harvard Medical
School; Associate Physician, Department of Medicine, Brigham
and Women's Hospital; Boston, Massachusetts

PHYLLIS JEN, MD
Assistant Professor, Department of Medicine, Division of General
Medicine, Harvard Medical School; Medical Director, Brigham
Internal Medicine Association, Brigham and Women's Hospital;
Boston, Massachusetts

PAULA A. JOHNSON, MD, MPH
Assistant Professor of Medicine, Department of Medicine,
Harvard Medical School; Director, Department of Quality
Management Services, Department of Medicine, Cardiovascular
Division, Brigham and Women's Hospital; Boston, Massachusetts

LEE M. KAPLAN, MD, PhD
Associate Professor of Medicine, Department of Medicine,
Harvard Medical School; Director, Massachusetts General
Hospital Weight Center, Massachusetts General Hospital; Boston,
Massachusetts

JEFFREY N. KATZ, MD, MS
Associate Professor of Medicine, Department of Medicine,
Harvard Medical School; Staff Physician, Co-Director Spine
Center, Department of Rheumatology, Immunology, and Allergy,
Brigham and Women's Hospital; Boston, Massachusetts

MARTHA ELLEN KATZ, MD
Clinical Instructor, Department of Medicine; Lecturer,
Department of Social Medicine, Harvard Medical School;
Associate Physician, Department of General Medicine, Brigham
and Women's Hospital; Assistant Physician, Department of
Medicine, Children's Hospital; Boston, Massachusetts

LAURENCE KATZNELSON, MD
Assistant Professor of Medicine, Department of Medicine,
Harvard Medical School; Assistant Physician, Department of
Medicine, Massachusetts General Hospital; Boston,
Massachusetts

JOHN M. KAUFFMAN, MD
Instructor in Medicine, Harvard Medical School; Associate
Physician, Gastroenterology Division, Brigham and Women's
Hospital; Boston, Massachusetts

POWELL H. KAZANJIAN, MD
Director of HIV/AIDS Program, Associate Professor of Internal
Medicine, University of Michigan Medical Center; Detroit,
Michigan

ROBYN S. KLEIN, MD, PhD
Instructor in Medicine, Department of Infectious Disease, Harvard
Medical School; Clinical Assistant in Medicine, Department of
Infectious Disease, Massachusetts General Hospital; Boston,
Massachusetts

ANNE KLIBANSKI, MD
Professor of Medicine, Department of Medicine, Harvard Medical
School; Chief Neuroendocrine Unit, Department of Medicine,
Massachusetts General Hospital; Boston, Massachusetts

ANTHONY L. KOMAROFF, MD, FACP
Professor of Medicine and Editor-in-Chief, Harvard Health
Publications, Department of Medicine, Harvard Medical School;
Senior Physician, Department of Medicine, Brigham and
Women's Hospital; Boston, Massachusetts

NICOLE B. KORBLY, BA
Research Coordinator, Anxiety Disorders Program, Department of
Psychiatry, Massachusetts General Hospital; Boston,
Massachusetts

IRENE KUTER, MD, DPhil
Assistant Professor, Department of Medicine, Harvard Medical
School; Associate Physician, Massachusetts General Hospital;
Boston, Massachusetts

JOSEPH C. KVEDAR, MD
Assistant Professor of Dermatology, Department of Dermatology,
Harvard Medical School; Assistant Dermatologist, Department of
Dermatology, Massachusetts General Hospital; Boston,
Massachusetts

CAROL LANDAU, PhD
Clinical Professor, Department of Psychiatry and Human
Behavior, Brown University School of Medicine; Consulting
Psychologist, Chair, Behavioral Sciences Committee, Division of
General Internal Medicine, Rhode Island Hospital; Providence,
Rhode Island

CAROLYN S. LANGER, MD, JD, MPH
Instructor in Occupational Medicine, Harvard School of Public
Health; Boston, Massachusetts

RUTH A. LAWRENCE, MD
Professor of Pediatrics and Obstetrics and Gynecology,
Department of Pediatrics, University of Rochester School of
Medicine and Dentistry; Physician, Department of Pediatrics,
Strong Memorial Hospital; Rochester, New York

MATTHEW H. LIANG, MD, MPH
Professor of Medicine, Department of Medicine, Harvard Medical
School; Staff Physician, Department of Medicine, Brigham and
Women's Hospital; Boston, Massachusetts

ROBERT C. LOWE, MD
Instructor, Harvard Medicine School; Associate Physician,
Department of Medicine, Brigham and Women's Hospital;
Boston, Massachusetts

JAMES A. MacLEAN, MD
Assistant Professor of Medicine, Harvard Medical School;
Assistant Chief, Allergy Unit, Massachusetts General Hospital;
Boston, Massachusetts

KATHRYN A. MARTIN, MD
Assistant Professor of Medicine, Department of Medicine,
Harvard Medical School; Director, Reproductive Endocrine
Medicine, Reproductive Endocrine Unit, Massachusetts General
Hospital; Boston, Massachusetts

KELLY A. McGARRY, MD
Assistant Professor, Department of Medicine, Brown University
School of Medicine; Associate Program Director of Residency,
Division of General Internal Medicine, Rhode Island Hospital;
Providence, Rhode Island

ROSEANNA H. MEANS, MD, MSC
Clinical Instructor, Harvard Medical School; Associate Physician,
Department of Medicine, Brigham and Women's Hospital;
Boston, Massachusetts

HAROLD MICHLEWITZ, MD
Clinical Instructor in Obstetrics, Gynecology, and Reproductive
Biology, Harvard Medical School; Department of Obstetrics,
Gynecology, and Reproductive Biology, Massachusetts General
Hospital; Boston, Massachusetts

FELISE B. MILAN, MD
Associate Professor of Clinical Medicine, Department of
Medicine, Albert Einstein College of Medicine, Montefiore
Medical Center; Bronx, New York

A. JACQUELINE MITUS, MD
Associate Physician, Hematology-Oncology Division, Department
of Medicine, Brigham and Women's Hospital; Instructor in
Medicine, Harvard Medical School; Boston, Massachusetts

ANNE W. MOULTON, MD
Associate Professor of Medicine, Brown University School of
Medicine; Associate Physician, Division of General Internal
Medicine, Rhode Island Hospital; Director, Fellowship in General
Internal Medicine, Division of General Internal Medicine, Rhode
Island Hospital; Providence, Rhode Island

TOUFIC I. NAKAD, MD
House Officer, Harvard Medical School, Harvard University;
Fellow, Reproductive Endocrinology and Infertility, Vincent
Centre of Reproductive Medicine, Massachusetts General
Hospital; Boston, Massachusetts

OLIVIA I. OKEREKE, MD
Clinical Fellow in Psychiatry, Harvard Medical School; Resident
in Psychiatry, Massachusetts General Hospital; Boston,
Massachusetts

LORI D. OLANS, MD, MPH
Assistant Professor of Medicine, Tufts University School of
Medicine; Assistant Physician, Department of Medicine, Division
of Gastroenterology, New England Medical Center Hospitals;
Boston, Massachusetts

L. CHRISTINE OLIVER, MD, MPH, MS
Assistant Clinical Professor, Department of Medicine, Harvard
Medical School; Associate Physician, Department of Medicine,
Massachusetts General Hospital; Boston, Massachusetts

RAPIN OSATHANONDH, MD
Associate Professor of Obstetrics and Gynecology, Harvard
Medical School; Department of Obstetrics and Gynecology,
Brigham and Women's Hospital; Boston, Massachusetts

KRISTINE PHILLIPS, MD, PhD
Clinical Fellow, Division of Rheumatology, Brigham and
Women's Hospital; Boston, Massachusetts

MAY C.M. PIAN-SMITH, MD, MS
Instructor, Department of Anesthesia and Critical Care, Harvard
Medical School; Attending Anesthesiologist/Assistant-in-
Anesthesiology, Department of Anesthesia and Critical Care,
Massachusetts General Hospital; Boston, Massachusetts

JOHN M. PONEROS, MD
Research Fellow in Gastroenterology, Department of Medicine,
Massachusetts General Hospital; Boston, Massachusetts

ATHENA POPPAS, MD
Assistant Professor, Section of Cardiology, Brown University; Co-
Director Echocardiography, Department of Cardiology, Rhode
Island Hospital; Providence, Rhode Island

JANEY S.A. PRATT, MD
Instructor in Surgery, Department of Surgery, Harvard Medical
School; Assistant in Surgery, Department of Surgery,
Massachusetts General Hospital; Boston, Massachusetts

DAVID M. RAPOPORT, MD
Associate Professor of Clinical Medicine, Department of
Medicine; Medical Director, Sleep Disorders Center, New York
University School of Medicine; New York, New York

NEERAJ RASTOGI, BE DNB
Research Fellow, Department of Urology, Massachusetts General
Hospital; Boston, Massachusetts

NANCY A. RIGOTTI, MD
Associate Professor, Department of Medicine, Harvard Medical
School; Director, Tobacco Research and Treatment Center,
Massachusetts General Hospital; Boston, Massachusetts

DOUGLAS S. ROSS, MD
Associate Professor of Medicine, Harvard Medical School; Co-
Director, Thurud Associates, Massachusetts General Hospital;
Boston, Massachusetts

RAJA A. SAYEGH, MD
Assistant Professor, Department of Medicine, Obstetrics and
Gynecology, Boston University School of Medicine; Department
of Obstetrics and Gynecology, Boston Medical Center; Boston,
Massachusetts

ISAAC SCHIFF, MD
Joe Vincent Meigs Professor of Gynecology, Harvard Medical School; Chief, Vincent Obstetrics and Gynecology Service, Massachusetts General Hospital; Boston, Massachusetts

ELLEN W. SEELY, MD
Assistant Professor, Department of Medicine, Harvard Medical School; Assistant Professor, Director of Clinical Research, Endocrine-Hypertension Division, Department of Medicine, Brigham and Women's Hospital; Boston, Massachusetts

JULIAN LAWRENCE SEIFTER, MD
Associate Professor of Medicine, Harvard Medical School; Department of Medicine, Brigham and Women's Hospital; Boston, Massachusetts

MARGARET SETON, MD
Assistant Professor of Medicine, Department of Medicine, Harvard University School of Medicine; Boston, Massachusetts; Chief of Rheumatology, Department of Medicine, Cambridge Health Alliance; Medical Director, Women's Health Task Force; Cambridge, Massachusetts; Staff Physician, Arthritis Unit, Massachusetts General Hospital; Boston, Massachusetts

LINDA SHAFER, MD
Instructor in Psychiatry, Department of Psychiatry, Harvard Medical School; Psychiatrist, Department of Psychiatry, Massachusetts General Hospital; Boston, Massachusetts

ELLEN ELIZABETH SHEETS, MD
Associate Professor, Obstetrics, Gynecology, and Reproductive Medicine, Harvard Medical School; Director, Pap Smear Evaluation Center, Associate Director, Gynecologic Oncology, Department of Obstetrics and Gynecology, Brigham and Women's Hospital; Boston, Massachusetts

JAN L. SHIFREN, MD
Assistant Professor, Department of Obstetrics, Gynecology, and Reproductive Biology, Harvard Medical School; Reproductive Endocrinologist, Vincent Obstetrics and Gynecology Service, Massachusetts General Hospital; Boston, Massachusetts

ROBERT H. SHMERLING, MD, FACP
Associate Professor of Medicine, Department of Medicine, Harvard Medical School; Associate Physician, Department of Medicine, Beth Israel Deaconess Medical Center; Boston, Massachusetts

IRIS SHUEY, MD
Clinical Assistant Professor, Department of Psychiatry and Human Behavior, Brown University School of Medicine; Providence, Rhode Island

LAWRENCE N. SHULMAN, MD
Associate Professor of Medicine, Harvard Medical School; Vice-Chair for Clinical Services, Department of Adult Oncology, Dana-Faber Cancer Institute; Boston, Massachusetts

NAOMI M. SIMON, MD
Instructor, Department of Psychiatry, Harvard Medical School; Associate Director, Anxiety Disorders Program, Department of Psychiatry, Massachusetts General Hospital; Boston, Massachusetts

DAVID M. SLOVIK, MD
Assistant Professor of Medicine, Harvard Medical School; Chief of Medicine, Department of Medicine, Spaulding Rehabilitation Hospital; Associate Physician, Department of Endocrinology, Massachusetts General Hospital; Boston, Massachusetts

BARBARA L. SMITH, MD, PhD
Assistant Professor of Surgery, Harvard Medical School; Co-Director Gillette Center for Women's Cancers, Massachusetts General Hospital; Chief Breast Surgery Service, Gillette Center for Women's Cancers, Dana Farber Cancer Institute; Boston, Massachusetts

OLGA SMULDERS-MEYER, MD
Instructor in Medicine, Department of Medicine, Harvard Medical School; Assistant in Medicine, Department of Medicine, Massachusetts General Hospital; Boston, Massachusetts

CAREN G. SOLOMON, MD, MPH
Assistant Professor, Department of Medicine, Harvard Medical School; Associate Physician, Brigham and Women's Hospital; Boston, Massachusetts

FARZANEH A. SOROND, MD, PhD
Stroke Fellow, Department of Neurology, Harvard Medical School; Stroke Fellow, Department of Neurology, Brigham and Women's Hospital; Boston, Massachusetts

EGILIUS L.H. SPIERINGS, MD, PRD
Associate Clinical Professor of Neurology, Department of Neurology, Harvard Medical School; Consultant in Neurology, Department of Neurology, Brigham and Women's Hospital; Boston, Massachusetts

MICHAEL R. STELLUTO, MD
Assistant Professor, Department of Obstetrics, Gynecology, and Reproductive Biology, Harvard Medical School; Obstetrician and Gynecologist, Department of Obstetrics and Gynecology, Brigham and Women's Hospital; Boston, Massachusetts

ANN E. TAYLOR, MD
Assistant Professor of Medicine, Harvard Medical School; Assistant Physician, Department of Reproductive Endocrine Unit, Massachusetts General Hospital; Boston, Massachusetts

KATHLEEN F. THURMOND, MD
Clinical Instructor in Obstetrics, Gynecology, and Reproductive Biology, Harvard Medical School; Consultant in Gynecology and Obstetrics, Vincent Memorial Gynecology Services, Massachusetts General Hospital; Boston, Massachusetts

ERIN E. TRACY, MD, MPH
Instructor, Obstetrics, Gynecology, and Reproductive Biology, Harvard Medical School; Attending Physician, Vincent Obstetrics and Gynecology, Massachusetts General Hospital; Boston, Massachusetts

KATHARINE K. TREADWAY, MD
Assistant Professor of Medicine, Department of Medicine,
Harvard Medical School; Physician, Department of Medicine,
Massachusetts General Hospital; Boston, Massachusetts

KATHLEEN HUBBS ULMAN, PhD
Instructor, Department of Psychiatry, Harvard Medical School;
Assistant in Psychology, Massachusetts General Hospital; Boston,
Massachusetts

ADELE C. VIGUERA, MD
Instructor, Department of Psychiatry, Harvard Medical School;
Associate Director of the Prenatal and Reproductive Psychiatry
Program, Massachusetts General Hospital; Boston, Massachusetts

MAY M. WAKAMATSU, MD
Clinical Instructor, Gynecology and Reproductive Biology,
Harvard Medical School; Assistant in Gynecology, Department of
Gynecology, Massachusetts General Hospital; Boston,
Massachusetts

JOYCE A. WALSLEBEN, RN, PhD
Research Associate Professor of Medicine, Department of
Medicine, New York University School of Medicine; Director,
New York University Sleep Disorder Center, Pulmonary
Department, New York University School of Medicine; New York,
New York

LOUISE WILKINS-HAUG, MD, PhD
Assistant Professor, Harvard Medical School; Medical Director,
Antenatal Diagnostic Center, Department of Obstetrics and
Gynecology, Brigham and Women's Hospital; Boston,
Massachusetts

JACQUELINE L. WOLF, MD
Associate Professor of Medicine, Harvard Medical School;
Director, Inflammatory Bowel Disease Center, Department of
Medicine, Gastroenterology Division, Brigham and Women's
Hospital; Boston, Massachusetts

BARBARA J. WOO, MD
Instructor, Harvard Medical School; Associate Physician in
Medicine, Department of Medicine, Massachusetts General
Hospital; Boston, Massachusetts

MYLENE W.M. YAO, MD
Clinical Fellow, Reproductive Endocrinology and Infertility,
Department of Obstetrics and Gynecology, Harvard Medical
School; Clinical Fellow, Reproductive Endocrinology and
Infertility, Department of Obstetrics and Gynecology, Brigham
and Women's Hospital; Boston, Massachusetts

Foreword

In the past 30 years there has been a remarkable growth of interest in the medical problems of women, as both the number of female physicians and the number of female patients who seek female physicians have increased. Thirty years ago in the United States, only 5% to 10% of medical school graduates were women, and most male and female patients (except black women) stated a strong preference for male physicians. Today, nearly one half of medical school graduates are women, and many women in the United States express a strong preference for female physicians. In addition, there is increased research support to study medical problems that predominate in or are exclusive to women, and a belated inclusion of women in studies of major diseases, such as coronary artery disease.

The past 30 years has also seen a resurgence of interest in primary care medicine. The explosion of knowledge generated by the growing investment in medical research and technology after the end of World War II led to a submersion of primary care medicine in the United States as specialties and subspecialties formed and grew. Whereas there were four primary care physicians for every specialist in the United States before World War II, there are now two specialists for every one primary care physician.

This proliferation of specialties created centrifugal forces in medicine and led to fragmentation of medical care as many patients sought and received care directly from specialized providers. For women, the fragmentation of care was compounded by very real needs for specialized care related to pregnancy and birth, menopause, cancers of the breast and reproductive organs, and other conditions that affect only women. As a result, primary care of women is provided in varied ways. Some women receive primary care from a general internist or family physician and one or more subspecialists. Other women (primarily healthy, premenopausal women) seek medical care primarily from a gynecologist and, during pregnancies, from an obstetrician. However, the growing body of knowledge about the medical problems of women is not comprehensively taught by training programs in internal medicine, family medicine, or obstetrics and gynecology.

This book successfully links and synthesizes knowledge from all of these disciplines. The section on medical disease will be of special interest to obstetricians and gynecologists, and the section on gynecology and obstetrics will be of special interest to internists and family physicians. The sections on behavioral medicine and prevention will be useful to doctors from all disciplines because these fields tend to be shortchanged in medical school and residency training.

The book also responds to another problem in women's health care. In this country and elsewhere, widespread variation in the treatment of conditions that are specific to women has been documented. Rates of hysterectomy vary fivefold or more from one geographic area to another. Similar variation has been documented for rates of cesarean section and for rates of mastectomy rather than breast-conserving surgery for women with early-stage breast cancer. Some nonsurgical treatment decisions are equally variable: whether a woman receives hormone replacement therapy may depend more on the training of the physician she sees than on her risk factors or personal preferences. Variations in medical practice and the questions these raise about the consistency and quality of medical decision making are not peculiar to women's health care. There is a general need for both better information about which interventions are most effective for different patients and better communication about the values and preferences of those who live with the results of medical care. However, gender differences between doctor and patient can impede effective communication about values and preferences, which is one factor behind many women's preference for female physicians. The authors of this book address this problem by being continually aware of the female patient's perspective.

The book is thorough and detailed in its treatment of all problems. It is well organized so that the reader can quickly find an answer to a particular question. The contributing authors, mostly from the faculties of two major teaching hospitals—Brigham and Women's Hospital and Massachusetts General Hospital, both major teaching hospitals of Harvard Medical School—have produced chapters of uniformly high quality. This book will provide an invaluable resource for any clinician who is committed to providing primary health care to women.

Anthony L. Komaroff, MD
Professor of Medicine and Editor-in-Chief, Harvard Health Publications, Department of Medicine, Harvard Medical School; Senior Physician, Department of Medicine, Brigham and Women's Hospital, Boston, Massachusetts

Albert G. Mulley, MD, MPP
Associate Professor of Medicine, Associate Professor of Health Policy, Harvard Medical School; Chief, General Medicine Division, Massachusetts General Hospital, Boston, Massachusetts

Preface

The first edition of *Primary Care of Women* was conceived in the midst of unprecedented transformation of the health care system in the United States and of the position of women within that system. A central feature of this transformation has been the recognition of the value of primary care and the importance of integrating the perspectives of multiple medical specialties to provide care for the whole woman. Particularly for women, the emphasis on specialization that dominated Western medicine since the 1950s has sometimes resulted in fragmentation of care. An interdisciplinary approach to health care is a core element of the new definition of women's health that has emerged in the past twenty years.

A second feature of this transformation of medical practice has been recognition of the gaps in scientific knowledge that underlie clinical practice; for women, these gaps are often particularly wide. In recent years government and scientific institutions have acknowledged the exclusion of women from much of past medical research. Many efforts are under way to establish a more scientific basis for clinical practice by studying disorders that manifest differently in or are exclusive to women.

Finally, medical practice has been changed by greater emphasis on the central role of the patient in the process of care. An important stimulus for this change was the lay women's health movement, which has critically questioned the scientific assumptions and social practices of medicine for over three decades. The concurrent infusion of female physicians into the medical profession has also had a major impact on this trend.

The purpose of this book is to provide a concise, practical reference for clinicians engaged in the primary care of women. Its subject matter includes the following:

1. Problems encountered in primary care practice that manifest differently, or respond differently to treatment, in women compared with men. Examples include coronary artery disease, human immunodeficiency virus infection, and alcohol abuse.
2. Problems that occur more commonly in women, such as osteoporosis, thyroid disorders, and gallstones.
3. Problems that occur exclusively in women, such as gynecologic and obstetric problems and certain endocrinopathies.

In addition to problems or diseases treated largely by the primary care clinician, the content includes problems about which the primary care provider must be knowledgeable even though care is managed by a subspecialist, for example, breast cancer. The book contains a section on psychology and behavior, which provides a framework for addressing many of the problems that prompt women to seek medical care, such as depression, obesity, and domestic violence. Finally, prevention and early detection of disease through screening, essential aspects of primary care practice, are reviewed.

An important feature is the inclusion of material on the interaction of pregnancy with medical illness. This material considers a range of issues relevant to the care of women in their childbearing years, including the effects of specific medical problems on fertility and on maternal and fetal health; the effects of pregnancy on existing diseases; the evaluation and management of problems in early pregnancy; and modification of treatment during pregnancy.

The second edition of *Primary Care of Women* expands substantially on the first edition. Material in original chapters has been carefully updated to reflect changes in scientific knowledge and clinical practice over the past five years. A significant number of new chapters have been added, covering a diverse group of subjects ranging from sports injuries to sleep disorders to care of women with disabilities. Finally, formatting has been improved throughout to allow greater accessibility of the material to the busy primary care practitioner.

This book is directed to all clinicians who provide primary care to adult female patients, including internists, family practitioners, obstetrician-gynecologists, nurse practitioners, physician assistants, medical subspecialists, and physicians-in-training. We recognize that the content of care varies in different settings; in some areas, obstetrician-gynecologists and medical subspecialists are important sources of primary care. In outlining recommendations regarding indications for referral, the convention in this book assumes that referral will be needed for many procedures, although some are routinely performed by some primary care clinicians.

We hope that the interdisciplinary and interinstitutional collaboration represented in this book will make it useful for a wide spectrum of clinicians and will promote more integrated, comprehensive, and effective care for women. For us, creating this book has been an opportunity to deepen our long-standing collaborations with our subspecialty colleagues, associate editors Dr. Fredric Frigoletto and Dr. Isaac Schiff. We are indebted to them for their essential role in shaping the sections on Obstetrics and Gynecology. We have worked side by side with most of the contributing authors in the care of patients at Massachusetts General Hospital and Brigham and Women's Hospital. To these valued colleagues, we owe our sincerest thanks for sharing their clinical expertise with the professional community through this book.

Our colleagues at Elsevier Science in St. Louis have remained exemplary in their professionalism and support. We thank our editor, Liz Fathman, and our developmental editor, Kristen Mandava, for their efforts in bringing the second edition to fruition.

The scientific basis for the clinical practice of primary care for women is an evolving body of knowledge. Current research related to women's health promises to provide new answers to clinical questions and to suggest new approaches to care. We welcome comments and questions from readers to ensure that future editions of this book further address the needs of clinicians engaged in the primary care of women.

Karen J. Carlson, MD
Stephanie A. Eisenstat, MD
Boston, Massachusetts

Contents

CARDIOVASCULAR DISORDERS

III PSYCHOLOGY AND BEHAVIORAL MEDICINE

COMMON PSYCHOLOGICAL PROBLEMS

IV PREVENTION

CANCER SCREENING

PART I
Medical Disease in Women

CHAPTER **1**

Chest Pain

Anne W. Moulton

▓ EPIDEMIOLOGY

Chest pain is a common outpatient medical problem, particularly in women. Approximately 200,000 new cases of noncardiac chest pain are identified each year in the United States. In one study of outpatient practices, two thirds of all chest pain diagnoses fell into one of three categories: angina, musculoskeletal chest pain, and pain related to the gastrointestinal tract.

Twenty percent of patients referred for cardiac catheterization for the evaluation of chest pain have normal coronary arteries; more than half are women. Most patients with normal coronary arteries at catheterization have a benign course, with a very low incidence of myocardial infarction (1%) or cardiac death (0.6%). Although the mortality rate is low, the morbidity associated with noncardiac chest pain can be high. Many patients may have an incomplete understanding of their diagnosis and may suffer persistent symptoms and decreased function because of fear of heart disease. One half regards themselves as disabled.

Patients who consult a primary care physician for symptoms of chest pain may describe an acute onset of pain, but more often it is chronic in nature. Although the initial goal in evaluating a woman with chest pain is to exclude coronary disease and other serious causes, it is also important to attempt to establish a specific diagnosis to guide therapy and provide reassurance. The history and physical examination have been shown to be sufficient for correctly diagnosing nonorganic chest pain (that is, not due to cardiac, gastrointestinal, or pulmonary disease) versus organic chest pain in almost 90% of cases.

Box 1-1 lists the various causes of chest pain in women, and Fig. 1-1 describes the evaluation of chest pain in women.

CARDIAC CAUSES

Ischemic chest pain resulting from epicardial coronary artery disease may present in women with classic symptoms of exertional chest pain, pressure, or heaviness lasting a few minutes, sometimes radiating to the neck, jaw, or shoulder. Women also more frequently experience nontypical angina,

including chest discomfort, nausea, or abdominal pain during rest, sleep, or mental stress. Age and the presence of cardiac risk factors (Box 1-2) can be used to estimate the likelihood of coronary artery disease in a woman presenting with chest pain. The effect of exercise test results on modifying these probabilities is discussed in Chapter 2.

A small minority of women with angina and normal coronary arteries may have myocardial ischemia caused by **microvascular angina.** Patients with this syndrome, the majority of whom are women, have angina-like chest pain, ischemic ST-segment depressions on electrocardiography during exercise testing, angiographically normal coronary arteries, normal ventricular function, and an excellent prognosis (see Chapter 2).

In patients who experience pleuritic chest pain the diagnosis of **pericarditis** must be considered. Potential causes of pericarditis include idiopathic (40%), viral (20%), connective tissue disease (16%), uremia (6%), bacterial infection (7%), and malignancy (7%). It is likely that the majority of cases of community-acquired idiopathic pericarditis are due to unrecognized viral infections. The seasonal peak of pericarditis is in the spring and fall. The most common viral causes are Coxsackie A and B, echovirus, and adenovirus. Other potential viruses include mumps, influenza, mononucleosis, varicella, rubella, hepatitis B, and HIV.

In about 50% of cases of pericarditis there is a prodrome of upper respiratory tract infection. Diagnosis can be made by the finding, in some cases, of a characteristic pericardial friction rub. Electrocardiographic changes are not specific but may include depressed PR segments and diffusely elevated ST segments. Echocardiographic documentation of a pericardial effusion is helpful. The illness, although short and dramatic, is usually self-limited, lasting 1 to 3 weeks.

Viral myocarditis can also present as chest pain, usually in the context of a recent febrile illness and often with significant myalgias. The most likely viruses are Coxsackie virus, echovirus, adenovirus, and influenza. Patients with **dilated cardiomyopathy** can present with chest pain, although symptoms of congestive failure predominate. Although about 50% of the cases of dilated cardiomyopathy are idiopathic, other potential etiologies include pregnancy, alcohol abuse, hypertension, and infection.

BOX 1-1
Causes of Chest Pain in Women

Cardiac
Ischemic heart disease
Mitral valve prolapse
Pericarditis
Hypertrophic cardiomyopathy
Aortic aneurysm
Microvascular angina
Abnormal cardiac sensitivity

Pulmonary
Pleurisy
Pneumonia
Pulmonary embolism
Pneumothorax

Gastrointestinal
Esophageal disorders
Nutcracker esophagus
Nonspecific esophageal motility disorders
Diffuse esophageal spasm
Hypertensive lower esophageal sphincter
Achalasia
Esophageal reflux
Peptic ulcer disease
Irritable bowel syndrome
Gallbladder disease

Musculoskeletal
Costochondritis/xiphoiditis
Cervical and thoracic osteoarthritis
Muscular strain
Fibromyalgia

Psychologic
Panic disorder
Anxiety and/or depression
Somatization
Hyperventilation
Substance abuse

Other
Chest pain associated with menopausal transition
Herpes zoster
Breast disorders

Chest pain, usually in association with dyspnea, may represent the relatively rare syndrome of **hypertrophic cardiomyopathy.** Diagnosis is suggested by a S4 or a systolic murmur at the left sternal border that is increased with the Valsalva maneuver.

An electrocardiogram (ECG) most often reveals left ventricular hypertrophy or an increased Q-wave suggestive of an old myocardial infarction (MI), with no clinical history to suggest prior infarction. Echocardiography is essential for making the diagnosis and assessing the severity of the condition.

The association of **mitral valve prolapse** (MVP) with chest pain is controversial. MVP occurs in 3% to 4% or

more of the population, making it one of the most common cardiovascular conditions. It is eight times more common in women than men, but complications are more common in men. Chest pain in association with MVP, although rare, has actually been reported as more common in both men and women. Diagnosis of MVP is suggested by a characteristic murmur or click, as well as echocardiography.

Dissecting **aortic aneurysm** is usually of acute onset, with a tearing pain noted in the anterior or posterior chest that radiates to the arms, legs, and abdomen. This process, which typically occurs in persons in their 60s and 70s, is more common in men, with a male/female ratio of 2:1. In most cases the pain is so severe that patients are taken immediately to an emergency setting, but in cases where there is a slow leak of blood through the intima, the presentation may be more subtle. Women who experience symptoms from an enlarging aneurysm are more likely to be older and to seek medical attention at the time of rupture of their aneurysm. Bilateral pulses and blood pressure measurements may be unequal, and there may be widening of the mediastinum indicated on chest radiograph. The definitive diagnosis is made with angiography.

PULMONARY CAUSES

Pleurisy appears to occur in women twice as much as in men. It is described as a sharp unilateral chest pain that may be referred to the shoulders, neck, or abdomen. It is often associated with splinting of the chest wall and shallow respiration. A pleural friction rub may occasionally be auscultated over the affected area. Pleurisy is caused by inflammation of the pleura, most often related to viral infection, but sometimes attributable to a collagen vascular disease.

Pneumonia should be considered in any patient who has chest pain accompanied by other symptoms, such as fever and persistent cough. Patients with bronchitis or acute exacerbation of asthma may also complain of chest pain with cough, presumed secondary to inflammation of the chest wall.

One of the most frequently underdiagnosed conditions, **pulmonary embolism,** must always be considered as a cause of chest pain. The classic presentation is acute pleuritic chest pain accompanied by shortness of breath, tachypnea, and tachycardia. When the presentation is atypical, a diagnosis of pulmonary embolism should be considered in women who have any risk factors, including estrogen use, current or recent pregnancy, a history of thrombophilia, previous deep vein thrombosis or pulmonary embolism, cancer, systemic lupus erythematosus, antiphospholipid syndrome, recent pelvic or orthopedic surgery, or prolonged immobility.

GASTROINTESTINAL CAUSES

Multiple gastrointestinal disorders have been associated with chest pain, but esophageal disorders are the most common, estimated to be up to 60% of patients with chest pain and normal coronary arteries.

Gastroesophageal reflux disease (GERD) is the most common cause of noncardiac chest pain in women. The patient may complain of angina-like substernal pain radiating to the back, arms, or jaw. Symptoms commonly occur after

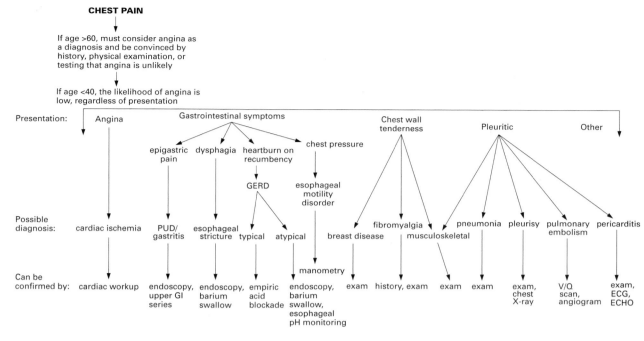

FIG. 1-1 Evaluation of chest pain in the female patient.

BOX 1-2

Risk Factors for Coronary Artery Disease in Women

Age over 55
Diabetes
Hypertension
Smoking
Dyslipidemia: high LDL and/or low HDL
Family history of premature CHD (first-degree male relative under age 55 or female under age 65)

LDL, Low-density lipoprotein; *HDL,* high-density lipoprotein; *CHD,* coronary heart disease.

---

meals or when recumbent and are relieved by exercise. Chest pain with GERD can increase with exercise. Although the majority of patients give a history of reflux symptoms, up to 20% of patients with GERD report none. Conditions that decrease lower esophageal sphincter pressure (e.g., pregnancy), as well as those that increase intraabdominal pressure (obesity), can predispose women to GERD.

Because there are no identifying features of GERD on examination, the history is an important tool in diagnosis. If the history is classic for GERD, the clinical consensus increasingly is to treat without further evaluation and evaluate only if there is no response to therapy. There is growing consensus that a trial of a protein pump inhibitor such as omeprazole may even be a more cost-effective tool for diagnosing acid-related chest pain. The absence of esophagitis on endoscopy does not rule out GERD. Two additional tests may be helpful in making the diagnosis in more complicated cases: esophageal acid perfusion, also known as Bernstein's test, and 24-hour esophageal pH monitoring (see Chapter 17).

The **esophageal motility disorders** are diagnosed by manometry, a procedure involving the placement of pressure transducers through the nose or mouth into the esophagus. Nutcracker esophagus is the most commonly diagnosed esophageal disorder associated with noncardiac chest pain. It is diagnosed by manometric findings of high-amplitude, peristaltic contractions in the distal esophagus. It is present in almost 50% of patients with abnormal motility on evaluation of chest pain.

Abnormal motility can be detected by manometry, but it is difficult to show that dysmotility itself is the cause of the chest pain. Frequently, the manometric abnormalities are not temporally related to the chest pain. Provocative testing can be done with pentagastrin, hot and cold liquids, vasopressin, ergotamine, edrophonium, bethanechol, and intraesophageal balloon distention in an attempt to reproduce chest pain. Achalasia is a syndrome characterized by increased tone in the lower esophageal sphincter with lack of normal peristalsis. It can progress to significant dilation of the esophagus and associated symptoms of chest pain, heartburn, and regurgitation. It is diagnosed by barium study or endoscopy.

Functional chest pain of presumed esophageal origin is defined as at least 12 weeks per year of midline chest pain and the absence of pathologic gastroesophageal reflux, achalasia, or other motility disorders with a recognized pathologic basis. There is substantial overlap of this syndrome with another functional gastrointestinal disorder, **irritable bowel syndrome.** Symptoms of irritable bowel syndrome are reported by 10% to 20% of adults. This syndrome has a marked female predominance. Women with noncardiac chest pain are more likely than age-matched control subjects to experience the constellation of symptoms compatible with irritable bowel syndrome. A large percentage of patients with irritable bowel syndrome report esophageal symptoms as well and on further evaluation are found to have esophageal motility abnormalities. Both irritable bowel and esophageal dysmotility may represent a spectrum of disease, the "irritable gut." Stress is known to exacerbate symptoms. Patients who seek medical attention for their symptoms have been shown to have a higher frequency of psychologic disturbances than those who do not seek medical care. Irritable bowel syndrome is discussed in Chapter 19.

Although epigastric pain is the more common presenting sign of **peptic ulcer disease** (PUD), duodenal or gastric ulcers and gastritis can manifest as a substernal chest pain. Duodenal ulcers cause pain 1.5 to 3 hours after eating. Pain is usually relieved by intake of food or antacids. Gastric ulcers may be worsened by eating. Nonsteroidal anti-inflammatory drugs, which are used commonly by older women for arthritis, can predispose to PUD. Smoking is the most common risk factor for ulcers in younger women. Alcohol may cause an erosive gastritis that may be accompanied by chest pain. PUD is discussed further in Chapter 17.

Gallbladder disease is rarely a cause of chest pain and symptoms are usually related to meals. The diagnosis of gallbladder disease is described in Chapter 16.

MUSCULOSKELETAL CAUSES

Disorders of the thoracic skeleton are among the most common causes of chest pain in the ambulatory setting. Most chest pain of musculoskeletal cause can be diagnosed by the history and physical examination alone.

Costochondritis is more common in women than men (with a ratio of 3:1). This condition may manifest as localized tenderness over the costochondral junctions, most commonly the second, third, and fourth. The pain is often described as gnawing, dull, and enduring for hours or days; but it can also be characterized as sharp and fleeting. Pain arises on pressure over the costochondral junctions or pectoralis muscle. **Xiphoiditis** may be manifested by a deep retrosternal ache that may radiate to the epigastrium or precordium. Chest pain will be reproduced on palpation of the xiphoid process.

Cervical and **thoracic osteoarthritis** can cause nerve root compression from narrowed foramina, leading to pain referred to the dermatomes innervated by the affected nerves. The C4-T7 nerve roots innervate the chest. The quality of the pain may be similar to angina, with radiation to the jaws, arms, and neck; and the pain may be precipitated by exertion—so-called cervicoprecordial angina. Usually the pain is precipitated by motion of the upper torso and arms, or by prolonged sitting or lying. Cervical spine radiographs may reveal osteoarthritis.

Muscular strain of the chest wall can be precipitated by unaccustomed exercise. The pain can be felt in the costochondral junctions or in the chest wall muscles. It is reproduced on movement of the torso, arms, or ribs (as in breathing). Palpation of trigger points may also elicit pain and muscle spasm.

Fibromyalgia is a chronic syndrome characterized by widespread pain, not explained by inflammatory or degenerative musculoskeletal changes, and mild or greater tenderness in at least 11 of 18 specified tender points on digital palpation. One of the classic trigger points is the second costochondral junction, which may be a source of chest pain. The prevalence of fibromyalgia in women in the primary care setting is estimated to be 3%, and up to 7% in women between 60 and 79 years old (see Chapter 33).

PSYCHOLOGIC CAUSES

Chest pain and palpitations constitute one of the top five symptom complexes that may be unexplained by physical illness. When no obvious explanation for continuing chest pain is discovered, a psychogenic diagnosis should be considered. Palpitations and atypical chest pain can be a prominent component of **panic disorder.** Although this entity is found in only 1.5% of the entire population, it occurs more commonly in women. The prevalence of panic disorder in primary care practice is considerably higher precisely because of associated somatic features. One half of women with panic disorder will also have agoraphobia. There is evidence that panic disorder is a biologic disorder with a strong genetic component, and there is considerable overlap of panic disorder with other causes of chest pain, including coronary artery disease (CAD), MVP, and hyperventilation syndrome, making diagnosis and treatment more difficult. The diagnosis of panic disorder is suggested by a history of atypical chest pain (i.e., long duration, unrelated to exertion, of varying quality) in association with chest pounding, shortness of breath, and dizziness in a young woman who is obviously healthy, or in an older woman when an extensive evaluation has been undertaken with no results. This diagnosis is confirmed when the patient describes chest pain as accompanied by recurrent, discrete attacks of intense fear and/or symptoms of extreme anxiety.

Chest pain and palpitations can occur as symptoms in patients with underlying **anxiety** and **depression.** Clues to diagnosis are the young age and general health of the patient or, in older women, a negative evaluation for medical causes. Detailed questioning regarding current stressors and a history of depression, anxiety, or physical or sexual abuse is essential.

Patients with **somatoform disorders** may have the symptom of chest pain in association with one or many ostensibly unrelated symptoms (i.e., no unifying diagnosis) in the presence of some degree of psychologic conflict. Somatization disorder in particular is much more common in women, whereas somatoform pain disorder is more common in men (see Chapter 82).

The symptom of chest pain in conjunction with breathlessness may be caused by **hyperventilation syndrome,** which occurs more commonly in women than in men. The diagnosis is suggested by an elevated respiratory rate and a shortened breath-holding time. A hyperventilation challenge test may be useful. Three minutes of forced overbreathing is followed by a 3-minute recovery period with a careful assessment of symptoms.

Any evaluation of intermittent chest pain, especially accompanied by palpitations, must include detailed questioning about **substance abuse,** particularly cocaine, alcohol, and benzodiazepines (see Chapter 91).

OTHER CAUSES

Symptoms of chest pain and palpitations are reported frequently by women going through **menopause.** The pain is somewhat atypical but is often brought on by exercise or episodes of stress and can occur in conjunction with hot flashes. This syndrome is thought to reflect a component of vasomotor instability that occurs as estrogen levels drop.

Herpes zoster is characterized by unilateral pain along thoracic dermatomes for a period of days followed by rash in the same distribution. Dormant varicella viruses are reactivated in the dorsal root ganglion. The pain and rash usually disappear in weeks, but the pain may persist in 10% of patients, especially in the elderly or immunocompromised, as postherpetic neuralgia.

EVALUATION

History and Physical Examination

A detailed **history** is the most important step in the evaluation of chest pain. Understanding the timing, precise location, and quality of the patient's pain and associated symptoms is essential. The clinician needs to obtain detailed information on medical history, cardiac risk factors (including clotting), pregnancy complications, menopausal status, dietary habits, and use of alcohol, nonsteroidal anti-inflammatory agents, aspirin, caffeine, or other medications. The information should include gentle questioning about a history of sexual or physical abuse, depression, anxiety, and any other current life stressors.

Knowledge of a woman's likelihood or **prior probability of significant cardiac disease at a given age** is useful. For example, women less than age 39 who exhibit typical angina have only a 26% pretest likelihood of CAD compared with men of the same age with typical angina who have a 70% pretest likelihood of CAD. Alternatively, a presentation of atypical angina in a woman older than 60 years represents a 54% pretest likelihood of disease, not markedly different from the 67% pretest likelihood in men of the same age with atypical angina. More extensive discussion of the diagnosis of coronary artery disease in women can be found in Chapter 2.

The **physical examination** should begin with vital signs including bilateral pulses and blood pressure if there is a concern about a dissecting aneurysm. Examination should include careful palpation of the chest wall and costochondral junctions, looking for musculoskeletal causes with palpation and specific maneuvers. Auscultation of the lungs may reveal findings of consolidation. A careful cardiac examination may reveal murmurs, clicks, or rubs. Pain on abdominal palpation may suggest gastrointestinal tract abnormality such as gallbladder disease or PUD. The clinician should note the patient's ability to assess depression or anxiety.

The differential diagnosis of chest pain poses a challenge to the primary care provider. Although some cases may be straightforward, others may involve overlapping causes and management may be more difficult. The way in which a woman expresses her complaints has been shown to influence decisions about further evaluation. A "business-like" rather than a "histrionic" style is more likely to lead to a cardiac evaluation. The medical literature also suggests that women with chest pain are less likely than men with a comparable likelihood of CAD to receive appropriate evaluation.

Once life-threatening causes of chest pain have been ruled out, careful observation over time may yield more insight into the cause of the chest pain and direct the evaluation and treatment. Reassurance about the absence of life-threatening abnormality is often not enough. Careful attention to the diagnosis of less serious causes is necessary so that appropriate treatment can be instituted.

BIBLIOGRAPHY

An exploratory report of chest pain in primary care: a report from ASPN, *J Am Board Fam Pract* 3:143, 1990.

Borzecki AM, Pedrosa MC, Prashker MJ: Should noncardiac chest pain be treated empirically? a cost-effectiveness analysis, *Arch Intern Med* 160:844, 2000.

Chambers J, Bass C, Mayou R: Non-cardiac chest pain: assessment and management, *Heart* 82(6):656, 1999.

Clouse RE et al: Functional esophageal disorders, *Gut* 45(11):II31, 1999.

Diamond GA, Forrester JS: Analysis of probability as an aide in the clinical diagnosis of coronary-artery disease, *N Engl J Med* 300:1350, 1979.

Freed LA, Levy D, Levine RA: Prevalence and clinical outcome of mitral-valve prolapse, *N Engl J Med* 341:1, 1999.

Gardner WN: The pathophysiology of hyperventilation disorders, *Chest* 109(2):516, 1996.

Goldenberg DL: Fibromyalgia syndrome a decade later, *Arch Intern Med* 159:777, 1999.

Locke GR III: The epidemiology of functional gastrointestinal disorders in North America, *Gastroenterol Clin* 25(1):1, 1996.

Richter JE: Cost-effectiveness of testing for gastroesophageal reflux disease: what do patients, physicians, and health insurers want? *Am J Med* 107(3):288, 1999.

Richter JE: Chest pain and gastroesophageal reflux disease, *J Clin Gastroenterol* 30(suppl):S39, 2000.

Sansone RA, Sansone LA, Righter EL: Panic disorder: the ultimate anxiety, *J Women's Health* 7(8):983, 1998.

CHAPTER 2

Coronary Artery Disease

Anne W. Moulton
Athena Poppas

Despite an overall reduction in mortality rates caused by cardiovascular disease (CVD), it remains the leading cause of death for women in the United States. It is responsible for almost 50% of all deaths in women, more than all cancer deaths combined. The death rate from CVD is one third higher in African-American women compared to white women. Rates in Hispanic and Asian women appear to be somewhat lower, although the data are limited and conflicting.

Coronary artery disease (CAD) develops approximately 10 to 15 years later in women than in men: by the age of 70, the male/female ratio approaches 1. Because of the aging "baby boom" population, the absolute number of deaths caused by CAD in women will continue to increase in the near future.

MAJOR RISK FACTORS

Risk factors for CAD in men have a similar predictive value in women. However, there are gender differences in the prevalence and magnitude of effects. Coronary atherosclerosis is a disease of older women, and thus **age** is the greatest predictor of the presence of CAD in women.

Diabetes mellitus is a particularly important risk factor in women. Women with diabetes have a greater risk of CAD than men with diabetes. Diabetes eliminates any female advantage in the development of heart disease. Even after adjustment for other risk factors, the relative risk of developing CAD in women with diabetes is twice that of nondiabetic women. Diabetes is closely linked to the development of atherosclerosis probably by way of its association with hyperinsulinemia, glucose intolerance, obesity (especially truncal), hypertension, lipid abnormalities, and clotting abnormalities. Insulin resistance, the earliest metabolic defect that can be detected in the clinical progression to type II diabetes, also confers an increased risk for CAD.

Hypertension is a powerful predictor of cardiovascular and cerebrovascular disease. It is the most prevalent major risk factor, present in 60% to 80% of women older than 45 years of age, the higher number being in black women. Isolated systolic hypertension occurs in 30% of women above the age of 65. The Systolic Hypertension in the Elderly Program (SHEP) confirmed that treatment of systolic hypertension reduced cardiovascular events in women, similar to studies of diastolic hypertension.

Differences in plasma **lipids** may partially explain the reported gender differences in CAD rates (see Chapter 4). *Low high-density lipoprotein (HDL)*, rather than high low-density lipoprotein (LDL), is more predictive of coronary risk in women. A low HDL is predictive of heart disease in both older and younger women. The Framingham Study has suggested that an *elevated triglyceride level* may also be independently associated with the development of coronary artery disease in women, although not in men. Preliminary studies suggest that *lipoprotein (a)* is strongly associated with the development of atherosclerosis and coronary artery disease, especially in women.

Smoking is an important risk factor for the development of CAD, especially in young females. A total of 50% of myocardial infarctions (MIs) among women are attributable to tobacco. From the Nurses Health Study, the risk for cardiovascular death and MIs for smokers of 25 or more cigarettes per day is known to be increased fivefold, even after controlling for other cardiac risk factors. When women quit smoking, their cardiovascular risk starts to drop and eventually approaches the risk for women who have never smoked, but those who continue to smoke even in small amounts (one to four cigarettes per day) have an elevated risk of CAD.

A **family history of premature MI** increases a woman's risk of CAD. The American Heart Association statement on cardiovascular disease in women defines premature CHD as a first-degree male relative under age 55 or a female under age 65.

OTHER RISK FACTORS

Obesity, in general, is a significant independent risk factor for the development of CAD in females only. This relationship is independent of other risk factors. One third of all adult American women are obese, defined as a body mass index (BMI) greater than 30. Abdominal or central obesity (waist to hip circumference ratio of >.9) appears to increase risk of CAD in women, as well as men. There is a strong relationship between truncal obesity and insulin resistance, another risk factor for the development of CAD.

A **sedentary lifestyle** increases the risk of CAD in both males and females. One survey revealed that more than 70% of US women are underactive, with even lower rates of activity in Black and Hispanic women and women of lower socioeconomic position. Regular exercise, even a moderate walking program, decreases risk of CAD in women of all age groups.

C-reactive protein is marker of systemic inflammation. In The Nurses Health Study, elevated levels were an independent predictor for CAD even in women with normal lipids (LDL cholesterol levels less than 130). At the present, this assay is neither widely available nor routinely recommended.

Studies suggest an increased risk of CAD (especially premature CAD) in patients with elevated **homocysteine** concentrations, independent of other risk factors. Indirect evidence in women from The Nurses Health Study reported lower rates of CAD in women with higher intake of vitamin B_6 and folate (both of which can decrease homocysteine levels).

Because data are limited, it has been difficult to determine the exact impact of **psychosocial factors** on the development of heart disease in women. There are some notable gender differences. Lower socioeconomic position and lower educational level are risk factors for CAD in women. Two possible mechanisms for this include differences in lifestyle and differences in social stress and support. Anger and "type A behavior" appear to be more significant risk factors for men. Depression, which is twice as common in women, is a risk factor for heart disease in both females and males.

GENDER-SPECIFIC RISK FACTORS

There is a 10- to 15-year lag in the manifestation of CAD in women, which has been attributed to the effects of estrogen. There is no association between reproductive experiences (e.g., parity, age at first birth) and risk of CAD. Recent data on low-dose **oral contraceptive pills** indicate that the incidence of cardiovascular disease is not increased by pill use in women under age 30 who smoke, or nonsmoking women without other cardiac risk factors over age 30. However, there is an increase in acute MIs in women above the age of 35 who smoke.

Women who experience **early menopause** (natural or surgical) are at greater risk of heart disease than age-matched premenopausal women. The normal age at menopause is not associated with an abrupt change in cardiac risk; rates increase constantly over the next 10 to 15 years. Although there is evidence that after menopause certain cardiac risk factors change and the rates of CAD increase, there is no direct evidence linking the decline in estrogen to these changes. The Women's Health Initiative and other ongoing studies should help clarify the role of HRT in the primary prevention of coronary disease.

PATHOPHYSIOLOGY

The pathophysiology of CAD in women is similar to that in men, with a few exceptions. Atherosclerotic lesions and adaptive remodeling to plaque deposition appear morphologically similar by intravascular ultrasound analysis. On the other hand, thromboembolic complications are more severe and platelet activity is greater in women. Pre-menopausal women, in particular, may have more vasospasm and thrombosis than fixed stenosis as a cause of MI and sudden death. On pathologic examination after sudden cardiac death, premenopausal women have more plaque erosion on mild luminal narrowing compared with men and older women, who have more calcified and narrowed arteries with plaque rupture. In nonhuman primate experiments, the presence or addition of estrogen influences the extent of atherosclerosis, but not its progression. Acute administration of estradiol to postmenopausal patients with CAD lowers systolic blood pressure, increases exercise time, and reduces anginal chest pain. These noted beneficial effects of estrogen on lipid profiles, coagulation, and vascular tone have been postulated to account for the 10- to 15-year lag time in the presentation of atherosclerosis in women.

CLINICAL ASPECTS

Differences Between Males and Females

There are certain anatomic, functional, and electrocardiographic characteristics that have some bearing on gender-related differences in clinical manifestations of CAD (Table 2-1). The heart of a normal woman is smaller and lighter than that of a normal man. Although the coronary arteries are smaller in women, this is attributable to differences in heart weight and body surface area. Women have a lower left ventricular end-diastolic pressure and volume, yet a higher resting ejection fraction. The ejection fraction response to exercise in healthy women is variable, with less of an increase than in men. In middle age, there is a higher

Table 2-1
Gender Differences in Clinical Manifestations of Coronary Artery Disease

Manifestation	Findings in Women Versus Men
Electrocardiography	Higher prevalence of primary ST-T abnormalities
Angina	More common as first presentation of CAD
	Stress- and rest-related angina more common than typical exercise-induced angina
	Vasospasm probably more common in women
Myocardial infarction	Less likely as first presentation of CAD
	Silent and non–Q-wave infarction more common
	Higher crude mortality and morbidity rates
	Early reinfarction and cardiac rupture more common
	Postinfarct congestive heart failure (with both systolic and diastolic dysfunction) more common
Sudden cardiac death	Overall incidence less
	No increase in risk of sudden death associated with frequent or complex ventricular ectopy after acute MI

CAD, Coronary artery disease; *MI,* myocardial infarction.

prevalence of primary ST-T abnormalities in women than in men. Suggested reasons for these differences include change in posture, hyperventilation, higher rates of mitral valve prolapse, and high estrogen levels.

The literature on the correlation between clinical presentation and prevalence of CAD in women is limited. The Coronary Artery Surgery Study (CASS) from the 1970s was the first to characterize patients according to the type of reported chest pain and then examine the prevalence of disease within these clinical subsets. The prevalence of obstructive coronary disease in women with definite angina, probable angina, and nonspecific chest pain was significantly different (58%, 35%, and 5%, respectively) from that noted in similar subsets for males (88%, 67%, and 22%). The recent NHLBI Women's Ischemia Syndrome Evaluation Study (WISE) found a similarly low prevalence of significant coronary disease in women with nonanginal chest pain.

Clinical Syndromes

The differential diagnosis of **chest pain** is discussed in greater detail in Chapter 1. Gastrointestinal and musculoskeletal causes are most commonly considered in the differential diagnosis of angina in women.

Angina is the most frequent first manifestation of CAD in women; in contrast, males are more likely to have acute MI as their first manifestation of CAD. There appear to be some clinical differences between angina in males and females. Women are more likely to have anginal patterns associated with mental stress, sleep, and rest, as opposed to men, whose angina is more likely to be associated with physical exertion.

Variant angina or **Prinzmetals angina** is quite rare. It is a syndrome defined as chest pain that occurs at rest associated with dramatic ST-segment elevations on electrocardiogram (ECG). Focal vasospasm occurs in normal or diseased arteries and is reversed with nitroglycerin. Patients with variant angina tend to be younger than those with chronic stable angina, and this syndrome occurs equally in males and females. The natural history of variant angina is periods of frequent spasm alternating with asymptomatic periods. The survival rate at 5 years is excellent (90%).

Microvascular angina, also rare, is more prevalent in women and is a diagnosis of exclusion in patients who have had extensive cardiac testing. Patients with this entity have angina-like chest pain, ischemic ST-segment depressions on electrocardiography during exercise testing, angiographically normal coronary arteries without coronary artery spasm, and normal ventricular function. The majority of patients have attenuated coronary flow with decreased vasodilator reserve in response to metabolic and pharmacologic vasodilator stimuli, thought to be secondary to endothelial dysfunction. There is some evidence that this syndrome may be more likely to occur in perimenopausal or postmenopausal women, suggesting a connection with fluctuating estrogen levels. The infarction-free survival rate is over 90% at 10 years, but a substantial number of patients with this syndrome continue to have symptoms of chest pain. Nonetheless, patients should be reassured that the absence of occlusive epicardial disease indicates a benign prognosis.

Women are less likely than men to have **acute MI** as their first manifestation of CAD and yet are more likely to experience silent MI. There is limited information about gender differences in presentation with acute MI. Although equal proportions of women and men with MI have chest pain, women have more associated symptoms such as gastrointestinal pain, nausea, dyspnea, and fatigue. Crude mortality and morbidity rates for acute MI show higher rates for women. However, these apparent gender differences appear to be secondary more to methodology than biology, as outcomes are equal when corrected for age and comorbidity.

Women are more likely to have non–Q-wave MI and more early reinfarction and cardiac rupture after MI. The overall risk for development of postinfarct congestive heart failure is greater in women than in men, despite having higher left ventricular ejection fraction post-MI. This has been ascribed to diastolic dysfunction with higher rates of coexisting systemic hypertension and diabetes.

The overall incidence of **sudden cardiac death** among women is less than in men. However, it still accounts for 37% of CAD deaths in women. Moreover, 67% of all sudden cardiac deaths among women occur without a previously known history of CAD.

▣ EVALUATION
Stress Electrocardiography

Numerous studies have shown limitations in the sensitivity and specificity of electrocardiographic stress testing (EST) for the diagnosis of CAD in women compared with men. Many studies, including the CASS study, noted a ***high false-positive rate,*** 22% to 37%, and hence ***reduced test specificity*** (Table 2-2). Confounding reasons for these findings are a marked difference in the prevalence of CAD in the populations studied and more abnormal resting ECGs in women, a factor known to reduce test specificity by half. Other non-Bayesian factors have been proposed, including digoxin-like effects of estrogen, catecholamine release and vasospasm, decreased intramyocardial potassium levels, and ECG changes associated with hyperventilation. More women show exercise-induced electrocardiographic evidence of ischemia (defined as 1 mm of ST-segment depression) but are less likely to have occlusive epicardial coronary artery disease.

Table 2-2 Evaluation of Coronary Artery Disease	
Test	**Operating Characteristics in Women**
Electrocardiographic stress test	Women more likely to have changes suggestive of ischemia, but less likely to have significant CAD
	False-positive rate 22%-37%
	False-negative rate 20%-50%
Thallium stress test	Higher sensitivity 87%
	Specificity 69%
	Breast attenuation artifacts
Exercise echocardiography	Sensitivity 85%
	Specificity 77%
	Obesity limits windows
Cardiac catheterization	Higher minor complication rates

CAD, Coronary artery disease; *ECG,* electrocardiogram.
From Fleischmann KE et al: *JAMA* 280:913, 1998.

There is conflicting information about the gender differences in the *sensitivity* of EST; the CASS study found no difference (80% vs 76%), but the Duke database noted a marked difference (72% vs 57%). One reason for a *higher false-negative rate* in women is the inability to complete a full exercise protocol (insufficient workload). In addition to ST-segment shift, other exercise testing parameters are important for prognostication in men and women and can enhance predictive estimates. These include duration of exercise, presence of angina, ability to reach target heart rate, and time to ST-segment depression and to normalization during recovery.

Stress Perfusion Imaging

When the resting ECG is abnormal or when there is an intermediate to high likelihood of disease by history, nuclear perfusion imaging improves the prognostic accuracy of stress testing (Table 2-3). Thallium-201 and technetium-99m sestamibi, the most commonly used radiotracers, are distributed according to regional blood flow in the myocardium.

The sensitivity and specificity of the nuclear stress test are not as high in women as in men. A recent evaluation of TI-201 SPECT in women compared with men found a reduced diagnostic accuracy, primarily resulting from smaller left ventricular chamber size in women. False-positive findings can result from attenuation of the radioactivity by breast tissue, which produces a fixed defect in the anteroseptal and anterolateral segments. Many experienced nuclear cardiologists recognize this common artifact and can "read around" it. ECG-gated imaging, which can correlate wall motion with perfusion abnormalities, and attenuation-correction algorithms are promising techniques to overcome this problem in women. Technetium, a higher energy agent, and single-photon emission computed tomographic (SPECT) scanning, which offers 32 images of the myocardium, provide better estimates of the extent and severity of disease and have improved the diagnostic accuracy. As with the routine exercise stress test, a common source of false-negative results is an inability to achieve adequate cardiac workload. For women who cannot exercise, pharmacologic stress with vasodilators, such as dipyridamole and adenosine, have been shown to be equally accurate for the detection of CAD in women.

Stress Echocardiography

When the resting ECG is abnormal or there is an intermediate to high likelihood of CAD by history, echocardiographic imaging improves the diagnostic accuracy of stress testing. With exercise echocardiography, the development of a new or worsening wall motion abnormality is diagnostic of myocardial ischemia. In a recent meta-analysis, the mean sensitivity for the diagnosis of CAD was 86% and specificity was 79%. Additionally, exercise echocardiography can provide information about cardiac structure and function that may cause chest pain or dyspnea, such as valvular stenosis or hypertrophic cardiomyopathy. In a contemporary meta-analysis comparing exercise SPECT with echocardiography in predominantly male populations with a high prevalence of CAD, the tests had equal sensitivity (85% vs 87%), but stress echo had a higher specificity (77% vs 64%).

Pharmacologic agents have been used in combination with echocardiography for patients who are unable to exercise. Dobutamine stress echocardiography (DSE) has been shown to be predictive of recovery of function when assessing myocardial viability before revascularization procedures. It has also been shown to provide good prognostic information for preoperative evaluation and post-MI risk stratification. The recent WISE study did raise concerns about DSE in low-risk women; of 92 women studied, 27% had CAD with a reported sensitivity of 50% overall, and 82% for multivessel disease.

In summary, available testing methods for suspected CAD in women all have some limitations in accuracy. The choice of testing method should be guided by local expertise and test availability.

Other Noninvasive Testing Modalities

Electron beam computed tomography (EBCT) has been shown to be a sensitive method of identifying coronary artery calcifications, a marker for subclinical atherosclerosis in men and older women. The AHA/ACC does not recommend EBCT for diagnosing obstructive CAD, because of its low specificity and because it has not been shown to be superior to other, established noninvasive methods.

Phosphorus-31 nuclear magnetic resonance spectroscopy is a promising noninvasive method of detecting myocardial ischemia. A recent substudy of the WISE trial utilized P31-NMR and found metabolic evidence of ischemia in 20% of women with chest pain syndromes and no angiographically significant coronary artery obstruction.

Cardiac Catheterization

There are abundant data indicating a gender bias in the evaluation of CAD: women are referred less often for noninvasive testing, for diagnostic and therapeutic catheterizations, and for bypass surgery. A recent computerized survey

Table 2-3
Probability of Coronary Artery Disease in Women According to History and Stress Test Results

History	Prevalence	Positive Results		Negative Results	
		EST	TST	EST	TST
Nonanginal chest pain	0.05	0.06	0.35	0.05	0.02
Atypical angina	0.35	0.54	0.85	0.20	0.14
Typical exertional angina	0.58	0.72	0.93	0.33	0.29

EST, Exercise electrocardiographic stress testing; *TST*, thallium exercise electrocardiographic stress testing.
Modified from Sox HC: *Postgrad Med* 743:333, 1983.

of 720 primary care physicians found that women and African Americans were less likely to be referred for cardiac catheterization than men and whites, respectively. A number of investigators have found lower rates of referral for cardiac catheterization in women for whom it is clearly indicated: those who have positive noninvasive test results, typical angina, and multiple cardiac risk factors. In a review of women with positive stress tests, fewer were referred for cardiac catheterization (38% vs 63%), but these women had a higher cardiovascular event rate (14% vs 6%). Women undergoing angiography have more total complications, dysrhythmias, and hemorrhage owing to older age and greater comorbidity. There is no difference in the incidence of death, MI, stroke, vascular complications, or contrast reactions between sexes undergoing diagnostic cardiac catheterization.

✖ MANAGEMENT

Medical Therapy

Limited data exist to clarify gender differences in pharmacologic therapy in acute MI. However, the efficacy overall appears similar for males and females (Table 2-4). Use of beta blockers in women is associated with a significant mortality reduction as it is in males. Use of calcium channel blockers does not decrease mortality or morbidity in women with acute MI. Studies in predominately male populations suggest that the use of angiotension-converting enzymes (ACE) inhibitors in post-MI in patients with a left ventricular ejection less than 40% reduces risk of cardiovascular death and complications. Several studies, including the Survival and Ventricular Enlargement (SAVE) trial suggest less benefit in women, although they are limited by small numbers. Nonetheless, experts recommend ACE inhibitor use in women. Nitrates do not affect mortality but are probably as effective for symptom relief in the acute MI setting in women as they are in men. Aspirin has been shown to be quite effective in reducing cardiovascular mortality in women post-MI. The clearest evidence of benefit post-MI is for the use of beta blockers and acetylsalicylic acid (ASA), yet some studies suggest these medications are used less commonly in women than in men.

In women with **angina,** beta blockers are most effective in reducing episodes of chest pain, as well as preventing cardiac death. There is no evidence of a mortality benefit in women or men with angina who use nitrates. A meta-analysis documented that ASA is effective in reducing cardiovascular events by 25% in women. Although lipid-lowering therapy has been shown to be more effective in secondary prevention than primary in women, (see Chapter 4) there is evidence that it is underused in women with existing CAD and elevated cholesterol.

From the Heart and Estrogen-Progestin Replacement Study (HERS), there is no evidence to support initiating estrogen therapy for secondary prevention in women. A recent angiographic study also revealed no change in established coronary arthrosclerosis after 3 years of estrogen.

The role of alcohol in the improvement of lipid profiles in women is somewhat controversial. Compared with nondrinkers, women who consume moderate amounts of alcohol (three to nine drinks per week) have been shown to have a decreased relative risk of CAD; this finding is consistent with those of previous studies in men. An elevation of HDL level with alcohol is the best documented mechanism for the positive effect of decreasing risk of heart disease. This potential beneficial effect of drinking on lipids needs to be weighed against the risk for alcohol-related morbidity in women, including hypertension, alcohol dependence with end-organ damage, and possible increase in breast cancer risk, which begins to increase significantly with more than seven drinks per week (see Chapter 90).

Thrombolytic Therapy

Thrombolytic therapy for acute MI has been shown to produce a similar reduction in early mortality rates in women. Women are less likely than men to be eligible for this therapy because of late or atypical presentation, comorbid conditions (e.g., hypertension), and more non-ST-elevation MI. Some studies show a lower reduction in 30-day mortality rates in women than in men with thrombolysis. Bleeding complications with thrombolysis are more common in women. Most studies demonstrate a twofold to threefold increase in the risk of hemorrhagic stroke in women even after adjusting for age,

Table 2-4
Gender Differences in Treatments for Coronary Artery Disease

Treatment	Differences in Women and Men
Medical therapy	Limited data on effectiveness in women
	ASA and beta blockers proven effective for acute MI and chronic stable angina
Thrombolytic therapy	Less reduction in mortality rates in women
	Higher rates of serious bleeding complications
Percutaneous transluminal coronary angioplasty	Lower clinical and angiographic success rates
	Better long-term outcome, lower restenosis rates
Coronary atherectomy	Higher acute complication rates (perforation, transfusion, Q-wave MI, death)
	Similar restenosis rates
Coronary artery bypass grafting	Higher perioperative mortality rates
	Less relief of angina
	Less graft patency
	Similar 5- to 10-year survival rates

MI, Myocardial infarction.

body surface area, or weight less than 70 kg. This may be secondary to the higher prevalence of hypertension in women.

Percutaneous Revascularization

There are numerous studies evaluating the outcome of percutaneous revascularization that have reported higher mortality and morbidity rates in women compared with men. The 1985-1986 NHLBI registry of 2136 patients undergoing angioplasty, 25% of whom were women, found increased complications (29% vs 20%) and periprocedural mortality (2.6% vs 0.3%) in women. This difference is partially explained by increased age and comorbidity and possibly by smaller vessel size. Despite having more risk factors and severe angina, the angiographic extent of CAD was less in women and the clinical and angiographic success was equal.

These statistics have improved with increased experience and better technology. In the 1993-1994 NHLBI registry of 274 women, a higher risk profile was noted in women, but clinical success was improved and major complications were less. The incidence of death/MI/coronary artery bypass graft (CABG) was 10% in 1985-1986 versus 4% in 1993 to 1994. A similar finding was noted in the BARI trial, which randomized 1829 patients with symptomatic multivessel disease, 27% of whom were women, to CABG or percutaneous transluminal coronary angioplasty (PTCA). Women, again, had more comorbidity but equivalent crude mortality at 5 years (12%). The long-term prognosis after angioplasty is similar among men and women, except that more women report recurrence of angina. In summary, the precise reason for women's increased morbidity rate at the time of angioplasty requires further study, but continually improving technology (such as intracoronary stents) and the favorable long-term outcome suggest that percutaneous interventions are an appropriate therapeutic option in women.

Coronary Artery Bypass Surgery

Older studies of CABG found that women had increased perioperative morbidity (bleeding, heart failure, and MI) and mortality. Factors explaining this include more advanced disease at presentation with more severe angina, left ventricular dysfunction, and emergent surgery. Some of the gender difference in mortality rates has been attributed to differences in body size, with smaller blood vessels and, thus, a reduced opportunity to obtain complete revascularization. Women referred for CABG are also more likely to have diabetes, hypertension, and congestive heart failure. Attempts to adjust for preoperative angina severity, number of diseased blood vessels, and body surface area have partially reduced the effect of gender on outcome.

Most of the original studies on CABG in women were made at a time before internal mammary artery grafting, advanced cardioplegic techniques, routine antiplatelet therapy, and aggressive lipid-lowering therapy were used. A recent single-center review of 1743 consecutive patients undergoing CABG between 1994 and 1997, 30% of whom were women, found equivalent morbidity and mortality between men and women. Although women were older, had more hypertension, diabetes, urgent surgeries, and fewer arterial grafts, the incidence of death, MI, and cerebrovascular events were not statistically significant. In the multicenter

BARI trial comparing multivessel angioplasty to CABG, similar positive findings were noted. There was similar 5-year mortality despite higher risk profiles in women, suggesting a change in outcomes with improved technology and techniques.

CARDIAC REHABILITATION

After an MI or CABG, women are more likely to report psychological symptoms, particularly anxiety and depression. This may be related to a variety of factors, including increased morbidity and disability after an MI, increased physical symptoms, and decreased activity. Women report longer recovery time and more days lost because of cardiac symptoms than men. Women return to paid employment less often than men after an MI, although return to work is not necessarily a reflection of disease or a suitable measure of recovery in women, many of whom work in the home. Domestic responsibilities are a source of concern for recovery in women, who may return to high-demand activities in the home sooner than is advisable. Women report having more fears about resumption of sexual activities. Finally, women are referred less often to cardiac rehabilitation programs, enroll less frequently, and have poorer attendance than men. As a recent American Heart Association panel noted, participation in a formal cardiac rehabilitation program, which usually includes risk factor modification, is critical for women post-MI. Postulated reasons for lack of attendance include lack of encouragement by the physician, depression, and older age. Some cardiac rehabilitation programs are now being developed with special attention to the exercise abilities and psychosocial needs of older women.

BIBLIOGRAPHY

Ades PA, Coello CE: Risk factor modification for cardiac disease. Effects of exercise and cardiac rehabilitation on cardiovascular outcomes, *Med Clin North Am* 84:254, 2000.

Aldea GS et al: Effect of gender on postoperative outcomes and hospital stays after coronary artery bypass grafting, *Ann Thorac Surg* 67:1097, 1999.

Buchthal SD et al: Abnormal myocardial phosphorus-31 nuclear magnetic resonance spectroscopy in women with chest pain but normal coronary angiograms, *N Engl J Med* 342:829, 2000.

Burke AP et al: Effect of risk factors on the mechanism of acute thrombosis and sudden coronary death in women, *Circulation* 97:2110, 1998.

Diamond GA, Forrester JS: Analysis of probability as an aid in the clinical diagnosis of coronary artery disease, *N Engl J Med* 300:1350, 1979.

Eaker ED: Psychosocial factors in the epidemiology of coronary heart disease in women, *Psychiatr Clin North Am* 12:167, 1989.

Eysmann SB, Douglas PS: Reperfusion and revascularization strategies for coronary artery disease in women, *JAMA* 268:1903, 1992.

Fleischmann KE et al: Exercise echocardiography or exercise SPECT imaging? A meta-analysis of diagnostic test performance, *JAMA* 280:913, 1998.

Hansen CL, Crabbe D, Rubin S: Lower diagnostic accuracy of thallium-201 SPECT myocardial perfusion imaging in women: an effect of smaller chamber size, *J Am Coll Cardiol* 28:1214, 1996.

Herrington DM et al: Effects of estrogen replacement on the progression of coronary-artery atherosclerosis, *N Engl J Med* 343:522, 2000.

Hulley S et al: Randomized trial of estrogen plus progestin for secondary prevention of coronary heart disease in postmenopausal women, *JAMA* 280:605, 1998.

Jacobs AK et al: Documentation of decline in morbidity in women undergoing coronary angioplasty (a report from the 1993-94 NHLBI Percutaneous Transluminal Coronary Angioplasty Registry), *Am J Cardiol* 80:979, 1997.

Kelsey SF et al: Results of percutaneous transluminal coronary angioplasty in women, *Circulation* 87:720, 1993.

Kornowski R et al: Comparison of men versus women in cross-sectional area luminal narrowing, quantity of plaque, presence of calcium in plaque, and lumen location in coronary arteries by intravascular ultrasound in patients with stable angina pectoris, *Am J Cardiol* 79:1601, 2000.

Kwork Y et al: Meta-analysis of exercise testing to detect coronary artery disease in women, *Am J Cardiol* 83:660, 1999.

Lewis JF et al: Dobutamine stress echocardiography in women with chest pain, *J Am Coll Cardiol* 33:1462, 1999.

Mosca L et al: Cardiovascular disease in women: a statement for healthcare professionals from the American Heart Association, *Circulation* 96:2468, 1997.

O'Rourke RA et al: ACC/AHA expert consensus document on electron-beam computed tomography for the diagnosis and prognosis of coronary artery disease, *J Am Coll Cardiol* 36:326, 2000.

Ridker PM et al: C-Reactive protein and other markers of inflammation in the prediction of cardiovascular disease in women, *N Engl J Med* 342:836, 2000.

Shaw LJ et al: Gender differences in the noninvasive evaluation and management of patients with suspected coronary artery disease, *Ann Intern Med* 120:559-566, 1994.

SHEP Cooperative Research Group: Prevention of stroke by antihypertensive drug treatment in older persons with isolated systolic hypertension. Final results of the systolic hypertension in the elderly (SHEP), *JAMA* 265:3255, 1991.

Schulman K et al: The effect of race and sex on physicians' recommendation for cardiac catheterization, *N Engl J Med* 340:618, 1999.

Sox H: Noninvasive testing in coronary artery disease, *Postgrad Med* 74:333, 1983.

Taillefer R et al: Comparison diagnostic accuracy of T1-201 and Tc-99m Sestamibi SPECT imaging (perfusion and ECG-gated SPECT) in detecting coronary artery disease in women, *J Am Coll Cardiol* 29:69, 1997.

Vaccarino V et al: Sex-based differences in early mortality after myocardial infarction, *N Engl J Med* 341:217, 1999.

Weiner DA et al: Exercise stress resting: Correlations among history of angina, ST-segment response and prevalence of coronary-artery disease in the Coronary Artery Surgery Study (CASS), *N Engl J Med* 301:230, 1979.

WHO Collaborative Study of Cardiovascular Disease and Steroid Hormone Contraception: Acute myocardial infarction and combined oral contraceptives: results of an international multicentre case-control study, *Lancet* 349:1202, 1999.

CHAPTER 3

Hypertension

Katharine K. Treadway

Hypertension occurs in approximately 25% of the American population. Despite the well-defined risks of untreated hypertension and the clear evidence that lowering blood pressure results in decreased cardiovascular morbidity and mortality, in the most recent National Health and Nutrition Survey only about 70% of patients with hypertension were aware they had it, only about 50% were treated, and only about 25% were adequately controlled according to current guidelines.

This chapter reviews the epidemiology, diagnosis, and management of hypertension in women, with particular attention to areas in which gender differences exist. Hypertension in pregnancy is discussed in Chapter 72.

DEFINITION

The risk of hypertension increases over all levels of diastolic and systolic blood pressure: a woman with a systolic blood pressure of 100 has a lower risk of cardiovascular mortality and morbidity than one with a systolic pressure of 120. The Joint National Commission on the Detection, Evaluation, and Treatment of Hypertension (JNC VI) has proposed the following definitions of hypertension:

	Systolic		Diastolic
Optimal	<120	and	<80
Normal	<130	and	<85
High Normal	130-139	or	85-89
Hypertension			
Stage 1	140-159	or	90-99
Stage 2	160-179	or	100-109
Stage 3	>180	or	>110

The high normal category consists of a group that is more likely to develop hypertension later and in whom primary prevention strategies should be considered. The former categories of mild, moderate, and severe hypertension have been renamed to emphasize the fact that Stage 1 (formerly mild) hypertension is anything but mild in its consequences, since it accounts for 58% of the excess cardiovascular mortality attributable to hypertension. Systolic pressure is as impor-

tant and as predictive of risk as diastolic pressure, and isolated systolic hypertension carries a significant risk of cardiovascular complications, especially in the elderly.

EPIDEMIOLOGY

Hypertension is less common in women than men. In the third and fourth decades, the incidence in men is more than twice that of women. With advancing age, the ratio decreases so that by age 60, there is only a slight male predominance. In both sexes the prevalence of hypertension rises with age and by the sixth decade approaches 50%.

In general women have a significantly lower complication rate from hypertension than men. The Framingham Study suggests that for all the major complications of hypertension (coronary disease, stroke, congestive heart failure, and peripheral vascular disease), mildly hypertensive women have about the same risk as normotensive men. African-American women are the exception in that their cardiovascular risk from hypertension is about the same as that of white men with hypertension. In addition, African-American women have about twice the prevalence of hypertension of white women.

Differences in hemodynamic profiles between men and women suggest some possible reasons for the relatively lower risk of hypertension in premenopausal white women. In comparison to men, women have a higher resting pulse rate, a higher pulse pressure, a higher cardiac output, and a lower peripheral resistance. In addition, women demonstrate less rise in blood pressure in response to stress.

The relatively lower risk of cardiovascular complications in white women tends to disappear after menopause, suggesting that estrogen may play a significant protective role. Estrogen has several direct effects on the vasculature. It inhibits inward calcium current in the vascular endothelium, which decreases vasoconstriction and resting tone. It increases endothelial production of nitric oxide and prostacyclin (both vasodilators and inhibitors of platelet aggregation) and reduces vascular growth. In addition, estrogen has indirect protective effects on the vasculature by increasing production of high-density lipoprotein (HDL) and increasing degradation of low-density lipoprotein (LDL).

Estrogen may also have direct blood pressure-lowering effects. In an intriguing study of estrogen replacement in menopausal women, Seely et al found that women repleted to premenopausal levels using transdermal estradiol had a significant decrease in nocturnal pressures and a nonsignificant trend toward reduction in daytime pressures. In addition, this study demonstrated an increase in total renin and prorenin, but not in active renin, in the treated women, suggesting that estrogen may have some inhibitory effect on the conversion of renin to active renin. These effects were not found using oral estrogens.

Natural History

Most patients with primary hypertension exhibit a labile phase in which blood pressure is elevated intermittently and often in the setting of stress. At this stage, blood pressure readings are typically in the high normal range, and there may be an exaggerated blood pressure response to exercise or an elevated resting heart rate. These signs typically occur in the fourth decade. Most persons with essential hypertension, excluding isolated systolic hypertension of the elderly, develop overt hypertension by the sixth decade. Left untreated, about 20% those with stage 1 hypertension will progress to stage 2 or 3. Less than 1% of those with hypertension will develop malignant hypertension. About 15% to 30% of patients with stage 1 hypertension will become spontaneously normotensive.

Systolic pressure tends to rise with age. Diastolic pressure also rises with age but peaks at about age 50. The complication rate increases linearly over all levels of pressure, such that for every 5 mm Hg rise in blood pressure, the risk of stroke increases by about 40% and the risk of coronary disease, by about 20%.

The risks of hypertension may be divided into those in which hypertension is the predominant causative factor—hypertensive risks—and those in which hypertension is one of several risk factors—atherosclerotic risks. Hypertensive risks include congestive heart failure, left ventricular hypertrophy, renal failure, and stroke. The major atherosclerotic risks are coronary artery disease and peripheral vascular disease.

Exacerbating Factors

Weight gain has a profound effect on the likelihood of developing hypertension. In a study of more than 16,000 women, Huang et al found that weight gain after age 18 dramatically increased the risk of subsequent hypertension so that women gaining 5 to 9.9 kg over several years had a 74% increase in the incidence of hypertension. Those who gained more that 25 kg had a fivefold increase. Conversely, women who were at a higher body mass index (BMI) at age 18 had a 15% reduction in the incidence of hypertension for a weight loss of 5 to 9.9 kg and a 26% reduction for a weight loss of 10 kg or greater.

In addition to total BMI, the distribution of fat also appears to influence the risk of developing hypertension, as well as the likelihood of subsequent complications. Women who have a waist/hip ratio of >0.85 are at higher risk than those with a lower ratio. The postulated mechanism for both weight gain and complications is an increase in insulin resistance, which has been demonstrated in this group.

The **excessive use of alcohol** is linked to the development of hypertension. Men who regularly drink more than 4 oz of hard liquor, 36 oz of beer, or 3 glasses of wine on a daily basis are at risk of developing hypertension; equivalent amounts for women should be assumed to be approximately half. The mechanism is probably related to the release by alcohol of corticotropin-releasing factor in the brain, which has been demonstrated to increase central sympathetic nervous system activity in mice.

There is a strong association between **high sodium intake** and the development of hypertension. Although studies of the effect of salt intake in the general population do not support the hypothesis that excessive salt alone can cause hypertension, there is substantial evidence that supports the impact of salt on the development of hypertension in susceptible individuals. It is reasonable to assume that most Americans eat an excessive amount of salt. Most Americans consume between 5000 and 10,000 mg of sodium daily, compared with 500 to 1000 mg of sodium in the diets of most non-Westernized cultures.

A variety of **medications** may cause a rise in blood pressure in susceptible persons. These include the sympathomimetics, such as decongestants, and caffeine. In a small proportion of women, oral contraceptives may cause a rise in blood pressure, although with current lower dose pills, this is less common. The mechanism is thought to be an increase in renin substrate. Postmenopausal hormone replacement therapy does not elevate pressures, presumably because of the significantly lower estrogen effect. Lastly, nonsteroidal anti-inflammatory drugs (NSAIDs) can cause the development of hypertension, especially in the elderly. The mechanism is blockade of vasodilator prostaglandins in the kidney, which leads to salt and water retention.

▣ EVALUATION
Diagnosis

It is important to make a diagnosis of hypertension based on multiple readings rather than a single reading as pressure measurements are variable, and, especially in the setting of an urgent or emergent visit, may be high, although subsequent readings are in the normal range. Except for the highest levels of blood pressure elevation or in the setting of acute cardiac disease, it is prudent to allow several readings before making a firm diagnosis. However, it is also important to realize that patients with transient elevations are much more likely to develop overt hypertension at a later time and should be considered for primary prevention measures. In either case, it is important to look for factors that may be exacerbating the elevated pressure.

Home blood pressure monitoring by the patient has been demonstrated to be accurate and effective. It should be noted that pressures at home are generally lower and thus 135/85 should be considered the upper limit of normal in home monitoring. Home blood pressure assessment is useful both in diagnosis and in following the response to treatment.

Twenty-four hour ambulatory blood pressure monitoring has been shown to be accurate and to correlate best with left ventricular mass. Its role in the treatment of hypertension has not yet been defined. For the present, ambulatory monitoring has not proven cost effective for routine use, although patients monitored this way have been shown to require fewer antihypertensive medications than those monitored in the office. Until its role is more clearly defined, ambulatory blood pressure monitoring should probably be reserved for patients in whom blood pressure seems poorly controlled without evidence of end-organ damage, or those who develop orthostatic symptoms despite seemingly poor control.

History

The goal of the history is to establish the cause of hypertension (>95% will be primary), to determine the presence of exacerbating factors, and to assess cardiovascular risk. Primary hypertension usually occurs between the ages of 35 and 55, is gradual in onset (frequently with a preceding period of lability), and is often associated with a family history of hypertension. Onset at extremes of age, rapid onset of stage 2 or 3 hypertension in a previously normotensive individual, or poor response to treatment should prompt a search for secondary causes.

It is important to assess the overall risk of each patient for developing the complications of hypertension, as this will determine treatment goals and the timing and aggressiveness of subsequent therapy. It is useful to divide risk into modifiable and nonmodifiable risk factors, to emphasize the importance of treating not only the hypertension but all treatable risks as well.

The Framingham Study has identified several risk factors that, when present in combination with hypertension, greatly increase the likelihood of developing cardiovascular complications. These include the presence of **diabetes, smoking, hypercholesterolemia, a low HDL,** and **left ventricular hypertrophy** on electrocardiography. The likelihood of developing clinically apparent coronary artery disease over a 10-year period in a 40-year-old woman with hypertension alone is about 5%. If that same woman has all of the listed risk factors, her risk increases to almost 70%.

Weight is a significant risk, not only for developing hypertension, but also for developing the complications of hypertension. Obese women, especially those with central obesity, tend to have higher LDL and triglyceride levels and to have a marked increase in the incidence of diabetes, thus significantly increasing their risk of atherosclerotic complications.

Women who have a **sedentary lifestyle** tend to have a higher incidence of hypertension and are more likely to develop complications of hypertension.

Finally, it is important to recognize that the presence of **target organ damage** is a marker for significant risk. Indicators of target organ damage include the presence of retinopathy, left ventricular hypertrophy, arterial bruits or evidence of peripheral vascular disease, congestive heart failure, coronary disease, stroke, or renal insufficiency.

Physical Examination

The measurement of blood pressure is susceptible to several errors, the most common of which is inappropriate cuff size. The cuff should be large enough that the bladder surrounds at least 80% of the arm circumference (within the index lines on the cuff). Pressures measured with a cuff that is too small are falsely elevated. The patient should be seated and comfortable and the arm supported with the cuff at heart level. The patient should not have recently exercised nor had caffeinated beverages.

The remainder of the examination is focused on looking for signs of target organ damage. This includes a careful examination of the optic fundi (for retinopathy), heart and lungs (for signs of congestive heart failure and left ventricular hypertrophy), pulses (for bruits), and abdomen (for renal masses or abdominal aneurysm). In addition, attention should be paid to signs of possible secondary causes of hypertension, including renal artery stenosis, hyperthyroidism, hypothyroidism, Cushing's syndrome, and coarctation of the aorta.

Laboratory Evaluation

The initial laboratory evaluation should include measurement of potassium, blood urea nitrogen and/or creatinine, glucose, cholesterol, a urinalysis, and electrocardiogram. More extensive testing is unnecessary unless the history or physical examination has suggested a need for further testing.

✳ MANAGEMENT

Treatment of women with hypertension has been demonstrated in numerous studies to reduce the risk of stroke, heart disease, and renal failure. A recent meta-analysis of 11 randomized controlled trials of primary treatment of hypertension showed that in women 55 years or older, treatment resulted in a 38% reduction in fatal and nonfatal cerebrovascular events, a 25% reduction in fatal and nonfatal cardiovascular events, and a 17% reduction in cardiovascular mortality. Treatment of hypertension in African-American women of all ages conferred even greater benefit, with reductions in risk of 53%, 45%, and 33%, respectively. The treatment of white women aged 30 to 54 did not show statistically significant benefit. Thus, although it is clear that white women 55 and older and African-American women of all ages should be treated, treatment of younger white hypertensive women should be individualized and should consider their complete risk profile.

In general the goal of therapy is to lower pressure to less than 140/90. In patients with diabetes, this goal is lowered to 130/85 because of the marked increase in cardiovascular risk in patients with both hypertension and diabetes. In patients with renal insufficiency and proteinuria >1 g, the target of <125/75 is even more stringent.

It has been increasingly recognized that the risk of developing cardiovascular complications can differ dramatically depending on the associated risk factors. The treatment recommendations of JNC VI reflect that awareness and differ in the speed and aggressiveness with which pharmacologic treatment is indicated depending on the risk profile of an individual patient. For specific recommendations, see Table 3-1.

Nonpharmacologic Treatments

A variety of nonpharmacologic interventions have proven efficacy in reducing hypertension. These should be used in all hypertensive patients, since they may reduce the number or level of medications needed and in addition promote a generally healthier lifestyle.

Not surprisingly given the clear relationship between weight gain and the development of hypertension, **weight loss** is quite effective in lowering blood pressure, and in some patients with stage 1 hypertension may lower it enough to avoid the need for medication. In the TAIM Study, which compared patients treated with chlorthalidone,

Table 3-1
Treatment of Hypertension According to Risk

Blood Pressure Stage, mm Hg	Risk Group A	Risk Group B	Risk Group C
	No risk factors,* target organ damage, or clinical cardiovascular disease	At least one risk factor* (not including diabetes), no target organ damage or clinical cardiovascular disease	Target organ damage and/or clinical cardiovascular disease and/or diabetes, with or without other risk factors
High Normal 130-139/85-89	Lifestyle modification	Lifestyle modification	Drug therapy if heart failure, diabetes, or renal insufficiency; lifestyle modification
Stage 1 140-159/90-99	Lifestyle modification for up to 12 months	Lifestyle modification for up to 6 months; initial drug therapy for patients with multiple risk factors	Drug therapy Lifestyle modification
Stages 2 and 3 >160/100	Drug therapy Lifestyle modification	Drug therapy Lifestyle modification	Drug therapy Lifestyle modification

From the Joint National Committee: *Arch Intern Med* 157:2413, 1997.
*Major risk factors include smoking, dyslipidemia, diabetes mellitus, age >60 years, postmenopausal status, and family history.

atenolol, or placebo to those treated with diet, patients who lost 4.5 kg or more had the same degree of reduction of their blood pressure as those treated with medication. Thus it is not necessary to reach ideal body weight to achieve significant results. In addition to the benefits of reducing blood pressure, weight loss also lowers the risk of developing diabetes and reverses some of the adverse lipid effects that may occur with weight gain. **Exercise** is a useful adjunct for weight loss, as well as for cardiovascular health and reducing blood pressure.

Salt restriction induces a modest reduction in blood pressure in most hypertensive individuals. Although it is clear that not all persons with hypertension are sodium sensitive, at present we have no simple means for identifying those who are. Thus it is reasonable to suggest moderate salt restriction for all patients with hypertension. Those most likely to benefit from salt restriction include the elderly, African Americans, and obese women. In addition to lowering blood pressure, salt restriction also tends to lessen the hypokalemia induced by thiazide diuretics by preventing a large load of sodium from being delivered to the distal tubule.

In general, people who eat a diet high in potassium, magnesium, and calcium tend to have lower pressures. Studies of the effects of supplementation of these ions have demonstrated a tendency toward lower pressures without reaching statistical significance. Use of the **DASH diet** (Dietary Attempts to Stop Hypertension), a diet high in grains, fruits, vegetables, and low-fat dairy products that was high in these elements, resulted in an 11.4/5.5 mm Hg reduction in systolic and diastolic pressures, respectively. The DASH diet in combination with sodium restriction produced even more impressive results.

Because of the potential of alcohol to induce or exacerbate existing hypertension, **moderation of alcohol** is another step in nonpharmacologic management of hypertension. Daily alcohol intake of more than 2 oz of hard liquor, 10 oz of wine, or 24 oz of beer has been shown to cause hypertension in men; safe levels are presumably lower in women, although the exact quantities have not been defined.

Pharmacologic Treatment

The JNC V and VI reports recommended use of thiazide diuretics and beta blockers as the preferred first-line agents, generally to be used before the use of angiotensin-converting enzyme (ACE) inhibitors, calcium channel blockers, or alpha blockers except in certain circumstances. This recommendation was based on the fact that, while all of these classes have been proven equally effective in lowering blood pressure, only thiazides and beta-blockers have been proven in clinical trials to improve cardiovascular mortality and lower the incidence of stroke and myocardial infarction. Trials to demonstrate the effectiveness of the other classes in this regard are currently in progress.

First-Line Agents

Thiazide diuretics inhibit sodium uptake in the distal tubule of the kidney, thus decreasing intravascular volume and sodium content. In addition, they appear to have some direct vasodilating effect. They block the excretion of calcium in the distal tubule, which has been shown to be somewhat protective against the development of osteoporosis in elderly women. The primary side effects are hypokalemia, hypomagnesemia, and occasionally hyponatremia. In addition, by blocking the excretion of uric acid thiazides can precipitate gout in susceptible individuals. Thiazides increase

Table 3-2
Agents of Choice in Patients with Concomitant Disease

Condition	First Choice	Alternative	Not Recommended
Angina	Beta blocker	CCB	
Recent MI	Beta blocker	Nondihydropyridine CCB	Dihydropyridine CCB
Heart failure	Diuretic / ACE inhibitor		Dihydropyridine CCB / CCB
Dyslipidemia	All		
Diabetes	ACE inhibitor	Low-dose thiazide	
Asthma			Nonselective beta blocker
Migraine	Beta blocker	Nondihydropyridine CCB	Beta blocker / Dihydropyridine CCB
Bradyarrhythmia	?Alpha blocker		Beta blocker / Nondihydropyridine CCB

CCB, Calcium channel blocker; *MI*, myocardial infarction; *ACE*, angiotensin-converting enzyme.

insulin resistance and at higher doses can precipitate overt glucose intolerance.

Despite the fact that **beta blockers** have been used to reduce blood pressure for decades, the exact mechanism of action remains elusive. Beta blockers have several effects that may lower blood pressure, all or some of which may be active. These include a decrease in cardiac output, a decrease in renin release, a decrease in central sympatholytic activity and catecholamine release, and a decrease in peripheral resistance.

Additional First-Line Agents

ACE inhibitors block the conversion of angiotensin I to angiotensin II by inhibiting angiotensin converting enzyme. The clinical advantages of ACE inhibitors for hypertension have been demonstrated only in particular subgroups of patients, namely, patients with diabetes and patients with congestive heart failure and poor systolic function. There are so far only two studies published comparing the results of treatment with an ACE inhibitor to diuretics or beta blockade. The CAPP study demonstrated no benefit in the captopril-treated group and an increase in the incidence of stroke, possibly related to higher baseline pressures in the captopril-treated group. The STOP trial from Sweden compared conventional therapy using thiazides and beta blockers to outcomes in those treated with enalapril, lisinopril, or felodipine. There was no advantage using the newer agents in lowering cardiovascular mortality.

In light of current knowledge, ACE inhibitors are the first-line agents of choice in types 1 and 2 diabetes, in non-diabetic glomerular disease, and in patients with congestive heart failure and poor systolic function. It should also be noted that the traditional view that these drugs are not effective in African Americans appears to be incorrect, although generally the doses used need to be higher in this population.

The most common side effect of ACE inhibitors is cough, which occurs in as many as 20% of users. If the cough is mild and not bothersome to the patient, there is no need to discontinue the drug. Other side effects include angioedema, renal failure in the presence of bilateral renal artery stenosis, rash, change in taste, and hyperkalemia alone or in the presence of NSAIDs or potassium-sparing agents. They are absolutely contraindicated in pregnancy (see Chapter 72).

Angiotensin receptor blockers (ARBs) block the action of angiotensin at the receptor site and thus share many of the properties of ACE inhibitors. They do not cause the cough that commonly occurs with ACE inhibitors, which is thought to be secondary to the effect of increased levels of bradykinin. They are effective antihypertensive agents, but whether the cardiac and renal-protective effects seen with ACE inhibitors occur with ARBs has not been established. Until further evidence is available, it is reasonable to reserve this class for patients who would benefit from ACE inhibitors but cannot tolerate them because of cough.

The short-acting forms of **calcium channel blockers** have been shown to increase cardiovascular mortality and should not be used. This effect is probably related to the rapid onset and offset of these drugs, resulting in wide swings in blood pressure. The long-acting forms appear to be safe.

Different members of this class have significantly different effects on cardiac contractility and conduction and on the gastrointestinal tract (Table 3-2). They all work by blocking the calcium-dependent contraction of vascular smooth muscle. For simplicity, they may be divided into the dihydropyridines (nifedipine-like) and the nondihydropyridines (verapamil-like). In general the dihydropyridines have no effect on the atrioventricular (AV) node, are not significant negative inotropes, and do not cause as much constipation. They do tend to lower blood pressure more and to cause associated peripheral edema, which is secondary to a change in hydrostatic forces rather than volume retention. They also relax the lower esophageal sphincter and may cause significant gastric reflux.

Alpha blockers inhibit the postsynaptic alpha-1 receptors, thereby preventing activation by circulating catecholamines. They have several actions that would suggest a beneficial effect on cardiovascular mortality, including lowering insulin resistance, lowering total cholesterol, and raising HDL levels. Despite this, the alpha-blocker arm of the Antihypertensive and Lipid-Lowering Treatment to Prevent Heart Attack Trial (ALLHAT) was discontinued early because of a marked increase in the rate of congestive heart failure in patients treated with alpha blockers. Their role in the treatment of hypertension remains to be defined; at present, alpha blockers should probably not be considered first-line agents.

⊞ APPROACH TO TREATMENT

Thiazide diuretics should be considered the first-line agents for most patients, except those with diabetes, for whom ACE inhibitors are the drug of choice, or in patients following myocardial infarction, for whom beta blockers should be used. If blood pressure is not controlled, the dose should be increased. If there is no response, that drug should be discontinued and another tried. If there is a partial response, a low dose of a second agent should be added and its dose increased as needed. All the first-line agents can be combined with one another. If a diuretic has not been used, it should almost always be added as a second agent, as it enhances the efficacy of all other antihypertensive medications.

If blood pressure remains poorly controlled, it is important to review the following issues. Is the patient taking the medication as prescribed? It is important to ensure that the regimen is not too complicated and that the patient can afford the drugs prescribed. Are there unacceptable side effects that have not been discussed? Is the patient using excessive amounts of salt or alcohol? In the presence of renal insufficiency, blood pressure becomes much more difficult to control, yet control is critically important to delay the onset of overt renal failure. In this instance, a loop diuretic in substantial doses is often needed, in addition to combination therapy with multiple agents. Lastly, in patients who are poorly responsive to a three-drug regimen, secondary causes of hypertension should be considered.

BIBLIOGRAPHY

ALLHAT Collaborative Research Group: Major cardiovascular events in hypertensive patients randomized to doxazosin vs chlorthalidone: the antihypertensive and lipid-lowering treatment to prevent heart attack trial (ALLHAT), *JAMA* 283:1967, 2000.

Blacher J et al: Pulse pressure not mean pressure determines cardiovascular risk in older hypertensive patients, *Arch Intern Med* 160:1085, 2000.

Hansson L et al for the Captopril Prevention Project (CAPPP) study group: Effect of angiotensin-converting-enzyme inhibition compared with conventional therapy on cardiovascular morbidity and mortality in hypertension: the Captopril Prevention Project (CAPPP) randomised trial, *Lancet* 353:611, 1999.

Hansson L et al: Randomised trial of old and new antihypertensive drugs in elderly patients: cardiovascular mortality and morbidity. The Swedish Trial in Old Patients with Hypertension (STOP)-2 study, *Lancet* 354:1751, 1999.

Huang Z et al: Body weight, weight change and risk for hypertension in women, *Ann Intern Med* 128:81, 1998.

Joint National Committee: The sixth report of the Joint National Committee on Detection, Evaluation, and Treatment of High Blood Pressure, *Arch Intern Med* 157:2413, 1997.

Kannel WB: Risk stratification in hypertension: new insights from the Framingham Study, *Am J Hypertens* 131:3S, 2000.

Kannel WB: Blood pressure as a cardiovascular risk factor: prevention and treatment, *JAMA* 275:1591, 1996.

LaCroix AZ et al: Low dose hydrochlorothiazide and preservation of bone mineral density in older adults, *Ann Intern Med* 133:516, 2000.

MacMahon S et al: Blood pressure, stroke and coronary heart disease. Part I. Prolonged differences in blood pressure, *Lancet* 335:765, 1990.

Messerli FH et al: Disparate cardiovascular findings in men and women with essential hypertension, *Ann Intern Med* 107:158, 1987.

Seely EW, Walsh B, Gerhard MD, Williams D: Estradiol with or without progesterone and ambulatory blood pressure in postmenopausal women, *Hypertension* 33:1190, 1999.

Staessen JA et al: Antihypertensive treatment based on conventional or ambulatory blood pressure measurement, *JAMA* 278:1065, 1997.

Wassertheil-Smoller S et al: The Trial of Antihypertensive Interventions and Management (TAIM) Study, *Arch Intern Med* 152:131, 1992.

CHAPTER 4

Hyperlipidemia

Paula A. Johnson

Although an elevated cholesterol level is a risk factor for development of coronary heart disease, the degree of elevation that requires medical intervention, the age at which intervention is beneficial, and the population that should be screened for the abnormality continue to be studied and debated. Previously, criteria for the evaluation and treatment of hyperlipidemia had resulted mainly from studies performed in men, such as the Lipid Research Clinics Coronary Primary Prevention Trial, the Helsinki Heart Study, and the Multiple Risk Factor Intervention Trial. It has only been in the past few years that major primary and secondary prevention trials have included women, such as in the Cholesterol and Recurrent Events (CARE) Trial, the Scandinavian Simvastatin Survival Study (4S), the Long-Term Intervention with Pravastatin in Ischemic Disease (LIPID) study, and the Air Force/Texas Coronary Atherosclerosis Prevention Study (AFCAPS/TexCAPS). As gender differences in epidemiology, biology, and outcomes are elucidated, the need for continued research that is inclusive of women grows.

This chapter addresses the following topics: the epidemiologic evidence relating cholesterol and lipoproteins to the development of coronary heart disease, screening and management of hyperlipidemia, the role of postmenopausal estrogen replacement in the hyperlipidemic patient, and the influence of oral contraceptive agents and progesterone agents on the lipid profile. A discussion of inherited forms of hyperlipidemias is beyond the scope of this chapter.

EPIDEMIOLOGY
RELATIONSHIP OF LIPIDS TO CORONARY HEART DISEASE

The Framingham Study proved the important relationship between increased total cholesterol level and increased risk of coronary heart disease (CHD). Over time it has become known that **low-density lipoprotein (LDL)** is the most atherogenic fraction of cholesterol. Oxidized LDL is considered significantly more atherogenic than its unoxidized precursor. This discovery has led to the investigation of antioxidants, such as vitamin E and folic acid, as agents that may be useful in primary and secondary prevention of CHD. The AFCAPS/TexCaps study showed a reduction in coronary events in a population of men and women with moderately elevated LDL and without coronary disease when treated with lovastatin. The inverse relationship between postmenopausal estrogen replacement and levels of LDL may constitute part of the basis for the finding of less CHD in women receiving postmenopausal estrogen replacement in observational studies. Elevated LDL levels are not as predictive of total cardiovascular mortality or all-cause mortality in women.

High-density lipoprotein (HDL), on the other hand, is protective against CHD. Apoprotein AI is the major component of HDL and is thought to act primarily as a transport molecule, removing cholesterol from tissue and delivering it to the liver. Data from the Framingham Study and the Lipid Research Clinics Follow-Up Study suggest that the level of HDL may be a particularly important risk factor for women and may be more predictive of the development of CHD than the level of LDL. Although the major focus in the AFCAPS/TexCAPS intervention was reduction in LDL, HDL increased as well. Therefore it is unclear how much of the decrease in coronary event rates should be attributed to LDL reduction versus increase in HDL. The lipid changes seen with the loss of endogenous estrogen, including a decrease in HDL and an increase in LDL, are believed to contribute to the increase in CHD observed in postmenopausal women. Lipid levels as predictors of cardiovascular death in white women were examined in the 14-year follow-up study of the Lipid Research Clinics Study. In women ages 50 to 69 years, HDL was an independent predictor of risk of cardiovascular disease (CVD) mortality. LDL was a poor predictor of CVD mortality.

The role of **triglycerides** in the development of CHD has not been fully defined. Data from several prospective studies, including the Framingham Study, identified elevated triglyceride levels as a univariate predictor for the development of CHD. This association does not persist in most studies once additional risk factors, LDL, and HDL are included in multivariate models. There was a small independent increase in the risk of mortality during 5 years of follow-up in a population of women with known coronary heart disease and elevated triglycerides who were screened for inclusion in a secondary prevention trial. A combined high triglyceride level and low HDL level may be a more important risk factor for the development of CHD in women.

Lipoprotein (a) (Lp [a]), a molecule with structural similarities to LDL and plasminogen, is associated with the development of atherosclerotic vascular disease. It is thought that the majority of the population has low Lp(a) levels (<0.2 g/L) and only a small proportion of the population has high (>1.0 g/L) levels that are associated with atherosclerotic disease. The presence of estrogen may lower Lp(a) levels, given that postmenopausal women have been found to have significantly higher levels than premenopausal women.

Women receiving postmenopausal estrogen replacement also have lower levels of Lp(a) than women not receiving hormone replacement. Data from the Heart and Estrogen/Progestin Replacement Study (HERS), a secondary prevention trial, showed that Lp(a) was an independent risk factor for recurrent coronary heart disease. A meta-analysis of 27 prospective studies in which the association of Lp(a) and CHD was evaluated showed that those in the top third of Lp(a) measurements had a 60% increase in risk of CHD death compared with those in the lowest third of Lp(a) measurement ($P < 0.00001$).

Whether there is a difference in the strength of the correlation between elevation in cholesterol levels and development or rate of progression of CHD in the elderly is also controversial. AFCAPS/TexCAPS, a study of primary prevention that included patients with a maximum age of 73 years, showed a 37% decrease in coronary events in patients with a moderately elevated LDL treated with lovastatin. A subanalysis of patients >65 years of age has not been published. It may be that in older patients other comorbid illnesses lead to a decrease in LDL and therefore weaken the association between LDL and cardiovascular events. It has been shown that when a low serum albumin and death within 1 year are taken into account, the relationship between an elevated cholesterol and the risk of death from coronary heart disease remains strong.

SCREENING

Cholesterol levels increase with age until one reaches the age group of 54 through 74 years, during which time the total cholesterol levels tend to decline. This trend holds true for women, although there is a delay of several years before the decrease is observed. In addition, levels of total cholesterol continue to decrease for the elderly population above 75 years of age. Men tend to have higher cholesterol levels than women until middle age (45 to 55 years of age), which coincides with menopause and the decline of endogenous estrogen levels in women.

Data from the National Health and Nutrition Examination Survey (NHANES) revealed the percentage of the population with total cholesterol levels greater than 240 mg/dl decreased from 26% in 1976 through 1980 to less than 20% for 1988 through 1994 (NHANES III). The decrease was similar for men and women. Although there has been a significant decrease in the proportion of the population with elevated cholesterol levels, a large number of people still required dietary and pharmacological intervention.

The Third Report of the National Cholesterol Education Program (NCEP) Expert Panel on Detection, Evaluation, and Treatment of High Blood Cholesterol in Adults (Adult Treatment Panel III [ATP III] recently issued May 2001) updated the recommendations for cholesterol screening and

management in its two previous reports, ATP I (1988) and ATP II (1993). It focuses on prevention of coronary heart disease in those with risk factors. These most recent guidelines still focus recommendations on the level of LDL, with <100 mg/dL defined as optimal for the entire population (Table 4-1), but lower the threshold for starting cholesterol-lowering agents and stratifies patients without CHD into risk categories, recommending that these "high risk" people be treated as if they had CHD (Table 4-2).

These changes have important implications for women. The panel identifies diabetes as significant a risk factor for coronary heart disease. Since women have a higher rate of diabetes, and women with diabetes suffer cardiac complications at a higher rate than men, all of their risk factors for heart disease—including elevated cholesterol—should be treated aggressively.

The guidelines also use Framingham projections of 10-year absolute CHD risk by gender (i.e., the percent probability of having a CHD event in 10 years, Fig. 4-1) to identify those patients with more than two risk factors for intensive treatment.

New is the recommendation that patients with "the metabolic syndrome" be considered as candidates for aggressive lifestyle changes and management (Box 4-1), a change that has implications for women.

The definition of low HDL has been modified from <35 mg/dL to <40 mg/dL and the cutoff for abnormal triglycerides has been lowered to focus treatment on modest elevations (both strong predictors for CHD in women; see Box 4-1).

By the new guidelines, patients at highest risk are defined as those with greater than 20% ten-year risk of coronary event by the Framingham global risk score, any atherosclerosis (peripheral arterial disease, abdominal aortic aneurysm, transient ischemic attacks, and/or stroke), and diabetes.

Treatment guidelines have also been modified with recommendations for cholesterol lowering medications in place of hormonal replacement therapy as primary intervention for high cholesterol in post-menopausal women and more aggressive lifestyle changes (lower intake of saturated fats and cholesterol, increased physical activity, and weight control) as the first line of intervention.

The panel recommends that *all adults aged 20 years or older undergo a fasting lipid profile (total cholesterol, LDL-C, HDL-C, and triglycerides) once every five years.* The results of the tests should be considered along with determinations for major risk factors (Box 4-2) and the 10-year CHD risk assessment (see Fig. 4-1).

✳ MANAGEMENT

Hypercholesterolemia

Goals of Therapy

Once the initial screening for hyperlipidemia is performed, intervention should be based on the patient's risk for CHD (or CHD-equivalents) (see Box 4-2). This is determined by identifying CHD or CHD risk equivalents, counting the risk factors and estimating the 10-year risk.

The NCEP also recommends that any person identified with an elevated LDL level or another form of hyperlipidemia should be screened for secondary dyslipidemia which includes screening for diabetes, hypothyroidism, obstructive

Table 4-1
Recommended Treatments of US NCEP Based on LDL Cholesterol Level

Risk Category	LDL Goal (mg/dl)	LDL Level at Which to Initiate Therapeutic Lifestyle Changes (mg/dL)	LDL Level at Which to Consider Drug Therapy (mg/dL)
CHD or CHD risk equivalents* (10-year risk >20%)	<100	≥100	≥130 (100-129: drug optional†)
2+ risk factors (10-year risk <20%)	<130	≥130	10-year risk 10%-20%: ≥130
0-1 risk factors‡	<160	≥160	10-year risk <10%: ≥160 ≥190 (160-189: LDL-lowering drug optional)

From Expert Panel on Detection, Evaluation, and Treatment of High Blood Cholesterol in Adults (Adult Treatment Panel III). *JAMA* 285:2486, 2001.
LDL, Low-density lipoprotein; *CHD,* coronary heart disease.
* See Box 4-3 for determination of risk equivalents.
† Some recommend use of LDL-lowering agents in this category if an LDL cholesterol of <100 mg/dL cannot be achieved by therapeutic lifestyle changes. Others prefer use of drugs that primarily modify triglycerides and HDL, for example, nicotinic acid of fibrate. Clinical judgment also may call for deferring drug therapy in this subcategory.
‡ Almost all people with 0-1 risk factors have a 10-year risk <10%; thus risk assessment in people with 0-1 risk factors is not necessary.

Table 4-2
Adult Treatment Panel III Serum Lipid Classification

Lipid Level (mg/dL)	Classification
LDL-cholesterol	
<100	Optimal
100-129	Near optimal or above optimal
130-159	Borderline high
160-189	High
≥190	Very high
HDL-cholesterol	
<40	Low (considered a risk factor for CHD)
≥60	High (protective against CHD)
Total cholesterol	
<200	Desirable
200-239	Borderline high
≥240	High
Triglycerides	
<150	Normal
150-199	Borderline high
200-499	High
≥500	Very high

From Expert Panel on Detection, Evaluation, and Treatment of High Blood Cholesterol in Adults (Adult Treatment Panel III): *JAMA* 285:2486, 2001.
LDL, Low density lipoprotein; *HDL,* high density lipoprotein.

liver disease, and renal failure. Drugs such as progestins, anabolic steroids and corticosteroids can increase LDL-C levels and lower HDL-C levels. Triglyceride levels may increase in women who receive oral contraceptives or postmenopausal estrogen replacement, given that exogenous oral estrogen can lead to elevation in triglyceride levels. Whereas initial treatment should be focused on the underlying abnormality, persisting lipid abnormalities should be managed according to NCEP guidelines.

Primary Prevention

The AFCAPS/TexCAPS study of lipid lowering with lovastatin in men and women with average LDL (150 mg/dl) and HDL (40 mg/dl for women and 36 mg/dl for men) showed a decrease in first acute major coronary events by 37% (RR 0.63 [95% CI 0.50 to 0.79]). This study did not stratify the results by gender (5608 men and 997 women). Several observational prospective studies that included women, such as the Framingham Heart Study, the Lipid Research Clinics Program Follow-Up Study, and the Rancho Bernardo Study, support that women benefit from lower levels of cholesterol with a decrease in morbidity and mortality rates from CHD. The effect of lowering cholesterol on overall mortality rate has been somewhat controversial. Data from the Cardiovascular Health Study show that low levels of total cholesterol (<160 mg/dl) have been associated with an increase in the rate of cancer diagnosed in the preceding 5 years in women. These data, combined with evidence suggesting that LDL may not be as strong a risk factor for CHD and that HDL may have a particularly strong protective effect in women compared with men, raise the question of whether treatment guidelines for hyperlipidemia should be the same for both genders.

For patients without known CHD, risk stratification is based on total cholesterol and HDL levels. A total cholesterol of 200 mg/dl is considered a desirable blood cholesterol level. A total cholesterol level of 200 to 239 mg/dl is considered borderline high and ≥240 mg/dl is considered a high blood cholesterol level. By the new guidelines an HDL level of ≤40 mg/dl is considered a risk factor for CHD. It is suggested that patients with low levels of HDL or high blood cholesterol levels have a lipoprotein analysis performed in the fasting state to quantify the level of LDL. Levels of LDL for patients without CHD are stratified as follows: optimal (<100 mg/dl), near optimal (100-129 mg/dl), borderline high risk (130 to 159 mg/dl, with or without two or more risk factors), high risk (≥160 mg/dl), and very high risk—aggressive (>190 mg/dl). Dietary therapy is recommended for patients in the borderline high-risk category with two or more risk factors for CHD and for those in the high-risk category. Given the results of AFCAPS/TexCAPS, these guidelines have been revised to reflect the benefit of treatment with HMA CoA reductase inhibitors in patients with borderline high-risk LDL (see Table 4-2).

Secondary Prevention

There are now good data to support the benefit of lowering cholesterol with HMA CoA reductase inhibitors in women with known coronary heart disease. The Cholesterol

Estimate of 10-Year Risk for Men
(Framingham Point Scores)

Age, y	Points
20-34	−9
35-39	−4
40-44	0
45-49	3
50-54	6
55-59	8
60-64	10
65-69	11
70-74	12
75-79	13

Total cholesterol, mg/dL	Points Age 20-39 y	Age 40-49 y	Age 50-59 y	Age 60-69 y	Age 70-79 y
<160	0	0	0	0	0
160-199	4	3	2	1	0
200-239	7	5	3	1	0
240-279	9	6	4	2	1
≥280	11	8	5	3	1

	Points Age 20-39 y	Age 40-49 y	Age 50-59 y	Age 60-69 y	Age 70-79 y
Nonsmoker	0	0	0	0	0
Smoker	8	5	3	1	1

HDL, mg/dL	Points
≥60	−1
50-59	0
40-49	1
<40	2

Systolic BP, mm Hg	If untreated	If treated
<120	0	0
120-129	0	1
130-139	1	2
140-159	1	2
≥160	2	3

Point total	10-year risk, %
<0	<1
0	1
1	1
2	1
3	1
4	1
5	2
6	2
7	3
8	4
9	5
10	6
11	8
12	10
13	12
14	16
15	20
16	25
≥17	≥30

A

Estimate of 10-Year Risk for Women
(Framingham Point Scores)

Age, y	Points
20-34	−7
35-39	−3
40-44	0
45-49	3
50-54	6
55-59	8
60-64	10
65-69	12
70-74	14
75-79	16

Total cholesterol, mg/dL	Points Age 20-39 y	Age 40-49 y	Age 50-59 y	Age 60-69 y	Age 70-79 y
<160	0	0	0	0	0
160-199	4	3	2	1	1
200-239	8	6	4	2	1
240-279	11	8	5	3	2
≥280	13	10	7	4	2

	Points Age 20-39 y	Age 40-49 y	Age 50-59 y	Age 60-69 y	Age 70-79 y
Nonsmoker	0	0	0	0	0
Smoker	9	7	4	2	1

HDL, mg/dL	Points
≥60	−1
50-59	0
40-49	1
<40	2

Systolic BP, mm Hg	If untreated	If treated
<120	0	0
120-129	1	3
130-139	2	4
140-159	3	5
≥160	4	6

Point total	10-year risk, %
<9	<1
9	1
10	1
11	1
12	1
13	2
14	2
15	3
16	4
17	5
18	6
19	8
20	11
21	14
22	17
23	22
24	27
≥25	≥30

B

FIG. 4-1 Estimating 10-year risk for women and men. Risk assessment for determining the 10-year risk for developing CHD is carried out using Framingham risk scoring (**A,** men and **B,** women). The risk factors included in the Framingham calculation of 10-year risk are age, total cholesterol, HDL cholesterol, systolic blood pressure, treatment for hypertension, and cigarette smoking. The first step is to calculate the number of points for each risk factor. For initial assessment, values for total cholesterol and HDL cholesterol are required. Because of a larger database, Framingham estimates are more robust for total cholesterol than for LDL cholesterol. Note, however, that the LDK and HDL cholesterol values should be the average of at least two measurements obtained at the time of lipoprotein analysis. The blood pressure value used is that obtained at the time of assessment, regardless of whether the person in on antihypertensive therapy. However, if the person is on antihypertensive treatment, an extra point is added beyond points for the blood pressure reading because treated hypertension carries residual risk (**A** and **B**). The average of several blood pressure measurements, as recommended by the Joint National Committee (JNC), is needed for an accurate measure of baseline blood pressure. The designation "smoker" means any cigarette smoking in the past month. The total risk score sums the points for each risk factor. The 10-year risk for myocardial infarction and coronary death (hard CHD) is estimated from total points, and the person is categorized according to absolute 10-year risk as indicated previously (see Table 4-2). (Expert Panel on Detection, Evaluation, and Treatment of High Blood Cholesterol in Adults: Summary of the Second Report of the National Cholesterol Education Program (NCEP) Expert Panel on Detection, Evaluation, and Treatment of High Blood Cholesterol in Adults (Adult Treatment Panel III), *JAMA* 285:2486, 2001.)

BOX 4-1
Metabolic Syndrome

Abdominal Obesity
   Waist circumference:
      Men   >102 cm (>40 in)
      Women >88 cm (>35 in)
Atherogenic dyslipidemia
    Elevated triglycerides   ≥150 mg/dL
    Small LDL particles
    Low HDL cholesterol   <40 mg/dL for men
                           <50 mg/dL for women
Hypertension   ≥130/>85 mm Hg
Insulin resistance (with or without
    glucose intolerance)   ≥110 mg/dL
Prothrombotic and proinflammatory states

BOX 4-2
Major Risk Factors (Exclusive of LDL) That Modify LDL Goals

CHD Risk Equivalents
Abdominal aortic aneurysm
Peripheral vascular disease
Symptomatic carotid artery disease
Diabetes

Major CHD Risk Factors
Cigarette smoking
Hypertension (blood pressure ≥140/90 mm Hg or on antihypertensive
   medication)
Low HDL cholesterol (<40 mg/dL)*
Family history of premature CHD (CHD in male first-degree relative
   <55 years; CHD in female first-degree relative <65 years)
Age (women ≥55 years; men ≥45 years)

Modified from Expert Panel on Detection, Evaluation, and Treatment of High Blood Cholesterol in Adults (Adult Treatment Panel III): *JAMA* 285:2486, 2001.
CHD, Coronary heart disease; *LDL*, low-density lipoprotein; *HDL*, high-density lipoprotein.
* HDL cholesterol ≥60 mg/dL is considered a negative risk factor removing one risk factor from the total count.

---

and Recurrent Events (CARE) Trial included 576 women with a history of myocardial infarction and a mean total cholesterol of <240 mg/dl and LDL of 115 mg/dl to 174 mg/dl. The treatment group received 40 mg of pravastatin with 5 years of follow-up. Women randomized to the study drug experienced a 43% decrease in coronary deaths or nonfatal MI and stroke, and a 46% decrease in all coronary events, including death, myocardial infarction (MI), stroke, percutaneous coronary transluminal coronary angioplasty (PTCA), and coronary artery bypass graft (CABG). The 46% decrease was significantly greater than the 20% decrease in coronary events seen in the male population that was randomized to pravastatin ($P = 0.001$). Similarly, the Scandinavian Simvastatin Survival Study (4S), that included 827 women (19% of the 4444 enrolled) who had a history of MI or angina with an elevated total cholesterol (213 mg/dl to 309 mg/dl) and triglycerides ≤220 mg/dl. Patients were randomized to simvastatin, 20 mg/day, with an increase to 40 mg/day, depending on the response to the lower dose. Although there were too few deaths in women to evaluate the effect of lipid lowering on mortality, there was a significant decrease in major coronary events (RR 0.66 [95% CI 0.48, 0.91]). The 34% decrease in major coronary events in women randomized to simvastatin was the same as the decrease seen in the male population. The Long-Term Intervention with Pravastatin in Ischemic Disease (LIPID) study randomized 9014 patients with ischemic heart disease to pravastatin or placebo. In all 17% of the population were women, with total cholesterol levels of 155 mg/dl to 271 mg/dl at baseline and an average LDL of 150 mg/dl. After 6 years of follow-up, there was a 24% decrease in nonfatal MI and CHD death in the total population. In addition, there was a 24% decrease in total death from any cause. This study has the largest number of women enrolled of the three main secondary prevention trials of lipid lowering with "statin" drugs.

For patients in whom secondary prevention is undertaken, intervention is based on LDL cholesterol level. An optimal level of LDL cholesterol is ≤100 mg/dl. Dietary therapy has been suggested for patients with LDL of 100 mg/dl and 130 mg/dl, with drug therapy suggested in those with LDL of ≥130 mg/dl. Recommendations for intervention are summarized in Table 4-2. The results of the CARE study, which

revealed positive benefits in women treated with a statin drug who had LDL levels of 115 to 174 mg/dl, provide data that may lead to revision of these guidelines. In addition, the NCEP II guidelines do not take into consideration HDL levels as part of the decision-making process regarding initiation of drug therapy.

Premenopausal women lose the protective effect of their premenopausal status if they have diabetes mellitus. The NCEP recommends that all patients with diabetes mellitus be screened and treated according to the guidelines developed for patients with established CHD. It is also important to note that diabetics frequently have elevated levels of triglycerides.

There is evidence that hyperlipidemia in women with known ischemic heart disease may be undertreated. In all, 90% of the women in HERS, a study of hormone replacement therapy in women with known ischemic heart disease, had an LDL >100 mg/dl.

Although HDL level may be a particularly important factor in the protection against CHD in women, it is not clear what steps should be followed in the case of patients with low levels of HDL and satisfactory levels of LDL. There are no good data to suggest that intervention in this population, beyond dietary and lifestyle changes, is beneficial. This is the case for both primary and secondary prevention. There is recent evidence that measurement of C-reactive protein in patients with normal levels of LDL may further refine risk for CHD events and CHD mortality. Statin drugs decrease the level of C-reactive protein. The use of statins in this population is under study.

Types of Therapy
Dietary Intervention
Change in diet is an important method of lowering cholesterol level. Although improved over the past 20 years, the average American diet leaves room for significant refine-

Table 4-3
Nutrient Composition of the Therapeutic Lifestyle Changes (TLC) Diet

Nutrient	Recommended Intake
Saturated fat*	<7% of total calories
Polyunsaturated fat	Up to 10% of total calories
Monounsaturated fat	Up to 20% of total calories
Total fat	25%-35% of total calories
Carbohydrate†	50%-60% of total calories
Fiber	20-30 grams/day
Protein	Approximately 15% of total calories
Cholesterol	<200 mg/dL
Total Calories‡	Balance energy intake and expenditure to maintain desirable body weight/prevent weight gain

From Expert Panel on Detection, Evaluation, and Treatment of High Blood Cholesterol in Adults (Adult Treatment Panel III): *JAMA* 285:2486, 2001.
* *Trans* fatty acids are another LDL-raising fat that should be kept at a low intake.
† Carbohydrates should be derived predominantly from foods rich in complex carbohydrates including grains, especially whole grains, fruits and vegetables.
‡ Daily energy expenditures should include at least moderate physical activity (contributing approximately 200 kcal/day).

ment with regard to fat intake. For example, an average daily US diet derives 37% of its caloric content from fat and 14% from saturated fat and contains 450 mg of cholesterol. Dietary cholesterol and saturated fats result in an increase in LDL level by suppressing hepatic LDL receptor activity and resulting in decreased clearance.

Diet therapy is described in Table 4-3. It is suggested that a 6-month trial of intensive dietary therapy, with nutritional consultation, be undertaken to achieve the desired LDL level (see Table 4-2). If dietary therapy is not successful after this period, drug therapy should be considered. Expected rates of success in dietary intervention are not well defined.

Weight reduction in overweight patients with abnormal lipid profiles is an essential element of the dietary intervention. In addition to lowering LDL levels, weight reduction leads to a decrease in triglyceride level and blood pressure. Data from the Third National Health and Nutrition Examination Survey (NHANES III) show that 43% of Caucasian women, 64.5% of African-American women, and 56.8% of Hispanic women are overweight. Interestingly the distribution of the overweight population differs for men and women, with the peak prevalence in men occurring from ages 45 to 54 years (31%). The prevalence in women continues to increase through later life, peaking at ages 65 through 74 years (39%). Because of the age distribution of overweight persons, the older female population may be more sedentary and less inclined or able to engage in regular physical exercise. It has been shown that a combination of dietary change, behavior modification, and physical exercise is the most successful strategy for achieving and maintaining weight loss. Assisting patients in achieving and maintaining weight loss is important, given that weight fluctuations (i.e., yo-yo dieting) may be an independent risk factor for mortality attributable to CHD.

A combination of weight reduction and physical exercise has been shown to lead to an improvement in the lipid profile with a decrease in LDL level, an increase in HDL level, and a decrease in triglyceride levels. Interestingly, calorie- and fat-restricted diets (NCEP Step I) and exercise may have differing effects on HDL level in women and men. Women may experience a lowering of HDL level with diet intervention alone. The addition of exercise may counter this decrease and result in an unchanged level of HDL. A combination of diet and exercise results in significant lowering of LDL levels.

Drug Therapy

Choice of Therapy. Cholesterol-lowering drugs can be divided into four main groups: 3-hydroxy-3-methylglutaryl coenzyme A (HMG CoA) reductase inhibitors or statins, bile acid sequestrants, nicotinic acid (niacin), and fibric acid derivatives. Although a detailed discussion of the mechanisms of cholesterol-lowering drugs is beyond the scope of this chapter, a brief description of the effects and side effects of the major drug classes can be found in Table 4-4.

HMG CoA Reductase Inhibitors (Statins). As discussed earlier in this chapter, statins have been shown to decrease cardiovascular mortality and/or cardiovascular events in women in both the CARE and 4S studies of secondary prevention. Pravastatin was shown to lead to a significant decrease in cardiovascular events, cardiovascular mortality, and total mortality in the LIPID study, although the data for women have not been published separately. Lovastatin was shown to be beneficial in decreasing cardiovascular mortality and events in study of primary prevention, but we do not have specific data for the women in the study. Statins effectively decrease LDL levels by 20% to 55% and slightly raise HDL level (5% to 15%). There is a slight effect on triglycerides (decrease 7% to 30%). The currently available statins include lovastatin (Mevacor), pravastatin (Pravachol), simvastatin (Zocar), fluvastatin (Lescol), and atorvastatin (Lipitor). Atorvastatin is the most potent of the statins and is thought to have some effect on lowering triglycerides. Statin drugs are well tolerated.

Nicotinic Acid (Niacin). Niacin lowers LDL by approximately 5% to 25%, lowers triglyceride levels by approximately 2% to 50%, and increases levels of HDL by 15% to 35%. Flushing is the most common side effect of niacin. An aspirin taken a half hour before the dose and dosing with meals may decrease cutaneous flushing and increase tolerability of the drug. Other side effects caused by niacin include elevated liver function tests, gout, and glucose intolerance. Niacin has not been well studied in women.

Bile Acid Sequestrants. Bile acid sequestrants, such as cholestyramine and colestipol, are among the oldest cholesterol-lowering agents. They can lead to a decrease in LDL by approximately 15% to 30%, with a small increase in HDL (3% to 5%). The bile acid sequestrants are often associated with no change or an increase in triglycerides. Constipation and bloating are common side effects.

Fibric Acid Derivatives. The fibric acid derivatives, such as gemfibrozil, have their main effect on lowering triglyceride level. These agents also lead to a modest decrease in LDL (5% to 20%) and a modest increase in HDL (10% to 20%). They are mainly used as a treatment for familial combined

Table 4-4
Lipid Lowering Agents

Drug Class	Dose	Effect	Side Effects	Indications
3-Hydroxy-3 Methylglutaryl Coenzyme A Reductase Inhibitors (Statins)				
Lovastatin	20-80 mg/day	Lowers LDL	Hepatitis, myositis and teratogenicity	High LDL level
Pravastatin	20-80 mg/day	Slightly increases HDL		
Simvastatin	20-40 mg/day	Slightly decreases		
Fluvastatin	20-80 mg/day	triglycerides		
Atorvastatin	10-80 mg/day			
Nicotinic Acid (Niacin)				
Immediate release (crystalline) nicotinic acid	1.5-3 gm/day	Lowers LDL Increases HDL Lowers TG	Hepatitis, gout, hyperglycemia. Ulcerogenesis, acanthosis nigricans, ichthyosis, atrial dysrhythmias, insomnia	High TG High LDL Low HDL
Extended release nicotinic acid	1-2 gm/day			
Sustained release nicotinic acid	1-2 gm/day			
Bile Acid Sequestrants				
Cholestyramine colestipol	8-12 gm bid 10 mg bid for colestipol	Lower LDL Slightly increases HDL	Constipation, abdominal pain, nausea, bloating, drug interactions and hypertriglyceridemia	High LDL
Fibric Acid Derivatives				
Gemfibrozil	600 mg bid	Lowers TG	Cholelithiasis, hepatitis, high LDL, decreased libido, myositis, ventricular dysrhythmia, increased appetite, abdominal pain, nausea	High TG Low HDL
Fenofibrate	200 mg	Increases HDL		
Clofibrate	1000 mg bid	May increase or lower LDL		

From Expert Panel on Detection, Evaluation, and Treatment of High Blood Cholesterol in Adults (Adult Treatment Panel III), *JAMA* 285: 2486, 2001.
LDL, Low-density lipoprotein; HDL, high-density lipoprotein; TG, triglycerides; CHD, coronary heart disease.

hyperlipidemia and hypertriglyceridemia, and decrease triglycerides by 20% to 50%. Side effects include dyspepsia, gallstones, myopathy, and unexplained non-CHD deaths in the WHO study.

Monitoring Therapy

The new NCEP guidelines recommend that after initiating LDL lowering drug therapy (generally a statin unless contraindications) to check the lipid profile and liver function tests after 6 weeks. If the LDL goal is not achieved then one should consider increasing the dose of a statin (if this was the initial therapy) or add a secondary agent such as a bile acid sequestrant or nicotinic acid. The lipid profile should then be checked again 6 weeks later and if the LDL is still not within recommended range a referral to a lipid specialist is warranted. It is important to continue with lifestyle changes and treatment of other CHD risk factors. Routine monitoring is then every 4 to 6 months to assure adherence to therapy.

Hypertriglyceridemia

Goals of Therapy

The role that triglycerides play in atherogenesis is still unclear. Fasting triglyceride levels are stratified into four categories: normal (<100 mg/dl), borderline high (150 to 199 mg/dl), high (200 to 499 mg/dl), and very high (<500 mg/dl). Patients with levels greater than 1000 have a significant risk of pancreatitis and should be treated. Drug treatment should be aimed at lowering both triglyceride and LDL levels for patients with known elevation in LDL level and high triglyceride level. Agents such as niacin or gemfibrozil are recommended especially for very high triglycerides (see Table 4-4). By new criteria more patients will be categorized with borderline high triglycerides, low HDL levels, and normal LDL. It is still unclear how best to treat them. Often, the borderline high triglycerides are seen in persons with the metabolic syndrome. Since all of these are independent risk factors for CHD, emphasis should be placed on weight reduction, modification of alcohol intake and increasing exercise.

Postmenopausal Hormone Replacement

Postmenopausal estrogen replacement is thought to decrease a woman's risk of morbidity and mortality from CHD. One mechanism through which estrogen replacement may provide protection is its beneficial effect on the lipid profile: a decrease in LDL level by 10% to 15% and an increase in HDL level by 10% to 15%. A first-pass effect through the liver is required for the effect on lipids. Therefore it is necessary that oral estrogen be used to achieve these benefits. Oral estrogen may also lead to a mild increase in triglyceride level. This effect may be problematic if the patient is hypertriglyceridemic before initiation of therapy. It may be beneficial to know a patient's triglyceride level before initiating estrogen therapy, although there are no published guidelines addressing this issue. Postmenopausal estrogen therapy may also improve the lipid profile by resulting in a decreased level of Lp(a).

A small study to evaluate the efficacy of hormone replacement therapy (HRT) in the treatment of hyperlipidemia was performed in postmenopausal women with coronary artery disease and LDL <130 mg/dl. Simvastatin, HRT, and the combination of the two decreased LDL by 45%, 20%, and 46%, respectively. Simvastatin was significantly more effective at reducing LDL and achieving a level of <100 mg/dl compared with HRT. The combination of HRT and simvastatin was well tolerated.

Most women with an intact uterus who are taking HRT receive a combination of estrogen and a progestin. The Postmenopausal Estrogen/Progestin Interventions (PEPI) trial showed that micronized progesterone had less of a detrimental effect on HDL compared with medroxyprogesterone.

The HERS study of HRT in secondary prevention of CHD in women revealed no significant difference in CAD deaths or nonfatal MI in the users of HRT. There was an increase in events during the first year after randomization in women receiving HRT. During years 4 and 5 after randomization, there was a statistically nonsignificant trend toward a decreased rate of fatal myocardial infarction and fatal cardiovascular events in women receiving HRT.

Despite the belief that estrogen provides a cardioprotective effect for women, the findings of these primary and secondary prevention trials have made the decision to use HRT even more complex. Statins, on the other hand, have been shown favorable effects on lowering cholesterol resulting in the new recommendation by the NCEP to use a cholesterol lowering drug rather than hormonal replacement therapy as the first line of pharmacological treatment aimed at lowering CHD risk.

Hormonal Contraception

Oral contraceptive agents provide an easy and highly effective form of birth control. The widespread use of these agents has raised questions regarding their impact on patients' risk for CHD. Most oral contraceptive agents contain a combination of synthetic estrogen and progesterone. The progesterone is usually one of the several available C-19 steroids that are thought to be more androgenic than the progesterone used in hormone replacement therapy. Over the past 20 years the dose of estrogen and progesterone contained in these preparations has decreased. Different types of progestins impact patients' lipid profiles differently. For example monophasic desogestrel and low-dose norethindrone, in combination with low-dose estrogen, may have the least negative impact on HDL and LDL levels. Overall, studies of lipid profiles of women taking oral contraceptives have shown that there is little impact on the lipid profile, except in elevations in triglyceride levels. Therefore underlying hypertriglyceridemia may be exacerbated by oral contraceptive agents. If a patient has a strong family history of hyperlipidemia, it may be worthwhile to screen for hypertriglyceridemia before initiating use of an oral contraceptive agent.

There is no evidence that oral contraceptives accelerate the rate of development of atherosclerotic vascular disease. Data from the Nurse's Health Study showed no association between past oral contraceptive use and development of coronary artery disease.

The impact on patients' lipid profiles of long-acting progestational agents, including levonorgestrel (Norplant) and injectable medroxyprogesterone acetate (Depo-Provera), has not been well described. Currently there are no guidelines for prescribing progestational agents in patients with preexisting lipid abnormalities.

■ PREGNANCY AND HYPERLIPIDEMIA

Total triglyceride and cholesterol levels (including all subfractions) increase during pregnancy. Hormonal changes, such as the rise of estrogen and progesterone levels during pregnancy and the relative insulin resistance that develops in the later half of pregnancy, may be factors in the observed lipid changes. Elevated cholesterol and triglyceride levels persist during pregnancy and can remain high up to 1 year after delivery. The LDL subfraction drops at 8 weeks gestation, but then continues to rise and remain elevated until 8 weeks postpartum with or without breastfeeding. The HDL subfraction rises until midgestation and then levels off or declines through the remainder of the pregnancy. Therefore measurement of a women's lipid profile should be delayed until at least 6 months postpartum. The effect of these lipid changes during pregnancy on development of atherosclerosis remains unclear.

BIBLIOGRAPHY

Baird DT, Glasier AF: Hormonal contraception, *N Engl J Med* 328:1543, 1993.

Bass KM et al: Plasma lipoprotein levels as predictors of cardiovascular death in women, *Arch Intern Med* 153:2209, 1993.

Blair SN: Evidence for success of exercise in weight loss and control, *Ann Intern Med* 119 (7, pt 2):702, 1993.

Braunwald E: *Heart disease: a textbook of cardiovascular medicine,* ed 6, Philadelphia, 2001, WB Saunders.

Castelli WP: Epidemiology of triglycerides: a view from Framingham, *Am J Cardiol* 70:3H, 1992.

Corti MC et al: Clarifying the direct relation between total cholesterol levels and death from coronary heart disease in older persons, *Ann Intern Med* 126:753, 1997.

Criqui MH et al: Plasma triglyceride level and mortality from coronary heart disease, *N Engl J Med* 328:1220, 1993.

Danesh J, Collins R, Peto R: Lipoprotein(a) and coronary heart disease: meta-analysis of prospective studies, *Circulation* 102:1082, 2000.

Downs JR et al: Primary prevention of acute coronary events with lovastatin in men and women with average cholesterol levels: results of AFCAPS/TexCAPS, *JAMA* 279:1615, 1998.

Ettinger WH et al: Lipoprotein lipids in older people: results from the Cardiovascular Health Study, *Circulation* 86:858, 1992.

Expert Panel on Detection, Evaluation, and Treatment of High Blood Cholesterol in Adults: Summary of the Second Report of the National Cholesterol Education Program (NCEP) Expert Panel on Detection, Evaluation, and Treatment of High Blood Cholesterol in Adults (Adult Treatment Panel III), *JAMA* 285:2486, 2001.

Foreyt JP, Goodrick GK: Evidence for success of behavior modification in weight loss and control, *Ann Intern Med* 119:698, 1993.

Godsland IF et al: The effects of different formulations of oral contraceptive agents on lipid and carbohydrate metabolism, *N Engl J Med* 323:1375, 1990.

Haim M et al: Elevated serum triglyceride levels and long-term mortality in patients with coronary heart disease: the Bezaibrate Infarction Prevention (BIP) Registry. *Circulation* 100:475, 1999.

Hulley S et al: Randomized trial of estrogen plus progestin for secondary prevention of coronary heart disease in postmenopausal women, *JAMA* 280:605, 1998.

Jacobs DR, Blackburn H, Higgins M: Low cholesterol: mortality associations, *Circulation* 86:1046, 1992.

Johnson CL et al: Declining serum total cholesterol levels among US adults: the National Health and Nutrition Examination Surveys, *JAMA* 269:3002, 1993.

Kannel WB, Wolf PA, Garrison RJ: Framingham Study: an epidemiological investigation of cardiovascular disease, Section 36: Means at each examination and inter-examination consistency of specified characteristics: Framingham Heart Study 30-year follow-up. National Heart, Lung, and Blood Institute Publication No NIH 88-2970, 1988.

LaRosa JC: Triglycerides and coronary risk in women and the elderly, *Arch Intern Med* 157:961, 1997.

Lewis SJ et al: Effect of pravastatin on cardiovascular events in women after myocardial infarction: the cholesterol and recurrent events (CARE) trial, *J Am Coll Cardiol* 32:140, 1998.

Lissner L et al: Variability of body weight and health outcomes in the Framingham population, *N Engl J Med* 324:1839, 1991.

The Long-Term Intervention with Pravastatin in Ischaemic Disease (LIPID) Study Group: Prevention of cardiovascular events and death with pravastatin in patients with CHD and a broad range of initial cholesterol levels, *N Engl J Med* 339:1349, 1998.

Manolio TA et al: Epidemiology of low cholesterol levels in older adults: the Cardiovascular Health Study, *Circulation* 87:728, 1993.

Miettinen T et al: Cholesterol-lowering therapy in women and elderly patients with myocardial infarction or angina pectoris: findings from the Scandinavian Simvastatin Survival Study (4S), *Circulation* 96:4211, 1997.

Mittelmark MB et al: Total blood cholesterol levels in older adult participants in community-wide screening programs, *J Am Geriatr Soc* 39:A7, 1991.

Rader DJ, Brewer HB Jr: Lipoprotein(a): clinical approach to a unique atherogenic lipoprotein, *JAMA* 267:1109, 1992.

Regnstrom J et al: Susceptibility to low-density lipoprotein oxidation and coronary atherosclerosis in man, *Lancet* 339:1183, 1992.

Ridker PM, Hennekins CH, Buring JE, Rifai N: C-reactive protein and other markers of inflammation in the prediction of cardiovascular disease in women, *N Engl J Med* 342:836, 2000.

Sbarouni E, Kyriakides ZS, Kremastinos DT: The effect of hormone replacement therapy alone and in combination with simvastatin on plasma lipids of hypercholesterolemic postmenopausal women with coronary artery disease, *J Am Coll Cardiol* 32:1244, 1998.

Shlipak MG et al: Estrogen and progestin, lipoprotein(a), and the risk of recurrent coronary heart disease events after menopause, *JAMA* 283:1845, 2000.

Stampfer MJ et al: A prospective study of past use of oral contraceptive agents and risk of cardiovascular disease, *N Engl J Med* 319:1313, 1988.

Stampfer MJ et al: Vitamin E consumption and the risk of coronary disease in women, *N Engl J Med* 328:1444, 1993.

Wood PD, Stefanick ML, Williams PT: The effects on plasma lipoproteins of a prudent weight-reducing diet, with or without exercise, in overweight men and women, *N Engl J Med* 325:461, 1991.

Writing Group for the PEPI Trial. Effects of estrogen or estrogenprogestin regimens on heart disease risk factors in postmenopausal women: the postmenopausal estrogen/progestin interventions (PEPI) trial, *JAMA* 273:199, 1995.

CHAPTER 5

Stroke

Barbara A. Dworetzky
Farzaneh A. Sorond
David M. Dawson

▦ EPIDEMIOLOGY

Stroke remains the third leading cause of death in the United States despite its decreasing incidence. Roughly 42% to 49% of strokes will occur in women this year. Overall, women have fewer strokes than men at every age group with the exception of those few cases occurring in patients younger than 45 years old. For the most part, risks, mechanisms, and treatments of stroke are similar in women and men, although there are certain conditions that predispose women to specific types of strokes that may be important in determining the pathogenesis of cerebrovascular disease. Pregnancy, use of birth control pills, and mitral valve prolapse are examples of such conditions and are addressed in this chapter. Although the incidence of intracerebral hemorrhage is roughly equal in women and men, subarachnoid hemorrhage occurs more frequently in women by as much as 50%. Most of these hemorrhages in women are caused by ruptured aneurysms, whereas in men they are more likely to be as a result of ruptured arteriovenous malformations. The topic of vascular malformations is beyond the scope of this chapter.

PATHOPHYSIOLOGY
Definition and Mechanism

Current approaches to stroke diagnosis and management focus on the mechanism of stroke. There are two basic types of infarction: hemorrhagic and ischemic. Hemorrhages can be intraparenchymal or subarachnoid. Ischemic events can be defined on a time continuum. Neurologic symptoms or signs (e.g., weakness, numbness, aphasia, slurred speech, double vision) that resolve in less than 24 hours suggest that a transient ischemic attack (TIA) has occurred. Neurologic deficits that last longer than 24 hours imply that an infarction or stroke has occurred. However, even at 2 hours, a stroke is often visible on neuroimaging. Ischemic infarctions can be the result of systemic hypoperfusion, emboli, or thrombosis. Emboli can originate from the heart, dislodge from plaques of proximal arteries, or arise paradoxically from peripheral venous clots that cross from the right atrium to the left via a septal defect, usually a patent foramen ovale (PFO). Arterial

thrombosis can occur in both large vessels (e.g., carotid, middle cerebral artery) and small vessels within the brain.

Gender Differences

Recent evidence demonstrates that risks, causes, and outcomes differ between the sexes. Counseling for prevention and treatment of strokes in women requires an understanding of these gender discrepancies. Cerebral angiograms and carotid ultrasounds, for example, have demonstrated increased intracranial atherosclerosis in women and blacks, and increased extracranial (carotid and vertebral) atherosclerosis in men and whites. Autopsy studies have indicated that between the fourth and sixth decades women are more likely than men not to have atherosclerosis. This difference disappears after age 65 years, suggesting a protective effect of estrogen on the development of atherosclerosis, possibly through favorable changes in the serum lipid ratio. Although the lifetime risk of having a stroke appears to be greater for men than for women, the lifetime risk of dying of a stroke is greater for women (16%) than for men (8%). A likely explanation for this observation is that women have longer life expectancies and have a later age of onset of stroke. Additionally, recent studies have shown that risk for ipsilateral stroke after nonelective endarterectomy is significantly higher for women and that men do better than women after this operation.

Risk Factors

Important risk factors for all strokes can be divided into nonmodifiable and modifiable ones. Nonmodifiable risk factors are male sex, race, family history of stroke, and prior stroke, TIA or myocardial infarction (MI) (especially if recent). Modifiable or treatable conditions that increase risk for stroke include hypertension, diabetes, hypercholesterolemia, obesity, physical inactivity, smoking, heavy alcohol use, and atrial fibrillation. Risk factors for stroke in general are additive, so that many victims of stroke have several determinants.

Race

Socioeconomic status, nutritional factors, access to health care, and lifestyle are a few of the confounding factors that make race a difficult risk factor to study. However, it seems clear that blacks have a higher death rate than whites from stroke, with black women faring the worst. Blacks and Japanese have more intracranial hemorrhages and less large vessel or extracranial disease.

Myocardial Infarction

The risk of stroke in individuals who have had a MI is approximately twice as high as in the general population of a comparable age. Patients with acute anterior MI are at even greater risk because of their propensity for formation of left ventricular thrombi, which can dislodge and lead to embolic stroke.

Carotid Stenosis

A substantially increased risk of stroke is associated with 60% to 99% narrowing of the cross-sectional area as measured by duplex ultrasound. This risk has been found even for patients who are asymptomatic.

Hypertension

The Multiple Risk Factor Intervention Trial (MRFIT) suggested that roughly 40% of strokes can be attributed to a systolic blood pressure of 140 or greater. Other studies have attributed elevated diastolic pressures to about 70% of strokes. Data from the Framingham Study prospectively demonstrated that hypertension, whether it was labile or fixed, systolic or diastolic, or even borderline, was the most frequent and most powerful predictor of stroke, providing a fourfold increase in risk over normotension. Even in the young, hypertension was the most potent contributing risk, associated with approximately one fourth of strokes.

Diabetes

The Nurses's Health Study cohort (made up largely of white women 30 to 55 years old) demonstrated a significantly increased risk of both fatal and nonfatal strokes among diabetic women. Most of these strokes were ischemic in origin, although a slight increase of hemorrhages was also seen. The adverse effect conferred by diabetes appeared to be compounded by the addition of smoking, hypertension, hypercholesterolemia, or obesity. Controlling for these added risks, diabetes still posed a threefold increase in cardiovascular risk when it was present for at least 15 years. There is no convincing evidence that attaining normoglycemia decreases the incidence of stroke; however, hyperglycemia has been shown to worsen the damage caused by cerebral infarction.

Cholesterol

The role that high cholesterol level has in stroke is not as clear as its role in heart disease. The MRFIT trial revealed a modest correlation between high serum cholesterol level and nonhemorrhagic strokes. Patients younger than age 40 who have strokes have been noted to have an elevated incidence of hypercholesterolemia. The recent CARE trial demonstrated a surprising 31% reduction in stroke events over 5 years in patients treated with pravastatin compared with placebo. Interestingly, it has been shown that low cholesterol is related to an increased incidence of intracranial hemorrhage.

Obesity

While obesity is highly correlated with many of the above risk factors for stroke, it still appears to be an independent contributor to stroke risk in younger men and older women. A recent study by Walker et al. showed that abdominal obesity, not elevated body mass index, was related to the increased risk. Future research in this area may be fruitful given the large differences in fat distribution between women and men.

Physical Activity

Recent evidence suggests that physical inactivity may lead to an increased risk of heart disease and stroke in men. Similar benefit was not found for women in the Framingham study, although it has been found in other studies. Added benefit was found with increased level of activity in a dose response way, but suggested that even walking helps.

Smoking

Smoking is a major risk factor for the development of both hemorrhagic and nonhemorrhagic strokes in women. More than one third of strokes can be attributed to cigarette smoking. In a prospective cohort study of women ages 30 to 55, the number of cigarettes smoked per day correlated with an increased risk of stroke, whereas the number of years of smoking did not correlate with risk. In fact, smokers had the same risk for strokes as nonsmokers within 2 years of quitting, thus emphasizing the importance of the major efforts to decrease the prevalence of smoking in the United States.

Alcohol

A prospective study by Stampfer et al. of female nurses showed that moderate alcohol intake significantly lessened the risk of ischemic stroke yet increased the risk of subarachnoid hemorrhage two to three times. In nonsmokers, the protective effect of alcohol was even more apparent. It has been shown that heavier alcohol use (more than 2 drinks/day) is associated with increased risk of hemorrhagic and ischemic stroke. The mechanisms for these observations are still incompletely understood.

Atrial Fibrillation

The Framingham data indicate that there is a 2% chance that atrial fibrillation (AF) will develop during a two-decade period, affecting 5 million people in the United States over the next 20 years. Nonvalvular AF increases the risk of embolic stroke sixfold over those without AF. AF, typically occurring in the elderly, will be increasingly important as the population ages.

Uncommon Risk Factors
Valvular Disease

In stroke registries, about 30% of cases are embolic. Valvular disease, such as rheumatic mitral stenosis or congenital bicuspid aortic valve, may be the source of emboli in any age group. In patients with idiopathic or alcoholic cardiomyopathy mural thrombi may form in the dilated left ventricle and be a source of emboli. Other less common causes include prosthetic heart valves, infective endocarditis, and Libman-Sacks endocarditis. In most instances, long-term anticoagulation with warfarin is the accepted mode of treatment to prevent cerebral embolism.

Mitral Valve Prolapse

Mitral valve prolapse (MVP) caused by myxomatous valve degeneration is a special example of cardiac valvular disease. It is common in younger individuals and is three times more common in women than in men. The risk of stroke rises fourfold in younger patients with MVP, although in older patients, as other causes of stroke rise in incidence, MVP is not a significant risk factor. Notably the subset of patients with severe MVP characterized by redundant leaflets or mitral regurgitation is at no more risk than those patients with mild disease. However, these patients are at higher risk for infectious or hemodynamic compromise. In patients without an apparent cause of stroke, patent foramen ovale leading to paradoxical embolization should be considered as the mechanism, especially if the history reveals that the onset of neurologic symptoms followed a Valsalva maneuver.

Migraine

Estimates of the frequency of migraine vary widely, but as many as 29% of women and 20% of men are subject to recurrent vascular headaches at some time in their lives. With such a high prevalence of migraine headaches in the population, it is hard to assess migraine as an independent risk factor for stroke, particularly in the middle-aged and elderly. Migraine and stroke occur as clinical features in certain genetic neurologic disorders such as cerebral autosomal dominant arteriopathy with subcortical infarcts and leukoariosis (CADASIL) and mitochondrial encephalopathy with lactic acidosis and stroke like infarcts (MELAS), suggesting this relationship is complex.

Two mechanisms may account for the few strokes that do occur in the migraine population: cardiogenic embolism and spasm of arteries or arterioles. Direct evidence for vasospasm in migraine, whether during the aura phase or the headache, is lacking. Cerebral blood flow is believed to be reduced during a migraine attack. Infarction, therefore, is a possible outcome. Many migraine researchers now believe that reduced blood flow is secondary, and that a biochemical event, involving serotonin and possibly other neurotransmitters, produces a zone of reduced metabolic activity preceding vascular changes.

Oral Contraceptives and Estrogen

In the 1960s, clinical data began to suggest a relationship between use of oral contraceptives and stroke. Estimates then indicated a fourfold to thirteenfold increased risk of stroke in young women, compared with that of women not exposed to oral contraceptives. Subsequent information suggested that the risk was multifactorial and was increased by high estrogen content pills, smoking, age above 35, and hypertension. There is some evidence that for women with migraines, there is a fourfold increased risk of ischemic stroke when placed on oral contraceptives. There is similar increased risk of subarachnoid hemorrhage in women who smoke while on the pill. The benefit of oral contraceptive use must be balanced against this increase in risk for women with migraine, women who smoke, women over 35, and

those with other vascular risk factors. The package inserts for implantable subcutaneous, as well as for oral agents, even those low in estrogen, advise caution in certain groups of patients:

1. Women who smoke
2. Women who have a prior history of venous or arterial thrombosis
3. Substance abusers, particularly users of cocaine and amphetamines

The risk of stroke in women who are postmenopausal and take estrogen is controversial. Most studies show no benefit or a modest protective effect.

Hypercoagulable State

Hypercoagulable states are usually inherited disorders of the hemostatic mechanism. There may also be excess coagulability in patients with cancer, disseminated intravascular coagulation, immobilization in bed, polycythemia, hyperviscosity, or pregnancy.

The **antiphospholipid syndrome** is an example of a hypercoagulable condition. Antibodies are formed against phospholipids and include lupus anticoagulant and anticardiolipin antibody. Patients may experience stroke at any age, as well as recurrent spontaneous abortion, venous thrombosis, migraines, thrombocytopenia, or livedo reticularis. Routine PTT may show elevation and be a clue that this condition exists. (See Chapter 37 for a more detailed discussion on this syndrome.)

Protein C, protein S, and **antithrombin III deficiencies, Factor V Leiden mutation, prothrombin 20210A mutation,** as well as **homocystinuria,** are all rare conditions but account for some instances of hypercoagulability. Unfortunately no direct treatment is available for any of these conditions.

Other blood abnormalities that increase the risk of stroke include sickle cell disease, polycythemia, hyperviscosity, leukemia, elevated fibrinogen levels, macroglobulinemia, thrombocytosis, and elevated C-reactive protein levels.

Dissection and Vasculitis

Spontaneous arterial dissection is believed to be initiated by an intimal tear, followed by entry of blood into the media and an upward migration of blood. These events cause the vessel to be narrowed. Dissection of a carotid or vertebral artery can lead to cerebral infarction in the territory of that artery. Dissection can occur at any age and should be considered after any trauma to the neck. It is more commonly seen in women than in men. Rarely intracranial vessels are affected by primary vasculitis and cause stroke.

DETECTION OF WOMEN AT RISK FOR STROKE

Women with a history of hypertension, diabetes, atrial fibrillation, MI, TIA, or stroke are at an increased risk for stroke and should be monitored closely, especially when pregnant. Asymptomatic carotid bruits are markers for vascular disease. Bruits can help identify women at risk for stroke, but are not necessarily indicative of a significant stenosis and may be associated with carotid stenoses varying from 30% to 99%. Such patients require evaluation by carotid ultrasound and electrocardiography.

EVALUATION OF STROKE IN WOMEN
History and Physical Examination

Not all neurologic deficits are strokes. It is often advisable to obtain a consultation with a neurologist early in a patient's presentation to aid with the diagnosis and management. Any history of trauma, alcoholism, or use of anticoagulant medication should bring subdural hematoma into the differential diagnosis. Fever and stiff neck make infection (e.g., abscess, meningitis, encephalitis) an important consideration because therapy with antibiotics may be lifesaving. Women with multiple sclerosis may have hemiparesis or unilateral numbness. Focal seizures can mimic stroke with prolonged focal symptoms postictally. Migraine can produce unilateral tingling, numbness, weakness, or aphasia. Hypoglycemia and hyperglycemia can unmask old strokes. Sudden confusion is usually not due to a stroke and should initiate a search for drugs, infections, or other metabolic processes.

Approach to Diagnosis
Imaging Studies
Computed Tomography and Magnetic Resonance Imaging

Once it is suspected that the patient may be having a stroke, it is important to determine whether there has been bleeding. A head computed tomographic (CT) scan (Fig. 5-1), without contrast, is indicated in practically all suspected strokes to rule out hemorrhage. In subarachnoid hemorrhage caused by aneurysm or arteriovenous malformations, blood surrounds the brain; with intraparenchymal hemorrhage, blood is visible as a bright white image. CT scan also can be useful to evaluate mass effect or shifting of brain contents from tumor or blood (raised intracranial pressure) and the need for urgent neurosurgical intervention. Bleeding into the cerebellum is particularly dangerous because the patient's condition can deteriorate quickly as a result of compression of the vital structures within the brainstem.

Magnetic resonance imaging (MRI) (Fig. 5-2) is superior to CT scan for diagnosing lacunae and posterior fossa abnormality. Newer MRI techniques are being used at major academic centers to aid in stroke diagnosis. Infarcts can now be visualized on diffusion weighted images (DWI scans), a new MRI technique that detects tiny random movements of water molecules in tissues. Acute brain ischemia can be detected within minutes of onset of deficits, whereas the CT scan can be normal in the first 24 hours. The combination of DWI and perfusion scans can identify diffusion-perfusion mismatches, identifying vulnerable tissue that may be salvaged by thrombolytics. MRI T_1- and T_2-weighted images can be used for diagnosis of hemorrhage. If a carotid or vertebral dissection is suspected, T_1-weighted image with fat suppression or CTA can aid in the diagnosis, although conventional angiogram is still the "gold standard." Vascular abnormalities can be diagnosed noninvasively by magnetic resonance angiography or CTA, and may ultimately replace conventional cerebral angiography. MRI is contraindicated in patients with pacemakers. It is not advised for critically ill patients, claustrophobic patients, or those with metallic clips, although it is best to discuss these particulars with the neuroradiologist.

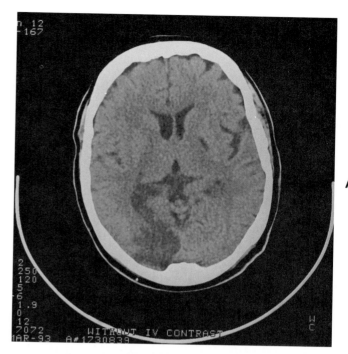

A

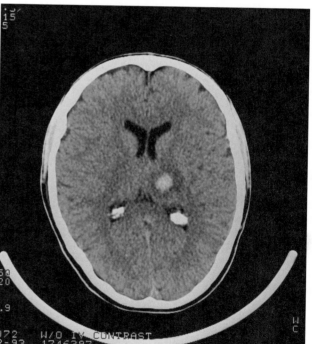

B

FIG. 5-1 A, Computed tomography (CT) scan without contrast showing a low-density zone in the right occipital lobe (left side of figure), resulting from prior embolic infarction. **B,** CT scan without contrast showing a small acute hemorrhage in the left thalamus. Calcification of the choroid plexuses within the lateral ventricles is also demonstrated.

If the scan does not show blood, the stroke is more likely ischemic in origin. It is important to remember that the CT result can be negative for the first 24 to 48 hours. If the patient experiences dizziness; is found to be pale, clammy, or near fainting; and has a history of heart disease, the differ-

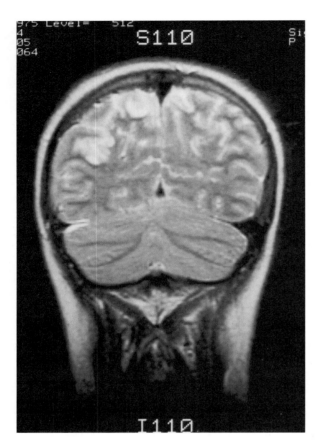

FIG. 5-2   MRI scan, T_2-weighted sequence, showing an infarction in the right parietooccipital region, caused by eclampsia in a 15-year-old patient at term.

ential should include dysrhythmia, sepsis, and MI. **Cerebral emboli** often appear with sudden neurologic deficits, but symptoms can improve once the embolus fragments. Transesophageal echocardiogram, 24-hour Holter monitoring, and serial blood cultures (if endocarditis is a concern) can identify heart disease and an embolic cause of the stroke. **Thrombotic strokes** usually manifest as the patient awakens from sleep, revealing neurologic deficits that may subside or progress. If symptoms are referable to the carotid artery, noninvasive carotid ultrasound can evaluate the patency of this vessel and can help determine the need for endarterectomy. Otherwise, transcranial Doppler ultrasonography allows visualization of the intracranial as well as posterior circulation. MRA of the carotid arteries eliminates the risk of dye used during conventional angiography and can be used in conjunction with the ultrasound information.

New Radiologic Tests

New radiologic tests study the flow of blood in the brain and make tissue viability estimates possible. These tests estimate cerebral territory that may be at risk for infarction even though no damage has yet been done. *Single-photon emission computed tomography* (SPECT) and *positron emission tomography* (PET) are two examples of these imaging techniques. *Diffusion-weighted MRI* is an even newer technique (see Imaging Studies). These studies are used primarily in major medical centers.

Other Diagnostic Testing

The abrupt onset of neurologic symptoms or signs should lead to suspicion of a stroke. These neurologic deficits can disappear, but the need for prompt evaluation is still critical because they may represent a TIA, a warning that the patient is at serious risk for stroke. Several screening blood tests should be completed on all patients with a suspected stroke or TIA. These include complete blood count, blood smear, platelets, protime, partial thromboplastin time, erythrocyte sedimentation rate (ESR), glucose, calcium, electrolytes, cholesterol, triglyceride, rapid plasma regain (RPR), blood urea nitrogen, creatinine, fibrinogen level, and, if the patient is of childbearing age, a pregnancy test. Serum and urine toxic screens should also be performed on women under 45 or those with a history of illegal drug use. Later, antinuclear antibody, rheumatoid factor, anticardiolipin antibody, antithrombin III, protein C, or protein S, factor V Leiden mutation and prothrombin 20210A mutation may be useful. Lumbar puncture can help diagnose vasculitis, infection, subarachnoid hemorrhage, and other more remote causes of stroke; however, it is rarely necessary. If a coagulopathy is suspected, blood coagulation factors should be drawn before heparin therapy is initiated.

MANAGEMENT
Goals of Management

The goal of treatment for bleeding in or around the brain is to prevent recurrence of hemorrhage and irreversible deterioration to coma and death from the increased pressure the blood exerts in the closed intracranial cavity. Early neurosurgical consultation for hemorrhage is extremely important to determine which patients will benefit most from surgical management.

The goal of treatment for acute ischemic stroke is fourfold: (1) restoration of cerebral blood flow (reperfusion), (2) prevention of recurrent thrombosis (antithrombotic therapy), (3) neuroprotection, and (4) supportive care. Reperfusion can be achieved by the administration of thrombolytic agents. Of the agents available, only *recombinant tissue plasminogen activator (t-PA)* is FDA approved. Timing of thrombolysis is critical, and the use of intravenous t-PA has been limited to the first 3 hours after the onset of symptoms. Candidates for intraarterial t-PA and pro-urokinase (r-proUK) may wait for up to 6 hours. Patient selection must rigidly adhere to the inclusion and exclusion criteria. In a patient with suspected stroke, hospitalization and consultation with a neurologist with specific expertise in acute diagnosis and therapy of ischemic stroke is essential for safe and effective management. The need for urgent carotid endarterectomy should be considered. Other issues in the management of acute stroke include risk for increased intracranial pressure in hemorrhages and large strokes, aggressive treatment of hyperglycemia and hyperthermia, and maintenance of adequate blood pressure to ensure cerebral perfusion. Rapid drop in blood pressure should be avoided because this can lead to progression of the stroke by decreasing cerebral perfusion. If embolism or large vessel stroke is suspected and the patient has no blood or risk for bleeding (no recent thrombolytics, anticoagulants, no large infarct), some neurologists begin heparin while searching for the source of embolus. Bed rest for the first 24 hours may improve blood flow to the brain in those patients whose symptoms worsen with postural changes.

Once the stroke is complete (symptoms no longer fluctuate), initiation of stroke prevention measures should be considered. Risk factor reduction, for example, cessation of smoking and normalization of blood pressure, are important goals. Within 2 years of smoking cessation, risk of stroke has declined to baseline value. Hypertension, the most potent risk for stroke, requires vigorous long-term management.

Choice of Therapy

Use of Antiplatelet Agents

Aspirin. The beneficial effects of antiplatelet agents are believed to be due to prevention of aggregation by inhibiting thromboxane A_2 synthesis. Aspirin or acetylsalicylic acid [ASA] has been used for this purpose since the mid-1970s. A meta-analysis by the Physician's Health Study Research Group has shown a slight reduction in stroke and death rate by approximately 20%. This is also noted in patients with a potential source of embolism. The ASA dose now commonly in use is one tablet a day (325 mg), although doses as low as 30 mg/day have proven effective for stroke prevention. It is not current practice to prescribe ASA for primary prevention of TIA or other cerebrovascular event. ASA is probably effective in both sexes, although some studies, at higher doses, have shown better response in men.

Dipyridamole Plus Aspirin (Aggrenox). Dipyridamole increases cyclic adenosine monophosphate (camp) in platelets and reduces platelet response to aggregating agents. Results from the European Stroke Prevention Study 2 (ESPS-2) suggest that the combination of extended-release dipyridamole (DP) plus aspirin (ASA) may be more effective than aspirin alone in preventing stroke. In a pairwise comparison by Diener et al., the relative risk reduction was 18% with aspirin alone, 16% with dipyridamole alone, and 37% with combination therapy. The fixed dose combination of DP/ASA was also twice as effective as either agent alone in secondary prevention of stroke. This combination drug seems to hold great promise, but additional confirmatory studies may be necessary before current practice is changed from the widespread use of aspirin as the standard therapy.

Thienopyridines. Clopidogrel and ticlopidine are inhibitors of platelet function in vivo. They are believed to inhibit platelet aggregation by noncompetitively inhibiting the platelet ADP receptor. These agents may be used as alternative therapy for recurrent stroke on ASA or for women who cannot tolerate the side effects.

Clopidogrel (Plavix). When compared to ASA, 325 mg/day, clopidogrel resulted in 9% relative risk reduction in ischemic events. It was shown to be at least as safe as aspirin and safer than ticlopidine. Its safety profile and once per day dosing make it a more attractive agent than ticlopidine. It is expensive and therefore has not replaced ASA.

Ticlopidine (Ticlid). Compared with ASA, 1300 mg/day, ticlopidine produced a further reduction of risk of stroke, in the overall range of 30%, and appeared to be effective in both sexes. It causes severe neutropenia in 1% to 3% of patients in the first 3 months of treatment, so blood counts need to be carefully monitored. Ticlopidine is no longer prescribed for new stroke patients since clopidogrel is nearly as effective, similar in cost, easier to dose, and safer.

Anticoagulation

Warfarin has been used for primary and secondary prevention of stroke for four decades. At the current time there is only one noncontroversial indication for the use of warfarin for stroke prevention, namely, for patients with suspected or proven cardiogenic source embolism. However, a recent retrospective study showed 47% reduction in major stroke risk in people on warfarin who had TIAs or prior strokes in the territory of a 50% to 99% stenotic intracranial vessel. Patients with AF who are over 65, or patients with AF and one risk factor for stroke, are recommended to use warfarin lifelong. Patients with acute stroke determined to need warfarin are usually started on heparin first. Low-molecular weight heparin and heparinoids have some advantages over heparin (higher bioavailability, more predictable anticoagulation effects, less platelet interaction) although neither has yet been proven effective. Only slight prolongation of the International Normalized Ratio (INR) of 2 to 3 is required. INR, a calculated value based on a standardized reagent, was adopted to correct inconsistencies in prothrombin time tests. The advantage of the INR is that it allows direct comparison of values obtained by different laboratories. Patients with hypercoagulable states may also be placed on warfarin therapy. For some of these patients, the INR may need to be as high as 3 to 4, depending on the specific disorder.

Surgical Intervention

Surgical removal of plaque from the carotid bifurcation is available as a method of prevention of stroke or prevention of recurrence. In patients with carotid symptoms (i.e., transient monocular blindness) and 70% to 99% stenosis, the absolute risk reduction after carotid endarterectomy (CEA) was 14% over a 2-year period. For asymptomatic patients with 60% to 99% stenosis, CEA provided an absolute risk reduction of 6% over 5 years compared with medical treatment alone. The current recommended management strategy from that trial is for carotid endarterectomy (if surgical risk <3%) for asymptomatic stenosis >60% and symptomatic stenosis >50%. Other surgical procedures with potential to prevent stroke include carotid stenting, patent foramen ovale (PFO) repair, carotid or basilar artery angioplasty, subclavian or vertebral endarterectomy.

Neuroprotective Agents

The ischemic cascade has been the target of many research trials in stroke. Medications such as calcium channel blockers, glutamate antagonists, and free radical scavengers have been tried, but none of these compounds has proven safe or effective for acute stroke. For now, effective neuroprotection must await newer agents and other trials.

Rehabilitation

Rehabilitation of stroke should include a multidisciplinary approach initiated early in treatment. Physical, occupational, and speech therapies can help to maximize functional recovery, allowing many patients to return to their former environment. Physicians should have a low threshold to treat for depression, which is quite common after stroke. Rehabilitation programs help to educate patients and families about stroke and teach prevention of common stroke complications such as limb contractures, decubitus ulcers, or deep vein thromboses.

■ PREGNANCY AND STROKE

Epidemiology

The risk of stroke during pregnancy or the puerperium is believed to be quite low. A recent study by Kittner et al. demonstrated that it is the postpartum period where most of these strokes occur. Fatal stroke, although rare, is a leading cause of nonobstetric maternal death. In addition, the social implications of puerperal strokes are devastating because they occur in younger women who have the major responsibility for providing care for their newborns. Still it is crucial to determine the cause of a stroke during or within 6 weeks after pregnancy because it carries implications for treatment and provides clues for counseling patients with regard to future pregnancies. It should not be assumed that pregnancy alone is a sufficient explanation for the stroke, and other causes should always be sought.

Pathophysiology

During pregnancy the mother undergoes hemodynamic and hemostatic changes that may increase the risk for stroke. Cardiac output rises 30% to 60%, peak effects occurring in the second trimester. Blood volume can rise as much as 45% through the middle of the third trimester. Coagulability of blood elements increases as a result of a rise in fibrinogen and clotting factor levels and a decline in fibrinolysis. Platelets are more aggregable as well. Given the increase in strokes during the postpartum period, there is the suggestion that the large decrease in blood volume or rapid change in hormone status may be causal.

There is a clear increase in hemorrhagic strokes in pregnant women. Women with aneurysms have a fivefold to eightfold increase in the rate of rupture, primarily during the third trimesters, when cardiac output and blood volume are maximal. These malformations can cause subarachnoid or intraparenchymal hemorrhages, either of which can have a devastating outcome. Most neurosurgeons would agree that surgical management of subarachnoid hemorrhage in pregnancy should be the same as in the nonpregnant state. A rare cause for stroke in pregnancy is eclampsia. Eclampsia can cause small hemorrhagic infarcts in the border zones between major arterial territories and in the occipital lobes. The mechanism is believed to be severe vasospasm that results from elevated blood pressure that overrides the upper limit of the cerebral autoregulatory system. This causes a breakdown of the blood-brain barrier with subsequent small hemorrhages and vasogenic edema.

Arterial occlusions and embolic phenomena are the most common cause of ischemic stroke during the puerperium, occurring during peak "hypercoagulability" in the third trimester of pregnancy. Deep vein thromboses are common in pregnancy and potentially could lead to embolic stroke via a patent foramen ovale. Cerebral venous thrombosis, associated with dehydration and hypercoagulation, is the most common stroke in the postpartum period. It can occur during the last week of pregnancy and up to 4 weeks postpartum. These

patients usually experience severe headache, nausea, vomiting, lethargy, seizure, or diminished visual acuity caused by papilledema. Diagnosis is made by brain MRI or CT scan, with contrast dye revealing the classic "empty delta" sign indicating a clot in the sagittal sinus. MR-venography or CT-venograms can be performed when the diagnosis is not apparent from the examinations described here. Bed rest, hydration, use of anticonvulsants, and heparinization are treatments for this entity. Mortality rate is about 25%. Fortunately those who survive usually have few sequelae. Extremely rare causes of embolic stroke are fat, air, and amniotic fluid emboli.

Stroke can also be caused by cerebral hypoperfusion from significant blood loss during delivery. Sheehan and Stanfield have described pituitary infarction by this mechanism. Peripartum cardiomyopathy, a disease more commonly seen with twin gestations, toxemia, hypertension, and births in older multiparous women of African descent, is also an important cause of stroke from hypoperfusion. Contractions of the uterus during labor and delivery further increase cardiac output from increased venous return to the heart and from increased cardiac demand secondary to pain. Women with cardiomyopathy manifesting heart failure or dysrhythmia should be treated with bed rest, digoxin, and diuretics. Subsequent pregnancy should be discouraged.

An extremely rare cause of stroke, also occurring in the postpartum period, is metastatic choriocarcinoma to the brain. This neoplasm can occlude an artery, thereby causing an infarct, or it can directly invade brain parenchyma, causing a hemorrhage. Although this neoplasm is rare, early diagnosis is crucial because it is curable with chemotherapy and whole brain radiation. Other tumors are hormonally stimulated and can appear with brain hemorrhage or infarct during pregnancy.

Evaluation of Stroke in Pregnancy

Imaging during Pregnancy

Increased risk for stroke is not the only important issue facing physicians caring for women who are pregnant. One question that recurs is, what is the risk to the fetus of imaging when a pregnant woman exhibits acute neurologic deficits? Because radiation is known to be hazardous during the implantation and organogenesis stages in fetal development, elective imaging should be avoided during this period. However, head CT scan provides less than 1 mrad radiation to the uterus and is relatively safe during pregnancy, with proper precautions. If a pregnant woman has a suspected stroke, MRI is the current study of choice, DWI, if available. There are no known biological risks associated with MRI, and it is generally accepted that the potential risk of delayed sequelae is extremely small or nonexistent. Women should be informed that, although to date there is no indication that the use of clinical MRI procedures during pregnancy produces deleterious effects, according to the US Food and Drug Administration, the safety of these procedures has not been definitely proved. Contrast agents cross the placenta and therefore should not be used if at all possible.

Management

Anticoagulation during Pregnancy

Another issue of concern is the use of anticoagulation for protection of stroke during pregnancy. Although no method of anticoagulation is entirely safe during pregnancy, chronic atrial fibrillation, a prosthetic valve, or an embolic source of stroke is more dangerous than the risks of anticoagulation therapy. Warfarin crosses the placenta and is known to be teratogenic, especially during the first trimester. The risk of fetal bleeding is increased. Heparin, a larger molecule, does not cross the placenta and is the preferred treatment for this reason. Subcutaneous low-molecular-weight heparin, enoxaparin (Lovenox) is preferred.

BIBLIOGRAPHY

Bogousslavsky J, Pierre P: Ischemic stroke in patients under age 45, *Neurol Clin* 10:113, 1992.

Bonita R: Epidemiology of stroke, *Lancet* 339:342, 1992.

Cardiovascular Disease Surveillance, Stroke, 1980-1989, Atlanta, GA: Centers for Disease Control 69, 1994.

CAPRIE Steering Committee: A randomized, blinded, trial of clopidogrel versus aspirin in patients at risk of ischaemic events (CAPRIE), *Lancet* 348:1329, 1996.

Diener HC et al: European Stroke Prevention Study 2: dipyridamole and acetylsalicylic acid in the secondary prevention of stroke, *J Neurol Sci* 143:1, 1996.

DiTullio M et al: Patent foramen ovale as a risk factor for cryptogenic stroke, *Ann Intern Med* 117:461, 1992.

Dunbabin DW, Sandercock PAG: Preventing stroke by the modification of risk factors, *Stroke* 21(suppl IV):iv36, 1990.

Ellekjaer H, Holmen J, Ellekjaer E, Vatten L: Physical activity and stroke mortality in women: ten-year follow-up of the Nord-Trondelag Health Survey, 1984-1986. *Stroke* 31:14, 2000.

European Carotid Surgery Trialist' Collaborative Group: Randomized trial of endarterectomy for recently symptomatic carotid stenosis: final results of the MRC European Carotid Surgery Trial (ECST), *Lancet* 351:1379, 1998.

Executive Committee for the Asymptomatic Carotid Atherosclerosis Study: Endarterectomy for asymptomatic carotid artery stenosis, *JAMA* 273: 1421, 1995.

Furlan A et al: Intra-arterial prourokinase for acute ischemic stroke. The PROACT II Study: a randomized controlled trial, *JAMA* 282:2003, 1999.

Gorelick PB et al: Prevention of first stroke: a review of guidelines and a multidisciplinary consensus statement from the National Stroke Association, *JAMA* 281:1112, 1999.

Kiely DK et al: Physical activity and stroke risk: the Framingham study, *Am J Epidemiol* 140:608, 1994.

Kittner SJ et al: Pregnancy and the risk of stroke, *N Engl J Med* 335:768, 1996.

Levine D, Barnes PD, Edelman RR: Obstetric MR imaging, *Radiology* 211:609, 1999.

Manson JE et al: A prospective study of maturity-onset diabetes mellitus and risk of coronary heart disease and stroke in women, *Arch Intern Med* 151:1141, 1991.

Manson JE et al: Physical activity and incidence of coronary heart disease and stroke in women, *Circulation* 91:927, 1995.

Mantello MT et al: Imaging of neurologic complications associated with pregnancy, *Am J Roentgenol* 160:843, 1993.

Marmot MG, Poulter NR: Primary prevention of stroke, *Lancet* 339:344, 1992.

Mas JL, Lamy C: Stroke in pregnancy and the puerperium, *J Neurol* 245:305, 1998.

McNally LE, Corn CR, Hamilton SF: Aspirin for the prevention of vascular death in women, *Ann Pharmacother* 26:1530, 1992.

North American Symptomatic Carotid Endarterectomy Trial Collaborators (NASCET): Beneficial effect of carotid endarterectomy in symptomatic patients with high-grade stenosis, *N Engl J Med* 325:445, 1991.

NASCET Collaborators: Final Results of the North American Symptomatic Carotid Endarterectomy Trial (NASCET). Twenty-third International Joint Conference on Stroke and Cerebral Circulation, Orlando, Fla, February 1998.

Pettiti DB et al: Stroke in users of low-dose oral contraceptives, *N Engl J Med* 335:8, 1996.

Pettiti DB, Sidney S, Quesenberry CP Jr, Bernstein A: Ischemic stroke and use of estrogen and estrogen/progestogen as hormone replacement therapy, *Stroke* 29:23, 1998.

Rosamond WD et al: Stroke incidence and survival among middle-aged adults: 9 yr follow-up of the atherosclerosis risk in communities (ARIC) cohort. *Stroke* 30:736, 1999.

Sacco RL et al: The protective effect of moderate alcohol consumption on ischemic stroke, *JAMA* 281:1112, 1999.

Sacks FM et al: The effect of pravastatin on coronary events after myocardial infarction in patients with average cholesterol levels, *N Engl J Med* 335:1001, 1996.

Schwartz RB: Neurodiagnostic imaging of the pregnant patient. Presented at New York University School of Medicine Conference on Neurologic Complications of Pregnancy, New York, Sept 18-19, 1992.

Steering Committee of the Physicians' Health Study Research Group: Final report of the aspirin component of the ongoing physicians' health study, *N Engl J Med* 321:129, 1989.

Tanne D et al: Frequency and prognosis of stroke/TIA among 4808 survivors of acute myocardial infarction, *Stroke* 24:1490, 1993.

Tretter JF et al: Perioperative risk and late outcome of nonelective carotid endarterectomy, *J Vasc Surg* 30:618, 1999.

Tzouio C et al: Case-control study of migraine and risk of ischemic stroke in young women, *BMJ* 310:830, 1995.

Walker SP et al: Body size and fat distribution as predictors of stroke among U.S. men, *Am J Epidemiol* 144:1143, 1996.

Warfarin-aspirin symptomatic intracranial disease (WASID) study group [abstract], *Stroke* 25:273, 1994.

Wolf PA, Abbott RD, Kannel WB: Atrial fibrillation as an independent risk factor for stroke: The Framingham Study, *Stroke* 22:983, 1991.

Wolf PA, D'Agostino RB: Epidemiology of stroke. In Barnett HJM, Mohr JP, Stein BM, Yatsu FM, editors: *Stroke: pathophysiology, diagnosis, and management,* ed 3, New York, 1998, Churchill Livingstone.

CHAPTER 6

Vascular Disease

Joshua A. Beckman
Marie Gerhard-Herman

Vascular disease represents a significant, but unrecognized source of morbidity in women. Further, peripheral arterial disease provides important prognostic information concerning a patient's risk of heart attack and death. Atherosclerosis, thrombosis, and vasculitis are commonly found, and, by instituting proven therapies, physicians may significantly improve the life expectancy and quality of life of their patients. This chapter describes the vascular disease that is commonly seen by primary care providers and creates a framework for diagnosis and treatment.

ARTERIAL SYSTEM

Symptomatic arterial occlusive disease begins when the diameter of the lumen is reduced to half normal. Acquired arterial stenoses and occlusions may be chronic or acute. The most common cause of peripheral arterial disease is atherosclerosis. Other etiologies must be considered in individuals without risk factors for atherosclerosis or in those with an unusual distribution of arterial occlusive disease (Box 6-1).

These entities affect the vessels of the upper and lower extremities. The majority of the patients with large vessel arteritis and up to 30% of individuals with thromboangiitis obliterans are female. Arterial occlusion also occurs as a consequence of embolism or thrombosis in situ. Emboli originating in the heart may travel to the aorta and distal sites in the extremities. Thrombosis can develop acutely in diseased arteries or occur in normal arteries in patients with hypercoagulable states or trauma.

Lower Extremity Atherosclerosis

Lower extremity atherosclerosis was once thought to be a disease exclusively affecting male patients. The most current data documents an increasing number of women with lower extremity atherosclerosis (peripheral arterial disease, PAD). By the year 2020, it is projected that women more than 65 years old will make up 15% of the population. The number of women with PAD will increase as these demographic changes occur. In the Framingham Study over a 20-year period, the biennial incidence rate of intermittent claudication was 3.5/1000 for women and 7.1/1000 for men.

The prevalence of claudication ranges from 1% to 14% in women compared with 2% to 14% in men.

The prevalence of PAD can also be measured using objective measures such as ankle brachial indices. The ankle brachial index is the ratio of ankle pressure divided by the highest arm pressure, and it is abnormal if the resulting ratio is less than 0.90. The Edinburgh Artery Study found that one fourth of the population 55 to 74 years of age had PAD, as determined by an ankle brachial index less than 0.9. Men and women were affected almost equally. In a recent observational study, 35% of all women over age 65 were found to have an ankle brachial index (ABI) less than 0.9.

One third of women with abnormal ABIs report symptoms of claudication. That means 60% of women with objective evidence of PAD do not have symptoms. Yet the diagnosis of even asymptomatic peripheral arterial disease identifies an individual with a fivefold increase in the risk of cardiovascular death. Atherosclerotic changes occur in all blood vessels, and it is the cardiac manifestations of this disease that are largely responsible for patient mortality. Symptoms of PAD can range from intermittent claudication, described as discomfort in the muscles of the legs with activity that disappears with rest, to critical limb ischemia, rest pain, and gangrene. Recent literature suggests that asymptomatic cases are more prevalent in women than men, and that women with critical limb ischemia may be more likely to progress to limb loss.

Risk Factors

Diabetes mellitus and cigarette smoking are the strongest risk factors for the development of atherosclerosis. Glucose intolerance is associated with a fourfold increase in risk in women for the development of atherosclerotic disease and only a 2.4-fold increase in risk in men. Even more disturbing is the observation that frank glycosuria increases the risk of intermittent claudication eightfold in women and fourfold in men. These findings suggest that diabetes may have a profound impact on the symptomatic progression of peripheral atherosclerosis in women. In addition, hyperlipidemia and hypertension are clear risk factors for PAD.

The impact of cigarette smoking on the incidence and progression of PAD in women cannot be overstated. As with diabetes, cigarette smoking has a profound impact on the duration of symptomatic disease, and the progression and extent of arterial stenoses. When women quit smoking, they have an improved prognosis as measured by stroke-free survival, decreased incidence of myocardial events, and limb salvage when compared to the prognosis of those who continue to smoke. It is quite ominous that the fastest growing population of cigarette smokers is teenage girls. Those women who smoke become symptomatic from PAD an average of 10 years earlier than nonsmoking women, and they appear to have more aortoiliac occlusive disease. The hypoplastic aortoiliac syndrome has been described as "an entity peculiar to women" and is the most severe example of this accelerated PAD in female cigarette smokers. This syndrome is characterized by disabling claudication occurring in women in their thirties and forties, and angiographic confirmation of marked narrowing of the distal aorta and severe stenosis of the iliac bifurcation.

The role of menopause and loss of ovarian function in the development and progression of peripheral atherosclerosis is not entirely understood. In animal models of atherosclerosis, ovariectomy is associated with accelerated atherosclerosis, whereas sham ovariectomy is not. In women, early menopause has been associated with an increased incidence of aortoiliac disease, an association first noted more than 30 years ago. The incidence of claudication increases in women in their postmenopausal years and is identical to that of men by the ninth decade. These findings suggest that there is decreased atherogenesis with intact ovarian function, perhaps via the hormones associated with intact ovarian function. In animal models of atherosclerosis, the increased atherosclerosis associated with ovariectomy is attenuated by replacing estrogen. In the first randomized controlled trial of hormone replacement in postmenopausal women, the Heart and Estrogen/Progestin Replacement Study (HERS), there was no difference in cardiovascular events at 5 years between the active and placebo treatments, and a trend toward less peripheral arterial procedures in the

women in the active treatment arm. This disparity between the animal observations and the first randomized clinical trial may be due in part to differences in replacement regimens used. Ongoing primary and secondary prevention trials of hormone replacement therapy in postmenopausal women, including those with soy and selective estrogen receptor modulators, may further clarify the role of estrogens in peripheral atherosclerosis.

APPROACH TO THE PATIENT WITH LOWER EXTREMITY ATHEROSCLEROSIS

MANAGEMENT

Medical Therapy for Peripheral Arterial Disease

Smoking cessation is associated with a significant decrease in the risk of cardiovascular events, but only a modest change in the symptoms of claudication and greater walking distance in women. Smoking cessation, however, does halt the progression of PAD (Box 6-2) (see Chapter 89). Aggressive blood sugar control in the treatment of diabetes has also had similar results. In the United Kingdom Prospective Diabetes Study, men and women receiving intensive therapy had fewer myocardial infarctions than those on diet therapy. Nonetheless, there was no change in limb loss or risk of PAD with intensive therapy. Clearly, the relationship of intensive blood glucose control to symptoms of PAD is poorly understood. (Diabetes is covered at length in Chapter 11.)

Patients with hypertension are treated to reduce systolic blood pressure to less than 130 mm Hg and diastolic blood pressure to less than 85 mm Hg to decrease cardiovascular risk. Unfortunately, large decreases in systemic blood pressure may cause large decreases in limb pressure and shorten pain-free walking distance. In contrast, supervised exercise training results in improved physical conditioning that may reduce blood pressure and yet results in improvement in pain-free walking distance.

Pharmacologic Therapy of Peripheral Arterial Disease

Cilostozol (therapy) results in improvement in both pain-free walking distance and ABI. The randomized trials of this medication have included women (up to 30%). The inclusion of women in significant numbers allows clinicians to make recommendations for women without extrapolating from exclusively male trials. One note of caution with cilostozol is that phosphodiesterase inhibitors such as cilostozol should not be administered to any patient with heart failure. This recommendation originates from the observed increase in mortality with other phosphodiesterase inhibitors administered to patients with heart failure.

Propionyl-L-carnitine improves muscle metabolism and has been observed to improve pain-free walking distance in men. It is approved for this indication in Europe and under investigation in the United States. Prostaglandins are also being evaluated in patients with critical limb ischemia and those with claudication. The intravenous preparations hold promise, but treatment is complicated by flushing, myalgias, headache, and gastrointestinal cramping.

Antiplatelet agents do not decrease claudication symptoms, but they have a profound beneficial effect on cardiovascular events in men with claudication. The trials of secondary prevention of vascular disease by antiplatelet treatment were reviewed by the Antiplatelet Trialists' Collaboration. Unfortunately, the impact of these agents on cardiovascular events and the secondary prevention of PAD in women is still unknown, as most of these trials excluded women. One exception is the randomized trial of clopidigrel versus aspirin in patients at risk of ischemic events (CAPRIE). More than 30% of the population in this trial were female. In this study the long-term administration of clopidigrel to patients with atherosclerotic vascular disease was slightly more effective than aspirin in reducing the combined cardiovascular endpoint. This suggests that both antiplatelet agents will decrease cardiovascular mortality in women with peripheral atherosclerosis.

Revascularization for Peripheral Arterial Disease

Women account for one third of all distal revascularization procedures and amputations. Women and men undergoing these procedures have similar risk factors, but the women are consistently 3 to 5 years older than their male counterparts. In a meta-analysis of population-based studies on limb ischemia, men were more likely to develop disease progression than women. The asymptomatic nature of limb ischemia in female patients did not indicate a benign disease process. Asymptomatic PAD patients appeared to have the same increased risk for cardiovascular morbidity and mortality as PAD patients with intermittent claudication. Despite the wealth of literature on the outcome of lower extremity revascularization and risk factor analysis for graft failure, few have clearly addressed the issue of gender. Two studies have identified female gender has an independent predictor of graft failure. Arterial size appears to have a significant impact on the success of these reconstructions. In a randomized multicenter controlled trial comparing prosthetic above knee femoropopliteal bypass grafting, the choice of smaller graft diameter was associated with a dramatic decrease in 5-year patency.

TAKAYASU ARTERITIS
Epidemiology and Pathophysiology

Takayasu arteritis is a chronic inflammatory disease with manifestations predominantly in the aorta and its branches (Box 6-3). This arteritis occurs predominantly in women less than 40 years old. It is a periarteritis that begins with inflammation throughout the vessel wall and occasional giant cells at sites where the elastic lamina is destroyed. Fibrosis of the vessel occurs in the chronic phase. The pattern of arteries that is affected varies according to the patient's geographic location. In North American and Japanese patients, the aortic arch and its branches are often involved, whereas in Indian and Mexican patients, the abdominal aorta and its branches are more often involved.

Clinical Presentation

The disease often begins with fevers, malaise, myalgias, and occasionally pain over the affected vessels (e.g., carotodynia). Over time symptoms of arterial occlusive disease with arterial insufficiency develop. These include claudication, cerebrovascular ischemia, and visceral pain. Aortic aneurysm or aortic dissection can also occur. Takayasu arteritis should be suspected in individuals with unequal pulses or blood pressures in their extremities, and in young women with carotid and subclavian bruits.

Diagnostic Tests

There is no laboratory test to diagnose Takayasu arteritis. The American College of Rheumatology has reporting criteria for studies of Takayasu arteritis. These include age less than 40, extremity claudication, diminished brachial pulse, significant systolic pressure difference between arms, subclavian or aortic bruit, and angiographic evidence of disease. Angiography can identify the long segmental narrowings that are typical of Takayasu's arteritis. Having three of the six criteria indicates high specificity and sensitivity for the diagnosis. In addition, angiography using computed tomography and magnetic resonance imaging can demonstrate artery wall inflammation. The erythrocyte sedimentation rate is a marker for disease activity. It is used in combination with systemic complaints or new symptoms of arterial insufficiency.

Management

Medical treatment with corticosteroids is effective in 60% of the patients. Methotrexate and cyclophosphamide can be added if prednisone is ineffective or poorly tolerated. These

---

BOX 6-3
Takayasu Arteritis

Female less than 40 years
8.5:1 female/male ratio
Propensity for aortic arch and branches, pulmonary artery, abdominal aorta, and branches
Complications:
　Cardiovascular/neurologic (hypertension/stroke)
Therapy: Corticosteroids for acute disease
Differential: Atherosclerosis
Diagnosis:
　Fever, myalgias, anorexia, cardiovascular symptoms, tapered narrowing on angiography

drugs may decrease clinical and angiographic evidence of Takayasu arteritis. Percutaneous transluminal angioplasty with stenting has been used successfully in few patients with short, concentric stenoses. Surgical arterial bypass is often used for patients with symptomatic ischemia. However, when surgery is performed during periods of active disease, there are dramatically higher complication and restenosis rates.

GIANT CELL ARTERITIS
Epidemiology and Pathophysiology

Giant cell arteritis, or temporal arteritis, occurs typically in individuals more than 50 years old (Box 6-4). The mean age of onset is 70 years, with the highest prevalence in Caucasian females of Northern European ancestry. It is found in the arteries throughout the body. This arteritis begins with lymphocyte infiltration throughout the arterial wall and intimal thickening. The classic pathologic findings are granuloma with multinucleated giant cells and focal necrosis in the region of the disrupted elastic lamina. The pattern is described as one of "skip" lesions. Therefore many arterial sections must be examined before excluding this diagnosis. Temporal, carotid, vertebral, subclavian, brachial, coronary arteries, and the aorta are often involved.

Clinical Presentation and Diagnosis

Symptoms of giant cell arteritis include visual changes, headache, scalp tenderness, fever, weight loss, and malaise. Claudication of the jaw, tongue, arms, and legs may occur. The presentation can be dramatic, as with aortic dissection. Half of these patients will have clinical findings of polymyalgia rheumatica. Elevated erythrocyte sedimentation rate is common, but not required to make the diagnosis. The diagnosis is based on clinical presentation, with confirmation by pathologic or angiographic examination.

Management

Steroids are the main treatment, and their use has dramatically decreased the incidence of blindness with temporal arteritis. Treatment begins with prednisone, 40 to 60 mg/day. The prednisone dose can typically be tapered in 2 to 4 weeks. Remission can occur and may not happen until after 1 to 2 years of therapy. Surgical intervention is indicated for limb salvage and may be needed to decrease mortality from aortic aneurysm or dissection. Death is rare and results from stroke, myocardial infarction, ruptured aortic aneurysms, and aortic dissection.

BOX 6-4
Giant Cell Arteritis

Elderly white female
3:1 Female/male ratio
Propensity for carotid artery and branches but may involve any artery
Complication: Visual disturbances and blindness
Therapy: Steroids
Differential: Atherosclerosis
Diagnosis: Elevated erythrocyte sedimentation rate, temporal artery biopsy

---

THROMBOANGIITIS OBLITERANS
Epidemiology and Pathophysiology

Thromboangiitis obliterans, also known as Buerger's disease, results in intimal inflammation and thrombosis in the small and medium arteries in the extremities. Migratory superficial thrombophlebitis also occurs. The disease historically affected young male cigarette smokers, but is now reported with increasing frequency in young female cigarette smokers.

Clinical Presentation

Patients present with a variety of symptoms including Raynaud's phenomenon, foot claudication, and digital gangrene. Severe ischemia may result in peripheral neuropathy. There are segmental occlusions of small and medium arteries on angiography. These are usually at the distal part of the upper and lower extremities and are accompanied by corkscrew collaterals.

Management

There is no effective treatment without abstinence from tobacco. New lesions develop less often if the patient stops smoking. Digital ulcers may require debridement. Pharmacologic therapy is designed to decrease the vasospasm that accompanies the arterial narrowings. It includes calcium channel blockers, alpha-adrenergic blockers, and vasodilator prostaglandin infusion to decrease vasospasm. The use of aspirin has also been advocated in these patients.

RAYNAUD'S PHENOMENON
Epidemiology and Pathophysiology

Raynaud's phenomenon refers to episodes of vasospasm resulting in digital ischemia. Episodes of well-demarcated digital cyanosis or pallor follow cold exposure and emotional distress. The diagnosis is based on the patient's history. Simple office maneuvers like cold water immersion do not reliably induce episodes of digital ischemia. Raynaud's phenomenon occurs in up to 20% of all women. The prevalence is highest in those populations living in colder climates. Unique features of digital arterial innervation contribute to the occurrence of Raynaud's phenomenon. The cutaneous vessels of the fingers and toes have only sympathetic adrenergic vasoconstrictor fibers. The increased sympathetic efferent activity that normally causes vasoconstriction can cause profound vasospasm in individuals with Raynaud's phenomenon. Decreased perfusion, digital arterial narrowing, and increased blood viscosity also alter digital blood flow and can contribute to Raynaud's phenomenon.

Classification

Raynaud's phenomenon is classified as primary (i.e., not associated with another disease) or secondary (i.e., occurring as a consequence of another disease or treatment). Criteria of primary Raynaud's phenomenon are given in Box 6-5 and include history of bilateral episodes of digital pallor or cyanosis; symptoms for longer than 2 years; strong, symmetric pulses on physical examination; and no digital pitting, ulcerations, or gangrene. The tests of antinuclear antibody, erythrocyte sedimentation rate, nail fold capillaroscopy are normal in primary Raynaud's phenomenon. Primary Raynaud's phenomenon is associated with a favorable prognosis.

BOX 6-5
Primary Raynaud's Phenomenon

Bilateral episodes of digital cyanosis or pallor
Absence of digital ulceration, pitting, or gangrene
Symmetric and strong peripheral pulses
Symptoms for more than 2 years
Evidence of disease or drugs associated with secondary Raynaudís
Normal ESR (erythrocyte sedimentation rate)
Normal ANA (antinuclear antibody test)
Normal nailfold capillaroscopy

BOX 6-6
Secondary Causes of Raynaud's Phenomenon

Occupational trauma
Collagen vascular diseases
   Scleroderma
   Dermatomyositis
   Systemic lupus erythematosus
Frostbite
Thoracic outlet syndrome
Thromboembolism
Thromboangiitis obliterans
Cryoglobulinemia
Cold agglutinins
Blood dyscrasias
Drugs (e.g., bromocriptive, ergot derivatives)
Toxins (e.g., vinyl chloride)
Chemotherapeutic agents (e.g., vinblastine, bleomycin)

A secondary cause of Raynaud's phenomenon is suggested by the presence of prolonged digital ischemia with findings such as digital ulcers (Box 6-6). These include connective tissue disease, thermal or vibration injury, arterial occlusive disease, blood dyscrasias, drugs, neurologic disorders, and toxins. Most secondary causes of Raynaud's phenomenon are obvious before the episodes of digital ischemia begin. One exception to this rule is scleroderma. In patients with scleroderma, the Raynaud's phenomenon can precede evidence of scleroderma by years.

Diagnostic Tests

In secondary Raynaud's phenomenon, the arterial supply to the digits can be evaluated to determine the degree of fixed arterial occlusion. Such testing includes digital systolic pressure measurements, digital plethysmography, or Doppler flow of the digits. When abnormal arterial flow is seen, the test can be repeated after warming of the patient. If the arterial flow appears normal after warming, vasospasm rather than fixed arterial occlusion is present. Arteriography is indicated only if an obstructive lesion requiring revascularization is suspected.

Management

The mainstay of treatment is teaching the patient to avoid stimuli that precipitate digital ischemic attacks. This includes instructions to dress warmly, and means not only wearing gloves, but also sweaters, coats, and hats. Reflex sympathetic vasoconstriction occurs in the digits in response to cold exposure in other parts of the body (e.g., head). Calcium channel blockers (except verapamil) and alpha-adrenergic blockers are used to decrease symptoms. Intravenous iloprost improves digital ulcer healing in patients with scleroderma. Selective digital sympathectomy and microarteriolysis may also result in ulcer healing and symptom improvement in severe cases. Cervical and lumbar sympathectomy have been performed, but with very limited long-term success.

ACROCYANOSIS
Epidemiology

Acrocyanosis is an unusual disorder in the general population, but is seen in 20% of the women with anorexia nervosa. Acrocyanosis presents as episodes of coldness and cyanosis in the hands and feet. Unlike Raynaud's phenomenon, the cyanosis extends beyond the digits to the palms and occasionally above the wrist.

Clinical Presentation

The clinical presentation is attributed to arteriolar spasm. The cyanosis increases with cold exposure and is relieved by warming. There may be mild edema and excess sweating of the hands and feet on physical examination. There are no trophic changes or ulceration of the digits. If the patient is examined during an episode, pallor is seen when the extremity is raised above the heart level, indicating that the findings are not attributable to venous obstruction. Patients with acrocyanosis have no physical evidence of central cyanosis, and routine laboratory evaluation is normal. The disorder is self-limited and does not indicate worsened prognosis from the underlying starvation. The acrocyanosis generally resolves as weight gain occurs in patients with anorexia nervosa.

VENOUS SYSTEM

In contrast to arterial disease, venous disease tends to be passive, providing the physician with a subtle complex of symptoms and signs from which to make a diagnosis. The venous system usually presents with one of two manifestations: thrombosis or insufficiency.

Venous Thrombosis

Thrombosis of the venous system most commonly occurs in the lower extremities. Our understanding of the pathogenesis of venous thrombosis is still founded on the tenet of hypercoagulability as described by Virchow, largely occurring as a result of venous stasis, venous endothelial cell injury, and activation of the clotting system. The more commonly encountered causes for venous thrombosis include pregnancy, contraceptives, surgery and postsurgical immobilization, cancer, age, and trauma. (For more details on venous thrombotic disease, see Chapter 7.)

Clinical Presentation

The patient with superficial thrombophlebitis may present with a warm, erythematous streak along the path of a superficial vein. This localized inflammation is responsible for the associated complaints including pain, tenderness, and swelling. Thrombosis is a common complication of venous varicosities. The presentation of multiple episodes of superficial phlebitis in multiple locations is suggestive of *Trousseau's syndrome,* a complication of pancreatic cancer.

In contrast to the superficial manifestation of venous thrombosis, deep vein thrombosis (DVT) may be more difficult to diagnose. The symptoms, present in approximately 50% of patients, may include pain with ambulation (most commonly at the ball of the foot) swelling, pain, pressure, or fullness. The vast majority of DVTs occur in the lower extremity and are a sequela of immobilization, trauma, or malignancy. Deep vein thromboses that occur in the absence of a precipitating factor are considered primary, the most common cause of which is activated protein C resistance, otherwise known as Factor V Leiden.

Physical Examination

Physical examination findings for patients with both superficial and deep vein thrombosis occur as a result of the decreased venous return and inflammation associated with the thrombosis. The patient with superficial thrombophlebitis may present with venous distention, a palpable venous cord, tenderness, warmth, or erythema. The physical findings in DVT are similar and include warmth, erythema, and swelling of the affected extremity. Venous cords, when palpable, are most often appreciated in the common femoral vein, just distal to the inguinal ligament. The extremity may become engorged, developing a change in the profile of the thigh or calf, and bogginess of the affected muscle.

Diagnostic Tests

The most commonly used modality for confirming the diagnosis of either superficial thrombophlebitis or deep vein thrombosis is duplex ultrasound. Using several diagnostic maneuvers including vein compression and examination of the respirophasic changes in venous flow, B-mode and Doppler ultrasonography, respectively, diagnose DVTs in the proximal circulation (at or above the knee) in nearly all cases. The smaller vein size and variations in venous anatomy decrease the sensitivity and specificity of the test in the calf; however, it is the appropriate first examination. Venography and magnetic resonance venography are rarely necessary for clinical management.

Differential Diagnosis

The differential diagnosis of deep vein thrombosis commonly made with duplex ultrasonography includes Baker's cyst, knee arthritis, cellulitis, muscular tears, and lymphangitis.

Management

The management of superficial thrombophlebitis is primarily palliative. Warm soaks, leg elevation, and nonsteroidal antiinflammatory medications are the mainstays of therapy. Thromboembolization is distinctly unusual in this setting, and there is no mandate for anticoagulation. In patients who remain symptomatic, heparin anticoagulation may relieve the inflammation and may be instituted for a several week course of therapy. In contrast, deep vein thrombosis in the proximal circulation carries a 1-year pulmonary embolism rate as high as 25%. To prevent these sequelae, anticoagulation must be instituted (refer to Chapter 7). Placement of inferior vena caval filters is necessary only in the setting of a contraindication to anticoagulation. Caval filters do not augment the protection of anticoagulation beyond 12 days and increase the risk of late DVT recurrence. Their use should be reserved for patients with a contraindication to anticoagulation and above-knee DVTs. Although not standard practice, thrombolytic therapy has been increasing in use. Currently thrombolytic therapy is recommended only for the severe deep vein thromboses that cause impairment of arterial blood flow.

The need for anticoagulation of calf vein deep vein thromboses is more controversial because of the much lower risk of thromboembolism. However, calf vein thromboses have a 15% to 20% chance of propagating proximally to the popliteal vein. Those that propagate to the level of the knee or above carry the same risk of thrombosis as primary proximal DVTs. Two strategies are acceptable. Patients may be anticoagulated as described previously. Alternately, ambulatory patients may have a repeat ultrasound 4 to 6 days later and, if the DVT has not changed in character at all, managed expectantly. Any extension proximally to the knee or within the calf to another vein is an indication for anticoagulation.

Varicose Veins

Epidemiology and Pathophysiology

Varicose veins are dilated, serpentine segments of superficial veins. Idiopathic or primary varicose veins are more common in women. About half these patients report a positive family history. The familial link implies a venous abnormality such as a structural abnormality of the vein wall or an incompetent venous valve. Progression is incremental, as valvular incompetence and structural abnormalities increase the pressure exerted on distal segments, thus causing new ectasia.

Secondary varicosities occur as a result of persistent elevations in intraluminal venous pressure, such as with compressive masses or pregnancy, or as a sequela of either superficial or deep vein thrombosis. With deep vein thrombosis, incompetence of the perforator veins, the veins that allow communication between the deep and superficial systems, subject the superficial veins to increased flow and pressure, causing dilation. Obesity, pregnancy, prolonged standing, and a sedentary lifestyle can exacerbate the progression of varicose veins.

Clinical Presentation

Patients may complain of burning, aching, or pruritus. Women may report symptomatic exacerbation premenstrually. In 80% of patients, the greater saphenous veins are involved. Patients will commonly report that symptoms are best in the morning and progress through the day. Leg dependence also worsens the symptoms while elevation provides relief. With inadequate care or disease progression, patients may develop ulceration, dermatitis, superficial thrombophlebitis, and venous hemorrhage. The hemorrhage

---

BOX 6-7
Management of Superficial Venous Disease

Exercise and weight loss
Control of blood pressure
Support stockings
Leg elevation
For progressive symptoms (painful thrombosis, bleeding varix, superficial phlebitis, leg ulceration):
    Sclerotherapy
    Laser therapy
    Support stockings
    Surgical intervention

---

tends to be without hemodynamic consequence, but may be dangerous, as it tends to be painless, delaying their recognition. The poor cosmetic appearance generates most physician appointments.

Physical Examination

On physical examination, the veins are superficial, dilated, and tortuous. Leg dependency augments blood reflux and increases the size of the veins. Balloting the veins may demonstrate a fluid wave. Thrombophlebitis is not an uncommon complication. Venous telangiectasis or "spider veins" are commonly mistaken for varicose veins. Spider veins are small, cutaneous veins that occur in a caput medusa pattern and may occur in clusters.

Management

Standard therapy for varicose veins includes weight loss, exercise, control of blood pressure, and the application of compression stockings (Box 6-7). Use of specially fit compression stockings, with an initial compression of 20 to 30 mm Hg, decreases the symptoms and progression of varicose veins. Stockings should be applied when the veins are empty. Thus, patients should get back into bed for several minutes before placing the stockings to maximize the benefit. Other recommendations include leg elevation and meticulous care of inflamed areas. Although some patients with frequent venous hemorrhage or intolerable symptoms may require surgical therapy, the majority of patients choose one of these therapies for cosmesis. Surgical therapies include compression sclerotherapy and ablative procedures for the superficial and perforator veins, such as venous stripping and ligation of incompetent communicating veins and laser therapy. These therapies effectively eliminate the treated veins, but a substantial number of patients develop recurrent disease.

Chronic Venous Insufficiency

Epidemiology and Pathophysiology

Chronic venous insufficiency (CVI) is present in up to 3% of the population and is a prominent source of functional limitation. The inciting abnormality in chronic venous insufficiency is increased intraluminal venous pressures, which most commonly occur as a result of outflow obstruction or increased reflux. The most common cause of obstruction is DVT, but other causes include congenital venous abnormalities, extraluminal compression such as bandages or tumors,

and intraluminal obstructions such as venous webs. Deep vein thrombosis is the most common cause of CVI and approximately 30% of all patients with DVT may develop symptoms or signs of CVI within 5 years. Venous reflux, or excess backflow, results from venous valve dysfunction. Valve dysfunction usually results from the scarring associated with thrombosis or a primary valvular insufficiency. The venous valvular incompetence exacerbates distal and perforator venous pressure and valvular competence. Perforating venous incompetence causes excess reflux into the superficial veins and may cause both varicose vein formation and fluid extravasation into the soft tissue.

Clinical Presentation

Although the inciting events occur in the large vessels, the clinical syndrome is usually the manifestation of small vessel effects. The syndrome is composed of edema, superficial venous dilation, leg pain, and skin changes. Edema is usually the first sign of CVI. Patients most commonly complain of leg swelling that is exacerbated by dependency. Venous dilation may begin during the second decade of life, but progresses most rapidly during pregnancy. Many patients complain of leg pain in CVI. Most commonly, patients have pain with long periods of standing and may improve with walking. The heaviness or aching is usually worse in the warm weather and during menstruation. Patients with obstruction to flow in the deep veins may develop venous claudication or reproducible deep pressure or bursting sensation within the calf with walking that improves with rest. *The primary skin manifestation, hyperpigmentation, stems from deposition of the hemosiderin of extravasated, lysed erythrocytes and results in the typical "brawny" appearance.* Other symptoms include burning, pruritus, pain, and eczema. Chronic edema reduces cutaneous nutrient vessel blood flow such that small injuries may cause ulcer formation, typically at the level of the malleolus.

Diagnostic Tests

Differentiating deep and perforator venous incompetence from superficial incompetence can be done in the office using the ***Brodie-Trendelenburg*** test. A tourniquet is applied after venous drainage with leg elevation (the patient's leg is placed on the examiner's shoulder). The leg is then put down and the patient is asked to stand. Superficial venous refill in under 30 seconds is evidence of deep and perforator venous incompetence. Calf tenderness, skin induration, cellulitis, and ulceration are not uncommon physical findings. Skin induration and fibrosis are a result of chronic inflammation. Venous insufficiency, in contrast to the well defined, pallid arterial ulcers, are large, erythematous, and moist and have irregular borders. The surrounding skin may be shiny.

Management

The management of CVI is aimed at decreasing intravenous pressures and treating the sequelae (Box 6-8). Similar to the treatment of superficial venous insufficiency, the application of graded elastic compression stockings, leg elevation periodically during the day and throughout the night, and medicated ulcer dressings form the triad of therapy. The use of graded pressure stockings, with the highest pressure at the ankle and lowest at the proximal segment, is required. A short course of diuretics may aid in the resolu-

---

BOX 6-8
Management of Chronic Venous Insufficiency

Exercise
Compression stockings
Leg elevation
Diuretics for edema
Progressive symptoms:
  Venogram
  If veins are incompetent, then surgical stripping of veins
  If veins are competent, the compression stockings

---

tion of chronic edema. The surgical options for deep vein thrombosis target the valvular incompetence. Surgical repair of valvular incompetence, a valvuloplasty, involves transposing a vein segment with incompetent valves to an adjacent segment with competent valves. A second surgical option is the transplant of a competent venous segment into an incompetent lower extremity vein. Patients with obstructive disease may benefit from a venous bypass procedure.

BIBLIOGRAPHY

Gerhard-Herman M, Thakore A: Lower extremity arterial occlusive disease in women, *Am J Med* Part II:14-20, 1998.

Hirsh, J, Hoak, J: AHA Medical/Scientific Statement. Management of deep vein thrombosis and pulmonary embolism, *Circulation* 93:2212, 1996.

Hyers TM et al: Antithrombotic therapy for venous thromboembolic disease, *Chest* 114:561S, 1998.

Kerr GS et al: Takayasu arteritis, *Ann Intern Med* 120:919, 1994.

Levine M et al: A comparison of low molecular weight heparin administered primarily at home with unfractionated heparin administered in the hospital for proximal deep vein thrombosis, *N Engl J Med* 334:667, 1996.

Mays BW et al: Women have increased risk of perioperative myocardial infarction and higher long-term mortality rates after lower extremity arterial bypass grafting, *J Vasc Surg* 29:807, 1999.

O'Donnell TF, McEnroe CS, Heggerick P: Chronic venous insufficiency, *Surg Clin North Am* 70:159, 1990.

Olin JW et al: The changing clinical spectrum of thromboangiitis obliterans, *Circulation* 82:IV3, 1990.

Prandoni P et al: Upper extremity deep vein thrombosis, *Arch Intern Med* 157:57, 1997.

Weitz JI et al: Diagnosis and treatment of chronic arterial insufficiency of the lower extremities: a critical review, *Circulation* 94:3026, 1996.

Wigley FM: Raynaud's phenomenon, *Curr Opin Rheumatol* 5:773, 1993.

CHAPTER 7

Venous Thromboembolic Disease

Samuel Z. Goldhaber

Venous thromboembolism (VTE), which comprises deep venous thrombosis (DVT) and pulmonary embolism (PE), poses special risks and dilemmas, especially for women. In collaboration with their primary care physicians, women must make important decisions at varying stages in their lives regarding oral contraception, pregnancy, and hormone replacement therapy—all of which increase the risk of VTE.

▦ EPIDEMIOLOGY

In the largest prospective registry of PE, which included 2454 subjects, 55% of PE patients were women. In a separate prospective cohort study of female nurses with more than 1,600,000 woman-years of follow-up, their three most frequent risk factors for PE were obesity, cigarette smoking, and hypertension.

Oral Contraceptives

First-generation oral contraceptives contained more than 50 μg of estrogen and were associated with an alarming increase in the frequency of VTE, especially massive PE. Second-generation low-dose oral contraceptives containing less than 50 μg, were introduced in the United States in 1967, and first-generation pills were withdrawn from the market in 1989. Third-generation oral contraceptives use the new progestogens—desogestrel or gestodene. They decrease the annoying side effects of acne and hirsutism and have a more favorable effect on carbohydrate metabolism and lipid profiles than second-generation pills. Ironically, they are associated with a doubling or tripling of the VTE rate compared with second-generation oral contraceptives. The explanation for this surprising finding is that third-generation oral contraceptives lead to acquired resistance to activated protein C, the most potent endogenous anticoagulant.

Despite the high relative risk of VTE from oral contraceptives, the absolute risk is low. A New Zealand study of oral contraceptives and fatal PE estimated the absolute risk of death from PE in current users as 1 per 10.5 million woman-years. In this study, the risk of fatal PE was double among those taking third generation pills.

Among women with inherited clotting disorders, those using oral contraceptives appear to be at especially high risk of VTE. For example, in a case-control study at Leiden University, women with the factor V Leiden mutation (which leads to resistance to activated protein C and enhances susceptibility to thrombosis) who used oral contraceptives were at a 35-fold greater risk of VTE than control subjects. In a subsequent analysis from the Leiden Thrombophilia Study, which included cases with factor V Leiden, protein C or S deficiency, the prothrombin gene 20210 A mutation, and antithrombin III deficiency, the overall risk of developing DVT during the first 6 months of oral contraceptive use was increased 19-fold compared with control subjects.

In summary, healthy women are excellent candidates for oral contraceptives. The initial prescription should be for a second-generation pill. Because of the increased risk associated with third-generation agents, they should be used only if acne or hirsutism become problematic. The standard of care dictates that women with prior VTE use alternative methods of contraception.

Whether women with a family history of VTE but no personal past history of VTE should be screened to help decide whether to use oral contraceptives is controversial. Generally, it is encouraged to avoid the use of oral contraceptives if thrombophilia is detected. For women with known thrombophilia but no prior VTE, the safest policy is to use alternative forms of contraception. However, no definitive ban on using oral contraceptives can be justified in this setting because the absolute risk of VTE remains very low.

Pregnancy

Discussion of venous thromboembolic disease in pregnancy is covered in Chapter 77.

Hormone Replacement Therapy

The traditional teaching for the past generation has been that hormone replacement therapy (HRT) does not predispose to VTE because the estrogen dose is much lower than that found in oral contraceptives. However, this concept had been widely accepted without substantial data. In 1996 this assumption was challenged when three separate large data sets implicated HRT as doubling, tripling, or even quadrupling the risk of VTE. As with oral contraceptives, the risk of VTE was highest during the first year of HRT.

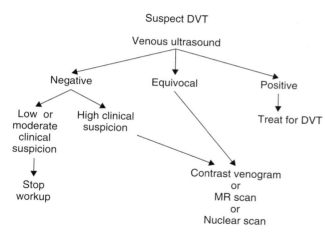

FIG. 7-1 Diagnosis of deep vein thrombosis.

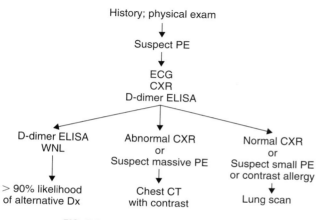

FIG. 7-2 Diagnosis of pulmonary embolism.

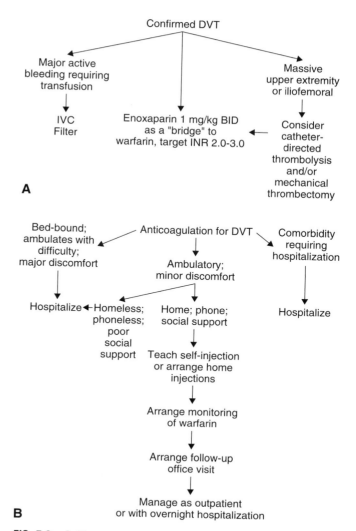

FIG. 7-3 **A,** Management of deep vein thrombosis. **B,** Deep vein thrombosis patient triage and disposition.

The Heart and Estrogen/Progestin Replacement Study was a randomized trial of 2763 postmenopausal women who had a history of coronary heart disease but no previous VTE. They were randomized to conjugated equine estrogens, 0.625 mg, plus medroxyprogesterone acetate, 2.5 mg, versus placebo. In results that shocked most of the medical community, the hypothesis that HRT would reduce the rate of new coronary events was not substantiated in this rigorous trial. Furthermore, the rate of VTE tripled among those women receiving HRT. Certain subgroups were at especially high risk of increased VTE, including women with lower extremity fractures (18-fold increase), cancer (fourfold increase), postoperative state (fivefold increase), or nonsurgical hospitalization (sixfold increase). Women with thrombophilia such as factor V Leiden seem to be at especially high risk of VTE if they take HRT.

Selective Estrogen Receptor Modulators

An alternative to HRT is raloxifene, a selective estrogen receptor modulator that has estrogenic effects on bone, lipid metabolites, and blood clotting but an estrogen antagonist effect on breast tissue. Raloxifene was touted as a "designer estrogen," and at the time of its release, expectations were widely held that it would quickly become a "billion dollar drug." Those who held out such high hopes were disappointed. In a randomized controlled trial of 7705 osteoporotic postmenopausal women, raloxifene decreased the risk of vertebral fractures, decreased the risk of breast cancer by 75% during 3 years of treatment, but tripled the rate of VTE.

Tamoxifen, another selective estrogen receptor modulator, also acts as an estrogen agonist on bone and an estrogen antagonist on breast tissue. In the British Cancer Prevention Trial of women at high risk of breast cancer, 55 months of treatment with tamoxifen 20 mg daily halved the rate of breast cancer. However, the DVT rate increased by 60%, and the PE rate tripled.

DIAGNOSIS AND TREATMENT OF VENOUS THROMBOEMBOLISM

There are no substantive differences in the diagnosis and treatment of DVT and PE (Figs. 7-1 to 7-4) between men and women. Women do seem more susceptible than men

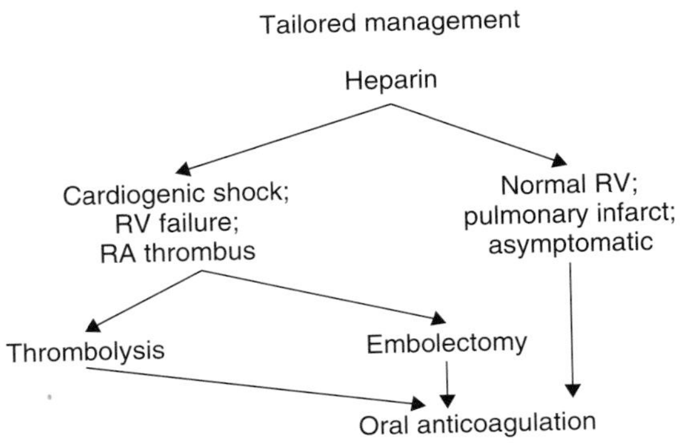

Tailored management

Heparin

FIG. 7-4 Tailored management of pulmonary embolism.

to varicose veins and venous insufficiency of the calf after DVT. Venous insufficiency can develop insidiously and first become symptomatic several years after the initial DVT. The frequency of developing venous insufficiency can be halved by prescribing prophylactically, at the time of the DVT, below-knee vascular compression stockings, 20 to 30 mm Hg or 30 to 40 mm Hg, to be worn during the day while ambulating; the stockings can be removed at night while in bed.

Women also seem to be more aware than men of the emotional and psychological burdens of VTE. Often, there is an initial bitterness at the health care system for overlooking the diagnosis of VTE. This feeling is followed, eventually, by fears of recurrent disease, occult cancer, and predisposition of apparently healthy siblings and children to VTE. Support groups, such as the Pulmonary Embolism Support Group, Brigham and Women's Hospital, Boston, Massachusetts, help women deal with these issues by having patients meet with clinicians once a month, compiling questions and answers in straightforward language, and utilizing an informational booklet on a website.

BIBLIOGRAPHY

Bloemenkamp KWM, Rosendaal FR, Helmerhorst FM, Vandenbroucke JP: Higher risk of venous thrombosis during early use of oral contraceptives in women with inherited clotting defects, *Arch Intern Med* 160:49, 2000.

Brandjes DPM et al: Randomised trial of effect of compression stockings in patients with symptomatic proximal-vein thrombosis, *Lancet* 349:759, 1997.

Brenner B et al: Gestational outcome in thrombophilic women with recurrent pregnancy loss treated by enoxaparin, *Thromb Haemost* 83:693, 2000.

Chan WS, Ray JG: Low molecular weight heparin use during pregnancy: issues of safety and practicality, *Obstet Gynecol* 54:649, 1999.

Chasan-Taber L, Stampfer MJ: Epidemiology of oral contraceptives and cardiovascular disease, *Ann Intern Med* 128:467, 1998.

Cummings SR et al: The effect of raloxifene on risk of breast cancer in postmenopausal women: results from the MORE randomized trial. Multiple Outcomes of Raloxifene Evaluation, *JAMA* 281:2189, 1999.

Daly E et al: Risk of venous thromboembolism in users of hormone replacement therapy, *Lancet* 348:977, 1996.

Douketis JD et al: The effects of long-term heparin therapy during pregnancy on bone density. A prospective matched cohort study, *Thromb Haemost* 75:254, 1996.

Fisher B et al: Tamoxifen for the prevention of breast cancer: report of the National Surgical Adjuvant Breast and Bowel Project P-1 Study, *J Natl Cancer Inst* 90:1371, 1998.

Gerhardt A et al: Prothrombin and factor V mutations in women with a history of thrombosis during pregnancy and the puerperium, *N Engl J Med* 342:374, 2000.

Goldhaber SZ, Visani L, De Rosa M: Acute pulmonary embolism: clinical outcomes in the International Cooperative Pulmonary Embolism Registry (ICOPER), *Lancet* 353:1386, 1999.

Goldhaber SZ et al: A prospective study of risk factors for pulmonary embolism in women, *JAMA* 277:642, 1997.

Grady D et al: Postmenopausal hormone therapy increases risk for venous thromboembolic disease. The Heart and Estrogen/progestin Replacement Study, *Ann Intern Med* 132:689, 2000.

Greer IA: Thrombosis in pregnancy: maternal and fetal issues, *Lancet* 353:1258, 1999.

Grodstein F et al: Prospective study of exogenous hormones and risk of pulmonary embolism in women, *Lancet* 348:983, 1996.

Hulley C et al: Randomized trial of estrogen plus progestin for secondary prevention of coronary heart disease in postmenopausal women. Heart and Estrogen/Progestin Replacement Study (HERS) Research Group, *JAMA* 280:605, 1998.

Hunt BJ et al: Thromboprophylaxis with low molecular weight heparin (Fragmin) in high risk pregnancies, *Thromb Haemost* 77:39, 1997.

Ito S: Drug therapy for breast-feeding women, *N Engl J Med* 343:118, 2000.

Jick H et al: Risk of hospital admission for idiopathic venous thromboembolism among users of postmenopausal oestrogens, *Lancet* 348:981, 1996.

Kupferminc MJ et al: Increased frequency of genetic thrombophilia in women with complications of pregnancy, *N Engl J Med* 340:9, 1999.

Lowe G et al: Thrombotic variables and risk of idiopathic venous thromboembolism in women aged 45–64 years. Relationships to hormone replacement therapy, *Thromb Haemost* 83:530, 2000.

Meinardi JR et al: Increased risk for fetal loss in carriers of the factor V Leiden mutation, *Ann Intern Med* 130:736, 1999.

Nelson-Piercy C, Letsky EA, de Swiet M: Low-molecular-weight heparin for obstetric thromboprophylaxis: experience of sixty-nine pregnancies in sixty-one women at high risk, *Am J Obstet Gynecol* 176:1062, 1997.

Parkin L et al: Oral contraceptives and fatal pulmonary embolism, *Lancet* 355:2133, 2000.

Ray JG, Chan WS: Deep vein thrombosis during pregnancy and the puerperium: a meta-analysis of the period of risk and the leg of presentation, *Obstet Gynecol Surv* 54:265, 1999.

Ridker PM et al: Factor V Leiden mutation as a risk factor for recurrent pregnancy loss, *Ann Intern Med* 128:1000, 1998.

Rosing J et al: Low-dose oral contraceptives and acquired resistance to activated protein C: a randomized cross-over study, *Lancet* 354: 2036, 1999.

Sanson BJ et al: Safety of low-molecular-weight heparin in pregnancy: a systematic review, *Thromb Haemost* 81:668, 1999.

Task Force on Pulmonary Embolism, European Society of Cardiology: Guidelines on diagnosis and management of acute pulmonary embolism, *Eur Heart J* 21:1301, 2000.

Toglia MR, Weg JG: Venous thromboembolism during pregnancy, *N Engl J Med* 335:108, 1996.

Vandenbroucke JP et al: Increased risk of venous thrombosis in oral-contraceptive users who are carriers of factor V Leiden mutation, *Lancet* 344:1453, 1994.

Walrath K, Berkovitz P, Morrison R, Goldhaber SZ: *Frequently asked questions of the Venous Thromboembolism Support Group*, 1999, Brigham and Women's Hospital. Available at: http://web.mit.edu.karen/www/faq.html/

Wellesley D, Moore I, Heard M, Keeton B: Two cases of warfarin embryopathy: a re-emergence of this condition? *Br J Obstet Gynaecol* 105: 805, 1998.

CHAPTER **8**

Common Dermatologic Problems

Olga Smulders-Meyer
Joseph C. Kvedar

Patients care deeply about their skin and often consult their primary care provider about any new or changing skin lesion. However, many, if not most, primary care physicians lack dermatology training during medical school and residency and are uncomfortable with a variety of presenting skin problems. In addition, because of managed care, primary care physicians are expected to diagnose and treat common dermatoses and screen for skin cancer rather than immediately referring patients to dermatologists.

This chapter provides a pragmatic review of common benign and malignant skin disorders that present throughout a lifetime. Disorders are commonly categorized by reproductive and life phases: adolescence and early adulthood, pregnancy, adulthood, and postmenopausal years.

COMMON DISORDERS DURING ADOLESCENCE AND EARLY ADULTHOOD

Although public awareness of the relationship between ultraviolet (UV) light exposure and skin cancer has increased, the primary physician should take every opportunity to remind young patients and their guardians that many potential skin changes in later life can be avoided by preventing sunburn during adolescence.

The application of sunscreen, topical agents that absorb and scatter UV radiation, is paramount. The SPF, or sunprotection factor on the product, for example 25, indicates that a person can stay exposed to the sun without developing an actual sunburn roughly 25 times as long as long as someone who is exposed to the sun without any protection. Pediatricians have recommended liberal application of sunscreen as standard procedure for every light-skinned child 6 months and older engaging in any type of prolonged outdoor activity. Yet, research has shown that adolescents often underutilize sunscreens and other protective modalities, such as wearing protective clothing, staying out of the sun mid-day, or seeking shade.

Sunscreens originally had only UVB-absorbing compounds, containing PABA esters or salicylates. More recent products containing benzophenone derivatives such as Parsol 1789 absorb some UVA radiation, usually the short-wavelength UVA range, leaving people exposed to the detri-mental effects of long-wave UVA, such as photoaging, without the warning signs of a burn. Physical sunscreens containing zinc oxide, red ferric oxide, or titanium dioxide offer broad-spectrum protection against all wavelengths of light. Unfortunately, these sunscreens often cause irritant reactions, particularly when applied near the eyes, but true allergic reactions are rare and sunscreens are not carcinogenic.

The use of tanning parlors should strongly be discouraged. The UVA radiation sources of these booths produce a tan that is not as protective against subsequent sunburn as UVB-induced tan. Tanning-booth lights often emit variable doses of UVB radiation, as well as UVA, and since these variables are poorly regulated the customer is at risk of being exposed to excessive and intense exposure to ultraviolet radiation.

Acne vulgaris affects millions of people in their teens and twenties, in varying degrees of severity. Adolescent acne develops in areas of high sebum production such as the T-zone of the face, the chest, and the back. Adult acne, on the other hand, is usually located in the perioral region of the face.

Mild acne is typically composed of comedones, scant papules, and pustules. The formation of acne is associated with increased sebum production, the formation of a closed comedo, overgrowth of anaerobic bacteria *Propionibacterium acnes (P. acnes),* and a subsequent inflammatory response. Mild acne can be treated with topical antibacterial agents, such as benzoyl peroxide preparations and retinoids. Retinoids (Table 8-1) are primarily comedolytic and enable other antiacne preparations to work more effectively. They cause dry skin and hypersensivity to the sun (although these symptoms tend to abate after a few weeks) and are contraindicated in pregnant or lactating patients. Treatment should be continued for at least 8 weeks to assess therapeutic effectiveness. If improvement is not forthcoming, topical antibiotic agents can be added (topical metronidazole, clindamycin, or erythromycin).

Moderate acne presents with more pustules, papules, and nodules. Oral antibiotics are the mainstream therapy based on their ability to decrease *P. acnes* in the skin. A trial of 2 to 3 months is required for a therapeutic response. Acne can become resistant to antibiotics, so switching to a

Table 8-1
Treatment for Acne

Severity	Therapy
Mild (comedones)	Tretinoin (Retin A) topical (0.05%, 0.1%) cream QD
	Topical antibiotics (erythromycin, clindamycin, metronidazole)
	Benzoyl peroxide (2.5%, 5%, 10%) lotion or gel
Moderate (comedones, papules)	Any of category 1 plus:
	Tetracycline 500 mg bid or
	Erythromycin enteric coated, 1 g/day
Severe (pustules, nodules, scarring)	Minocycline 100 mg bid or
	Doxycycline 100 mg bid or
	Isotretinoin 0.5–1 mg/kg/day for 20 weeks

different class of oral antibiotic every 6 to 12 months increases effectiveness.

Oral contraceptives, particularly those containing a hypoandrogenic progestin, are another option. This is the treatment of choice for patients with polycystic ovary syndrome who tend to have irregular menses, elevated androgen levels, and moderate to severe acne. Even without a hyperandrogenic state, women with regular menstrual cycles often experience improvement of their acne on oral contraceptives.

Severe acne is nodular cystic acne. This has all the features of mild and moderate acne and deep cystic inflammatory lesions that may lead to scarring. The most effective treatment of this disfiguring form of acne is oral isotretinoin (Accutane) for 20 weeks. It decreases plugging of the follicle, *P. acnes* counts, and sebum production in the entire skin. As isotretinoin decreases sebum production, a side effect may be a marked dryness of lips, scalp, and face. Patients must be informed of this, as well as other potential dose-related side effects, such as myalgias, headaches, and even acute worsening of depression. Suicide is an extreme but not insignificant potential side effect. Accutane is teratogenic. These issues should be a part of the informed consent process.

Monthly office visits and routine laboratory evaluation, including B-HCG, CBC, LFTs, and a cholesterol profile to exclude significant hypertriglyceremia are recommended for any patient on isotretinoin. Because of the teratogenicity, patients must consent to a reliable form of contraception while on this medication. Table 8-1 summarizes the treatment for the various forms of acne.

Atopic dermatitis is a skin disorder that is associated with an atopic diathesis and commonly occurs in patients with a history of asthma and allergic rhinitis. Although it can happen at any age, atopic dermatitis often presents in early childhood but flares during adolescence. The presenting complaints include pruritis, erythema, thickening of the skin from repeated scratching, excoriations, and erosions. The lesions then become infected with common skin flora such as *Staphylococcus aureus*. Untreated, atopic dermatitis results in thickening of the skin and painful fissures on fin-

gers and soles. Treatment consists of topical steroids, antipruritic medications (such as oral antihistamines and H-2 blockers), and often antistaphylococcal antibiotics. Because of the sensitivity of the skin, patients should avoid harsh soaps and apply unscented emollients after daily baths or showers.

Keratosis pilaris is a skin problem that is more common and more extensive in patients with an atopic diathesis. Patients present with tiny papules and pustules, without much surrounding erythema, on the posterior aspect of the upper arms and on the anterior thighs. Although this condition sometimes persists into adulthood, it usually fades with time. Hydrating lotions such as 12% ammonium lactate (Lac-Hydrin) offer the most benefit. Oral antibiotics and hydrocortisone cream are not indicated for this condition.

The skin manifestations of **sexually transmitted diseases** are important to recognize (see Chapter 22 for complete discussion of sexually transmitted diseases).

Herpes simplex virus (HSV) and *molluscum contagiosum* are cutaneous infections frequently encountered in primary care. Herpes simplex virus is the most common cause of chronic genital ulceration in the United States, with sexually active young adults being at highest risk for contracting the infection. In the United States, one in every five persons is seropositive for HSV2 even though less than 10% of these patients actually report a history of genital lesions. Moreover, HSV1 is a significant cause of genital herpes infection, implicated in 5% to 10% of all first-episode cases. Therefore current HSV2 seropositivity underestimates the actual prevalence of genital herpes and illustrates that the majority of infections are asymptomatic. Asymptomatic viral shedding may occur at any time, thus exposing their sexual partner(s) to infection. Because of this, it is important to reinforce the protective effect of condoms in preventing infection.

Symptoms of a primary outbreak of HSV2 usually occur within 2 weeks of exposure. Patients report painful red macules that later blister and ulcerate. Erosions heal spontaneously without scarring, typically within 2 weeks. Active HSV lesions shed the virus with greater efficiency than an asymptomatic infection. Associated symptoms of primary genital herpes infection include lethargy, fever, headache, and inguinal lymphadenopathy. Recurrences can present as fissures, edema, dysuria, and myalgia. Treatment with valacyclovir twice a day for 5 days has been shown to shorten the duration of symptoms and the viral shedding but has no effect on recurrence rates.

Molluscum contagiosum presents with multiple umbilicated dome-shaped papules, in varying stages of development, on the skin of the genital area, lower abdomen, and upper thighs. The disease is self-limited and in a normal host resolves in 6 to 9 months. However, any mechanical trauma to the skin, such as shaving, may promote autoinoculation and thus prolong the condition. Treatment is usually destructive with liquid nitrogen, or with Tretinoin cream. Imiquimod 5% cream induces a number of proinflammatory cytokines, such as interferon alpha, that enhance the immune response against the virus and help to clear the lesions. Unlike HSV, molluscum contagiosum does not have latency, and once lesions have been treated, the patient is considered cured.

COMMON DISORDERS DURING ADULTHOOD

Adult acne, rosacea, and *perioral dermatitis* are related disorders that require different treatments respectively and occur during adulthood.

Although **acne** is thought of as an adolescence disease, it is also quite common in adulthood. Unlike adolescent acne, adult acne extends beyond the T-zone of the face to the cheeks, the jaw line, and the perioral area. For this condition in adulthood, treatment is similar to that for adolescent acne and is summarized in Table 8-1.

Rosacea, in contrast to acne, rarely presents in adolescence and is common for middle-aged and older adults. Although both dermatoses feature inflammatory papules and pustules, comedones are not characteristic of rosacea, and oily skin is seen only in the most severe of cases. Patients with rosacea have lesions typically localized on the central part of the face and not on the chest and back as seen with acne. Since the condition is vascular in etiology, it is commonly associated with diffuse facial erythema, often transient in early stages and becoming more pronounced and permanent as the disease progresses. This skin "redness" intensifies with alcohol intake, eating spicy foods, and drinking hot beverages. The "flush and blush" response may precede the development of the papules and pustules. Telangiectases, which are blanching, permanently dilated small blood vessels consisting of either venules, capillaries, or arterioles, are located over the nasal bridge and cheeks and are common as well. Other associated features include ocular dryness that can lead to chronic conjunctivitis (red eye syndrome), blepharitis, and episcleritis. Eye involvement warrants a referral to an ophthalmologist. The development of nasal enlargement (rhinophyma) in severe cases of rosacea is rare in women.

Mild rosacea is treated with topical antibiotics, such as metronidazole 0.75% cream, or with sulfa-containing applications, such as Sulfacet lotion. Azelaic acid 20% cream is another treatment option that is usually as effective as metronidazole. Moderate to severe rosacea is treated with systemic antibiotics such as tetracycline, erythromycin, and minocycline. The aim is to induce remission in 4 to 6 weeks and then use these topical agents as maintenance therapy. To decrease the facial erythema, patients should avoid alcoholic and hot beverages.

Perioral dermatitis afflicts young women in their 20s and 30s. Tiny papules and pustules, usually 2 to 3 mm, develop an erythematous and sometimes scaly base. The lesions are mostly present on the nasolabial folds and chin but can also affect the medial side of the cheeks abutting the nose. These lesions can itch and burn. Perioral dermatitis is associated with an atopic diathesis. It is also associated with excessive use of moisturizers. Treatment consists of systemic antibiotics for 1 month and can be repeated in case of recurrences. Low-potency steroid creams can be used in the short term to decrease the erythematous base, but high-potency steroids should be avoided altogether as these exacerbate and prolong this condition. Topical metronidazole or erythromycin creams are treatment options for mild cases of perioral dermatitis.

Hidradenitis suppurativa is a chronic skin disorder of the apocrine glands that affects the axillae, groin, and the inframammary folds. Recurrent painful large abscesses develop in areas where previously several large interconnected comedones were located. Like acne, there may be plugging of apocrine sweat glands, rupture, and bacterial overgrowth. These in turn can cause the formation of painful abscesses. In hidradenitis suppurativa, the inflammatory process is deeper than in acne, involving the entire dermis and subcutaneous tissues. This can produce pronounced scarring once the lesion has healed. This disease tends to run in families whose members have also often been afflicted with nodular acne. Symptoms are often worse in obese patients. Treatment consists of high-dose antibiotics during an acute exacerbation. In certain cases of hidradenitis suppurativa, surgical incision and drainage can relieve the pain. Frequent sitz baths help promote spontaneous drainage of lesions in the groin. Oral antibiotics, intralesional steroid injections, and oral isotretinoin have all been used to prevent recurrences of this chronic malady.

Vulvar pruritus, intense itching of the genitalia and perineum, can be devastating and difficult for patients to discuss with their medical provider. The woman presenting with vulvar itching requires a careful history and physical examination. Initial attention must be paid to the diagnosis of common conditions that lead to genital pruritus including moniliasis, chlamydia, and eczematous dermatitis. The history should include asking about sexual contacts, and physical examination should focus on identification of any cutaneous findings and microscopic examination of any discharge. Occasionally a skin biopsy is helpful.

Patients with vulvar pruritus are grouped according to the presence or absence of physical findings and vaginal discharge and symptoms such as vulvodynia and pruritus vulvae.

Management should be directed to treatment of the identified etiology in those with clear findings on physical examination or microscopic evaluation of the discharge. The most challenging patients are those with symptoms and no physical or laboratory findings. A careful history often reveals that these women are distraught over their malady and spend a great deal of their conscious time worrying about their symptoms. There is often a sense of "uncleanliness" that can lead to overuse of cleansers, as well as vigorous scrubbing behavior, when washing. This combined with scratching and any irritation from bodily fluids can exacerbate symptoms greatly.

Initial treatment in patients who have no physical or laboratory findings are listed in Box 8-1.

BOX 8-1

Treatment of Vulvar Pruritis Without Physical or Laboratory Findings

- No use of soap. Use mild lotion cleanser such as Balneol.
- No use of dry paper for wiping after urinating. Use the mild lotion cleanser on a cotton ball to decrease friction during wiping.
- Apply a fragrance-free moisturizer as needed to decrease scratching.
- Use a mild corticosteroid to help heal inflamed or excoriated skin. Some patients benefit from a lotion containing pramoxine and hydrocortisone, either 1% or 2.5%.

Treatment protocols need to be tried for at least 2 to 3 weeks and, if unsuccessful, referral to a specialist in dermatology or gynecologic vulvar disorders may be warranted. See Chapter 44 for further discussion.

Urticaria, or hives, is the abrupt onset of intensely pruritic polymorphic erythematous plaques that change in size and shape. Most cases are acute, lasting from a few hours to a few weeks. Urticaria can be caused by food additives, medications, viral infections, or by emotional stress. Chronic hives, present for more than 6 weeks, can be associated with hepatitis C infection, parasitic infections, and sometimes underlying malignancies such as lymphoma. In most cases, however, the cause remains unknown. Hives can be treated with systemic antihistamines, such as hydroxyzine, 10 to 25 mg, or with second-generation nonsedating antihistamines. Oral doxepin has been a useful adjunct to the treatment protocol because it contains both H_1 and H_2 properties. Menthol lotions can be soothing and cool on the skin. Topical and oral steroids have little therapeutic effect on urticaria. For a more in-depth discussion on allergic disorders and evaluation of urticaria, see Chapter 9.

Androgenetic alopecia is the result of the transformation of thick, pigmented hair follicles into vellus follicles under the influence of androgen. As a result of estrogen withdrawal, there appears to be a relative increase in the level of androgen in middle-aged women. Women present with vertex thinning. The temporal and frontal hairlines are usually maintained. While tumors of the ovary and adrenal gland that produce androgen can cause androgenetic alopecia, other symptoms indicating an elevated androgen level such as acne vulgaris, hirsutism, and menstrual abnormalities are often present. Diagnostic evaluation should include a determination of free testosterone and dehydroepiandrosterone (DHEAS) (see Chapter 14). Androgenetic alopecia often runs in certain families. Treatment with minoxidil 2% lotion twice a day for 8 to 10 months can improve hair thickness.

Telogen effluvium presents as diffuse hair loss, occurring 2 to 4 months after a stressful event of significant magnitude. Examples of events that have been associated with telogen effluvium are childbirth, severe blood loss, myocardial infarction, high fever, and shock. Patients report rather sudden onset of dramatic thinning as evidenced by clumps of hair in the shower and on the hairbrush. On examination, one can often find a widened frontal hair part, evidence of generalized thinning in the absence of scalp pathology and a positive pull test (the examiner goes over the scalp gently pulling hairs to see the frequency with which they can be extracted). On a normal scalp, one or two hairs can be removed in this way. In the height of an episode of telogen effluvium, the majority of the hairs will be easily removed.

Although the differential diagnosis of diffuse thinning can be broad and beyond the scope of this chapter, in the case of women in the postpartum period, telogen effluvium is common. It is prudent to check for iron deficiency and subclinical thyroid disease in these patients. Treatment is largely in the form of psychological support. The "shedding" phase of the disease lasts about 4 months. After that, new hairs will grow in where each has shed. The appearance of a full head of hair is slow in coming and patients may not feel "back to normal" for about 1 year after the initial event.

COMMON DISORDERS DURING PREGNANCY

In pregnancy, both physiologic and pathologic skin changes can occur. The former include hyperpigmentation caused by increased levels of the melanocyte-stimulating hormone and occurs in approximately 90% of pregnant women. These changes are usually most notable around the areola, genital skin, and linea alba with the coloration fading during the postpartum period.

Melasma is characterized by a centrofacial, malar, and mandibular distribution of hyperpigmentation, which causes cosmetic concern in pregnant women. Sun exposure tends to exacerbate the condition, so these patients should be advised to use sunscreens that block both UVB and UVA.

Unlike hyperpigmentation during pregnancy, which resolves postpartum, that associated with oral contraceptives can be permanent. It is unclear whether those women who have melasma during pregnancy are at increased risk of hyperpigmentation with the oral contraceptive postpartum. If the woman is not pregnant, persistently discolored patches can be treated with depigmenting agents such as hydroquinone or with tretinoin cream. Chemical peels with trichloracetic acid in water or glycolic acid can be effective as well. Cosmetic covering agents can be a last resort.

Striae ("stretch marks") develop on the distended abdomen and legs most often in pregnant women under 30. Initially, these present as pink or purplish longitudinal bands that fade postpartum into pale atrophic bands. Regardless of advertising claims, there is no current treatment to reverse stretch marks.

The **hormonal/vascular changes of pregnancy** can result in increased size and number of cherry hemangiomas, palmar erythema, and spider nevi. Worsening varicose veins, both in lower extremities and in the rectum (hemorrhoids), are common. Pigmented nevi may change, enlarge, and become more numerous, sometimes requiring biopsy to exclude dysplasia or cancer. Although many women complain of hair changes throughout pregnancy, usually a frontotemporal hair loss, or diffuse thinning is noted after delivery and early in the postpartum period. Hair growth is restored to prepregnancy thickness within the first year postpartum.

Pruritis gravidarum is a benign disorder that often affects pregnant women during the third trimester. The intense pruritis can be associated with temporary hepatic dysfunction induced by high levels of estrogen. This condition is not associated with infant morbidity or mortality and rapidly clears postpartum. Antipruritic lotions such as Sarna and oatmeal baths may provide some relief. Antihistamines such as diphenhydramine are considered safe in late pregnancy. In severe cases of pruritis, bile acid binders such as cholestyramine can be therapeutic.

Pruritic urticarial papules and plaques of pregnancy (PUPPP) cause patients severe discomfort. It presents with the development of various pruritic lesions, including vesicles, erythematous papules, and plaques within the striae of the abdomen. These lesions may then spread to the breasts, thighs, and arms. Fortunately, the face is rarely affected. A primipara in the third trimester of pregnancy is usually affected by this condition. Recurrence in subsequent pregnancies is rare. Mild cases are treated similarly to those with pruritis gravidarum. However, relief from severe pruritis can often be found only in liberal application of topical gluco-corticoid cream or by prescribing oral glucocorticoids. If medically safe, early delivery of the child is another option to end suffering from extreme PUPPP.

Erythema nodosum is an inflammatory skin disorder characterized by a symmetric, painful nodular erythematous eruption on the extensor aspects of both arms and legs with an increased incidence in young pregnant women and those women taking oral contraceptive agents. High levels of circulating estrogen may play a role in the pathogenesis. Erythema nodosum is also associated with certain infections such as tuberculosis and beta-hemolytic streptococcus infection and drugs such as sulfonamides. In half the cases, the etiology remains unclear. Fatigue, myalgia, arthralgia, and fever often precede the eruption of inflammatory papules by 1 or 2 weeks. Over the course of 2 or 3 weeks after the occurrence of these lesions, they become less tense and painful and gradually fade and resolve spontaneously within 2 to 3 months. Bed rest, leg elevation, and antiinflammatory medications provide relief during the painful stages of this disease.

COMMON SKIN DISORDERS OF THE ELDERLY

Chronological aging induces changes both in the epidermal and dermal skin layers. The epidermis consists primarily of keratinocytes that differentiate as they move from the basal layer of the epidermis to its outermost layer, the stratum corneum. This forms a smooth layer of cells that protect the skin against physical and chemical insults.

In the aging skin, there is a decrease in the turnover rate of keratinocytes resulting in a thinner epidermis and poor differentiation of the keratinocytes. The result is dryer and rougher skin, increased scale formation, and decreased barrier function. Older patients are therefore more prone to develop a "winter itchiness" of the skin and should be advised to avoid using harsh soaps and bathing in hot water. Studies are inconclusive as to whether hormone replacement therapy affects the decrease of epidermal thickness with age.

The epidermis also contains melanocytes that synthesize melanin. Within the epidermis lie the Langerhans' cells that play a role in immunologic reactions. As a person ages, the synthesis of melanocytes decreases and as a result older people will develop fewer new pigmented moles. Melanocyte decrease also causes patches of hypopigmented skin amidst areas of normal skin. Aging results in fewer Langerhans' cells, which makes the skin more prone to inflammatory processes such as contact dermatitis.

The dermis contains collagen, elastic fiber, and glycosaminoglycans that provide it with tensile strength, elasticity, and turgor. The dermis also contains hair follicles, oil and sweat glands, nerve endings, and a network of blood vessels. Dermal thickness decreases at a rate of 6% per decade, containing less collagen, fewer fibroblasts, and fewer blood vessels. All of these changes may result in slower wound healing.

Estrogen withdrawal is associated with these atrophic changes. Studies have shown that hormone replacement therapy can counteract the gradual decline in dermal thickness, because estrogen stimulates collagen synthesis and preserves collagen content. Physical exercise also has a pos-itive effect on skin thickness. In contrast, high caffeine ingestion, hyperthyroidism, and oral prednisone therapy have a detrimental effect on skin thickness.

Photoaging accelerates the decline of the dermis and causes further degeneration of collagen. The result is increased wrinkle formation. There is some evidence that fine wrinkles are responsive to long-term therapy with topical tretinoin cream. This enhances the turnover rate of the epidermal keratinocytes and stimulates collagen synthesis in the dermis. Larger wrinkles and furrows can be treated with dermal injections of bovine collagen or with injections of *Botulinum neurotoxin.* Botox is an exotoxin that prevents the release of acetylcholine from the presynaptic neuron of the striated muscles of the face. It essentially paralyses the injected facial muscle. After an injection, this muscle atrophies, the facial skin relaxes, and the wrinkle fades. However, the effect only lasts between 3 and 6 months after which the facial nerves and muscles regenerate and the wrinkles recur unless treated again. Too many treatments with Botox can induce ptosis.

Excess UV exposure accelerates the appearance of **solar lentigines,** often called "liver spots." These are large, brownish macules on the face and dorsum of the hands and lower arms. Liver spots can be treated with liquid nitrogen, bleaching agents, or chemical peels. Topical retinoids have been shown to improve the hyperpigmentation but this treatment may take months.

Papular changes can also occur. These include the appearance of **seborrheic keratoses,** which are benign epidermal growths that are usually tan-brown-black in color with a waxy appearance and a sharply demarcated border. They are often present in sun-exposed areas and patients may have multiple lesions. Diagnosis of seborrheic keratosis can be confused with a malignant melanoma because both share similar coloration. However, the sharply demarcated border of the seborrheic keratosis is clearly different from that of melanoma. Some seborrheic keratoses have an outer surface that resembles a wart. These pseudohorn cysts are the defining characteristic of seborrheic keratoses. Both cryosurgery and shave excision are effective treatments if seborrheic keratosis becomes cosmetically unacceptable or if the lesions get irritated from rubbing against clothing.

Cherry (senile) hemangiomas are small vascular tumors that range in size from a pinpoint to 5 mm. These are completely benign and are often run in families. Patients may have multiple lesions scattered over trunk and extremities. In rare instances, cherry hemangiomas bleed spontaneously.

Sebaceous hyperplasia cause common, yellowish papules that often occur in multiples on the face. They can be difficult to differentiate from basal cell carcinoma. Often they will have a central dell and will express sebaceous material on gentle pressure.

Skin tags are completely benign, small, soft, tan-colored tumors. These often appear to grow on a thin stalk and are usually found in sites of friction such as the neck, chest, axillae, and, in women, in the inframammary folds. Treatment is simple—scissor excision with or without lidocaine, or cryosurgery.

Dermatofibromas are benign lesions that often appear on the anterior parts of legs. These are often a cause for concern for patients. Dermatofibromas tend to develop in response to trauma to a skin area, including folliculitis, insect bites, or shaving accidents. As a result, a fibrous, hard, hyperpigmented nodule can be palpated. Removing these lesions rarely gives a satisfactory result, since the subsequent scar may be as offensive to the patient as the initial dermatofibroma.

SUN-RELATED SKIN CANCERS
Basal Cell Carcinoma and Squamous Cell Carcinoma

Most adult Caucasian women who are seen in the primary care setting have had ample sun exposure throughout their life owing to a variety of cultural factors. They are generally at risk for sun-induced skin cancers. Individuals of Asian, African-American, Muslim and southern European extractions are generally less at risk for these types of cancers.

The early signs of precancerous sun damage are a roughening and drying of the skin texture, marked freckling, mottled hyperpigmentation and hypopigmentation and telangiectasia formation. Many individuals consider these findings to be "normal" aging, but in fact those same individuals, if they compare non–sun-exposed areas to those areas with sun damage will readily see the effects of years of sun exposure.

The cardinal premalignant skin lesion is the **actinic keratosis.** This lesion is often more easily palpated than seen. The skin, often with the appearance noted previously, has a sand-papery feel to it. Occasionally one will see yellowish, rough, adherent scale as well. These are the findings of actinic keratosis. When examined by routine histology, actinic keratoses have the characteristic of having marked keratinocyte atypia of the lower one half to one third of the epidermis and hyperkeratotic scale formation.

Actinic keratoses occur primarily on sun-exposed areas and most often in fair-haired and blue-eyed individuals. However, with prolonged exposure all patients are at risk to develop these precancerous lesions. It is thought that the excessive UV radiation induces chromosomal abnormalities in keratinocytes, which can lead to an altered immune response to factors that promote carcinogenesis. At this point an actinic keratosis develops, presenting as a hyperkeratotic, flesh-colored papule or plaque that varies in size. Stopping further exposure to sun, the actinic keratoses may stay constant or even regress completely. However, with repeated insults from sun exposure, carcinogenesis is stimulated and the actinic keratosis develops into a squamous cell cancer. Bleeding, ulceration, and infection are all signs that should set of the alarm of a potential conversion of actinic to squamous cell carcinoma. The rate of malignant transformation of actinic keratoses is debated, but most authorities believe that approximately 1:1000 will progress to squamous cell carcinoma. In addition, some of the lesions spontaneously regress. Still, actinic keratosis and squamous cell carcinoma are often very hard to tell apart.

Actinic keratoses can be treated in several ways. One important therapy is compulsive sunscreen use. It has been observed that use of sunscreen leads to fewer lesions. The most common treatment is focal, superficial epidermal destruction with liquid nitrogen. Multiple lesions can be treated during the same office visit. Another common treatment is curettage, with or without electrosurgery. This, however, requires subcutaneous lidocaine before the procedure.

For those cases where there is marked involvement, therapy with 5% fluorouracil applied topically may be considered. This destroys the lesion by interfering with the DNA synthesis of the atypical cell. The cream should be applied twice a day on the entire area that is affected for two to four weeks. Patients must be carefully selected for this treatment. It uniformly results in edema, pain, and a characteristic brick-red erythema. Therapy with 5-FU should not be attempted during spring and summer, since it will lead to increased sun sensitivity.

Some patients present with more substantive lesions that appear as either well-demarcated pink plaques with a fine adherent scale or erythematous, keratotic nodules. The former are suggestive of squamous cell carcinoma in-situ and the latter are suggestive of invasive squamous cell carcinoma. Squamous cell carcinoma, arising in sun-damaged skin, generally carries a good prognosis. The diagnosis should be confirmed by biopsy and therapy usually consists of local excision.

The relationship between actinic keratosis and basal cell carcinoma is unclear. *Basal cell carcinoma* has unique clinical and histologic features. It appears to arise spontaneously. The most common clinical appearance is that of a shiny, telangiectatic nodule of gelatinous, translucent appearance. Basal cell carcinoma can also appear as described previously for squamous cell carcinoma in situ. This presentation is particularly prevalent on the trunk. More rarely, basal cell carcinoma presents as an atrophic enlarging scar (the morpheaform type). Most basal cell carcinomas are treated by excision, either primarily or with frozen section control of margins (Mohs technique). Occasionally, these cancers can be removed by electrodessication and curettage or cryotherapy.

Melanoma and Precursor Lesions

The most important risk factor for melanoma is a changing mole. Those patients who present with a history of a changing mole must be carefully evaluated. Other risk factors are listed in Box 8-2.

Caucasian patients presenting for advice on sun exposure and skin cancer should be screened for these historical features. Anyone with one or more risk factors should have a thorough examination of the entire skin surface and biopsy of any dysplastic-appearing lesions. It is important for patients with risk factors to be aware of the appearance of dysplastic nevi, the importance of routine self-examination of the skin, and the importance of changing moles.

Dysplastic melanocytic nevi are defined by their appearance. They are more than 6 mm in diameter and have indistinct borders, irregular pigmentation, and marked asymmetry. The appearance of multiple nevi of this type defines a

---

BOX 8-2
Risk Factors for Melanoma

- Family history of melanoma or dysplastic nevi
- Personal history of melanoma or dysplastic nevi
- Numerous common nevi
- History of blistering sunburns as a child

syndrome, and those patients are of increased risk for developing superficial spreading melanoma. This phenotype in a patient with a family history of melanoma or a personal history of melanoma is indicative of a high degree of risk for developing melanoma. These patients must be careful about sun exposure, do frequent self-skin examinations, and report any new or changing lesions. They are often seen in the office on a quarterly basis and are often followed by a dermatologist.

Most **melanomas** arise de novo in patients at increased risk. The dysplastic nevus is therefore more of a marker of risk than an actual premalignant lesion. Melanomas are of four general types. The most common is the superficial spreading melanoma. This lesion has much the same appearance as a dysplastic nevus, but is often more dramatic in its characteristics. In addition, one often sees an unusual blending of colors (red, blue, silver, black, white) and occasionally erosion. The prognosis of these lesions can be predicted by the thickness in millimeters. In the last 30 years, there has been a tremendous public health effort in the area of melanoma awareness. As a result, most tumors diagnosed these days are thin and have a good prognosis.

Other less common types of melanoma include nodular melanoma, lentigo maligna melanoma and acral lentiginous melanoma.

The therapy for melanoma is primary surgical excision. The surgical margin size varies according to the thickness of the lesion. The first excision is often one with narrow margins and is used for histopathologic diagnosis to confirm the need for a wider excision.

BIBLIOGRAPHY

Bolognia, J: Dermatologic and cosmetic concerns of the older woman, *Clin Geriatr Med* 209:1, 1993.

Birthisle K, Carrington D: Molluscum contagiosum, *J Infect* 34:21, 1997.

Brown T et al: Overview of sexually transmitted diseases. Part 2, *J Am Acad Dermatol* 4:661, 1999.

Callen J et al: Actinic keratosis, *J Am Acad Dermatol* 36:4, 1997.

Carruthers A: Cosmetic uses of botulinum A exotoxin, *Adv Dermatol* 12:325, 1997.

Dinehart D: The treatment of actinic keratoses, *J Am Acad Dermatol* 42:1, 2000.

Greendale G: The menopause transition, *Endocrinol Metab Clin North Am* 26:2, 1997.

Habif TP: *Clinical dermatology: a color guide to diagnosis and therapy,* ed 3, St Louis, 1997, Mosby.

Lim HW et al: The health impact of solar radiation and prevention strategies, *J Am Acad Dermatol* 41:1, 1999.

McLean DI et al: Sunscreens: use and misuse, *Dermatol Clin* 16:2, 1998.

Pereira FA: Herpes simplex evolving concepts, *J Am Acad Dermatol* 35:5, 1996.

Schomogyi M et al: Herpes simplex 2 infection: an emerging disease, *Infect Dis Clinic North Am* 12:47,1998.

Vaughan-Jones SA et al: Pregnancy dermatoses, *J Am Acad Dermatol* 40:2, 1999.

Whitmore ES et al: Risk factors for reduced skin thickness and bone density, *J Am Acad Dermatol* 38:2, 1998.

CHAPTER **9**

Allergic Disorders

James A. MacLean

Allergic diseases are among the most common illnesses seen in the primary care setting. Two of the most common allergic conditions seen by the practicing generalist are allergic rhinitis and chronic urticaria. These two disorders will be reviewed in this chapter with emphasis on etiology, appropriate diagnostic evaluation, and current management strategies. A less common disorder, but one that has emerged as an important cause of occupation-related illness in the last decade, is latex allergy. The final section of this chapter presents an encapsulated review of this condition.

ALLERGIC RHINITIS
Definitions and Epidemiology

Rhinitis is defined as inflammation of the mucous membranes of the nasal passages. Allergic rhinitis is the most common cause of rhinitis, affecting an estimated 10% to 20% of the adult population. Prevalence studies indicate that males and females are affected equally.

Allergic rhinitis may be seasonal or perennial depending on individual sensitivity and allergen exposure. Both genetic and environmental factors play a role in determining the expression of allergic rhinitis. A positive family history of atopy is a risk factor for the development of rhinitis, as is a history of exposure to indoor allergens. In most cases of allergic rhinitis, the onset of disease occurs before 20 years of age and persists throughout adulthood. Allergic rhinitis is frequently seen in association with asthma. Recent epidemiologic studies suggest that the prevalence of asthma is increasing in industrial nations; the same may be true for allergic rhinitis.

Pathophysiology

Allergic rhinitis occurs after immunologic sensitization to specific airborne allergens. Sensitization occurs after repeated exposure to allergens on mucosal surfaces (e.g., ocular and nasal epithelium) and results in the production of allergen-specific IgE antibodies, which bind to the surface of mast cells. Mast cells with surface-bound IgE reside in the mucosa lining the nasal passages. Subsequent exposure to allergen leads to cross-linking of the IgE on the mast cell surface, which triggers the release of a variety of mediators

of inflammation including histamine, leukotrienes, and neuropeptides. These mediators cause immediate vasodilatation and fluid leakage from vessels, with resultant clinical symptoms of rhinorrhea and congestion. The mediators may also act on nerve fibers to induce symptoms of pruritis and sneezing. Other mediators (e.g., cytokines and chemokines) induce the migration of leukocytes to the nasal mucosa and establish a localized allergic inflammation. Repeated exposure to antigen may establish a chronic inflammatory state in the nasal mucosa resulting in perennial symptoms.

Allergens

The major inhalant allergens associated with allergic rhinitis are listed in Box 9-1. The major seasonal allergens responsible for allergic rhinitis are the pollens of trees, grasses, and weeds. The timing and length of the pollen season for any given plant vary considerably with geographic location.

The major indoor allergens include dust mites, cockroach, and animal antigens. Dust mites are among the most important indoor allergens. Dust mites are microscopic insects that feed on human skin scales. They are found in greatest abundance in bedding material (pillows and mattresses), but may also be found in other woven materials such as carpets, upholstered furniture, and children's stuffed animals. Dust mites proliferate in areas of high relative humidity (>40%). Cockroach antigens are important indoor inhalant allergens particularly in urban settings. Allergens from cats, dogs, and pet rodents account for perennial and sporadic symptoms in sensitive individuals. Animal allergens are present in dander (epidermal antigens), saliva, and urine.

Fungal spores may be found in both outdoor and indoor environments. Outdoors, airborne levels of spores vary seasonally and affected individuals may present with symptoms suggestive of a seasonal allergic rhinitis. Indoor mold exposure occurs in areas of high humidity (e.g., cellars and bathrooms) or in residential or office buildings that are contaminated with mold from water damage. Workplace exposure to allergens may occur in a variety of industries (e.g., laboratory animals and latex) and may result in an occupational rhinitis in some individuals.

BOX 9-1
Allergens Associated with Allergic Rhinitis

Seasonal (Outdoor)
Tree pollen
Grass pollen
Weed pollen
Mold spores

Nonseasonal (Indoor)
House dust mites
Cockroach
Antigens from household pets
Mold spores
Occupational antigens (e.g., laboratory animals, latex)

BOX 9-2
Etiology of Rhinitis

A. Allergic rhinitis
 1. Seasonal
 2. Perennial
 3. Occupational
B. Nonallergic rhinitis
 1. Infectious rhinitis
  a) Viral
  b) Bacterial
  c) Fungal
 2. Drug-induced rhinitis
  a) Antihypertensives
   Angiotensin-converting enzyme inhibitors
   Beta-blockers
   Guanethidine
   Methyldopa
   Prazocin
  b) Nonsteroidal anti-inflammatory medications and acetylsalicylic acid
  c) Oral contraceptives
 3. Rhinitis medicamentosa
  a. Topical alpha-adrenergic nasal sprays
 4. Endocrine associated rhinitis
  a. Hypothyroidism
  b. Pregnancy
  c. Menstrual cycle
 5. "Nonallergic rhinitis with eosinophilia syndrome" (NARES) syndrome
 6. Nonallergic vasomotor rhinitis
 7. Reflex rhinitis
   Gustatory rhinitis
   Chemical or irritant rhinitis (may be occupational)
C. Other conditions
 1. Inflammatory diseases
   Wegener's granulomatosis
   Sarcoidosis
   Ciliary dysmotility syndromes
 2. Tumors
   Benign
   Malignant
 3. Structural abnormalities
   Deviated septum
   Hypertrophic turbinates
   Nasal polyps
   Foreign body

Etiology

Rhinitis may be broadly classified as either allergic or nonallergic (Box 9-2). Although the majority of patients presenting with symptoms of rhinitis have an allergic etiology, nonallergic causes must also be considered in the differential diagnosis. **Allergic rhinitis** is usually classified as seasonal, perennial, or occupational, depending on the allergen that is eliciting the symptoms.

Nonallergic rhinitis encompasses a heterogeneous group of conditions with multiple etiologies. Infectious rhinitis is most commonly caused by viruses; rhinitis caused by bacteria or fungi is much less common and occurs primarily in immunocompromised individuals. Drug-induced rhinitis occurs with antihypertensives, nonsteroidal anti-inflammatory drugs (NSAIDs), and oral contraceptive medications. Rhinitis medicamentosa is a unique form of drug-induced rhinitis, which occurs after the repeated use of topical alpha-adrenergic nasal decongestant sprays (oxymetazoline and phenylephrine). Hormonally induced rhinitis may occur in association with hypothyroidism, pregnancy, or with the menstrual cycle (i.e., premenstrual) and is believed to result from vasodilatation of the nasal blood vessels.

The "nonallergic rhinitis with eosinophilia syndrome" (NARES) is characterized by rhinitis in association with nasal eosinophilia in the absence of skin test reactivity to inhaled allergens. The mechanism of the eosinophilia is not known but is not believed to result from allergic sensitization to airborne allergens.

Vasomotor rhinitis is a chronic perennial rhinitis that is not due to allergy, infectious, inflammatory, structural, or other abnormality. The name implies a vascular or neurogenic cause, but the true pathophysiology of this condition remains unknown. Reflex-induced rhinitis includes gustatory rhinitis induced by consumption of spiced foods or alcohol and irritant rhinitis.

Other conditions that should be considered in the differential diagnosis of rhinitis include systemic inflammatory diseases and structural abnormalities. Inflammatory conditions that may involve the nose include Wegener's granulomatosis and sarcoidosis. Ciliary dysmotility syndromes may present as a chronic rhinosinusitis. Benign or malignant tumors of the nasopharynx and structural abnormalities of the nose such as a deviated septum, hypertrophic nasal turbinates, nasal polyps, and foreign bodies may mimic rhinitis.

Clinical Presentation

Differentiating allergic rhinitis from other forms of rhinitis relies on an accurate history and physical examination. Allergic rhinitis typically presents with nasal pruritis, clear watery rhinorrhea, and sneezing. Postnasal drip and nasal congestion may also be presenting complaints. Associated symptoms of ocular itching and redness and itchiness of the palate may accompany allergic rhinitis. Historical features that may suggest an allergic etiology are a seasonal or perennial occurrence or an association with a specific exposure (e.g., an animal).

Vasomotor rhinitis is usually triggered by nonspecific irritants or changes in environmental conditions (e.g., temperature and humidity). Congestive symptoms are a prominent component of vasomotor rhinitis. In drug-induced and hormonally associated rhinitis, nasal congestion is also usually the predominant complaint.

Routine physical examination should include visualization of the nasal vault by anterior rhinoscopy using either a nasal speculum or otoscope. Allergic rhinitis is frequently associated with pale and edematous turbinates. In contrast, the turbinates in vasomotor rhinitis appear dusky and red. Anatomic defect such as nasal septal deviation, hypertrophic turbinates, and nasal polyps can frequently be visualized by anterior rhinoscopy.

Diagnostic Testing

Skin testing or the radioallergosorbent test (RAST) is used to detect the presence of immunoglobulin E (IgE) antibodies to specific allergens. Skin testing is the preferred method for most patients as it is simple and efficient and has a higher sensitivity than RAST testing. Skin testing involves the introduction of antigens into the skin by the epicutaneous or intradermal route. Positive reactions manifest as a wheal and flare reaction 15 to 20 minutes after application of the antigen. Rarely, a systemic reaction may occur after skin testing. For this reason, skin testing should be performed only by trained personnel with experience in the management of anaphylaxis.

Allergen-specific IgE can also be measured serologically by RAST testing. RAST testing is less sensitive than skin testing and is usually reserved for special circumstances such as patients with extreme sensitivity to an antigen (e.g., food anaphylaxis), extensive dermatitis, or inability to discontinue a medication that interferes with skin testing.

Additional tests used in the evaluation of rhinitis include radiographic imaging and flexible or rigid rhinoscopy. Radiographic imaging may be used to confirm structural abnormalities or to demonstrate coexistent sinusitis. Computed tomography is preferred to standard sinus radiographs to evaluate the sinuses and other paranasal structures. Endoscopic visualization of the nasal vault is useful in evaluating suspected anatomic defects and structural abnormalities or tumors, as well as to visualize the patency of sinus ostia.

MANAGEMENT

Environmental Control and Allergen Avoidance

Environmental control and allergen avoidance are important adjunctive treatment measures used in the management of allergic rhinitis. Air conditioning is an effective method of reducing pollen exposure during the warmer months, with the added benefit of temperature control. Air-filtration units (e.g., high-efficiency particulate arresting [HEPA] filters) can reduce airborne particles, but their efficacy may not always translate into a dramatic clinical response. Humidification or dehumidification may be required depending on the ambient environment to achieve an optimum humidity (i.e., between 30% and 40%). Excessive humidity may promote mold and dust mite proliferation, and excessive dryness may aggravate preexisting symptoms of rhinitis.

Measures to reduce exposure to pollen allergens include remaining indoors and in air-conditioned environments (home or work). Providing patients with education regarding seasonal variation in pollen counts is helpful. Local media and Internet sources provide pollen forecasts for most geographic regions (e.g., www.aaaai.org/nab/pollen.stm). Specific measures directed against indoor allergens include dust-mite control, cockroach eradication, reduction in animal dander exposure, and mold control. Dust-mite control should include encasing the pillow and mattress with impermeable covers. Noncovered bedding should be laundered in hot water (130° F) to kill the mites. If possible, carpets should be removed, particularly from the bedroom. Commercially available acaricides may be used to eliminate mites, but studies suggest that this type of elimination is only temporarily effective. Control of cockroach allergens depends on standard hygienic measures. Eradication of cockroach infestation can be difficult, and the irritating fumes from some insecticides can aggravate underlying respiratory symptoms. The ideal control measure for animal dander sensitivity is removal of the animal from the home, but patients often fail to comply with this recommendation. Restriction of the animal from the bedroom may ameliorate some symptoms. Contrary to popular belief there are no "hypoallergenic" cat or dog breeds. Controlling indoor mold exposure relies on the reduction of humidity and areas of water damage. Heavily contaminated areas may require treatment with fungicides.

Medication

The pharmacologic treatment of allergic rhinitis includes the use of antihistamines, decongestants, mast cell stabilizing agents, and inhaled and systemic steroids. Table 9-1 lists the classes of **first-generation antihistamines,** with a representative medication from each class. Although the first generation antihistamines are effective antagonists of histamine, their major limitation is sedation and anticholinergic side effects.

Second-generation antihistamines are listed in Table 9-2. These medications are effective antagonists of histamine with fewer side effects. Loratadine and fexofenadine are nonsedating antihistamines, which have no anticholinergic side effects. Cetirizine, the active metabolite of hydroxyzine (Atarax), has significantly less sedative properties than the parent molecule but is labeled as "low-sedating" because some individuals experience sedation with this drug. Azelastine is a newer antihistamine that is delivered topically to the nose. This medication has sedating properties like the first-generation antihistamines.

Oral decongestants include phenylephrine and pseudoephedrine. These agents act via alpha-adrenergic receptors in the nose and are effective in reducing the nasal congestion associated with many forms of rhinitis. Side effects include insomnia, palpitations, headache, and nervousness. These medications should be used with caution in patients with hypertension and glaucoma. Oral decongestants should be avoided in patients on monoamine oxidase inhibitors (MAOIs).

Topical nasal decongestants include phenylephrine and oxymetazoline. Although these medications are potent vaso-

Table 9-1
First-Generation Antihistamines: Major Classes

Drug	H$_1$ Antagonism	Sedation	Anticholinergic Effect	Pregnancy Category	Dosing
Ethylenediamine (e.g., tripelennamine—PBZ)	+++	++	++	B	25-50 mg q4-6h Max. dose: 600 mg/day
Ethanolamine (e.g., diphenhydramine—Benadryl)	+++	+++	+	C	25-50 mg q4-6h Max. dose: 300 mg/day
Alkylamines (e.g., chlorpheniramine—Chlor-Trimeton)	+++	+	+	B	4 mg q4-6h Max. dose: 24 mg/day
Piperazine (e.g., hydroxyzine—Atarax)	+++	+++	+	C	25-100 mg tid-qid Max dose: 400 mg/day
Piperidine (e.g., azatadine—Trinalin)	+++	++	+	C	1-2 mg bid

Table 9-2
Second-Generation Antihistamines

Drug	H$_1$ Antagonism	Sedation	Anticholinergic Effect	Pregnancy Category	Dosing
Loratadine—(Claritin)	+++	−	−	B	10 mg qd
Fexofenadine (Allegra)	+++	−	−	C	60 mg bid or 180 mg qd
Cetirizine (Zyrtec)	+++	+	−	B	5-10 mg qd
Azelastine (Astelin)	+++	++	−/+	C	137 μg/spray 2 sprays bid each nostril

constrictors and rapidly reduce nasal congestion, they are associated with tachyphylaxis with repeated use and may lead to severe rebound nasal congestion termed *rhinitis medicamentosa* (see Box 9-2). Use of topical decongestants should be discouraged. Limited short-term courses (<5 days) may be used in sinusitis to improve drainage.

Topical nasal anticholinergic medication (Atrovent) is useful in reducing symptoms of rhinorrhea but is not effective in treating pruritis, sneezing, and nasal congestion. Topical anticholinergics may be used to treat the rhinorrhea that accompanies allergic, vasomotor, or infectious rhinitis.

Topical antiinflammatory medication for the treatment of allergic rhinitis includes cromolyn sodium and corticosteroids. Cromolyn sodium is less effective than corticosteroids in the treatment of allergic rhinitis but has the advantage of having few side effects. Topical corticosteroids are highly effective for the treatment of allergic rhinitis (Table 9-3). They are also effective in vasomotor rhinitis and NARES. Topical steroids may cause excessive dryness in the nose and occasional epistaxis. Nasal septal perforation may occur with the use of topical nasal steroids. Topical nasal steroids are locally active and rapidly metabolized and therefore do not lead to any significant systemic steroid effect. Both cromolyn sodium and topical steroids may be used alone or in combination with oral antihistamines. Patients should be instructed that symptom reduction may take several days to occur with the topical antiinflammatory medications. Oral corticosteroids may used to treat severe allergic rhinitis; prolonged use is rarely if ever indicated and should be avoided because of possible side effects.

Allergen Immunotherapy

Immunotherapy ("allergy shots") is a treatment method that involves the administration of increasing subcutaneous doses of allergenic proteins to reduce an individual's sensitivity to a given allergen. Immunotherapy has been shown to be effective for the treatment of allergic rhinitis caused by tree, grass and weed pollen, dust mite, and animal dander sensitivity. Its efficacy in mold sensitivity is still being established. Approximately 80% of individuals undergoing immunotherapy will have symptomatic improvement and a reduced need for medication. Allergen immunotherapy requires weekly visits during the phase of immunotherapy when doses are being escalated. Once a maintenance dose is achieved, injections are given biweekly to monthly for 3 to 5 years.

ALLERGIC RHINITIS AND PREGNANCY

The decision to use pharmacotherapy in the treatment of rhinitis in pregnancy depends on the severity of the symptoms. Ideally, all medication should be avoided during the first trimester. If medications are used, the safety of the medications should be discussed with the patient. Traditionally, the first-generation antihistamines chlorpheniramine and tripelenemine (both Pregnancy Class B) have been suggested as the antihistamines of choice in pregnancy (Table 9-1). Of the second-generation antihistamines, loratadine and cetirizine are Class B drugs (Table 9-2), but their use has not been as widespread as chlorpheniramine and tripelenemine. Cromolyn may be used as an antiinflammatory medication for allergic rhinitis that occurs during pregnancy (Class B).

Table 9-3
Topical Nasal Corticosteroids

Drug	Formulations	Dosing	Pregnancy Category
Beclomethasone (Beconase, Vancenase)	42 μg/spray 84 μg/spray (double strength)	84 μg each nostril qd-bid 84 μg each nostril qd	C
Budesonide (Rhinocort)	32 μg/spray	64 μg each nostril bid	C
Flunisolide (Nasalide)	25 μg/spray	50 μg each nostril qd	C
Fluticasone (Flonase)	50 μg/spray	100 μg each nostril qd	C
Mometasone (Nasonex)	50 μg/spray	100 μg each nostril qd	C
Triamcinolone (Nasacort)	55 μg/spray	110 μg each nostril qd	C

All of the topical nasal corticosteroids are listed as Class C drugs (Table 9-3). If topical steroids are used, beclomethasone is recommended. Pseudoephedrine is the recommended decongestant for use in pregnancy (Class C); however, there are studies that suggest that abdominal wall defects may occur with exposure in the first trimester. Therefore oral decongestants should probably be avoided in the first trimester. Immunotherapy that was initiated before pregnancy may be continued without any harmful effects to the fetus. Initiating immunotherapy during pregnancy is not recommended.

URTICARIA AND ANGIOEDEMA
Definitions and Epidemiology

Urticaria is an intensely pruritic rash consisting of a centrally blanched wheal surrounded by an erythematous flare. The lesions result from dilated blood vessels and edema in the superficial dermis. Urticaria may range in size from a few millimeters to several centimeters. Angioedema is a well-demarcated swelling of the skin and soft tissue resulting from dilated blood vessels in the deep dermis. Angioedema is often painful rather than pruritic, may occur in nondependent areas (e.g., eyelids, lips, and tongue), and is frequently asymmetric in its distribution.

Urticaria is usually classified as either acute or chronic. Urticaria is considered acute if the lesions are present for less than 6 weeks. Acute urticaria may occur at any age, but has a peak incidence in childhood and young adulthood. Males and females are equally affected. Urticaria that lasts longer than 6 weeks is termed *chronic urticaria*. Chronic urticaria is most often seen in adulthood, and women are more commonly affected than men. Angioedema accompanies chronic urticaria in 50% of the cases, 40% will have urticaria alone, and only 10% will have isolated angioedema. The true prevalence of urticaria is unknown, but it has been estimated that 10% to 25% of the population experience urticaria at some time in their lives, and a quarter of all urticaria becomes chronic. The natural history of chronic urticaria is variable. Some individuals will have persistent lesions for years.

Pathophysiology

Chronic urticaria represents a heterogeneous group of disorders with differing pathophysiologic mechanisms. The mast cell is felt to play a central role in many forms of urticaria. The mast cell releases a variety of both preformed and newly synthesized mediators, resulting in vessel dilatation, edema, and perivascular inflammation that is characteristic

BOX 9-3
Etiology of Urticaria

Acute
Drug allergy
Food allergy
Insect stings and bites
Contactants (e.g., latex allergy)
Infections

Chronic
Systemic medical illness
  Infections
  Malignancy
  Connective tissue disease
  Thyroid disease
Complement deficiency syndrome
  Hereditary deficiency of the C1 inhibitor (hereditary angioedema)
    Type I—Diminished production
    Type II—Defective protein
  Acquired deficiency of the C1 inhibitor
    Type I—Lymphoproliferative disease
    Type II—Autoantibody to C1 INH
Mastocytosis
Autoimmune urticaria
Chronic idiopathic urticaria

Physical Urticaria
Cold urticaria
Cholinergic urticaria
Exercise-induced urticaria
Symptomatic dermatographism
Aquagenic urticaria
Solar urticaria
Vibratory urticaria

of urticarial lesions. Mast cells may be activated by a variety of factors including allergens, endogenous agents (including anaphylatoxins, histamine-releasing factors, hormones, and neuropeptides), exogenous agents such as drugs, and direct physical stimuli (light, heat, cold, pressure, or vibration).

Etiology

The etiologic classification of urticaria and angioedema is presented in Box 9-3. Acute urticaria is often associated with an antigenic exposure. The most commonly associated antigens are drugs and foods. Injected (e.g., insect venom) or contact (e.g., latex) allergens can also cause urticaria in sensitized individuals. Acute urticaria may accompany viral infections. Many cases of acute urticaria remain idiopathic.

Chronic urticaria presents a greater diagnostic challenge than acute urticaria. The concern is that urticaria may be a presenting or an accompanying feature of an underlying systemic medical illness. The major medical illnesses that have been associated with chronic urticaria include systemic infections, malignancy, connective tissue disease, and thyroid autoimmunity. As mentioned previously, urticaria may be seen in association with viral **infections** (e.g., hepatitis, mononucleosis). Urticaria with bacterial, fungal, and helminth infections has been reported. Recently, infection with *Helicobacter pylori* has been suggested as a possible cause of urticaria; this association still needs to be established.

The association of **malignancy** with chronic urticaria has been suggested, but a clear association is lacking. A retrospective study of 1155 patients with chronic urticaria revealed that malignancy was no more likely to occur than would have been expected based on standardized incidence data. The exception is an acquired deficiency of the C1 inhibitor protein, which may be associated with certain lymphoproliferative disorders (see later discussions).

Urticaria as a manifestation of **immune complex** or **connective tissue disease** is well established. Urticaria may be a presenting complaint of serum sickness, systemic lupus erythematosus (SLE), or cryoglobulinemia. Urticarial vasculitis is a distinct entity that may present as either cutaneous or multisystem disease. The urticarial lesions on biopsy demonstrate leukocytoclastic vasculitis, distinguishing these lesions from ordinary urticaria. When multisystem disease is present there is usually associated hypocomplementemia.

An association between chronic urticaria and **thyroid autoimmunity** was reported by Leznoff in 1989, based on an examination of 624 cases of chronic urticaria. Thyroid autoimmunity was demonstrated in 14% of the chronic urticaria patients versus 6% of controls. The association of thyroid autoimmunity and urticaria was more common in women than men (ratio 7:1). Of those with thyroid autoimmunity, most were euthyroid. The association led to the identification of previously undiagnosed thyroid disease in many cases and argues for the serologic assessment for thyroid disease in patients with chronic urticaria. The mechanism of chronic urticaria in thyroid disease has not been elucidated.

Acquired and hereditary **deficiencies of the inhibitor of the first component of complement (C1 INH)** represent rare but important causes of episodic angioedema. The C1 INH is a serine protein inhibitor that plays a role in regulating the complement, coagulation, and kinin-forming systems. Hereditary angioedema results from either reduced C1 INH production (type I, 85% of cases) or the production of a defective protein (type II, 15% of cases). Hereditary angioedema is inherited as an autosomal dominant trait and usually presents as recurrent episodes of painful swelling without urticaria. Laryngeal involvement may result in airway obstruction. Angioedema of the bowel presents as abdominal pain and cramping and may mimic an acute abdomen. Trauma is a frequent precipitant. The serum C4 complement level is usually depressed and is a useful screening test for this disorder. A C1 INH protein level and function is performed to confirm the diagnosis.

Acquired C1 INH deficiency results from either an exaggerated activation of C1 by abnormal proteins (globulins or immune complexes) in the blood (type I) or from the development of an autoantibody to the C1 inhibitor (type II). Type I acquired C1 INH deficiency results in the overconsumption of the C1 INH. This form of C1 INH deficiency is seen most commonly with B cell lymphoproliferative diseases such as chronic lymphocytic leukemia, multiple myeloma, Waldenstrom's macroglobulinemia, and cryoglobulinemia. Type II acquired C1 INH deficiency results from the formation of an autoantibody to the C1 INH and has been described with connective tissue disorders (e.g., SLE). As in the hereditary forms of C1 INH deficiency, acquired forms of deficiency manifest with both a diminished C4 level and C1 INH function. The hereditary deficiencies of C1 INH usually present before the third decade of life. The acquired forms should be suspected in older patients presenting with isolated angioedema.

Mastocytosis should be considered in patients with chronic urticaria. Mastocytosis encompasses a spectrum of illness characterized by an abnormal collection of mast cells at various tissue sites. Mastocytosis is classified as either aggressive or indolent depending on the presence or absence of associated hematologic disorders. *Urticaria pigmentosa* is the term used to described the skin lesions of mastocytosis. These lesions appear as reddish-brown macules and represent collections of dermal mast cells. Stroking these lesions will cause the mast cells to degranulate and cause a wheal and flare around the macule (Darier's sign). Urticaria pigmentosa is present in 90% of patients with indolent mastocytosis but only 50% of aggressive forms of disease.

The **physical urticarias** are a group of disorders that share as a common feature urticaria or angioedema after exposure to a physical or mechanical stimulus (Box 9-3). Cold urticaria is important to recognize because while localized exposure to a cold stimulus may result in localized hives, complete immersion of the body in cold water (i.e., ocean swimming) can result in massive mediator release resulting in anaphylaxis and death. Cold urticaria can be confirmed in many cases by a localized challenge test. Rarely, cold urticaria is found in association with a serum cryoglobulin.

Cholinergic urticaria is associated with increases in the body core temperature, usually after exercise or heat exposure (e.g., sauna). Individuals present with small, punctate lesions with an erythematous flare. Exercise-induced urticaria/anaphylaxis syndrome is a separate condition that manifests with urticaria, angioedema, and/or anaphylaxis after exercise. These individuals will not manifest symptoms on raising their core body temperature. Exercise-induced urticaria/anaphylaxis may depend on the prior ingestion of foods to which the patient has IgE antibodies (i.e., food-associated, exercise-dependent anaphylaxis). These patients must be cautioned not to ingest food 4 to 6 hours before exercising.

Symptomatic dermatographism is a common physical urticaria that presents with linear wheals that occur after stroking of the skin. Dermatographism frequently accompanies chronic idiopathic urticaria. Elicitation of the dermatographism can be performed in the office by stroking the skin with a tongue blade; wheal formation will occur within minutes and generally resolves within a half hour.

Pressure urticaria occurs after the application of direct pressure without mechanical stroking. Lesions are usually red and burn rather than itch. There may be associated swelling of the affected area. Pressure urticaria occurs over weight-bearing areas such as the feet and buttocks and may be associated with pressure from clothing such as waist belts or bra straps. Lesions may be delayed several hours after the stimulus has been removed.

A cause for chronic urticaria is found in only 5% to 10% of cases. The remaining cases are termed *chronic idiopathic urticaria.* The true prevalence of chronic idiopathic urticaria is unknown but has been estimated to occur in approximately 0.1% of the population. Although chronic urticaria is rarely life threatening, it does have a significant impact on quality of life. Recent investigations into the etiology of chronic urticaria suggest that in approximately one third of patients diagnosed with chronic idiopathic urticaria, an autoimmune pathogenesis may be the cause. These individuals develop autoantibodies directed against the high affinity receptor for IgE (FcεRI) present on mast cells. These autoantibodies can cross-link adjacent receptors on the mast cell surface and induce mast cell degranulation and mediator release. At the present time there is no serologic test available to detect the presence of these antibodies. At some academic centers autologous serum skin testing is used to confirm the diagnosis.

Evaluation

Evaluation of patients with urticaria and angioedema requires a careful history and physical examination. Drug, food, and contact allergy are usually suggested by the history. The physical urticarias are suggested by the physical stimuli eliciting the hives or swelling. Challenge tests for the physical urticarias have been developed and can be performed in consultation with an allergist to confirm a diagnosis of physical urticaria.

Concern arises over the possibility of the urticaria being a manifestation of an underlying systemic illness. Laboratory investigations should be directed at excluding underlying systemic medical illness suggested by the history and physical examination. Extensive laboratory investigations of individuals with longstanding urticaria without accompanying symptoms is unlikely to reveal an etiologic cause and is not warranted.

There is debate about what constitutes appropriate screening tests for chronic urticaria. A complete blood count, erythrocyte sedimentation rate (ESR), urinalysis, and thyroid-stimulating hormone (TSH) are warranted for most patients. Microbiologic and serologic tests and possibly imaging studies should be ordered for suspected underlying infections. For patients with a history suggesting an underlying immune complex or connective tissue disease, complement studies, cryoglobulins, and antinuclear antibody testing should be performed. If the urticaria lasts for more than 24 hours or if lesions leave a hemosiderin deposit in the skin, a skin biopsy should be performed to rule out an urticarial vasculitis. Isolated angioedema should prompt an investigation for either a hereditary or acquired form of the C1 INH with a measurement of the C4 level and a determination of the C1 INH protein level and function.

MANAGEMENT

Urticaria that occurs from an exposure to a specific antigen, as in the case of food, drug or contact allergy, is treated by avoidance. An adrenaline auto-injector and Medic-Alert bracelet should also be considered for those with more severe reactions or reactions that involve swelling of the oropharynx. The physical urticarias require education regarding avoidance. Antihistamines are frequently needed as adjunctive therapy for the physical urticarias. For those physical urticarias that may present with systemic anaphylaxis, (e.g., cold urticaria and exercise-induced urticaria/anaphylaxis) adrenaline and a Medic-Alert bracelet should also be prescribed.

Antihistamines are the mainstay of treatment for chronic urticaria. Antihistamine choice is frequently governed by patient tolerance. Because chronic urticaria may persist for long periods and because high doses of antihistamines are often required to control pruritis, second-generation antihistamines with less sedation and anticholinergic side effects are usually the treatment of choice (see Table 9-2). **Doxepin,** a tricyclic antidepressant, is a potent inhibitor of H_1 and H_2 receptors and may be used in combination with other antihistamines. The major side effect of doxepin is sedation; therefore evening dosing is often used (10 to 75mg). **H_2 blockers** have an additive effect with H_1 antagonists in the treatment of urticaria and are used as adjunctive therapy. **Oral corticosteroids** are effective in the treatment of chronic urticaria; but their use should be discouraged because of the potential for significant side effects with long-term use. The **leukotriene antagonists** have been suggested for use in chronic urticaria; however, their effectiveness is still being evaluated. The antiinflammatory medications dapsone, colchicines, and Plaquenil have been used successfully in the treatment of urticarial vasculitis. Anabolic steroids (danazol and stanozolol) are used for the maintenance treatment of hereditary C1 INH deficiency. Acquired forms of C1 INH deficiency are best managed by treating the underlying illness. For patients with refractory autoimmune urticaria, there have been reports of temporary success with cyclosporine, intravenous immunoglobulin, and plasmapheresis; these treatments should be regarded as experimental.

LATEX ALLERGY

Definitions and Epidemiology

The term *latex* refers to the milky white sap produced by the cells of various plants. The latex from certain plants contains cis 1,4 polyisoprene ("natural rubber") as a major constituent. The manufacturing of natural rubber products from latex is a complex multi-step process. Manufactured rubber products may be contaminated by two major constituents: (1) plant-derived proteins and (2) compounding agents (e.g., accelerants, antioxidants, and cross-linking agents) that are added to raw latex during manufacturing. Individuals exposed to rubber products may become sensitized to either the protein or chemical contaminants in rubber products. Individuals with sensitivity to latex proteins manifest with IgE-mediated or immediate-type hypersensitivity reactions and are often referred to as having type I latex allergy (Gell and Coombs classification). Individuals with reactivity to the compounding chemicals present with a cell-mediated delayed type-hypersensitivity reaction and are designated as having type IV latex allergy.

Epidemiologic studies have identified several groups that are at high risk for developing IgE-mediated reactions to natural rubber latex. The occupational use of rubber gloves is the most often cited risk factor for IgE-mediated latex allergy and health care workers represent the largest group of affected individuals. The prevalence of latex allergy among health care workers in Europe and North America is between 2% and 12%. Individuals with spina bifida represent the second major risk group for IgE-mediated reactions to natural rubber latex with prevalence rates between 18% and 50%. Affected individuals are believed to become sensitized by repeated exposures to latex gloves and medical products during surgical procedures and through the use of indwelling latex catheters. Rubber factory workers represent another defined risk group with a prevalence rate of immediate hypersensitivity to latex proteins of approximately 10%. The prevalence of immediate-type hypersensitivity to latex proteins in the general population is unknown but has been estimated to be between 0.1% and 1%.

Pathophysiology

Sensitization to natural rubber latex proteins occurs after repeated exposures in susceptible individuals. There are multiple potential routes of exposure to latex proteins including cutaneous (e.g., gloves), mucosal (e.g., dental procedure or indwelling urinary catheter), percutaneous (e.g., surgical procedure), and inhalant (e.g., inhalation of latex protein on an airborne carrier). The major route of sensitization currently remains unknown. The importance of glove powder in the pathobiology of latex allergy needs to be emphasized. Cornstarch powder can bind latex proteins and act as a carrier for both airborne and contact dispersal of latex allergens. Studies in hospital centers have identified high levels of latex aeroallergens in areas with extensive use of powdered gloves, whereas areas with minimal use of powdered gloves have substantially lower concentrations of latex aeroallergens. These data suggest that glove powder acts as a major contributor to airborne latex proteins in hospital environments. Further studies have documented a substantial reduction in latex aeroallergens in the hospital setting, with the removal of high-protein, powdered gloves.

Clinical Presentation

The spectrum of hypersensitivity reactions to natural rubber latex is outlined in Table 9-4. The most common reaction to rubber products is irritant contact dermatitis. This is a non-immunologically mediated irritation of the skin often seen with extended use if rubber gloves. Irritant contact dermatitis may be aggravated by abrasive glove donning powder or by defatting of the skin, through the use of detergents and alcohol. Irritant contact dermatitis may range from mild erythema and pruritis to chronic fissuring and hyperkeratosis.

Allergic contact dermatitis is an immunologically mediated cutaneous eruption that is a manifestation of a cell-mediated immune response. When seen in association with rubber products, the immune response is directed against one of the chemical additives that exist as contaminants in the end products. Allergic contact dermatitis may be difficult to distinguish from irritant contact dermatitis. Irritant reactions predominantly affect the dorsum of the hand and spare the palmar surface. Weeping, vesiculation, and lichenification of the skin are seen more commonly with allergic contact reactions. Both allergic and irritant reactions localize to the area of contact and often have well-defined borders that suggest a contactant as the cause. Individuals with preexisting hand eczema secondary to atopic dermatitis may have an aggravation of their dermatitis when their hands are placed under occlusion or are exposed to irritants.

Contact urticaria is an immunologically mediated cutaneous eruption that is a manifestation of an IgE-mediated immune response. Affected individuals make IgE antibodies to protein contaminants in manufactured latex products. In contrast to irritant and allergic contact reactions, which have a delayed onset (usually days), contact urticaria usually manifests within minutes of exposure. The symptoms consist of erythema, pruritis, and the development of wheals on areas of contact. Angioedema may be the presenting complaint with contact on mucosal surfaces. Contact urticarial lesions tend to resolve quickly (minutes to hours) after removal of the inciting agent, in contrast to allergic contact dermatitis, which may persist for days to weeks. IgE-mediated reactions to natural rubber latex proteins may also manifest as inhalant disease (i.e., rhinitis or bronchospasm). If there is significant systemic exposure or absorption of latex protein through a mucosal surface, anaphylaxis may occur. Individuals with IgE-mediated sensitivity to natural rubber latex proteins have an increase prevalence of food-related reactions. The prevalence of food-related syndromes in latex-allergic individuals has been estimated to be between 20% and 40%. The foods most commonly associated

Table 9-4
Spectrum of Reactions to Natural Rubber

Clinical Entity	Immunologically Mediated	Mechanism	Causative Agent
Irritant contact dermatitis	No	Irritant	Irritants
Aggravation of atopic dermatitis	No	Irritant on preexisting eczema	Irritants
Allergic contact dermatitis	Yes	Cell-mediated	Chemical additives
Contact urticaria/angioedema	Yes	IgE-mediated	Rubber proteins
Inhalant disease	Yes	IgE-mediated	Rubber proteins
Rhinitis			
Conjunctivitis			
Bronchospasm			
Anaphylaxis	Yes	IgE-mediated	Rubber proteins
Food related oral symptoms and anaphylaxis	Yes	IgE-mediated	Plant proteins with homology to rubber proteins

with this condition are chestnuts, bananas, avocados, and kiwi fruit. The food-related reactions occur as a result of cross-reacting IgE antibodies that recognize proteins in foods that share homology with natural rubber latex proteins.

EVALUATION

Laboratory tests available for use in the diagnosis of IgE-mediated latex allergy include skin testing, serologic testing, and provocative testing. Cell-mediated immune reactions to rubber chemicals are confirmed by patch testing.

Skin Testing

Skin testing is the preferred diagnostic procedure for individuals with suspected IgE-mediated latex allergy. Latex extracts are currently available in Canada and some European countries and are under development in the United States.

Serologic Testing

In the absence of a commercially available skin test reagent, serologic testing for the presence of latex-specific IgE can be performed. Comparison studies suggest that skin testing is more sensitive and specific than serologic testing. Latex-specific IgE may be measured by enzyme-linked immunosorbent assay (ELISA) or RAST. The sensitivity of most commonly used tests is less than 80%, indicating that ~20% of individuals with clinical latex allergy may be missed by serologic testing alone.

Provocative Tests

Use-testing has been reported as an alternate diagnostic test for individuals with suspected immediate-hypersensitivity to latex. The glove-use test procedure involves placing glove material on a finger or hand and assessing for evidence of immediate sensitivity. Glove-use testing has been reported to correlate well with results of skin prick testing in diagnosing individuals with immediate hypersensitivity to latex. As with skin testing, use testing should be performed by experienced personnel.

Patch Testing

Individuals with suspected latex-associated allergic contact dermatitis should be referred for patch testing. The Standard Allergen Series for patch testing includes the chemicals that are most commonly associated with allergic contact dermatitis.

MANAGEMENT

Contact Dermatitis

Individuals with irritant cutaneous reactions should be treated with topical emollients and reduction in exposure to strong detergents, irritating chemicals, and abrasives. Allergic contact dermatitis can be managed by identifying the causative chemical and eliminating exposure. Therapy directed at the ongoing dermatitis may include drying compresses, oral antihistamines, topical corticosteroids, and occasionally oral steroids. Emollients are used for desiccated and lichenified skin. Significant eczematous dermatitis (cracking and weeping of the skin) may require temporary work restriction. For individuals with reactions to the chemi-cals in latex gloves, non-chemical-containing latex gloves may be used as substitutes. Other alternatives include polyvinyl chloride, or non-latex synthetic gloves. It should be noted that some non-latex synthetic gloves still contain chemicals that may result in allergic contact dermatitis reactions.

IgE-Mediated Reactions

Treatment of an ongoing immediate allergic reaction to latex depends on the manifestations and severity but conforms to the standard treatment of IgE-mediated reactions. Latex allergic individuals should obtain a Medic-Alert bracelet and self-injectable adrenaline. The mainstay of the long-term treatment of immediate reactions to latex products is avoidance. Affected individuals should be educated about avoidance both at home and in the workplace. Lists of latex-containing devices have been compiled, with suitable non-latex-containing alternatives (Spina Bifida Association of America, Washington, DC).

Careful preparation is needed for latex-sensitive individuals who require hospitalization or dental or surgical procedures. All procedures on latex-sensitive individuals should be performed in a "latex-safe" environment, which is defined as one in which no natural rubber latex product is brought in direct contact with the affected individual. Guidelines for the prevention of reactions to natural rubber products in the workplace have also been established. These guidelines stress the importance of appropriate barrier protection for workers exposed to infectious or other hazardous material. The use of reduced-chemical and reduced-protein gloves that are powder free is recommended.

BIBLIOGRAPHY

Task Force on Allergic Reactions to Latex. American Academy of Allergy and Immunology. Committee report, *J Allergy Clin Immunol* 92:16, 1993.

NIOSH alert: preventing allergic reactions to natural rubber latex in the workplace, *Hosp Technol Ser* 16:10, 1997.

Bensch G, Borish L: Leukotriene modifiers in chronic urticaria, *Ann Allergy Asthma Immunol* 83:348, 1999.

Davis AED: C1 inhibitor and hereditary angioneurotic edema, *Annu Rev Immunol* 6:595, 1988.

Dykewicz MS et al: Diagnosis and management of rhinitis: complete guidelines of the Joint Task Force on Practice Parameters in Allergy, Asthma and Immunology. American Academy of Allergy, Asthma, and Immunology, *Ann Allergy Asthma Immunol* 81:478, 1998.

Fisher AA: Allergic contact reactions in health personnel, *J Allergy Clin Immunol* 90:729, 1992.

Greaves M: Chronic urticaria, *J Allergy Clin Immunol* 105:664, 2000.

Greisner WA, Settipane RJ, Settipane GA: Natural history of hay fever: a 23-year follow-up of college students, *Allergy Asthma Proc* 19:271, 1998.

Hamann C: Natural rubber latex protein sensitivity in review, *Am J Contact Dermatol* 4:4, 1993.

Hunt LW et al: A medical-center-wide, multidisciplinary approach to the problem of natural rubber latex allergy, *J Occup Environ Med* 38:765, 1996.

Kulp-Shorten CL, Callen JP: Urticaria, angioedema, and rheumatologic disease, *Rheum Dis Clin North Am* 22:95, 1996.

Leznoff A, Sussman GL: Syndrome of idiopathic chronic urticaria and angioedema with thyroid autoimmunity: a study of 90 patients, *J Allergy Clin Immunol* 84:66, 1989.

Lindelof B et al: Chronic urticaria and cancer: an epidemiological study of 1155 patients, *Br J Dermatol* 123:453, 1990.

Markovic SN et al: Acquired C1 esterase inhibitor deficiency, *Ann Intern Med* 132:144, 2000.

Mazzotta P, Loebstein R, Koren G: Treating allergic rhinitis in pregnancy. Safety considerations, *Drug Saf* 20:361, 1999.

Metcalfe D: Mastocytosis syndromes. In Middleton E et al, editors: *Allergy: principles and practice,* St Louis, 1998, Mosby.

Schatz M: Special considerations for the pregnant woman and senior citizen with airway disease, *J Allergy Clin Immunol* 101:S373, 1998.

Schnyder B, Helbling A, Pichler WJ: Chronic idiopathic urticaria: natural course and association with *Helicobacter pylori* infection, *Int Arch Allergy Immunol* 119:60, 1999.

Schoenwetter WF: Allergic rhinitis: epidemiology and natural history, *Allergy Asthma Proc* 21:1, 2000.

Slater JE: Latex allergy, *J Allergy Clin Immunol* 94:139, 1994.

Slavin RG: Occupational rhinitis, *Ann Allergy Asthma Immunol* 83:597, 1999.

Stafford CT: Urticaria as a sign of systemic disease, *Ann Allergy* 64:264, 1990.

Sussman GL, Beezhold DH: Allergy to latex rubber, *Ann Intern Med* 122:43, 1995.

Tharp MD: Chronic urticaria: pathophysiology and treatment approaches, *J Allergy Clin Immunol* 98:S325, 1996.

Weber RW: Immunotherapy with allergens, *JAMA* 278:1881, 1997.

CHAPTER **10**

Temporomandibular Joint Syndrome

Meredith August
Julie Glowacki

Temporomandibular joint (TMJ) syndrome is a collective term that includes a number of disorders affecting both the joint itself and the associated muscles and ligaments used in jaw movement and stability. The most common presenting complaint, despite etiology, is pain. Occlusal abnormalities and TMJ parafunction (such as tooth grinding and clenching) are often cited as causes of TMJ syndrome. In addition, stress and somatization appear to play a mediating role in pathogenesis.

▦ EPIDEMIOLOGY

It is estimated that up to 90% of people diagnosed with TMJ syndrome are women. Signs and symptoms of TMJ syndrome usually increase in frequency and severity beginning in the second decade. Although joint noise, such as clicking, is a common complaint for many people, in only a small percentage does this progress to pain requiring treatment or other jaw function abnormalities. Degenerative changes in the joint begin to occur in response to repetitive overload in excess of functional capacity, or when a normal load is applied to a joint whose functional capacity is reduced.

Epidemiologic studies suggest that female sex hormones play a role in the pathophysiology of temporomandibular dysfunction. Estrogen receptors have been found in the TMJ complex in the baboon and the human disc. Studies with ovariectomized rats have attempted to examine direct effects of estrogen on the TMJ, but there are concerns about the significance in humans. The complex relationships between endogenous hormones and pharmacologic effects, differences between surgical and natural menopause and cartilage versus bone effects, and the unique aspects of the human TMJ anatomy complicate the interpretation of existing experimental studies.

ANATOMY

The temporomandibular joints are responsible for articulating the mandible to the cranium (Fig. 10-1). Each TMJ provides for both a hinging movement and a gliding movement. The joint is formed by the mandibular condyle fitting into the glenoid fossa of the temporal bone. Interposed between these two structures is an articular disc or meniscus that is composed of dense fibrous connective tissue. This is distinct from other joints in which disc tissue is primarily composed of hyaline cartilage. This is an important difference because fibrous tissue possesses more reparative and adaptive properties than does hyaline cartilage.

Both movement and stability of the temporomandibular joints are provided by a group of muscles known as the muscles of mastication (Fig. 10-2). These include the masseter, medial pterygoid, and temporalis muscles, which are predominantly involved with mouth closure; the lateral pterygoid muscle, which assists in protrusive movements; and the digastric muscles, which aid in mouth opening.

CLASSIFICATION

Abnormalities of the TMJ are commonly described as being either extracapsular or intracapsular; understanding this distinction is important because treatments differ. Extracapsular disorders most commonly affect the masticatory muscles and are broadly described as "myofascial" in nature. Intracapsular disorders encompass TMJ arthritis, as well as abnormalities in the articular disc/condyle relationship (internal derangements).

Myofascial Pain Dysfunction

Myofascial pain dysfunction (MPD) is perhaps the most common disorder associated with the TMJ syndrome. It is characterized by a dull, aching, and radiating pain involving the muscles of mastication and is generally described as being exacerbated by jaw function. An associated limitation of mandibular motion is commonly found. Pain is described as being worse on awakening in the morning, especially in patients with a nocturnal grinding or clenching habit.

Patients with MPD initially have no clinical and radiographic evidence of TMJ pathology. Although it begins as a functional muscular disorder, MPD can lead to degenerative changes, as well as internal derangements. The pain associated with MPD is secondary to hyperactivity and spasm of the facial muscles and, in susceptible patients, appears to be exacerbated by stressful situations.

Intracapsular Disorders

Various systemic disease processes, particularly rheumatologic and autoimmune disorders, may be associated with **TMJ arthritis.** In addition, the effect of aging on the bony condyle of the joint, the meniscus, and the muscles of mastication has ramifications on changing jaw function and may result in degenerative arthritis at the TMJ.

The correct management of **internal derangements** requires both an accurate diagnosis, as well as an appreciation for the natural history and progression of this process. Abnormal disc/condyle relationships are often accompanied by various joint noises, especially clicking or popping. However, it is well known that the presence of chronic, unchanging, and asymptomatic clicking is not always progressive. In fact, only joint sounds associated with pain or limitation of function should be considered for treatment. This becomes an even more important point in the era of magnetic resonance imaging (MRI) where discal position can be imaged in a noninvasive way and a tendency to overtreat such anatomic findings may result. In general, internal derangements may be classified as either reducing or nonreducing, based on the initial displacement of the disc and the capacity of the condyle to reestablish a position beneath it during opening.

EVALUATION
History

A thorough understanding of the nature of the pain is a critical part of the evaluation of TMJ syndromes. Pain is often localized to the preauricular area and the muscles of mastication and is commonly described as being worse with jaw function, especially chewing. A pattern of pain more prominent in the morning suggests the presence of a nighttime habit such as bruxism.

Other frequent complaints include limited jaw function, asymmetric movement, and various TMJ noises such as popping, clicking, or crepitation. Stiffness and locking of the jaw often correlate with meniscal dislocation. Because of the anatomic proximity of the TMJ to the external auditory canal, as well as the rich and shared neuronal pool between the fifth cranial nerve and upper cervical spine, referred pain is frequently described. Ear symptoms such as pain and blockage, as well as headaches and other facial

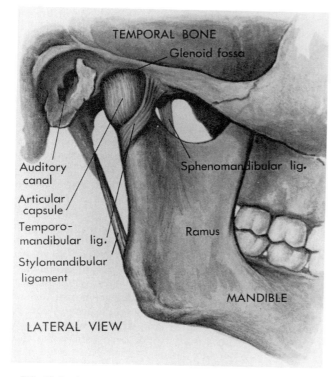

FIG. 10-1   Lateral view of the anatomy of the temporomandibular joint.

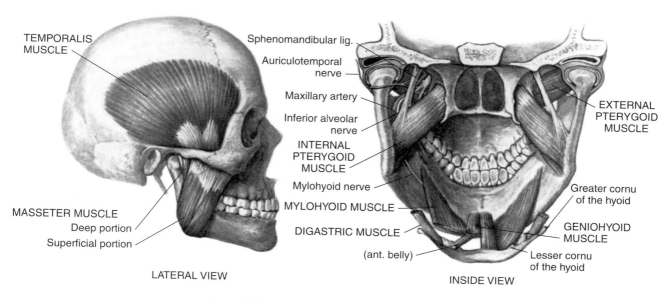

MUSCLES ACTING ON THE MANDIBLE

FIG. 10-2   The muscles of mastication and their relationship to the temporomandibular joint.

pain complaints, are commonly encountered. Complaints of an inability to occlude posterior teeth on the affected side suggest the presence of a joint effusion.

Onset of TMJ problems may be related to a specific event. For example, a traumatic injury to the chin may result in intraarticular bleeding or a condylar fracture. Prolonged dental visits or recent general anesthesia may be associated with ligamental tearing and a sprain-type injury. Specific questions regarding tooth grinding (bruxism) or other oral habits should be made, although patients are often unaware of such habits unless informed by a spouse or roommate. Often, severe attrition of the teeth is the only indication that bruxism is ongoing.

Psychosocial factors may impact directly on TMJ syndrome or influence a patient's ability to adapt. A concurrent history of anxiety, stress-related disorders, depression, and major life-altering events should be gently explored.

Physical Examination

Examination of the TMJ includes an evaluation of the muscles of mastication, direct palpation of the joint and associated capsule, assessment of mandibular function (extent and symmetry of opening), and a thorough intraoral examination. The masseter and temporalis muscles are easily palpated through the skin, and the medial pterygoid muscle is palpated intraorally on the medial aspect of the mandible. Muscle spasm is associated with a patient's complaint of soreness when these muscles are examined and often a tightness can be appreciated. Accessory muscles such as the sternocleidomastoid and trapezius muscles are often secondarily involved. Direct capsular tenderness when palpating the TMJ is usually indicative of an inflammatory process. Synovitis may be caused by infection, inflammation, or trauma. Capsulitis, an inflammation of the capsule itself, may be related to a sprain injury and can be difficult to distinguish from synovitis.

Diagnostic Tests

Various radiologic studies may be helpful. As a baseline, plain films of the bony portion of the joint will demonstrate degenerative changes such as bony spurs and erosions. Other more subtle radiographic changes may suggest a history of parafunction. Other bony pathology, such as condylar mass lesions or destructive bony processes in the area, can be ruled out as well. When an internal derangement is suspected, an MRI is a noninvasive and sensitive method of determining disc morphology, position, and function.

Applications of biochemical assays for synovial fluid samples from patients with TMJ disorders have been correlated with arthroscopic documentation of osteoarthritis or disc displacement. There has been intense activity to develop biochemical markers of joint disorders. Serum markers of cartilage turnover have been developed; these appear to be more relevant in rheumatoid than in osteoarthritic changes.

CHANGES IN THE TEMPOROMANDIBULAR JOINT ASSOCIATED WITH AGING

Although the TMJ is not a weight-bearing joint per se, it is the recipient of significant loading forces secondary to both normal masticatory function and various parafunctional habits. Manifestations of osteoarthrosis and bony degeneration, as well as alterations in soft tissue and bite force generation, are seen as sequelae of aging. Postmortem studies of the TMJ demonstrate meniscal perforations in one fourth of people over age 65. Some experts believe that discal thinning and ultimate perforation are an anticipated part of aging and are not pathologic. Mild degenerative changes in the condyle itself are common, but gross degenerative changes are rare.

One of the more commonly described symptoms associated with TMJ dysfunction is the presence of joint noise (clicking and/or crepitation) that is secondary to meniscal movement and degenerative changes. Most studies indicate that the presence of joint sounds increases with age and with the progressive tooth loss that occasionally accompanies aging. Mandibular dysfunction, as well as crepitation, is most common in edentulous individuals.

Maximal interincisal opening is measured as the vertical distance between the maxillary and mandibular central incisors. This measurement is usually greater in men than in women and ranges from 40 to 55 mm. Studies on large elderly populations have shown significant decreases with age for both sexes.

A progressive decrease in bite force with aging has also been shown and likely results from a decrease in the cross-sectional area of the both the masseter and medial pterygoid muscles. These changes seem to correlate with the general age-related changes seen in other muscles of the body. The clinical implication of this reduction in bite force and masticatory ability is that older patients may self-impose dietary restrictions that may compromise overall nutritional status.

Despite the anatomic changes and degenerative changes noted in the TMJ with aging, the natural history of internal derangements and associated pain tends to be one of improvement in postmenopausal populations of women. The reason for this is not well understood.

ASSOCIATION OF TEMPOROMANDIBULAR JOINT DISORDERS WITH SYSTEMIC DISEASE

Involvement of the TMJ in **rheumatoid arthritis** (RA) seems to become more common as the disease progresses. It is estimated that between 50% and 75% of patients will have some involvement during the course of the disease. When the TMJ is involved with RA, symptoms are commonly bilateral. Patients often complain of a dull, aching pain in the preauricular distribution that is worsened with function. In addition, the associated masticatory muscles are tender, and patients often describe morning stiffness. As involvement progresses, there is a demonstrable decrease in biting force and limitation in jaw movement. Severe end-stage involvement may lead to either fibrous or bony ankylosis and a progressive bite alteration caused by loss of mandibular ramus height (Fig. 10-3).

Juvenile rheumatoid arthritis (JRA) is commonly diagnosed before the age of 16 years. A disproportionate number of patients are female. Involvement of the TMJ is variable. Joint involvement during periods of facial growth has important implications on both facial morphology and jaw function. TMJ manifestations are similar to those described for RA.

Other connective tissue disorders are also associated with TMJ involvement. **Systemic lupus erythematous** (SLE) is

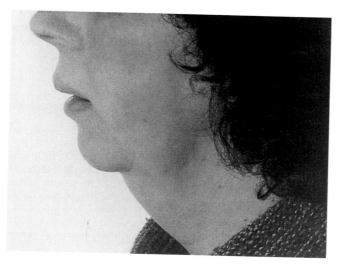

FIG. 10-3   Lateral photograph demonstrating severe retrognathia in a patient with rheumatoid arthritis affecting the temporomandibular joints.

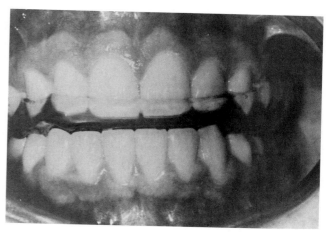

FIG. 10-4   Hard acrylic splint fitted to the maxillary teeth and worn at night in a patient with a parafunctional habit.

BOX 10-1
Treatment of Temporomandibular Joint Syndrome

Bite appliance therapy
Medication
    Nonsteroidal antiinflammatory drugs
    Muscle relaxants
    Antidepressants
Physical therapy
    Massage
    Exercises
    Biofeedback
    Relaxation techniques
Psychotherapy
Arthroscopic or open surgery

---

associated with symmetrical polyarthritis and the development of articular osteoporosis and soft tissue swelling. Tenderness in the muscles of mastication is commonly found and joint deformity resulting from capsular laxity, ligamentous destruction, and degenerative arthritis may ensue. Approximately two thirds of patients with SLE have pain referable to the TMJ on careful examination. **Scleroderma** may also be associated with complaints of TMJ pain and/or crepitation, as well as bony changes on radiograph.

Fibromyalgia is a nonarticular rheumatism characterized by diffuse musculoskeletal aches, stiffness, and exaggerated tenderness at multiple defined anatomic sites. Recent studies have indicated an increased association between fibromyalgia and TMJ complaints. In as many as 97% of patients with a diagnosis of fibromylagia, pain in the muscles of mastication is found. The response of these patients to conservative measures to decrease muscle spasm is less predictable than in patients with myofascial pain dysfunction without a diagnosis of fibromyalgia.

MANAGEMENT

Therapy for MPD is aimed at muscle relaxation and often involves several modalities (Box 10-1). **Bite appliance therapy** is important in those in whom occlusal forces and habits are identified or suspected. The stabilization or muscle relaxation appliance is used for most cases of MPD. It provides stabilization of the joints, protection of the teeth, redistribution of occlusal forces, and reduction in bruxism with consequent relaxation of the involved musculature. The stabilization appliance is made of hard acrylic and is usually fitted to the maxillary teeth (Fig. 10-4). Generally, the appliance is worn only during sleep. Abatement in symptoms is frequently seen within the first month of use. The goal is to wean patients from appliance therapy as soon as possible, although this is often difficult and long-term use is common.

Various medications are used in the treatment of MPD. **Nonsteroidal antiinflammatory agents** (NSAIDs) are helpful in the treatment of acute symptoms. Although the inflammatory component of this problem may be minimal, the analgesia provided is helpful. Muscle relaxants are indicated in cases of severe muscle spasm. These drugs are often associated with sedation and therefore need to be titrated to effect. Very often, even a small dose of a benzodiazepine will be helpful if taken before sleep to both relax the facial muscles and as an anxiolytic. Proper patient selection and short-term use are important in this setting. Care should be taken in prescribing any type of narcotic medication to patients with MPD or chronic facial pain.

A well-documented relationship between chronic pain and depression exists, although whether one is a consequence of the other is not known. Evidence shows that various **antidepressants** are helpful in the management of chronic pain even in the absence of depressive symptoms. Tricyclics and selective serotonin-reuptake inhibitors (SSRIs) are prescribed most commonly, and the dose must again be titrated to maximize therapeutic benefit and minimize the more commonly described side effects. Evidence suggests that the tricyclics are effective at decreasing bruxism.

The application of **heat** to the muscles of mastication and aggressive **physical therapy** play an important part in the management of MPD. Deep massage, ultrasound, therapeutic exercise, and electrical stimulation all have demonstrable efficacy. In addition, a home therapy program can be used to maintain the progress made during formal physical therapy sessions. **Biofeedback, relaxation techniques,** and **psychotherapy** may also play a role in long-term management.

Failure of conservative therapy and medical management of TMJ problems often leads to more invasive procedures whose aim is to correct various anatomic conditions that are felt to be responsible for the patient's symptom complex. As **arthroscopic evaluation** of the TMJ has become more sophisticated, this modality is used for diagnostic purposes as well. The most common arthroscopic procedures are biopsy, lavage, lysis of adhesions, smoothing of bony irregularities, and discal repositioning.

Open arthrotomy is used to treat TMJ problems that have been refractory to other therapeutic maneuvers. Because TMJ complaints are multifactorial, anatomic correction of abnormalities in the face of ongoing parafunction has only guarded success. Thus, even in postsurgical patients, continued treatment of muscular complaints and parafunction is imperative.

BIBLIOGRAPHY

Agerberg G, Carlsson GE: Functional disorders of the masticatory system. Distribution of symptoms according to age and sex as judged from investigation by questionnaire, *Acta Odontol Scand* 30:597, 1972.

August M, Kaban LB: The aging maxillofacial skeleton. In Rosen CJ, Glowacki J, Bilezikian JP, editors: *The aging skeleton,* San Diego, 1999, Academic Press.

Bush FM et al: Analysis of gender effect on pain perception and symptom presentation in temporomandibular pain, *Pain* 53:73, 1993.

Funch DP, Gale EN: Biofeedback and relaxation therapy for chronic temporomandibular joint pain: predicting successful outcomes, *J Clin Consult Psychol* 52:928, 1984.

Green CS, Laskin DM: Long-term status of TMJ clicking in patients with myofascial pain dysfunction, *J Am Dent Assoc* 117:461, 1988.

Green CS et al: The TMJ pain-dysfunction syndrome. Heterogenicity of the patient population, *J Am Dent Assoc* 79:1168, 1969.

Huber MA, Hall EH: A comparison of the signs of temporomandibular joint dysfunction and occlusal discrepancies in a symptom-free population of men and women, *Oral Surg Oral Med Oral Pathol* 70:180, 1990.

Laskin DM: Diagnosis and etiology of myofascial pain and dysfunction, *Oral Maxillofac Surg Clin North Am* 7:73, 1995.

LeResche L et al: Use of exogenous hormones and risk of temporomandibular disorder pain, *Pain* 69:153, 1997.

Okeson JP: Nonsurgical treatment of internal derangements, *Oral Maxillofac Surg Clin North Am* 7:63, 1995.

CHAPTER **11**

Diabetes

Linda S. Jaffe
Caren G. Solomon
Ellen W. Seely

The prevalence of type 2 diabetes mellitus (DM), which represents 90% of all diabetes, is increasing dramatically in the United States in both women and men. Some of this increase is due to increased screening and a change in threshold of diagnosis, but major contributors are the rising rates of obesity and physical inactivity. As a result, the primary care provider is seeing increasing numbers of patients with or at risk for diabetes and needs to understand gender differences in the care of diabetes.

Apart from the management of diabetes during pregnancy (see Chapter 71), many of the complications and treatment approaches in diabetic women are similar to those in men. However, there are some clear differences in risk factors for, and complications of, diabetes (Table 11-1). This chapter focuses on issues that are unique or particularly relevant to the care of women with diabetes.

EPIDEMIOLOGY

Type 1 Diabetes Mellitus

In childhood there is an increased incidence of type 1 DM compared with that in adulthood in both women and men with a peak just before puberty. Between ages 12 and 14 years, the incidence declines; the decrease occurs approximately 1 to 2 years earlier in girls than in boys. From this age until approximately age 30, there is a slightly lower incidence of type 1 DM in women (12/100,000 per year) compared to men (15/100,000 per year), with men exceeding women by approximately 25% (Fig. 11-1).

The reason for this sex difference is unclear. After age 30 incidence rates appear to be similar. However, the incidence in both sexes has decreased dramatically by this time. Little information is available about the potential sex differential during the second peak of increased incidence of type 1 DM in the sixth and seventh decades.

Type 2 Diabetes Mellitus

The incidence of type 2 DM according to gender is less well established than that of type 1 DM. Some studies using a physician diagnosis of diabetes without specific laboratory criteria reported a higher annual incidence in women. However, other studies using more well-defined laboratory criteria show a lower incidence in women (Fig. 11-2).

Many risk factors for type 2 DM are shared between both genders. However, there are several risk factors unique to women including polycystic ovarian syndrome (PCOS) (see Chapter 46) and prior history of gestational diabetes (see Chapter 71). Women with PCOS have an increased risk for type 2 DM of up to 10% to 20%. Women with a history of gestational DM have up to a 40% risk of developing type 2 DM within 5 years and even higher with longer follow-up.

EFFECT OF DIABETES ON NORMAL FEMALE PHYSIOLOGY

Menstrual Function

Menstrual irregularity may be seen in women with both type 1 and type 2 diabetes. Up to one third of women with type 1 DM of reproductive age experience irregular menstrual cycles. A delay in menarche may be seen when the onset of type 1 DM occurs during pubertal development. Oligomenorrhea may also occur as a result of hypothalamic-pituitary-ovarian dysfunction. Other autoimmune disorders such as primary ovarian failure and Graves' disease that may affect menses should also be considered in women with type I DM. Ovarian versus hypothalamic dysfunction can be distinguished on the basis of a high follicle-stimulating hormone (FSH) and low estradiol level in the former and a low to normal FSH and low estradiol in the latter condition. Pregnancy and hyperprolactinemia should be excluded in all women of reproductive age presenting with oligomenorrhea.

Women with type 2 DM may often present with the syndrome of obesity, hirsutism, and oligomenorrhea, consistent with an insulin-resistant state and the clinical syndrome of polycystic ovarian syndrome (PCOS) (see Chapter 46). Correcting the insulin-resistant state in these women with diet, exercise, and in some cases insulin sensitizers is critical in the management of this disorder.

Insulin Sensitivity

Insulin sensitivity may vary with phase of the menstrual cycle with a luteal phase-related decrease in insulin sensitivity. The cause of this decrease in insulin sensitivity is not certain but may relate to effects of progesterone, which increases during the luteal phase, and has insulin antagonizing

Table 11-1
Medical Disorders of Increased Frequency in Diabetic Women

Complication	RR*	Treatment Considerations
Cardiovascular disease		Screen for and treat cardiac risk factors; consider converting enzyme inhibitors and aspirin
Myocardial infarction	7-8	
Congestive heart failure	3-5	
Cardiovascular mortality	4.5	
UTI	2-3	7-day course of antibiotics
Vaginal candidiasis	†	Improvement in glycemic control
		Topical (or oral) antifungal agents
Eating disorders	†	Preventive counseling
		Metabolic stabilization to prevent/correct DKA and caloric loss via glycosuria
		Psychiatric referral
Necrobiosis diabeticorum	3-4	Effectiveness of topical steroids controversial

*Relative risk compared to that of nondiabetic women.
†Has not been directly determined (see text for details).
UTI, Urinary tract infection; *DKA,* diabetic ketoacidosis.

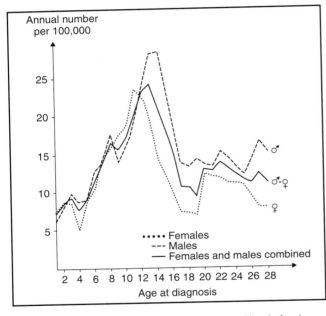

FIG. 11-1 Incidence of insulin-dependent diabetes mellitus in females and males age 0 to 29 years in Denmark. (From Christau B et al: *Acta Med Scand* 6724:54, 1979.)

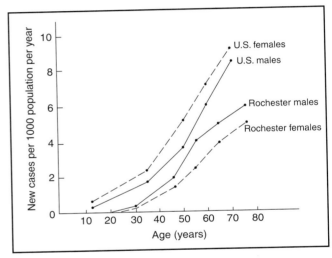

FIG. 11-2 Incidence of non-insulin-dependent diabetes mellitus (NIDDM) in females and males in the 1975-1981 National Health Interview Surveys (US females and US males) versus Rochester, Minnesota, in 1945-70 NIDDM, non-insulin-dependent diabetes mellitus. (Modified from Everhart J et al: *Diabetes in America,* NIH Publication No. 85-1468, Bethesda, Md, 1985, National Diabetes Data Group.)

effects when given exogenously. This normal physiologic change may be more obvious in the woman with diabetes, who may observe higher glucose levels and resultant increases in insulin requirements in the luteal phase. The potential importance of this deterioration in glucose control was demonstrated by studies in the 1970s that showed women in diabetic ketoacidosis were more likely to present during or at the end of the luteal phase. Furthermore, at the time of menopause some women note a decrease in their insulin requirements. However, such variation is not uniform and some women note no changes.

The observed effects of the menstrual cycle on glucose homeostasis underscore the need for a careful menstrual history in all female diabetics with erratic glycemic control. Recognition of menstrual cycle effects on glucose levels may enable the patient and provider to improve control by allowing for treatment changes according to the phase of the menstrual cycle.

EFFECT OF DIABETES ON REPRODUCTION
Preconception and Pregnancy

Pregnancy in diabetic women with complications may be associated with an increase in risk to the mother, and conception during poor glycemic control is associated with a significantly increased risk of congenital malformations in the fetus. Family planning for the female diabetic patient is thus of paramount importance and should be a routine part of care for these patients. Pregnancy should be planned months in advance to achieve glucose levels as normal as possible

Table 11-2
Contraceptive Methods

Method	Advantages	Disadvantages	Comments
Barrier	No effect on glycemic control	Motivation required for compliance	First-line method for patients able to comply
IUD	No effect on glycemic control	Inflammation, infection, bleeding	
OCP	Relative ease of use vs barrier	Possible deterioration in glucose control	For use in women with no other cardiac risk factors or micro-angiopathy, or risk of thrombotic complications
Tubal ligation	Single procedure	Surgical procedure, permanent	For women who have completed permanent childbearing or at very high risk for pregnancy-related complications

IUD, Intrauterine device; *OCP*, oral contraceptive pill.

before conception. For a more detailed discussion refer to Chapter 71.

Contraception

Of the contraceptive methods available today, use of the oral contraceptive pill has been the most controversial in the diabetic woman because of possible effects on carbohydrate and lipid metabolism and potential for increased vascular disease risk. The effects of oral contraceptive pills (OCPs) on lipid metabolism are discussed in Chapter 4.

Glycemic Control

Although some recent data suggest that estrogens may affect insulin resistance, many of the alterations in carbohydrate tolerance with OCP use have been attributed to the progestational component of these pills. Typical effects of OCP use in the nondiabetic woman include an increase in insulin levels but maintenance of normal glucose levels suggestive of insulin resistance. Data from insulin sensitivity studies indicate that some progestins, such as norgestrel and levonorgestrel, lead to an increase in insulin secretion after an oral glucose load. The effects on insulin levels may differ among progestins. For example norgestrel, a gonane progestin, may lead to a greater increase in insulin levels after an oral glucose load than norethindrone, an estrane progestin. Other progestins, such as gestodene and desogestrel, increase insulin levels by prolonging the half-life of insulin. Progestins may also lead to a decrease in glucose metabolism, as demonstrated by the euglycemic insulin clamp technique. Whether this effect involves a postreceptor defect in insulin action has not been determined. Data from studies of diabetic women suggest that several progestin-only pills (including norethindrone 300 mg, lynestrenol 500 mg, and norethisterone 350 mg) have no significant effect on daily insulin requirements, despite the increase in insulin resistance demonstrated in the experimental setting.

Since there are many OCP preparations available, most have not been studied directly in diabetic women. However, several commonly used monophasic and triphasic preparations, as well as some preparations available only in Europe, have been directly studied and suggest that these preparations have no significant impact on glycemic control in diabetic women. Specifically, commonly used monophasic and triphasic preparations have resulted in no clinically significant changes in 24-hour insulin requirements, hemoglobin A1c levels, fasting blood glucose, free fatty acids, or lipid profiles over 6 months of use.

The prior use of combination OCPs by nondiabetic women has generally not been associated with an increase in subsequent risk for the development of diabetes. However, in one study of women with a prior history of gestational diabetes, there was a threefold increase in the subsequent development of overt diabetes with the use of a progestin-only pill (norethindrone 0.3 mg).

Vascular and Endothelial Effects

Macrovascular complications, particularly cardiac, central nervous system, and retinal, have been of concern in diabetic women on OCPs. The higher doses of estrogen in earlier OCP preparations were considered to underlie these complications. Limited data suggest an increase in markers of coagulability in diabetic women on OCPs. Despite these biochemical changes, short-term prospective studies of 6 to 12 months have not demonstrated increases in thrombotic complications, development or worsening of microalbuminuria, or deterioration in renal function with OCP therapy.

Of concern was a retrospective population study that demonstrated an increase in stroke and venous thrombosis in 120 diabetics who used OCPs compared with 156 diabetics who did not. Of note, the incidence was not compared with that of the nondiabetic population using OCPs. In six of the OCP users, proliferative retinopathy developed, and in three a rapidly progressive form developed. However, another retrospective population study of 432 diabetic women found no association between past or current OCP use, or the number of years of use, and the severity of retinopathy. None of the OCPs studied have been demonstrated to have a significant impact on blood pressure in women with diabetes.

Approach to Contraception for the Diabetic Woman

A careful assessment of the risks and benefits of each type of contraception should be made on an individual basis (Table 11-2).

Barrier methods should be strongly considered as first-line contraceptive methods for women who are able to comply with these methods because of the absence of effect on glycemic control and potential complications. The IUD also has this advantage and is a good alternative for the multiparous woman. In one controlled study using the copper IUD, the pregnancy rate of approximately 1% per year was the same in diabetics and control subjects. Furthermore, discontinuation rates for infection, inflammation, bleeding, and other medical conditions were similar in diabetic and nondiabetic women. Whether IUDs should be used as first line in nulliparous women intending future pregnancy is controversial.

The use of OCPs has generally been reserved for those patients with otherwise low cardiovascular risk profiles, including young age, normal blood pressure, normal lipid profiles, nonsmoking, and no evidence of microangiopathy or microalbuminuria. Although data for women with diabetes are limited, none of the agents studied has had any clinically significant influence on daily insulin requirements or renal complications.

Because any given individual may differ in her response to an OCP, diabetic women should be counseled to monitor blood glucose levels closely while initiating an OCP to assess any changes in glycemic control and insulin requirements. Furthermore, the patient should be examined before initiation of OCPs and followed regularly for increases in blood pressure, development or acceleration of microalbuminuria and deterioration in renal function, unfavorable alterations in lipid profiles, and development or acceleration of retinopathy.

Finally, for the very high-risk patient or the patient who has completed a family or does not wish to have children, tubal ligation should be considered after careful counseling of the patient by her physician.

DIABETES AND MENOPAUSE
Hormone Replacement Therapy

The decision to use hormone replacement therapy (HRT) is complex for most women (see Chapter 48). The decision is even more difficult for women with DM given the paucity of data addressing risks and benefits in this population. The relief of menopausal symptoms such as hot flushes with HRT is a benefit to women with DM. Estrogen decreases urogenital symptoms, which may be particularly important to the woman with diabetes who is already prone to more urinary tract infections. Although cardiovascular disease (CVD) affects women with DM to a greater degree, it is not clear at present whether HRT decreases this risk in women with or without diabetes (see Chapter 48).

Risks associated with HRT may differ in women with diabetes. Women with type 2 DM have an increased baseline risk of endometrial cancer, which may be increased further by HRT; hence additional careful monitoring may be indicated with a lower threshold for endometrial evaluation. Likewise diabetic women are at high risk for gallstones, which also are further increased by HRT. HRT may also increase the hypertriglyceridemia seen in DM, although the use of a transdermal preparation may minimize this side effect. Some data have suggested increased breast cancer risk in women with diabetes, but most studies fail to support this. There is a theoretical concern that some formulations of HRT might worsen glycemic control, but data do not suggest an increase risk of development of diabetes among nondiabetic women using HRT.

Approach to Hormone Replacement Therapy in the Diabetic Woman

Women with either type 1 or type 2 DM who start HRT should be counseled that the therapy may affect their glucose control, and diabetic medications must be adjusted accordingly. In a woman who experiences a deterioration in her glucose control with HRT, the use of natural progesterone or a more estrogenic progestin should be considered. Women with DM who experience an elevation in triglycerides with HRT may benefit from a change to a transdermal estrogen.

Bone Health in the Postmenopausal Woman with Diabetes

Although bone loss is a hallmark of menopause (see Chapter 48), women with type 2 diabetes appear to have less osteoporosis than women of the same age who do not have diabetes. Possible explanations for this reduced risk include the frequent coexistence of obesity, which is associated with greater bone mass, higher androgen and estrogen levels, or a trophic effect of hyperinsulinemia on bone. In contrast, women with type 1 DM may have a greater risk for osteoporosis than age- and weight-matched healthy women. This increase in risk may be related to failure to attain peak bone mass when the diabetes presents early in life. Women who have diabetes secondary to corticosteroid use are at high risk for osteoporosis and fracture. Regardless of bone density, fracture risk is increased in diabetics who have disease complications that increase the chance of falling, such as sensory and autonomic neuropathy and amputation. To date, there are no studies of osteoporosis prevention or treatment that specifically address the issue of diabetes.

DIABETES AND CARDIOVASCULAR DISEASE

CVD is the leading cause of death in women and men patients with DM. Diabetic individuals have approximately three times the risk of coronary heart disease as those without diabetes, even after adjusting for other coronary risk factors that are commonly associated with diabetes such as hypertension and hypercholesterolemia. Diabetic individuals without a history of myocardial infarction (MI) have a subsequent coronary event rate similar to nondiabetic individuals who have previously had an MI.

Women with diabetes are at particular risk, essentially losing the cardiovascular protection that is typically associated with female gender. Women with diabetes have higher rates of MI, higher complication rates (including congestive heart failure and reinfarction), and higher fatality rates than nondiabetic women or men.

Pathophysiology

Women and men with diabetes commonly have other associated coronary risk factors, including hypertension, dyslipidemia (increased low-density lipoprotein [LDL] cholesterol and triglycerides and low high-density lipoprotein), and a tendency to hypercoagulability, as evidenced by increased levels of plasminogen activator inhibitor (PAI)-1 and increased platelet aggregability. Type 2 diabetes is commonly associated with obesity, and particularly central obesity, both of which are independent risk factors for CVD. Hyperinsulinemia, a marker for insulin resistance, has been associated with CHD risk in men, although data are lacking in women. Hyperglycemia is also predictive of CHD and may contribute to endothelial dysfunction in diabetic patients. The presence of other coronary risk factors, such as hypertension, smoking, dyslipidemia, and poor glycemic control, markedly increases risk for CHD in diabetic patients greater than that seen with diabetes alone.

Some metabolic derangements may be particularly relevant in women and may contribute to their relatively higher CVD risks. Women with diabetes appear to have higher levels of dense LDL, which is considered more atherogenic, than both diabetic men and nondiabetic individuals. Recent data suggest that endothelial dysfunction is especially common in diabetic women.

Clinical Presentation

Atypical presentations of coronary disease, including "silent" MI, are more common in patients with diabetes and in women in particular. Thus coronary disease needs to be considered when a diabetic woman presents with atypical symptoms such as mental status change, deterioration in glycemic control, congestive heart failure, or stroke. Because women with diabetes do not share the relative premenopausal protection from coronary disease observed in nondiabetic women, coronary disease must be considered even in relatively young diabetic women presenting with typical or atypical symptoms.

Management

Primary Prevention

In view of the high CVD risk in diabetes, preventive strategies should be a part of routine care. Given the synergistic effect of other risk factors on CVD risk in diabetes, aggressive management of these other factors is indicated. Diabetic women should be encouraged to avoid smoking, and current smokers should be offered aids for smoking cessation. Counseling (see Chapter 85) regarding weight control and exercise is routinely warranted in view of data demonstrating improvements in insulin sensitivity, glycemic control, lipids, and blood pressure with exercise and weight reduction.

Hypertension

Several studies, which have included sizable numbers of women, have confirmed the benefit of blood pressure control in reducing CVD risk in diabetes. In the Hypertension in Diabetes Study, tight blood pressure control with atenolol or captopril significantly reduced risk of stroke, as well as microvascular complications, compared with less intensive therapy. Although this study did not find differences in outcome between these two medications, more recent data have suggested a particular value to angiotensin-converting enzyme inhibition even in the nonhypertensive diabetic population (see following discussion).

Hyperlipidemia

Management of hyperlipidemia is critical in the care of diabetic women. Subgroup analyses of diabetics enrolled in two large studies of cholesterol reduction and coronary risk have confirmed a significant reduction in CHD morbidity and mortality with statin therapy. Diabetic women treated with pravastatin or simvastatin had reductions in CVD risk comparable to their nondiabetic counterparts.

Glycemic Control

The microvascular benefits of improved glycemic control have been clearly demonstrated in women with type 1 and type 2 diabetes, but the role of glycemic control in reducing macrovascular disease risk is presently less clear. The observation of a 16% reduction in risk for MI among women and men randomized to tight glycemic control in the United Kingdom Prospective Diabetes Study raises the question of benefit, but this finding was of borderline statistical significance.

Aspirin

Subgroup analyses of diabetic men and women in secondary prevention trials of aspirin have demonstrated significant risk reductions in CHD with aspirin therapy. In the Early Treatment of Diabetic Retinopathy Study, a placebo-controlled trial involving diabetic patients with and without a history of CVD, men and women randomized to aspirin therapy had a 28% reduction in risk of MI, although this association was not statistically significant in subgroup analysis limited to women. Randomized clinical trial data on primary prevention are presently available only for diabetic men, among whom aspirin reduces CVD risk similarly to nondiabetic persons. The American Diabetes Association recommends routine use of aspirin therapy in diabetic women and men with known macrovascular disease and consideration of aspirin therapy for primary prevention in the absence of contraindications to this therapy.

Angiotensin-Converting Enzyme Inhibitors

In addition to their recognized renal benefits angiotensin-converting enzyme inhibitors have recently been shown to reduce risks for MI and CVD mortality among diabetic women and men even in the absence of concomitant hypertension or known CVD. The use of these agents should be considered broadly in the diabetic population, although care must be taken to avoid use during pregnancy.

Beta Blockers

Beta blockers have documented benefit in the diabetic population not only in the treatment of hypertension but also for cardioprotection after MI. Although the clinician must be aware of possible adverse effects of this class of medication on glucose tolerance and hypoglycemic symptomatology, in the absence of clear contraindications, beta blockade is indicated after MI and also may have a role in hypertensive therapy.

Invasive Treatment of Coronary Artery Disease

After CAD is established, women have traditionally been considered less optimal surgical candidates for coronary artery bypass grafting (CABG), possibly because of the smaller caliber of their native vessels; they may experience less symptomatic relief and have greater operative mortality rates than men. Some, but not all, studies suggest that diabetics are also high-risk candidates for CABG and have higher morbidity and mortality rates than nondiabetic patients. This may in part be attributed to more diffuse and distally located atherosclerotic lesions found in diabetics, although this finding has not been confirmed in all studies. Whereas there appear to be more complications from percutaneous transluminal coronary angioplasty in women, it is not yet clear to what extent diabetic women differ from nondiabetic women or diabetic men in this regard. See Chapter 2 for further discussion of coronary artery disease.

DIABETES AND GENITOURINARY PROBLEMS
Urinary Tract Infections

Although there is some controversy, many studies report a twofold to threefold increased frequency of urinary tract infection (UTI) in diabetic compared with nondiabetic women. In men in contrast, diabetes does not appear to confer increased risk for UTI. Similarly, an increased frequency of asymptomatic bacturia has been found in diabetic women but not in diabetic men. While *Escherichia coli* is the most commonly isolated organism in both diabetics and nondiabetics, *Pseudomonas* and *Klebsiella* sp. are found in much greater frequency in diabetics.

The cause of this increase in frequency of UTI in diabetic women is not clear, although it is often ascribed to hyperglycemia and glycosuria. Low urinary leukocyte counts and low cytokine levels may also contribute. Risk factors that have been identified for asymptomatic bacturia in diabetes include increased age, peripheral neuropathy, and macroalbuminuria. Other contributing factors may include prior instrumentation and bladder dysfunction secondary to autonomic neuropathy.

Because of the possibility of more serious sequelae if pyelonephritis develops, including urosepsis, papillary necrosis, and perinephric abscess, there is a tendency to be more aggressive in the treatment of UTIs in diabetic women. Three-day regimens for UTIs have not been well studied in this population, and therefore a 7-day course of antibiotic therapy may be advisable. Because not all asymptomatic bacteriuria (without pyuria) progresses to frank UTI, it remains controversial whether this condition requires treatment in the diabetic woman (see Chapter 23).

Candida Vaginitis

Vaginal candidiasis is common even in the absence of diabetes, but there is an increased incidence in the diabetic woman. However, candidiasis is so prevalent in premenopausal women that its presence does not appear to warrant testing for diabetes if it is the only suggestive symptom. However, it is important to question women with recurrent *Candida* infections as to other possible symptoms of diabetes. Given the decreased incidence of vaginal candidiasis in postmenopausal women, recurrent infections in this population should prompt consideration of diabetes, although there are no studies to our knowledge addressing the cost-effectiveness of this strategy.

Candida growth and adherence to vaginal epithelial cells increase in the presence of glucose. Increased glucose levels in vaginal secretions and urine may thus underline the high propensity for *Candida* infections among diabetic women.

Antifungal treatment is indicated for symptomatic infections. Improvement in glucose control may reduce recurrence risk.

DIABETES AND EATING DISORDERS
Epidemiology

Eating disorders are more common in female than male adolescents and young adults (see Chapter 84). Recent studies suggest that whereas the incidence of anorexia nervosa is similar in diabetic and nondiabetic women, bulimia nervosa may be more common in diabetic women. Furthermore, diabetic women may have a twofold increase in the risk of binge eating and a higher risk of subclinical eating disorders (which fail to meet all of the DSM-IV criteria). Diabetics on insulin may utilize a unique "purge" technique of omitting or underdosing insulin, which leads to glycosuria and calorie loss in the urine. This phenomenon has now been included among DSM-IV criteria for purging. Intentional insulin omission for the purpose of weight control has been estimated to occur in 10% to 40% of diabetic women; in diabetic women with diagnosed eating disorders, the rate may be as high as 75%. These rates are probably underestimated given patients' concerns about revealing this information to their doctors. In contrast, intentional insulin omission appears infrequent among male diabetics (Fig. 11-3).

Eating disorders may also be a concern in women with type 2 DM. Limited data in type 2 DM suggest an increase in disordered eating, particularly binge eating disorders associated with increased body mass index (BMI). Omission of oral agents for the purpose of weight loss has been reported in this setting.

Pathogenesis

In general, young women are at greatest risk for the development of eating disorders. Several factors related to diabetes may make these women even more susceptible to these disorders. The treatment of diabetes places great emphasis on weight, dietary habits, and food. Furthermore, the onset of type 1 DM often occurs during adolescence, a time of increased vulnerability to the development of an eating disorder. Women who have experienced weight loss before diagnosis often gain weight with the initiation of insulin, which may precipitate disordered eating.

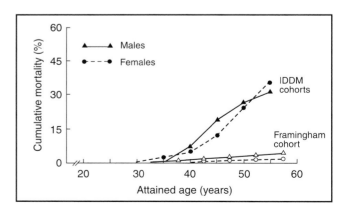

FIG. 11-3 Coronary artery disease cumulative mortality rate in females and males with insulin-dependent diabetes mellitus (IDDM) compared to the nondiabetic population in the Framingham Heart Study. IDDM, insulin-dependent diabetes mellitus. (From Krowleski AS et al: *Am J Cardiol* 59:750, 1987.)

Clinical Presentation

Detection of an eating disorder in a diabetic patient can be challenging for the clinician. Many symptoms, such as difficulty in concentrating, decreased energy level, and sleep disturbances, are also common with erratic glycemic control alone. However, significant changes in weight, persistently erratic glycemic control, and recurrent episodes of hypoglycemia or diabetic ketoacidosis should alert the physician to the possibility of an eating disorder. This possibility should be distinguished from diabetic gastropathy, which can also present with nausea, vomiting, anorexia, and fluctuations in weight and glycemic control.

Diagnosis

Approaches to diagnose eating disorders in the nondiabetic population may not be directly applicable to diabetic women. For example, diagnostic instruments such as the Eating Attitude Test include questions on whether one follows a diet, as a way to identify a possible eating disorder; however, following a prescribed diet is a standard component of the treatment of diabetes. Detection of eating disorders may be improved by ascertaining a history of insulin manipulation and intentional insulin omission, behavior that may be the single most important piece of information suggesting an eating disorder. This information is also critical for management, since this behavior results in impaired glycemic control and increased risk of diabetic complications. Psychiatric consultation is often useful to confirm the diagnosis of an eating disorder and to rule out coexisting psychiatric disorders such as depression and anxiety, which are more common in patients with eating disorders; depression may also be more common in diabetes.

Complications

Most, although not all, studies show that insulin omission and formal eating disorders are associated with an elevated hemoglobin A1C (Hb A1C). Given the recognized association between elevated Hb A1C and risk of microvascular disease, it is not surprising that eating disorders are associated with an increased risk in complications including retinopathy and neuropathy, especially painful peripheral neuropathy.

Management

As with nondiabetic patients, the management of eating disorders or subclinical eating disorders requires a multidisciplinary approach involving the primary physician, psychiatrist, family, and patient. Patients should be educated regarding complications of eating disorders, including potential or increased diabetic complications. Insulin must also be managed carefully with the recognition that restoration of appropriate insulin dosage will predispose to weight gain, which then can lead to further disordered eating behavior.

In general, management of the young diabetic female patient should emphasize prevention of eating disorders. The physician should routinely inquire about dietary habits, stress-related eating, and binging. Patients should also be warned about the dangers of strict dieting and should be taught how to manage eating and drinking in social situations in the context of diabetes. Chapter 84 discusses eating disorders in greater detail.

OTHER COMPLICATIONS

Microvascular Disease

Major complications of diabetes include retinopathy, nephropathy, and neuropathy. In contrast to macrovascular complications, these complications appear to occur with similar frequency in women and men with comparable duration of diabetes. However, it should be recognized that pregnancy may exacerbate preexisting proliferative retinopathy, and women should be screened before and carefully monitored through pregnancy (see Chapter 71).

Necrobiosis Diabeticorum

Necrobiosis diabeticorum is a skin lesion uniquely associated with diabetes, whose pathogenesis is poorly understood. Women with diabetes have twice to four times the risk of this condition as diabetic men.

MANAGEMENT OF DIABETES MELLITUS

The goal of treatment of diabetes mellitus is to normalize sugars as much as possible with avoidance of recurrent hypoglycemia. Improved glucose control is associated with a significant reduction in microvascular complications in both type 1 and type 2 diabetes. The Diabetes and Control and Complications Trial (DCCT) included relatively young patients with type 1 DM, randomized to frequent insulin injections (to maintain or normalize Hb A1C) as compared with conventional therapy. Benefits of intensive insulin therapy, including delay in the onset and progression of retinopathy and proteinuria and delay in the onset of neuropathy, were similar in magnitude for women and men, as was the risk of hypoglycemia. The United Kingdom Prospective Diabetes Study (UKPDS) studied type 2 diabetic patients, randomized to sulfonylurea insulin, metformin, or diet therapy and demonstrated how improved glucose control with any of the medications was associated with a significant reduction in risk of microvascular complications over a 10-year period.

Studies of glycemic control have not been specifically designed to address a gender difference. Glucose control is known to be important for women with both type 1 and type 2 diabetes surrounding conception and the first trimester to reduce risk of birth defects (see Chapter 71).

Choice of Therapy

The treatment options available are listed in Table 11-3. The treatment, goals, and options are not different for women and men with the exception of a few issues discussed later.

All type 1 diabetics must be treated with insulin to prevent hyperglycemia and ketogenesis. Type 2 diabetic women on oral agents who are contemplating pregnancy should be switched over to insulin therapy if adequate glycemic control cannot be achieved with diet alone. Whether oral agents can be used safely in pregnancy is under study. In addition, angiotensin-converting enzyme inhibitors and angiotensin-2 receptor blockers must be discontinued to avoid the risk of both morbidity and mortality in the developing fetus that can occur during all trimesters of pregnancy.

For nonpregnant type 2 diabetics, a number of pharmacologic agents are available for patients who require drug therapy in addition to diet. The **sulfonylureas** increase the

Table 11-3
Drug Treatment Options for Diabetes

Insulin	For all type 1 diabetics, and type 2 diabetics contemplating pregnancy or pregnant, or inadequately controlled on oral agents
NPH	Delivered subcutaneously usually in 2-4 injections per day, usually with combination of longer acting NPH and shorter acting regular insulin
Ultralente	Longer acting insulin with less peaking effect. May be used as basal insulin with premeal dosing of regular insulin. Allows for greater flexibility.
Glargine	New once a day basal insulin with no peaking effect. Used in combination with oral agents for type 2 or Lis-pro with meals
Regular	May be used alone as basal insulin via continuous subcutaneous insulin infusion, plus premeal boluses via insulin pump. Allows for greater flexibility.
Lis-pro	Very short onset of action and t 1/2 that more closely mimics the physiologic release of insulin
Sulfonylureas (Second generation most commonly used)	Risk of hypoglycemia and weight gain
Glyburide	
Glipizide	Shorter half life than glyburide; may be safer for the elderly
Biguanides	Minimal risk of hypoglycemia when used as monotherapy
Metformin	Risk of lactic acidosis in setting of renal insufficiency.
	Do not use if creatinine >1.4 mg/dl in women, or if creatinine clearance <60 mL/min; discontinue before use of iodinated contrast dye or in setting of dehydration or illness associated with decreased intravascular volume.
	May be beneficial in improving the insulin resistant state and clinical features of PCOS, including infertility; therefore contraception must be addressed when used in this setting. Gastrointestinal side effects may limit use
Thiazolidinediones	No risk of hypoglycemia when used as monotherapy
Rosiglitazone	Must monitor LFTs at baseline and q2 months at least for first year and
Pioglitazone	periodically thereafter. Must monitor hemoglobin, hematocrit periodically, given possible risk of anemia. Use with precaution in patients with CHF. May be beneficial in improving the insulin resistant state and clinical features of PCOS, including infertility; therefore contraception must be addressed when used in this setting; however, unlike metformin, may be associated with weight gain
Alpha-glucosidase inhibitors	Inhibit gastrointestinal conversion of carbohydrates to monosaccharides
Acarbose	Greatest effect is on lowering postprandial rise in glucose; may be used in both
Miglitol	type 1 and type 2 diabetic patients; severe gastrointestinal side effects with flatulence and diarrhea limit its use. Acarbose may have favorable lipid effects

release of insulin from the pancreas and may therefore be associated with weight gain. **Insulin sensitizers,** such as metformin (a biguanide), and rosiglitazone and pioglitazone (thiazolidinediones) improve the action of insulin. The exact mechanisms are not fully understood; however, metformin has been shown to decreases hepatic glucose output, and the thiazolidinediones have been demonstrated to enhance glucose transport into muscle and liver cells. These latter agents may improve the insulin-resistant state seen in type 2 diabetics and tend to have more favorable effects on lipids than the sulfonylureas. In addition, they are not associated with the side effect of hypoglycemia. In women with diabetes mellitus, insulin resistance and polycystic ovarian syndrome (PCOS), insulin sensitizers may also improve hirsutism, acne and oligomenorrhea. These classes of drugs may lead to ovulation and pregnancy in previously anovulatory women. Therefore contraception should be carefully addressed when treating diabetic women with these agents. The sulfonylureas and insulin sensitizers may be used in

combination or added to insulin (in type 2 diabetics) when one agent is not effective alone in achieving adequate glycemic control. The **alpha-glucosidase inhibitors,** on the other hand, may be used in both type 1 and type 2 diabetics. Severe gastrointestinal side effects, however, limit their use in practice.

Surgical treatment options for type 1 diabetes include pancreas transplantation and pancreatic islet cell transplantation. Both procedures require lifelong use of immunosuppressants. According to the American Diabetes Association position statement published in 2001 pancreas transplantation is a viable treatment option for diabetic patients with end-stage renal disease who are also undergoing or have undergone renal transplantation. The survival of each organ graft may actually be enhanced by the transplantation of the second organ. For patients not undergoing renal transplantation, pancreas transplantation may be considered for patients who experience frequent, acute, and severe complications; when insulin usage fails to prevent these complications; and for severe clinical and emotional difficulty with insulin usage. Islet cell transplantation, a less invasive technique, is currently considered experimental. Unfortunately, the majority of allografts fail. There are no specific guidelines with either procedure with respect to gender.

BIBLIOGRAPHY

Affenito SG et al: Subclinical and clinical eating disorders in IDDM negatively affects metabolic control, *Diabetes Care* 20(2):182, 1997.

Barrett-Coimor E, Holbrook TL: Sex differences in osteoporosis in older adults with non-insulin-dependent diabetes mellitus, *JAMA* 268:3333, 1992.

Bloomgarden ZT: American Diabetes Association Annual Meeting, 1999. New approaches to insulin treatment and glucose monitoring. *Diabetes Care* 22(12):2078, 1999.

Christau B et al: Incidence of insulin-dependent diabetes mellitus (0-29 years at onset) in Denmark, *Acta Med Scand* 624(Suppl):54, 1979.

Cohn BA et al: Gender differences in hospitalization for IDDM among adolescents in California, 1991. Implications for prevention, *Diabetes Care* 20(11):1677, 1997.

Consensus opinion of the North American Menopause Society: Effects of menopause and estrogen replacement therapy or hormone replacement therapy in women with diabetes mellitus, *Menopause* 7:87, 2000.

Crow SJ, Keel PK, Kendal D: Eating disorders and insulin dependent diabetes mellitus, *Psychosomatic* 39:233, 1998.

Diabetes Control and Complications Trial Research Group: The effect of intensive treatment of diabetes on the development and progression of long-term complications in insulin-dependent diabetes mellitus, *N Engl J Med* 329:977, 1993.

Diamond MP, Simonson DC, DeFronzo RA: Menstrual cyclicity has a profound effect on glucose homeostasis, *Fertil Steril* 52:204, 1989.

Elkind-Hirsch KE, Sherman LD, Malinak R: Hormone replacement therapy alters insulin sensitivity in young women with premature ovarian failure, *J Clin Endocrinol Metab* 76:472, 1993.

Everhart J, Knowler WC, Bennett PH: Incidence and risk factors for non-insulin-dependent diabetes. In *Diabetes in America*, NIH Publication No. 85-1468, 1985, Bethesda, Md, 1985, National Diabetes Data Group.

Geerlings SE et al: Asymptomatic bacteriuria may be considered a complication in women with diabetes, *Diabetes Care* 23:744, 2000.

Godsland IF et al: Insulin resistance, secretion and elimination in postmenopausal women receiving oral or transdermal hormone replacement therapy, *Metabolism* 42:846, 1993.

Griffin ML et al: Insulin-dependent diabetes mellitus and menstrual dysfunction, *Ann Med* 26:331, 1994.

Jones JM et al: Eating disorders in adolescent females with and without type 1 diabetes: cross-sectional study, *BMJ* 320(7249):1563, 2000.

Kaplan RC et al: Postmenopausal hormones and risk of myocardial infarction in diabetic women, *Diabetes Care* 21:1117, 1998.

Kjos SL et al: Contraception and the risk of type 2 diabetes mellitus in Latina Women with prior gestational diabetes mellitus, *JAMA* 280(6): 533, 1998.

Kjos SL et al: Hormonal choices after gestational diabetes: subsequent pregnancy, contraception, and hormone replacement. *Diabetes Care* 2l(25)(suppl): SOB-57B, 1998.

Klein BEK, Moss SE, Klein R: Oral contraceptives in women with diabetes, *Diabetes Care* 13:895, 1990.

Krolewski AS et al: Magnitude and determinants of coronary artery disease in juvenile-onset, insulin-dependent diabetes mellitus, *Am J Cardiol* 59:750, 1987.

Manson IL et al: A prospective study of postmenopausal estrogen therapy and subsequent incidence of non-insulin-dependent diabetes mellitus, *Ann Epidemiol* 2:665, 1992.

Marcus MD, Wing RR: Eating disorders and diabetes. In Holmes CS, editor: *Neuropsychological and behavioral aspects of diabetes*, New York, 1990, Springer-Verlag.

Nabulsi AA et al: Association of hormone replacement therapy with various cardiovascular risk factors in postmenopausal women, *N Engl J Med* 328:1106, 1993.

Petersen KR, Skouby SO, Vedel P, Haarber AB: Hormonal contraception in women with IDDM: influence on glycometabolic control and lipoprotein metabolism, *Diabetes Care* 8(6):800, 1995.

Piepkorn B et al: Bone mineral density and bone metabolism in diabetes mellitus, *Horm Metab Res* 29:584, 1997.

Pyorala K et al: Cholesterol lowering with simvastatin improves prognosis of diabetic patients with coronary heart disease, *Diabetes Care* 20:641, 1997.

Rao SV, Bethel MA, Feinglos MN: Treatment of diabetes mellitus: implications of the use of oral agents, *Am Heart J* 138:334, 1999.

Rimm EB et al: Oral contraceptive use and the risk of type II (non-insulin dependent diabetes mellitus) in a large prospective study of women, *Diabetologica* 35:967, 1992.

Robertson RP, Larsen DC, Sutherland SR: *Diabetes Care* 23:112, 2000.

Sattar N, Jaap AJ, MacCuish AC: Hormone replacement therapy and cardiovascular risk in postmenopausal women with NIDDM, *Diabetic Med* 13:782, 1996.

Shapiro AM et al: Islet transplantation in seven patients with type 1 diabetes mellitus using a glucocorticoid-free immunosuppressive regimen, *N Engl J Med* 343(4):230, 2000.

Skouby SO et al: Mechanism of action of oral contraceptives on carbohydrate metabolism at the cellular level, *Am J Obstet Gynecol* 163:343, 1990.

Stampfer MJ et al: Postmenopausal estrogen therapy and cardiovascular disease, *N Engl J Med* 325:756, 1991.

UK Prospective Diabetes Study (UKPDS) Group: Intensive blood-glucose control with sulphonylureas or insulin compared with conventional treatment and risk of complications in patients with type 2 diabetes, *Lancet* 352:837, 1998.

UK Prospective Diabetes Study Group: Tight blood pressure control and risk of macrovascular and microvascular complications in Type 2 diabetes: UKPDS 38, *Br Med J* 317:703, 1998.

Widom B, Diamond MP, Simonson DC: Alterations in glucose metabolism during menstrual cycle in women with IDDM, *Diabetes Care* 15:213, 1992.

CHAPTER 12

Osteoporosis

David M. Slovik

Osteoporosis is a major public health problem that leads to increased morbidity and mortality, loss of function, and long-term physical and emotional suffering. It is estimated that 10 million Americans have osteoporosis (8 million women and 2 million men), and 18 million more have low bone mass, placing them at increased risk for osteoporosis and fractures.

Osteoporosis is a systemic skeletal disease characterized by low bone mass and microarchitectural deterioration of bone tissue, with a consequent increase in bone fragility and susceptibility to fracture. Osteoporotic bone has a normal ratio of mineral to matrix. **Osteomalacia** refers to a group of disorders characterized by an abnormality in bone mineralization. The ratio of mineral to matrix is diminished as a result of an excess of unmineralized osteoid. **Osteopenia** is a general term referring to bone density that is lower than that seen in healthy young adults. Osteopenia can be caused by many disorders, including osteoporosis, and predisposes bone to fragility fractures. A **fragility fracture** is one that occurs without any trauma, or it can occur after a fall from a height of less than 12 inches or after abrupt deceleration from a speed slower than a run.

EPIDEMIOLOGY

The hip, vertebrae, and distal portion of the forearm are the most common sites of osteoporotic fractures, although fractures of other sites, including the pelvis, femur, tibia, and humerus, also occur with increased frequency.

At 50 years of age, the average white woman has a lifetime risk of 18% for hip fracture, and the lifetime risk for any fracture of the hip, spine, or distal forearm is almost 40%. After the age of 60 years, the age-specific incidence of proximal femur fractures increases almost exponentially. The increase in hip fractures with advancing age is due to a combination of factors, including low bone mass, increased falls, and decreased protection from falls.

PATHOPHYSIOLOGY OF AGE-RELATED BONE LOSS

Most of the bone mass in adults is laid down during adolescence. Even though bones have stopped growing in length after puberty with closure of the growth plates, radial bone growth continues, the bone mineral content increases, and bones become stronger.

Trabecular (cancellous) bone attains its peak bone mass in the 20s and cortical (compact) bone shortly thereafter. After a transient period of equilibrium, bone loss may begin sometimes by the late 30s or early 40s and accelerates for several years after the menopause. Thus the amount of bone later in life represents a combination of the amount achieved at skeletal maturity and the amount lost since that time.

Age-related bone loss occurs in both genders and affects trabecular and cortical bone, although at different rates and to different degrees.

Risk Factors for Bone Loss (Box 12-1)

Genetics

The prevalence of osteoporosis and incidence of fracture vary by gender, race, and ethnicity. Postmenopausal women have the highest incidence of hip fractures. Both men and women sustain an age-related decline in bone density; however, women have a more rapid rate of bone loss and lower peak bone mass. African-American women have higher bone mineral density than white non-Hispanic women throughout life and have lower hip fracture rates. Mexican-American women have bone density intermediate to these two groups. Japanese women have lower peak bone mineral density than white non-Hispanic women but a lower hip fracture rate, for unclear reasons.

Bone density is more highly correlated in monozygotic than in dizygotic twins. Daughters of women with osteoporosis have lower spinal bone mass than normal control subjects of similar age.

Aging

A steady age-related decline in bone mass occurs in all persons after skeletal maturity, although the rates vary.

Fracture History

Women who have sustained a fracture as an adult or who have first-degree family members who have had fractures are at greater risk.

Peak Bone Mass

The amount of bone attained at the time of skeletal maturity is very important. If the rate of bone loss with age is constant, then those women with the lowest bone density at skeletal maturity will be at greatest risk for sustaining fractures later in life.

Nutrition and Lifestyle Factors

Good nutrition is important to bone health. Adequate calcium is especially important in the years of growth and development and also in the postmenopausal years. Diets high in protein, phosphorus, fat, fiber, sodium, and caffeine may be harmful, either by increasing the excretion of calcium in the urine or interfering with the intestinal absorption of calcium. Alcohol abuse and cigarette smoking also are harmful to bone.

Exercise and Physical Activity

Immobilization can cause significant bone loss.

Hormones

Many hormones are important in bone development and maintaining a normal skeleton. These include estrogens, androgens, parathyroid hormone, vitamin D and its metabolites, calcitonin, insulin, glucocorticoids, prolactin, growth hormone, and thyroid hormone.

Deficiencies of gonadal steroids during the time of bone development will lead to thinner bones later in life; deficiencies later in life will produce severe bone loss and osteoporosis. Estrogen deficiency in premenopausal women as a result of gonadal dysgenesis, anorexia nervosa, prolonged amenorrhea, excessive exercise, or gonadotropin-releasing hormone (GnRH) therapy may reduce peak bone mass. Excesses of thyroid hormone or glucocorticoids can lead to bone loss.

Medications

Exogenous glucocorticoid administration and excessive thyroid hormone can cause bone loss. Cyclosporine, especially in conjunction with glucocorticoids after organ transplantation, can cause rapid and severe bone loss.

Bone Remodeling

Bone remodeling is the cellular process that allows continuous removal of old bone by osteoclasts and replacement with new bone by osteoblasts. In remodeling there is cyclic erosion and repair of microscopic cavities, with long periods of quiescence between cycles. The adult skeleton is composed of two types of bone tissue: cortical (compact, lamellar) or trabecular (spongiosa, cancellous). Cortical bone constitutes approximately 80% of the total skeletal mass but only one third of the total surface. It forms the outer wall of all bones, but the bulk of cortical tissue is in the shafts of long bones of the appendicular skeleton. Trabecular bone provides the remaining 20% of total skeletal mass and about two thirds of its surface. Trabecular bone consists of plates that are distributed in relatively uniform manner. In osteoporosis there is a reduction in the number of plates, and there is conversion of plates to rods. Trabecular bone is found mainly in the bones of the axial skeleton and in the ends of the long bones.

Bone remodeling is a complex process regulated by hormones and growth factors. Any time that bone resorption is greater than bone formation, bone loss occurs.

CLASSIFICATION

Age-related osteoporosis accounts for 80% to 90% of osteoporosis in women. However, there are many medical disorders and secondary causes of osteoporosis that may affect the amount of bone seen at the time of skeletal maturity or the amount of bone that subsequently is lost (Box 12-2).

EVALUATION

Two groups of patients usually seek medical evaluation:
- Those with no history of osteoporosis. These women are usually young and healthy and are either premenopausal or in their early menopausal years. They are concerned about developing osteoporosis and want to know whether they are at risk and what they can do to prevent it.
- Those with evidence of osteoporosis on the basis of clinical problems (e.g., fractures), bone density measurements, or radiographs.

In women with vertebral fractures, the most frequent symptoms are back pain, loss of height, and the development of a dorsal kyphosis. Back pain may be of acute onset following ordinary physical activity such as bending or lifting. The pain may be severe and usually is located over the fractured vertebrae. It often radiates in a radicular pattern laterally and is accompanied by severe paraspinal muscle spasm. The pain may be sufficient to produce shortness of breath and may be increased by minimal movements such as turning in bed, flexing the spine, or taking a deep breath. On examination, a dorsal kyphosis usually is evident, especially if prior fractures have occurred, and spasm with guarding may significantly limit spinal motion. Additional problems include nausea, anorexia, abdominal distention, and constipation.

The acute pain usually subsides after 1 to 2 weeks but is often present for as long as 4 to 6 weeks, and it may take even longer before normal activities can be resumed. Chronic back pain in these patients can be very troublesome. It is usually more diffuse and difficult to localize compared with the acute pain and is often described as a dull ache. This chronic pain usually is due to muscle strain and results from changes in the normal structure of the back with the development of a kyphosis and an increased lumbar lordo-

---

BOX 12-2
Classification of Osteoporosis

Unknown Causes
Primary osteoporosis (postmenopausal, senile)
Juvenile osteoporosis
Idiopathic osteoporosis

Endocrine Causes
Hypogonadism
Glucocorticoid excess (endogenous or exogenous)
Hyperthyroidism (endogenous or exogenous)
Primary hyperparathyroidism
Diabetes mellitus

Hematologic Malignancies
Multiple myeloma
Leukemia
Lymphoma

Systemic Mastocytosis

Heritable Disorders of Connective Tissue
Osteogenesis imperfecta
Homocystinuria
Ehlers-Danlos syndrome

Immobilization

Drugs
Alcohol
Chronic heparin administration
Anticonvulsants
Antimetabolites: Methotrexate, cyclosporine

Nutrition
Calcium deficiency
Scurvy
Malnutrition

Localized
Posttraumatic (Sudeck's osteodystrophy)
Postfracture
Regional (migratory) osteolysis

Miscellaneous
Postorgan transplantation
Primary biliary cirrhosis
Rheumatoid arthritis
Chronic obstructive pulmonary disease

From Slovik DM: In Barbieri R, Schiff I, editors: *Reproductive endocrine therapeutics*, New York, 1988, Alan R Liss.

BOX 12-3
Classification of Rickets and Osteomalacia

I. Vitamin D deficiency
  A. Dietary
  B. Insufficient sunlight exposure
II. Gastrointestinal disorders
  A. Postgastrectomy
  B. Small intestinal diseases with malabsorption (e.g., celiac disease)
  C. Hepatobiliary disease (e.g., biliary atresia)
  D. Pancreatic insufficiency
III. Disorders of vitamin D metabolism
  A. Pseudovitamin D deficiency (vitamin D dependent)
  B. Anticonvulsants
IV. Hypophosphatemic rickets and osteomalacia
  A. X-linked hypophosphatemic rickets (vitamin D resistant)
  B. Sporadic or adult-onset
  C. Fanconi syndrome
  D. Tumor-induced
  E. Phosphate depletion
V. Acidosis
  A. Distal renal tubular acidosis
  B. Ureterosigmoidostomy
  C. Drug-induced (e.g., chronic acetazolamide therapy)
VI. Chronic renal failure
VII. Mineralization defects
  A. Hypophosphatasia
  B. Aluminum
  C. Medications: fluoride, bisphosphonates
VIII. Defective matrix synthesis
  A. Fibrogenesis imperfecta ossium
IX. Miscellaneous
  A. Axial osteomalacia

From Slovik DN, Ritter JS: In Aronoff GM, editor: *Evaluation and treatment of chronic pain*, Baltimore, 1992, Williams & Wilkins.

History and Physical Examination

A detailed history and physical examination is necessary to identify risk factors and the secondary causes of osteoporosis. This should include looking for evidence of disorders that cause osteomalacia (Box 12-3). Other causes of chronic low back pain, including degenerative arthritis and disk disease, should be sought. An extensive history of medications, diet and exercise, and activity level should be obtained. The medication history should also include those that may increase the likelihood of falling (e.g., diuretics and psychotropic agents). Height should be measured initially and on follow-up visits.

Laboratory Tests

Selective laboratory tests should be obtained to help in the differential diagnosis of osteoporosis and osteomalacia (Box 12-4). Initial screening tests include a complete blood count, chemistry profile, and thyroid stimulating hormone level.

Second-level tests include a serum 25-hydroxyvitamin D level, which should be obtained in those women suspected of having vitamin D deficiency. This group most commonly

---

sis. Acute sudden back pain may be caused by additional fractures, microfractures, or muscle spasm. Progressive loss of height occurs as a result of these fractures. In severe cases the rib cage may come to rest on the iliac crest. Loss of height may also be seen as a result of narrowing of the intervertebral disc space, and back pain may be caused by problems such as spinal stenosis and disc disease.

In evaluating patients for osteoporosis, it is important to diagnose treatable and reversible causes, determine the extent of bone loss, and establish baseline data that can be followed.

Table 12-1
Approximate Proportions of Cortical and Trabecular Bone at Various Sites in the Skeleton

Site	Cortical (%)	Trabecular (%)
Hip		
Trochanteric region	50	50
Femoral neck	75	25
Vertebrae	40-60	40-60
Forearm		
Shaft	95	5
Distal	30-50	50-70

Modified from Cummings SR et al: *Epidemiol Rev* 7:178, 1985.

includes elderly persons living in northern climates, those with evidence of malabsorption, and those taking medications known to affect vitamin D metabolism, for example, phenytoin (Dilantin). A parathyroid hormone level should be obtained in suspected cases of primary (high serum calcium) or secondary (low serum calcium) hyperparathyroidism.

Blood and urine test results usually are normal in uncomplicated cases of osteoporosis. After a fracture the alkaline phosphatase level may be elevated. Very high levels of alkaline phosphatase suggest other metabolic bone diseases, including Paget's disease and osteomalacia. A small group of patients with osteoporosis has hypercalciuria; a 24-hour test of urine calcium will help to identify such patients.

Biochemical markers of bone remodeling are available. These include bone-specific alkaline phosphatase and osteocalcin, indices of bone formation, and urinary levels of pyridinolines and deoxypyridinolines (DPD) and serum and urine levels of type I procollagen telopeptides (CTX, NTX), indices of bone resorption. As yet they have not gained wide clinical utility because of lack of demonstration in individuals of predictive value for fracture risk or response to therapy.

However, biochemical markers of bone turnover including urine N-telopeptide (NTX) may be helpful in selected patients to assess bone turnover. For example, in a menopausal woman with a normal bone density who elects no specific treatment for osteoporosis prevention, a measurement of NTX indicating a low rate of bone turnover provides reassurance that this strategy of "watchful waiting" is reasonable. Baseline and follow-up measurement of urinary NTX may also be helpful in assessing response to antiresorptive therapy. A fall in urinary NTX excretion of 40% or more a few months after starting treatment suggests that significant bone loss during treatment is unlikely.

Radiologic Evaluation

Osteopenia is difficult to diagnose on spine radiographs because a decrease of at least 30% of bone mass may be necessary before osteopenia is evident. In osteoporosis, thinning and accentuation of the cortex and a relative increase in the vertical trabeculae (caused by a relatively greater loss of the horizontal trabeculae) may be evident. If a fracture is evident on x-ray film, then severe bone loss already has occurred unless the fracture was traumatic in nature. A radiograph of a tender area of the spine may show a fracture, but

other vertebrae also may show deformities. The types of fractures identified are (1) anterior wedge fractures caused by loss of anterior height, (2) biconcave fractures caused by the expansive forces of the intervertebral disks, primarily in the lumbar region, and (3) compression fractures with loss of both anterior and posterior height of the vertebrae.

Bone Density Measurements

Bone mineral density (BMD) measurements are the standard for assessing future fracture risk, and for diagnosing and monitoring patients with osteoporosis. Several techniques are available. Because the amount of cortical and trabecular bone and the rate of bone loss vary in different parts of the body (Table 12-1), it is helpful to have BMD measurements available for testing at various sites of the body. There is a more rapid loss of trabecular bone in the vertebrae in the early menopausal years compared with cortical bone loss in other sites of the body.

Dual-energy x-ray absorptiometry (DXA) is the most widely used technique. DXA has gained wide acceptance because of its accuracy, precision, low radiation exposure, fast scan time, and ease of measurement. Measurements of the lumbar spine (in the anteroposterior, and lateral projection), hip, total body, and forearm can be made using this technique. Because of its excellent reproducibility, DXA is preferred for the follow-up of BMD measurements. Peripheral DXA for appendicular measurements is also available.

Quantitative computed tomography (QCT) has been adapted to measure the mineral content in the axial skeleton. A conventional CT scanner with a calibration phantom and special software is used. This technique measures trabecular bone. Because trabecular bone is lost most rapidly after the menopause, QCT is a good technique for diagnosing osteopenia. QCT is not appropriate for long-term follow-up because of poorer reproducibility and higher radiation dose and cost. Peripheral QCT for appendicular measurements is also available.

Quantitative ultrasound methods are increasingly being used to assess skeletal status. Peripheral measurements especially of the calcaneus have been reported to be useful in diagnosing osteoporosis and fracture risk prediction. Its clinical utility in the general setting is currently being assessed.

Bone density measurements can be used to diagnose osteopenia before a fracture has occurred and can identify patients at risk of developing future fractures. Bone density tests cannot distinguish osteoporosis from osteomalacia.

BOX 12-5
Bone Mineral Density Reporting

T-Score
Standard deviations (SD) above or below peak bone mass in young normal sex-matched adults

Z-Score
Standard deviations (SD) above or below level in age-and-sex-matched adults

Bone density measurements can be compared with those of a young, normal population **t-score** (to determine if significant osteopenia has developed); to age-matched control subjects **z-score** (to determine if there has been excessive loss of bone); or to a **fracture threshold** (defined as 2.5 standard deviations below the mean for young adults of the same sex and race), a level below which fractures are more likely to occur.

When to Obtain Bone Mineral Density Measurements

Bone density measurements should be obtained when the results will influence the physician's therapeutic recommendations or the patient's compliance with them.

Recently, the National Osteoporosis Foundation in collaboration with many subspecialty societies published clinical guidelines for bone density testing. They suggest that BMD testing be obtained for the following groups:

- All postmenopausal women under age 65 who have one or more additional risk factors for osteoporosis (besides menopause)
  - Weight less than 127 lbs (58 kg)
  - Personal or family history of fracture
  - Current cigarette smoking
- All women aged 65 and older regardless of additional risk factors
- Postmenopausal women who present with fractures (to confirm diagnosis and determine disease severity)
- Women who are considering therapy for osteoporosis if BMD testing would facilitate the decision
- Women who have been on hormone replacement therapy for prolonged periods.

In addition, in 1998 the Bone Mass Measurement Act (BMMA) went into effect. This was federal legislation to standardize Medicare reimbursement for bone density. Eligible beneficiaries included:

- Estrogen-deficient women at clinical risk for osteoporosis
- Individuals with vertebral abnormalities
- Individuals receiving chronic glucocorticoid therapy
- Individuals with primary hyperparathyroidism
- Individuals being monitored to assess response to or efficacy of any FDA-approved osteoporosis drug therapy.

Bone mass measurements need not be obtained (1) for women who are on or are about to be placed on long-term hormone replacement therapy unless changes in therapy are being considered, (2) as an isolated screening program without an organized plan for patient management, or (3) for patients with established osteoporosis unless the measurement is being used as a baseline to evaluate subsequent treatment.

Table 12-2
World Health Organization Criteria for Diagnosing Osteoporosis

	T-Score
Normal: A value for bone mineral density (BMD) or bone mineral content (BMC) that is not more than on SD below the young adult mean value.	>-1
Osteopenia (low bone mass): A value for BMD or BMC that lies between one and 2.5 SD below the young adult mean value.	-1 to -2.5
Osteoporosis: A value for BMD or BMC that is more than 2.5 SD below the young adult mean value.	<-2.5
Severe osteoporosis (or established osteoporosis): A value for BMD or BMC more than 2.5 SD below the young adult mean value *in the presence of one or more fragility fractures.*	<-2.5

How to Interpret Bone Mineral Density Measurements

Measurements of bone density at any site can be used as a predictor of fracture risk at other sites. However, it appears that site-specific measurements are better; for example, DXA measurements of the proximal femur predict hip fracture risk better than measurements at other sites.

The T-score is the best measurement for risk assessment and can help confirm a diagnosis of osteoporosis (Box 12-5). The lower the T-score, the higher the risk for subsequent fractures. However, it will not predict who will fracture since other factors come into play (e.g., fall velocity, type of fall, direction of fall, protective padding).

The World Health Organization has used bone density measurements to establish diagnostic criteria for osteoporosis (Table 12-2). Although there may be some controversy as to the accuracy and validity of these definitions, it at least allows for a quantitative framework to discuss bone density measurement with patients.

How Often to Obtain Bone Density Measurements

According to the BMMA, the frequency of testing should be every 2 years, but more frequent BMD testing may be covered if determined to be medically necessary by the treating physician. There is some evidence that use of bone density testing as early as 1 year after initiation of treatment may be misleading.

PREVENTION AND TREATMENT

Any agent or means of achieving the maximum amount of bone at the time of skeletal maturity, reducing postmenopausal bone loss, or lowering the risk of falling will have long-term beneficial effects.

In establishing a program to prevent and treat osteoporosis, the approach should be divided into two parts: nonpharmacologic intervention (calcium, vitamin D, nutrition, lifestyle changes, exercise, and fall prevention) and pharmacologic options (hormone-replacement therapy, selective estrogen receptor modulators, bisphosphonates, and calcitonin).

Table 12-3
Calcium Supplements

Recommended intake of elemental calcium:	
Non–estrogen-deficient women: 1000 mg/day	
Estrogen-deficient women: 1500 mg/day	
Maximum intake in one dose for optimal absorption:	500 mg

Calcium Preparation	% Elemental Calcium
Calcium carbonate	40%
(e.g., Tums, Os-Cal, Viactiv, Caltrate)	
Calcium citrate (e.g., Citra-Cal)	21%

Nonpharmacologic

Calcium and Nutritional Factors

Calcium is essential for the development of a normal skeleton and for achieving peak bone mass. Inadequate calcium can reduce peak bone mass and hasten bone loss later in life. With advancing age, there is (1) a decrease in the dietary intake of calcium, (2) a decrease in intestinal absorption of calcium, and (3) a decreased ability to adapt to the low-calcium diets common in the postmenopausal years by increasing $1,25-(OH)_2$ vitamin D production and intestinal calcium absorption. The usual dietary calcium intake for postmenopausal American women ranges from 400 to 500 mg/day. This is much below the recommended daily allowance of 1000 mg/day for premenopausal or estrogen-treated postmenopausal adults and 1200 to 1500 mg for estrogen-deficient postmenopausal women. There is increasing evidence that calcium supplementation, together with vitamin D, may slow down bone loss and reduce fractures, especially in elderly women. To achieve adequate calcium intake, consumption of foods with a high calcium content such as milk and dairy products is recommended.

If sufficient calcium cannot be obtained from food sources, then calcium supplementation is necessary. The amount of elemental calcium varies with the different calcium salts (Table 12-3).

Many calcium preparations are poorly absorbed, especially in older persons. Calcium supplements are best taken with meals since food helps absorption. Calcium carbonate preparations are the most commonly used because they provide the highest amount of element calcium in each tablet and cost less, thus making compliance easier. However, they have limited solubility and absorption in patients with high gastric pH (e.g., elderly women taking antacid medication or with achlorhydria). If the calcium carbonate preparations are taken with food, absorption should be adequate. Other preparations such as calcium citrate may be better absorbed.

In healthy persons with no personal or family history of nephrolithiasis and who are not hypercalciuric, calcium supplements appear to be associated with minimal risk of nephrolithiasis. Patients with a personal or family history of calcium-containing kidney stones need to be evaluated before increasing their calcium intake.

Vitamin D

Numerous factors and disorders affect vitamin D metabolism in postmenopausal women. Any factor that reduces skin exposure to sunlight will diminish endogenous vitamin D synthesis. In elderly persons, vitamin D ingestion may be insufficient to compensate for the reduced exposure to sunlight. In addition, vitamin D deficiency may result from interference with the intestinal absorption of vitamin D.

Vitamin D deficiency is common in postmenopausal women with hip fractures and in elderly persons, especially those who are chronically ill, housebound, and poorly nourished.

Many therapeutic programs for osteoporosis include vitamin D in various doses, although its use in osteoporosis is based on scant scientific data. High doses of vitamin D can increase the intestinal absorption of calcium, but when it is given along with calcium supplementation, the risk for developing hypercalcemia and hypercalciuria is increased. Lower doses of vitamin D in the range of 400 to 800 IU (10 to 20 μg) per day should generally be sufficient to prevent vitamin D deficiency.

In contrast to calcium, which is quite abundant in foods, vitamin D is not generally available in sufficient quantities in unfortified foods. Thus, in postmenopausal women, especially older women, 400 to 800 units of vitamin D in the form of multivitamins is appropriate, especially if they receive insufficient sunlight exposure.

Nutrition

In addition to calcium and vitamin D, other nutrients are important for bone health. These include protein, calories, phosphorus, vitamins, and trace minerals. Adequacy of protein and calories is important to also maintain adequate nutrition, since malnutrition can be associated with decreased muscle mass, predisposition to fall, and less padding at the hip to absorb the energy if one fell on the hip. In addition, low serum albumin level is associated with poorer prognosis after hip fracture.

Lifestyle

It is important to stress the need to avoid excess alcohol and cigarette smoking.

Exercise

Physical exercise is important both in bone development and in the maintenance of the skeleton. Immobilization can produce rapid and significant bone loss. There is increasing evidence that exercise is beneficial to bone in helping achieve peak bone mass and preserving bone later in life. Bone adapts to physical and mechanical loads that are placed on it by altering its mass and strength. Exercise also helps strengthen back muscles, improve agility and mobility, and helps one develop a sense of well-being. There is no consensus as to which exercise programs are best, or how frequently and for how long one should participate in them. High-impact exercises (weight training), if tolerated, may stimulate new bone. Weight-bearing exercises are important, although water exercises or swimming can be helpful if the patient has a vertebral fracture associated with pain.

A referral to a physical therapist is sometimes necessary to initiate a program and ensure that it is properly instituted. This program should include gentle abdominal and back-strengthening exercises but should avoid exercises that produce flexion and sudden rotational movement of the spine. An exercise program for 30 minutes, three times a week if tolerated, would seem appropriate, but this regimen must be individualized. Walking briskly for 1 hour, three or four times weekly, also may help. Older postmenopausal women and even the frail elderly can tolerate and potentially show improvements in muscle strength, BMD, and balance in response to strength training and resistance exercise program.

Fall Prevention

Many factors can lead to falls including poor vision, frailty, medication (especially hypotensive agents and psychotropic agents), and balance disturbance. Each needs to be addressed appropriately. Padded hip protectors that can dissipate the energy generated from a fall may be helpful in preventing hip fractures in some patients. In addition, a safety check of the home is very important to remove objects that can lead to falls (Box 12-6).

Pharmacologic

Estrogen Replacement Therapy

Estrogen replacement therapy continues to be the primary means used to treat menopausal symptoms and prevent early postmenopausal bone loss. The beneficial effect of estrogen is most dramatic when instituted as close to the onset of the menopause as possible. Most studies have shown a reduction in bone loss and maintenance of bone mass when estrogen therapy is instituted, but there may be a small transient increase in bone mass within the first year when previous activated bone remodeling units are filled in.

Estrogen replacement therapy may slow down bone loss when instituted many years after the menopause and in women with established osteoporosis. Thus, even when postmenopausal women begin hormone therapy later in life, the rate of bone loss can be reduced. In this setting, estrogen is not really a "replacement" as it may be when instituted close to the menopause but acts rather as a pharmacologic antiresorptive agent.

Bone loss may begin several years before the actual menopause, but estrogen-replacement therapy should not be started in the premenopausal years unless there is evidence of estrogen deficiency or bone loss with repeated bone density measurements. Estrogen-replacement therapy will maintain the structural integrity and architecture of bone. Epidemiologic studies have reported a reduction of 50% to 60%

in hip, distal forearm, and vertebral fractures in women receiving estrogen-replacement therapy.

The minimum dose of estrogen to prevent bone loss has been thought to be 0.625 mg of conjugated equine estrogen daily or equivalent doses of other estrogen preparations. Several recent studies have shown that 0.3 mg of conjugated estrogens *with* calcium are effective in maintaining bone mass. The beneficial effect of estrogen on bone is independent of its route of administration.

The risks, benefits, indications, and various estrogen treatment regimens are discussed in Chapter 48.

Selective Estrogen Receptor Modulators

Selective estrogen receptor modulators (SERMs) represent a group of compounds, distinct from estrogen, that bind and interact with estrogen receptors. They thus have both estrogen agonist and antagonist properties depending on the target tissue.

Early studies with tamoxifen, a synthetic antiestrogen used for the treatment of breast cancer, showed a reduction in trabecular bone loss. Several years ago raloxifene (Evista) was approved by the Food and Drug Administration (FDA) for the prevention of osteoporosis and more recently for the treatment of osteoporosis. The Multiple Outcomes of Raloxifene (MORE) trial showed that raloxifene produced modest increases in BMD and reduced new vertebral fractures by 40% to 50%. In another report from the MORE trial, among postmenopausal women with osteoporosis the risk of invasive breast cancer was decreased by 76% during 3 years of treatment with raloxifene. Raloxifene does not produce endometrial hyperplasia but does lower low-density lipoprotein cholesterol; its effect on cardiovascular disease is not clear.

Raloxifene is taken orally in a dose of 60 mg/day for both the prevention and treatment of osteoporosis. It has no beneficial effects on menopausal symptoms and indeed sometimes causes hot flashes. Like estrogen, raloxifene increases the risk of deep vein thrombosis twofold to threefold.

Bisphosphonates

The bisphosphonates are potent inhibitors of osteoclastic bone resorption. They appear to bind to hydroxyapatite crystals, and when these crystals are taken up by osteoclasts, the osteoclast's ability to resorb bone is impaired. The various bisphosphonates currently in clinical use are formed by the addition of different side chains, thus effecting their biologic potency. They are resistant to biologic degradation, can be administered orally, and have a long skeletal half-life.

In addition to their use in osteoporosis, the bisphosphonates have been used for years in the treatment of disorders characterized by increased bone turnover including Paget's disease, malignancy-associated hypercalcemia, and skeletal complications from breast cancer and multiple myeloma.

Over a decade ago, etidronate (Didronel), a first-generation bisphosphonate, was reported in several studies to significantly increase vertebral BMD and lower the rate of new vertebral fractures. In these studies, etidronate, 400 mg/day, was administered for 2 weeks and then followed by an 11- to 13-week period in which no drug was administered but 1000 to 1500 mg calcium was given. This cycle was repeated for

24 to 36 months. However, etidronate was never approved by the FDA for use in the management of osteoporosis.

In 1995 alendronate (Fosamax) became the first bisphosphonate approved by the FDA for the treatment of osteoporosis (10 mg/day or more recently 70 mg once weekly). It has subsequently been approved for osteoporosis prevention in postmenopausal women (5 mg/day or 35 mg once weekly), fracture prevention (10 mg/day), for the treatment of glucocorticoid-induced osteoporosis (5 mg/day), and for the treatment of osteoporosis in men (10 mg/day).

In the 3-year multicenter study of postmenopausal women with osteoporosis, alendronate 10 mg/day significantly increased BMD of the spine (9%), femoral neck (6%), and trochanter (8%). There was a 48% reduction in the proportion of women with new vertebral fractures, a decreased progression of vertebral deformities, and a reduced loss of height. Subsequently, in the Fracture Intervention Trial (FIT) alendronate reduced the incidence of vertebral (47%), hip (50%), and wrist (47%) fractures and in the Early Postmenopausal Intervention Cohort (EPIC), alendronate (5 mg) prevented bone loss in early menopausal women.

Recently, risedronate (Actonel) was approved by the FDA for the prevention and treatment of postmenopausal osteoporosis and glucocorticoid-induced osteoporosis with an oral dose of 5 mg/day. In a large 3-year multicenter study postmenopausal women with osteoporosis and at least one vertebral fracture in response to risedronate, 5 mg/day, significantly increased BMD compared with placebo at the spine (4%), femoral neck (3%), and femoral trochanter (4%). There was a decreased cumulative incidence of new vertebral fractures by 41% and nonvertebral fractures by 39%.

The bisphosphonates are poorly absorbed (often <1%) and must be given on an empty stomach to maximize absorption. Alendronate and risedronate must be taken 30 minutes before the first food, beverage, or medication with 6 to 8 ounces of plain water. The patient must then avoid lying down for at least 30 minutes. Although in the clinical trials there was no increased incidence of gastrointestinal (GI) side effects with the bisphosphonates compared with placebo, there is the potential for developing upper GI symptoms and esophagitis, thus the need to remain upright after taking the drug and to avoid giving it to patients with GERD (gastroesophageal reflux).

Calcitonin

Calcitonin is a peptide hormone secreted by the parafollicular cells of the thyroid gland. Its physiologic role in calcium metabolism is unclear, but as a therapeutic agent it inhibits osteoclast function. Injectable synthetic salmon calcitonin was approved for the treatment of Paget's disease over 25 years ago and by the FDA for the treatment of postmenopausal osteoporosis over 15 years ago.

Several years ago nasal spray calcitonin (Miacalcin) was approved for the treatment of postmenopausal osteoporosis. The dose is 200 units (one spray) daily (alternating nostrils). Recently, the PROOF (Prevention Recurrence of Osteoporotic Fractures) study reported a 36% reduction in new vertebral fractures at the 200 IU dose, but other fracture data are not available, and a positive effect on hip fracture incidence has not been reported.

Other Potential Therapies

There are many pharmacologic agents under active investigation for the treatment of osteoporosis. Some of these are approved by the FDA for indications other than osteoporosis. Until they are proved to be effective in the treatment of osteoporosis and approved by the FDA, they should be considered experimental.

Combination Regimens

There is some evidence suggesting that combining estrogen or raloxifene with bisphosphonate therapy may produce changes in bone density greater than with either agent alone. Combinations of antiresorptive and anabolic agents would be ideal but are not available as yet.

Fluoride

The skeletal effects of excessive fluoride have been known for 60 years and include sclerosis of bones, ligaments, and muscle attachments. Fluoride has the potential for being an anabolic agent for the treatment of osteoporosis. Large increases in trabecular bone density have been reported with fluoride therapy. However, this is not accompanied by a decrease in vertebral fractures, and there may be an increase in nonvertebral fractures. Stress fractures are increased. Perhaps the problems are related to a combination of calcium deficiency and high fluoride levels in bone, thus producing osteomalacic bone with poor mineralization.

Parathyroid Hormone

Parathyroid hormone (PTH) produces an increase in osteoblastic activity and has a beneficial effect on the skeleton. In humans, studies with intermittent administration of human PTH have consistently shown a significant increase in trabecular bone mass of the spine, with no consistent change in cortical bone. The work with PTH fragments in the treatment of osteoporosis is experimental, but evidence of its beneficial effect is accumulating. This agent has potential for being an activator of bone and beneficial for the treatment of osteoporosis.

Growth Hormone and Growth Factors

Bone turnover and bone mass are increased in acromegaly. Growth hormone administration has been shown to increase skeletal remodeling in humans, and early results suggest it may have a positive effect on bone mass. With recombinant human growth hormone available, studies are underway evaluating this agent as a potential activator and beneficial agent for the treatment of osteoporosis.

Anabolic Steroids

A reduction in the blood levels of weak androgens has been reported with aging and in women with osteoporosis. Anabolic steroids or synthetic derivatives of testosterone appear to inhibit bone resorption and may weakly stimulate bone formation.

Vitamin D Analogs

Active metabolites of vitamin D have been synthesized and used in clinical trials for postmenopausal osteoporosis. Some reports suggest a beneficial effect with agents such as 1,25-dihydroxy vitamin D (calcitriol). The results, however, have not been consistent, and one of the major drawbacks is the potential development of hypercalciuria and hypercalcemia.

Thiazide Diuretics

These agents reduce urinary calcium excretion, and in some patients a positive effect on calcium balance and a reduction in bone loss and fractures have been reported. Thiazide diuretic therapy is indicated in patients with hypercalciuria but should not be instituted at this time specifically to prevent bone loss. Caution should be used in hypertensive, osteoporotic persons who may be receiving high doses of calcium and vitamin D in addition to a thiazide diuretic, because hypercalcemia may occur in this setting.

Statins

Some recent epidemiologic studies have reported an increase in bone formation and reduction in fracture risk associated with use of statins for lipid lowering.

SUMMARY RECOMMENDATIONS
Universal Recommendations: Nonpharmacologic

- Calcium 1000 mg/day: premenopausal women or postmenopausal women on HRT
- 1200 to 1500 mg/day in estrogen-deficient women
- Vitamin D: 400 to 800 IU/day
- Regular weight-bearing exercise
- Good nutrition
- Avoidance of tobacco use and alcohol abuse
- Fall prevention strategies

Pharmacologic

The lower the T-score with BMD measurements, the higher the risk for future fractures.

For women without established osteoporosis who are seeking risk assessment (early postmenopausal women):

- Clinical risk factors are not sensitive for detection of women with low bone mass who may be at increased fracture risk. Therefore bone density measurements can be used to assess for subsequent fracture risk inasmuch as low bone mass is a major determinant of fracture. However, bone density measurements should be obtained only when the results would influence treatment.
- Universal recommendation as above
- Pharmacologic options
  - Estrogen-replacement therapy is first choice in appropriate women (although many are starting to use raloxifene)
  - For women who cannot or will not take estrogen consider:
    Raloxifene: 60 mg/day
    Alendronate: 5 mg/day or 35 mg once weekly
    Risedronate: 5 mg/day

For women with established osteoporosis:

- Although 80% to 90% have age-related osteoporosis, it is important to consider other causes.
- Bone density measurements are helpful to follow so that changes in treatment can be made when necessary.

- Universal recommendation as above
- Avoid medications that can increase the tendency to fall, and survey the home to remove hazards
- Pharmacologic options
  - Bisphosphonates are first choice
    Alendronate (most experience) 10 mg/day or 70 mg once weekly
    Risedronate 5 mg/day
  - Other agents
    Raloxifene 60 mg/day
    Intranasal calcitonin 200 IU/day
    Estrogen-replacement therapy

BIBLIOGRAPHY

Black DM et al: Randomized trial of effect of alendronate on risk of fracture in women with existing vertebral fractures, *Lancet* 348:1535, 1996.

Bone Mass Measurement Act: *Federal Register* 63:121 (HCFA-3004-IFC), 1998.

Cosman F, Lindsay R: Selective estrogen receptor modulators: clinical spectrum, *Endocr Rev* 20:418, 1999.

Cummings SR et al: The effect of raloxifene on risk of breast cancer in postmenopausal women: results from the MORE randomized trial, *JAMA* 281:2189, 1999.

Dawson-Hughes B, Harris SS, Krall EA, Dallal GE: Effect of calcium and vitamin D supplementation on bone density in men and women 65 years of age or older, *N Engl J Med* 337:670, 1997.

Ettinger B et al: for The Multiple Outcomes of Raloxifene Evaluation (MORE) Investigators: Reduction of vertebral fracture risk in postmenopausal women with osteoporosis treated with raloxifene: results from a 3-year randomized clinical trial, *JAMA* 282:637, 1999.

Finkelstein JS et al: Prevention of estrogen deficiency-related bone loss with human parathyroid hormone (1–34): a randomized controlled trial, *JAMA* 280:1067, 1998.

Fleisch H: Bisphosphonates: mechanism of action, *Endocr Rev* 19:80, 1998.

Greenspan SL et al: Fall direction, bone mineral density, and function: risk factors for hip fracture in frail nursing home elderly, *Am J Med* 104:539, 1998.

Harris ST et al: The Vertebral Efficacy with Risedronate Therapy (VERT) Study Group: Effects of risedronate treatment on vertebral and nonvertebral fractures in women with postmenopausal osteoporosis: a randomized, controlled trial, *JAMA* 282:1344, 1999.

Hosking D et al: Prevention of bone loss with alendronate in postmenopausal women under 60 years of age, *N Engl J Med* 338:485, 1998.

Hulley S et al for the Heart and Estrogen/Progestin Replacement Study (HERS) Research Group: Randomized trial of estrogen plus progestin for secondary prevention of coronary heart disease in postmenopausal women, *JAMA* 280:605, 1998.

Kannus P et al: Prevention of hip fracture in elderly people with use of a hip protector, *N Engl J Med* 343:1506, 2000.

Kleerekoper M, Avioli LV: Osteoporosis: pathogenesis and therapy. In Avioli LV, Krane SM, editors: *Metabolic bone disease and clinically related disorders,* San Diego, 1998, Academic Press.

Layne JE, Nelson ME: The effects of progressive resistance training on bone density: a review, *Med Sci Sports Exerc* 31:25, 1999.

Leboff MS et al: Occult vitamin D deficiency in postmenopausal US women with acute hip fracture, *JAMA* 281:1505, 1999.

Liberman UA et al: Effect of oral alendronate on bone mineral density and the incidence of fractures in postmenopausal osteoporosis, *N Engl J Med* 333:1437, 1995.

Lindsay R et al. Addition of alendronate to ongoing hormone replacement therapy in the treatment of osteoporosis: a randomized, controlled clinical trial, *J Clin Endocrinol Metab* 84:3076, 1999.

National Osteoporosis Foundation: *Physician's guide to prevention and treatment of osteoporosis,* Belle Mead, NJ, 1999, Excerpta Medica.

Nelson ME with Wernick S: *Strong women, strong bones,* New York, 2000, G.P. Putnam's Sons.

Orwoll E et al: Alendronate for the treatment of osteoporosis in men, *N Engl J Med* 343:604, 2000.

Reginster JY et al: Long-term (3 years) prevention of trabecular post-menopausal bone loss with low-dose intermittent nasal salmon calcitonin, *J Bone Miner Res* 9:69, 1994.

Reid DM et al: Efficiency and safety of daily risedronate in the treatment of corticosteroid-induced osteoporosis in men and women: a randomized trial, *J Bone Miner Res* 15:1006, 2000.

Rosen CJ, Glowacki J, Bilezikian JP, editors: *The aging skeleton,* San Diego, 1999. Academic Press.

Saag KG, Emkey R, Schnitzer TJ et al for the Glucocorticoid induced osteoporosis intervention study group: Alendronate for the prevention and treatment of glucocorticoid-induced osteoporosis, *N Engl J Med* 339: 292, 1998.

Slovik DM: Osteoporosis. In Frontera WF, Dawson DM, Slovik DM, editors: *Exercise in rehabilitation medicine,* 1999, Human Kinetics.

Wang PS, Solomon DH, Mogun H, Avorn J: HMG-CoA reductase inhibitors and the risk of hip fractures in elderly patients, *JAMA* 283:3211, 2000.

Wasnich RD, Miller PD: Antifracture efficacy of antiresorptive agents are related to changes in bone density, *J Clin Endocrinol Metab* 85:231, 2000.

CHAPTER 13

Thyroid Disease

Douglas S. Ross

▦ EPIDEMIOLOGY

Virtually all types of thyroid dysfunction are more common in females than in males. Hypothyroidism resulting from autoimmune thyroiditis is three to five times more common in women than in men. Population surveys indicate a prevalence of hypothyroidism of 6% to 7% in older women, whereas up to 17% of women over age 60 have been reported to have positive antithyroid antibodies. Data on the true prevalence of hyperthyroidism are more difficult to interpret, since sensitive thyroid-stimulating hormone (TSH) measurements have only recently allowed for the detection of mild hyperthyroidism. Prevalence estimates have varied from 0.4% to 2.0% of the female population. Hyperthyroidism is 5 to 10 times more common in females than in males. Postpartum thyroid dysfunction occurs in 4% to 7% of women. Sporadic goiter or clinically solitary thyroid nodules are present in 5% to 7% of women in the United States and are at least four times more common in women than men. Differentiated thyroid cancer accounts for 1.6% of cancers in women and is three to four times more common than in men.

THYROID FUNCTION TESTS

The introduction and widespread use of sensitive TSH assays over the past several years have made the correct interpretation of thyroid function considerably more reliable than in the past. TSH is the pituitary hormone that regulates thyroid hormone production through negative feedback. The relationship between TSH and free thyroxine (T_4) concentrations is log-linear. Therefore relatively small changes in free T_4 concentrations are associated with large changes in serum TSH concentrations. With rare exceptions in ambulatory patients, elevated serum TSH concentrations indicate hypothyroidism, and subnormal or undetectable TSH concentrations indicate hyperthyroidism.

Screening Thyroid Function

The most precise single test to screen thyroid function is a serum TSH level. Many laboratories measure TSH and automatically add a free T_4 level if the TSH level is high to assess the degree of hypothyroidism, or add free T_4 and T_3 lev-

els if the TSH level is subnormal to assess the degree of hyperthyroidism. TSH levels alone are not a reliable indicator of thyroid function if the patient has pituitary or hypothalamic disease. Patients with a TSH-producing pituitary adenoma or partial pituitary resistance to thyroid hormone may have a normal or elevated TSH level associated with hyperthyroidism. Patients with non-thyrotropin-producing pituitary tumors or hypothalamic disease may have secondary or central hypothyroidism with subnormal, normal, or even elevated TSH values. Therefore some recommend that both TSH and free T_4 be measured as screening tests. A more cost-effective approach is to add free T_4 measurements to TSH levels only when there is a strong suggestion of thyroid dysfunction in a patient with a normal TSH level, or when there is a history suggestive of past or present pituitary or hypothalamic dysfunction. For example, TSH alone would be an inappropriate screening test in a woman complaining of fatigue who has galactorrhea or amenorrhea.

Free T_4 Measurements

Measurement of serum T_4 and triiodothyronine (T_3) concentrations is complicated by protein binding to thyroxine-binding globulin (TBG), transthyretin, and albumin. The free hormone hypothesis states that only the unbound or free hormone is readily available for uptake into tissues. Because more than 99% of T_4 is bound, the free hormone level is a very small fraction of the total hormone level and is difficult to measure. Free T_4 and T_3 measurements are estimated by several different techniques. Equilibrium dialysis is too tedious for routine measurements. Commercial kits estimating "direct" free hormone levels may give misleading values for patients with nonthyroidal illness or unusual binding protein abnormalities. The free T_4 index is calculated by multiplying the total T_4 by the T_3 uptake, a measure of the inverse of unoccupied sites on T_4-binding proteins. Because this test has been confused with serum T_3 measurements, it has been renamed the thyroid hormone-binding ratio (THBR), or index (THBI). This ratio is the patient's T_3 uptake divided by the average T_3 uptake for the laboratory.

$$\text{Free } T_4 \text{ index} = \text{Total } T_4 \times \frac{\text{Patient's } T_3 \text{ uptake}}{\text{Average normal } T_3 \text{ uptake}}$$

BOX 13-1

Causes of Abnormal Serum T_4 Values in Euthyroid Patients

Euthyroid Hyperthyroxinemia
TBG excess
Hereditary, estrogens, hepatitis, acute intermittent porphyria
Drugs (5-FU, perphenazine, clofibrate, heroin, methadone)
Familial dysalbuminemic hyperthyroxinemia
Abnormal transthyretin
Autoantibodies to thyroxine
Peripheral resistance to thyroid hormone
High altitude
Amphetamines
Inhibition of T_4 to T_3 conversion
    Amiodarone, ipodate, iopanoic acid, propranolol

Euthyroid Hypothyroxinemia
TBG deficiency
Hereditary, androgens, glucocorticoids, acromegaly
Nephrotic syndrome, drugs (danazol, colestipol-niacin,
    L-asparaginase), nonthyroidal illness
Displacement of T_4 from binding proteins
    Phenytoin, salicylates, fenclofenac, furosemide, phenylbutazone
Triiodothyronine (T_3) therapy

T_4, Thyroxine; *5-FU*, 5-fluorouracil; T_3, triiodothyronine; *TBG*, thyroxine-binding globulin.

The free T_4 index corrects abnormal total T_4 values caused by high or low serum levels of the major binding protein, TBG. TBG excess, the most common abnormality, is seen in hyperestrogenic states including pregnancy and in oral contraceptive or estrogen replacement therapy. TBG excess is associated with a normal serum TSH level, a high total T_4 level, a low THBI, and a normal free T_4 index. In contrast hyperthyroidism is associated with a subnormal TSH level, a high total T_4 level, a high THBI, and a high free T_4 index. Box 13-1 lists other causes of hyperthyroxinemia and hypothyroxinemia seen in euthyroid patients.

Thyroid Function in Hospitalized Patients

Assessment of thyroid function is considerably more difficult in critically ill hospitalized patients. Such patients have reductions in serum T_4 and T_3 values, and estimates of free T_4 levels are frequently unreliable. Serum TSH values may be subnormal in severely ill patients and may be slightly elevated during recovery from severe illness. Therefore both TSH and thyroid hormone measurements are required, and mild abnormalities in test results warrant repeat testing after full recovery from the acute illness.

HYPERTHYROIDISM
Clinical Presentation

Few women with moderate to severe hyperthyroidism delay seeking medical advice. However, mild and subclinical hyperthyroidism may be unnoticed for years. The most common complaints are weight loss, palpitations, tremulousness, heat intolerance, and sweating. Increased cardiac output may aggravate angina or congestive heart failure. Up to 20% of older patients may have atrial fibrillation, and such patients should have anticoagulation to prevent embolic sequelae.

Dyspnea may result from increased oxygen consumption and CO_2 production, respiratory muscle weakness, congestive heart failure, exacerbation of asthma, or tracheal narrowing caused by goiter. Increased gut motility results in hyperdefecation, malabsorption, and steatorrhea. Rarely anorexia or vomiting may occur.

A normochromic normocytic anemia develops primarily as a result of increased plasma volume. Ferritin levels are elevated. Graves' disease may be associated with leukopenia caused by antineutrophilic antibodies, idiopathic thrombocytopenic purpura, or pernicious anemia.

Hyperthyroidism increases the level of sex hormone-binding globulin, which increases the total estradiol level but decreases the unbound estradiol level. LH level is increased, but the midcycle LH surge is reduced and oligomenorrhea is common.

Thyroid hormone has a direct resorptive effect on bone, increasing the serum ionized calcium level and suppressing parathyroid hormone and 1,25-dihydroxyvitamin D levels; the result is a negative calcium balance. Alkaline phosphatase level may rise and remain elevated for months during and after treatment, presumably reflecting remineralization of osteoporotic bone.

Tremor, hyperactivity, emotional lability, insomnia, and proximal muscle weakness are commonly seen. Diagnosis of elderly patients may be difficult because conduction system disease masks the tachycardia; they may be more apathetic than hyperactive, and a goiter may not be readily appreciated.

Ophthalmopathy occurs in Graves' disease. Most patients have mild periorbital swelling and proptosis. More severe orbitopathy results in limitation of extraocular muscles and diplopia. Corneal ulceration from exposure and loss of vision caused by compression of the optic nerve are rare severe manifestations of autoimmune ophthalmopathy.

Differential Diagnosis

Conceptually there are two groups of disorders: hyperthyroidism caused by de novo synthesis of thyroid hormone associated with a *high* radioiodine uptake, and hyperthyroidism caused by release of preformed hormone from an inflamed gland associated with a *low* radioiodine uptake. Because treatment of these two groups of disorders differs, it is critical to obtain a radioiodine uptake in most hyperthyroid patients to prevent inappropriate therapy (Table 13-1).

Hyperthyroidism with an Elevated Radioiodine Uptake

Graves' disease is the most common form of hyperthyroidism in all age groups in the United States. It is due to stimulation of the TSH receptor by a specific thyroid-stimulating immunoglobulin (TSI). Some patients with autoimmune thyroiditis initially have a short-lived hyperthyroid phase presumably mediated by TSI ("Hashitoxicosis"). Toxic adenoma and toxic multinodular goiter are more common in older patients and result from autonomy of thyroid follicular cells. TSH-producing pituitary adenomas, partial pituitary resistance to thyroid hormone, and trophoblastic disease are rare causes of hyperthyroidism with an elevated radioiodine uptake.

Table 13-1
Differential Diagnosis of Hyperthyroidism

Disorder	Radioactive Iodine Uptake	Confirmatory Findings
Graves' disease	Increased	Thyroid scan: diffuse bilateral homogeneous uptake
Autoimmune thyroiditis ("Hashitoxicosis")	Increased	Clinical course: hypothyroidism follows
Toxic adenoma	Increased	Thyroid scan: focal uptake corresponding to a palpable nodule
Toxic multinodular goiter	Increased	Thyroid scan: patchy areas of increased and decreased uptake, possibly corresponding to palpable nodules

Rare causes
  TSH-producing pituitary adenoma
  Partial pituitary resistance to thyroid hormone
  Trophoblastic disease
	Increased	

Subacute granulomatous thyroiditis	Decreased	Tender thyroid, fever, elevated ESR
Subacute lymphocytic thyroiditis (painless thyroiditis)	Decreased	Nontender thyroid; may occur postpartum

Rare causes
  Factitious ingestion of thyroid hormone
  Struma ovarii
  Metastatic follicular thyroid carcinoma
	Decreased	

Iodine-induced hyperthyroidism	May be decreased if history of recent iodine load: radiocontrast dye, kelp tablets, povidone-iodine (Betadine) douche, amiodarone use	

TSH, Thyroid-stimulating hormone; *ESR,* erythrocyte sedimentation rate.

Hyperthyroidism with a Low Radioiodine Uptake

Hyperthyroidism produced by inflammation and destruction of thyroid parenchyma with release of stored hormone is associated with a low radioiodine uptake (usually <1%). Subacute granulomatous thyroiditis (de Quervain's thyroiditis) frequently follows a viral respiratory illness; the patient is acutely ill with fever and elevated sedimentation rate, and the thyroid is exquisitely tender. Subacute lymphocytic thyroiditis (silent or painless thyroiditis) is part of the spectrum of autoimmune thyroid disease, is not associated with thyroid tenderness, and may occur in the postpartum period or may recur in the same patient. Both classically appear with a hyperthyroid phase, followed by a hypothyroid phase and then recovery (Fig. 13-1). Occasionally the hyperthyroid or hypothyroid phase is mild and asymptomatic. In the absence of ophthalmopathy, it is impossible to differentiate painless thyroiditis from mild Graves' disease without radioiodine uptake testing. Other rare causes of hyperthyroidism with a low radioiodine uptake are factitious ingestion of thyroid hormone (thyroglobulin will be suppressed), struma ovarii (the uptake is elevated over the pelvis), and large deposits of metastatic thyroid follicular carcinoma.

Iodine-Induced Hyperthyroidism

The mechanism of iodine-induced hyperthyroidism is a substrate-induced increase in hormone synthesis, usually occurring in a nodular goiter with areas of autonomous function. If the iodine load was recent, however, the radioiodine uptake may be low as a result of washout of the tracer by the nonradioactive iodine. It is unusual for the uptake to be less

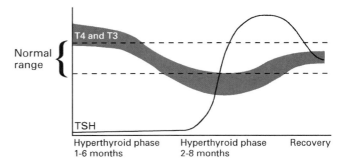

FIG. 13-1 Time course of changes in thyroid function test results in patients with subacute thyroiditis. A similar course is seen in patients with subacute granulomatous thyroiditis (de Quervain's thyroiditis), subacute lymphocytic thyroiditis (painless, silent, or postpartum thyroiditis), or radiation-induced thyroiditis.

than 1%, however. Common causes of iodine loads include radiocontrast dye, kelp tablets, povidone-iodine (Betadine) douches, iodine-containing expectorants, and amiodarone.

Diagnostic Tests

The diagnosis of hyperthyroidism is made by measuring serum TSH and thyroid hormone levels as described previously. A radioiodine uptake is necessary to distinguish hyperthyroidism caused by new hormone synthesis from hyperthyroidism caused by subacute thyroiditis. This may be inconvenient in the postpartum period, since it would interrupt nursing. The serum T_3/T_4 ratio ([ng/mg]) is usually

Table 13-2
Management of Hyperthyroidism

Disorder	Choice of Therapy
Graves' disease	
Young women	Radioactive iodine often preferred; thionamides or surgery
Young women anticipating pregnancy	Radioiodine or surgery to ensure euthyroidism before pregnancy
Pregnant women	Propylthiouracil
Toxic multinodular goiter or **toxic adenoma**	Usually radioactive iodine preferred
	Surgery if nodule or goiter presents cosmetic or obstructive problem
	Thionamides only as adjunctive therapy before or after ablative procedure
Subacute granulomatous or **lymphocytic thyroiditis**	No therapy or beta-blockers only
	Steroids and ipodate or iopanoic acid possibly helpful in severe cases
Iodine-induced hyperthyroidism	Discontinuation of iodides
	Beta-blockers if mild; thionamides if moderate to severe

greater than 20 in hyperthyroidism caused by Graves' disease or toxic goiter, and usually less than 20 in hyperthyroidism caused by subacute thyroiditis. Therefore one could defer the radioiodine uptake test in a mild case of suspected postpartum lymphocytic thyroiditis and follow the patient's course. A thyroid scan is necessary if one wishes to differentiate Graves' disease (diffuse bilateral homogeneous uptake) from a toxic nodule (focal uptake corresponding to a palpable nodule) or toxic multinodular goiter (patchy areas of increased and decreased uptake, possibly corresponding to palpable nodules).

Management

Beta-blockers are useful in all causes of hyperthyroidism unless contraindicated. Hyperthyroidism causes an increased number of beta-adrenergic receptors, and beta-blockers reduce tachycardia and tremulousness (Table 13-2).

Graves' Disease

The three major treatment options for Graves' disease are antithyroid drugs, radioiodine, or surgery. Antithyroid drugs are administered for one of two reasons. Most patients opting for surgery are pretreated with antithyroid drugs so that they are euthyroid preoperatively. Many patients opting for radioiodine are also pretreated with antithyroid drugs to alleviate symptoms more rapidly and prevent a transient radiation-induced exacerbation of hyperthyroidism. Alternatively one can take antithyroid drugs for 1 to 2 years or longer with the hope of obtaining a remission.

Propylthiouracil (PTU) and **methimazole** (Tapazole), the two antithyroid drugs available in the United States, inhibit iodination of tyrosyl residues on thyroglobulin, thus preventing new hormone synthesis. Therefore 2 to 8 weeks of therapy is necessary to exhaust preformed thyroid hormone stores and control hyperthyroidism. Initial doses are high

(PTU 100 mg tid or Tapazole 10 mg tid or 20 to 30 mg qd) to be certain that iodination is inhibited. Doses are then reduced to maintenance levels (PTU, 50 to 100 mg bid or methimazole, 5 to 15 mg qd), allowing some hormone to be synthesized to maintain a euthyroid state. Both drugs are poorly tolerated by 5% to 10% of patients because of nausea, vomiting, rashes, hives, joint pains, or fevers. There is a 0.25% or less risk of reversible agranulocytosis, and rarely PTU causes hepatocellular necrosis and methimazole causes cholestatic jaundice. Many physicians prefer methimazole to PTU because of its longer half-life, once-daily dosing regimen, and possible lower incidence of serious toxicity. Radioiodine therapy may also be less successful after PTU than methimazole. Methimazole has been associated with a rare scalp defect, aplasia cutis, if administered during pregnancy, and PTU is therefore preferred for the pregnant hyperthyroid patient (see Chapter 76). PTU, unlike methimazole, is protein bound; it crosses the placenta less readily and is poorly concentrated in breast milk. It is therefore also preferable for a mother who wishes to nurse while on antithyroid medication.

Patients who have been taking antithyroid drugs for 1 to 2 years have a 20% to 30% remission rate in the United States. This rate is as high as 40% for women with small glands, mild hyperthyroidism, high antimicrosomal antibody titers, and glands that shrink on antithyroid drug therapy. Remission rates are higher if antithyroid drugs are taken for 10 years.

Radioiodine is widely used in the United States. The only known complication of therapy is a 1% risk of radiation thyroiditis. This results in 2 to 3 weeks of thyroid pain, as well as exacerbation of the hyperthyroidism as a result of release of hormone stores from the radiation-induced inflammation. Patients with cardiovascular disease, elderly patients, or patients who are not tolerating the hyperthyroidism well are pretreated with antithyroid drugs to deplete hormone stores and ameliorate symptoms more rapidly. Radioiodine averages 8 to 16 weeks or longer for its full therapeutic effect. There is no increased risk of cancer after radioiodine treatment of hyperthyroidism; the dose to the ovaries is similar to that of pelvic computed tomography (CT), barium enema, or other diagnostic procedures; and a small study failed to show any increased risk in birth defects in babies of mothers who had previously received radioiodine. However, radioiodine cannot be administered during pregnancy since it would ablate the fetal thyroid tissue.

Surgery has become an unpopular treatment for Graves' disease. There is a 1% risk of hypoparathyroidism or recurrent laryngeal nerve damage; it requires general anesthesia and a hospital admission, and it leaves a scar. Patients allergic to antithyroid drugs can be safely operated on by using beta-blockade, ipodate, or iopanoic acid for 5 to 7 days preoperatively to reduce T_4 to T_3 conversion, and 10 days of saturated solution of potassium iodide (SSKI) treatment preoperatively to reduce gland vascularity.

Many centers consider the goal of radioiodine or surgical therapy to be permanent hypothyroidism. When this approach is taken, recurrent hyperthyroidism is rare, and thyroid hormone levels are easily controlled by levothyroxine administration. Some centers attempt to maintain a functioning remnant so that the patient is euthyroid. Many such patients may become asymptomatic but have persistent subclinical hyperthyroidism with its associated risks (see later discussion). Treatment failure, recurrent hyperthyroidism, or late development of hypothyroidism is more likely when a partially ablative approach is chosen.

Choice of Therapy. Young women with hyperthyroidism should be encouraged to avoid pregnancy until the condition has resolved. If they opt for a trial of antithyroid drugs, it is optimal that they wait for a year after stopping therapy to prevent recurrent hyperthyroidism during a pregnancy. Thus the onset of Graves' disease could delay a desired pregnancy for 3 years or longer, and women should consider more definitive therapy. It is generally advised that women wait for 6 months after receiving radioiodine before conceiving; however, this recommendation is not based on any data. Pregnancy plans can proceed shortly after a thyroidectomy.

New mothers may want to delay definitive therapy, since surgery and radioiodine treatment both result in a short absence from their baby and interrupt nursing. Patients who receive radioiodine are advised to avoid close contact with children and pregnant women for about 5 days.

Very large goiters may best be approached surgically. Very small glands and mild hyperthyroidism are more likely to be associated with a remission after a course of antithyroid drugs. Otherwise the choice of initial therapy is best discussed with the patient and many find one approach more attractive than another.

Toxic Nodules and Toxic Multinodular Goiter

Unlike Graves' disease, autonomous thyroid function rarely goes into remission (although iodine-induced hyperthyroidism may resolve). Ablative therapy is therefore offered early. When appropriate, patients are pretreated with antithyroid drugs, and when euthyroidism is achieved, one can proceed with surgery or radioiodine. For large goiters, especially if there is substernal extension, surgery may be more appropriate than radioiodine. Hypothyroidism after radioiodine administration is uncommon after ablation of a toxic nodule and is less commonly seen in patients with toxic nodular goiter.

Subacute Thyroiditis

Spontaneously resolving hyperthyroidism from subacute thyroiditis does not respond to antithyroid drugs or radioiodine because there is no de novo hormone synthesis. Beta-blockers are usually sufficient to ameliorate the symptoms of hyperthyroidism. In subacute granulomatous thyroiditis, pain is best treated with salicylates or nonsteroidal anti-inflammatory agents; however, severe pain and hyperthyroidism respond to a course of steroids. Steroids may also ameliorate the course of subacute lymphocytic thyroiditis in the rare patient who is not tolerating the hyperthyroidism, and ipodate or iopanoic acid may also be used to reduce T_4 to T_3 conversion. The hypothyroid phase is treated with levothyroxine.

Management of hyperthyroidism in pregnancy is discussed in Chapter 76.

HYPOTHYROIDISM
Clinical Presentation

Hypothyroid symptoms frequently have an insidious onset and the diagnosis may be delayed for years. Most commonly patients complain of weight gain, fatigue, cold intolerance,

and muscle cramps. These complaints are sufficiently nonspecific that many euthyroid patients are screened for possible hypothyroidism. Hypothyroidism is associated with a reduced cardiac output. Serum cholesterol and triglyceride levels are markedly elevated, thereby increasing the risk of atherosclerosis. In severe myxedema there may be pericardial and pleural effusions. Alveolar hypoventilation caused by a blunted response to both hypercapnia and hypoxia occurs. Sleep apnea may develop.

Decreased gut motility leads to constipation. Anemia may be normochromic as a result of hypoproliferation or may be related to iron malabsorption or associated pernicious anemia. Decreased free water clearance may lead to hyponatremia. Abnormal luteinizing hormone and follicle-stimulating hormone dynamics result in menorrhagia. In severe hypothyroidism increased prolactin and galactorrhea levels may be present.

Patients may be hypothermic and lethargic, with severe myxedema leading to coma. Peripheral neuropathies, abnormal visual-evoked responses, neurosensory deafness, carpal tunnel syndrome, and myopathies are all common. Patients characteristically have facial puffiness, hyperkeratosis and carotenemia, hair loss including the lateral third of the eyebrows, and brittle nails.

Differential Diagnosis

Worldwide the most common cause of hypothyroidism is iodine deficiency. However, endemic goiter is no longer found in the United States because of the iodination of the food supply. Virtually everyone in the United States with hypothyroidism has chronic lymphocytic thyroiditis (Hashimoto's disease), or the hypothyroidism is due to prior treatment of hyperthyroidism. Most patients with Hashimoto's thyroiditis have a characteristic symmetric and rubbery goiter, frequently with a palpable pyramidal lobe. Some patients, however, have an atrophic variant. Dietary goitrogens are not a cause of hypothyroidism in the United States but may play an important role in Third World countries. Lithium may cause goiter and hypothyroidism, frequently with positive titers of antithyroid antibodies. It is controversial as to whether all such patients have underlying autoimmune thyroid disease. Patients taking lithium should be monitored periodically with serum TSH level determinations. Iodine in large doses can also cause hypothyroidism in patients with underlying autoimmune thyroid disease. Amiodarone and other iodine-containing medications may be the cause of iodine-induced hypothyroidism (Box 13-2). (Note that iodine can cause hyperthyroidism in nodular goiter with autonomy and can cause hypothyroidism in autoimmune thyroiditis.)

Rarely patients with partial biosynthetic defects in thyroid hormone biosynthesis have goiter and mild hypothyroidism. The thyroid can be damaged through external radiation therapy. Hypothyroidism may be secondary or central, caused by pituitary or hypothalamic disease. Because subacute lymphocytic thyroiditis (silent thyroiditis) may present minimal symptoms, one should also consider the possibility that the hypothyroidism is transient, especially if it occurs in the postpartum period.

Diagnostic Tests

The evaluation of hypothyroidism is straightforward. If there is no history of radioiodine therapy, surgery, external radiation, or pharmacologic intervention; an elevated TSH

Differential Diagnosis of Hypothyroidism

More Common Causes
Chronic lymphocytic thyroiditis (Hashimoto's thyroiditis)
Prior treatment of hyperthyroidism (radioactive iodine or surgery)

Less Common Causes
Lithium
Iodine-containing medications (in setting of underlying autoimmune thyroid disease)
Congenital thyroid hormone biosynthetic defects
External radiation therapy
Transient hypothyroid phase of subacute granulomatous or lymphocytic thyroiditis

Table 13-3
L-thyroxine Therapy

Type of Therapy	Indications	Clinical Guidelines
Replacement	Hypothyroidism	Average replacement dose is 0.112 mg Aim for normal TSH level; T_4 level may be modestly elevated
Suppression	Thyroid nodule	Use lowest dose necessary to suppress TSH level to subnormal values Aim for TSH level 0.05-0.5 mU/L (third-generation TSH assay)
	Thyroid cancer	Generally suppress TSH level to 0.01 mU/L

TSH, Thyroid-stimulating hormone; T_4, thyroxine.

level; and a low free T_4 level strongly suggest autoimmune (Hashimoto's) thyroiditis. Antimicrosomal or antithyroid peroxidase (anti-TPO) antibodies (TPO is the microsomal antigen) are inexpensive and confirm the diagnosis of autoimmune thyroiditis. If the thyroid is symmetric and nonnodular, a thyroid scan adds little information and is not necessary. Although many "nodules" in a patient with hypothyroidism represent focal thyroiditis or fibrosis, both nodular goiter and Hashimoto's thyroiditis are common and can coexist. Hypothyroid patients with nodular thyroids therefore require further evaluation.

Management

Most endocrinologists prefer to use levothyroxine (T_4) preparations to treat hypothyroidism (Table 13-3) because their long half-life (6 to 7 days) results in very stable serum levels, even when a dose is inadvertently omitted. In contrast the half-life of T_3 is about 1 day, and frequently patients who are taking T_3 or T_3-containing preparations (thyroid extract or liotrix) have hypertriiodothyronemia shortly after ingestion of the hormone and may have subnormal concentrations before the next dose. Occasionally patients who take their medication in the morning may note palpitations or tremulousness. However, patients taking levothyroxine have on average slightly lower serum T_3 concentrations than euthyroid control subjects, and some patients taking a combination of levothyroxine with T_3 may feel better and do better on psychometric tests when 12.5 μg of T_3 is substituted for 50 μg of levothyroxine.

Conflicting recommendations relate to the rapidity with which thyroid hormone replacement is initiated. The degree of myxedema is not solely dependent on the measurement of free T_4 and TSH levels, but rather is assessed clinically on the basis of the duration and end-organ effects of hypothyroidism. One patient with a T_4 level of 0.5 μg/ml and a TSH level of 80 mU/L may have minimal symptoms, whereas another with similar values may be nearly comatose. Patients with more severe symptoms, elderly patients, and those with coexisting cardiopulmonary or other complicating illness are started gradually on thyroid hormone, whereas younger patients may be started on close to full replacement doses. For example, an 80-year-old hypothyroid woman with con-

gestive heart failure and coronary artery disease might be started on 0.025 mg of levothyroxine, with 0.025-mg increments every 3 to 6 weeks. A 65-year-old woman with no known cardiac disease might be started on 0.050 mg of levothyroxine with 0.025- to 0.050-mg increments every 4 to 6 weeks. In contrast, a healthy 21-year-old woman discovered to have hypothyroidism can safely be started on 0.100 mg of levothyroxine that is then titrated to achieve a normal TSH concentration. Changes in serum TSH level after a dose adjustment may take 4 to 6 weeks before a steady state is obtained. More frequent adjustments in levothyroxine dose can be made, but TSH values obtained earlier than 4 to 6 weeks after a dose adjustment do not fully reflect the effects of the prior change in dose. Levothyroxine dose should be titrated to normalize serum TSH concentrations to prevent subclinical hyperthyroidism and adverse skeletal and cardiac effects.

Management of hypothyroidism in pregnancy is discussed in Chapter 76.

SUBCLINICAL THYROID DISEASE
Subclinical Hyperthyroidism

Subclinical hyperthyroidism is a subnormal or undetectable serum TSH concentration with normal serum free T_4 and T_3 concentrations in an asymptomatic patient. The largest group of these patients is receiving thyroid hormone preparations. Many are being inappropriately treated with overzealous replacement therapy for hypothyroidism. Others are purposely given suppressive doses of levothyroxine to prevent growth of goitrous tissue.

Patients taking levothyroxine in doses that result in subclinical hyperthyroidism may have a reduction in bone density of 5% to 15% after 5 to 10 years. These changes are most pronounced in postmenopausal women who are not taking estrogens. The femoral neck, femoral trochanter, and radius are affected more than spinal trabecular bone. It is therefore critical that women receiving replacement doses of thyroid hormone have the dose titrated to normal serum TSH concentrations. Measurement of serum T_4 concentration alone is inadequate, as changes in serum free T_4 concentrations are insensitive and may not detect even 40% overtreatment with levothyroxine.

Another group of patients with subclinical hyperthyroidism includes those with very mild endogenous hyperthyroidism. Some of these patients have autoimmune thyroid disease; however, the majority are older women with multinodular goiters and autonomous function. In addition to reduction in bone density, older patients with subclinical hyperthyroidism have an increased risk of atrial fibrillation, and subclinical hyperthyroidism may also exacerbate angina or congestive heart failure. Thus it appears appropriate to consider treatment of patients with endogenous subclinical hyperthyroidism, especially in the presence of coexisting cardiovascular disease, osteoporosis, or a well-defined autonomous nodule.

SUBCLINICAL HYPOTHYROIDISM

Asymptomatic patients with an elevated TSH and normal free T_4 levels have subclinical hypothyroidism. In the United States most of these patients have Hashimoto's thyroiditis. In two randomized trials women with subclinical hypothyroidism did better on symptom scoring and psychometric testing when treated with levothyroxine. A subgroup with initial abnormal systolic time intervals became normal with treatment. There was no change in cholesterol levels, although subsequent studies have reported an improvement in high-density lipoprotein and low-density lipoprotein cholesterol levels in patients with subclinical hypothyroidism after treatment. If a patient with subclinical hypothyroidism caused by Hashimoto's thyroiditis also has a goiter, suppression of the TSH level to normal values will usually cause regression of the goiter.

SPORADIC NONTOXIC GOITER AND THYROID NODULES

Nodular thyroid disease is extremely prevalent in women. By palpation 6% of women have thyroid nodules. However, ultrasound demonstrates nodules in 21% to 28% of patients, and an autopsy series reports nodularity in 57% of patients. Unselected series suggest that the risk of cancer in a thyroid nodule is about 5%. The risk may be slightly less in patients with multinodular goiter. Therefore any solitary nodule or any palpable nodule within a multinodular goiter requires further evaluation. Controversy exists as to whether nonpalpable nodules less than 10 mm found on ultrasound require further evaluation; such nodules are found in more than 25% of women; however, in a recent study using ultrasound-guided needle biopsy, up to 4% of these nodules were malignant.

Diagnostic Tests

Fine needle aspiration (FNA) is frequently the initial diagnostic procedure. FNA is an office procedure done with local (Xylocaine) anesthesia and generally uses a 25-gauge needle. An adequate cytologic specimen is obtained in 90% of aspirates. *Macrofollicular lesions* (which include normal thyroid, colloid goiter, and true macrofollicular neoplasms) are benign and do not require surgery unless they are large and cause obstructive symptoms or are cosmetically unacceptable. Papillary cancer is readily diagnosed by needle aspirate and accounts for about 4% of nodules. *Microfollic-*

ular or *cellular lesions* are problematic, since they may represent benign microfollicular adenomas, well-differentiated follicular carcinomas, or benign hyperfunctioning adenomas. Therefore a thyroid scan is needed to distinguish the hyperfunctioning ("hot") nodules. Nonfunctioning ("cold") microfollicular lesions are excised to exclude capsular or vascular invasion consistent with the diagnosis of follicular carcinoma.

Alternatively (although less cost effective) one can start the evaluation with a thyroid scan. A total of 5% or more of thyroid nodules may be hyperfunctioning, and these nodules do not require further evaluation by needle aspiration. Nodules that are indeterminate on thyroid scan can be rescanned while the patient is taking levothyroxine ("suppression scan") to determine whether they are truly autonomous. Ultrasound adds little to the initial evaluation of the thyroid nodule. It is useful, however, in following nodule size when the examination is difficult or in defining anatomic characteristics in a multinodular goiter.

Management

Until recently levothyroxine has been widely used to suppress pituitary TSH production and to reduce or inhibit growth of goitrous tissue. Suppressive therapy by definition results in subclinical hyperthyroidism and may therefore be a risk for reduced bone density or atrial fibrillation (see previous discussion). Randomized trials have supported the use of suppressive therapy for nontoxic goiter. However, several short-term trials have failed to demonstrate a reduction in the size of solitary nodules in patients taking suppressive doses of levothyroxine. A meta-analysis suggests that slightly less than 20% of nodules regress as a result of levothyroxine therapy. Because many apparent solitary nodules are associated with multinodularity, when the thyroid is examined by ultrasound, it is possible that suppressive therapy may interrupt further goitrogenesis, and studies have demonstrated that patients taking levothyroxine are less likely to develop new nodules than patients receiving no treatment. If used, levothyroxine should be given in doses that result in subnormal but detectable TSH concentrations with the hope of minimizing any adverse effects of subclinical hyperthyroidism (Table 13-3).

BIBLIOGRAPHY

Arem R, Munipalli B: Ipodate therapy in patients with severe destruction-induced thyrotoxicosis, *Arch Intern Med* 156:1752, 1996.

Bunevicius R et al: Effects of thyroxine as compared with thyroxine plus triiodothyronine in patients with hypothyroidism, *N Engl J Med* 340:424, 1999.

Carr D et al: Fine adjustment of thyroxine replacement dosage: comparison of the thyrotropin-releasing hormone test using a sensitive thyrotropin assay with measurement of free thyroid hormones and clinical assessment, *Clin Endocrinol* 28:325, 1988.

Cooper DS: Subclinical hypothyroidism. In Mazzaferri EL, Bar RS, Kreisberg RA, editors: *Advances in endocrinology and metabolism*, vol 2, St Louis, 1991, Mosby.

Franklyn JA: The management of hyperthyroidism, *N Engl J Med* 330:1731, 1994.

Leenhardt L et al: Indications and limits of ultrasound-guided cytology in the management of nonpalpable thyroid nodules, *J Clin Endocrinol Metab* 84:24, 1999.

Ross DS: Subclinical thyrotoxicosis. In Mazzaferri EL, Bar RS, Kreisberg RA, editors: *Advances in endocrinology and metabolism*, vol 2, St Louis, 1991, Mosby.

Ross DS: Evaluation of the thyroid nodule, *J Nucl Med* 32:2181, 1991.

Ross DS: Thyroid hormone suppressive therapy of sporadic nontoxic goiter, *Thyroid* 2:263, 1992.

Schneider DL, Barrett-Connor EL, Morton DJ: Thyroid hormone use and bone mineral density in elderly women. Effects of estrogen, *JAMA* 271:1245, 1994.

Uzzan B et al: Effects on bone mass of long term treatment with thyroid hormones: a meta-analysis, *J Clin Endocrinol Metab* 81:4278, 1996.

Zelmanovitz F, Genro S, Gross JL: Suppressive therapy with levothyroxine for solitary thyroid nodules: a double-blind controlled clinical study and cumulative meta-analyses, *J Clin Endocrinol Metab* 83:3881, 1998.

CHAPTER 14

Hirsutism and Ovarian Endocrine Disorders

Ann E. Taylor

The definitions of hirsutism and acne vary for an individual woman, depending on her personal interpretation of normal. Hirsutism, acne, and irregular menstrual cycles are the most common manifestations of excess androgen effects in women. Some hyperandrogenic women have pathologically elevated androgen levels, some have a benign functional elevation of androgen levels, and some have normal androgen levels with either increased production and clearance of androgens, increased biologic sensitivity to circulating androgens, or increased personal sensitivity to the cosmetic impact of normal androgens. Because any woman who perceives herself to have excess androgenic effects may request a hormonal evaluation for reassurance, all disorders of hyperandrogenism in women will be considered together in this chapter.

The clinician's role in the management of such women includes the identification of pathologic hyperandrogenism in women who have not complained of symptoms; the exclusion of pathologic causes of hyperandrogenism; the choice of appropriate treatment with consideration of the woman's preferences; and the prevention of other disorders that are frequently associated with hyperandrogenism (Box 14-1).

▦ EPIDEMIOLOGY

The overall prevalence of hyperandrogenism in women is unknown, as excess androgens have previously been defined simply from the 95% confidence limits of levels in apparently normal women. Similarly, symptoms of hyperandrogenism such as hirsutism have also been defined from population studies. Determination of the prevalence of a subjective condition such as hirsutism is difficult as a result of ethnic variation and sometimes unrealistic social norms. Ferriman and Gallwey's study of 430 women in London indicated that normal women almost never had terminal hair on the upper back or upper abdomen, and only 3% and 10% had terminal hair on the sternum and chin, respectively. Conversely, a significant number of normal women have terminal hair on the upper lip and linea alba.

The majority of women with hirsutism have at least one elevated androgen level or an increased androgen production rate, if one looks hard enough. Because of more recent evidence of potential adverse consequences of hyperandro-

genism, new studies are needed to determine whether there is a "safe" level of androgens for women, above which one should definitely treat the condition.

The prevalence of hyperandrogenism in specific clinical conditions has been studied recently. In populations of women of reproductive age in the southern United States, Greece, and Spain, the prevalence of polycystic ovary syndrome (PCOS) ranges from 4% to 7%, respectively. Of those women, 10% to 38% were significantly obese, with a body mass index greater than 30 kg/m^2. Approximately 5% of amenorrhea and approximately 15% of female infertility in premenopausal women are estimated to be attributable to hyperandrogenism. Up to 38% of women with diffuse alopecia have evidence of hyperandrogenism, as do up to 50% of women with acne.

The distribution of hyperandrogenic symptoms varies with race. Asian and Native American women have relatively little body hair of any type, whereas women of Mediterranean extraction frequently have moderately heavy facial and body hair. Certain racial groups, particularly African-American and Hispanic women, appear to have a greater frequency of the metabolic abnormalities such as acanthosis nigricans and insulin resistance that are associated with hyperandrogenism, whereas other groups, such as Asians, appear to have a higher frequency of acne.

PATHOPHYSIOLOGY

Androgenic steroids include **testosterone,** the most potent androgen; **dihydrotestosterone,** a more potent tissue metabolite of testosterone derived especially from skin and skeletal muscle; and the weaker androgenic precursors androstenedione, dehydroepiandrosterone **(DHEA),** and its sulfoconjugate **DHEA-S.** Normal women secrete testosterone in approximately equal amounts from the adrenal glands and the ovaries; the result is a serum level that is 5% to 20% that of men. Testosterone and other androgens circulate bound to both sex hormone–binding globulin (SHBG) and other binding proteins, including albumin, so that increased amounts of SHBG result in less free and biologically available hormone. SHBG is produced in the liver, increased by estrogens, and decreased by androgens and insulin. Thus free testosterone levels are a better marker of

---

BOX 14-1
Management Goals

Identify women with hyperandrogenism
  Exclude pathologic causes of hyperandrogenism
Prevent secondary disease
  Endometrial hyperplasia and endometrial cancer
Ameliorate associated diseases
  Obesity
  Insulin resistance
  Hyperlipidemia
Regulate menses
Treatment cosmetic complaints and infertility

BOX 14-2
Differential Diagnosis of Excess Hair in Women

Hirsutism (Increased Sexual Hair)
Common
Idiopathic hirsutism   60%
Polycystic ovary syndrome   30%
Rare   10%
Medications
    Androgenic oral contraceptives
    Danazol
Hyperprolactinemia
Hyperthecosis
Congenital adrenal hyperplasia
Ovarian tumors
Adrenal tumors
Severe insulin resistance syndromes

Hypertrichosis (Increased Total Body Hair)
Drugs
    Dilantin
    Minoxidil
    Cyclosporine
Systemic illness
    Hypothyroidism
    Anorexia nervosa
    Malnutrition
    Porphyria
    Dermatomyositis

---

androgenic activity than is total testosterone. Androgens are aromatized to estrogens in peripheral tissues, especially fat.

The **effects of increased androgens** increase with the severity of the defect. Sebum production is increased at relatively low androgen levels; and *acne, hirsutism, oligomenorrhea, male-pattern balding, deepening of the voice, increased muscle mass,* and *clitoromegaly* sequentially become more apparent as androgen levels increase to more pathologic levels. Body hair can be classified as androgen-dependent hirsutism, including dark terminal hairs on the face, chest, abdomen, and back, and androgen-independent hypertrichosis, as on the scalp, arms, and legs. Once androgen levels are sufficient to cause differentiation of soft vellus hair to darker, thicker terminal hair, those follicles remain more sensitive to androgens thereafter.

Androgen excess in women has several **pathophysiologic consequences** in addition to the cosmetic manifestations. The prolonged amenorrhea is associated with chronic endometrial stimulation by unopposed estrogens and an increased risk of *endometrial hyperplasia* and *endometrial cancer.* Most of the cases of endometrial cancer in young women occur in association with oligomenorrhea and evidence of hyperandrogenism.

DIFFERENTIAL DIAGNOSIS

The differential diagnosis of hirsutism is outlined in Box 14-2. The most important differentiation for the clinician to make is between malignant and benign disease.

After idiopathic hirsutism, **PCOS** is the most common cause of hirsutism and other hyperandrogenic symptoms in women. PCOS can be diagnosed when women have signs or symptoms of androgen excess, whether or not serum androgen levels are elevated, in association with menstrual irregularity and in the absence of any of the pathologic processes described. Both the ovaries and adrenal glands can contribute to the excess androgen level in this heterogeneous syndrome. Obesity tends to make the hirsutism, menstrual irregularity, and insulin resistance worse; and weight loss will improve menstrual function and hirsutism in at least some women (see Chapter 46).

Hyperprolactinemia has been associated with elevated DHEA-S levels and hirsutism. Typically the prolactin level

elevations are mild, and there is no evidence of pituitary tumor on scans. Prolactin may increase adrenal androgen production, if adrenocorticotropic hormone (ACTH) secretion is intact.

Exogenous hormone administration should be easily determined by the clinician; it includes covert or overt androgen ingestion for muscle building or for female to male transsexual conversions. Some medications given for other purposes may have androgenic side effects. For example, the progestin norgestrel, commonly used in oral contraceptives, is particularly androgenic.

Genetic defects in the androgen synthesizing enzymes of the ovary and adrenal gland that cause a clinical picture indistinguishable from that of PCOS have been identified. The most common of these is 21-hydroxylase deficiency, also known as **congenital adrenal hyperplasia** or adrenogenital syndrome. The classic form may cause salt wasting and an adrenal insufficiency crisis in a newborn female with ambiguous genitalia, whereas the nonclassic form typically presents at puberty with excess androgen production with or without menstrual irregularities. The phenotype appears to depend on both the alleles acquired and on predisposing factors, as affected members of the same family may have very different symptoms. Other forms of congenital adrenal hyperplasia involving other enzymes in the cortisol production pathway are rare but should be considered in a woman with a known family history, in a high-risk ethnic group such as the Ashkenazi Jews, or in cases of unexplained hypertension.

Perhaps the most difficult differential diagnosis to make is in the woman who clearly develops new onset hirsutism after the menopause. This is exactly the situation in which one is most concerned about the development of an androgen-secreting ovarian tumor. However, in many cases, it appears that these patients instead have **hyperthecosis,** with exaggerated androgen secretion from the remaining ovarian thecal cells in response to stimulation by postmenopausal levels of gonadotropins. Many patients, if not all, with premenopausal hyperthecosis also have insulin resistance, such that this condition overlaps with PCOS in the younger age group. The condition in postmenopausal women is rare enough that it is unclear whether it merely represents unmasking of prior PCOS or is a separate entity without the associated insulin abnormalities. Unfortunately, at this time, the only way to definitively establish the diagnosis is to perform oophorectomy and careful pathology to exclude an ovarian tumor.

Fortunately **androgen-secreting tumors** are rare. Steroid-secreting ovarian tumors represent approximately 5% of all ovarian tumors. Androgen-secreting adrenal tumors are similarly rare. Adrenal tumors may appear with signs and symptoms of Cushing's syndrome caused by coincident excess of cortisol production as well as of androgens. Ovarian or adrenal tumors should be suspected when the onset of hyperandrogenic symptoms is abrupt, rapid, and not associated with puberty, and when symptoms are especially severe when compared to the woman's family history.

⚕ EVALUATION OF HYPERANDROGENISM
History and Physical Examination

All women who have hyperandrogenic complaints require a detailed history and physical examination designed to elicit symptoms or signs suggestive of more sinister causes of hyperandrogenic symptoms, establish a primary diagnosis, and evaluate associated conditions and long-term risk factors. The **history** should focus on the *time course of the symptoms,* including the age at onset and the rate of progression. A *menstrual history,* including menarche, regularity, conceptions, use of oral contraceptives, and symptoms of ovulation (cervical mucus, mittelschmerz, molimina), helps determine the severity of the hyperandrogenism. Also important are fluctuations and *correlations of symptoms and menstrual regularity with body weight,* as well as a history of all *medications* that might have androgenic side effects or cause hypertrichosis. Lastly, a *family history* of ethnic background, hirsutism, oligomenorrhea, infertility, diabetes, obesity, and insulin resistance can be helpful in ruling out pathologic conditions, in indicating an increased likelihood of congenital adrenal hyperplasia, and in identifying long-term cardiovascular risk factors.

Important **physical examination** features include *height, weight, waist-to-hip ratio,* and *pattern of body fat distribution* (abdominal, buffalo hump, supraclavicular fat). In the examination of the skin, the location and quantity of *terminal hair and acne* should be carefully documented, so that response to therapy can be more objectively assessed. Other signs of virilization include deepening of the *voice,* temporal or crown *balding,* increased *muscle mass,* and *clitoromegaly.* A clitoral index (length $\times$ width) >35 mm^2 is above the normal range. In addition, a careful examination

should include consideration of associated abnormalities, including elevated *blood pressure, xanthomas,* and *acanthosis nigricans,* which may be seen at the axillae, knuckles, knees, elbows, inguinal crease, and nape of the neck. Evidence of excess cortisol production, such as wide purple *abdominal striae, thin skin, bruising,* and *proximal muscle weakness,* should be documented. The breasts should be examined for *galactorrhea.* Finally, *adrenal and ovarian masses* should be ruled out by careful abdominal and pelvic examinations.

Diagnostic Tests

The laboratory evaluation for androgen excess symptoms depends on the clinical course, the clinician's concern about possible sinister causes, and the risk factors for other conditions. The mildly hirsute woman with a gradual onset of symptoms and perfectly regular menstrual cycles may need no evaluation at all. A woman with peripubertal onset of hirsutism and acne who also has menstrual dysfunction should have a simple evaluation for the other known causes of menstrual dysfunction, including a pregnancy test, prolactin, thyroid-stimulating hormone, and follicle-stimulating hormone.

Only for those women in whom virilization is significant, or in whom one is concerned about a change in clinical course, may serum androgen testing be necessary. The only validated tests to rule out androgen-secreting tumors are total testosterone and DHEA-S. Further testing, as follows, or referral to an endocrinologist is advised if there is evidence of more serious disease or if the androgen levels are excessive testosterone greater than 150 ng/ml or DHEA-S greater than 800 μg/dl (Boxes 14-3 and 14-4).

The best validated screening test for ovarian androgen-secreting tumors is serum **total testosterone** levels. Several investigators have shown that total testosterone levels above 150 to 200 ng/dl are relatively sensitive, but are not specific tests for identifying androgen-secreting tumors. In one series all women with tumors had a total testosterone level greater than 200 ng/dl, but only 2 of 11 women with such high testosterone levels had tumors.

The androgen precursor **DHEA-S** derives at least 95% from the adrenal gland and therefore is considered a good marker for adrenal androgen hypersecretion. The upper limit of DHEA-S for normal young women is about 500 μg/dl. Women with PCOS can have DHEA-S levels up to about 900 μg/dl without evidence of tumor. However, DHEA-S is typically suppressed in patients with adrenal adenomas, and the level is often normal in patients with adrenal carcinoma. Also adrenal androgen secretion decreases after about age 30, so age-related normal subjects must be studied to determine elevated levels in older women (Fig. 14-1).

All women with menstrual irregularities should have a screening **prolactin** level. Because the prolactin level is increased by food, stress, and breast examinations, any woman with an elevated level should have the prolactin determination repeated at a time when she is fasting and has not had an examination. Hyperprolactinemia is discussed in detail in Chapter 15.

A **24-hour urine collection for 17-ketosteroids,** which will detect androgen precursors, is an important part of the evaluation for pathologic hyperandrogenism, because some tumors may not be sufficiently differentiated to synthesize

---

BOX 14-3
Diagnostic Tests

Screening Laboratory Tests
Free testosterone
DHEA-S
24-hour urine collection for creatinine and 17-ketosteroids (add urine free cortisol when symptoms of Cushing's syndrome present)

Second-Level Tests
LH and FSH
Prolactin
Pelvic ultrasound to evaluate endometrial thickness, ovarian size, presence of abnormal ovarian masses
Oral glucose tolerance test for glucose and insulin (especially if obesity or acanthosis present)
Fasting lipids
Liver function tests if planned oral contraceptive therapy

Third-Level Tests (Usually by an Endocrinologist or Gynecologist)
ACTH stimulation test for cortisol and 17-OH progesterone (to screen for congenital adrenal hyperplasia)
Dexamethasone suppression test (to screen for adrenal tumor)
Abdominal CT (to screen for adrenal tumor)
Ovarian and adrenal vein sampling
Müllerian-inhibiting substance level as a marker for sex-cord tumors
Laparoscopy or laparotomy

DHEA-S, Dehydroepiandrosterone sulfate; *LH,* luteinizing hormone; *FSH,* follicle-stimulating hormone; *ACTH,* adrenocorticotropic hormone; *CT,* computed tomography.

BOX 14-4
Evaluation of Hyperandrogenism

Initial Screening
Free testosterone level
DHEA-S level
Prolactin level (if oligorrhea or amenorrhea present)

Indications for Further Evaluation or Referral
History
Abrupt, rapid onset of symptoms
Symptoms of Cushing's syndrome or malaise suggestive of a tumor
Severity out of proportion to family history
Strong family history suggestive of steroidogenic enzyme dysfunction
Menstrual irregularity or infertility
Significant patient concern
Physical examination
Evidence of higher androgen levels
  Terminal hair on chin, sternum, upper back, or upper abdomen
  Clitoral index (height × width) >35mm^2
  Temporal balding
  Deepening of voice
Evidence of associated diseases
  Abdominal or pelvic mass
  Acanthosis nigricans
  Obesity
Galactorrhea
Diagnostic testing
Free testosterone level greater than 2 ng/dl

DHEA-S, Dehydroepiandrosterone sulfate.

---

the more potent androgens at the final steps of the pathway. Fewer than 1% of normal women under age 30 will have a 17-ketosteroid level greater than 17 mg/24 hr. Abdominal computed tomography (CT) may be indicated to rule out an adrenal mass. Because nonfunctioning and benign adrenal adenomas are so common, an abdominal CT should not be done unless there is a significant elevation of an adrenal androgen level. Just as with DHEA-S levels, it is critical to evaluate 17-ketosteroid levels on a nomogram that adjusts for age, because of the gradual decline in normal levels after about age 30 (Fig. 14-1).

If an ovarian tumor is suspected, high-resolution **pelvic ultrasonography,** often with a transvaginal probe that gets closer to the ovaries than previous transabdominal transducers, allows identification of ovarian cysts as small as 2 to 3 mm. The sensitivity and specificity of ultrasound for the diagnosis of ovarian tumors in hyperandrogenic women are unknown, as hyperandrogenic women are typically young and intermittently grow normal physiologic cysts. Suspicious findings include large cysts and complex cysts that do not resolve spontaneously over 2 to 4 weeks. However, small hilar cell ovarian tumors can produce large amounts of androgens and still be invisible on ultrasound, and even on direct ovarian visualization at surgery.

Ultrasound can also be used to identify the classic ovarian morphology of PCOS. This morphology is identified by a ring of small peripheral follicles, typically each less than 8 mm, with an increased amount of central stroma. Such ovaries are typically, but not always, enlarged. Of a large series of women with hirsutism, 83% had the classic appearance of polycystic ovaries on ultrasound. In addition, 23% of regularly menstruating women also had this characteristic, raising the possibilities that either the predisposition for PCOS is much more common than previously believed or that the morphology is merely a variant of normal. The ultrasound characteristics of PCOS cannot be used to rule out other causes of hyperandrogenism, however, because the same ovarian morphology has been seen in women with hyperandrogenism of different primary causes, including exogenous androgen administration and congenital adrenal hyperplasia.

Although the "gold standard" for screening for congenital adrenal hyperplasia (CAH) is still the 1-hour ACTH-stimulation test, recent studies have demonstrated that a single **17-hydroxyprogesterone level,** if obtained in the morning and in the follicular phase (around day 21), is adequate to rule out CAH if the value is less than 2 ng/ml. As a rule, a stimulated 17-OH progesterone level greater than 20 ng/ml is most consistent with homozygous enzyme deficiency, whereas stimulated levels less than 4 ng/ml are normal. Stimulated levels between 4 and 10 ng/ml are indeterminate: some such women are heterozygotes for 21-OH deficiency, and some have a functional abnormality of androgen production that may be reversible.

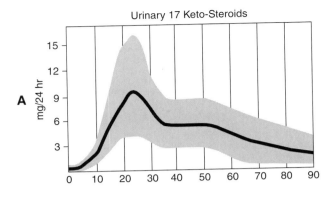

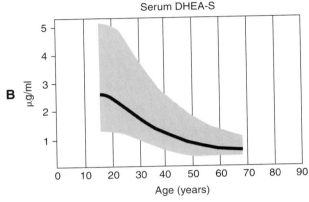

FIG. 14-1 Urinary 17-ketosteroids (mg/24 hr) **(A)** and serum DHEA-S levels **(B)** in normal women with aging. Note that there is a significant decline in both measures of adrenal androgens after age 30, long before the menopause. **A,** The shaded area represents 97% to 98% of the values in normal women. **B,** The shaded area represents the log equivalent of the mean ± 2 SD and represents about 90% of the measured values. (**A,** Modified from Hamburger C: *Acta Endocrinol* 1:19, 1948; **B,** Modified from Orentreich N et al: *J Clin Endocrinol Metab* 59:551, 1984.)

✴ MANAGEMENT
Goals of Management

The woman who has hirsutism or acne generally has one goal in mind, the clarification of her skin and normalization of her menses. The health professional has several additional management goals including primarily the exclusion of pathologic causes of hyperandrogenism. Women with a rapid onset of symptoms, a strong family history suggestive of a steroidogenic enzyme dysfunction, free testosterone levels greater than 2 ng/dl, or refractory response to initial treatment should be referred to an endocrinologist for further evaluation.

In the majority of women who do not have these features, the primary care provider must next consider the secondary health effects associated with hyperandrogenism such as endometrial cancer, insulin resistance, and cardiovascular risk factors. A careful history of menstrual frequency and abnormal vaginal bleeding should be obtained. Women with oligomenorrhea will need to be treated to prevent endometrial hyperplasia.

All women with PCOS should also be assessed for cardiovascular risk factors, including family history, waist-to-

---

BOX 14-5
Therapy

Drugs
Oral contraceptives: Ethinyl estradiol 20 to 35 μg plus low dose of weakly androgenic progestin (0.4 to 1 mg norethindrone or ethynodiol diacetate, 0.15 mg desogestrel, or 0.18 to 0.25 mg norgestimate)

Antiandrogens: Spironolactone 50 to 100 mg bid
Progestins: Medroxyprogesterone acetate 5 mg qd for 10 to 14 days/month
Oral micronized progesterone 200 mg qd for 10 to 14 days/month
Vaginal progesterone gel (4%) (Crinone) qod × 6 doses/month

Other
Weight loss
Cosmetic (electrolysis, bleaching, tweezing, shaving)

---

hip ratio, blood pressure, and fasting lipid levels. It may be advisable to perform an oral glucose tolerance test for insulin levels in women who are obese or have other cardiovascular risk factors, if such information will improve a woman's motivation to lose weight or change her diet. However, the predictive value of such testing in women with PCOS has yet to be established.

Choice of Therapy

Women with hirsutism or acne and regular menses may be satisfied with cosmetic approaches such as tweezing, bleaching, and electrolysis once pathologic causes have been ruled out. Women whose primary concern is menstrual irregularity can be treated with cyclic progestins or oral contraceptives. Women with elevated adrenal androgen levels associated with elevated prolactin levels may improve with low-dose bromocriptine therapy.

Most other women can be treated with one or more of the specific antiandrogen therapies available. In general these therapies can be initiated by the primary care physician, if there is no evidence of a pathologic cause of the hyperandrogenism. All treated women should be advised that the hair follicle is viable for up to 6 months, and therefore a full 6-month trial of medication will be required before an appropriate cosmetic response can be assessed.

Because of their effect of regulating menses as well as reducing androgen levels, **oral contraceptives** remain the drug of choice in women not currently desiring pregnancy (Box 14-5). Combined pills work by several additive mechanisms, including both suppression of gonadotropins leading to secondary suppression of ovarian androgen production, and increase of estrogen levels leading to increased SHBG levels and decreased free androgen levels.

In general the lowest dose pills (such as Ovcon and Modicon or Brevicon, which contain 0.4 and 0.5 mg norethindrone, respectively, with 35 μg of ethinyl estradiol) or the multiphasic pills should be tried first. In addition, pills containing the least androgenic progestins should be used. Thus pills (such as Ortho-Cept, Desogen, Ortho-Tricyclen, and Ortho-Cyclen) containing desogestrel or norgestimate that have the least androgenic effect on lipids may also be the best for women with PCOS, although this assumption has not yet been formally tested. Some women with PCOS who have relatively large and active ovaries, as well as elevated luteinizing hormone (LH) levels, may need slightly higher dose pills to prevent breakthrough bleeding. For these women, higher progestin doses (such as found in Norinyl or Ortho-Novum 1/35) or the more estrogenic progestin ethynodiol diacetate (found in Demulen 1/35) are more effective. Pills containing the more androgenic progestins levonorgestrel, norgestrel, and norethindrone acetate (such as Nordette, Lo-Ovral, and Lo-Estrin, respectively) should be avoided.

The use of oral contraceptives should be carefully considered in women with hyperprolactinemia, as estrogen tends to increase prolactin levels and could induce tumor growth. The suppression of androgen levels by oral contraceptives does not eliminate the possibility of an ovarian or adrenal tumor.

Women with irregular menses and fewer cosmetic symptoms may prefer **cyclic progestin therapy** to daily oral contraceptives. Medroxyprogesterone acetate (Provera) 10 mg/day for 10 to 14 days per month should induce a withdrawal bleeding in most women with PCOS because they have sufficient peripheral conversion of androgens to estrogens to induce endometrial proliferation. Some women prefer to take progestins once every 3 months, but no controlled studies have been performed to determine whether such intermittent therapy is adequate to prevent endometrial hyperplasia. Highly androgenic women may have sufficient endometrial atrophy that bleeding in response to a progestin alone will not occur and estrogen supplementation will be required.

Antiandrogens must be administered with an effective contraceptive because of their ability to cross the placenta and potentially block the normal androgen-dependent virilization of the male fetus. **Spironolactone** is the most potent antiandrogen currently available in the United States. Dosages to improve hirsutism are at least 50 to 100 mg twice a day. These dosages have been surprisingly well tolerated in normal young women, but women should have their potassium level checked within a few weeks of initiating therapy and be advised to increase their fluid intake. Spironolactone can induce menstrual irregularity in women who had previously been regular but can help normalize menses in some oligomenorrheic women, presumably by normalizing androgenic effects. The addition of an oral contraceptive to spironolactone will synergistically suppress androgens, as well as regularize menses and ensure contraception, making the combination an excellent option for many women.

The optimal management of the insulin resistance associated with female hyperandrogenism has not yet been established. Since obese women with PCOS are more insulin resistant and weight loss will improve insulin resistance as well as hyperandrogenism and menstrual irregularity, they should be targeted for serious weight management. Other cardiovascular risk factors such as hypertension and hyper-lipidemia should be treated directly, as potential responses to antiandrogen treatment are not yet known. For some women, drugs that lower insulin levels may be appropriate.

Indications for Referral

Referral to an endocrinologist is appropriate when a woman does not respond to the initial treatments described previously.

The initial choice of therapy for women with **congenital adrenal hyperplasia** is probably best determined in conjunction with an endocrinologist. Although classic therapy with glucocorticoids probably requires endocrinologic supervision, new data suggest that antiandrogens and oral contraceptives may be just as efficacious for late-onset congenital adrenal hyperplasia in women who do not desire immediate pregnancy.

Women whose primary complaint is **infertility** also need referral to a reproductive endocrinologist. The major cause of infertility in hyperandrogenic women is anovulation, and up to 80% of anovulatory women with PCOS respond well to oral ovulation induction therapy with clomiphene citrate. Because of the risk of multiple gestations and hyperstimulation of the ovaries, the primary provider is advised to consult a specialist before considering such treatment.

Treatment for women with identified **ovarian** or **adrenal tumors** is surgical resection, which usually results in complete cure. Many small ovarian tumors can now be removed by laparoscopy, avoiding the prolonged recovery associated with laparotomy.

PROGNOSIS

Women with PCOS should be reassured that their prognosis is excellent, especially if they are vigilant about health maintenance habits to reduce cardiovascular risk. The majority of androgen-secreting tumors have a relatively benign course. Late onset congenital adrenal hyperplasia also has a good prognosis. Many women with PCOS are concerned that their menstrual irregularity or amenorrhea represents permanent infertility, and they are therefore reluctant to use oral contraceptives. All women should be reassured that the prospects for eventual fertility are actually quite good. One recent retrospective study of women who had had ovarian wedge resections for PCOS 20 years previously demonstrated no difference in their eventual fertility compared with that of control subjects.

BIBLIOGRAPHY

Adams J, Polson DW, Franks S: Prevalence of polycystic ovaries in women with anovulation and idiopathic hirsutism, *Br Med J* 293:355, 1986.

Dahlgren E et al: Women with polycystic ovary syndrome wedge resected in 1956 to 1965: a long-term follow-up focusing on natural history and circulating hormones, *Fertil Steril* 57:505, 1992.

Dewailly D et al: Clinical and biological phenotypes in late-onset 21-hydroxylase deficiency, *J Clin Endocrinol Metab* 63:418, 1986.

Dunaif A et al: Profound peripheral insulin resistance, independent of obesity in polycystic ovary syndrome, *Diabetes* 38:1165, 1989.

Ferriman D, Gallwey JD: Clinical assessment of body hair growth in women, *J Clin Endocrinol Metab* 21:1440, 1961.

Friedman CI et al: Serum testosterone concentrations in the evaluation of androgen-producing tumors, *Am J Obstet Gynecol* 153:44, 1985.

Futterweit W et al: The prevalence of hyperandrogenism in 109 consecutive female patients with diffuse alopecia, *J Am Acad Dermatol* 19:831, 1988.

Hamburger C: Normal urinary excretion of neutral 17-ketosteroids with special reference to age and sex variations, *Acta Endocrinol* 1:19, 1948.

Higuchi K et al: Prolactin has a direct effect on adrenal androgen secretion, *J Clin Endocrinol Metab* 59:714, 1984.

Hull MGR: Epidemiology of infertility and polycystic ovarian disease: endocrinological and demographic studies, *Gynecol Endocrinol* 1:235, 1987.

Hull MG et al: Population study of causes, treatment, and outcome of infertility, *Br Med J* 291:1693, 1985.

Laue L et al: Adrenal androgen secretion in postadolescent acne: increased adrenocortical function without hypersensitivity to adrenocorticotropin, *J Clin Endocrinol Metab* 73:380, 1991.

Maroulis GB: Evaluation of hirsutism and hyperandrogenism, *Fertil Steril* 36:273, 1981.

Meldrum DR, Abraham GE: Peripheral and ovarian venous concentrations of various steroid hormones in virilizing ovarian tumors, *Obstet Gynecol* 53:36, 1979.

Orentreich N et al: Age changes and sex differences in serum dehydroepiandrosterone sulfate concentrations throughout adulthood, *J Clin Endocrinol Metab* 59:551, 1984.

Pang S et al: Worldwide experience in newborn screening for classical congenital adrenal hyperplasia due to 21-hydroxylase deficiency, *Pediatrics* 81:866, 1988.

Pasquali R et al: Clinical and hormonal characteristics of obese amenorrheic hyperandrogenic women before and after weight loss, *J Clin Endocrinol Metab* 68:173, 1989.

Polson DW et al: Polycystic ovaries—a common finding in normal women, *Lancet* 1:870, 1988.

Seppala M, Hirvonen E: Raised serum prolactin levels associated with hirsutism and amenorrhoea, *Br Med J* 18:144, 1975.

Stuart CA et al: Insulin resistance with acanthosis nigricans: the roles of obesity and androgen excess, *Metabolism* 35:197, 1986.

Tagatz GE et al: The clitoral index: a bioassay of androgenic stimulation, *Obstet Gynecol* 54:562, 1979.

Wild RA, Bartholomew MJ: The influence of body weight on lipoprotein lipids in patients with polycystic ovary syndrome, *Am J Obstet Gynecol* 159:423, 1988.

Yen SSC: Chronic anovulation caused by peripheral endocrine disorders. In Yen SSC, Jaffe JB, editors: *Reproductive endocrinology: physiology, pathophysiology and clinical management,* ed 3, Philadelphia, 1991, WB Saunders.

Zawadzki JK, Dunaif A: Diagnostic criteria for polycystic ovary syndrome: towards a rational approach. In Dunaif A et al, editors: *Polycystic ovary syndrome,* Boston, 1992, Blackwell Scientific.

CHAPTER **15**

Hyperprolactinemia and Galactorrhea

Laurence Katznelson
Anne Klibanski

In 1954 Forbes and co-workers hypothesized that the syndrome of amenorrhea and galactorrhea was caused by a lactogenic pituitary hormone. This anterior pituitary hormone was later identified to be prolactin, and we have since learned a great deal regarding both its normal physiologic function and its pathologic disorders. Prolactin has a major role in lactation and affects gonadal function. The pathologic hypersecretion of prolactin is the cause of secondary amenorrhea in approximately 20% of women and may be associated with galactorrhea. This chapter summarizes the normal physiologic control of prolactin secretion, actions of prolactin, and evaluation and management of women with hyperprolactinemic disorders.

PATHOPHYSIOLOGY
Normal Control of Prolactin Secretion

Prolactin secretion is controlled by dual inhibitory and stimulatory factors (Fig. 15-1). Prolactin is unique among anterior pituitary hormones because it is primarily regulated through tonic inhibition. Two decades of investigation have shown the presence of one or more prolactin-inhibiting factors (PIFs). Dopamine is the most important PIF described. Multiple studies support this hypothesis, all pointing to a direct effect of dopamine on the pituitary lactotrophs. In addition, most pharmacologic agents that cause prolactin release act by either blockade of dopamine receptors (haloperidol and phenothiazines) or dopamine depletion in the tuberoinfundibular neurons (reserpine and α-methyldopa).

Stimulatory factors also regulate prolactin secretion. Estrogens are important physiologic stimulators of prolactin release. Thyrotropin-releasing hormone (TRH) stimulates both the synthesis and release of prolactin in vivo and in vitro from normal, as well as tumor, lactotrophs. However, the physiologic role of TRH in prolactin secretion is unclear. Hypothyroidism results in an increase in both the thyroid-stimulating hormone and prolactin responses to TRH, and elevations in basal prolactin levels may be seen in primary hypothyroidism. Vasoactive intestinal polypeptide may potentiate prolactin release, although the clinical significance is unknown. GnRH may also have stimulatory

properties; its administration induces the acute release of prolactin in both women with normal cycles and hypogonadal subjects.

Clinical Aspects of Prolactin Physiology

Physiologic causes of hyperprolactinemia are summarized in Box 15-1. The following discussion summarizes specific clinical aspects of prolactin physiology.

Diurnal and Menstrual Cycle Variation

Prolactin is secreted in a pulsatile fashion with 4 to 9 pulses per day (60% occur during sleep). The amplitude of pulses is highly variable among individuals, with peak levels occurring during the late hours of sleep. Such rises are not associated with any specific stage of sleep. Although some studies have suggested that prolactin level varies during the menstrual cycle, the precise nature of this relationship remains unclear. Several investigators have shown that prolactin levels are significantly higher during the ovulatory and luteal phases, particularly at midcycle. This midcycle rise may be due to increased circulating periovulatory estradiol levels. Other studies have not confirmed this finding. Prolactin is probably not necessary for ovulation, since ovulatory periods may occur in females taking bromocriptine, a medication that suppresses prolactin.

Food

Abrupt rises in serum prolactin level occur within an hour of eating in normal and pregnant hyperprolactinemic individuals, but not in individuals with prolactinomas.

Stress

Prolactin rises during stress, including physical exertion, surgery, sexual intercourse, insulin hypoglycemia, and seizures. The significance of these changes is not known. Nipple stimulation, chest wall trauma or surgery, and herpes zoster infection of the breast may result in increases in prolactin levels.

Age

Mean levels of prolactin are slightly higher in premenopausal women than in men, probably as a result of a

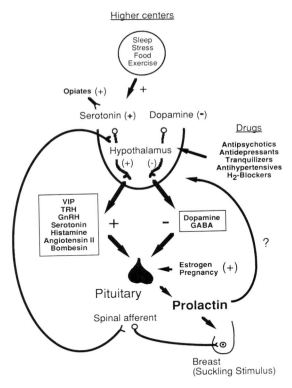

FIG. 15-1 Regulation of prolactin secretion. Prolactin release is under tonic inhibition by PIFs, predominantly dopamine. Prolactin release is stimulated by a number of factors, including VIP, TRH, and GnRH. Estrogens, pregnancy, and breast suckling stimulate prolactin release. Within the hypothalamus serotonergic and dopaminergic pathways are stimulatory and inhibitory, respectively, to prolactin release. *PIFs,* Prolactin inhibiting factors; *VIP,* vasoactive intestinal peptide; *TRH,* thyrotropin-releasing hormone; *GnRH,* gonadotropin releasing hormone. (Modified from Molitch ME: *Endocrinol Metab Clin North Am* 21:877, 1992.)

BOX 15-1
Physiologic Causes of Hyperprolactinemia

Pregnancy
Postpartum
Nonnursing: days 1-7
Nursing: with suckling
Newborn
Estrogens

Stress
Sleep
Hypoglycemia
Sexual intercourse
Nipple stimulation
Exercise

BOX 15-2
Clinical Manifestations of Hyperprolactinemia

Amenorrhea-galactorrhea syndrome
Oligomenorrhea
Altered luteal phase function
Hypogonadism
Hyperandrogenism
Osteopenia

---

direct effect of estrogen on pituitary prolactin secretion. Some studies suggest that there is a progressive decline in prolactin levels in women with aging, particularly after the menopause. Responsiveness of prolactin to various pharmacologic agents (e.g., TRH) declines with age in women. This decline is probably due to postmenopausal estrogen deficiency.

Function of Prolactin in Normal States

The only established role of prolactin is to initiate and maintain lactation. Prolactin levels increase progressively with pregnancy. Estrogens play a major role in stimulation of prolactin levels. Prolactin levels rise progressively, peaking at term (100 to 300 ng/ml). Lactation begins when estradiol levels fall at parturition. Prolactin levels increase to 60 times higher than baseline levels in the circulation within 20 to 30 minutes of nursing. The nursing stimulus effectively promotes acute prolactin release via afferent spinal neural pathways. With continued nursing the nipple stimulation itself elicits progressively less prolactin release, and in the weeks after initiation of lactation, both basal and nursing-induced prolactin pulses decrease, although lactation continues. Within 4 to 6 months postpartum, basal prolactin levels are normal without a nursing-induced rise.

EVALUATION OF HYPERPROLACTINEMIA
Clinical Manifestations (Box 15-2)

The **amenorrhea-galactorrhea syndrome** is the classic description of the clinical manifestation of hyperprolactinemia. However, a spectrum of reproductive disorders may be seen. Prolactin level elevations are found in approximately 20% of patients with secondary amenorrhea. Women with hyperprolactinemia may have more subtle abnormalities in gonadal function, including **oligomenorrhea** or **alterations in luteal phase function.** A subset of infertile women have been described with mild or intermittent hyperprolactinemia in whom fertility was restored with bromocriptine therapy. Galactorrhea is present in only approximately 30% of female patients with hyperprolactinemia, but the presence of galactorrhea in a woman with an ovulatory disorder greatly increases the chance that hyperprolactinemia is the underlying cause of the amenorrhea.

Hypogonadism (decreased gonadal steroid levels) frequently occurs in patients with hyperprolactinemia. There are multiple potential mechanisms hypothesized for the induction of hypogonadism by prolactin, and the antigonadotrophic actions of prolactin may occur at multiple levels. Frequently the hypogonadism is associated with decreased or inappropriately normal luteinizing hormone (LH) and follicle-stimulating hormone (FSH) levels relative to the state of estrogen deficiency. Several investigations suggest that prolactin may have a suppressive effect on spontaneous LH release via decreases in endogenous GnRH levels. Prolactin appears to affect its own secretion via a short-loop negative feedback at the level of the hypothalamus. This feedback may be mediated through an increase in dopamine inhibitory tone. This increased hypothalamic dopamine tone, along with opiates and other factors, may suppress GnRH with a resultant decrease in LH pulses. The restoration of ovulatory menstrual periods in hyperprolactinemic women with pulsatile exogenous GnRH administration confirms the importance of endogenous GnRH abnormalities as the key mechanism of hypogonadism in these women.

In addition, prolactin may modulate androgen secretion at the level of both the adrenal gland and the ovary, resulting in increased secretion of dehydroepiandrosterone sulfate and testosterone. Therefore altered ratios of estrogens and androgens may further result in abnormal gonadal function, with evidence of **hyperandrogenism** (e.g., hirsutism). If the underlying cause of the increased prolactin level is a pituitary macroadenoma, then the adenoma could cause compression of the normal, adjacent pituitary gland with a resultant decrease in gonadotroph activity.

Hyperprolactinemia is also associated with both trabecular and cortical **osteopenia.** Hyperprolactinemic women may have trabecular osteopenia with spinal bone density ranging from 10% to 25% below normal. Studies have shown that the bone density in such patients may increase with normalization of prolactin levels with therapy; however, the bone density typically still remains lower than that of normal control subjects. The cause of this decrease in bone density is thought to be the hypogonadism resulting from the hyperprolactinemic state, and not the prolactin per se. Hyperprolactinemic women with normal menstrual function do not have associated bone loss.

History and Physical Examination

The history and physical examination should include investigation into potential causes of hyperprolactinemia in addition to its clinical manifestations. The history should therefore screen for causes of hyperprolactinemia (Box 15-3). It is important to consider primary hypothyroidism and pregnancy as causes. Chronic renal disease may be associated with prolactin level elevations, likely caused by altered metabolism/clearance of prolactin and/or decreases in dopaminergic tone. A detailed history of medications may elicit a pharmacologic cause of hyperprolactinemia. Medications associated with hyperprolactinemia include calcium channel blockers, α-methyldopa, cimetidine, phenothiazines and other neuroleptics, and opiates. Atypical neuroleptics such as risperidone frequently cause hyperprolactinemia as do a number of antidepressants that affect serotonergic tone such as SSRIs (selective serotonin reuptake inhibitors). Estrogen therapy may lead to increases in prolactin levels, as are seen in pregnancy. However, estrogen concentrations in typical oral contraceptives (e.g., 35 mg ethinyl estradiol) are not associated with hyperprolactinemia, and there is no evidence that postmenopausal replacement estrogen causes elevations in serum prolactin concentration.

In women hypogonadism related to hyperprolactinemia may cause abnormal menstrual function. The presence of oligomenorrhea or amenorrhea will have an impact on therapy. A history of infertility caused by altered luteal phase function may be present. Other hypogonadal symptoms include vaginal dryness, dyspareunia, fatigue, and diminished libido. The physical examination should include assessment of galactorrhea, which may be unilateral or bilateral.

The evaluation should also include assessment of the presence of a pituitary tumor. Hyperprolactinemia may be detected in up to 25% of patients with acromegaly and has been reported in Cushing's disease. Therefore acromegaly and Cushing's disease should be evaluated in those hyper-

---

BOX 15-3
Pathologic and Pharmacologic Causes of Hyperprolactinemia

Pituitary Disease
Prolactin-secreting tumors
Acromegaly
Cushing's disease
Empty sella syndrome

Pituitary Stalk Section
Clinically nonfunctioning pituitary tumors
Trauma

Hypothalamic Infiltrative or Degenerative Disease
Craniopharyngiomas
Meningiomas
Dysgerminomas
Gliomas
Lymphoma
Metastatic disease
Tuberculosis
Sarcoidosis
Eosinophilic granuloma
Irradiation

Neurogenic
Chest wall trauma
Chest wall lesions
Herpes zoster
Breast stimulation

Medications
Phenothiazines
Tricyclic antidepressants
Metocloproamide
Cimetidine
Methyldopa
Reserpine
Calcium-channel blockers
Cocaine

Other
Renal failure
Liver disease
Primary hypothyroidism
Ectopic hormone production
Seizures

Modified from Molitch ME: *Endocrinol Metab Clin North Am* 21:877, 1992.

---

prolactinemic patients with suggestive clinical manifestations. Pituitary and nonpituitary tumors may cause local mass effects, and symptoms such as headaches, diplopia, and blurry vision are common. Careful visual field examination by confrontation may reveal evidence of visual field deficits, including bitemporal hemianopsia or quadrantanopsia. These findings suggest the presence of compression of the optic chiasm by a tumor. Compression of the adjacent, normal pituitary gland may result in hypopituitarism. Symptoms attributable to hypopituitarism may include fatigue, anorexia, weight loss, dizziness, and polyuria (suggesting the presence of diabetes insipidus). Therefore in consideration of the presence of a sellar mass, a careful history and physical examination should be performed to evaluate for the presence of thyroid, adrenal, and antidiuretic hormone function.

Diagnostic Testing

As shown in Box 15-3, there are several causes of hyperprolactinemia. First, the prolactin level should be remeasured in a nonstimulated state, and, if possible, we recommend measuring a morning prolactin level after an overnight fast in a nonstressed state. For example, prolactin may be secreted to a modest degree after a breast examination, so a mild increase in prolactin levels after such an examination warrants a repeat prolactin determination.

Although a number of pathologic causes can elevate prolactin level, pituitary tumors are clinically the most important. Prolactin-secreting pituitary adenomas are the most common type of pituitary tumor and may account for up to 40% to 50% of all pituitary tumors.

Substantial elevations in prolactin level, greater than 150 ng/ml, in a nonpuerperal state are usually indicative of a pituitary tumor. There is a good correlation between radiographic estimates of tumor size and prolactin levels, and very high levels of prolactin are associated with larger tumors. Prolactinomas are classified as microadenomas (<10 mm) and macroadenomas (>10 mm). Therefore the finding of a substantial elevation in serum prolactin level in association with a pituitary lesion greater than 10 mm by radiographic analysis supports the diagnosis of a macroprolactinoma.

The majority of women with prolactinomas have microadenomas; in contrast, the majority of tumors in men are macroadenomas. This difference may occur because women may seek earlier evaluation than men because of menstrual disturbances.

Modest levels of prolactin elevation (e.g., 25 to 100 ng/ml) may be associated with a number of diagnoses. All causes of hyperprolactinemia should be excluded before a tumor is considered. Pregnancy should be excluded. Medications, including phenothiazines, metoclopramide, cimetidine, and calcium channel blockers, may be associated with hyperprolactinemia.

Any intrasellar or suprasellar mass may lead to modest prolactin level elevations through stalk compression. Therefore any patient with hyperprolactinemia and no clear secondary cause, such as pregnancy or medication use, should undergo radiographic analysis. These masses include primary pituitary tumors, meningiomas, and craniopharyngiomas. In addition, hypothalamic disorder including destructive (tumors, granulomatous diseases) lesions may lead to hyperprolactinemia by interfering with normal dopaminergic tone. When an elevated serum prolactin level is not associated with primary hypothyroidism, pregnancy, or use of pharmacologic agents, a pituitary radiographic scan should be performed to rule out the presence of either a prolactin-secreting pituitary tumor or other lesions. In addition, as described later, it is important to distinguish microprolactinomas from macroprolactinomas. Magnetic resonance imaging (MRI) is a more sensitive tool than computed tomography for evaluating the sellar and suprasellar areas. If the scan shows normal sellar and extrasellar contents and there is no clear secondary cause of the elevated prolactin level, then the diagnosis of idiopathic hyperprolactinemia is made. These cases may represent microprolactinomas, and a small tumor may be beyond the sensitivity of the scanning technique.

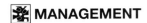 **MANAGEMENT**

Treatment depends on whether the woman has hyperprolactinemia resulting from an underlying cause, such as drug use or hypothyroidism, or a prolactinoma. If the preceding evaluation suggests the presence of a microprolactinoma, there are three available treatment options: careful follow-up without treatment, medical therapy with a dopamine agonist, and, rarely, surgery. All patients with macroadenomas should be treated.

Close Follow-Up Observation Without Treatment

Patients with a microadenoma and those without evidence of a pituitary tumor can sometimes be monitored without therapy if fertility is not an issue, tumor size has not increased, and normal menstrual function is not disrupted. Studies evaluating the natural history of microprolactinomas have generally shown that prolactin level elevations may remain stable and in some cases spontaneously normalize. Martin and co-workers studied 41 patients over 5.5 years of follow-up observation and showed that 67% of patients whose initial prolactin values were less than 57 ng/ml had normalization of the prolactin level, whereas none of the patients with initial prolactin values greater than 60 ng/ml reached normal values. These and other data suggest that the degree of prolactin level elevation is a prognostic factor for spontaneous resolution. Schlechte and co-workers showed that basal menstrual function is an important variable in determining progression of the prolactin level. In this study patients with normal initial menstrual function were more likely to experience normalization of prolactin values, whereas those with oligomenorrhea or amenorrhea were more likely to have no change or increases in prolactin values.

In terms of tumor size, most studies show that the majority of microprolactinomas do not increase in size. Many of these studies are not recent and must be interpreted in light of the use of less sensitive radiographic techniques such as skull films and tomograms. Studies show that tumors in patients with microprolactinomas or no radiographic evidence of tumor increase in size in 0% to 22% of patients. In a study by Webster and colleagues, of 43 patients with presumed microadenomas with a mean follow-up period of 5 years, only two patients showed evidence of tumor progression. Tumor progression was not necessarily accompanied by an increasing serum prolactin level. Follow-up evaluation of untreated patients should include both serial prolactin levels and periodic MRI scans.

Medical Therapy

Medical therapy for a patient with microprolactinomas is based on the effects of hyperprolactinemia in that patient. Patients with hyperprolactinemia usually have accompanying menstrual irregularities. Dopamine agonist therapy results in a return of menstrual function in the majority of patients with amenorrhea. Luteal phase defects associated with hyperprolactinemia also reverse with dopamine agonist therapy. Ovulation rates in excess of 90% have been reported, with induced pregnancy rates in greater than 80% of patients. The presence of galactorrhea itself is not an absolute indication for dopamine agonist therapy, unless the degree of galactorrhea is significantly bothersome to the patient. Hyperprolactinemia has also been associated with headaches or hirsutism, which may resolve with prolactin level normalization. If there is no evidence of hypogonadism in patients with microprolactinomas, then having no therapy is an option for some women with microadenomas who do not desire fertility.

Almost all patients with hyperprolactinemia caused by pituitary disease can be effectively treated with the dopamine agonist bromocriptine mesylate (Parlodel). Bromocriptine lowers serum prolactin levels in patients with pituitary tumors and all other causes of hyperprolactinemia. Bromocriptine is very effective in rapidly decreasing prolactin levels and both normalizing reproductive function and reversing galactorrhea. It is also useful in treating galactorrhea in patients with normoprolactinemic galactorrhea. Bromocriptine decreases prolactin production and secretion with consequent reduction in prolactin cell size. This often results in decreased tumor size.

Therapy should be initiated slowly because side effects, including nausea, headache, dizziness, nasal congestion, and constipation, may occur. Gastrointestinal side effects may be minimized by starting with a very low dose at night (e.g., 1.25 mg [½ tablet]) and increasing the dosage by 1.25 mg over 4- to 5-day intervals. This is continued until a dose that normalizes prolactin levels is reached. Taking the medication at bedtime with a snack initially helps minimize the gastrointestinal symptoms. These side effects usually improve with either continuing at the same dose or temporarily reducing the dose. If patients stop taking the medication for a few days, they may need to restart therapy at a lower dose, since these side effects may return. Rarely, chronic therapy may result in side effects, including painless cold sensitive digital vasospasm, alcohol intolerance, dyskinesia, and psychiatric reactions, such as fatigue, depression, and anxiety.

Cabergoline (Dostinex), an ergoline derivative, is a potent and long-lasting dopamine agonist that is highly effective in the management of hyperprolactinemia. Compliance rates with cabergoline are high, because of the ease of administration (0.5 to 1.0 mg once or twice a week) and its improved side effect profile compared to bromocriptine. In addition, cabergoline is more effective than bromocriptine in normalizing serum prolactin levels. In one study in 113 patients with microprolactinomas, cabergoline administration resulted in normalization of serum prolactin in 95%. In addition, cabergoline may be effective in patients resistant to bromocriptine. Therefore, cabergoline should be considered as medical therapy for all patients with hyperprolactinemia, including use as primary therapy or as secondary therapy in subjects intolerant of or resistant to bromocriptine.

Surgery

Although surgery is not a primary mode of management for patients with prolactinomas, in a few cases it may be useful. There are several indications for surgery, including large tumors with visual field deficits unresponsive to dopamine agonists, inability to tolerate medical therapy as a result of side effects, cystic tumors that do not to respond to medical therapy, and apoplexy of the prolactinoma. A transsphenoidal approach is almost exclusively used. When surgery is performed by an experienced surgeon, the morbidity rate is negligible. The main advantage of curative surgery is avoidance of long-term medication. Serri and colleagues reported

that of 28 patients with microprolactinomas, 24 were cured with transsphenoidal surgery as determined by normalization of serum prolactin levels. However, after approximately 4 years, 50% of these initially cured patients experienced a recurrence of hyperprolactinemia, although there was no radiographic evidence of tumor. Another group reported more recently that recurrence rates as low as 26% can be achieved. These data suggest that although surgery may normalize prolactin levels initially in patients with microprolactinomas, there is a relatively high recurrence risk.

Conventional radiotherapy (4500 to 5000 rad), proton beam therapy, or gamma knife may be indicated in patients with larger tumors in whom immediate control of symptoms and fertility is not a high priority and in those who are not able to tolerate medical therapy.

Macroprolactinomas

In contrast to patients with microprolactinomas, patients with macroprolactinomas need more definitive therapy. Patients with macroadenomas may have evidence of local mass effects caused by the expanding tumor, with resultant visual field abnormalities and hypopituitarism resulting from compression of the normal pituitary gland. Therefore it is important to be aggressive in management to prevent or reverse these complications. Bromocriptine produces significant tumor shrinkage in up to 75% of patients. Size reduction may occur in weeks or over many months. This is frequently accompanied by improvement in visual field abnormalities and pituitary function. Molitch and co-workers treated 27 such patients with bromocriptine and found reduction in tumor size by at least 50% in 64% of patients. Tumor shrinkage often occurred within 6 weeks in this study. A total of 66% of patients had normalization of prolactin levels, but the fall in prolactin level did not necessarily correlate with reduction in tumor size. Cabergoline administration may also result in tumor shrinkage, a decrease in prolactin levels, and restoration of gonadal function in subjects with macroprolactinomas. Biller and co-workers administered cabergoline to 15 patients with macroprolactinomas and noted normalization of serum prolactin in 73% and a reduction in tumor size by 31%. Therefore, cabergoline may be useful as first-line therapy in the management of macroprolactinomas.

Transsphenoidal surgery is not used as a primary therapy for patients with macroprolactinomas except in neurosurgical emergency. Surgical cure is inversely proportional to serum prolactin levels and tumor size. There are no data directly comparing medical therapy to surgery as primary therapy for macroadenomas. Specific circumstances, such as the presence of a cystic prolactinoma (which often does not respond fully to dopamine agonist therapy), may predict a poor initial response to medical therapy in all such patients. Dopamine agonists are a useful adjunct therapy in patients with large tumors when complete resection has not been possible.

◼ PREGNANCY AND PROLACTINOMAS

Many women with hyperprolactinemia are infertile. Bromocriptine is typically used to normalize prolactin levels and allow normal ovulation to occur. We recommend discontinuing bromocriptine when pregnancy is detected. There is concern, however, that during pregnancy the high levels of estrogens may lead to lactotroph stimulation and tumor growth. Pregnancy in a normal woman will lead to increased pituitary size through estrogen-stimulated lactotroph hyperplasia. Therefore pituitary enlargement may lead to local complications including visual field deficits, headaches, and diabetes insipidus. Molitch reviewed the series on pregnancy outcomes in hyperprolactinemic patients. Up to 5% of patients with microprolactinomas experience clinically significant tumor enlargement (headaches or visual deficits or both). Therefore patients with microprolactinomas may be followed carefully without therapy during pregnancy. Patients should receive close follow-up observation, and visual field analysis performed at monthly intervals is recommended.

In contrast, 15% to 36% of patients with macroadenomas are at risk for clinically significant tumor enlargement in any trimester. Some centers therefore recommend transsphenoidal resection of the macroadenomas before conception. However, prior surgery does not prevent tumor enlargement during pregnancy. We do not recommend a preventive surgical approach and instead follow these patients closely, as noted for patients with microprolactinomas. Monitoring of serum prolactin levels throughout pregnancy is not clinically useful because prolactin levels increase markedly during pregnancy, and a decision to reinstitute therapy is dependent on clinical symptoms. The published data suggest that if a complication does occur, it is rapidly reversible with the reinstitution of bromocriptine, which is then continued through term.

The outcome of bromocriptine-induced pregnancies is comparable to that of normal pregnancies. A large international experience with bromocriptine and pregnancy suggests that bromocriptine therapy does not result in complications for the fetus. Breastfeeding after delivery appears to be safe. Patients with macroadenomas should continue to be followed closely, and the decision to institute therapy is based on tumor size and clinical symptoms.

Data on the safety of cabergoline in pregnancy are more limited. In a review of 226 pregnancies induced by cabergoline, no evidence of pregnancy-associated complications or birth defects were detected. However, until further information is available regarding use of cabergoline in pregnancy, bromocriptine is recommended as first choice therapy for hyperprolactinemic women seeking pregnancy.

Indications for Referral

The routine evaluation and management of hyperprolactinemia may be performed by the primary caregiver. There are several indications for referral to an endocrinologist; the presence of a macroprolactinoma is one. These patients often have visual field dysfunction, cranial nerve deficits, and hypopituitarism. The urgency of these situations dictates that the therapy be managed by a clinician experienced in dopamine-agonist dosing and monitoring of side effects. In addition, medical therapy may be complicated by the presence of anterior and posterior pituitary insufficiency, and management may require an endocrinologist with experience in such therapy. Hyperprolactinemia that does not respond to dopamine agonist therapy should also be an indication for referral. Again, use of dopamine agonists should be administered by physicians with experience with such medications. Finally, patients considered for surgery should also have the indications for surgery reviewed with an endocrinologist.

BIBLIOGRAPHY

Bassetti M et al: Bromocriptine treatment reduces the cell size in human macroprolactinomas: a morphometric study, *J Clin Endocrinol Metab* 58:268, 1984.

Biller BM et al: Treatment of prolactin-secreting macroadenomas with the once-weekly dopamine agonist cabergoline, *J Clin Endocrinol Metab* 81:2338, 1996.

Carlson HE: Prolactin stimulation by protein is mediated by amino acids in humans, *J Clin Endocrinol Metab* 69:7, 1989.

Colao A et al: Prolactinomas resistant to standard dopamine agonists respond to chronic cabergoline treatment [see comments], *J Clin Endocrinol Metab* 82:876, 1997.

Feigenbaum SL et al: Transsphenoidal pituitary resection for preoperative diagnosis of prolactin-secreting pituitary adenoma in women: long term follow-up, *J Clin Endocrinol Metab* 81:1711, 1996.

Forbes AP et al: Syndrome characterized by galactorrhea, amenorrhea and low urinary FSH: comparison with acromegaly and normal lactation, *J Clin Endocrinol Metab* 14:265, 1954.

Katznelson L et al: Prolactin pulsatile characteristics in postmenopausal women, *J Clin Endocrinol Metab* 83:761, 1998.

Kleinberg D et al: Prolactin levels and adverse events in patients treated with risperidone, *J Clin Psychopharmacol* 19:57, 1999.

Klibanski A et al: Effects of prolactin and estrogen deficiency in amenorrheic bone loss, *J Clin Endocrinol Metab* 67:124, 1988.

Klibanski A, Greenspan SL: Increase in bone mass after treatment of hyperprolactinemic amenorrhea, *N Engl J Med* 315:542, 1986.

Klibanski A et al: Decreased bone density in hyperprolactinemic women, *N Engl J Med* 303:1511, 1980.

Klibanski A, Zervas NT: Diagnosis and management of hormone-secreting pituitary adenomas, *N Engl J Med* 324:822, 1991.

Koppelman MC et al: Vertebral body bone mineral content in hyperprolactinemic women, *J Clin Endocrinol Metab* 59:1050, 1984.

Martin TL, Kim M, Malarkey WB: The natural history of idiopathic hyperprolactinemia, *J Clin Endocrinol Metab* 60:855, 1985.

Molitch ME: Pathologic hyperprolactinemia, *Endocrinol Metab Clin North Am* 21:877, 1992.

Molitch ME: Pregnancy and the hyperprolactinemic woman, *N Engl J Med* 312:1364, 1985.

Molitch ME et al: Bromocriptine as primary therapy for prolactin-secreting macroadenomas: results of a prospective multicenter study, *J Clin Endocrinol Metab* 60:698, 1985.

Polson DW et al: Ovulation and normal luteal function during LHRH treatment of women with hyperprolactinaemic amenorrhoea, *Clin Endocrinol* 24:531, 1986.

Robert E et al: Pregnancy outcome after treatment with the ergot derivative, cabergoline, *Reprod Toxicol* 10:333, 1996.

Scheithauer BW et al: The pituitary gland in pregnancy: a clinicopathologic and immunohistochemical study of 69 cases, *Mayo Clin Proc* 65:461, 1990.

Schlechte J et al: The natural history of untreated hyperprolactinemia: a prospective analysis, *J Clin Endocrinol Metab* 68:412, 1989.

Serri O et al: Recurrence of hyperprolactinemia after selective transsphenoidal adenomectomy in women with prolactinoma, *N Engl J Med* 309:280, 1983.

Sisam DA, Sheehan JP, Sheeler LR: The natural history of untreated microprolactinomas, *Fertil Steril* 48:67, 1987.

Turkalj I, Braun P, Krupp P: Surveillance of bromocriptine in pregnancy, *JAMA* 247:1589, 1982.

Webster J et al: A comparison of cabergoline and bromocriptine in the treatment of hyperprolactinemic amenorrhea, *N Engl J Med* 331:904, 1994.

Webster J et al: Dose-dependent suppression of serum prolactin by cabergoline in hyperprolactinaemia: a placebo controlled, double blind, multicentre study. European Multicentre Cabergoline Dosefinding Study Group, *Clin Endocrinol* 37:534, 1992.

CHAPTER **16**

Gallstones

John M. Kauffman
David L. Carr-Locke

Gallbladder and biliary tract diseases that result from gall-stones are major causes of morbidity and mortality in the United States and other industrialized countries and are twice as common in women as in men. As epidemiologic observations have suggested and as clinical studies have confirmed, estrogens and progesterones potentiate forma-tion of cholesterol stones.

Cholecystectomy represents one of the most common op-erations on women, with approximately 500,000 performed annually in the United States. This chapter outlines the pathophysiologic and epidemiologic characteristics and treatment of gallstones, with particular emphasis on why women are more prone to the development of cholesterol stones.

PATHOPHYSIOLOGY

Bile formation and secretion represent the primary mecha-nism for elimination of cholesterol from the body. The functions of bile secretion are twofold: to eliminate lipids, principally bile salts and cholesterol, along with detoxified xenobiotics from the body, and to assist in the absorption of lipids in the small intestine.

Types of Gallstones

Cholesterol stones, which constitute more than 80% of gallstones in the United States, are composed predominantly of crystalline cholesterol, together with small amounts of inorganic and organic calcium salts. In Western cultures, cholesterol stones display a 2 to 1 female preponderance. **Black pigment stones** are largely composed of polymerized calcium bilirubinate (unconjugated bilirubin), together with inorganic calcium salts. Clinical risk factors for black pig-ment stones include conditions in which increased quanti-ties of conjugated bilirubin are excreted into bile, such as hemolytic anemia and cirrhosis. Cholesterol and black pigment stones are formed exclusively in the gallbladder, although their clinical presentations may occur after migra-tion to the cystic or common bile ducts. **Brown pigment stones** are formed almost exclusively in the bile ducts, are associated with bacterial infection of the biliary tree, and are predominantly formed of bacterial degradation products.

Mechanisms of Gallstone Formation

Several defects interact to initiate gallstone formation: the presence of cholesterol-supersaturated bile, rapid formation of cholesterol crystals, and gallbladder hypomotility. Be-cause of its extreme insolubility in water, cholesterol is excreted from the body almost entirely via biliary secretion, as cholesterol or after transformation into bile salts.

Cholesterol Hypersecretion

Cholesterol homeostasis is controlled by hepatocytes, which synthesize cholesterol and regulate its secretion into bile, either as free cholesterol or bile salts. Biliary choles-terol supersaturation can be produced by imbalances in the enzymes regulating cholesterol flux. The sensitivity of these processes to hormonal regulation accounts for an excess of gallstone disease in women, as well as higher high-density lipoprotein (HDL) levels, one of the factors associated with a decreased risk of cardiovascular disease in women.

Effects of Estrogen and Progesterone

Several of the enzymes regulating cholesterol homeosta-sis are affected by either endogenous and exogenous estro-gens or progesterone. However, their net effect on biliary cholesterol secretion depends on the dose and differs for acute and chronic exogenous administration. Estrogens, whether in oral contraceptives, at puberty, or as estrogen re-placement therapy, increase biliary cholesterol saturation. Estrogen-mediated increases in hepatic cholesterol uptake via low-density-lipoproteins (LDL) and chylomicrons are largely matched by increases in biliary cholesterol secretion, but not bile salt synthesis. Progesterones increase the biliary free cholesterol pool and, consequently, biliary cholesterol secretion. Although HMG CoA reductase is not affected by sex hormones, its activity is increased in obesity and hyper-triglyceridemia, with consequent increases in cholesterol synthesis and secretion into bile.

Biliary Sludge

An important intermediate step in the formation of gall-stones is the development of biliary sludge. Sludge can be detected ultrasonographically (Fig. 16-1) and is composed of microcrystals of cholesterol and calcium bilirubinate in a

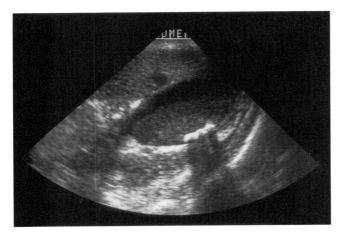

FIG. 16-1 Ultrasonographic appearance of hyperechoic gallbladder sludge without acoustic shadowing, layering above three stones with distinct acoustic shadows.

<table>
<tr><td>

BOX 16-1

Risk Factors for Gallbladder Disease in Women

- Ethnic origin: Native American
- Age
- Estrogen
  Pregnancy
  Parity
  Exogenous estrogen
    Oral contraceptives
    Postmenopausal estrogen
- Hypertriglyceridemia
- Drugs
  Fibric acid derivatives
  Nicotinic acid
- Obesity and rapid weight loss
- Gallbladder stasis

</td></tr>
</table>

thick mucin gel. Although sludge may evolve to gallstone formation, in the majority of cases it disappears spontaneously. Occurrence of biliary sludge is more common in pregnancy, and its clinical implications are discussed later in this chapter.

Gallbladder Hypomotility and Emptying

Gallbladder hypomotility prevents the complete clearance of cholesterol crystals by the gallbladder and can predispose to cholesterol gallstone formation. In a vicious cycle, cholesterol-supersaturated bile itself induces gallbladder hypomotility. Progesterones, but not estrogens, directly impair both the rate of gallbladder emptying and the maximum ejection fraction. Gallbladder volume is increased and ejection fraction is impaired in pregnancy, but both return to normal in the postpartum period.

EPIDEMIOLOGY AND RISK FACTORS

In general, the clinical groups at risk for gallstones reflect the pathophysiologic processes of gallstone formation (Box 16-1). Although ultrasound studies have shown a great deal of geographic and ethnic variation in the prevalence of gallstone disease, the overall prevalence of gallstones in women is about twice that in men in all ethnic groups.

Native American populations, in particular the Pima, constitutionally hypersecrete biliary cholesterol and hyposecrete bile salts. Consequently, cholesterol gallstone disease is frequent in this population, reaching a prevalence of about 80% in older women. In Asian and African black populations, gallstone disease is much rarer, with prevalence of less than 10%. European populations have intermediate prevalence of 10% to 25%.

Such differences in prevalence among ethnic groups, along with the high incidence of familial occurrence, have led to the search for a genetic basis for cholesterol gallstone disease. Studies of mouse models have revealed at least two *Lith* genes associated with cholesterol gallstone disease. Because of the similarity of the human and murine genomes, some of these genes may be responsible for cholesterol gallstones in humans.

After childhood, when gallstones are equally rare in both sexes, gallstone prevalence increases sharply with **age,** as shown in Fig. 16-2. In all postpuberty age groups the relative risk of gallstones in women exceeds that in men, but in younger age groups the relative risk is greater.

Gender differences in the prevalence of gallstones are largely attributable to the consequences of **pregnancy.** As shown in Fig. 16-3 the risk of gallstone disease rises with each pregnancy, and the relative risk is highest for younger women. Although parity is a strong risk factor for gallstone disease in young women, the relative risk diminishes in the postmenopausal age group.

Exogenous estrogens also promote the development of gallstones in females as well as males treated with supraphysiologic estrogen doses. Shortly after the introduction of oral contraceptives, case-control studies noted a twofold to threefold increase in the incidence of gallstone disease, but more recent studies have shown a lower relative risk of 1.1 (age-adjusted), with the highest relative risks in the youngest women. The effect of pregnancy is confounding, as initiation of oral contraceptives may follow recent pregnancy, and studies did not use ultrasound to detect asymptomatic gallstones. However, a dose-related response was demonstrated, with the risk for use of products with more than 50 μg of estrogen daily of 1.21, and a risk of 0.97 for those with less than 50 μg estrogen. Prospective ultrasound studies of prevalence have shown an elevated risk for users of oral contraceptives, but the effect was not significant after multivariate analysis. With current use of lower estrogen doses, the relative risk for users of oral contraceptives is thought to be minimal.

Postmenopausal estrogen replacement therapy is associated with a 2.5-fold increase in surgical gallstone disease. The risk of gallstone disease persists after stopping estrogen therapy, as gallstones seldom spontaneously dissolve or pass. In contrast to oral estrogens, which undergo first pass metabolism in the liver, transdermal estrogens do not increase biliary cholesterol saturation and probably do not increase the risk of gallstones.

Because the body's cholesterol is almost exclusively excreted through the bile, there has been much study on the

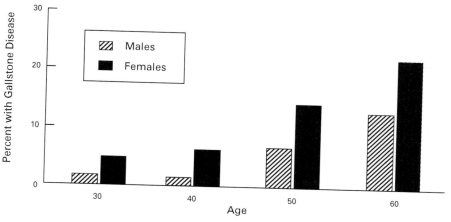

FIG. 16-2   Gallstone prevalence in a large prospective ultrasound survey of over 4500 adult Danish subjects increases sharply with age. At younger ages there is a female preponderance that narrows in older age groups. (From Jorgensen T: *Am J Epidemiol* 126:912, 1987.)

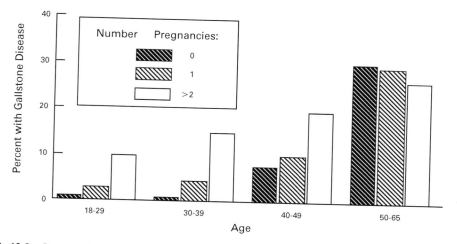

FIG. 16-3   Pregnancy is a risk factor for the development of gallstones, as shown in this prospective study of Italian women. The relative risk is highest for young women but increases in all premenopausal groups with each successive pregnancy. (From Barbara L et al: *Hepatology* 7:913, 1987.)

interrelationship between serum lipid levels and cholesterol gallstones. **Hypertriglyceridemia** is associated with an increased risk of gallstones. Increased total serum cholesterol level is not associated with an increased risk, but high levels of HDL cholesterol and low levels of total cholesterol are probably associated with a decreased risk of gallstone disease. Not surprisingly, pharmacologic agents that alter serum lipid levels have important effects on biliary cholesterol secretion and hence on cholesterol gallstone formation. The fibric acid derivatives **clofibrate** and **gemfibrozil** both increase the amount of cholesterol secreted into bile and have been associated with statistically significant differences in the prevalence of gallstone disease and biliary tract complications. **Nicotinic acid** has also been associated with a modest increase in biliary tract disease. In contrast, HMG-CoA reductase inhibitors such as mevinolin or lovastatin decrease cholesterol synthesis and also markedly reduce cholesterol secretion into bile. Biliary cholesterol saturation therefore decreases markedly, and preliminary studies show that HMG-CoA reductase inhibitors accelerate pharmacologic dissolution of gallstones.

Obesity is considered an independent risk factor for cholesterol gallstones, independent of the effect on serum lipids. In the Nurses' Health Study cohort, relative weight was associated with an increased incidence of symptomatic gallstones (sixfold higher for the highest quintile) for women, but not for men. A confounding factor in the association of obesity with gallstones is that **reducing diets** are associated with a very high risk of development of gallstones. Patients undergoing rapid weight loss, of more than 15 kg over several weeks, are at extremely high risk of development of gallstones, with gallstones developing in 20% in this short time. Increased biliary cholesterol excretion, as well as failure of low levels of dietary fat to contract the gallbladder, interact synergistically to accelerate formation of cholesterol gallstones. Ursodiol has been successful in preventing the formation of biliary sludge and gallstones, suggesting that prophylaxis of gallstone formation in this very-high-risk group is warranted.

Gallbladder stasis potentiates gallstone development by preventing clearance of biliary sludge and microgallstones. Patients with subnormal cholecystokinin release caused by decreased duodenal stimulation (e.g., those on total parenteral nutrition or fat-restricted diets) or with neuropathy (e.g., spinal cord injury patients and diabetics with autonomic dysfunction) have impaired gallbladder motility. Progesterone, but not estrogen, impairs gallbladder emptying and acts synergistically to accelerate gallstone development while cholesterol secretion is increased during pregnancy.

NATURAL HISTORY OF GALLSTONES

The natural history of gallstones has been studied in asymptomatic and symptomatic patients. In several studies subjects have been retrospectively identified with gallstones, and the risk of development of symptoms or biliary complications such as acute cholecystitis or cholangitis, common duct obstruction, or pancreatitis was determined. The risk of symptom development is from 20% to 40% over 20 years, with the highest risk in the first 5 years and decreasing risk the longer the stones remain asymptomatic. Patients did not have complications as their initial manifestation of gallstones.

In several studies, gallstones appear to have a higher risk of causing symptoms in women than in men. Although this effect has been ascribed to the greater use of ultrasonography in women, with incidental identification of gallstones, prospective studies have also observed higher rates of development of symptoms, but not complications, in women. The number or size of stones does not appear to correlate with the development of symptoms.

Patients who are already symptomatic are more likely to continue to have symptoms than those who were initially asymptomatic. Moreover, the risk of complications in previously symptomatic patients, including common bile duct obstruction, cholecystitis, cholangitis, and pancreatitis, is 15% to 20% over 5 years. Gallbladder nonvisualization on oral cholecystogram confers an additional risk of worsening symptoms or biliary complications.

Pancreatitis is a well-known complication of gallstones. In contrast to other causes of pancreatitis that are more common in males, gallstone pancreatitis has the same epidemiologic patterns as gallstones and is twice as common in women as in men. Recently it has been established that biliary sludge is present in the majority of patients with recurrent idiopathic pancreatitis. Although follow-up evaluation has been limited, cholecystectomy or treatment with ursodiol may be successful in preventing further recurrences.

A rare but significant long-term complication is gallbladder carcinoma, which accounts for about 2% of all malignancies in the United States. The majority of patients with gallbladder cancer have gallstones, usually of the cholesterol type. Common risk factors for gallstones and gallbladder cancer include older age, female sex, and American Indian ancestry. The highest risk is found in gallbladders harboring large gallstones, with the size of the largest gallstone correlating with the risk of development of gallbladder cancer. The relative risk rises for stones from 1 to 2 cm in

diameter and reaches a relative risk of about 10 for gallstones greater than 3 cm in diameter. It should be noted that very large gallstones are relatively rare, constituting only 6% of all gallstones in one study in the Native American Indian and white populations. However, because of the high relative risk of gallbladder cancer in patients with large stones, about one third of all gallbladder cancers have been estimated to occur in patients with stones greater than 3 cm. In populations in whom cholesterol stones are less common, a disproportionate number of patients with gallbladder cancer harbor cholesterol stones. The actual risk of cholesterol versus pigment stones is unknown. However, since cholesterol stones form at a younger age, the duration of gallstone disease may be the important variable, and gallstone size may simply be a marker for duration of gallstone disease.

CLINICAL PRESENTATION

History and Symptom Presentation

Gallstones cause symptoms only when migration occurs into the cystic or common bile duct. Biliary pain, caused by stones intermittently obstructing or passing through the cystic duct, bile duct, or papilla, is a constant, noncolicky, abdominal pain lasting from 30 minutes to several hours. The location is most often epigastric, rather than right upper quadrant, and may radiate to the back or scapulae. A history of postprandial or nocturnal symptoms is helpful. There is no correlation between the presence of gallstones and symptoms such as nausea, dyspepsia, diarrhea, constipation, heartburn, irregular bowel habits, or bloating. Additional symptoms are present when gallstone disease has led to complications, including acute cholecystitis, biliary obstruction, pancreatitis, and cholangitis.

Physical Examination

Physical examination is most helpful during an acute attack of biliary colic or cholecystitis. Abdominal tenderness localized to the midclavicular line below the costal margin has been termed *Murphy's sign*. Ultrasonic demonstration of tenderness over the gallbladder, the radiographic equivalent of Murphy's sign, is very helpful in confirming the diagnosis. Cholecystitis or cholangitis is typically accompanied by fever, but in cholangitis localizing abdominal signs may be absent.

Diagnostic Tests

The logical application of diagnostic tools for the documentation of suspected gallstone disease naturally depends on the correct recognition of clinical presentation. It cannot be overemphasized that a carefully taken history is essential before embarking on what should be a thorough assessment of the biliary tract when indicated. Technology should complement, not substitute for, good clinical practice.

Laboratory Tests

During biliary pain, results of laboratory tests may be entirely normal. Transient partial or complete obstruction of the biliary tree may produce abnormalities in levels of serum transaminase, alkaline phosphatase, and bilirubin. After passage of a gallstone serum transaminase levels may be elevated to 10 to 20 times normal but rapidly decrease to normal. Alkaline phosphatase level is characteristically disproportionately elevated during partial or complete biliary obstruction. Serum bilirubin level rises during complete biliary obstruction, but the rise occurs more slowly over days.

Imaging Tests

The **plain abdominal radiography (KUB)** will detect between 10% and 30% of gallstones within the gallbladder and 2% or less in the bile duct. This simple procedure carries no risk. It has a very low sensitivity but high specificity, making this an initial investigation of limited benefit. Detection of calcification in gallstones, however, has implications for nonoperative therapy.

Oral cholecystography (OCG) was the principal method for gallstone evaluation until the advent of ultrasound. Radiographic imaging of the gallbladder area is obtained 12 to 15 hours after ingestion of contrast medium and is usually followed by induction of gallbladder contraction achieved by ingestion of fat or by intravenous injection of cholecystokinin or its octapeptide, sincalide. Serious morbidity from orally administered contrast agents is rare, but minor symptoms of nausea, vomiting, and diarrhea occur in up to 50%. Renal toxicity may occur in patients receiving large doses or a simultaneous intravenous agent, and this combined examination is therefore contraindicated. A technically satisfactory OCG will allow diagnosis of radiolucent gallstones with a sensitivity of more than 90%. In the absence of interfering factors, a nonopacified gallbladder has a positive predictive value of disease of more than 90%. However, at least 10% of patients with complete nonopacification and 60% with poor opacification after single-dose OCG have normal gallbladders. Nonopacification may result from failure of contrast medium absorption, uptake or excretion by the liver, or failure of entry into the gallbladder, implying mechanical obstruction of the cystic duct. OCG is now commonly used to assess cystic duct patency for proposed medical therapy.

Transcutaneous ultrasound now represents the first-line investigation of suspected biliary disease and uses high-frequency sound of 3.5 to 5 MHz for imaging by reflection. Gallbladder stones have a characteristic appearance of high-amplitude intraluminal reflections casting acoustic shadows with gravity-dependent movement (Fig. 16-1). The patient must fast for at least 8 hours before the examination to allow maximal distention of the gallbladder. Ultrasound detects gallbladder stones with sensitivity and specificity of more than 95% but is somewhat less sensitive for biliary sludge. Nonimaging of the gallbladder may be due to its being packed with stones with very little surrounding bile, a small contracted gallbladder, lack of fasting, obesity, or an atypical gallbladder position. Ultrasound is far less sensitive (40% to 70%) for bile duct stones because of the relative inaccessibility of the lower bile duct to sound waves that results from surrounding structures and bowel gas.

Radionuclide scanning (scintigraphy) with a technetium-labeled derivative of iminodiacetic acid (IDA) injected intravenously has become the most popular form of radionuclide scanning. After an interval of 20 to 60 minutes the radionuclide is taken up by the liver and excreted into bile, where it readily produces a representation of the biliary tract on gamma camera imaging. Patient preparation is minimal as the test is used only in suspected acute cholecystitis. In the absence of chronic liver disease and parenteral feeding, the sensitivity exceeds 95% and the specificity approaches 100% for cystic duct obstruction if the gallbladder fails to image. The presence of mild cholestasis with bilirubin levels up to 4 mg/dl does not preclude use of this technique, and some IDA analogs are excreted in the presence of a level greater than 15 mg/100 ml. The negative predictive value of a normal scan finding is greater than 98%.

Computed tomography (CT) is capable of demonstrating the biliary tree and gallstones, but pure cholesterol stones may not be distinguishable from surrounding bile by CT. Diagnosis of gallbladder disease is likely to be 80% accurate, and in the presence of jaundice the distinction between a dilated and a nondilated system is possible with a sensitivity of up to 88% and a specificity of up to 97%. Sensitivity and specificity of identification of the cause of obstruction are equivalent to those of ultrasound, although CT shows the lower bile duct more accurately. CT assessment of stone density has improved the results of medical dissolution with bile acids with or without shock-wave lithotripsy. Recent software developments and the ability to acquire volume data by helical CT scanning have made CT cholangiography possible.

Endoscopic retrograde cholangiopancreatography (ERCP) was developed in the early 1970s as a method for direct cholangiography by instillation of radiographic contrast medium across the papilla and directly into the biliary tree. Its advantages over percutaneous transhepatic cholangiography are the additional information gained from endoscopic examination of the upper gastrointestinal tract and papilla, the ability to perform biopsy, the concomitant pancreatogram, and the potential for immediate biliary therapy. Endoscopy also allows collection of bile for microscopic examination for cholesterol crystals or bilirubin granules and is the most sensitive method for diagnosing biliary sludge. Attention to detail and the need for high-quality radiographs make for improved accuracy in the diagnosis of calculous disease, and it is vital that no barium studies have been undertaken within 3 days of the ERCP as residual barium in the colon commonly overlies the pancreas and lower bile duct. In experienced hands successful cholangiography should be achieved in more than 95% of cases irrespective of bile duct diameter and is a highly accurate method for identifying stones in the bile ducts and gallbladder. Sensitivity and specificity for stone disease exceed 90%. ERCP fails in a small number of attempts because of inaccessibility of the duodenal papilla, presence of pyloric or duodenal stenosis, and some cases of duodenal diverticulum or Billroth II partial gastrectomy. Morbidity rate for diagnostic ERCP should be less than 10% with a mortality rate of less than 0.1%. Sepsis was once the most serious complication but has been minimized by the introduction of immediate endoscopic therapy. Acute pancreatitis now represents the most common complication, but no preprocedure pharmacologic manipulations have proved effective in preventing it.

Magnetic resonance imaging (MRI) has been applied to the evaluation of the biliary tract in recent years, particularly since the development of software allowing reconstruction of the biliary tract and pancreatic ductal system as a two-dimensional projection, **magnetic resonance cholangiopancreatography (MRCP).** No oral or intravenous contrast administration is required, and its popularity is growing as MRI scanners become faster and capable of creating MRCP images automatically with less dependence on the radiologist's expertise and enthusiasm. Detection of bile duct stones carries a sensitivity of up to 100% and a specificity of 73% with a positive predictive value of 63% and a negative predictive value of 100%. There is a limitation in imaging small stones, but this is likely to improve with evolution of the technology. MRCP is a realistic and safe alternative to diagnostic ERCP, but its exact role in different clinical situations is still being evaluated.

Endoscopic ultrasound (EUS) is a method of intracorporeal ultrasound whereby an ultrasound transducer mounted on the tip of a flexible endoscope can be placed very close to the organs under examination, such as the bile duct. It is an invasive procedure performed under sedation but carries no greater risk in the majority of patients compared with standard upper gastrointestinal endoscopy. An experienced endosonographer may detect bile duct stones with a sensitivity of more than 95%, and EUS is therefore comparable with ERCP without the risk of post-ERCP complications. This imaging modality is not widely available, requires considerable training, and has no current therapeutic ability for bile duct stones.

APPROACH TO THE PATIENT WITH GALLSTONES

For a patient with a history of recurrent biliary pain without jaundice, ultrasound is likely to be the only modality needed. ERCP may occasionally be required when abdominal ultrasound does not show gallstones and symptoms continue. OCG and CT may be useful for assessment before nonoperative therapy (Fig. 16-4).

For the woman with suspected cholecystitis, urgent ultrasound and/or radionuclide scanning has a high success rate for diagnosis. Only in the presence of significantly abnormal liver function test results or overt jaundice is cholangiography necessary. The presence of a gallbladder mass may be further defined by CT or MRI.

Characterization of obstructive jaundice is now possible in all patients by logical and judicious use of initial noninvasive studies such as ultrasound, CT, MRI/MRCP followed by direct cholangiography by percutaneous trans-

hepatic cholangiography or ERCP with a view to therapy if indicated. In a patient with acute pancreatitis without obvious cause the diagnosis of gallstones is important, and urgent ultrasound combined with biochemical predictive tests allows a diagnosis in up to 80%. This allows selection of patients for emergency ERCP when appropriate and elective treatment for those who recover from the initial attack.

Today few cases of gallstone disease are not amenable to modern imaging methods, but all modalities have some limitations, and clinical suspicion remains imperative in pursuing the correct diagnosis.

MANAGEMENT

Once clinical symptoms of gallstones develop, treatment algorithms, as summarized in Fig. 16-4, are the same for both sexes, with the exception of treatment during pregnancy. Treatment options range in degrees of invasiveness from oral pharmacologic dissolution with ursodiol, extracorporeal shock-wave lithotripsy with ursodiol, endoscopic interventions and percutaneous techniques, to surgery.

Choice of Therapy

Ursodiol, or ursodeoxycholic acid, is a naturally occurring bile acid, is present in minor quantities in bile, and dissolves cholesterol gallstones when given in doses of 8 mg/kg/day. Only selected patients are suitable candidates for dissolution therapy. The stones must be cholesterol, as determined by their ability to float on an OCG, and demonstrate no calcification on KUB or CT; the cystic duct should be patent (gallbladder opacification on OCG) for the bile salts to reach the gallstones; and ideally the stones should be less than 1 cm in diameter. Although larger stones have been successfully treated, the success rate is much lower, and these patients should be treated by lithotripsy followed by dissolution therapy.

For patients who meet these criteria, dissolution is successful in about two thirds but takes up to 2 years, typically proceeding at 1 mm per month. Dissolution is monitored by abdominal ultrasound, and ursodiol is continued for 3 months after a negative ultrasound result to ensure dissolution of small fragments. During ursodiol administration intestinal cholesterol absorption and biliary cholesterol secretion decrease, but bile salt synthesis and serum lipoprotein levels are unchanged. Ursodiol has no significant toxicity and only occasionally causes diarrhea. Only patients with infrequent symptomatic biliary pain, without urgent complications of gallstones, should be considered for dissolution therapy.

Extracorporeal shock-wave lithotripsy fragments cholesterol gallstones by high-energy shock waves into smaller fragments that can either pass spontaneously through the cystic and common bile ducts or dissolve with ursodiol 45. Postlithotripsy treatment with ursodiol must be continued until 3 months after the gallbladder is clear of fragments. For the ideal candidate with a single gallstone of less than 2 cm in diameter, the success rate approaches 80%. Lithotripsy can also be used for patients with up to three stones with a total diameter of 2 cm, but with a lower success rate. The rate of complications, including common bile duct obstruction or pancreatitis secondary to fragment passage, is less than 5%.

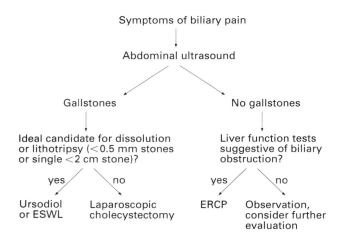

FIG. 16-4 Approach to the woman with uncomplicated gallstones. *ESWL,* Extracorporeal shock-wave lithotripsy; *ERCP,* endoscopic retrograde cholangiopancreatography.

After lithotripsy or dissolution therapy, the risk of gallstone recurrence is high, up to 50% after 5 years. Patients should be monitored with periodic ultrasound every 6 months, and therapy with ursodeoxycholic acid should be reinstated if asymptomatic gallstones recur, as dissolution is more rapid for small stones.

The use of **ERCP** for choledocholithiasis has gained widespread acceptance since the first independent reports of endoscopic sphincterotomy in 1974. Endoscopic sphincterotomy was initially considered justifiable only in elderly postcholecystectomy patients with recurrent or retained common bile duct stones who were at high risk of serious complications from conventional surgical common bile duct exploration. With improved efficacy, demand, and training in therapeutic biliary endoscopic techniques, however, there has been an expanding role for the endoscopic management of choledocholithiasis.

There is now general agreement among surgeons and gastroenterologists that endoscopic removal of common bile duct stones is preferable to surgery in the following patients:

- Patients who have undergone previous cholecystectomy.
- High-risk surgical patients when the gallbladder is still present.
- Patients with severe acute cholangitis.
- Selected patients with acute biliary pancreatitis.
- Special circumstances for the average risk surgical patient with suspected choledocholithiasis before laparoscopic cholecystectomy (Fig. 16-4).

Up to 15% of patients undergoing cholecystectomy have common duct stones. Unlike those with gallbladder stones, the majority of individuals with asymptomatic common duct stones will ultimately become symptomatic, in either the early or the late perioperative period, with the development of one or more symptoms, including biliary pain, jaundice, cholangitis, or pancreatitis. The natural history supports an active treatment approach rather than expectant management for all patients with common bile duct stones. Endoscopic sphincterotomy is the procedure of choice for common bile duct stones that appear in the late perioperative period.

Laparoscopic cholecystectomy has largely replaced conventional **open cholecystectomy** because of the short hospitalization and rapid return to normal activities as the standard. Advances in surgical technique and equipment have made possible laparoscopic transcystic stone extraction and exploration of the common duct, although these techniques are not yet routine in all hospitals. Laparoscopic cholecystectomy has a 5% rate of conversion to open cholecystectomy that is primarily due to local complications, usually bleeding, or to technical difficulties that prevent adequate dissection. Common bile duct injuries are currently more frequent than in open cholecystectomy, 0.2% to 0.5%; most occur during the first 25 procedures by an individual surgeon. The introduction of laparoscopic cholecystectomy should not alter the indications for cholecystectomy, but overall numbers of cholecystectomies have increased.

PREGNANCY AND GALLSTONES
Epidemiology

Prospective ultrasonographic study has shown that the incidence of sludge and gallstone formation increases progressively with each trimester of pregnancy (Fig. 16-5). During pregnancy biliary cholesterol saturation increases, mediated at least partly through the effects of estrogens. Gallbladder stasis also occurs secondary to the effects of high progesterone levels. The additive effects contribute to a very high incidence of cholesterol gallstone formation during pregnancy that is several times that for age-matched women. Stones tend to be multiple and small.

Natural History

The natural history of gallstones in pregnant and postpartum women differs from that in the general population. In contrast to longitudinal studies in the general population suggesting that the annual incidence of new symptoms is 2% to 3%, symptoms develop in about one third of pregnant women with gallstones. Moreover, the most common cause of pancreatitis during pregnancy is gallstone or biliary sludge. Hence biliary disease should be high on the differential diagnosis of abdominal pain during pregnancy.

In the first postpartum month approximately one half of women have either gallbladder sludge or stones. However, in the next year at least the gallbladder reverts to normal in at least 75% of women with biliary sludge, and about one third of women with gallstones spontaneously pass or dissolve the gallstones.

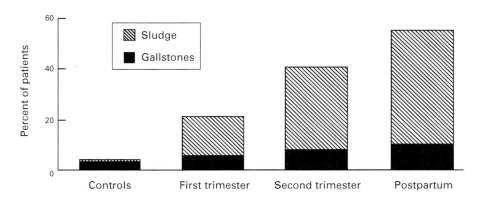

FIG. 16-5 The development of sludge and gallstones during pregnancy. The incidence of sludge increases with each trimester, and gallstones developed in almost 10% by delivery. (From Maringhini A et al: *Gastroenterology* 95:1160, 1988.)

Management

During Pregnancy

In general, therapy is aimed at temporizing and delaying surgical intervention until the postpartum period. Patients with symptoms thought to be due to common bile duct stones causing cholangitis, obstruction, or severe pancreatitis should be treated without delay by ERCP and sphincterotomy, using appropriate radiologic safety precautions to the fetus. In experienced hands the risk of complications is low. If unavoidable, conventional cholecystectomy does not seem to pose significant risks to the pregnancy in the first or third trimester. Surgery during the second trimester has been associated with premature labor. Laparoscopic cholecystectomy has been undertaken during pregnancy but may be limited by technical considerations as pregnancy advances and, if possible, should be deferred until the postpartum period.

Postpartum

In view of their high frequency of spontaneous clearance of gallstones, women with postpartum biliary pain may be considered for ursodiol therapy if they have small (<5 mm) gallstones or biliary sludge as documented by ultrasound. Once the high-risk period of pregnancy has passed, these women are most likely at lower risk of gallstone recurrence. Case reports have shown that ursodiol is not excreted in breast milk, although no controlled data are available.

BIBLIOGRAPHY

Barbara L et al: A population study on the prevalence of gallstone disease: the Sirmione study, *Hepatology* 7:913, 1987.

Braverman DZ, Johnson ML, Kern F Jr: Effects of pregnancy and contraceptive steroids on gallbladder function, *N Engl J Med* 302:362, 1980.

Carey MC: Pathogenesis of gallstones, *Am J Surg* 165:410, 1993.

deLedinghen V et al: Diagnosis of Choledocholithiasis: EUS or magnetic resonance holangiography? A prospective controlled study, *Gastrointest Endosc* 49:26, 1999.

Diehl AK: Epidemiology and natural history of gallstone disease, *Gastroenterol Clin North Am* 20:1, 1991.

Everson GT, McKinley C, Kern F Jr: Mechanisms of gallstone formation in women: effects of exogenous estrogen (Premarin) and dietary cholesterol on hepatic lipid metabolism, *J Clin Invest* 87:237, 1991.

Friedman GD: Natural history of asymptomatic and symptomatic gallstones, *Am J Surg* 165:399, 1993.

Grodstein F et al: A prospective study of symptomatic gallstones in women: relation with oral contraceptives and other risk factors, *Obstet Gynecol* 84:207, 1994.

Janowitz P et al: Gallbladder sludge: spontaneous course and incidence of complications in patients without stones, *Hepatology* 20:291, 1994.

Jorgensen T: Gallstones in a Danish population: fertility period, pregnancies, and exogenous female sex hormones, *Gut* 29:433, 1989.

Jorgensen T: Prevalence of gallstones in a Danish population, *Am J Epidemiol* 126:912, 1987.

Lowenfels AB et al: Gallstone growth, size, and risk of gallbladder cancer: an interracial study, *Int J Epidemiol* 18:50, 1989.

Maclure KM et al: Weight, diet, and the risk of symptomatic gallstones in middle-aged women, *N Engl J Med* 321:563, 1989.

Maringhini A et al: Biliary sludge and gallstones in pregnancy: incidence, risk factors, and natural history, *Ann Intern Med* 119:116, 1993.

May GR, Sutherland LR, Shaffer EA: Efficacy of bile acid therapy for gallstone dissolution—a meta-analysis of randomized trials, *Aliment Pharmacol Therapeut* 7:139, 1993.

NIH Consensus conference: Gallstones and laparoscopic cholecystectomy, *JAMA* 269:1018, 1993.

O'Donnell LDJ, Heaton KW: Recurrence and re-recurrence of gallstones after medical dissolution: a longterm follow-up, *Gut* 29:655, 1988.

Petitti DB, Sidney S, Perlman JA: Increased risk of cholecystectomy in users of supplemental estrogen, *Gastroenterology* 94:91, 1988.

Ransohoff DF, Gracie WA: Treatment of gallstones, *Ann Intern Med* 119:606, 1993.

Ros E et al: Symptomatic versus silent gallstones—radiographic features and eligibility for nonsurgical treatment, *Dig Dis Sci* 39:1697, 1994.

Sackmann M et al: The Munich gallbladder lithotripsy study: results of the first five years with 711 patients, *Ann Intern Med* 114:290, 1991.

Schoenfield LJ: Oral and contact dissolution of gallstones, *Am J Surg* 165:427, 1993.

Strasberg SM, Clavien PA: Overview of therapeutic modalities for the treatment of gallstone disease, *Am J Surg* 165:420, 1993.

Valdivieso V et al: Pregnancy and cholelithiasis: pathogenesis and natural course of gallstones diagnosed in early puerperium, *Hepatology* 17:1, 1993.

CHAPTER 17

Gastroesophageal Reflux and Peptic Ulcer Disease

John M. Poneros
Lawrence S. Friedman

GASTROESOPHAGEAL REFLUX DISEASE

Gastrointestinal disorders are among the most common conditions for which women seek medical attention. Heartburn caused by gastroesophageal reflux disease (GERD) is estimated to occur daily in 7% and monthly in 44% of adults in the United States. Although men experience symptoms of GERD more frequently than women, GERD and associated complications are particularly common in women who are pregnant, take oral contraceptives, or have certain rheumatologic conditions such as scleroderma.

Pathophysiology

Factors that promote GERD include increased gastric volume after meals, gastric stasis, and recumbency. Most reflux episodes are associated with transient relaxations of the lower esophageal sphincter (LES). Resting LES pressure is also decreased by smoking, anticholinergic medications, calcium channel antagonists, pregnancy, progesterone, and scleroderma. Esophagitis occurs when caustic gastric contents remain in contact with the esophageal mucosa for a sufficient amount of time to overwhelm esophageal defenses, including salivary bicarbonate and esophageal peristalsis. Certain medications can also cause esophagitis; these include alendronate in women with osteoporosis, nonsteroidal anti-inflammatory drugs (NSAIDs), tetracyclines, quinidine, and potassium chloride preparations. The role of a hiatal hernia in the pathophysiology of GERD has long been debated; hiatal hernias appear to promote esophagitis as a result of a decrease in the LES pressure and an increase in contact time between refluxed gastric acid and the mucosa in the hernia.

Clinical Features

The most common clinical manifestation of GERD is heartburn, most often after meals or on reclining. Chest pain resulting from GERD may also result from esophageal spasm and must be distinguished from cardiac pain. Other possible symptoms include regurgitation, "water brash" as a result of increased salivary secretion, and dysphagia as a result of an esophageal stricture or diminished esophageal peristalsis. Extraesophageal manifestations of GERD include cough, laryngitis, asthma, and aspiration pneumonia. The possibility of underlying GERD should be considered in patients with asthma who present in adulthood, lack a history of atopy, and have predominantly nocturnal symptoms. Reflux-induced asthma generally responds poorly to bronchodilator and corticosteroid therapy.

Diagnosis

In patients presenting with symptoms of GERD, a characteristic history often permits diagnosis and initiation of treatment. Moreover, there is little correlation between the severity of symptoms and the presence of mucosal disease (esophagitis).

Physical examination is generally unrevealing, although findings associated with extraesophageal manifestations (e.g., hoarseness, wheezing) should be sought. Additional diagnostic testing should be performed only in patients with persistent symptoms despite therapy or with signs suggestive of esophagitis or other complications, including dysphagia, a positive fecal occult blood test, or anemia.

Commonly used diagnostic tests include upper endoscopy, barium swallow, 24-hour ambulatory pH monitoring, and the Bernstein test. Endoscopy is more sensitive and specific than barium-based upper gastrointestinal radiography in demonstrating esophageal mucosal injury. However, in patients with dysphagia, a barium swallow is a useful initial test for demonstrating a stricture and assessing its length and severity. Endoscopy permits detection of not only esophagitis but also Barrett's esophagus, or metaplastic transformation of the esophageal mucosa (see following discussion). Although considered the "gold standard" for the diagnosis of GERD, 24-hour ambulatory pH recording is indicated only to (1) evaluate patients with symptoms of GERD in whom esophagitis is absent on upper endoscopy and symptoms fail to improve on a proton pump inhibitor, (2) confirm abnormal esophageal acid exposure in a patient being considered for antireflux surgery without endoscopic evidence of esophagitis, and (3) evaluate patients after antireflux surgery who are suspected of having persistent reflux. The Bernstein test assesses whether symptoms are reproduced on infusion of 0.1N hydrochloric acid into the esophagus to determine whether atypical chest pain is related to acid reflux.

A recent study found the "omeprazole test" to have a high positive predictive value in determining that noncardiac chest pain is secondary to GERD. This test consists of assessing symptomatic improvement after a 7-day course of oral omeprazole, 40 mg orally every morning and 20 mg orally every evening. If validated, the "omeprazole test" may result in improved diagnostic capability and potential cost savings compared with traditional diagnostic strategies for GERD.

✳ MANAGEMENT

The goals of therapy for patients with GERD are to ameliorate symptoms and heal esophagitis, if present. Many patients with GERD can be treated with modifications in lifestyle and over-the-counter medications, generally antacids or histamine H-2-receptor antagonists. Beneficial lifestyle modifications include elevating the head of the bed, reducing the size of meals, avoiding recumbency after eating, and avoiding tobacco and alcohol. Foods that exacerbate symptoms of GERD should be avoided; common offenders include fatty foods, chocolate, carminatives (peppermint, spearmint), onion, garlic, coffee (caffeinated and decaffeinated), and citrus fruit juices. Obese patients may be aided by losing weight. Patients with severe GERD should avoid the following medications, if possible: anticholinergics, theophylline, diazepam, narcotics, and calcium channel blockers.

Medical Therapy

Antacids, such as Mylanta, Maalox, and Gelusil, may be used on an as-needed basis for rapid relief of heartburn. Their efficacy stems from their ability to buffer acid. Patients should be made aware of potential complications, particularly diarrhea with magnesium-containing products and constipation with aluminum-containing agents. Excessive, long-term use may lead to milk-alkali syndrome.

If lifestyle modifications and over-the-counter medications fail to control symptoms, more potent antisecretory or prokinetic agents (or both) may be prescribed. H-2-receptor antagonists, including cimetidine, ranitidine, famotidine, and nizatidine, are generally effective for symptomatic GERD. These agents inhibit gastric acid secretion and thereby raise the gastric pH to levels that are less harmful to the esophageal mucosa. Because GERD is a chronic condition, long-term treatment is often necessary. For maximum benefit, the H-2-receptor antagonists should be administered at least twice a day and in an "antireflux dosage." Ranitidine in doses of 150 mg twice a day has been approved by the Food and Drug Administration (FDA) for maintenance therapy of GERD, but some patients require higher than standard doses for the control of symptoms (e.g., 300 mg twice a day, or higher) (Table 17-1).

In patients with mild to moderate GERD, two prokinetic agents are available for treatment: metoclopramide, a dopamine antagonist, and bethanecol, a cholinergic agonist that is now rarely used. These agents increase LES pressure, enhance esophageal peristaltic amplitude, and promote gastric emptying. However, prokinetic agents must be used with caution owing to their serious side effects and potential complications. Metoclopramide may cause muscle hypertonia, extrapyramidal reactions, and acute dystonic reactions.

Table 17-1
Medical Therapy of Gastroesophageal Reflux Disease and Peptic Ulcer Disease in Pregnancy

Acid-Suppressing Agents		Category*
H-2-receptor antagonists:	Cimetidine	B
	Ranitidine	B
	Famotidine	B
	Nizatidine	C
Proton pump inhibitors:	Omeprazole	C
	Esomeprazole	C
	Lansoprazole	B
	Pantoprazole	B
Drugs that increase mucosal resistance:	Sucralfate	B
Promotility agents:	Metoclopramide	B

*FDA Designations of Drugs for Use in Pregnancy.

Category	Designation
A	Controlled studies show no risk to fetus
B	Human trials demonstrate no risk to the fetus, animal studies show some risk, or no adequate human trials but animal trials demonstrate no risk to the fetus
C	Human studies unavailable, but animal studies demonstrate increase fetal risk or are unavailable
D	Experimental or marketing information demonstrate fetal risk, but possible benefit of drug outweighs risk

Neuroleptic malignant syndrome has also been seen with use of metoclopramide.

Proton pump inhibitors (PPIs) are indicated for the treatment of erosive esophagitis and GERD refractory to H-2-receptor antagonists. Proton pump inhibitors block gastric acid secretion and raise gastric pH more effectively than H-2-receptor antagonists by irreversibly inhibiting the $H+-K+$ adenosine triphosphatase (ATPase) of the parietal cell, the final common pathway for gastric acid secretion. Omeprazole is approved by the FDA for use as first-line therapy in patients with heartburn; both omeprazole, 20 mg/day, and lansoprazole, 15 mg/day, are approved for maintenance therapy. The long-term safety of PPIs continues to be debated; however, to date no data have emerged to support initial concerns raised about the possibility of gastric neoplasia with long-term use.

Surgical Therapy

Antireflux surgery for GERD may be considered as an alternative to lifelong medical therapy or in patients with symptoms or esophagitis refractory to medical treatment. Surgery may also be considered after the occurrence of reflux-induced aspiration pneumonia or the failure of medical therapy to control reflux-related extraesophageal disease, such as asthma or laryngitis.

First performed laparoscopically in 1991, the Nissen fundoplication is the most commonly performed antireflux surgery and consists of a 360-degree wrap of the gastric fundus around the distal esophagus. The Toupet partial fundoplication consists of a 270-degree posterior partial wrap and is used in patients with diminished esophageal peristaltic activity. Numerous studies have shown that the outcomes associated with laparoscopic Nissen or Toupet fundoplication are equal or superior to those obtained with open procedures. Mortality rates for laparoscopic fundoplication have been low as a result of careful patient selection and the avoidance of an open abdominal incision. Contraindications to laparoscopic antireflux surgery are similar to those for the open operation and include poor general anesthesia risk, coagulopathy, severe chronic obstructive pulmonary disease, and pregnancy. In addition, these procedures are technically more difficult in obese patients and in patients with large paraesophageal hernias.

Complications

The primary complications of esophagitis include stricture formation, Barrett's esophagus, bleeding, and, rarely, perforation. Strictures develop at sites of recurrent inflammation and manifest clinically as progressive dysphagia for solid foods. The length and degree of narrowing of a stricture are best assessed by barium swallow. Endoscopy should be performed to confirm the benign nature of the stricture and perform dilatation. Failure to dilate a stricture successfully or to prevent its recurrence is an indication for surgery.

Barrett's esophagus is characterized by the replacement of the normal squamous epithelium in the distal esophagus with specialized columnar epithelium, also described as intestinal metaplasia. Barrett's esophagus occurs in approximately 12% of patients with chronic GERD, and affected patients are predominately white men between the ages of 40 and 60. The yearly incidence of adenocarcinoma in patients with Barrett's esophagus is thought to be on the order of 0.5% to 1%, and regular endoscopic surveillance is recommended in these patients.

Patients with severe GERD may have mucosal injury associated with esophageal ulceration and erosions. Occasionally, inflammation is severe enough to result in chronic bleeding and anemia. Rarely, deep ulcerations have been reported to cause perforation.

Gastroesophageal Reflux Disease and Women

There is experimental and clinical evidence that estrogens and particularly progesterone lower LES tone, and women taking oral contraceptives may note worsening of GERD symptoms. If the onset or worsening of GERD symptoms relates temporally to hormonal therapy, adjustment of the dose or discontinuation should be considered initially. However, if this is not possible or desired, acid suppressive therapy may control the symptoms.

Esophageal involvement results in motility abnormalities in 75% to 85% of patients (often women) with scleroderma. Scleroderma may result in a patulous LES and aperistalsis of the distal esophagus. The severity of esophageal involvement does not correlate with the extent of cutaneous changes or other systemic manifestations. There is no effective treatment to prevent esophageal involvement in scleroderma, and GERD associated with scleroderma must be treated aggressively. Stricture formation is a common complication and may require repeated dilatations.

■ GASTROESOPHAGEAL REFLUX DISEASE AND PREGNANCY

Symptoms of GERD are frequent in pregnant women. In a recent large study of pregnant women, the frequency and severity of heartburn increased steadily throughout pregnancy: 22% of women complained of heartburn in the first trimester, 39% in the second trimester, and 72% in the third trimester. On regression analysis, the risk of heartburn was found to increase directly with gestational age, the presence of prepregnancy heartburn, and parity and to decrease with maternal age. Body mass index before pregnancy, weight gain during pregnancy, and race did not predict the frequency or severity of heartburn.

GERD in pregnancy may be severe enough to interfere with sleep and the intake of food and poses a risk for malnutrition. Therapy is generally the same as for any patient with GERD, but conservative measures, specifically lifestyle modifications, dietary changes, and nonsystemic therapies, such as antacids, should be attempted before systemically absorbed drugs are prescribed. Antacids containing magnesium or aluminum or a combination of antacids and alginic acid (Gavison) are acceptable first-line therapy early in pregnancy; these drugs are not absorbed by the intestine and have shown no teratogenic effects in animals. In a British study, a twice-daily dose of magnesium trisilicate or a combination of an alginate preparation with aluminum hydroxide improved daily and nocturnal symptoms in 47% of 157 pregnant patients with GERD at the end of 2 weeks. Magnesium-containing antacids should be avoided in the latter part of pregnancy because magnesium sulfate may slow down or arrest labor and may cause convulsions. Antacids containing sodium bicarbonate should be avoided throughout pregnancy because they can lead to metabolic alkalosis and fluid overload. Antacids may also interfere with iron absorption.

Although it is likely that cimetidine, ranitidine, and possibly famotidine are safe if needed in pregnancy, these medications should be used only when absolutely necessary. Cimetidine crosses the placenta, but there have been no reports of fetal harm, and administration of cimetidine was not associated with teratogenic effects in a study of 460 newborns exposed to the drug in the first trimester (Table 17-1).

Although the antiemetic and prokinetic agent metoclopramide has been designated a category B agent because no fetal abnormalities have been reported in animal studies, the drug is not recommended in pregnancy because of frequent side effects, including drowsiness, anxiety, insomnia, and dystonic and parkinsonian-like reactions.

Omeprazole has been classified as a category C drug (Table 17-1) and has resulted in teratogenesis in rabbits when administered at 17 to 172 times the standard dose in humans. Individual patients given the drug during pregnancy have not been reported to experience adverse effects. One patient with Zollinger-Ellison syndrome delivered three healthy infants after continuous treatment with omeprazole, 60 mg twice a day, or ranitidine,150 mg twice a day, throughout all three pregnancies. Lansoprazole has been designated a category B drug on the basis of animal studies in which 40 to 60 times the recommended dose in humans did not result in impaired fertility or fetal harm. However, there are no clinical studies of lansoprazole in pregnant women, and the drug should be used only if absolutely necessary.

■ ENDOSCOPY AND PREGNANCY

When complications of GERD are suspected, upper endoscopy is the diagnostic procedure of choice, because barium radiography must be avoided in pregnancy, particularly during the first trimester. When indicated, upper endoscopy appears to be safe in pregnancy. Sedation and analgesia with meperidine and midazolam or diazepam is likely to be safe, particularly after the first trimester (although not approved by the FDA). However, midazolam and diazepam are designated category D drugs (Table 17-1), and meperidine (and fentanyl) are designated category C drugs during the first, second, or third trimester of pregnancy. In a retrospective study of upper endoscopy performed in 20 women for a range of indications, no significant complications occurred, and labor was not induced. In this study, 65% of the patients received meperidine and 20% received midazolam or diazepam; 95% of the women delivered healthy infants, a rate equal to that for age-matched controls. Premature delivery or fetal distress did not occur, and Apgar scores at delivery were uniformly 8 or higher. In general, it is recommended that, when possible, endoscopy be postponed until after the first trimester.

PEPTIC ULCER DISEASE

Peptic ulcer disease (PUD) develops in approximately 10% of adults in the United States during their lifetimes and is the most common cause of upper gastrointestinal bleeding, accounting for half of all cases. Physiologic studies have reported no difference in gastric acid secretion or fasting gastric and duodenal pH between women and men. The incidence of ulcers increases with age in both women and men. The prevalence of ulcers for women aged 25 to 29 years, 35 to 39 years, and greater than 50 years is reported to be 0.3, 0.62, and 0.84 per 1000, respectively. The increased prevalence of ulcers in elderly women has been attributed to increased use of NSAIDs in this population.

Pathophysiology

Peptic ulcer disease results from an imbalance between "aggressive" factors such as gastric acid and pepsin and "defensive" factors involved in mucosal resistance such as gastric mucus and bicarbonate. It is thought that infection with *Helicobacter pylori* may promote loss of the protective barrier provided by the mucous layer and epithelium, allowing acid and pepsin damage and ulceration. *H. pylori* is a spiral urease-producing organism that colonizes gastric antral mucosa, usually in childhood, and invariably results in active chronic gastritis but leads to ulcer disease in only about 15% of infected persons. Normally, active gastric and duodenal mucosal bicarbonate secretion creates a pH gradient from the luminal acid to near neutrality at the mucosal epithelial cells. Bicarbonate secretion is inhibited by alpha-adrenoceptor agonists, indomethacin, bile acids, smoking, and possibly *H. pylori* infection. Peptic ulcers most commonly occur in the stomach (gastric ulcers) or the duodenum (duodenal ulcers).

Risk Factors and Associations

Approximately 90% to 100% of patients with duodenal ulcers and 70% to 90% of patients with gastric ulcers (not associated with NSAIDs) are infected with *H. pylori*. In the United States, about 30% of the population is infected with *H. pylori*, with higher rates in certain minority and lower socioeconomic groups. However, the risk of *H. pylori* infection is not related to gender. Multiple prospective trials have demonstrated that the therapeutic eradication of *H. pylori* is associated with cure of ulcer disease and a marked decrease in ulcer recurrence.

The risk of gastric and duodenal ulcers associated with long-term use of NSAIDs ranges from 9% to 31% and 0% to 19%, respectively. A prior history of ulcer disease, advancing age, a higher dose of NSAID, use of more than one NSAID, and concurrent use of corticosteroids all increase the incidence of NSAID-induced ulcerations. Certain NSAIDs, such as piroxicam, indomethacin, ketoprofen, and naproxen, in particular, have a higher risk of gastrointestinal complications. The risk of gastrointestinal hemorrhage resulting from NSAID use is highest in the first 1 to 3 months after the initiation of NSAID therapy. One meta-analysis has suggested that women may be at greater risk than men for NSAID-induced ulcerations. Recently, a new group of highly selective cyclo-oxygenase (COX)-2 inhibitors has been introduced and has been shown to cause less gastroduodenal ulceration than traditional NSAIDs (see later discussion).

There is a strong positive correlation between tobacco use and the incidence, mortality, complication, recurrence, and delayed healing rates for ulcer disease. The role of stress in the development of PUD remains controversial.

Clinical Presentation

Dyspepsia is the most frequent presenting symptom of a peptic ulcer. The sensation is often described as a burning discomfort localized to the epigastrium. In the case of duodenal ulcer, dyspepsia often occurs preprandially or at night and is relieved by food intake or antacid therapy. The pain of gastric ulcer may be worsened by food intake and associated with nausea or weight loss. Patients with gastrointestinal hemorrhage may present with melena, hematemesis, or anemia.

Complications

Gastrointestinal hemorrhage occurs in approximately 10% to 15% of patients with a peptic ulcer. Hemorrhage is more common in patients over age 50 and may be more common in elderly women, perhaps because of a high frequency of NSAID use in this population. Approximately 10% to 20% of patients who bleed from gastric or duodenal ulcers do not have antecedent ulcer symptoms.

Perforation complicates approximately 0.7% of ulcers, more commonly in duodenal than gastric ulcers. The increased use of NSAIDs has led to an increased incidence of perforation, which is particularly apparent in the geriatric population. Duodenal ulcers can penetrate into the pancreas, resulting in acute pancreatitis.

Gastric outlet obstruction occurs in approximately 2% to 5% of ulcer patients as a result of acute pyloric inflammation and edema. When scarring has resulted in gastric outlet obstruction, endoscopic balloon dilatation can be attempted; surgery is reserved for refractory cases. Nowadays, gastric outlet obstruction is more likely to be caused by gastric cancer than PUD.

Diagnosis

The differential diagnosis of chronic dyspepsia includes PUD, gastric cancer, GERD, cholelithiasis, pancreatitis, gastroparesis, and chronic functional, or nonulcer, dyspepsia. Functional dyspepsia accounts for 60% of patients with chronic dyspepsia and is characterized by absence of an ulcer or other lesion to explain the symptoms. As in the general population, a substantial number of patients with functional dyspepsia are infected with *H. pylori,* but it is still unclear whether *H. pylori* gastritis in the absence of an ulcer causes dyspepsia.

Consensus statements from the United States and Europe recommend diagnostic endoscopy for patients with dyspepsia who are older than 45 years of age (the age at which the risk of gastric cancer generally begins to rise) or dyspeptic patients of any age with unexplained weight loss, vomiting, dysphagia, gastrointestinal bleeding, or anemia. Endoscopy is also recommended for persons of any age with dyspepsia who are at increased risk for gastric cancer because of their ethnic, socioeconomic, or familial background. For patients 45 years or younger, decision analysis suggests that the least expensive approach is to perform serologic tests for *H. pylori* and prescribe eradication therapy for those with positive results. This strategy will benefit the 15% to 25% of

H. pylori-positive patients who have an ulcer (or in whom ulcers are destined to develop), as well as about 20% of patients with nonulcer dyspepsia, whose symptoms resolve (Fig. 17-1). Treatment of *H. pylori* may also reduce the risk of gastric cancer.

Upper endoscopy is the preferred diagnostic test when PUD is strongly suspected. Upper endoscopy allows direct visualization of the gastroduodenal mucosa and biopsies to confirm that a gastric ulcer is benign. Mucosal biopsies are also the "gold standard" to diagnose *H. pylori.* A barium upper gastrointestinal series is less expensive than endoscopy but has a lower diagnostic yield, does not provide the prognostic information afforded by visualization of the ulcer base, and does not allow application of hemostatic therapy.

Many diagnostic methods have been developed to detect *H. pylori* infection, some of which rely on endoscopy (i.e., rapid urease test, histology, culture, and polymerase chain reaction) and others of which are noninvasive (i.e., serology, urea breath test, and, more recently, detection of *H. pylori* antigen in feces). A comparison of the available tests to diagnose *H. pylori* is shown in Table 17-2.

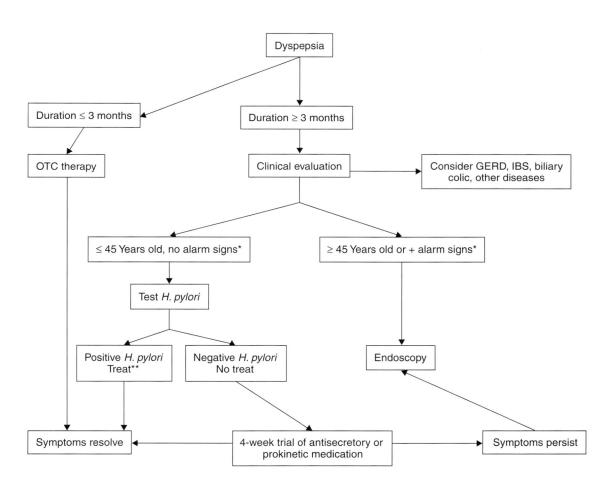

* Alarm symptoms: unexplained weight loss, vomiting, dysphagia, gastrointestinal bleeding, anemia.
** See Table 17-3.

FIG. 17-1 Management of the patient with dyspepsia.

Table 17-2
Diagnostic Tests for *Helicobacter pylori*

Diagnostic Test	Sensitivity, %	Specificity, %
Rapid urease tests (e.g., CLOtest, Hp*fast,* PyloriTek)	88-90	95-100
Histology	93	99
Culture	80-95	100
Antibody detection tests		
ELISA	94	78
Serum immunoassay	89	74
Urea breath test	90	96

ELISA, Enzyme-linked immunosorbent assay.

✴ MANAGEMENT

The goals of medical treatment for PUD are to relieve pain, expedite healing, prevent complications, and prevent recurrences. Ulcer healing may be maximized by using a proton pump inhibitor (e.g., omeprazole, 20 mg/day) for 6 to 8 weeks or an H-2-receptor antagonist for 10 to 12 weeks. In patients with a gastric ulcer, follow-up endoscopy in 8 to 12 weeks is recommended to confirm healing and exclude malignancy.

Numerous prospective trials have shown that the eradication of *H. pylori* will prevent ulcer recurrence in 90% to 100% of patients with *H. pylori*-associated ulcers. A 1994 National Institutes of Health Consensus Conference Panel concluded that all patients with a history of PUD and *H. pylori* infection should receive treatment to eradicate the organism (Table 17-3). In light of the rising incidence of metronidazole resistance in the United States, use of clarithromycin and amoxicillin in combination with a proton pump inhibitor is recommended as first-line therapy.

In ulcer patients taking NSAIDs, the NSAID should be discontinued if possible. Otherwise, high-dose proton pump inhibitor therapy should be continued with the NSAID. Patients with NSAID-associated ulcers who test positive for *H. pylori* should also be treated for *H. pylori.*

The advent of effective acid suppression and therapy to eradicate *H. pylori* has made surgical intervention for PUD much less frequent now than in the past. Still, approximately 5% of patients with peptic ulcers ultimately require surgery, often for a complication of PUD.

Patients with clinical evidence of gastrointestinal bleeding should undergo urgent endoscopy after hemodynamic stabilization. Two recent meta-analyses showed a 30% to 60% decrease in the mortality rate for patients treated endoscopically compared with those who did not undergo endoscopic therapy. An NIH Consensus Conference concluded that endoscopic hemostatic therapy should be used in patients at high risk for persistent or recurrent bleeding and death, specifically those with a large initial blood loss and evidence of active bleeding or a nonbleeding visible vessel in the ulcer base. There is limited evidence that administration of proton pump inhibitor therapy may have some efficacy in stopping active bleeding. Eradication of *H. pylori* markedly reduces the risk of recurrent ulcer bleeding in patients with an *H. pylori*-induced ulcer.

Table 17-3
Frequently Used Treatment Options for *Helicobacter pylori*

	Duration
Bismuth-Based Regimens	
Bismuth subsalicylate 302 mg QID	14 days
Clarithromycin 500 mg TID	
Tetracycline 500 mg QID	
Bismuth subsalicylate 302 mg QID	14 days
Metronidazole 500 mg TID	
Amoxicillin 500 mg TID	
Triple Therapy	
Omeprazole 20 mg BID	7-14 days
Amoxicillin 1g BID	
Clarithromycin 500 mg BID	
Lansoprazole 30 mg BID	7-14 days
Amoxicillin 1 g BID	
Clarithromycin 250 mg BID	
Metronidazole 500 mg BID	7-10 days
Omeprazole 20 mg BID	
Clarithromycin 500 mg BID	
Metronidazole 250 mg QID	14 days
Omeprazole 20 mg BID	
Amoxicillin 1 g TID	
Lansoprazole 30 mg BID	7-14 days
Clarithromycin 250 mg BID	
Metronidazole 400 mg BID	
Ranitidine Bismuth Citrate-Based Therapy	
Tritec* 400 mg BID	14 days
Clarithromycin 500 mg TID	14 days
Tritec* 400 mg BID	7 days
Clarithromycin 500 mg BID	7 days
Metronidazole 500 mg BID	7 days
Quadruple Therapy	
Helidac†	14 days
H-2-receptor antagonist	28 days

*Ranitidine bismuth citrate.
†Bismuth subsalicylate 525 mg po QID. Metronidazole 250 mg po QID. Tetracycline hydrochloride 500 mg po QID.

Nonsteroidal Anti-Inflammatory Drugs and Ulcer Prevention

The best way to prevent mucosal injury secondary to NSAIDs is to substitute an analgesic that is less toxic to the gastroduodenal mucosa, such as acetaminophen, salsalate, or magnesium salicylate. If continuation of an NSAID is preferred, however, prophylactic therapy with a proton pump inhibitor, or prostaglandin may be administered concurrently or a newer COX-2 inhibitor may be substituted.

Large randomized trials have shown that sucralfate and H-2-receptor antagonists are ineffective in preventing NSAID-associated gastric ulcers. Although the prostaglandin misoprostol is effective in preventing NSAID-induced ulcers and is the only drug approved by the FDA for prophylaxis against NSAID-related gastroduodenal ulcers, misoprostol has a number of side effects including diarrhea and abdominal pain. In a recent study that compared omeprazole

(20 mg/day) and misoprostol (200 μg given twice a day) for the prevention of recurrent ulcers in arthritis patients receiving NSAIDs, omeprazole was more effective.

Highly selective COX-2 inhibitors have become available and have been found to cause significantly less gastroduodenal ulceration than nonselective cyclooxygenase inhibitors. However, as yet no trial has shown a decrease in the rate of ulcer complications (i.e., hemorrhage and perforation) with these new NSAIDs, and further long-term studies are needed.

◾ PREGNANCY AND PEPTIC ULCER DISEASE

Multiple epidemiologic studies have shown that the incidence of PUD is decreased during pregnancy. Whether this decrease in incidence relates to a reluctance to order definitive diagnostic tests, increased levels of sex hormones, or maternal avoidance of ulcerogenic factors is unknown.

Complications such as bleeding, obstruction, and perforation occur less frequently in pregnant than in nonpregnant ulcer patients, and less than 100 cases of complicated peptic ulcers have been reported during pregnancy. When they do occur, complications are generally in the third trimester and are associated with eclampsia.

The medications available for the treatment of PUD in pregnant women are limited. Antacids are generally considered safe during pregnancy; as noted earlier, magnesium-containing antacids may be used during the second and early third trimesters, and aluminum-containing antacids may be used during the second and third trimesters.

Sucralfate, a sulfated polysaccharide complex with aluminum oxide, is also an acceptable therapy for peptic ulcers. The drug is thought to act by attaching to the proteinaceous surface of an ulcer, thereby protecting the mucosa against further injury by acid, pepsin, and bile salts. In a randomized, controlled trial of 66 pregnant patients with heartburn, sucralfate was found to be safe, effective, and not teratogenic. Sucralfate is a category B drug (Table 17-1) and considered by many authorities to be a preferred drug for PUD during pregnancy.

H-2-receptor antagonists should be used in pregnancy only when safer drugs such as antacids or sucralfate have failed. Ranitidine is preferable to cimetidine during pregnancy because of the possibility that cimetidine may have antiandrogenic effects on the male fetus. Nizatidine should not be used.

Omeprazole is a category C drug (Table 17-1). The accumulated data indicate that omeprazole is not teratogenic when administered at term, but fetal safety during early pregnancy is not established. Lansoprazole lacks terato-

genicity in animal models, but there are few data on its safety in pregnant humans.

Misoprostol and other prostaglandin analogs are contraindicated during pregnancy because of abortifacient effects. Eradication of *H. pylori* may generally be deferred until after pregnancy.

BIBLIOGRAPHY

Cappell MS, Garcia A: Gastric and duodenal ulcers during pregnancy, *Gastroenterol Clin North Am* 27:169, 1998.

Chae FH, Stiegmann GV: Current laparoscopic gastrointestinal surgery, *Gastrointest Endosc* 47:500, 1998.

The European *Helicobacter pylori* Study Group: Current European concepts in the management of *Helicobacter pylori* infection, *Gut* 41:8, 1997.

Fass R et al: The clinical and economic value of a short course of omeprazole in patients with noncardiac chest pain, *Gastroenterology* 115:42, 1998.

Feldman M, McMahon AT: Do cyclooxygenase-2 inhibitors provide benefits similar to those of traditional nonsteroidal anti-inflammatory drugs, with less gastrointestinal toxicity? *Ann Intern Med* 132:134, 2000.

Fendrick AM et al: Alternative management strategies for patients with suspected peptic ulcer disease, *Ann Intern Med* 123:260,1995.

Friedman LS: *Helicobacter pylori* and nonulcer dyspepsia, *N Engl J Med* 339:1928, 1998.

Graham DY, Malaty HM, Evans DG: Epidemiology of *Helicobacter pylori* in an asymptomatic population in the United States: effect of age, race, and socioeconomic status, *Gastroenterology* 100:1495, 1991.

Harper MA et al: Successful pregnancy in association with Zollinger-Ellison syndrome, *Am J Obstet Gynecol* 173:863, 1995.

Hawkey CJ et al: Omeprazole compared with misoprostol for ulcers associated with nonsteroidal antiinflammatory drugs, *N Engl J Med* 338:719, 1998.

Kaneshmend TK et al: Omeprazole versus placebo for acute upper gastrointestinal bleeding: randomized double blind controlled trial, *Br Med J* 304:143, 1992.

Marrero JM et al: Determinants of pregnancy heartburn, *Br J Obstet Gynaecol* 99:731, 1992.

NIH Consensus Conference: Therapeutic endoscopy and bleeding ulcers, *JAMA* 262:1369, 1989.

NIH Consensus Conference: *Helicobacter pylori* in peptic ulcer disease, *JAMA* 272:65, 1994.

Ofman JJ et al: Management strategies for *Helicobacter pylori*-seropositive patients with dyspepsia: clinical and economic consequences, *Ann Intern Med* 126:280, 1997.

Ott DJ: Gastroesophageal reflux: what is the role of barium studies? *AJR Am J Roentgenol* 162:627, 1994.

Sampliner RE: Adenocarcinoma of the esophagus and gastric cardia: is there progress in the face of an increasing cancer incidence? *Ann Intern Med* 130:67, 1995.

Talley NJ et al: AGA technical review: evaluation of dyspepsia. American Gastroenterological Association, *Gastroenterology* 114:582, 1998.

Talley NJ et al: Functional gastroduodenal disorders, *Gut* 45 (suppl II): II 37, 1999.

Wolfe MM, Lichtenstein DR, Singh G: Gastrointestinal toxicity of nonsteroidal antiinflammatory drugs, *N Engl J Med* 340:1888, 1999.

CHAPTER 18

Liver Disease

Robert C. Lowe

▦ EPIDEMIOLOGY

Abnormal liver function tests (LFT) are a common clinical problem in primary care for both men and women, occurring in 0.5% to 4% of asymptomatic patients. Although the majority of hepatic disorders are not gender-specific, several common diseases of the liver such as autoimmune hepatitis, primary biliary cirrhosis, and nonalcoholic steatohepatitis are more prevalent in women and require careful consideration in the female patient with liver enzyme abnormalities. In addition, certain forms of drug-induced liver disease are more commonly observed in women. Finally, some disorders, although no more prevalent in women, may have different implications for female patients. In particular, alcoholic liver disease may take a more aggressive course in women, whereas hepatitis C may be less aggressive and more amenable to treatment in female patients.

For the purposes of discussion, the common hepatic disorders are divided into those that primarily cause elevations of the serum transaminases (aspartate aminotransferase [AST], alanine aminotransferase [ALT]) and those that more commonly induce elevations of the alkaline phosphatase.

▨ APPROACH TO THE ASYMPTOMATIC PATIENT WITH ABNORMAL SERUM TRANSAMINASES

Elevations of the AST and ALT are commonly seen in the primary care setting, and may be the only sign of significant hepatic disease in an otherwise asymptomatic patient. A basic differential diagnosis of elevated transaminases is given in Box 18-1. The history and physical examination may give clues to some of these disorders, but the origin of the LFT abnormalities is often found after further laboratory testing or, in some cases, after liver biopsy.

History

Alcoholic liver disease can often be diagnosed after a careful history; the CAGE questions provide a sensitive and specific means of assessing for alcohol abuse (see Chapter 90). Since alcoholic liver damage occurs only after significant alcohol ingestion (80 g/day in men and 20 g/day in women,

for >10 years), this simple tool can be quite useful in implicating alcohol in the etiology of elevated transaminases.

Autoimmune liver disease may be associated with a personal or family history of other autoimmune disorders, particularly autoimmune thyroid disease, sicca syndrome, ulcerative colitis, and rheumatoid arthritis.

Chronic viral hepatitis (both B and C) is associated with a history of blood exposure via transfusion (before 1990) or intravenous (IV) drug use. Hepatitis B is also commonly contracted through sexual activity, but this is much less common for the transmission of hepatitis C. A prior history of acute hepatitis is helpful but often absent. This is especially true in cases of hepatitis C, in which only 30% of patients have symptomatic acute hepatitis with jaundice.

Drugs and toxins are a common cause of elevated transaminases, and questions regarding medications should always include a discussion of dietary supplements (such as vitamin A), herbal preparations, and over-the-counter medicines in addition to the standard questions regarding prescription drugs. In particular, commonly used medications including acetaminophen and nonsteroidal antiinflammatory drugs can cause significant liver damage in a small number of patients. Patients need to be questioned regarding illicit drug use, as such drugs as cocaine, ecstasy, and PCP are associated with hepatic toxicity. Drug-induced hepatitis may be associated with fever and skin rash, but in many cases hepatic inflammation is the only manifestation of an adverse drug reaction.

Several metabolic disorders can manifest as elevated transaminases. The most common of these is hereditary hemochromatosis; features of the history that point toward this disorder are symptoms of other end-organ dysfunction, including impotence or loss of libido (in both men and women), arthritis, symptoms of diabetes, and gradual darkening of skin pigmentation. Other more rare disorders to be considered in the diagnosis of elevated transaminases include Wilson's disease and alpha-1 antitrypsin deficiency. The former condition principally affects men 20 to 30 years old and is associated with derangement of personality, movement disorders, and progressive dementia in some cases. The latter disease affects men and women equally and is often associated with a family history of either liver disease or pulmonary icterus. The neck examination may reveal an enlarged thyroid that can signify autoimmune thyroiditis, which can occur concomitantly with autoimmune hepatitis.

The abdominal examination is clearly important, with hepatomegaly or hepatic tenderness providing a clue to a number of liver diseases. The presence of splenomegaly or ascites suggests more chronic and severe liver disease. Rarely, a nest of dilated veins is visible around the umbilicus. This sign, the *caput medusae*, indicates advanced portal hypertension. The lower extremities can manifest edema, suggesting fluid overload from portal hypertension, and the upper extremities can show clubbing (in cirrhosis or in chronic cholestatic disorders), palmar erythema (in cirrhosis), or leukonychia (whitening of the nails seen in low albumin states). Finally, the skin can be revealing in hepatic disease; in addition to jaundice, the presence of spider angiomata on the neck and upper chest may indicate portal hypertension. Lichen planus may be a sign of hepatitis C, and petechiae may signify cryoglobulinemia, a sequela of chronic hepatitis C. In addition, ecchymoses may signify a coagulopathy associated with chronic liver disease. The neurologic examination may reveal asterixis in cases of hepatic encephalopathy, a sign of advanced liver dysfunction.

Diagnostic Tests

A basic panel of laboratory tests are useful in the initial workup of elevated transaminases (Box 18-3). Serologic evaluation of hepatitis B should begin with determination of surface antigen (HBsAg), surface antibody (HBsAb), and core antibody (HBcAb) status. A positive HBsAb indicates resolution of a prior infection and confers immunity from reinfection. Nearly all patients with acute or chronic active hepatitis B will be HBsAg positive; testing for HBcAb is helpful in diagnosing hepatitis B infection in a subset of patients whose testing is done during the so-called "window period" of infection. During this period, which lasts days to weeks, the patient will have cleared HBsAg from serum, but will not yet have mounted a detectable surface antibody titer. A positive HBcAb indicates infection with hepatitis B, and fractionation of the antibody is often useful in that IgM antibody is associated with acute infection, whereas IgG antibody indicates a chronic or past infection.

Hepatitis C antibody (anti-HCV) testing is indicated in all patients with elevated transaminases, as chronic hepatitis C is a major cause of chronic hepatitis in the United States and Western Europe. The third-generation enzyme-linked

disease, as smokers with deficient A-1 antitrypsin will have an early onset of emphysema (median age 35 to 40 years).

Fatty liver and steatohepatitis are disorders that have engendered a great deal of clinical and research interest in recent years. Although these conditions were thought to affect women disproportionately, recent prospective series have called this into question, reporting male/female ratios of nearly 1:1. Gender aside, there is a clear correlation between the fatty liver disorders and the presence of diabetes, obesity, and hypercholesterolemia; and a history of any of these conditions in a patient with abnormal liver chemistries should raise the possibility of steatosis or steatohepatitis.

Physical Examination

The physical examination in patients with abnormal liver enzymes should be geared toward the findings of chronic liver disease or cirrhosis, but in some cases the examination reveals important clues to the etiology of hepatic disease (Box 18-2). The eye examination, in addition to revealing scleral icterus or the conjunctival pallor of anemia, can show scarring from prior episodes of iritis or episcleritis that can suggest a predisposition to autoimmune disorders. The Kayser-Fleischer rings of Wilson's disease are often difficult to recognize on examination and often require a slit-lamp evaluation. The oral examination may reveal oral aphthous ulcers (associated with immune disorders) or lichen planus (associated with chronic hepatitis C). The buccal mucosa and frenulum of the tongue may be the first areas to display immunosorbent assay (ELISA) antibody test is 97% sensitive for detecting HCV antibody. In high-risk groups, including former IV drug users, recipients of transfusions, and patients with elevated ALT levels, the positive predictive value of an ELISA test is approximately 80% to 85%. In a low-risk population, however, only 25% of positive ELISA tests are true positives, and population screening is not effective owing to the high false-positive rate. All positive tests should be followed with a highly sensitive and specific molecular biologic test (PCR or bDNA assay) to detect HCV RNA in serum. Not only does RNA testing eliminate false-positive antibody tests, but it also identifies the 15% of patients who spontaneously clear HCV after an acute infection. These patients will remain HCV antibody positive for life, but they do not have active liver disease, and their prognosis is no different from that of the general population.

Diagnostic testing for autoimmune hepatitis should include determination of both antinuclear antibody (ANA) and antismooth muscle antibody (ASMA). Both tests are useful as an initial screen, as many patients will express one, if not both, of these antibodies. Iron studies, consisting of serum iron, total iron binding capacity (TIBC), and ferritin, are useful in diagnosing hereditary hemochromatosis. As an initial screen, the serum iron and TIBC should be determined, and the iron/TIBC ratio should be calculated. A ratio higher than 45% should be followed with a serum ferritin and a genetic test for the mutations associated with hemochromatosis.

When these initial tests are unrevealing, a serum ceruloplasmin to screen for Wilson's disease and an alpha-1 antitrypsin level are obtained to exclude these rare but possible causes of elevated transaminase levels. In addition, disorders of thyroid function may affect transaminase levels (by an unknown mechanism), and a screening TSH may be helpful. Recently, celiac sprue has been associated with liver enzyme abnormalities in the absence of other symptoms or laboratory abnormalities, and an antiendomysial antibody determination is obtained in otherwise obscure cases of elevated transaminases, with or without associated symptoms of malabsorption. A liver ultrasound, although most useful in the evaluation of jaundice or elevation of the alkaline phosphatase, can also be helpful in evaluating elevated transaminases. The finding of fatty liver on ultrasound in the appropriate clinical setting may confirm a diagnosis of steatosis/steatohepatitis. If the imaging is not diagnostic, it is still useful in locating hemangiomas or other anatomic abnormalities, which aids in the planning of a percutaneous liver biopsy, the next step in evaluation if laboratory and radiologic studies are unrevealing or inconclusive.

SPECIFIC DISORDERS WITH AN INCREASED INCIDENCE IN WOMEN
Autoimmune Hepatitis

▦ EPIDEMIOLOGY

Autoimmune hepatitis is an uncommon disorder that occurs with a frequency of roughly 50 to 200 cases per million in the Northern Europe and North America and accounts for approximately 20% of chronic hepatitis in these populations. The female/male ratio for this disease is estimated at 4:1, and the average age of onset is between 20 and 40 years.

Clinical Presentation
Many patients with autoimmune hepatitis are diagnosed after the discovery of elevated transaminases by a primary physician. The disease is often insidious and without symptoms until late in its course, and 30% to 80% of patients will have progressed to cirrhosis by the time of presentation. Patients may describe fatigue and anorexia, and up to 40% complain of vague discomfort or pain in the right upper quadrant. On physical examination, most patients have hepatomegaly, and many will have concomitant splenomegaly.

Uncommonly, autoimmune hepatitis can present as fulminant hepatic failure, with markedly elevated transaminases, hepatic synthetic dysfunction (elevated prothrombin time), and encephalopathy. It is important to consider autoimmune disease in the differential of acute liver failure, especially in a young or middle-aged woman.

Extrahepatic features of autoimmune hepatitis include arthralgias of both small and large joints, skin rashes (including lichen planus), and leg ulcers. Several autoimmune conditions are associated with this disorder, including autoimmune thyroiditis, Sjögren's, and inflammatory bowel disease.

Diagnostic Tests
The diagnosis of autoimmune hepatitis is made on the basis of several clinical and laboratory criteria, and a scoring system for diagnosis has been devised. In addition to elevated transaminases, most patients with autoimmune hepatitis have an elevated serum globulin level and at least one of the characteristic autoantibodies. A serum protein electrophoresis is not required, but if performed, it demonstrates a polyclonal immunoglobulin G (IgG) band. Both the ANA and the ASMA (antismooth muscle antibody) should be measured, and titers of greater than 1:80 are highly suggestive of this disorder. Patients may have lower titers, but nearly all cases have at least one antibody present in a titer of greater than 1:40. In rare cases, patients with findings on liver biopsy that suggest autoimmune disease have no detectable serum antibodies. The LKM-1 antibody (liver-kidney microsomal) is associated with type 2 autoimmune hepatitis, which is seen primarily in female children. It is rarely seen in the United States, and LKM antibody testing is not recommended as an initial screening test for autoimmune hepatitis. The diagnostic criteria for autoimmune hepatitis also include testing to exclude other forms of liver disease, including viral serologies, iron studies, and assessment of alcohol consumption and possible toxic exposures.

Once the diagnosis of autoimmune hepatitis is suspected, a liver biopsy is indicated to assess the grade of inflammation and the stage of fibrosis. This information is useful both for planning possible treatment and estimating prognosis.

Prognosis
The prognosis of untreated autoimmune hepatitis depends on the severity of the inflammatory process within the liver. Patients with ALT levels > 10 times normal, or those with ALT > 5 times normal coupled with a serum globulin level > 2 times normal, have a 3-year mortality rate of 50%. Biopsy findings of bridging necrosis or severe lobular inflammation also portend a poor prognosis, with over 80% of patients developing cirrhosis within 5 years. More mild inflammation (periportal hepatitis), however, is associated with a good prognosis and uncommonly progresses to frank cirrhosis.

Treatment

The use of immunosuppressive therapy in autoimmune hepatitis has markedly improved the prognosis in this disease. Treatment is reserved for patients with severe inflammation on liver biopsy; patients with mild or moderate inflammation and no significant fibrosis do not require therapy. The most often used regimens consist of either prednisone alone or a combination of prednisone and azathioprine. Combination therapy is preferred, since the azathioprine serves as a steroid-sparing agent, allowing steroids to be tapered off completely or reduced to a low level that minimizes systemic side effects.

Remission induction is possible in approximately 65% of patients, and therapy may be discontinued after 2 years if a complete remission is achieved (defined as the absence of symptoms, normal transaminases, and a biopsy showing normal histology). Unfortunately, up to 80% of patients relapse after cessation of therapy and require retreatment and subsequent maintenance therapy with azathioprine and/or low-dose steroids.

In addition to immunosuppressive therapies, patients should receive vitamin D (50,000 units every week) and calcium supplementation (at least 1 g/day) to prevent steroid-induced osteoporosis. If bone disease is documented, then treatment with bisphosphonates or calcitonin is recommended.

Patients who develop cirrhosis and end-stage liver disease from autoimmune hepatitis are candidates for orthotopic liver transplantation, with reported 5-year survival rates of nearly 90%. Autoimmune hepatitis may recur in the graft, however, despite the immunosuppressive regimen used in the post-transplant period.

Nonalcoholic Steatohepatitis

Nonalcoholic steatohepatitis (NASH) is a condition characterized by elevated transaminases in a patient without a history of significant alcohol consumption but whose liver biopsy demonstrates fatty infiltration and inflammation that appear similar to the changes seen in alcoholic liver disease.

EPIDEMIOLOGY

NASH is thought to have a female predominance, since roughly 75% of cases in early series were women. These data, however, were from retrospective autopsy series, and recent prospective studies in patients evaluated for abnormal liver enzymes report a more nearly equal gender ratio. Significant risk factors for NASH include diabetes mellitus, obesity, and hypercholesterolemia, although these factors may be absent in a significant number of patients with biopsy-proven NASH. The histologic picture of NASH may also be seen in drug-induced hepatotoxicity states; among the medications that induce this form of liver injury are amiodarone, tamoxifen, nifedipine, and diltiazem.

Clinical Presentation

Most patients with NASH are asymptomatic, and the disease is often discovered when an elevation of serum transaminases is detected. A minority of patients complain of fatigue or vague right upper quadrant discomfort. Physical examination is generally unremarkable with the exception of hepatomegaly, which is reported in up to 75% of cases. Splenomegaly has been reported in about 25% of patients. Stigmata of portal hypertension are usually absent.

Diagnostic Tests

There is no definitive diagnostic test for NASH. Patients usually manifest elevated transaminases with nearly equal AST and ALT values; this is in contrast to alcoholic liver disease, in which the AST/ALT ratio is usually 2:1 or greater. There may be mild elevations of alkaline phosphatase levels; but an abnormal bilirubin, albumin, or prothrombin time is uncommon. Given the association between NASH and both diabetes and hyperlipidemia, it is not surprising that elevated glucose and lipid levels are reported in 25% to 75% of patients with NASH. Viral serologies and autoimmune markers are negative, but iron studies may be abnormally elevated in a minority of patients, and there is evidence that these patients may have more severe hepatic fibrosis than those with normal iron studies.

Radiologic imaging can identify fatty infiltration of the liver in some cases, and ultrasound, computed tomography (CT), and magnetic resonance imaging have all been used in this capacity. Unfortunately, these are relatively insensitive for diagnosing hepatic steatosis, and more important, these imaging studies are unable to distinguish simple steatosis from steatohepatitis, which is associated with progressive hepatic fibrosis and cirrhosis.

Liver biopsy is currently the only definitive method of diagnosing NASH; in addition to confirming the presence of steatohepatitis, biopsy allows assessment of the level of inflammation and fibrosis in the liver (disease staging). The utility of biopsy is debated, since there is no effective therapy for NASH at this time except weight loss, which can be recommended in patients with suspected NASH without their undergoing the risk of liver biopsy. The counterargument is that patients with cirrhosis on biopsy (7% to 16% in case series) will benefit from closer follow-up and should have an esophagogastroduodenoscopy (EGD) to identify possible esophageal varices. In addition, such patients should be screened periodically for hepatocellular carcinoma with liver ultrasound examination every 6 months and serum alpha fetoprotein determination two to four times a year.

Prognosis

There is controversy over the prognosis of NASH, since good natural history studies have not yet been conducted. In existing series, severe fibrosis is seen on initial biopsy in 15% to 50% of patients, and frank cirrhosis in 7% to 16%. The time course of the development of cirrhosis and the clinical course of NASH-induced cirrhosis are not yet known, but it is clear that progressive liver disease will occur in a fraction of patients with steatohepatitis.

MANAGEMENT

Currently, the mainstays of therapy for NASH include treatment of diabetes and hyperlipidemia and a program of weight loss in obese individuals. In some cases, a loss of as little as 10% of body weight can lead to an improvement in transaminase levels. Unfortunately, there is no data on whether these therapies change the natural history of steatohepatitis. Pharmacologic therapy with agents such as ursodiol, metronidazole, and glutamine have been reported to improve liver enzymes in very small numbers of selected patients, but there is not yet any clear indication for specific drug therapy in NASH. Avoidance of alcohol and known hepatotoxic agents is generally recommended.

APPROACH TO THE PATIENT AN ELEVATED ALKALINE PHOSPHATASE LEVEL

An elevation of serum alkaline phosphatase is a commonly seen liver enzyme abnormality, with a well-defined differential diagnosis and several diagnostic modalities involved in determining its origin. Sources of alkaline phosphatase include bone, liver, and placenta, with a smaller fraction present in kidney. Normally, the presence of placental alkaline phosphatase is not difficult to tease out of the clinical scenario, and the clinician is more often faced with deciding whether an elevated alpha lipoprotein is of bone or liver origin. The best tests for confirming hepatic origin of alkaline phosphatase are the gamma glutamyl transpeptidase (GGT) and the 5′-nucleotidase (5′-NT). The GGT lacks specificity and can be elevated after alcohol use or in patients taking a variety of medications (phenytoin and carbamazepine being the most common confounders). Elevation of 5′-NT is more specific, but may lag behind the alkaline phosphatase in cases of biliary duct obstruction.

Once the alkaline phosphatase is found to be of hepatic origin, the basic differential diagnosis is as shown in Box 18-4. At this point, radiologic imaging with either an ultrasound or computed tomography (CT) (with IV contrast) is indicated. If a mass lesion is seen on imaging, a directed biopsy should be obtained. If dilated intrahepatic and/or extrahepatic bile ducts without an obvious mass are seen, endoscopic retrograde cannulation of the pancreatic duct (ERCP) is the next diagnostic modality, searching for large duct obstruction from stone disease, malignancy, or a benign stricture. ERCP also permits examination of the intrahepatic biliary ducts for evidence of primary sclerosing cholangitis, a rare disorder occurring more commonly in men and usually in association with inflammatory bowel disease. If there is no evidence of mass lesion or obvious ductal pathology on imaging, then parenchymal liver disease must be considered. At this point, an antimitochondrial antibody test (AMA) is indicated to rule out primary biliary cirrhosis. The patient's medication list should be carefully reviewed for possible hepatotoxins, and a careful listing of all over-the-counter and herbal supplements must be obtained. If any potential toxins are identified, a trial of drug withdrawal may be made. If there is no identifiable toxic insult, a liver biopsy is indicated to search for other parenchymal disorders.

Disorders more common in women include primary biliary cirrhosis, certain liver masses including hepatic adenomas and focal nodular hyperplasia, and a number of drug effects (oral contraceptives, estrogen preparations).

PRIMARY BILIARY CIRRHOSIS

Primary biliary cirrhosis (PBC) is an autoimmune disorder primarily affecting women, characterized by progressive destruction of intrahepatic bile ducts by an inflammatory process that leads to fibrosis and eventual cirrhosis.

EPIDEMIOLOGY

PBC is an uncommon disease, with a prevalence estimated at 4 to 15 cases per 100,000. It is largely a disease of women, with only 10% of cases occurring in men, and most cases are diagnosed in middle age. There is a clear genetic component to PBC, with first-degree relatives having a relative risk of PBC that is greater than 500 times that of the general population.

Several autoimmune diseases are associated with PBC. Thyroid disorders (most often Hashimoto's thyroiditis) are seen in 15% of patients with PBC. Sjögren's syndrome is seen in 50% to 75% of cases, and features of CREST scleroderma are reported in up to 15% of patients. A total of 10% of PBC patients develop an inflammatory arthritis.

Clinical Presentation

The classic description of PBC is of a middle-aged woman who complains of generalized pruritus; however, only 55% of patients present with this symptom. Up to a quarter of patients are asymptomatic at diagnosis, and the disease is often recognized after an elevated alkaline phosphatase level is found on testing for some other reason. In patients who are symptomatic, fatigue is reported in 65% of patients. A minority of patients (10%) present with jaundice, a sign of more advanced disease. Physical examination reveals hepatomegaly in a quarter of patients. Skin findings include hyperpigmentation (25%) and xanthelasma (10%).

Diagnostic Tests

Nearly all patients with PBC have an alkaline phosphatase level three to four times normal. Serum bilirubin levels are usually normal at diagnosis, with only 10% of patients displaying frank jaundice. Serum transaminase levels are normal or slightly elevated. Diagnosis is confirmed by determination of a serum antimitochondrial antibody (AMA) level, which is elevated to a titer of greater than 1:40 in 90% to 95% of patients with PBC. Elevated AMA levels may also be seen in a minority of patients with autoimmune hepatitis, and rarely in primary sclerosing cholangitis or drug-induced liver disease. Although very sensitive for the diagnosis of PBC, the AMA test may be negative in a variant form of disease with characteristic histologic findings of PBC but with negative serologic testing; this entity is called *AMA-negative PBC* or, more recently, *autoimmune cholangiopathy*.

Imaging studies are unrevealing in PBC, with ultrasound, CT scanning, and ERCP typically normal. These studies

---

BOX 18-4
Differential Diagnosis of an Elevated Alkaline Phosphatase

Common bile duct obstruction (stone, tumor)	Primary biliary cirrhosis
Drug effect	Primary sclerosing cholangitis
Malignancy	Infiltrative diseases (amyloidosis, TB)
Granulomatous disorders	Variant autoimmune hepatitis

may be useful early in the diagnostic evaluation of PBC to rule out a mass lesion or large duct obstruction as a cause for an elevated alkaline phosphatase level.

Once the diagnosis of PBC is made on the basis of a positive AMA test, a liver biopsy is indicated both to confirm the diagnosis and to stage the disease, as staging has important implications for prognosis in PBC.

Prognosis

Primary biliary cirrhosis is a slowly progressive disease that leads to hepatic cirrhosis 10 to 20 years after diagnosis. Patients who are diagnosed in an asymptomatic phase have a longer time between diagnosis and development of cirrhosis than symptomatic patients, but this is a function of earlier diagnosis and not a sign of slower progression. For patients with PBC, a number of predictive models have been developed to aid in predicting survival, with most models including age, bilirubin level, prothrombin time, and serum albumin, among other variables.

✸ MANAGEMENT

Many agents have been evaluated for the treatment of primary biliary cirrhosis, but only ursodeoxycholic acid (ursodiol, Actigall) has been proven efficacious in slowing the progression of this disease. At doses of 13 to 15 mg/kg/day, oral ursodiol induced clinical and biochemical improvement, and significantly increased survival free of liver transplant in three randomized controlled trials.

For patients with advanced liver disease from PBC, liver transplantation is the treatment of choice. Prognosis after transplant is excellent, with 5-year survival rates of greater than 70%. Although PBC recurs in the transplanted liver in up to 15% of cases, it does not appear to adversely affect survival.

Primary biliary cirrhosis is associated with a number of complications common to the cholestatic liver disorders. Osteoporosis is seen in 30% to 50% of patients with PBC, and it is recommended that all patients receive supplemental calcium and vitamin D after diagnosis, in doses similar to those used in postmenopausal women. When osteoporosis is evident, bisphosphonate therapy with alendronate appears to be beneficial; this therapy should be used with caution in patients with cirrhosis and portal hypertension, since alendronate can induce esophageal ulceration and promote hemorrhage from esophageal varices.

Pruritus is a significant problem in many patients with PBC; ursodiol therapy may reduce symptoms, but this effect has been inconsistent. Agents that have been used successfully to ameliorate itching include antihistamines, cholestyramine, and rifampin. Recently, opioid antagonists such as naltrexone and nalmephene have shown promise in the treatment of cholestasis-induced pruritus.

Hypercholesterolemia is present in 85% of patients with PBC. Levels of high-density lipoprotein (HDL) are elevated early in the disease, but with time low-density lipoprotein (LDL) levels also rise; however, patients with PBC do not appear to have an increased risk of atherosclerosis or coronary artery disease. A number of patients will develop xanthelasma as a result of hyperlipidemia. The lipid disorder in PBC is often treated with cholestyramine, which may also ameliorate pruritus in symptomatic patients. Other cholesterol-lowering agents may be used in patients with PBC, with the usual recommended monitoring for hepatotoxicity depending on the agent used.

Although frank steatorrhea occurs uncommonly in PBC, fat-soluble vitamin deficiency occurs in up to 20% of patients, with deficiencies of vitamins A, D, and K occurring most commonly.

DRUG-INDUCED LIVER DISEASE

The incidence of drug-induced liver disease is, in general, greater in women than in men. Toxic hepatitis in response to certain drugs, such as alpha methyldopa, nitrofurantoin, tetracycline, chlorpromazine, diclofenac, and halothane, is clearly more common in women; data regarding gender specificity for most other agents are limited. However, certain medications merit discussion, since they are used primarily in women, and their adverse effects are, therefore, seen most commonly in women.

Oral Contraceptives and Estrogen Preparations

Oral contraceptive (OCP) use has been associated with the development of hepatic dysfunction, with jaundice occurring in 1 in 4000 to 10,000 women. Particularly at risk for OCP-induced jaundice are patients with a personal or family history of cholestasis of pregnancy. The estrogen component of OCPs is responsible for the hepatic toxicity, with progesterone having no effect on liver function. Estrogen replacement therapy has also been associated with cholestasis and jaundice. The mechanism of hepatic dysfunction is unclear, but a defect in canalicular secretion of bile has been reported.

OCP-induced jaundice usually occurs within the first six cycles of use and may occur during the first cycle. Serum bilirubin is moderately elevated, but usually less than 10 mg/dl, and patients may experience malaise, nausea and vomiting, and pruritus in addition to jaundice. Discontinuation of the estrogen-containing agent reverses the LFT abnormalities, with jaundice typically resolving within 1 month.

BIBLIOGRAPHY

Bach N, Schaffner F: Familial primary biliary cirrhosis, *J Hepatol* 20:698, 1994.

Bacon BR et al: Nonalcoholic steatohepatitis: an expanded clinical entity, *Gastroenterology* 107:1103, 1994.

Bardella MT et al: Chronic unexplained hypertransaminasemia may be caused by occult celiac disease, *Hepatology* 29:654, 1999.

Culp KS et al: Autoimmune associations in primary biliary cirrhosis, *Mayo Clin Proc* 57:365, 1982.

Czaja AJ et al: Autoimmune features as determinants of prognosis in steroid-treated chronic active hepatitis of uncertain etiology, *Gastroenterology* 85:713, 1983.

Czaja AJ: Drug therapy in the management of type 1 autoimmune hepatitis, *Drugs* 57:49, 1999.

Dickson ER et al: Prognosis in primary biliary cirrhosis: model for decision making, *Hepatology* 10:1, 1989.

Diehl AM: Nonalcoholic steatohepatitis, *Semin Liver Dis* 19:221, 1999.

Heathcote EJ et al: Combined analysis of French, American, and Canadian randomized controlled trials of ursodeoxycholic acid therapy in primary biliary cirrhosis, *Gastroenterology* 108:A1082, 1995.

James OFW, Day CP: Nonalcoholic steatohepatitis (NASH): a disease of emerging identity and importance, *J Hepatol* 29:495, 1998.

Kundrotas LW, Clement DJ: Serum alanine aminotransferase (ALT) elevation in asymptomatic US Air Force basic trainee blood donors, *Dig Dis Sci* 38:2145, 1993.

Manns MP, Rambusch EG: Autoimmunity and extrahepatic manifestations in hepatitis C, *J Hepatol* 31(Suppl 1):9, 1993.

Palmer JM et al: Antimitiochondrial antibody negative primary biliary cirrhosis: a distinct syndrome of autoimmune cholangitis, *Gut* 35:260, 1994.

Ratziu V et al: Long-term follow-up after liver transplantation for autoimmune hepatitis: evidence of recurrent primary disease, *J Hepatol* 30:131, 1999.

Seeff LB: Drug-induced chronic liver disease with emphasis on chronic active hepatitis, *Semin Liver Dis* 1:104, 1981.

Sheth S, Gordon FD, Chopra S: Nonalcoholic steatohepatitis, *Ann Intern Med* 126:137, 1997.

Teli MR et al: The natural history of nonalcoholic fatty liver: a follow-up study, *Hepatology* 22:1714, 1995.

CHAPTER 19

Bowel Function

Jacqueline L. Wolf

Normal bowel functions elicits little attention. However, alterations in bowel function may consume inordinate amounts of time and energy. Such focused attention on the bowels often results in frequent consultations with physicians. In the United States, Canada, and Northern Europe, women are more likely than men to seek the advice of their physicians for changes in bowel function.

Women report many changes in bowel function throughout their lives. Anecdotal reports of variations during the perimenstrual period, in pregnancy, and posthysterectomy have stimulated clinical and basic research studies on the effect of these states and concomitant changes in female sex hormone levels on normal gastrointestinal physiologic processes. Two disorders of bowel function—irritable bowel syndrome and intractable constipation—are more common in women than in men, lending further support to the possible effect of female hormones on bowel function.

This chapter focuses on (1) two disorders that are more common in women than in men (irritable bowel syndrome and intractable slow transit constipation); (2) the effect on bowel function of three states with different levels of sex hormones (the menstrual cycle, pregnancy, and posthysterectomy); and (3) the effect of sexual and physical abuse on symptoms of abdominal and pelvic pain.

DEFINITION OF NORMAL BOWEL FUNCTION

Normal bowel function is quite difficult to define and varies greatly from person to person. In the general population normal bowel frequency varies from three times per week to two to three times per day. However, to an individual, abnormal bowel function may mean a change in the frequency of stool; a change in the consistency or ease in elimination of the stool; the occurrence of gas, cramping, or pain; or a general belief that the bowel movements should be different from what they are.

SYNDROMES THAT ARE MORE COMMON IN WOMEN
Irritable Bowel Syndrome

EPIDEMIOLOGY

Irritable bowel syndrome (IBS) occurs in about 10% to 20% of the population. However, the exact incidence is difficult to estimate because most people with symptoms do not consult a physician. In industrialized countries female patients predominate; twice as many women as men report symptoms in large studies. In less developed countries such as India, males constitute the majority of patients. Cultural biases in the use of the health care system raise the question of the true incidence and gender frequency of IBS. In the United States, IBS accounts for 12% of primary care practices and 28% of gastroenterology practices.

Definition of Irritable Bowel Syndrome
Definitions for IBS vary from physician to physician and from study to study. In an attempt to standardize the definition, a consensus conference held in Rome in 1989 developed a formal classification system for all of the functional gastrointestinal (GI) conditions. The Rome I criteria updated in 1999 and called Rome II, is the current standard for diagnosing functional GI disorders. The diagnostic criteria specify that within the past year a patient must have had more than 12 weeks (not necessarily consecutively) of abdominal discomfort or pain accompanied by two of three of the following features: (1) pain or discomfort relieved by defecation, (2) onset of pain or discomfort associated with a change in stool frequency, or (3) onset of pain or discomfort associated with a change in stool appearance or form. Additional symptoms, which are supporting evidence for IBS are abnormal stool frequency (>3/day or <3/wk), abnormal stool form (lumpy/hard or loose/watery), abnormal stool passage (straining, urgency, feeling of incomplete evacuation, passage of mucus, bloating or feeling of abdominal distention).

Pathogenesis
The cause of IBS has not been determined but is multifactorial and includes a number of abnormalities and differences in visceral sensitivity, motor function, brain activation,

psychosocial factors, and the enteric nervous system in IBS patients compared with women without IBS. A subgroup of IBS patients clearly have increased visceral sensitivity. Balloon distention of different colonic segments causes pain in about 50% of IBS patients compared with only 10% of control subjects. However, with balloon distention in the rectum, only IBS patients who predominantly have diarrhea experience gas, distention, urgency, and the desire to evacuate.

During a normal day some patients with IBS are aware of distal and proximal small bowel contractions. Occasionally when patients with IBS undergo a routine colonoscopy, they are aware of the exact position of the colonoscope and actually feel the pinch of the biopsy (personal observation). Whether this sensation is more common in IBS patients than in the general population is not known. Visceral pain that occurs with rectal distention is associated with increased prefrontal cortex activation. In the anterior cingulate gyrus and insula of the limbic system, correlation of activation and subjective pain intensity are abnormal. Colonic and small bowel motility abnormalities have been noted in some patients who meet all the criteria for IBS. However, colonic motility abnormalities do not correlate well with clinical findings. Small bowel motility abnormalities correlate better with symptoms. There is a strong association of altered jejunal and ileal motility with abdominal pain and of small bowel transit time with constipation or diarrhea.

Stress clearly exacerbates symptoms of IBS and may be important in its onset. After an episode of infectious gastroenteritis, up to one third of patients may develop IBS-like symptoms. Those who develop IBS are more likely to have stressful life events preceding and 3 months after the infection and are more likely to have had more anxiety, depression, somatization, and neurotic traits at the time of the infection. Comorbid anxiety and depression occur in 42% to 61% and fibromyalgia in 32% to 70%. It is postulated that many hormones and peptides, such as serotonin, vasoactive intestinal polypeptide, substance P, cholecystokinin, and enkephalins, found in both gut and brain play a role in the exacerbation of symptoms.

Clinical Presentation

History and Symptom Presentation. Although IBS is defined by lower abdominal complaints (Box 19-1), there is an increased incidence (25% to 50%) of upper gastrointestinal complaints such as reflux, heartburn, and dyspepsia. Delayed gastric emptying occurs in as many as 30% of IBS pa-

---

BOX 19-1
Definition of Irritable Bowel Syndrome

Continuous or recurrent symptoms for at least 12 weeks in the last year
Abdominal discomfort or pain accompanied by two of three of the following features:
- Pain or discomfort relieved by defecation
- Onset of pain or discomfort associated with a change in stool frequency
- Onset of pain or discomfort associated with a change in stool appearance or form

From Drossman DA et al: *Functional GI disorders. Irritable bowel syndrome.* Part 2: Diagnosis and Treatment, 2000, American Digestive Health Foundation. Monograph.

---

tients. Respiratory and urinary tract symptoms such as frequency, nocturia, and urgency are common in patients with IBS. To determine the cause for these urinary tract symptoms, urodynamic studies were done in 30 patients with IBS and 30 matched control subjects. Bladder distensibility was the same in both IBS and control patients. Detrusor instability, which is involuntary detrusor muscle contractions, appeared to play a major causative role; it occurred in 30% of IBS patients but only 3% of control subjects.

Abdominal pain is the major criterion for IBS. Distinguishing a GI from a gynecologic source of abdominal pain can be difficult. In one study up to 60% of women who reported pain to a gynecologist and had a negative laparoscopy had symptoms suggestive of IBS. In a 12-month study of 71 women complaining of abdominal pain who sought medical attention at gynecology clinics in Manchester, England, those with symptoms of IBS were less likely to have had a definitive diagnosis made or have resolution of their pain during the study period. In the study 52% of the patients had IBS. Only 8% of the women with IBS compared with 44% of those without it had a definitive gynecologic diagnosis. At the end of the year, 65% of women with and 32% of women without IBS still had abdominal pain. Determining how far to pursue a definitive diagnosis with costly and invasive tests in patients with IBS requires a careful history, physical examination, and clinical acumen.

History that would rule out the diagnosis of IBS and should prompt further evaluation includes unexplained weight loss, abdominal pain or diarrhea that awakens the patient from sleep, steatorrhea, melena, hematochezia except when documented from hemorrhoids or fissure, and fever. Onset in old age does occur, but IBS should be a diagnosis of exclusion in this population. A careful history of drug (laxatives and other medications) ingestion should be obtained.

Physical Examination. The physical examination by itself is not helpful in making the diagnosis of IBS but may help by arousing suspicion of another diagnosis. Findings incompatible with the diagnosis of IBS are rebound tenderness, involuntary abdominal boardlike rigidity, an abdominal mass, a succussion splash, high-pitched tinkling bowel sounds in rushes, fever, or guaiac-positive stool.

Diagnostic Tests. There is no test for diagnosing IBS. As with the physical examination, the tests are useful for ascertaining that another diagnosis is not more likely. The routine blood tests that should be done in most patients are a complete blood count, which includes a white blood cell count, hemoglobin, hematocrit, and platelet count; an erythrocyte sedimentation rate; and certain chemical determinations, including glucose, electrolytes, amylase, lipase, and liver function tests. A protime and partial thromboplastin time are helpful in patients with diarrhea. Tests for malabsorption should be individualized. A urinalysis is useful for patients with urinary tract symptoms. A stool volume greater than 200 ml is inconsistent with IBS. In patients with frequent stools, an examination of stool for leukocytes, ova and parasites (three samples), culture and sensitivity (three samples), and Sudan stain for qualitative stool fat should be done. If a patient has taken antibiotics recently, a stool test for *Clostridia difficile* toxin should be done. A flexible sigmoidoscopy should be done in all patients with hematochezia, sudden constipation, or diarrhea and in all patients more than 50 years old. A barium enema or colonoscopy is indicated for some patients to exclude neoplastic or obstructive lesions or colitis. An oral lactose tolerance test or hydrogen breath test for lactase deficiency may be indicated in patients with bloating or frequent stools. Further diagnostic tests may be indicated, but a detailed discussion is beyond the scope of this chapter.

Differential Diagnosis. The final diagnosis of IBS is one of exclusion. Other identifiable and potentially specifically treatable causes should be excluded, including neoplasm, inflammatory bowel disease, endometriosis, sorbitol intolerance, malabsorption, pseudoobstruction, and pancreatic and hepatic disease. A full differential diagnosis is beyond the scope of this chapter. However, the diagnosis of lactose intolerance is worth special consideration.

LACTOSE INTOLERANCE. In patients with bloating the clinician should first ascertain that the patient does not have a lactose intolerance. In those with a lactase deficiency the onset of bloating with or without abdominal pain may occur several minutes to hours after lactose ingestion. For diagnosis, a 1- to 2-week trial of a completely lactose-free diet, a hydrogen breath test after lactose ingestion, or serial blood glucose levels after lactose ingestion can be done. If the patient is lactose-intolerant, avoidance of lactose-containing foods and medications should help decrease or eliminate flatulence. Foods with lactose are milk, cream, cheese, butter, whey, casein, lactalbumin, milk solids, yogurt, ice cream, ice milk, and prepared foods that contain these substances. If lactase deficiency is not complete many patients tolerate milk products pretreated with or ingested with exogenous lactase (Lactaid and Dairyease) and yogurt.

✳ MANAGEMENT

Goals of Therapy

Because of the probable multifactorial causes of IBS, treatment is directed toward symptomatic relief and stress management. New therapies are being developed to inhibit or stimulate the serotonin receptors 5HT3 or 5HT4, which are important for gut motility and function. No one therapy will help all patients. Some need no therapy, since they spontaneously become asymptomatic without treatment.

Most IBS patients continue to have intermittent symptoms for years. Many require therapy for their symptoms.

Choice of therapy

Fiber Therapy. One of the mainstays of therapy is fiber. A good healthy diet should contain 25 to 30 g/day of fiber, but many people eat far less fiber. Dietary manipulation with the aim of increasing the fiber intake to 25 to 40 g of fiber should be one of the first treatments undertaken for both constipation and diarrhea, although most studies show fiber is not helpful for diarrhea. The increased stool fiber content results in increased water retention and in bulkier stool. There are two sources of fiber: *insoluble* (wheat bran, lignin, methylcellulose, hemicellulose, or calcium polycarbophil) and *soluble* (oat bran, psyllium, gums, or pectin). Many over-the-counter preparations contain these fiber sources and are useful for fiber supplementation. Box 19-2 lists some of the more common preparations. Patients may tolerate one type of fiber and not others. Bloating and gas are common after ingestion of some sources of fiber, but it is difficult to predict which source of fiber will produce no or minimal side effects in an individual. Personal observation suggests that methylcellulose (Citrucel) or pectin may be better tolerated, but this has not been proven.

Therapy for Bloating. Bloating may respond to elimination of foods likely to cause gas. These include beans, brussel sprouts, carrots, celery, onions, apricots, bananas, prunes, raisins, pretzels, and wheat germ (Box 19-3). Beano, an over-the-counter preparation of the enzyme alpha-galactosidase, may partially metabolize the insoluble sugar racinose, in beans and peas, thereby decreasing the amount of sugar available for bacterial fermentation in the colon.

Because bacterial fermentation of the sugar causes gas, a decrease in available sugar should decrease flatulence. Decreased flatulence may also follow ingestion of *activated charcoal,* which may absorb gas, and *simethicone,* which changes the surface tension of liquids, allowing easier elimination of gas bubbles (Table 19-1).

Prokinetic Agents. In some patients with constipation and/or bloating, the prokinetic agents *cisapride* (recently

---

BOX 19-2
Fiber Preparations

Content	Preparation
Psyllium	Fiberall: powder, wafers
	Konsyl
	Maalox daily fiber
Metamucil: powder, wafers, effervescent, sugar-free	
Mylanta natural fiber	
Methylcellulose	Citrucel
Pectin Certo, Sure-Jell, pectin powder, pectin capsules	
Calcium Fibercon tablets polycarbophil	
Flax seed	

BOX 19-3
Fiber Preparations

Foods Likely To Produce Flatulence
Beans
Apricots
Pretzels
Brussels sprouts
Bananas
Wheat germ
Carrots
Prunes
Milk and milk products
Celery
Raisins
Onions

Modified from Sutalf LO, Levitt MD: *Dig Dis Sci* 248:652, 1979.

removed from the market, except by protocol, in the United States), *metoclopramide,* and *domperidone* (not available in the United States) may be helpful (Table 19-2). Metoclopramide increases upper GI tract motility but does not affect colonic motility. A new class of medications that acts as agonists for the serotonin receptors $5HT_3$ and $5HT_4$ will soon be available for therapy of constipation.

Anticholinergic Agents. Anticholinergic agents are the most frequently used agents for the treatment of IBS (Table 19-3). They may be beneficial for abdominal pain and diarrhea associated with IBS. Doses of anticholinergics should be small and administered 30 minutes before meals and at bedtime.

Anticholinergics exist alone or as combination medication. They are often combined with a mild tranquilizer in a single tablet or capsule.

Antidiarrheal Agents. For chronic diarrhea or frequent stools, cholestyramine (a binder of bile acids), diphenoxylate, and loperamide may be useful (Table 19-4). Lactose-intolerant patients should ascertain that the medication is lactose-free. The loperamide liquid preparation (Imodium) is lactose-free.

Anxiolytics and Antidepressants. Anxiolytic medications such as buspirone HCL (Buspar), chlordiazepoxide (Lithium), lorazepam (Ativan), and diazepam (Valium) may help diminish IBS symptoms associated with stress and anxiety, but their use poses the risk of dependency (Table 19-5). Tricyclic antidepressants in low doses may help abdominal pain. The usual doses for this use are smaller than for treating depression: amitriptyline or nortriptyline, 25 to 75 mg at bedtime, and desipramine, 50 mg at bedtime. Selective serotonin reuptake inhibitors have been used successfully in IBS by treating symptoms of concurrent anxiety and depression. Trials are currently underway to assess their utility in IBS. Dosages used are the same as those for depression.

$5\text{-}HT_3$ Antagonists and $5\text{-}HT_4$ Agonists. Seratonin receptors are important participants in gut motor and sensory physiology. The first available drug of this class, alosetron, a 5-hydroxytryptamine$_3$ (5-HT_3) antagonist, was effective in treating a large percentage of women (not men) with diarrhea-predominant IBS, but the report of 5 deaths, 49 cases of ischemic colitis, and 21 cases of severe constipation necessitated withdrawal of the drug from the market. Cilansetron or cilasetron, which was in clinical trial, were temporarily halted because of potential side effects of constipation and ischemic colitis. $5\text{-}HT_4$ agonists may accelerate orocecal transit and thereby improve constipation. A drug application for tegaserod, a selective $5\text{-}HT_4$ agonist, was recently rejected by the Food and Drug Administration (FDA) for clinical trial because of similar concerns.

Table 19-1
Preparation for Controlling Flatulence

Generic	Brand	Dose
α-Galactosidase	Beano	3-8 drops with food
Activated charcoal	Charcoal Plus	400mg (2 tabs) tid
Simethicone	Gas X chewables	80-160 mg tid or
	Mylicon	125 mg qid
	Phazyme	

Table 19-2
Prokinetic Agents

Drug	Dosing	Precautions
Cisapride	5-20 mg tid-qid	Diarrhea, cardiac arrhythmias. Only available in US on protocol from manufacturer.
Metoclopramide	10 mg qid	Restlessness, drowsiness, fatigue, lassitude in 10%; dizziness, insomnia, headache, confusion, depression, acute dystonic reactions

Table 19-3
Anticholinergic Agents*†

Agent	Dose	Side Effects (for all medications)
Belladonna	5-10 GTT PO tid	Dry mouth, decreased sweating, blurred vision, mydriasis, cycloplegia, increased ocular tension, drowsiness, urinary hesitancy and retention, tachycardia, palpitations, loss of taste, headache, nervousness, dizziness, insomnia, nausea, vomiting, constipation, bloating, decreased lactation, allergic reactions.
Clidinium bromide (Quarzan)	2.5-5 mg PO tid to qid	
Dicyclomine hydrochloride (Bentyl)	10-20 mg PO qid	
Hyoscyamine sulfate (Levsin)	0.125-0.25 mg SL or PO q4h or time released 0.375-0.75 mg PO q12h	
Propantheline bromide (Pro-Banthine)	7.5-15 mg PO qid	

*For tid or qid dosing give 3 doses 15-30 min before meals.
† Note: use with care in the elderly and patients with other diseases.

Complimentary and Alternative Health. A well-controlled trial of Chinese herbs in IBS showed improvement on bowel and global symptom scores. Ayurvedic (traditional Indian) herbs were beneficial in the diarrhea of IBS. Acupuncture has been used, but more studies need to be done.

Psychological Treatments. Many psychotherapeutic approaches are often effective in the treatment of IBS either alone or in conjunction with other therapies. These include cognitive behavioral therapy, interpersonal psychotherapy, hypnosis, and stress management.

Intractable Constipation

Definition and Pathogenesis

Constipation causes much consternation and often results in a significant amount of time spent in trying to produce a bowel movement. Patients with severe, intractable idiopathic constipation are predominantly young women of reproductive age. These patients have one or fewer bowel movements per week and a colon of normal diameter. Their GI motility is less than those of normal women or men.

GI transit can be determined by measuring the amount of time radiopaque markers take to traverse the distance from mouth to anus. After ingestion of 20 radiopaque markers, 95% of normal people eliminate all markers by 5 days. In contrast, patients with slow transit constipation retain more than four or five markers at 5 days and may retain markers at 8 days. As in IBS, women with intractable constipation have had reported associated abnormal bladder function and esophageal motility.

Table 19-4
Antidiarrheal Agents for Treatment of Irritable Bowel Syndrome

Agent	Dose
Cholestyramine	1/2 to 1 scoop or packet (4 g) qd-qid
Loperamide	2 mg qd-qid
Diphenoxylate HCl	2.5 mg qid

Table 19-5
Anxiolytics and Antidepressants Used in the Treatment of Irritable Bowel Syndrome

Medication	Dose
Anxiolytics	
Buspirone HCL (Buspar)	5-10 mg tid
Diazepam (Valium)	2-5 mg bid-qid
Chlordiazepoxide (Librium)	5-10 mg tid or qid
Lorazepam (Ativan)	0.5-2 mg bid-tid
Phenobarbital	15 mg tid
Antidepressant	
Amitryptyline	25-125 mg qhs
Imipramine	25-125 mg qhs
Desipramine	25-125 mg qhs
Nortriptyline	25-125 mg qhs
SSRIs	Psychiatric dosing
Fluoxetine	
Paroxetine	

Clinical Presentation

The evaluation of patients with intractable constipation is similar to that of patients with constipation predominant IBS. The diagnosis is one of exclusion and demonstration of abnormal gut transit time. A history of drug ingestion, age of onset of symptoms, speed of onset (i.e., sudden versus progressive), and other associated symptoms should be elicited. GI bleeding and weight loss are incompatible with the diagnosis. The physical examination is remarkable for palpable stool in the colon. Diagnostic tests should center around excluding the diagnosis of obstructing lesions, volvulus, pseudoobstruction, hypothyroidism, and chronic laxative abuse. A barium enema and sigmoidoscopy or colonoscopy with or without biopsy is usually done. A sitzmaker study should be done as follows: A patient is given a sitzmaker capsule at night. Abdominal supine and lateral radiographs are taken to enumerate and locate the markers the next day (optional), at 5 days, and, if any marker remains, at 7 to 8 days after ingestion. To exclude other motility disorders, which are common, rectal and esophageal studies may be helpful.

✵ MANAGEMENT

Choice of Therapy

Treatment is difficult and often meets with limited success (Table 19-6). Increased fiber should be the first line of therapy, but fiber use alone may not be successful. Adequate hydration and exercise are important. Avoidance of bowel stimulating laxatives, which when used may result in dependence, should be the aim of therapy but usually cannot be avoided. Treatment trials with a nonabsorbable sugar or short-term therapy with mineral oil should precede treatment with milk of magnesia, magnesium citrate, castor oil, bisacodyl USP (Dulcolax), senna, cascara sagroda. Polyethylene glycol preparations, such as MiraLax, and other herbal teas may be helpful. Although the prokinetic 5-HT$_4$ receptor agonists may be useful, but they have serious side effects. Why slow transit constipation occurs more commonly in young women is unknown and under investigation.

MENSTRUAL CYCLE AND GI FUNCTION

Menstruating women undergo many physiologic changes throughout the month. Recent studies have examined the effects of the variable levels of estrogen and progesterone on GI function. Based on the results of these studies, however, whether GI function is altered during different phases of the menstrual cycle is controversial.

Small Intestinal Transit

One parameter that has been examined is small intestinal transit. Small intestinal transit affects bowel frequency and consistency of stool. Measurement of expired breath hydrogen after ingestion of lactulose estimates the length of time a substance takes to reach the proximal colon. As lactulose is not absorbed in the small intestines, it passes unchanged into the colon. It is metabolized by colonic bacteria, releasing H$_2$ gas that is absorbed through the colonic wall, is exhaled by the lungs, and then can be measured. That this assessment mainly determines small intestinal transit is based on the assumption that there is not delayed gastric emptying. Wald and colleagues found significantly increased small intestinal

Table 19-6
Choice of Therapy for Intractable Constipation

Drug	Dose	Side Effects/Precautions
Fiber (including supplements)	25-40 g/day	
Beano or activated charcoal (for gas)	(See Table 13-1)	
Lactulose	1-2 Tbsp qd-qid	Bloating
Mineral oil	1-2 Tbsp qd-tid	Do not use in the elderly, or patients with reflux (because of lipoid pneumonia associated with reflux). Use over long period may interfere with absorption of fat-soluble vitamins.
Cisapride	10-20 mg tid	Diarrhea, arrhythmias. (Available in U.S. only on protocol from manufacturer).
Laxatives	Use sparingly	Bowel may become dependent on laxatives
Milk of magnesia	Begin with minimum dose	
Magnesium citrate		
Castor oil	PO	
Bisacodyl (sodium or calcium)	Suppositories or tablets	
Senna	PO, tablets or tea	
Cascara sagrada	PO	
Glycerin	Suppositories	
Isosmotic electrolyte solution	17-34 g qd-bid	
Oral prostoglandin (Misoprostil)	200-400 mg qd-tid	

transit time in the luteal phase compared to that in the follicular phase in 15 women who ingested lactulose mixed in water. Although the mean transit times were 25% longer, five women had no prolongation of the transit times in the luteal phase. Turnbull and colleagues could not confirm these results. Measurements of intestinal transit after ingestion of a test meal mixed with lactulose showed no variations with the menstrual cycle.

Colonic Motility

The effect of the menstrual cycle on colonic motility has also been examined. In the colon water is absorbed from the intestinal contents, decreasing stool volume. Hence colonic motility may affect the volume and frequency of the stool. The measurement of whole gut transit using unabsorbable markers is mainly a measurement of colonic motility. Because the solid markers mixed with feces reside in the colon for a significantly longer period than in the rest of the GI tract, investigators use the time taken to eliminate the markers after their ingestion as a gross estimate of colonic transit. Colonic transit has been reported to be both equal in men and women and slower in women. Measurements of colonic transit during the menstrual cycle of women have shown both slowing and no change in the luteal phase compared with that in the follicular phase.

Common Bowel Complaints

Normal menstruating women often report periods of constipation or diarrhea that seem to fluctuate with the menstrual cycle. However, these symptoms are often subjective and cannot be confirmed in prospective studies. Whitehead attempted to estimate bowel complaints at menstruation in patients from a family planning clinic and women referred to a gastroenterology clinic with IBS or functional bowel disorder (FBD), a term used when not all but some of the symptoms used for the definition of IBS were met. In all, 34% of Planned Parenthood subjects without IBS or FBD reported one or more bowel symptoms with menstruation. These included increased gas (14%), increased diarrhea (19%), and increased (11%) and decreased (16%) constipation. Significantly more patients with FBD and IBS than control subjects had increased gas at menstruation, and significantly more patients with IBS than control subjects had increased diarrhea or constipation at menstruation. In smaller studies, 64% and 96% of women reported a change in bowel habits with menses. A more recent retrospective study confirmed these results and found significantly more complaints of diarrhea and constipation in women with IBS.

To determine whether the retrospective recall of menstrual symptoms was accurate, Heitkemper and Jarrett prospectively examined GI symptoms and select mood and somatic symptoms in a small number of women with and without FBD. Confirming the observations of Whitehead and colleagues, they found a significant increase in abdominal pain at menses compared with that in the follicular or luteal phases in both groups. Patients with FBD had increased abdominal pain, nausea, and diarrhea compared with women without FBD. No significant differences were noted in stool consistency and frequency across the menstrual cycle, although in a previous study Heitkemper and colleagues found decreased consistency of the stool in women at menses. Bloating and cramping abdominal and pelvic pain were worse during menses in the FBD group. Other complaints of poor work or school performance and backache paralleled the increase in abdominal pain in the premenstrual period through the third day of menses. More women with FBD (39%) than control subjects (28%) had sought health care for perimenstrual distress. Dysmenorrheic women report more menses-related GI symptoms than do control subjects.

HYSTERECTOMY AND BOWEL FUNCTION

If bowel function is affected by the hormonal state of a woman, changes in bowel function should follow hysterectomy. In a case-control study of Scottish women with and without hysterectomy, Taylor and colleagues found that women who had had a hysterectomy reported less frequent bowel movements than control subjects. They also reported more laxative use, harder stools, and constipation, but these findings were not statistically significant. Increased urinary frequency concomitant with decreased bowel frequency was noted in 10 of 91 women after hysterectomy. A criticism of the study is that no control was included for patients with IBS. Because IBS patients have an increased risk of hysterectomy, this may have biased the findings.

A prospective study of bowel function in 205 women before, 6 weeks after, and 6 months after hysterectomy examined the effect of hysterectomy on bowel function. Only 13 women had bilateral oophorectomy. A total of 22% of patients had symptoms of IBS before surgery. After surgery 10% of normal women complained of new GI symptoms occurring more than once per week, and 5% of the women experienced constipation. Of the women with preexisting IBS 6 months after hysterectomy, 33% were asymptomatic, 27% had improved symptoms, and 20% complained of increased symptoms. Although no relationship could be found between the development of de novo constipation and de novo urinary dysfunction, 29 of the 205 women had an increase in frequency, urgency, and/or incontinence. The cause of development of constipation after hysterectomy is unclear. It is thought to be caused by injury of the autonomic nerves that are located on the lateral side of the rectum, cervix, and vaginal fornix. However, constipation not only occurs after a radical hysterectomy, in which the nerves may be damaged, but also after a simple hysterectomy, in which presumably the nerves are left intact.

The effect of hysterectomy on sphincter and colonic motility has been examined and the results are controversial. One report noted failure of the internal anal sphincter to relax to baseline in 60% of patients after radical or simple hysterectomy for cervical cancer, whereas others found no change in the sphincter. Barnes and Smith reported increased rectal volume required to trigger the rectal-anal sphincter inhibitory response; however, a study by Roe did not. An increased paradoxical reaction of the colonic motility gradient to the prokinetic agent neostigmine methylsulfate (Prostigmin) that created a functional obstruction was found in patients after hysterectomy with ovaries left in situ. From the data obtained from these small studies, it would appear that women may experience constipation and urinary symptoms after hysterectomy, but they occur only in a minority of patients.

RELATIONSHIP BETWEEN ABUSE AND PELVIC AND ABDOMINAL PAIN

Physical and sexual abuse not only affect the psychologic well-being of a patient but often result in gynecologic and GI symptoms. Abuse is a major epidemic in the United States. Estimates of the incidence of childhood sexual abuse in the United States vary from 15% to 38%. Women outnumber men by 2:1 to 4:1. Physician awareness of the abuse is poor; as few as 2% of physicians in one study and

17% in another were cognizant of the abuse. Only 20% to 50% of abuse episodes come to the attention of authorities. Because the history is rarely volunteered and may affect medical therapy, physicians should routinely ask patients about abuse. Suspicion of possible abuse (sexual or physical) should be aroused by a patient who has chronic pelvic or abdominal pain, frequent visits to a physician for seemingly minor or unexplained complaints, drug abuse, panic attacks, or frequent ecchymoses. Up to 80% of severely sexually abused girls report sexual abuse as women. The risk of sexual abuse appears to be higher in patients with IBS than in the general population. In a referral-based gastroenterology clinic practice, Drossman and colleagues found a 44% incidence of abuse. In a university GI clinic they found 53% of women with FBD reported past sexual abuse and 37% past physical abuse. In a random sampling of healthy residents of Olmsted County, Minnesota, in which 70% of the queried group responded, 28% of 830 residents reported abuse and 23% reported sexual abuse. Those who reported sexual abuse were twice as likely to have IBS or FBD as those without abuse. All patients with abuse were more likely to have seen a physician within the past year than nonabused patients. In another large study in which members of a health maintenance organization in California were queried, sexual abuse was reported by 19% of women and 6% of men. Sexual abuse was reported in 10% of the population without IBS, in 21% of IBS patients who reported constipation or diarrhea as predominant symptoms, and in 36% of IBS subjects with pain as the predominant symptom. Most studies report significantly more physician visits by both IBS patients and subjects reporting sexual abuse and increased surgical procedures among patients who have been abused. For more detailed discussion of abuse see Chapters 87 and 88.

Knowing about abuse can potentially affect decisions about surgery, endoscopy, and other invasive tests. Every patient, male or female, should be asked whether he or she has ever had unwanted sexual attention, been forced to perform sexual acts, or has had physical acts of abuse such as hitting, pushing, or kicking directed against him or her. Posttraumatic syndrome can develop after either physical or sexual abuse. Psychologic intervention may be of benefit for such patients.

◼ PREGNANCY AND BOWEL FUNCTION
Epidemiology

It is commonly believed that constipation is a frequent complaint in pregnancy. However, many studies have failed to show that a majority of women have constipation. In a study by Levy of bowel function in 1000 healthy pregnant Israeli women, 55% had no change in bowel frequency, 34% had increased frequency, and 11% had decreased frequency. Other surveys showed an increase in constipation. In Anderson's study of 200 British women interviewed in the third trimester, 38% of women reported having had constipation sometime during their pregnancy and 18% still had it at the time of the interview. Because of constipation and other ill-defined GI complaints, 70% of women reported dietary modification, primarily increasing fiber intake, which likely improved the symptoms of constipation.

Physiologic Changes in Gastrointestinal Function During Pregnancy

Small bowel transit time appears to be prolonged in pregnancy. In a study using mercury-filled balloons, small intestinal transit time was longer in 12- to 20-week pregnant women than in control subjects (58 ± 12 hours versus 52 ± 10 hours, respectively). Use of H2 breath tests after lactulose ingestion in 15 women revealed prolongation of transit time in the third trimester compared with the postpartum period (131 ± 14 minutes versus 93 ± 7 minutes). Lawson and colleagues found a statistically significant increase in the mean transit time from the first to the second trimester with an increase that was not significant in the third trimester and a subsequent fall in the postpartum period. Although the postpartum mean transit time was less than in the first trimester, the difference was not significant. Transit times increased as progesterone levels increased from <1 ng/mg to 80 ng/ml but not as levels increased further.

Colonic motility or transit in pregnant women has not been evaluated, but studies in rats have examined the effects of hormones and pregnancy on colonic transit. Rats that are in a high estrogen-progesterone state or that have been ovariectomized and pretreated with estrogen and progesterone show significantly slower transit times than animals in a low hormonal state or ovariectomized without hormone replacement. Pregnant rats have transit times similar to those of the ovariectomized animals pretreated with hormones.

Management

Treatment of constipation in pregnancy should be aimed at dietary modification through increased fiber intake and adequate liquid consumption. Supplementation of fiber ingested in the diet with psyllium (Metamucil, Konsyl, Effersyllium), methylcellulose (Citrucel), calcium polycarbophil (Fibercon), or pectin to 25 to 40 g/day of fiber is safe and often effective. Bloating may occur with some sources of fiber but not others. Therefore, if bloating occurs, changing the source of fiber may be beneficial. Nonabsorbable sugars such as lactulose, sorbitol, and glycerin are safe if dietary manipulation fails. Use of mineral oil should be limited to short periods because of the possibility of malabsorption of vitamins and nutrients, only in patients without a risk of aspiration and only in the morning or at lunch. Saline solutions containing laxatives may result in sodium retention in the mother. Other laxative use should be limited because of the risk of dependence. Laxatives to avoid are castor oil, which may induce uterine contractions in the mother; cascara sagrada, which may cause diarrhea in the neonate, and the anthraquinones. The other stimulant laxatives appear to be safe. Although many women attribute some of their constipation to the use of prenatal vitamins that contain iron, the vitamins should be continued if at all possible.

Hormonal fluctuations throughout the menstrual cycle and in pregnancy may affect bowel function, causing changes in frequency of bowel movements and periodic complaints of abdominal discomfort and bloating.

BIBLIOGRAPHY

Anderson AS: Constipation during pregnancy: incidence and methods used in its treatment in a group of Cambridgeshire women, *Health Visit* 12: 363, 1984.

Arthan D et al: Segmental colonic transit time, *Dis Colon Rectum* 24:625, 1981.

Bachmann GA, Moeller TP, Benett J: Childhood sexual abuse and the consequences in adult women, *Obstet Gynecol* 71:4:631, 1988.

Barnes W et al: Manometric characterization of rectal dysfunction following radical hysterectomy, *Gynecol Oncol* 42:116, 1991.

Baron TH, Ramirez B, Richter JE: Gastrointestinal motility disorders during pregnancy, *Ann Intern Med* 118:366, 1993.

Bensoussan A et al: Treatment of irritable bowel syndrome with Chinese herbal medicine: a randomized control trial, *JAMA* 280:1585, 1998.

Camilleri M: Therapeutic approach to the patient with irritable bowel syndrome, *Am J Med* 107:27S, 1999.

Davies GJ et al: Bowel function measurements of individuals with different eating patterns, *Gut* 27:164, 1986.

Drossman DA, Thompson WG: The irritable bowel syndrome: review and a graduated multicomponent treatment approach, *Ann Intern Med* 116: 1009, 1992.

Drossman DA et al: Bowel patterns among subjects not seeking healthcare: use of questionnaire to identify a population with bowel dysfunction, *Gastroenterology* 83:529, 1990.

Drossman DA et al: Sexual and physical abuse in women with functional or organic gastrointestinal disorders, *Ann Intern Med* 113:828, 1990.

Drossman DA et al: Health status by gastrointestinal diagnosis and abuse history, *Gastroenterology* 110:999, 1996.

Drossman DA, Whitehead WE, Camilleri M: Irritable bowel syndrome: a technical review for practice guideline development, *Gastroenterology* 112:2120, 1997.

Drossman DA et al: Irritable Bowel Syndrome, ADHF Part 1: Nosology. Epidemiology and Pathophysiology, 1999. Monograph.

Drossman DA et al: Irritable Bowel Syndrome, ADHF Part 2: Diagnosis and treatment. Epidemiology and Pathophysiology 2000. Monograph.

Everson GT: Gastrointestinal motility in pregnancy. In Reily CA, Abell TL, editors: *Gastroenterology clinics of North America,* Philadelphia, 1992, WB Saunders.

Heitkemper MM, Jarrett M: Pattern of gastrointestinal and somatic symptoms across the menstrual cycle, *Gastroenterology* 102:505, 1992.

Heitkemper MM, Shaver JF, Mitchell ES: Gastrointestinal symptoms and bowel patterns across the menstrual cycle in dysmenorrhea, *Nurs Res* 37:108, 1988.

Hinds JP, Stoney B, Wald A: Does gender or the menstrual cycle affect colonic transit? *Am J Gastroenterol* 84:123, 1989.

Kamm MA, Farthing MJG, Lennard-Jones JE: Bowel function and transit rate during the menstrual cycle, *Gut* 30:605, 1989.

Kane SV, Sable K, Hanauer SB: The menstrual cycle and its effect on inflammatory bowel disease and irritable bowel syndrome: a prevalence study, *Am J Gastroenterol* 93:1867, 1998.

Lawson M, Kern F Jr, Everson GT: Gastrointestinal transit time in human pregnancy: prolongation in the second and third trimesters followed by postpartum normalization, *Gastroenterology* 89:996, 1985.

Leserman J et al: The relationship of abuse history with health status and health care use in a referral GI clinic, *Gastroenterology* 104:A541, 1993.

Levy N, Lemberg E, Sharf M: Bowel habit in pregnancy, *Digestion* 4:216, 1971.

Lind CD: Motility disorders in the irritable bowel syndrome. In Friedman G, editor: *Gastroenterology clinics of North America,* vol 20, Philadelphia, 1991, WB Saunders.

Longstreth GF, Shragg GP: Irritable bowel syndrome and childhood abuse in HMO health examiners, *Gastroenterology* 102:A477, 1992.

Lynn RB, Friedman LS: Current concepts: irritable bowel syndrome, *N Engl J Med* 329:1940, 1993.

Mayer EA: Emerging disease model for functional gastrointestinal disorders, *Am J Med* 107:125, 1999.

Metcalf AM et al: Simplified assessment of segmental colonic transit, *Gastroenterology* 92:40, 1987.

Preston DM, Lennard-Jones JE: Severe chronic constipation of young women: idiopathic slow transit constipation, *Gut* 27:41, 1986.

Prior A, Marton DG, Whorwell PJ: Anorectal manometry in irritable bowel syndrome: differences between diarrhea and constipation predominant subjects, *Gut* 31:458, 1990.

Prior A, Whorwell PJ: Gynaecological consultation in patients with the irritable bowel syndrome, *Gut* 30:996, 1989.

Prior A et al: Relation between hysterectomy and the irritable bowel: a prospective study, *Gut* 33:814, 1992.

Rao SSC et al: Studies on the mechanism of bowel disturbance in ulcerative colitis, *Gastroenterology* 93:934, 1987.

Rees WDW, Rhodes JWT: Altered bowel habit and menstruation, *Lancet* 2:475, 1976.

Roe AM, Bartolo DCC, Mortensen NJM: Slow transit constipation: comparison between patients with or without previous hysterectomy, *Dig Dis Sci* 33:1159, 1988.

Ryan JP, Bhojwani A: Colonic transit in rats: effect of ovariectomy, sex steroid hormones, and pregnancy, *Am J Physiol* 251:G46, 1986.

Schmulson MW, Chang L: Diagnostic approach to the patient with irritable bowel syndrome, *Am J Med* 107:20S, 1999.

Schuster MM: Diagnostic evaluation of the irritable bowel syndrome. In Friedman G, editor: *Gastroenterology clinics of North America,* 1991, vol 20, Philadelphia, 1991, WB Saunders.

Springs FE, Friedrich WN: Health risk behaviors and medical sequelae of childhood sexual abuse, *Mayo Clin Proc* 67:527, 1992.

Smith AN et al: Disordered colorectal motility in intractable constipation following hysterectomy, *Br J Surg* 77:1361, 1990.

Stanhope CR: editorial, *Gynecol Oncol* 42:114, 1991.

Sutalf LO, Levitt MD: Follow-up of a flatulent patient, *Dig Dis Sci* 248:652, 1979.

Talley NJ, Zinsmeister AR, Melton LJ III: Sexual abuse is linked to functional bowel disorders in the community, *Gastroenterology* 104:A590, 1993.

Taylor T, Smith AN, Fulton PM: Effect of hysterectomy on bowel function, *Br Med J* 299:300, 1989.

Turnbull GK et al: Relationships between symptoms, menstrual cycle and orocaecal transit in normal and constipated women, *Gut* 30:30, 1989.

Wald A et al: Effect of pregnancy on gastrointestinal transit, *Dig Dis Sci* 27:1015, 1982.

Walker EA et al: Medical and psychiatric symptoms in women with childhood sexual abuse, *Psychosom Med* 54:658, 1992.

Whitehead WE et al: Evidence for exacerbation of irritable bowel syndrome during menses, *Gastroenterology* 98:1485, 1990.

Whorwell PJ et al: Bladder smooth muscle dysfunction in patients with irritable bowel syndrome, *Gut* 27:1014, 1986.

Wingate DL: The irritable bowel syndrome. In Friedman G, editor: *Gastroenterology clinics of North America,* vol 20, Philadelphia, 1991, WB Saunders.

Yadav SK et al: Irritable bowel syndrome: therapeutic evaluation of indigenous drugs, *Indian J Med Res* 90:496, 1989.

Zighelboim J, Talley NJ: What are functional bowel disorders? *Gastroenterology* 104:1196, 1993.

CHAPTER **20**

Blood Disorders

Margaret H. Baron
A. Jacqueline Mitus

The general approach to hematologic problems is the same in men and women. However, certain of these disorders occur more frequently in women than in men and, therefore, their special clinical implications form the main focus of discussion. Abnormalities unique to pregnancy are addressed at the end of this chapter. Hematologic malignancies (leukemias, lymphomas) and certain premalignant conditions (e.g., myelodysplastic syndromes, polycythemia vera) are not discussed here.

ABNORMALITIES OF RED BLOOD CELLS
Anemia
Definition and Epidemiology

A useful operational definition of anemia is a reduction in one or more of the major red blood cell (RBC) measurements: hemoglobin concentration, hematocrit, or RBC count. The mean normal value and lower limits of normal for these measurements depend on age, gender, race, and altitude of residence. The lower limits of hemoglobin (Hb) and hematocrit (Hct) for women are Hb 12 g/dl; Hct 36%. Anemia is more prevalent among women of childbearing age than in men of this age group, in part because iron deficiency resulting from blood loss is more common. Previous studies reporting lower hemoglobin levels in the elderly are controversial. Anemia in these patients is most likely due to disease and warrants careful clinical investigation. Although population-based data can be valuable, it is critical that the physician consider factors of relevance to a particular patient.

Pathophysiology

Analysis of the cause of anemia may be approached by focusing on kinetics (decreased RBC production, increased RBC destruction, or RBC loss) or cell morphology (normocytic, microcytic, or macrocytic anemia). The kinetic approach is discussed first. Morphologic classification of anemia is covered in the following discussion.

Anemia results from decreased red cell production or increased destruction as a consequence of hemolysis or blood loss. These two fundamental pathophysiologic processes are distinguished by the reticulocyte count, a marker of red cell proliferative activity (Box 20-1). The hypoprolifer-

ative anemias (low reticulocyte count) can be classified into different categories, including metabolic deficiency (iron, folate, vitamin B_{12}, erythropoietin deficiency), infiltrative marrow processes (fibrosis, metastatic cancer, granuloma), marrow suppression (toxin, virus), and primary hematologic conditions (aplastic anemia, myelodysplasia, leukemia).

In acute bleeding or hemolysis, compensatory erythroid hyperplasia is reflected in an elevated reticulocyte count. Hemolysis may result from a defect in the red blood cell itself or from some alteration in the red cell environment. Intrinsic erythrocyte abnormalities generally are inherited, and comprise disorders of hemoglobin (the hemoglobinopathies), the red cell membrane (e.g., hereditary spherocytosis), and cellular enzymes (e.g., glucose-6-phosphate dehydrogenase deficiency [G6PD]). Environmental changes leading to premature destruction of an otherwise normal erythrocyte tend to be acquired. Hypersplenism, antierythrocyte antibodies, red cell parasites, and mechanical fragmentation are some examples of these "extrinsic" red cell abnormalities (Box 20-1).

Clinical Presentation

The clinical manifestations of anemia depend on the rate of its development and its causative factors. Specific findings particularly relevant to women are discussed later in the chapter. In general, however, most patients complain of fatigue or decreased tolerance for work or physical activity. Others may report no change in energy level or stamina but have come to the attention of a physician because of pallor noted by friends or family. Cardiopulmonary symptoms reflect the degree of anemia, the rapidity of its onset, and the compensatory capacity of the cardiovascular system. A sudden drop in the hematocrit level precipitates dizziness, light-headedness, and, when the person stands, syncope. Symptoms of chronic anemia, in contrast, are dyspnea on exertion or at rest and palpitations.

History

The history is directed at ascertaining the duration and onset of anemia. Prior blood counts or a history of blood donation (implying normal blood counts at that time) may prove invaluable in dating onset. Questions regarding the patient's general health, with specific emphasis on signs or

---

BOX 20-1
Approach to Anemia

Decreased Production (Low Reticulocyte Count)
Metabolic deficiency
Iron
Folate
Vitamin B_{12}
Erythropoietin
Infiltrative marrow processes
Metastatic cancer
Fibrosis
Granuloma
Necrosis
Bone marrow suppression
Toxin
Virus
Radiation
Primary hematologic conditions
Aplastic anemia
Acute leukemia
Myelodysplastic syndromes

Increased Destruction (Elevated Reticulocytes)
Intrinsic red blood cell abnormalities
Hemoglobinopathies (structural variant hemoglobins, thalassemias)
Enzymopathies (e.g., glucose-6-phosphate dehydrogenase [G6PD] deficiency)
Membrane defects (e.g., hereditary spherocytosis)
Extrinsic red blood cell defects
Hypersplenism
Antibody deposition
Mechanical fragmentation
Intraerythrocytic infection (e.g., malaria)

BOX 20-2
Mean Corpuscular Volume ●nd Anemia

Decreased (MCV<80 fl)
Iron deficiency
Thalassemia
Anemia of chronic disease (25%)
Sideroblastic anemia
Lead poisoning

Normal (MCV 80-100)
Infiltrative processes
Anemia of chronic disease (75%)
Bleeding

Increased (MCV>100 fl)
Folate deficiency
Vitamin B_{12} deficiency
Hypothyroidism
Drugs (e.g., alcohol)
Liver disease
Aplastic anemia
Myelodysplasia
Reticulocytosis

---

symptoms of bleeding, should be explored. Dietary habits, hobbies, and occupational and social history may provide important clues concerning possible toxic suppression of the marrow, nutritional deficiency, risk for human immunodeficiency virus (HIV) infection, and other relevant findings. A hereditary anemia may become obvious with a careful family history. Even if the patient is unaware of the genetic disorder, splenectomy and/or cholecystectomy in multiple members of earlier generations point to an inherited hemolytic process.

Physical Examination

Pallor and icterus—indicative of hemolysis—are best detected by examination of the conjunctiva, mucous membranes, and palmar creases. Glossitis suggests an underlying vitamin deficiency (e.g., vitamin B_{12} deficiency) and should prompt careful neurologic testing of the posterolateral columns (position and vibratory sense). The spleen enlarges in an inferomedial direction and is best detected with the patient in the right lateral decubitus position.

Diagnostic Tests

As previously noted, the reticulocyte (retic) count is pivotal in classifying anemias as a process of decreased pro-

duction or accelerated destruction. Generally reported as a percentage of total red cells, this value should be corrected in an anemic patient to account for a decrease in the absolute erythrocyte number and is termed the *reticulocyte index:*

$$\text{retic (corrected)} = \text{retic (observed)} \times \text{(patient's Hct/normal Hct)}$$

Without this adjustment, a mild reticulocytosis may be misinterpreted as an elevation, whereas in fact it may be inappropriately low for the degree of anemia present.

Red Blood C●ll Indices. An assessment of erythrocyte size, Hb concentration, and shape is useful in the evaluation of anemia. Automated cell counters have the capacity to directly measure mean corpuscular volume (MCV), mean corpuscular hemoglobin (MCH), and mean corpuscular hemoglobin concentration (MCHC). The normal MCV ranges from 80 to 100 fl, and diagnostic possibilities are refined on the basis of the MCV value—whether it is normal (normocytic), microcytic (MCV 80 fl), or macrocytic (MCV 100 fl) (Box 20-2). Hypochromia (decreased erythrocyte hemoglobin content, MCH or MCHC) results from a defect in hemoglobin synthesis—abnormal or reduced globin chain production or decreased iron availability. Less commonly, hyperchromia implies loss of red cell membrane and ensuing rise in surface/volume ratio. Many automated blood counters also report an RBC distribution width (RDW), an assessment of size variation. The RDW is abnormal when greater than 14, a value that indicates a wide range in erythrocyte size. Examination of the blood smear should be performed whenever possible as important changes in erythroid size and morphology may escape detection by an automated blood counter. Infiltration of the bone marrow (tear drop cells), disturbance of the vascular endothelium (fragmentation), and congenital hemolysis (bite cells) are but a few of the many disorders that can be diagnosed by careful review of the peripheral smear (Box 20-2).

Serum Chemistry Tests. Several serum chemistry tests are helpful as general screens for hemolysis. Destruction of red cells occurs most commonly in the reticuloendothelial system (extravascular hemolysis) but also may develop within the vascular tree (intravascular hemolysis). In both instances, there is elevation of indirect bilirubin and serum lactate dehydrogenase (LDH) and depression of haptoglobin. In contrast, detection of free hemoglobin in the plasma (hemoglobinemia) or urine (hemoglobinuria) or the presence of iron-laden tubular epithelial cells in the urine sediment (urine hemosiderin) is specific for intravascular lysis of erythrocytes. More refined studies then follow to delineate the specific cause of hemolysis.

Specific Types of Anemia
Iron Deficiency
Pathogenesis
Iron stores are meticulously conserved by the body and represent a carefully regulated balance between dietary intake and physiologic requirements. There is no specific normal mechanism for excretion; daily losses of approximately 1 mg result from sloughing of epithelial cells from the skin and from the gastrointestinal and genitourinary tracts. Iron is best absorbed as the heme moiety found in meats and fish. Vegetables and grain products provide small amounts of ferrous (Fe^{2+}) and ferric (Fe^{3+}) iron, the absorption of which is less efficient than heme iron and is dependent on intestinal pH and food ligands. Despite iron fortification in many commercial food products, only 10% of ingested iron is absorbed, even with a normal, well-balanced diet. Consequently, individuals with restricted dietary intake (e.g., vegetarians) may consume an inadequate amount of this element.

Although decreased oral intake, increased demand (pregnancy), abnormal absorption (achlorhydria), and urinary loss of iron (chronic hemolysis) should be considered in the differential diagnosis, by far the most common cause of iron deficiency is bleeding—physiologic or pathologic. Men and women enter adulthood with marginal iron reserves because of the demands imposed by growth spurts during childhood and adolescence. In women, obligatory iron loss is compounded by menstrual bleeding, which claims an additional 20 to 40 mg per month (40 to 80 ml blood). As a result, monthly requirements for women approach 50 to 70 mg compared with only 30 mg for men. Most menstruating women, if not overtly iron deficient, will have borderline iron stores. In a postmenopausal woman, the presence of iron deficiency mandates a search for occult blood loss.

Clinical Presentation. Absence of iron leads to decreased manufacture of hemoglobin, as well as abnormal epithelial growth. Glossitis, angular cheilosis, and koilonychia (spooned, ridged, and brittle nails) signal advanced deficiency. Dysphagia can result from the unusual development of an esophageal web, the Plummer-Vinson syndrome, which usually does not reverse itself with iron replacement.

Pica, the abnormal craving of anything, remains a puzzling but at times dramatic symptom in some patients. Although ice craving (pagophagia) is most common and benign, ingestion of clay-rich soils (geophagia) or starch (amylophagia) is particularly hazardous because these materials interfere with normal iron absorption.

Diagnostic Tests. Microcytic, hypochromic erythrocytes with occasional "pencil" and target forms are hallmarks of iron deficiency. Laboratory confirmation of iron deficiency (Table 20-1) includes the finding of depressed serum iron and ferritin levels. Of these, the serum ferritin value is both more sensitive (90%) and specific (100%) for iron deficiency. The total iron-binding capacity (TIBC), a reflection of transferrin level, is elevated in a compensatory response. Because these laboratory values can be altered by concomitant systemic illness (see following discussion), a bone marrow examination for assessment of iron stores may be helpful. However, the absence of stainable iron in a bone marrow aspirate is not necessarily diagnostic of iron deficiency. Less commonly relied on, an elevated RDW also has been shown to aid in the diagnosis of iron deficiency.

Differential Diagnosis. Two clinical situations may be mistaken for iron deficiency, thalassemia trait and anemia of chronic disease (Table 20-1). The **thalassemias** make up a remarkably diverse group of monogenic disorders caused by deficient or absent production of alpha or beta globin chains (alpha- or beta-thalassemia, respectively). Imbalanced globin synthesis leads to hypochromic cells and precipitation of unmatched chains within the erythrocyte, leading to its premature destruction. This process occurs both within the peripheral circulation and in the bone marrow (ineffective erythropoiesis). The clinical manifestations of alpha-thalassemia, prevalent in black and Asian individuals, depend on how many of the four alpha-globin genes have been deleted. One gene deletion is phenotypically silent. When two genes are affected, microcytosis is observed, which can be misinterpreted as a sign of iron deficiency. Three- and four-gene deletion leads to more pronounced clinical and laboratory findings, rendering the correct diagnosis more obvious. In beta-thalassemia trait, common in persons of Mediterranean descent, microcytosis and mild anemia also are potentially confused with iron deficiency anemia. For the purposes of genetic counseling and because it may be harmful to prescribe iron for patients with thalassemia (who have a tendency to overabsorb iron), it is important to distinguish between these processes (Table 20-1). In addition to obtaining iron studies (iron, TIBC, and ferritin), the RDW can be helpful in this distinction; it is elevated in iron deficiency and typically normal in thalassemia trait. Although findings on Hb electrophoresis confirm the presence of beta-thalassemia (elevated levels of hemoglobin A_2 and hemoglobin F), results may be normal in alpha-thalassemia, which therefore remains a diagnosis of exclusion.

Chronic disease also gives rise to a hematologic profile easily confused with iron deficiency. Through mechanisms incompletely defined, chronic inflammation leads to sequestration of iron within reticuloendothelial tissue, thereby rendering it unavailable for incorporation into hemoglobin. Consequently, the terms *anemia of ineffective iron reutilization* and *anemia of inflammation* are better reflections of the

Table 20-1
Differential Diagnosis of Iron Deficiency: Clinical and Laboratory Features

History/Physical Examination	Iron	Total Iron-Binding Capacity	Ferritin	Smear	Red Cell Distribution Width	Marrow Iron
Iron Deficiency Bleeding Pica Angular cheilosis Koilonychia Dysphagia	↓	↑	↓	Microcytosis Hypochromia Pencil shapes	↑	Absent
Anemia of Chronic Disease Chronic infection or inflammation	↓	↓	↑	RBC normal (1/4 micro-cytosis)	Normal	↑ (in reticulo-endothelial system, not RBC precur-sors)
Thalassemia Trait Family history Splenomegaly (±)	Normal/↑	Normal	↑	Microcytosis Targets Hypochromia	Normal	↑

RBC, Red blood cells.

true pathophysiologic mechanism. Anemia is usually mild (Hct in the low 30s) and, although usually normocytic, may be microcytic in up to one fourth of cases. Even though distinctions are not always straightforward, differentiation of iron deficiency from anemia of chronic disease can be accomplished from review of laboratory data (Table 20-1). In both situations, the serum iron level is depressed, but the TIBC typically is high in iron deficiency and low in anemia of chronic disease. Although determination of the serum ferritin level remains the best noninvasive test, it is an acute-phase reactant and may be mildly elevated even in the setting of low iron stores. It has been argued, however, that ferritin levels greater than 50 mg/L rarely indicate iron deficiency. In equivocal cases, an empiric trial of iron therapy may be warranted before a bone marrow examination is performed.

✳ MANAGEMENT

In addition to replacing lost iron, thus improving the patient's well-being, the most important aspect in the assessment of iron deficiency is defining the source of blood loss. In premenopausal women, menstrual bleeding is the likely cause; however, further evaluation may be dictated by the clinical, social, and family history. The gastrointestinal tract is a common site of hemorrhage, and the finding of iron deficiency in postmenopausal women (or men) warrants a thorough radiographic or endoscopic evaluation.

Iron Supplementation. Iron stores usually can be replenished by oral supplementation. Many iron preparations are poorly tolerated because of bloating, constipation, and/or diarrhea; however, ferrous gluconate or polysaccharide-iron complexes seem to cause fewer side effects than does ferrous sulfate. For optimal absorption, patients should be ad-

Table 20-2
Oral Iron Supplements

Iron Preparation	Elemental Iron	Dose
Polysaccharide iron complex (Niferex)	150 mg	1 tablet per day
Generic ferrous sulfate 300 mg	60 mg	2-3 tablets per day
Generic ferrous gluconate 300 mg	27 mg	4 tablets per day

vised to take iron with citrus juice or 250 mg ascorbic acid, but without food. However, gastrointestinal side effects may be diminished by taking iron with a meal. Extended release formulations are less well absorbed, but may improve adherence by lessening side effects. Side effects can be minimized by gradual titration of the dosage over a few weeks.

Peak reticulocytosis occurs at variable time periods after institution of therapy, and complete correction of anemia and restoration of iron reserves requires up to 8 or 9 months (Table 20-2).

Alternatively, total body iron can be rapidly replaced by a single intravenous administration of iron. Peak reticulocytosis occurs after about 10 days; although normalization of the Hct level takes 4 to 5 weeks, most patients experience symptomatic improvement within 1 to 2 weeks. Because the major drawback of this approach is the small risk of anaphylaxis and transient arthralgias, intravenous dosing should be reserved for patients whose condition is refractory to oral replacement, who are unable to absorb iron, or in whom a more rapid normalization of Hb and Hct levels are desired.

Pernicious Anemia

Epidemiology

Pernicious anemia (PA) traditionally has been regarded as a disorder affecting older persons of northern European descent. As a result, it probably has been underrecognized in other populations, in particular, young black women.

Pathogenesis. Because of the abundance of cobalamin (vitamin B_{12}) in red meats and dairy products, deficiency of this vitamin on a dietary basis is extremely rare, occurring only in fastidious ovolactovegetarians (vegans). Instead, depletion usually results from defective absorption. Once ingested, cobalamin binds to intrinsic factor, produced by gastric parietal cells, whereby it is protected from enzymatic degradation until it reaches its site of absorption in the terminal ileum. Any disturbance along this pathway can lead to vitamin B_{12} deficiency; these include surgical absence of the stomach or ileum, inflammation (e.g., sprue), or bacterial overgrowth of the ileal mucosa. Antibodies produced against intrinsic factor or parietal cells also interfere with cobalamin absorption and result in a condition named for its formerly lethal potential, pernicious anemia.

Absence of cobalamin, a critical cofactor in DNA synthesis, leads to arrest of nuclear division that is most apparent in tissues with rapid turnover. In the bone marrow, these effects are striking. While cytoplasmic maturation proceeds unimpaired, nuclear division comes to a halt (nuclear-cytoplasmic dysynchrony), leading to the formation of large cells with an immature and noncondensed nucleus (megaloblasts). These abnormal cells are destroyed within the marrow cavity, resulting in ineffective erythropoiesis. Although morphologic findings are most pronounced in the erythroid lineage, all marrow elements are affected, resulting in anemia, leukopenia, and thrombocytopenia; *megaloblastic pancytopenia* is perhaps a more accurate description of this disorder.

Clinical Presentation (Box 20-3)

HISTORY. Because anemia develops slowly in PA, compensatory cardiac mechanisms often protect the patient from symptoms until the hematocrit has fallen to very low levels. Easy bruising and bleeding may be noted. A number of patients report glossitis, diarrhea, heartburn, and bloating, which reflect changes in gastrointestinal epithelial division. Abnormal cervical Pap results also may be found. Neurologic abnormalities develop in a percentage of individuals with cobalamin deficiency, but these do not correlate with the severity of anemia. Bilateral, symmetric paresthesias of the fingers and toes, imbalance, and ataxia reflect classic involvement of the posterolateral columns (subacute combined system disease). Less commonly, slowed mentation, irritability, depression, and impaired memory mimic dementia. Other autoimmune disorders such as vitiligo and hypothyroidism are diagnosed with increased frequency in patients with PA and in their relatives.

PHYSICAL EXAMINATION. Jaundice as a result of intramedullary hemolysis superimposed on the pallor of anemia explains the unusual lemon-yellow hue of persons with untreated cobalamin deficiency. The tongue typically is depapillated, smooth, and shiny, producing a classic "beefy red" appear-

---

BOX 20-3
Clinical Presentation of Pernicious Anemia

History
Fatigue
Dyspnea
Bleeding
Gastrointestinal complaints

Examination
Lemon-colored skin
Glossitis
Neurologic changes (combined system disease)

Laboratory Tests
Pancytopenia
Macrocytosis
Hypersegmented neutrophils
Elevated indirect bilirubin level
Elevated lactic dehydrogenase level
Low vitamin B_{12} level
Abnormal bone marrow (megaloblasts)

---

ance. Abnormal position and vibratory sense point to nervous system involvement.

DIAGNOSTIC TESTS. The peripheral blood smear findings are characteristic, revealing large, oval-shaped red cells (macro-ovalocytes) and hypersegmented neutrophils. Indirect hyperbilirubinemia and markedly elevated serum lactic dehydrogenase (LDH) levels attest to the profound intramedullary hemolysis underlying this condition. The availability of serum B12 assays has largely replaced the need for bone marrow examination.

A Schilling test can be performed to help define the cause of cobalamin deficiency and establish a diagnosis of PA. Vitamin B_{12} stores are replaced by intramuscular injection, and then oral radiolabeled B_{12} is administered. The presence of radioactivity in the urine confirms absorption and subsequent excretion of the vitamin. A patient with PA is unable to absorb vitamin B_{12} when it is given alone (the first phase of the test), which is corrected by coadministration of intrinsic factor (second phase). Rarely, bacterial overgrowth of the ileum accounts for malabsorption, and if findings of the first two parts of the Schilling test are abnormal, a course of antibiotics is prescribed as a last measure (third phase). Because the Schilling test is somewhat cumbersome (requiring several 24-hour urine collections) and irrespective of causative factors, parenteral B_{12} administration is the therapy of choice; thus, most practitioners treat empirically without obtaining this study.

Therapy. Replacement of vitamin B12 is accomplished by intramuscular injection (1000 mg cobalamin), initially weekly for 4 weeks, and then monthly for life.

Anemia of Starvation: Eating Disorders

The hematologic changes associated with anorexia nervosa have been recognized for decades but remain unexplained. Anemia can be profound and is characterized by prominent acanthocytsis (spiculation of red cells). Varying degrees of leukopenia and thrombocytopenia also are noted. Gelatinous degeneration of the bone marrow with focal cellular necrosis appears to underlie these hematologic abnormalities, all of which improve on increase in caloric intake and weight gain. (Chapter 84 covers anorexia and bulimia in detail.)

Hemolytic Anemia

Infrequently, disorders inherited as sex-linked recessives may affect women. One of the more common of these is G6PD deficiency. Because of unequal inactivation of the X chromosome (lyonization), some women have a relative deficiency of this enzyme. As a result, hemoglobin is abnormally susceptible to oxidative stress such as occurs on exposure to certain medications (e.g., antimalarial agents, dapsone). When oxidized, hemoglobin denatures, forming rigid aggregates, termed Heinz bodies, that impede the red cell's pliability and are removed in the macrophage-lined sinusoids of the spleen. Bitelike deformation of the erythrocyte and extravascular hemolysis ensue.

Polycythemia and Erythrocytosis

The term *polycythemia* loosely refers to any elevation above normal in RBC number in the circulating blood. Usually, although not always, the increase is accompanied by increases in Hb and Hct. Because the total body RBC number may or may not be elevated, it is important to distinguish between *absolute* polycythemia (increased total RBC mass) and *relative* polycythemia. In the latter condition, the concentration of RBCs increases as the result of plasma volume (as in abnormally lowered fluid intake, loss of fluid into interstitial spaces, or significant loss of body fluids through persistent vomiting, severe diarrhea, copious sweating, acidosis, etc.).

The more specific, and preferred, terms for absolute polycythemia are *erythrocytosis* and *erythremia*. Erythrocytosis signifies absolute polycythemia that occurs in response to a known stimulus (thus, a secondary polycythemia). In general, this condition is a physiologic response to conditions of hypoxia such as those found at high altitude, in certain cardiopulmonary diseases, in patients who smoke, and in response to inappropriate production or therapeutic administration of steroid hormones. The term *erythremia* is used to denote polycythemia of unknown etiology (polycythemia vera).

ABNORMALITIES OF THE PLATELET COUNT

Thrombocytopenia

Pathophysiology

Thrombocytopenia on the basis of underproduction results from megakaryopoiesis that is ineffective (e.g., myelodysplasia) or that has been disrupted by infiltration of the marrow by malignant or infectious processes. Isolated absence of platelet precursors (amegakaryocytosis) is extremely rare. In contrast, increased destruction of platelets accompanies a variety of clinical situations, including hypersplenism, disseminated intravascular coagulation (DIC), immune thrombocytopenic purpura (ITP), and thrombotic thrombocytopenic purpura (TTP). Because the last two con-ditions appear to affect women disproportionately compared with men (3:1), they are discussed in greater detail later in this section.

Clinical Presentation

Normal hemostasis hinges on complex interactions among platelets, coagulation proteins, and the vessel wall. Platelets play a central role in this process through the formation of a hemostatic plug that subsequently is stabilized by the coagulation proteins to produce a firm fibrin clot. In patients with thrombocytopenia, bleeding occurs immediately on injury and typically involves mucocutaneous surfaces: epistaxis, oral and gastrointestinal hemorrhage, menorrhagia, petechiae, and ecchymoses. Deep-seated bleeding (e.g., hemarthrosis) is unusual and suggests a factor deficiency such as hemophilia. Platelet counts greater than $50,000/mm^3$ rarely are associated with spontaneous bleeding, and patients usually have no symptoms or note only mild excessive bruising after trauma. In contrast, when severe depression occurs (platelets $20,000/mm^3$), pronounced and often unprecipitated hemorrhage ensues.

History

All patients with thrombocytopenia should be carefully queried as to symptoms of underlying illness; collagen vascular diseases and human immunodeficiency virus (HIV) infection may first occur with ITP. A meticulous list of all medications must be obtained (prescription and nonprescription), inasmuch as both immune thrombocytopenia and, less commonly, direct suppression of megakaryopoiesis have been reported with myriad drugs. Rarely, a family history may suggest a form of congenital thrombocytopenia.

Physical Examination

Physical findings depend on the degree of thrombocytopenia. With significant platelet depression, petechiae, mucosal bullae, and hematomas, as well as retinal and gastrointestinal bleeding, may be noted. Evaluation of a patient with thrombocytopenia should include careful palpation for the presence of an enlarged spleen and a search for stigmata of underlying systemic illness.

Specific Causes

Immune Thrombocytopenic Purpura. ITP results from deposition of antibody or antigen-antibody complexes on the platelet and their subsequent consumption within the reticuloendothelial system. Women, particularly in their childbearing years, appear to have a higher incidence of idiopathic autoimmune thrombocytopenia for reasons that remain unclear. The degree of thrombocytopenia is variable as is the propensity for bleeding. Often a diagnosis is made incidentally after a complete blood count has been obtained for unrelated purposes.

The diagnosis of ITP remains one of exclusion, resting on the careful consideration of other causes of thrombocytopenia and the finding of normal or increased numbers of megakaryocytes in the bone marrow. The peripheral smear typically reveals decreased numbers of platelets, some of which appear larger than normal. Assays for antiplatelet antibodies may help confirm the diagnosis but are neither specific nor sensitive enough to stand alone as a diagnostic test.

MANAGEMENT. No therapy is required when thrombocytopenia is mild. If the platelet count falls below 50,000/mm³ or if bleeding develops, treatment with corticosteroids is initiated. Although usually effective, steroids rarely are curative, and relapse often occurs after the drug is discontinued. Splenectomy is generally the next step, resulting in remission in about 70% of cases. Infusion of intravenous gammaglobulin, another therapeutic option, is highly likely to improve platelet number, but its effects are transient and a treatment course very expensive. Therefore, it is best reserved for the setting of acute bleeding refractory to steroids. Management of pregnancy in a women with ITP poses additional considerations and therapeutic dilemmas (see later discussion).

Thrombotic Thrombocytopenic Purpura

DEFINITION. TTP is a rare condition with a classic pentad of fever, neurologic change, uremia, microangiopathic hemolysis, and thrombocytopenia. For reasons that are poorly understood, as with ITP, woman are affected about two to three times more frequently than are men.

PATHOPHYSIOLOGY. The cause of TTP remains unknown. Widespread thrombotic occlusion of arterioles and capillaries involves predominantly the brain, kidneys, heart, pancreas, spleen, and adrenal glands. It is presumed that after some inciting event, endothelial damage results in the formation of platelet-rich microthrombi that occlude vascular flow and cause shearing fragmentation or red blood cells. TTP has been associated with a variety of systemic conditions, including infection, pregnancy, and collagen vascular illness, as well as the use of such drugs as cyclosporine.

CLINICAL PRESENTATION. Clinical symptoms can be subtle or absent at onset. Vague neurologic findings are often present at some point during the course of the disease and include headache, visual changes, neuropathies, seizures, and coma. Fever and bleeding are variable in severity. Although the diagnosis may be apparent when all symptoms are present, the full pentad occurs in only 30% of cases; especially when complaints are mild, this disorder can be overlooked.

DIAGNOSTIC TESTS. Thrombocytopenia, abnormal renal function, and hemolytic anemia are the hallmarks of TTP. Examination of the peripheral smear is pivotal inasmuch as it will reveal fragmentation of red cells consistent with microangiopathic destruction. Intravascular hemolysis is confirmed by the finding of an elevated indirect bilirubin and LDH, depressed haptoglobin, presence of plasma, and urine-free hemoglobin.

MANAGEMENT. Immediate recognition of TTP is crucial because delay in therapy results in significant mortality. Although the pathogenesis of this condition remains largely unknown, empiric treatment with plasma infusion or plasma exchange results in remission in about 80% of instances.

Thrombocytosis. Thrombocytosis is a normal response to a number of systemic conditions, including iron deficiency, chronic inflammation, infection, and hyposplenism. However, an elevated platelet count may indicate aberrant marrow production and suggest a disorder such as essential thrombocythemia (ET).

Essential Thrombocythemia

EPIDEMIOLOGY AND DEFINITION. ET is a chronic myeloproliferative disease characterized by marked elevation in platelet number and an unpredictable pattern of hemorrhage or thrombosis. Although it affects older men and women equally, it seems to be more common in young females.

CLINICAL PRESENTATION. Hemorrhage and recurrent thrombosis punctuate the course of patients with ET. Bleeding tends to occur at mucocutaneous surfaces, reflecting the defect in primary hemostasis. Thrombosis can develop in the venous or arterial tree and involves large and small vessels. Although deep venous thrombosis and pulmonary embolus are most common, occlusion at unusual sites (sagittal and portal vein, subclavian and coronary artery) has been described. Headache, transient ischemic attack, and other neurologic symptoms represent microthrombotic obstruction. Previously regarded as a benign condition in young persons, several studies have documented severe and life-threatening complications in this cohort. Splenomegaly is present in one third of cases; otherwise, findings on physical examination are unremarkable.

DIAGNOSTIC TESTS. Platelets typically exceed 1 million and exhibit a variety of functional abnormalities. No single clinical finding is specific for ET, and thus diagnosis remains one of exclusion. First, reactive causes of thrombocytosis must be eliminated. Among laboratory data helpful in this regard are iron studies (normal in ET), sedimentation rate (often very low in ET), and fibrinogen level (normal in ET). Elimination of other myeloproliferative conditions is the next step, and more detailed hematologic testing is required.

THERAPY. Management of patients with ET remains controversial. In the absence of symptoms, it is reasonable to monitor clinical developments carefully without intervention. Platelet-lowering agents such as hydroxyurea, anagrelide, and interferon are reserved for the development of hemorrhage or thrombosis. Aspirin and other antiplatelet drugs should be used with caution, inasmuch as they can exacerbate the underlying hemorrhagic diathesis.

ABNORMALITIES OF WHITE BLOOD CELLS
Leukopenia

Normal white blood cell (WBC) count and granulocyte number differ among races; approximately one fourth of African Americans are neutropenic. Although it has been demonstrated that granulocyte reserve (as measured by neutrophil increment after hydrocortisone administration) is depressed in this group, neutropenia does not correlate with an increased risk of infection and represents a normal variant.

Immune Neutropenia

As with anemia and thrombocytopenia, neutropenia results from decreased production or increased destruction. Rare congenital disorders and primary bone marrow diseases (e.g., myelodysplasia, leukemia) are the major conditions leading to diminished synthesis of granulocytes. More often, neutropenia arises from increased clearance by an autoantibody and, occasionally, a drug may be implicated. Idiopathic neutropenia is of particular relevance to women inasmuch as it may be the first sign of an underlying illness such as systemic lupus erythematosus. When it is accompanied by rheumatoid arthritis and splenomegaly, the triad of Felty's syndrome is met. Although many patients with neutropenia remain asymptomatic, the risk of life-threatening bacterial infection mandates close observation and the immediate institution of antibiotics in the presence of fever. Bone marrow examination is indicated to exclude a primary hematologic condition. Tests for antineutrophil antibodies are unreliable; therefore, the diagnosis of immune neutropenia remains one of exclusion.

Leukocytosis

Although leukocytosis usually implies infection, it may be noted in otherwise healthy women. Significant elevations in WBC have been detected in women who are obese, smoke, and use oral contraceptives. Of these associations, smoking causes the most marked abnormalities and has a dose-dependent effect. However, a recent study suggests that higher WBC counts are a predictor of mortality from coronary heart disease (CHD), independent of the effects of smoking and other traditional cardiovascular risk factors. These findings suggest a role for inflammation in the pathogenesis of CHD, but whether interventions aimed at decreasing inflammation can reduce the risk for CHD associated with elevated WBC is unknown.

PREGNANCY AND BLOOD DISORDERS

Normal pregnancy results in expected alteration of the hematologic profile (Box 20-4). Some changes, however, are not benign and reflect pathologic developments during gestation.

Physiologic Changes
Red Blood Cell Changes

Hb concentrations fall during normal pregnancy because of a disproportionate rise in plasma volume over red cell mass. Between weeks 34 and 36, plasma volume has expanded by about 1250 ml, whereas red cell mass increases more slowly and less dramatically, 250 to 400 ml at term. This physiologic or dilutional change accounts for second and third trimester Hct values in the low-30 range (Hb 10 to 11 g/dl), although 3% to 5% of apparently healthy women have even lower levels. The MCV typically rises 1 to 4 fl in pregnancy and can mask underlying iron deficiency.

BOX 20-4
Normal Hematologic Changes During Pregnancy

Red Blood Cells
Dilutional anemia
Elevated MCV (1-4 fl)

White Blood Cells
Leukocytosis
Early myeloid forms

Platelets
Mild thrombocytopenia

Pregnancy places extreme demands on the iron reserves of women: approximately 250 mg of iron is used by the developing fetus and an additional 100 mg is sequestered in the placenta. Expansion of maternal red cell mass consumes another 500 mg, with variable amounts lost at delivery. Overall, about 1 g of iron is required for normal gestation. Consequently, iron supplementation is mandatory during routine prenatal care and should be continued for many months thereafter.

White Blood Cell Changes

Nearly 50% of women develop leukocytosis (WBC 10,000) or some abnormality of the white cell differential during pregnancy. Circulating myelocytes and metamyelocytes are noted in 25% of complete blood counts (CBCs) even when the absolute white count is normal. These changes seem to be most prominent during the third trimester and resolve postpartum.

Changes in Platelets

Thrombocytopenia in the pregnant woman presents a complex series of diagnostic and management issues that have been summarized in a recent review by Burrows. Mild depression in platelet number can accompany normal, uncomplicated gestation. A total of 8% of healthy women have platelet counts that range between 100,000 and 150,000/mm^3, and a small percentage drop below 50,000/mm^3. Infants born to these women are at low risk for complications, as neonatal thrombocytopenia and bleeding are rare. The cause of thrombocytopenia during pregnancy remains unclear but probably represents accelerated activation and consumption of platelets in the uteroplacental circulation. Benign pregnancy-associated thrombocytopenia must be distinguished from other conditions in which depressed platelet number can lead to serious hemorrhage.

Pathologic Processes
Folate Deficiency

Folate is second only to iron as the most common cause of nutritional anemia in the gravid female. Derived from green leafy vegetables and legumes, folate stores are depleted within weeks to months if intake is restricted or demand is increased. In pregnancy, minimal daily requirements rise twofold or higher over nongravid needs and thus exogenous supplementation should be provided. Except for the absence of neurologic abnormalities, the clinical and hematologic findings in folate deficiency are identical to those of megaloblastic anemia caused by vitamin B_{12} deficiency.

Preeclampsia

Preeclampsia, defined by hypertension and proteinuria during pregnancy, is accompanied by thrombocytopenia in 15% to 50% of cases. Probably a variant of this condition, the HELLP syndrome (hemolysis, elevated liver enzymes, and low platelet count) also is characterized by microangiopathic hemolytic anemia and accelerated consumption of platelets. Because of high maternal and fetal mortality, these disorders must be promptly recognized and treated. Expeditious delivery of the fetus and aggressive transfusional support form the mainstay of therapy. These syndromes are covered in detail in Chapter 69.

Immune Thrombocytopenic Purpura

As previously noted, ITP is particularly common in women of childbearing years. Because maternal antiplatelet antibodies can cross the placenta, management is complicated by the additional risk posed to the fetus. The optimal mode of delivery in these cases remains controversial. It has been argued that because passage through the birth canal places the thrombocytopenic infant at risk for intracranial hemorrhage, cesarean section should be performed in this setting. However, C-section may be unnecessary in the woman whose fetus is unaffected. Neither maternal platelet count nor antibody titer reliably predicts thrombocytopenia in the neonate, further complicating delivery decisions. Consequently, some clinicians advocate obtaining fetal blood (via fetal scalp vein or percutaneous umbilical blood sampling). If thrombocytopenia is absent in the neonate, normal vaginal delivery can be undertaken.

Antiphospholipid Antibodies and Habitual Abortion

The antiphospholipid antibodies make up a heterogeneous family of proteins associated with recurrent arterial and venous thrombosis. Although involvement of the uteroplacental vessels has been implicated in habitual abortion, the precise risk of miscarriage in this setting is not known. Clinical studies are hampered by fluctuating antibody titers and imperfect assays. It does appear, however, that those women with repeatedly positive assay results incur an increased risk of fetal loss (see Chapter 37).

BIBLIOGRAPHY

Barron BA, Hoyer JD, Tefferi A: A bone marrow report of absent stainable iron is not diagnostic of iron deficiency, *Ann Hematol* 80:166, 2001.

Bini EJ, Micale PL, Weinshel EH: Evaluation of the gastrointestinal tract in premenopausal women with iron deficiency anemia, *Am J Med* 105:281, 1998.

Black RE: Micronutrients in pregnancy, *Br J Nutr* 85:S193, 2001.

Brown DW, Giles WH, Croft JB: White blood cell count: an independent predictor of coronary heart disease mortality among a national cohort, *J Clin Epidemiol* 54:316, 2001.

Burrows RF: Platelet disorders in pregnancy, *Curr Opin Obstet Gynecol* 13:115, 2001.

Clarke GM, Higgins TN: Laboratory investigation of hemoglobinopathies and thalassemias: review and update, *Clin Chem* 46:1284, 2000.

Eliason BC: RDW to detect iron deficiency, *J Fam Pract* 43:223, 1996.

Handin RI: Bleeding and thrombosis. In Braunwald E et al, editors: *Harrison's principles of internal medicine*, ed 5, New York, 2001, McGraw-Hill.

Lee GR: Anemia: general considerations. In Lee GR et al: Wintrobe's clinical hematology, ed 10, Baltimore, 1999, Lippincott, Williams & Wilkins.

Liu TC, Seong PS, Lin TK: The erythrocyte cell hemoglobin distribution width segregates thalassemia traits from other nonthalassemic conditions with microcytosis, *Am J Clin Pathol* 107:601, 1997.

Olivieri N: Thalassemia: clinical management, *Baillieres Clin Haematol* 11:147, 1998.

Rockey DC: Gastrointestinal tract evaluation in patients with iron deficiency anemia, *Semin Gastrointest Dis* 10:53, 1999.

Schilling RF: Anemia of chronic disease: a misnomer, *Ann Intern Med* 115:572, 1991 (editorial).

Swain RA, Kaplan B, Montgomery E: Iron deficiency anemia. When is parenteral therapy warranted? *Postgrad Med* 100:181, 1996.

Tefferi A, Hoagland HC: Issues in the management of essential thrombocytosis, *Mayo Clin Proc* 69:651, 1994.

van Zeben D et al: Evaluation of microcytosis using serum ferritin and red blood cell distribution width, *Eur J Haematol* 44:105, 1990.

Weatherall DJ: The phenotypic diversity of monogenic disease: lessons from the thalassemias, *Harvey Lect* 94:1, 1998.

Wians FH, Urban JE, Keffer JH, Kroft SH: Discriminating between iron deficiency anemia and anemia of chronic disease using traditional indices of iron status vs transferrin receptor concentration, *Am J Clin Pathol* 115:112, 2001.

Williams WJ, Morris MW, Nelson DA: Examination of the blood. In Beutler E et al, editors: *Williams' Hematology*, ed 5, New York, 1995, McGraw-Hill.

CHAPTER **21**

Human Immunodeficiency Virus

Robyn S. Klein
Powell H. Kazanjian
Stephanie A. Eisenstat

EPIDEMIOLOGY

Worldwide, approximately 47% of the 33 million adults living with human immunodeficiency virus/acquired immunodeficiency syndrome (HIV/AIDS) are women. In the year 2000, of the 2.5 million adults who died from AIDS, 1.3 million were women. In the United States, women are the fastest growing segment of AIDS cases, their proportion more than tripling from 7% in 1985 to 20% in 1999 (Table 21-1).

Minority women are disproportionately represented among these new infections. Although African-American and Hispanic women together represent less than 25% of all US women, they account for 77% of all AIDS cases reported to date in this country. Currently, the Centers for Disease Control and Prevention (CDC) estimates that 650,000 to 900,000 Americans are living with HIV infection, with an estimated 40,000 new infections each year, 30% of which occur in women. Although AIDS-related deaths among all persons are decreasing as a result of advances in HIV treatment, HIV/AIDS remains among the leading causes of death for American women aged 25 to 44 years (Table 21-2).

This chapter reviews the epidemiology, demographics, and natural history of HIV infection in women and offers management strategies for the asymptomatic HIV-infected woman. Indications for immunizations, antiretroviral agents, and medications used for prophylaxis against opportunistic infections are summarized. In addition, information regarding psychosocial issues affecting HIV-positive women is provided.

DEMOGRAPHIC FEATURES

The demographic features of women with HIV infection differ from those of HIV-infected men. More women with AIDS are persons of color than are men with AIDS (76% versus 49%), with African-American women accounting for the gap in numbers between women and men of color with AIDS (56% versus 32%) (Fig. 21-1). Risk behaviors also differ somewhat between the genders. In 1998 equal numbers of women with AIDS were infected via heterosexual exposure to HIV or injection drug use (41% versus 40%; Fig. 21-2), whereas most heterosexual men with AIDS were exposed to

HIV via injection drug use (30% versus 4.5%). In addition, seropositive women are much more likely than seropositive men to be the sex partners of intravenous drug users (IVDUs) (16% versus 1%). Thus, intravenous drug use, by itself and through contact with drug using partners, appears to account for approximately 57% of HIV infection in women.

Most women infected with HIV are of reproductive age, married, monogamous, and poor. A 10-year study of heterosexual HIV transmission in HIV-serodiscordant couples found male-to-female transmission to be eight times more likely than female-to-male transmission. Heterosexual transmission has increased from 3% of all AIDS cases among women in 1983 to approximately 38% in 1998. Factors associated with increased transmission include lack of condom use, anal intercourse, numbers of contacts, advanced disease state of partner, and genital ulcerative disease (Box 21-1).

The incidence of transmission of HIV from an infected man to a female partner in a fixed relationship after unprotected sex over a sustained period of time is approximately 20%.

CLINICAL PRESENTATION

Important gender differences exist in the presentation and complications of HIV infection. Women have been reported to have lower viral loads with equal disease progression or faster progression with equivalent viral loads when compared with men. Thus HIV-infected women generally meet criteria for AIDS earlier in their illness and develop different complications early in the course of their infection than do men. Psychosocial variables such as lack of access to health care, young age, poverty, and attention to the health care needs of children over self-care may contribute to later detection and intervention.

Many manifestations of HIV infection are similar in men and women. Signs of systemic illness, such as low-grade fevers, night sweats, fatigue, and weight loss, may appear early in the course of HIV infection in both sexes. However, given the differences in demographic data between HIV-infected women and men, chronic consequences of HIV infection may affect women more adversely because they are more likely to be nonwhite, poor, and using intravenous

Table 21-1
Number and Percentage of Reported Cases and Male/Female Ratio for Women and Heterosexual Men with AIDS in the United States

	NO. (%) OF ALL AIDS CASES		
Year	Women	Heterosexual Men	Ratio
1981	6 (3.2)	24 (12.7)	4.0
1987	1701 (8.1)	4127 (19.7)	2.4
1990	4890 (11.5)	11632 (27.3)	2.4
1999	64082 (20.0)	88300 (27.6)	1.4

Modified from Ellerbrock TV: *JAMA* 265:2971, 1991.
With CDC AIDS Surveillance Report, June 1999.

Table 21-2
Death Rates and Leading Causes of Death Among Women Ages 15 to 44 Years

Rank	Cause of Death	Numbers
New Jersey, 1998		
1	AIDS	117
2	Cancer	77
3	Heart disease	58
4	Injuries	51
5	Homicide	28
New York, 1998		
1	AIDS	261
2	Cancer	195
3	Heart disease	111
4	Injuries	82
5	Homicide	50

CDC, National Center for Injury Prevention and Control, 1998.

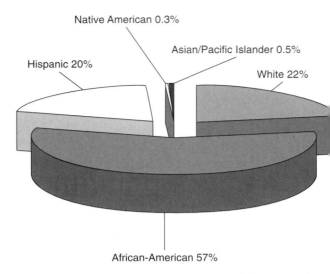

FIG. 21-1 AIDS in women by ethnicity. (From CDC, June 2000.)

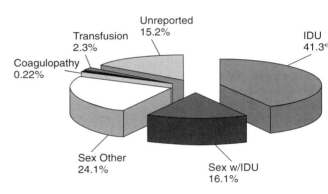

FIG. 21-2 AIDS in women by exposure category. (From CDC, June 2000.)

BOX 21-1

Risk Factors Correlated with Increases in Male to Female Sexual Transmission Rate of HIV

Viral load of male partner >1500 copies/ml
History of genital discharge or dysuria in male partner
Presence of AIDS-defining diagnoses
History of syphilis, genital warts, or vaginitis in female partner
No condom usage
No oral contraceptive usage
Intrauterine device usage
Anal intercourse

From Lazzarin A: *Arch Intern Med* 1991; Quinn TC: *N Engl J Med* 2000.

drugs. These risk factors have been associated with low quality-of-life scores on the Medical Outcomes Study Short Form Health Survey.

Most of the information regarding the natural history of HIV infection and management of the HIV-infected patient is derived from studies of infected homosexual men (Fig. 21-3). Symptoms of acute HIV infection occur 2 to 6 weeks after viral transmission. Most patients experience a flulike illness with fever, rash, pharyngitis, and lymphadenopathy (Table 21-3).

Viral loads at this time are usually in the range of millions of copies per milliliter and occasionally signs of severe immunosuppression can occur owing to an acute drop in CD4+ T cells to <200/mm^3 (Fig. 21-3, Table 21-3). These patients may present with opportunistic infections including oral candidiasis and *Pneumocystis carinii* pneumonia (PCP) and often progress rapidly. Many patients seek medical attention, and this acute retroviral syndrome is often missed or dismissed as an acute viral syndrome of unknown etiology. Since there is increasing evidence that treating HIV during acute infection may provide significant immunologic benefits, clinicians should measure plasma HIV RNA in patients who present with a flulike illness and have risk factors for exposure to HIV. Positive HIV serology (enzyme-linked immunosorbent assay [ELISA] and Western blot) will first appear 1 to 3 months later, and viral load will decline to a viral "set point" that remains essentially static until later stages of the disease. After rebounding from the transient drop seen in acute infection, CD4+ T cells will decline an average of 50 to 80 cells/mm^3 a year.

Surveillance data from the CDC of more than 16,000 diagnosed cases of AIDS in women (1981 through 1990

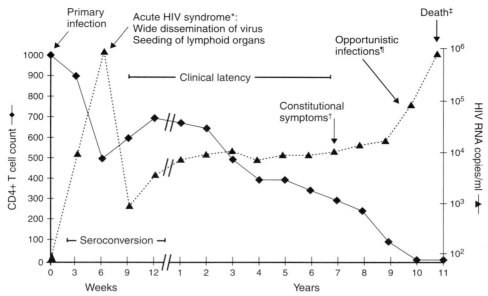

*Acute HIV: self-limited viral illness with fever, adenopathy, splenomegaly, rash, leukopenia; may
   see aseptic meningitis.
†Constitutional symptoms: thrush, hairy leukoplakia, ITP, bacterial infections, vaginal candidiasis,
   cervical cancer, recurrent HSV.
¶Opportunistic infections: PCP, *Candida* esophagitis, *Mycobacterium avium* complex, wasting
   syndrome, recurrent pneumonia.
‡Death usually 8-12 months after AIDS-defining diagnosis.

FIG. 21-3   Natural history of HIV infection. (Modified from Fauci AS: *Ann Intern Med* 1996.) *AIDS-defining diagnoses
from *MMWR,* March 1999.

Table 21-3
Acute Retroviral Syndrome

Symptom	Percentage
Fever	96
Lymphadenopathy	74
Pharyngitis	70
Rash (erythematous/maculopapular; on face and trunk)	70
Myalgias/arthralgias	54
Diarrhea	32
Headache	32
Nausea/vomiting	27
Hepatosplenomegaly	14
Weight loss	13
Thrush	12
Neurologic symptoms	12

Modified from Rodriguez, W: *IDSE,* 3:12, 2000.

BOX 21-2

**Opportunistic Infections in Women and Men: CDC AIDS
Surveillance Data: 1992-1997 (10,353 Cases; 1542 Women)**

Five Most Common Infections in Women with AIDS
Pneumocystis carinii pneumonia
Esophageal candidiasis
Mycobacterium avium complex
Wasting syndrome
Recurrent pneumonia

From *MMWR* 48:14, 1999.

reveal a different spectrum of opportunistic infections commonly seen in women with AIDS. The five most common are listed in Box 21-2.

For the clinician caring for women at all stages of HIV infection, it is important to recognize that many gynecologic conditions are not only more common in women with HIV but also may take a more aggressive course and require more intensive intervention (Box 21-3).

Cervical dysplasia, recurrent vaginosis caused by *Candidia albicans,* and sexually transmitted diseases (STDs) (including herpes) that are unusually severe, recurrent, or resistant to treatment are all associated with the early stage of HIV infection (CD4+ T cell count as high as $500/mm^3$).

Clinical studies have demonstrated up to fourfold increases in cervical neoplastic disease in HIV-infected women compared with noninfected control subjects. Thus in 1993 the CDC designated invasive cervical cancer, but not carcinoma in situ, as a diagnostic criteria for AIDS in HIV-infected women (Box 21-4).

The definitions are important for reporting statistics and for classification. Once classified as having AIDS, the patient may be eligible for disability compensation. HIV appears to accelerate the pathogenesis of cervical neoplasia at the molecular level, although clinical evidence of disease progression is limited. The disease is more often multifocal

---

BOX 21-3

Common Gynecologic Problems in HIV-Infected Women

Candidal vaginitis
Genital herpes
Human papillomavirus disease
    Condyloma acuminatum
    Cervical dysplasia
    Cervical carcinoma
Syphilis
Pelvic inflammatory disease
Primary HIV ulcers
Chancroid
Menstrual irregularities
Amenorrhea
Dysmenorrhea

BOX 21-4

AIDS-Defining Gynecologic Diagnoses

Invasive cervical cancer
Severe ulcerative genital lesions from herpes simplex virus

BOX 21-5

When to Refer for HIV Counseling and Testing

Persistent/recurrent/severe vaginal candidiasis
Recurrent/severe genital herpes simplex infection
Genital ulcer disease (syphilis, chancroid)
Recalcitrant or multisite condyloma acuminatum
Abnormal Pap smear result (moderate to severe cervical dysplasia, carcinoma in situ, or squamous cell carcinoma)
Persistent/recurrent pelvic inflammatory disease
Pregnancy

---

and more likely to involve the vagina and vulva, with more rapid progression and higher rates of recurrence after treatment. Vaginal candidiasis is a frequent disorder in women and is especially prevalent in HIV-infected women. Women with HIV and vaginal candidal infection have been found to have higher CD4+ T cell counts than those with esophageal candidal infection (means: 504 versus 30/mm^3). New and unexpected or more frequent or refractory candidal infection in the absence of antibiotic treatment, as well as other STDs and abnormal Pap smear results, should prompt physicians of these affected women to recommend HIV testing.

Severe ulcerative genital lesions secondary to herpes simplex virus (HSV) infection was the AIDS-defining illness in 18% of women followed in a prospective study who developed AIDS (Box 21-5).

Genital HSV infections are prevalent in the general population and may be particularly refractory to treatment in HIV-infected women and men. Idiopathic genital ulcers are also a manifestation of HIV disease and can be confused with those caused by HSV. Current studies are assessing the prevalence of idiopathic genital ulcer disease in HIV-infected women and the effect of thalidomide on these lesions. Menstrual irregularities are frequently reported by HIV-infected women. Although a recent WIHS survey found that menstrual irregularities were equally common in HIV-infected women and at-risk HIV-negative women, women with CD4+ T cell counts below 50/mm^3 were more likely to report amenorrhea than uninfected women or HIV-infected women with higher cell counts. In addition, megestrol, which is often prescribed for HIV-associated wasting, can cause irregular vaginal bleeding. Pelvic inflammatory disease (PID) is also more common and more severe in HIV-infected women and may

become chronic as a function of an immunocompromised state.

Diffuse lymphadenopathy is often present during moderate stages of immunosuppression (CD4+ T cell count of 300/mm^3). The enlarged glands are nontender, persist for a minimum of 3 months, and are characterized by the presence of two or more extrainguinal sites of involvement. Other diseases that occur during the middle stage of HIV infection include extrapulmonary *Mycobacterium tuberculosis* infections, recurrent herpes zoster, persistent mucocutaneous herpes simplex infections and recurrent bacteremias by *Streptococcus pneumoniae* and *Salmonella* sp. The oral manifestations of HIV infection—candidiasis and hairy leukoplakia—make their first appearance at this time. These manifestations of HIV disease are similar in women and men.

Many conditions associated with progression to AIDS occur in different frequencies in women and men. HIV-infected men are eight times more likely than HIV-infected women to develop Kaposi's sarcoma (KS). The etiologic agent of KS, human herpes virus 8 (HHV-8) has been detected in the peripheral blood of patients with KS, and its presence in KS-negative, HIV-positive persons is predictive of subsequent development of the disease. Seropositivity for HHV-8 is associated with high-risk sexual activity. Thus, when KS does occur in women, it is associated with having multiple or bisexual male partners. As described previously, women who are immunosuppressed also have an increased risk of developing cervical intraepithelial neoplasia (CIN) and possibly invasive squamous cell carcinoma of the lower anogenital tract. CIN and isolation of the likely etiologic agent, human papillomavirus, have been shown to be associated with CD4+ T cells <200/mm^3.

PCP is the dominant infection in men with AIDS, whereas women appear more likely to develop bacterial pneumonias caused by *S. pneumoniae* or *Haemophilus influenzae*. In some studies, women have had higher rates of esophageal candidiasis and herpes simplex infections than men. Other opportunistic infections occurring in the late stage of HIV infection in women or men include cerebral toxoplasmosis and cryptococcal meningitis. Disseminated cytomegalovirus infection and *Mycobacterium avium* complex infection occur at the most terminal stage, when the CD4+ T cell count falls below 50/mm^3. No significant differences between the sexes exist in the clinical presentations of any of these opportunistic infections or, on the basis of present data, in the response to therapy for these conditions.

APPROACH TO THE WOMAN WITH ASYMPTOMATIC HIV

Although self-reported barriers to obtaining HIV care have decreased significantly over time, HIV-infected women utilize HIV-related services less often than men, receiving medical care later in the course of their illness. As antiretroviral treatment has been shown to slow the course of HIV disease when begun early, it is important to diagnose and treat all HIV-infected patients during the first stage of the disease. Inasmuch as women frequently use emergency rooms, family planning clinics, sexually transmitted disease clinics, youth guidance centers, jail clinic facilities, and drug treatment units, these are the sites at which to target efforts at early diagnosis and use of early intervention. Most important, the treatment of HIV infection in pregnant women should not differ from that for nonpregnant women (see later discussion).

History and Physical Examination

A thorough history and physical examination are important for all women whose test results are positive for HIV, not only to identify the stage of the disease but to aid prognosis. The history should focus on HIV exposure, signs, and symptoms of systemic disease and gynecologic complaints. Since greater than 90% of HIV-infected women report histories of sexual and physical abuse, documentation of ongoing domestic violence should be included in the history; disclosure of HIV status is also associated with worsening of violent relationships (see Chapter 87). The initial physical examination should include a vaginal examination and Pap smear, as well as a complete physical.

Diagnostic Tests

Initial testing helps in staging of the disease because the risk of developing opportunistic infections is closely associated with the fall in CD4+ T cell counts. Plasma HIV RNA levels indicate the magnitude of HIV replication, whereas CD4+ T cell counts indicate the extent of HIV-induced damage to the immune system. The plasma HIV RNA level and CD4+ T cell count should be measured every 3 to 4 months, depending on the response to antiretroviral therapy, to determine the risk for disease progression, the need for prophylactic medications, and to assess whether the antiretroviral regimen needs modification. A Pap smear is repeated every 6 to 12 months because HIV infection has been shown to accelerate the progression of cervical neoplastic disease. In addition, initial testing should identify infections previously acquired by the patient that may be reactivated as a result of loss of immune function. Tests such as serologic reactions to *Toxoplasma gondii* and cytomegalovirus (CMV), treponemal serologies for syphilis (VDRL), and a purified protein derivative (PPD) skin test may reveal a latent infection that could progress. Hepatitis B (HBV) serologic testing for surface or core antibodies (anti-HBs or anti-HBc) hepatitis C serologic testing and baseline liver enzyme analyses should be performed. Finally, a baseline fasting lipid profile and glucose level should be obtained for all candidates for highly active antiretroviral therapy (HAART), which has been associated with an increase in lipid abnormalities and insulin resistance (Box 21-6).

BOX 21-6
Initial Evaluation of Women with Positive HIV Serology

Complete physical examination and Pap smear
Baseline CBS and LFTs
CD4+ T cell count
Serology for *Toxoplasma gondii, syphilis,* cytomegalovirus
PPD
Hepatitis B (anti-HBs and anti-HBc) and C serologies
Baseline fasting lipid profile (cholesterol, LDL, HDL)
Glucose level

CBS, Conjugated bile salts; *LFT,* liver function test; *PPD,* purified protein derivative; *LDL,* low-density lipoprotein; *HDL,* high-density lipoprotein.

MANAGEMENT

Gynecologic Complications

Vaginal Candidiasis

Intravaginal miconazole or clotrimazole are sometimes effective in the treatment of vaginal infections caused by *Candida* spp. Some antifungal preparations with a broader spectrum of activity against yeast species (*C. glabrata,* as well as *C. albicans*), such as butoconazole (Femstat) or terconazole (Terazol), may be more effective (see Table 21-3). Cases refractory to topical treatment occur with a greater frequency than in HIV-negative women, and oral fluconazole or ketoconazole have been shown to be effective in these patients. Some patients may require continuous treatment with oral antifungal medications to prevent relapse. Weekly fluconazole (200 mg) appears to be effective without risk of azole resistance in women with CD4+ T cell count > 300/cu mm (Table 21-4).

Candida prophylaxis is not recommended even in patients with CD4+ T cell counts < 100/mm^3 because studies showed no survival benefit and there is concern for azole-resistant *Candida* infections.

Genital Herpes

Infection with herpes simplex is extremely common in the general population. Suspected infections should be confirmed with viral culture or antibody staining of tissue specimens. For severe (urinary retention, fever, or signs of encephalitis) or refractory cases, the clinician should administer acyclovir intravenously (15 mg/kg/day) for at least 7 days. Otherwise, for acute infection, oral famciclovir (500 mg twice a day) or valacyclovir (1000 mg twice a day) for 7 to 10 days is recommended. For recurrent herpes simplex infections, oral famciclovir or valacyclovir can be administered for 5 days. The efficacy of acyclovir ointment (5% ointment applied topically every 8 hours) is dubious; however, patients with recognizable prodrome symptoms (burning, tingling before the onset of lesion formation) may obtain some benefit. Depending on the frequency of recurrences, the clinician may opt to treat each episode or use famciclovir or valacyclovir prophylactically. It is important to monitor renal function while the patient is on therapy. Refractory cases should be tested for acyclovir sensitivity, since resistant

Table 21-4
Treatment for Common HIV-Related Gynecologic Condition: HSV Infection

		Dose	Comments
Acute (mild)	Acyclovir	400 mg tid × 7-10d	Side effects: leukopenia
	Famciclovir	250 mg tid × 7-10d	Anemia, renal dysfunction
	Valacyclovir	1 gm bid × 7-10d	
Recurrent	Acyclovir	400 mg bid-tid 800 mg bid	
	Famciclovir	125 mg bid	
	Valacyclovir	500 mg bid	
Resistant	Acycolovir	15 mg/kg iv qd × 7d	Side effects: hypocalcemia renal failure, leukopenia
	Foscarnet	40 mg/kg iv q8h or 60 mg/kg q12h × 3wk	
Prevention	Acyclovir	400 mg bid	

Table 21-5
Treatment of Human Papillomavirus-Related Conditions

Condition	Therapy
Condyloma acuminatum Vaginal flat condyloma	Topical 5-fluorouracil cream once a week for 10 wk or qd for 5d
Vulvar/perianal lesions < 2 cm	Trichloroacetic acid (95%) topically
Cervical lesions	Topical 5-fluorouracil, then if not effective
	Consider cryosurgery or laser treatment
Abnormal Pap smear Atypia, koilocytosis, inflammation or dysplasia, cervica intraepithelial neoplasia	Refer for colposcopy; after treatment, repeat Pap smear q3 mo

strains can emerge in immunocompromised patients on chronic suppressive therapy. For resistant recurrent herpes simplex infections, intravenous foscarnet (40 mg/kg every 8 hours) can be used for 3 weeks. Foscarnet is extremely nephrotoxic and the patient should be monitored carefully during treatment. Relapses after treatment of acyclovir-resistant herpes simplex infections often involve acyclovir-sensitive strains (Table 21-4).

Menstrual Irregularities
Intervention for menstrual irregularities is covered in Chapter 52.

Human Papillomavirus (HPV)
ABNORMAL PAP SMEAR FINDINGS. The current recommendations for Pap smear screening in the woman with HIV infection is a baseline test, at 6 months, and then annually if negative. Any evidence of abnormal results on a Pap smear, including atypia, koilocytosis, or inflammation, should be referred to a gynecologist for further evaluation and consideration of colposcopy. After colposcopic examination, careful screening with Pap smears should be performed every 3 months (see Chapter 97 for more details on management of abnormal Pap smear results).

CONDYLOMA. Cervical and vaginal warts (or condyloma) are very common in HIV-infected patients, and various treatment options are available for these epithelial manifestations of HPV infection. These are summarized in Table 21-5. (Chapter 22 covers the management of sexually transmitted diseases.)

Pelvic Inflammatory Disease
PID is highly associated with HIV infection; therefore women presenting with PID should be offered HIV testing. The course of the disease varies, depending on the degree of immunocompetence reflected by the CD4+ T cell count. Women with lower CD4+ T cell counts (<200/mm^3) have a more aggressive course than those with lesser degrees of immunosuppression. Among women with HIV infection who have PID, there is a higher incidence of abscess formation and surgical intervention (see Chapter 23).

Prophylaxis for Latent Opportunistic Infections
Prevention of reactivation of a latent infection may be possible with the use of specific agents (Table 21-6). Guidelines established for prophylaxis against PCP and other opportunistic infections are derived from large national studies conducted on women and men. Although men predominate in these studies, the results led to licensure of these agents and established recommendations for persons of both genders. More recent studies that suggest that there are gender differences in initiation of, compliance with, and medical response to antiretroviral therapies are discussed.

PCP Prophylaxis
Prophylaxis against PCP is indicated in HIV-infected patients with either a prior history of PCP, a CD4+ T cell count < 200/mm^3 or a history of oral candidiasis or fevers of unknown origin. Three prophylactic regimens have been shown to dramatically reduce the incidence of PCP in HIV-infected persons with CD4+ T cell counts < 200/mm^3. However, the most cost-effective regimen with the most reduced morbidity and mortality is TMP-SMX (1 double-strength tablet daily), which is recommended by the CDC as the first-line prophylaxis for PCP. As a single agent, TMP-SMX also provides protection against reactivation of latent *T. gondii* infections (see later discussion). On the basis of in vitro data, TMP-SMX may also provide protection against infections caused by *Nocardia* sp., *Salmonella* sp., *H. influenzae,* and *Listeria monocytogenes.* Unfortunately, the incidence of severe adverse reactions to TMP-SMX, including fever, rash, leukopenia, and gastrointestinal distress, is estimated to be as high as 40% to 60% and results in cessation of drug administration in half of those who experience an

Table 21-6
Prophylaxis Against Some Important Opportunistic Infections in Women

Infection	First Choice	Alternatives
Vulvovaginal candidiasis	Daily or weekly fluconazole	
Esophageal candidiasis	Fluconazole 100 mg qd or 200 mg 3 ×/wk	Ketoconazole 200 mg qd
		Itraconazole 200 mg qd
Herpes simplex	Acyclovir 400 mg bid	
PCP	CD4 < 200, thrush, or unexplained fevers > 2 wk	Dapsone 50 mg bid or 100 mg qd
		Dapsone + pyrimethamine
	TMP-SMX 1 DS qd or TMP-SMX 1 SS qd	Aerosolized pentamidine 300 mg q30d
		Atovaquone 1500 mg qd
	Consider d/c when pts on HAART have CD4 > 200 For 3-6 mos.	TMP-SMX 1 DS thrice weekly
mTB	TST rxn ≥ 5 mm or exposure to mTB INH 300 mg + pyridoxine 50 mg qd × 9 mo	Rifabutin 300 mg + PZA 20 mg/kg qd × 2 mo or RIF 600 mg qd × 4 mo
MAC	CD4 < 50	
	Azithromycin 1200 mg q7d	Rifabutin 300 mg qd
	Clarithromycin 500 mg bid	Azithromycin 1200 mg q7d + Rifabutin 300 mg qd

adverse reaction. One double-strength tablet taken three times a week may reduce the incidence of adverse reactions, although adherence may be more problematic. Alternative regimens include dapsone (100 mg/day), atovaquone (750 mg twice a day), or aerosolized pentamidine (300 mg/month). None of these regimens have been shown to be as effective as TMP-SMX in preventing PCP and pentamidine has been shown to increase the incidence of extrapulmonary *pneumocystis* and threatens the transmission of *M. tuberculosis* from patient to health care worker. The use of these agents is not contraindicated in pregnancy. In patients receiving HAART, the clinician may consider discontinuing primary prophylaxis against PCP when the CD4+ T cell count is > $200/mm^3$ for 3 to 6 months.

Toxoplasmosis

The indications for prophylaxis against *Toxoplasmosis* include a positive serum IgG to *T. gondii* and a CD4+ T cell count < $100/mm^3$. It has been estimated that one third of patients with reactive serology to *T. gondii* will experience a recrudescence of their chronic latent infection. The reactivation of toxoplasmosis may be prevented by trimethoprim-sulfamethoxazole (TMP-SMX) used as prophylaxis for PCP. Patients with intolerance to TMP-SMX may use an alternative regimen (dapsone, pyrimethamine, and leukovorin).

Syphilis

Patients co-infected with HIV and *Treponema pallidum* experience a more rapid progression to neurosyphilis than HIV-negative patients with syphilis. Thus HIV-positive patients with a positive blood VDRL should undergo lumbar puncture to rule-out central nervous system involvement. Benzathine penicillin should be administered only to those whose cerebrospinal fluid (CSF) is entirely normal. Treatment for neurosyphilis with intravenous penicillin G (18 to 24 μ/day) for 10 to 14 days is recommended for any CSF abnormalities in the context of an untreated positive blood VDRL.

Mycobacterium Tuberculosis

HIV-positive patients with PPD positivity (induration of 5 mm or greater) and no evidence of active mycobacterium tuberculosis (mTB) should receive isoniazid (INH) (300 mg/day) plus pyridoxine (50 mg biweekly) for 9 months. With INH resistance, INH intolerance or INH-induced hepatitis, oral rifampin (600 mg/day) plus pyrazinamide (20 mg/day) for 2 months is recommended.

Mycobacterium Avium *Complex*

Prophylaxis against complications of infection with *mycobacterium avium* complex (MAC) is recommended in HIV-infected patients with CD4+ T cell counts < $50/mm^3$ and consists of azithromycin (1200 mg) every 7 days. In patients receiving HAART, the clinician may consider discontinuing primary prophylaxis against MAC when CD4+ T cell counts remain > $100/mm^3$ for more than 6 months.

Highly Active Antiretroviral Therapy (HAART)

HIV replication leads to immune system damage and progression to AIDS. Thus suppression of replication and consequent decrease in HIV virions is the goal of antiretroviral therapy. Three classes of potent antiretroviral drugs have been developed, aimed at inhibiting two enzymes essential for HIV replication and virion formation: reverse transcriptase and viral protease. When used in combination, nucleoside and nonnucleoside reverse transcriptase (NRTIs and NNRTIs), and protease inhibitors (PIs) have been definitively shown to delay the onset of opportunistic infections in persons with CD4+ T cell counts less than $500/mm_3$ and to prolong survival in patients with AIDS.

Because the rapid rate of HIV replication leads to a high incidence of mutations, drug-resistant variants rapidly emerge in patients on antiretroviral monotherapy. Multiple studies have examined various combinations of antiretroviral medications for their efficacy in viral suppression, improvement in CD4+ T cell numbers, and prolonged survival of patients with HIV infection and/or AIDS. The overall conclusion is that several different combinations of antiretroviral drugs have been proven effective in suppressing viral replication long term, preventing loss of CD4+ T cells and immune function. Current guidelines emphasize the importance of using combination therapy to treat all patients who show signs of progressive or symptomatic disease. Antiretroviral regimens are complicated, pose difficulties with compliance, have major side effects, and carry potential consequences in terms of viral resistance when not implemented or adhered to properly. For these reasons, the panel on clinical Practices for the Treatment of HIV Infection convened by the Department of Health and Human Services recommends that care of HIV-infected persons be supervised by an expert, particularly when monitoring the effects of antiretroviral agents.

Initiation of HAART

HAART should be offered to all patients with the acute HIV syndrome, those within 6 months of HIV seroconversion and to all patients with symptoms ascribed to HIV infection. Women should receive optimal antiretroviral therapy regardless of pregnancy status (see later discussion).

Initiation of therapy for asymptomatic HIV-infected patients is based on measures of plasma HIV RNA and CD4+ T cell counts and differs for women versus men (see later discussion and Table 21-7).

Initiation of therapy with combinations of antiretrovirals that have not been used previously to treat HIV in the patient and do not demonstrate cross-resistance patterns with antiretrovirals already used in the patient is the most effective way to suppress viral replication. In general, the recommendation to initiate therapy in the asymptomatic patient depends critically on the commitment of the patient to adhere to a prescribed regimen. It is crucial that patients understand the relationship between noncompliance with drug regimens and viral resistance so that they can participate in the design of their regimen. HIV therapy needs to be individualized since rates of disease progression differ among HIV-infected persons, and the ability to adhere to prescribed regimens differs among patients. Therapeutic decision making regarding antiretroviral therapy requires mutual understanding and frank discussions between the patient and health care provider regarding risks and benefits of treatment. Recommended antiretroviral agents for the initial treatment of HIV infection are presented in Table 21-8.

Response to Treatment of HIV Infection

The goal of antiretroviral therapy is maximal and durable suppression of viral replication with restoration and/or preservation of immune function resulting in improved quality of life and reduced HIV-related morbidity and mortality. Patients for whom treatment is considered appropriate should be started on combination antiretroviral medications that suppress viral replication to below the limit of detection of sensitive HIV RNA assays. This level of suppression limits the emergence of antiretroviral-resistant HIV variants. Although several combinations can be effective, combina-

---

Table 21-7
Ranges of CD4+ T Cell Count and Viral Load Levels for Initiation of Therapy in Women

Plasma HIV RNA Level, Copies/ml	CD4 + T Cell Count <5000 5000 to 15,000 >15,000
<350	Recommend therapy Recommend therapy Recommend therapy
350-500	Consider therapy Recommend therapy Recommend therapy
>500	Defer therapy Consider therapy Recommend therapy

Table 21-8
Recommended Antiretroviral Agents for Initial Treatment of Established HIV Infection: Choose One Choice Each from Columns A and B

	Column A	Column B
Strongly recommended	Efavirenz Indinavir Nelfinavir Ritonavir + saquinovir	Stavudine + lamivudine Stavudine + didanosine Zidovudine + lamivudine Zidovudine + didanosine
Recommended as alternative	Abacavir Amprenovir Delavirdine Nelfinavir + saquinovir Ritonavir Saquinavir-SGC*	Didanosine + lamivudine Zidovudine + zalcitabine
No recommendation	Hydroxyurea in combination with other antiretrovirals	
Insufficient data	Ritonavir + indinavir Ritonavir + nelfinavir	
Not recommended; Should not be offered	Saquinavir-HGC†	Stavudine + zidovudine Zalcitabine + lamivudine Zalcitabine + stavudine Zalcitabine + didanosine

*SGC, Soft gel capsule.
†HGC, Hard gel capsule.

tion therapy should optimally include 2 NRTIs plus either a PI or the NNRTI efavirenz. Features of the 15 antiretroviral medications now available are presented in Table 21-9.

Treatment decisions should be based on the level of plasma HIV RNA and CD4+ T cell counts, which both influence the risk of progression to AIDS-defining illnesses. After initiation of therapy, HIV RNA levels should fall by one-$\log_{10}$ by 2 to 8 weeks and no virus should be detectable (<50 copies/ml) by 4 to 6 months.

Patients with undetectable plasma levels of HIV RNA remain potentially infectious and should be counseled to avoid sexual and drug-use behaviors that foster transmission of HIV. Failure to reach undetectable levels of virus may be as a result of a variety of variables including nonadherence, inadequate potency or suboptimal levels of drugs, and/or viral resistance. Various studies in treatment experienced patients have demonstrated a strong association between viral resistance and failure to suppress HIV replication. Thus failure of therapy despite adherence should prompt changes in the antiretroviral regimen based on drug resistance testing (genotyping and phenotyping resistance assays) and the prior history of antiretroviral usage. It is recommended that interpretation of genotypic test results be facilitated by consultation with an expert in HIV drug resistance. Changes in therapy for a failing regimen can be difficult owing to limitations in alternative medications, problems with adherence, toxicity, and viral resistance. In some cases, patients may benefit from participation in a clinical trial with or without access to new drugs or the clinician may opt to use a regimen that does not achieve complete suppression of viral replication but instead ensures a low steady state level.

Considerations for HAART in Women

Multiple studies have examined differences in viral load and CD4+ T cell counts in women compared with men at various stages of HIV disease. In general, HIV RNA levels are 32% to 50% lower in women then in men at CD4+ T cell counts > 200/mm^3 but not at CD4+ T cell counts < 200/mm^3. Thus, when CD4+ T cells are still in the normal range, plasma HIV RNA levels in women correlate with similar numbers of CD4+ T cells found in men at higher levels of viral RNA. Based on clinical guidelines for the initiation of HAART therapy derived from studies of T cell counts and viral load in men, women have experienced a delay in initiation of therapy because of their lower viral loads. In some studies, this delay has been shown to unfavorably influence disease progression with women progressing to AIDS at lower HIV RNA levels than men do. Thus newer guidelines suggest that clinicians may wish to consider lower plasma HIV RNA thresholds when determining whether to initiate therapy in women with CD4+ T cell counts > 350/mm^3 (Table 21-7). In patients with CD4+ T cell counts < 350/mm^3, very small gender-based differences in viral load have been detected;

Table 21-9
Summary of Antiretroviral Therapy

Drug (abbrev.)	Dose	Food Effect	Major Side Effects
Nucleoside Reverse Transcriptase Inhibitors (NRTIs)			
Zidovudine (ZDV or AZT)	200 mg tid or 300 mg bid	No regard	Leukopenia, anemia, headache, N/V, elev. LFTs, LA/HS
Stavudine (d4T)	30-40 mg bid	No regard	Peripheral neuropathy, N/V, elev. LFTs, LA/HS
Didanosine (ddI)	250-400 mg qd	Take 30-60 min before meal	Peripheral neuropathy, pancreatitis, N/D, rash, fever, LA/HS
Zalcitabine (ddC)	0.75 mg tid	No regard	Anemia, thrombocytopenia, peripheral neuropathy, pancreatitis, elev. LFTs, apthous ulcers, LA/HS
Lamivudine (3TC)	150 mg bid	No regard	Headache, rash, LA/HS
Abacavir (ABC)	300 mg bid	No regard	hypersensitivity rxn, LA/HS
Non-Nucleoside Reverse Transcriptase Inhibitors (NNRTIs)			
Efavirenz (EFV)	600 mg qhs	No regard	Rash, Stevens-Johnson, insomnia, nightmares, mood disturbance, hallucinations, elev. LFTs
Nevarapine (NVP)	200 mg qd × 2w Then 200 mg bid		Rash, Stevens-Johnson, elev. LFTs
Delavirdine (DLV)	400 mg tid	Separate from ddI by 1h	Same
Protease Inhibitors (PIs)			
Indinavir (IDV)	800 mg q8h	Take 1h before meals	Nephrolithiasis, elev. indirect bili., hyperglycemia, fat redistribution, abnormal lipids
Ritonavir (RTV)	600 mg q12h	Take with food	GI intolerance, perioral paresthesias, hepatitis, hyperglycemia, fat redistribution, abnormal lipids
Saquinovir (SQV)	1200 mg tid 400 mg with RTV	Take with food	Same
Nelfinavir (NFV)	750 mg tid or 1250 mg bid	Take with food	Diarrhea, hyperglycemia, fat redistribution, abnormal lipids
Amprenavir (APV)	1200 mg bid 1400 mg bid	Avoid after high fat meal	GI intolerance, rash, paresthesias, hyperglycemia, fat redistribution and abnormal lipids

N/V, Nausea and vomiting; *LFTs,* liver function tests; *LA/HS,* lactic acidosis/hepatic steatosis; *N/D,* nausea and diarrhea; *GI,* gastrointestinal.

therefore no changes in guidelines for initiating therapy in women are recommended for this group.

Toxicity Issues of HAART

Various HAART-associated adverse clinical events have been reported. Severe lactic acidosis and hepatomegaly with steatosis is a rare side effect associated with the use of NRTIs that has a high fatality rate. Women appear to be at higher risk for development of this toxicity for unknown reasons. Additional risk factors include obesity and prolonged usage of NRTIs. Patients may present initially with nonspecific gastrointestinal symptoms before the onset of abdominal distention, nausea, vomiting, diarrhea, abdominal pain, anorexia weight loss, and hepatomegaly. Laboratory evaluation may reveal hyperlactatemia, increased anion gap, elevated aminotransferases, creatine phosphokinase, lactate dehydrogenase, lipase and amylase. CT scan may demonstrate an enlarged fatty liver, whereas biopsy of the liver reveals microvesicular steatosis. Mitochondrial injury is one proposed mechanism of toxicity and may be responsible for other adverse events associated with NRTI usage including myopathy, cardiomyopathy, pancreatitis, and peripheral neuropathy. Antiretroviral treatment should be suspended if clinical and laboratory evidence of lactic acidosis occurs. Resumption of HAART should include only NRTI-sparing regimens.

Hyperglycemia, diabetes mellitus, diabetic ketoacidosis, and exacerbation of preexisting diabetes mellitus have all been reported in patients receiving HAART, especially those on regimens that include PIs. The pathogenesis of these abnormalities is unknown; however, they appear to be reversible on discontinuation of PI therapy. Changes in fat distribution ("lipodystrophy") have been observed in 6% to 80% of patients receiving HAART (the wide range of estimates reflects the lack of a uniform case definition), especially those using PIs or NRTIs. Clinical findings include central obesity, peripheral fat wasting, and lipomas. Hyperlipidemia and insulin resistance can be associated with lipodystrophy. NRTI-associated syndromes are more likely to be associated with fatigue and nausea, weight loss, higher levels of lactate and alanine aminotransferase, and lower levels of albumin, cholesterol, triglycerides, glucose, and insulin. Use of PIs has also been implicated in dysregulation of lipid metabolism with subsequent elevations in triglycerides and/or cholesterol, raising concern because of the association of these lipids with cardiovascular events and pancreatitis. Some experts recommend monitoring of serum cholesterol and triglycerides at 3- to 4-month intervals during PI therapy and use of lipid-lowering agents in patients with significant alterations in lipid profile. Important major side effects associated with antiretroviral usage are summarized in Table 21-9.

Psychosocial Issues

The success of prophylactic medications and HAART in maintaining prolonged inhibition of opportunistic infections and viral replication, respectively, depends on strict adherence to medication regimens essentially for the remainder of the HIV-infected patient's life. Multiple studies have shown that nonadherence to HAART is the strongest prediction of failure to achieve virologic suppression and is associated with the development of drug resistance. For most patients, imperfect adherence is common; and many predictors of poor adherence have been identified including poor clinician-patient relationship, active drug and alcohol use, depression, lack of patient education, and lack of access to primary medical care or medication. These predictors are similar to risk factors associated with HIV infection in women. Clinicians caring for HIV-infected women are encouraged to address these various psychosocial issues to increase compliance with medication regimens. Clinicians should consider psychiatric referral in patients with serious signs of substance abuse and depression. Some of the predictors of good adherence to HIV medications include strong support systems, compatible daily routines, understanding the relationship between poor adherence and viral resistance, and keeping clinic appointments. A variety of HIV/AIDS support groups provide information and support networks for women. Patients should be encouraged to make contact with such groups and individuals.

Considerations for Discontinuing Therapy

Patients begun on HAART with CD4+ T cell counts > $350/mm^3$ may wish to discontinue treatment because of toxicity issues. There are no data addressing whether this is advisable or safe. However, potential benefits include a reduction in toxicities, drug interactions, viral drug resistance, and a general improvement in quality of life. Clinicians should be advised that poor adherence with subsequent viral resistance in asymptomatic HIV-infected patients reduces medication options for later and should be avoided. Adverse responses to loss of control of viral replication include high viremia, further destruction of CD4+ T cells, and progression of HIV-induced immunosuppression. Close monitoring of patients who discontinue HAART is recommended.

Preventive Interventions

The primary care of women with HIV infection is important. Box 21-5 summarizes the basic primary care management for these patients.

Immunizations

HIV-infected persons should receive annual influenza vaccine in November. Because the frequency of *S. pneumoniae* and *H. influenzae* infections are increased in HIV-infected persons, Pneumovax and recombinant *H. influenzae* type B (HIB) vaccine are recommended by the Advisory Committee on Immunization Practices (ACIP) and the CDC for all persons with HIV infection. Revaccination should be administered every 3 years. Hepatitis B vaccine is recommended for persons who lack evidence of HBV markers and have any of the following risk factors: active intravenous drug use, sexually active women, and household or sexual contacts of HBV surface antigen carriers. Tetanus-diphtheria vaccine boosters should be given every 10 years. Mumps, rubella, and varicella zoster virus vaccines are recommended for susceptible HIV-positive adults. Vaccine to hepatitis A virus is recommended for HIV-infected patients who are coinfected with hepatitis C.

Other Strategies

All sexually active people are potentially at risk for contracting HIV. Some people, however, are at higher risk than others. Although it is important to discuss safe sex practices with all patients, particular patients should be offered HIV testing as well. Box 21-5 summarizes current recommendations concerning when to refer women for HIV testing. It is important to counsel the patient so as to ensure confidentiality in testing.

Surveys of low-income women have identified AIDS as their most serious health, social, or relationship concern. Half of those surveyed stated they would attend risk reduction programs to learn how to avoid infection with HIV. Clinicians may wish to refer interested patients to the CDC National AIDS Hotline (1-800-342-AIDS) for more information about HIV prevention.

A vaginal sheath, or female condom, has been licensed for use as a contraceptive device that a woman controls. It has been shown to provide contraceptive efficacy in the same range as other barrier methods and has the added benefit of protecting against STDs including HIV. Usage of the detergent-type spermicide, nonoxynol-9, which is the only microbicide known to protect against sexual transmission of HIV, has been shown to cause lesions in vaginal and cervical epithelia, which may leave women more vulnerable to HIV infection and is no longer recommended.

■ PREGNANCY AND HIV DISEASE

One study of HIV-infected women who became pregnant after diagnosis suggested that CD4+ T cell counts fall more during pregnancy than in the nonpregnant state. A study on HIV-infected women in India concluded that pregnancy increased maternal mortality owing to opportunistic illnesses. However, evidence from two large Swiss cohort studies indicates that acceleration of disease progression is inconsistent among HIV-infected women who become pregnant during follow-up monitoring. Although it is unclear how pregnancy affects the progression of HIV disease, it is clear that all women should receive optimal antiretroviral therapy regardless of their pregnancy status. Recent studies also indicate that the risk of maternal-fetal transmission is directly correlated to the level of maternal viremia. Thus control of HIV replication is in the best interest of both mother and infant.

Guidelines for optimal antiretroviral therapy and initiation of therapy in HIV-infected pregnant women are the same as those for nonpregnant adults with one caveat: The impact of antiretroviral therapy during pregnancy on the fetus and infant is unknown. Thus the decision to treat HIV during pregnancy should be made by the woman after a full discussion of potential risks. Women in their first trimester of pregnancy who are not currently receiving antiretroviral medications may consider postponing initiation of treatment until the second trimester, after organogenesis, since the teratogenic effects of antiretroviral medications are not completely known except for efavirenz, which is a known teratogen in primates. Along the same lines, women already receiving antiretroviral therapy, when they learn of their pregnancy, may consider temporarily stopping their medications until after the first trimester. However, most experts recommend continuation or initiation of maximally suppressive therapy even during the first trimester because uncontrolled viremia increases the risk of both progression of HIV disease in the mother and transmission of HIV to the fetus.

There is limited data on the pharmacokinetics and safety of antiretroviral medications during pregnancy for drugs other than zidovudine (AZT). The FDA pregnancy classification for all currently approved antiretroviral medications and additional information regarding the use of these drugs during pregnancy is shown in Table 21-10.

AZT has been demonstrated to reduce the risk of perinatal HIV transmission by 66% when oral administration (200 mg three times a day or 300 mg twice a day), begun after 14 weeks gestation, is accompanied by intravenous administration during the intrapartum period and to the newborn for the first 6 weeks of life. Comparisons of children born to HIV-infected mothers from 1985 to 1990 to those born between 1990 and 1997 demonstrates a decline in risk of vertical transmission from 20.7% to 6.5% owing to the actions of intrapartum and neonatal treatment AZT. There are no data to support the substitution of any other antiretroviral medication for the purpose of reducing perinatal HIV transmission. Thus AZT should be included as a component of the prenatal HAART regimen for the treatment of HIV infection. If AZT is not included in the regimen of the pregnant patient or during the intrapartum period for reasons of toxicity or drug interactions (i.e., D4T is a preferred nucleoside for treatment of the pregnant patient), it should still be administered to the newborn as recommended.

Several studies in Africa have shown that intrapartum/ postpartum administration of AZT plus 3TC or nevirapine alone combined with similar antiretroviral treatment of the newborn reduced neonatal HIV transmission by 38% and 50%, respectively. Thus, if HIV infection is not diagnosed

Table 21-10
FDA Pregnancy Categories for Antiretrovirals

Drug	FDA Category*	Placental Passage
Zidovudine	C	Yes
Zalcitabine	C	Yes
Didanosine	B	Yes
Stavudine	C	Yes
Lamivudine	C	Yes
Abacavir	C	Yes
Saquinavir	B	Unknown
Indinavir	C	Yes
Ritonavir	B	Yes
Nelfinavir	B	Unknown
Amprenavir	C	Unknown
Nevirapine	C	Yes
Delavirdine	C	Yes
Efavirenz	C	Yes

*FDA Pregnancy Categories are:

A—Adequate and well-controlled studies of pregnant women fail to demonstrate a risk to the fetus during the first trimester of pregnancy and there is no evidence of risk during later trimesters.

B—Animal reproduction studies fail to demonstrate a risk to the fetus and adequate but well-controlled studies of pregnant women have not been conducted.

C—Safety in human pregnancy has not been determined, animal studies are with positive for fetal risk or have not been conducted, and the drug should not be used unless the potential benefit outweighs the potential risk to the fetus.

D—Positive evidence of human fetal risk based on adverse reaction data from investigational or marketing experiences, but the potential benefits from the use of the drug in pregnant women may be acceptable despite its potential risks.

until the onset of labor, it is still possible to reduce neonatal HIV transmission.

Although perinatal AZT therapy was implemented in 1994 and resulted in a dramatic decline in perinatal transmission of HIV, 300 perinatally infected infants are born annually in the United States. High maternal weight and conditions associated with fetal exposure to maternal blood or cervicovaginal secretions may diminish the efficacy of AZT chemoprophylaxis. To further reduce this number, the CDC recommends improving prenatal care, routine prenatal HIV testing, treatment for HIV infected pregnant women, and follow-up HIV care. Clinicians treating HIV-infected pregnant women are strongly encouraged to report cases of prenatal exposure to antiretroviral agents to the Antiretroviral Pregnancy Registry (1-800-258-4263). This registry collects observational, nonexperimental data regarding anteroviral exposure during pregnancy for the purpose of assessing teratogenicity. The registry allows patient anonymity and uses the information gathered to help clinicians develop guidelines for the treatment of individual pregnant patients with antiretroviral medications.

Although the agents used to treat opportunistic infections in pregnancy are potentially teratogenic, the benefits of treatment to the mother outweigh the potential risk to the fetus. At present, standard use of CD4+ T cell counts for initiation of prophylaxis against opportunistic infections is recommended, as many of these infections are life-threatening (e.g., *P. carinii, T. gondii,* and *Cryptococcus neoformans*). Others may result in significant morbidity to the mother and devastation to the fetus (e.g., cytomegalovirus and syphilis). TMP-SMX is safe and effective for both prophylaxis and therapy of PCP in pregnancy.

BIBLIOGRAPHY

Adachi A et al: Women with human immunodeficiency virus infection and abnormal Papanicolaou smears: a prospective study of colposcopy and clinical outcome, *Obstet Gyncol* 81:372, 1993.

Anastos K et al: Association of race and gender with HIV-1 RNA levels and immunologic progression, *J Acquir Immune Defic Syndr* 24:218, 2000.

Bartlett JG: *The Johns Hopkins Hospital guide to medical care of patients with HIV infection,* ed 4, Baltimore, 2000, Williams & Wilkins.

Bartlett JG: *1999-2000 recommendations for the medical care of persons with HIV infection,* Baltimore, 1992, Critical Care Co.

Biggar R et al: Immunosuppression in pregnant women infected with HIV, *Am J Obstet Gyncol* 161:1239, 1989.

Brettle RP, Leen CLS: The natural history of HIV and AIDS in women, *AIDS* 5:1283, 1991.

Carey MP et al: HIV and AIDS relative to other health, social, and relationship concerns among low-income urban women: a brief report, *J Women Health Gend Based Med* 8:657, 1999.

Carpenter CJ et al: Human immunodeficiency virus infection in North American women: experience with 200 cases and a review of the literature, *Medicine* 70:307, 1991.

Centers for Disease Control: 1993 revised classification system for HIV infection and expanded surveillance: case definition for AIDS among adolescents and adults, *MMWR* 41(PR-17), Dec 18, 1992.

Centers for Disease Control: *HIV/AIDS Surveillance Reports* 9:1, 1997, 12:1, 2000.

Centers for Disease Control: *MMWR* 44:81, 1995.

Centers for Disease Control and Prevention. Focus on women and HIV. *HIV/AIDS Prev* 1:2, 1997.

Cotton D: AIDS in women. In Broder S, Merrigan T, Bolognesi D, editors: *Textbook of AIDS medicine,* Baltimore, 1994, William & Wilkins.

Dattel BJ et al: AIDS (HIV) risk assessment in an inner city women's clinic, *J Reprod Med* 37:821, 1992.

Davidson AJ et al: Comparison of health status, socioeconomic characteristics, and knowledge and use of HIV-related resources between HIV-infected women and men, *Med Care* 36:1676, 1998.

Ellerbrock TV et al: Epidemiology of women with AIDS in the United States, 1981-1990: a comparison with heterosexual men with AIDS, *JAMA* 265:2971, 1991.

Farr G et al: Contraceptive efficacy and acceptability of the female condom, *Am J Public Health* 84:1960, 1994.

Friedland GH et al: Survival differences in patients with AIDS, *AIDS* 4:144, 1991.

Fiore JR et al: Biological correlates of HIV-1 heterosexual transmission, *AIDS* 11:1089, 1997.

Greenblatt RM et al: Lower genital tract infections among HIV-infected and high-risk uninfected women: findings of the Women's Interagency HIV Study (WIHS), *Sex Transm Dis* 26:143, 1999.

Hankins CA, Handley MA: HIV disease and AIDS in women: current knowledge and a research agenda, *J AIDS* 5:957, 1992.

Jewett JF et al: High risk of human papilloma virus infection and cervical squamous intraepithelial lesions among women with symptomatic human immunodeficiency virus infection, *Am J Obstetrics and Gynecology,* 165(2):392, 1991.

Jewett JF, Hecht FM: Preventive health care for adults with HIV infection, *JAMA* 269(9):1143, 1993.

Kaplan JE et al: Epidemiology of human immunodeficiency virus—associated opportunistic infections in the United States in the era of highly active antiretroviral therapy, *Clin Infect Dis* 30:S5, 2000.

Kaufman GR et al: Rapid restoration of CD4 T cell subsets in subjects receiving antiretroviral therapy during primary HIV-1 infection, *AIDS* 14:2643, 2000.

Kumar RM, Uduman SA, Khurrana AK: Impact of pregnancy on maternal AIDS, *J Reprod Med* 42:429, 1997.

Lazzarin A et al: Italian study group on HIV heterosexual transmission man-to-woman sexual transmission of the human immunodeficiency virus, *Arch Intern Med* 151:2411, 1991.

Masur H: Prevention and treatment of *Pneumocystis* pneumonia, *N Engl J Med* 327:1853, 1993.

McDonnell M, Kessenich CR: HIV/AIDS and women, *Lippincotts Prim Care Pract* 4:66, 2000.

Minkoff ML, DeHovir JA: Care of women infected with the human immunodeficiency virus, *JAMA* 266:2253.

Padian NS, Shiboski SC, Jewell NP: Female to male transmission of human immunodeficiency virus, *JAMA* 226:1664, 1991.

Prins M et al: Do gender differences in CD4 cell counts matter? *AIDS* 13:2361, 1999.

Quinn TC et al: Viral load and heterosexual transmission of human immunodeficiency virus type 1, *N Engl J Med* 342:921, 2000.

Robinson W: Invasive and preinvasive cervical neoplasia in human immunodeficieny virus-infected women, *Semin Oncol* 27:463, 2000.

Roddy RE et al: A controlled trial of nonoxynol 9 film to reduce male-to-female transmission of sexually transmitted diseases, *N Engl J Med* 339:504, 1998.

Rodriguez W, Sax PE: Treatment of HIV and opportunistic infections. *IDSE* 3:12, 2000.

Rogers MF, Stockton PL: Organizational approaches to the HIV/AIDS crisis, *Ann NY Acad Sci* 918:188, 2000.

Rompalo A, Anderson J, Quinn T: Reproductive tract infections and their management in women infected with the human immunodeficiency virus, *Infectious diseases in clinical practice,* p 277, 1992.

Rosenberg ES et al: Immune control of HIV-1 after early treatment of acute infection, *Nature* 407:523, 2000.

Sambamoorthi U et al: Antidepressant treatment and health services utilization among HIV-infected medicaid patients diagnosed with depression, *J Gen Intern Med* 15:311, 2000.

Safrin S et al: Seroprevalence and epidemiologic correlates of human immunodeficiency virus infection in women with acute pelvic inflammatory disease, *Obstet Gynecol* 75:666, 1990.

Shapiro DE et al: Risk factors for perinatal human immunodeficiency virus transmission in patients receiving zidovudine prophylaxis. Pediatric AIDS Clinical Trials Group protocol 076 Study Group, *Obstet Gynecol* 94:897, 1999.

Simpson BJ, Shapiro ED, Andiman WA: Prospective cohort study of children both to human immunodeficiency virus-infected mothers, 1985 through 1997: trends in the risk of vertical transmission, mortality and acquired immunodeficiency syndrome indicator diseases in the era before highly active antiretroviral therapy, *Pediatr Infect Dis J* 19:618, 2000.

Spence MR, Reboli AC: Human immunodeficiency virus infection in women, *Ann Intern Med* 115:827, 1991.

St Louis ME et al: Human immunodeficiency virus infection in disadvantaged adolescents: findings from the US Job Corps, *JAMA* 226:2387, 1991.

Uckun FM, D'Cruz OJ: Prophylactic contraceptives for HIV/AIDS, *Hum Reprod Update* 5:506, 1999.

Valleroy LA et al: HIV infection in disadvantaged out-of-school youth: prevalence for U.S. Job Corps entrants, 1990 through 1996, *J Acquir Immune Defic Syndr* 19:67, 1992.

Wachtel T et al: Quality of life in persons with human immunodeficiency virus infection: measurement by the medical outcomes study instrument, *Ann Intern Med* 116:129, 1992.

Weisser M et al: Does pregnancy influence the course of HIV infection? Evidence from two large Swiss cohort studies. *J Acquir Immune Defic Syndr Hum Retrovirol* 17:404, 1998.

Wofsy C: Therapeutic issues in women with HIV disease. In Sande MA, Volberding PA, editors: *The medical management of AIDS,* Philadelphia, 1992, Saunders. www.Hopkins-AIDS.edu

www.hivatis.org

CHAPTER 22

Sexually Transmitted Disease

Donna Felsenstein

Each day approximately 40,000 persons in the United States (15 million annually) contract one or more sexually transmitted infections. Of these infections 25% occur in adolescents, an age-group of persons who will be entering the reproductive years. Women are at greater disadvantage than men are; because the infections can be asymptomatic, most women who are infected do not realize that they need medical help. In addition, physical examination may reveal no signs of infection. Unless screening techniques are used to identify infection, these women are at significant risk for the development of complications, including infertility, adverse pregnancy outcomes, chronic abdominal pain, and cervical cancer. The primary care clinician needs to know who to screen, which tests to use, and how to interpret the test results. In addition, practitioners must know how to educate their patients regarding the modes of transmission of infection and methods to decrease the risk of acquiring a sexually transmitted disease (STD).

The list of sexually transmitted pathogens is long (Box 22-1). Several of the major pathogens are discussed here; *human papillomavirus* is discussed in Chapter 96 and *human immunodeficiency virus* in Chapter 21.

RISK FACTORS

Although a woman may contract a sexually transmitted infection at any age, the incidence of STD is greatest in those younger than 25 years old. Any woman in this age group who has had at least one sexual encounter should undergo the appropriate screening tests for STD. Regardless of age, other risk factors include a history of multiple partners, a previous STD, a sex partner with other partners in the preceding 3 months, use of illicit drugs, and use of nonbarrier contraceptives. To identify those women at risk, the practitioner must use a frank, nonjudgmental approach in obtaining a sexual history. Unfortunately, clinicians often are uncomfortable asking patients about numbers of sexual partners, sexual preferences, and sexual practices and thus prevent their patients from feeling free to respond truthfully. In addition, many professionals use terminology that their patients may neither understand nor interpret correctly. Questions should be phrased simply to avoid misinterpreta-

tion. Giving patients latitude in answering the questions facilitates obtaining more truthful responses. Being specific as to a patient's actual sexual practices helps the practitioner determine from which areas of the body to obtain a specimen to rule out potential infection (Box 22-2).

APPROACH TO THE WOMAN AT RISK

All women whose sexual history determines them to be at risk for an STD should receive appropriate screening. The physical examination should include evaluation of the oral cavity, skin, lymph nodes, and external genitalia, as well as a pelvic and bimanual examination. A wet preparation of the vaginal secretions should be obtained to search for hyphae, *Trichomonas* organisms, clue cells, and polymorphonuclear leukocytes (PMNs). Specimens should be obtained from the cervix for identification of gonorrhea and chlamydia. A Gram stain of the cervical secretions allows identification of mucopurulent cervicitis by the presence of at least 10 to 20 PMNs per oil-immersion field (1000) in an area of cervical mucus and a minimal number of epithelial cells. A positive Gram stain or the finding of mucopus on a cotton swab of the cervical os has been shown to correlate with infection caused by *Chlamydia trachomatis*. Alternatively, it may indicate the presence of infection with organisms such as *Neisseria gonorrhoeae,* or *Herpes simplex virus.* In some patients no organism is identified. Specimens from the oral cavity and rectum should be obtained when indicated by the sexual history or dictated by signs or symptoms. All women at risk for an STD should be screened for syphilis (see later discussion). Human immunodeficiency virus (HIV) testing should be offered.

NEISSERIA GONORRHOEAE

Gonorrhea is caused by the bacteria *N. gonorrhoeae,* a gram-negative diplococcus. Approximately 600,000 cases of gonorrhea occur annually in the United States. Transmission of infection with *N. gonorrhoeae* occurs readily. There is a 20% risk of a man acquiring urethral infection after one exposure to an infected woman. The likelihood of transmission from a man to a woman is probably higher.

BOX 22-1
Pathogens

- Bacteria—*Neisseria gonorrhoeae, Haemophilus ducreyi* (chancroid), *Calymmatobacterium granulomatis* (granuloma inguinale, donavanosis), *Gardnerella vaginalis, Chlamydia trachomatis*
- Mycoplasma—*Mycoplasma hominis, Mycoplasma genitalium, Ureaplasma urealyticum*
- Fungi—*Candida albicans* and other candida species
- Spirochetes—*Treponema pallidum*
- Viruses—Herpes simplex virus, human papillomavirus (warts), hepatitis A, B, and C, cytomegalovirus, human immunodeficiency virus (HIV)
- Protozoa—*Trichomonas vaginalis, Entamoeba histolytica, Giardia lamblia*
- Ectoparasites—*Phthirus pubis* (crab louse), *Sarcoptes scabiei* (scabies)

BOX 22-2
Taking a Sexual History

1. Do you have sex with men or women, or both?
2. How many different people do you have sex with at present, for example, 1, 2, 5, 10?
3. How many people have you had sex with in the past 6 months? year? lifetime? 1, 5, 10, 50?
4. How old were you when you first had sex?
5. When did you have sex last, including "oral sex" (i.e., your mouth on someone's penis, rectum, vagina).
6. Do you put your mouth on someone's penis? rectum? vagina?
7. Does someone put his penis in your vagina? mouth? rectum?
8. Do you use birth control? What kind? Do you use birth control all the time?
9. Do you use condoms? Do you use them all the time and with every partner?
10. Have you ever had a sexually transmitted infection such as gonorrhea, herpes, chlamydia, warts, syphilis, or pelvic inflammatory disease?

Clinical Presentation

The incubation period for gonorrhea is difficult to define in women, but symptoms may occur within 10 days. Unlike men, most infected women have no symptoms. Although the endocervical canal is the primary site of infection in women, colonization of the urethra also occurs in up to 70% to 90% of women. In women who have undergone a hysterectomy, the urethra is the primary site of infection. Gonococcal **urethritis** is one of the causes of the sterile pyuria syndrome. Symptoms may include dysuria and urinary frequency. Discharge may be expressed from the infected urethra.

Women with symptomatic **cervical infection** may report vaginal discharge, dysuria, abnormal uterine bleeding, or labial pain or swelling (Bartholin's gland abscess). The cervix may be normal in appearance, or there may be evidence of mucopurulent cervicitis, including edema, erythema, friabil-

ity, or a discharge from the cervical os. **Endometritis** results from ascension of infection from the cervical canal.

Fitz-Hugh–Curtis syndrome, or **perihepatitis,** is an inflammatory process involving the surface of the liver. Patients have right upper quadrant abdominal pain that can be pleuritic. Fever, nausea, and symptoms of lower tract infection may be present. The liver is tender on examination. Evidence of salpingitis sometimes is present. The white blood cell (WBC) count and erythrocyte sedimentation rate (ESR) may be elevated. Liver function tests reveal elevated levels in 50% of patients. Normal findings on a right upper quadrant ultrasound can help distinguish this syndrome from acute cholecystitis. A culture specimen of the cervix may be positive for *N. gonorrhoeae*. A definitive diagnosis is established by laparoscopic findings of patchy purulent or fibrinous deposits on the surface of the liver.

N. gonorrhoeae causes 20% to 40% of cases of **salpingitis** (**pelvic inflammatory disease** [PID]). Other causes of PID include *Chlamydia trachomatis* and anaerobic bacteria. The role of other organisms such as *Trichomonas vaginalis, Gardnerella vaginalis, Ureaplasma urealyticum, Mycoplasma genitalium,* and *Mycoplasma hominis* has yet to be clarified. Regardless of the cause, the signs and symptoms generally are similar (see discussion under *C. trachomatis*). Complications of salpingitis include infertility, an increased propensity for ectopic pregnancies, and chronic pelvic pain as a result of scarring and adhesions. One episode of PID can predispose a patient to recurrent episodes of PID caused by vaginal flora, presumably because of an alteration of host defense mechanisms within the salpinx.

Pharyngeal infection is more readily transmitted by fellatio than by cunnilingus. Of heterosexual women with gonorrhea, 10% to 20% have infection of the pharynx. The sexual history and results of subsequent screening cultures are important in making this diagnosis because more than 90% of cases are asymptomatic. Patients with symptoms often report a mildly to moderately sore throat. Cervical lymph nodes may be painful. The pharynx may be normal in appearance or mildly inflamed, or an exudative pharyngitis may be present. The anterior cervical nodes may be enlarged and tender on examination. Indeed, it is difficult to distinguish gonococcal pharyngitis from that caused by group A streptococcus. The diagnosis of gonococcal pharyngitis must be specifically sought by obtaining a sexual history from patients with a sore throat. The diagnosis of pharyngeal gonococcal infection can be made by placing a specimen from the posterior pharynx on a culture plate containing Thayer-Martin or modified Thayer-Martin (MTM) medium. Culture media used to diagnose group A streptococcal infection do not permit the growth of the gonococcus.

If untreated, pharyngeal infection will resolve spontaneously within 12 weeks. Treatment, however, is necessary to eliminate the pharynx as a reservoir of infection. More important, treatment can prevent dissemination of the organism, a complication of pharyngeal infection.

Infection of the rectum occurs in 30% to 50% of women with gonorrhea. The most common cause is contamination of the rectum by infected vaginal secretions, and in a smaller percentage of women, by rectal intercourse. Although most infected women are asymptomatic, symptoms of proctitis can occur. These include constipation, tenesmus, anorectal pain, and anorectal bleeding or discharge. The discharge may be purulent or mucoid. On examination, there may be mild erythema around the anus. Findings on anoscopic or proctoscopic examination may be insignificant or may reveal involvement of the lower end of the rectum. The mucosa may show inflammatory changes, may be friable, and may bleed easily. A mucopurulent exudate may be present. Gonococcal proctitis should be differentiated from infection caused by *Chlamydia trachomatis, Herpes simplex virus, Treponema pallidum,* and *Entamoeba histolytica.*

A positive Gram stain of a rectal smear can be found in 60% to 80% of infected patients. Although this smear is difficult to read, its specificity is extremely high. Diagnosis also can be made by obtaining a specimen for culture.

Gonococcal ophthalmia neonatorum, a severe, bilateral purulent conjunctivitis, occurs in the neonate 1 to 7 days after the infant's passage through an infected birth canal. This infection is prevented by the instillation of 1% silver nitrate in each conjunctival sac at birth. Adult **ocular infection** often is due to autoinoculation. Both infections require treatment with systemic antibiotics.

Disseminated gonococcal infection (DGI) occurs in 1% to 3% of infected patients. The incubation period is variable, ranging from 7 to 30 days after mucosal infection. In women, DGI often occurs around the time of menses or during pregnancy. Women may be at greater risk for dissemination than are men. Other risk factors include pharyngeal infection and complement deficiency. Patients have symptoms of systemic illness, including fever, anorexia, and malaise. Skin lesions are the most common manifestation of DGI. They occur predominantly on the extremities and range in number from 5 to 30. The upper extremities are involved more often than the lower extremities. The lesions occur most often near the joints of the hands and feet. Their initial appearance is nonspecific, beginning as an erythematous macule or papule, which evolves into a pustule that ultimately may develop a hemorrhagic or necrotic center.

Infection with *N. gonorrhoeae* is the most common cause of acute septic arthritis in young adults and most often involves the knees, elbows, ankles, and wrists. Migratory polyarthralgias are more common in DGI than is septic arthritis. Tenosynovitis may occur at one or several sites. Other manifestations of DGI include hepatitis, myopericarditis, and, rarely, endocarditis, meningitis, osteomyelitis, and pneumonia.

Blood cultures are positive in only 25% of patients with DGI. Cultures of skin lesions may be positive in a small percentage of patients. The diagnosis is made by culturing all potentially infected sites, including the cervix, urethra, rectum, and pharynx.

Diagnostic Tests

Gram stain remains the most rapid and inexpensive method of diagnosing gonococcal infection; it is highly sensitive in specimens obtained from men with symptomatic urethritis. Although the sensitivity of Gram stain is only 40% to 60% for cervical and anal specimens, the specificity of this test is 95%.

Culture remains the "gold standard" of diagnosis. The bacteria *N. gonorrhoeae* are small gram-negative diplococci with flattened abutting sides that on a Gram-stained smear have the appearance of a pair of kidney beans. The organism is extremely sensitive to drying and temperature. Specimens must be placed on the appropriate medium within minutes; the organism will die on the tip of a cotton swab. Specimens should be plated on culture plates that are at room temperature. Planted cultures will not survive unless they are rapidly placed at 35° to 37° C in 3% to 5% carbon dioxide. When a carbon dioxide environment is not readily available, the planted specimen can be put in a candle jar and placed in an incubator. Selective culture media, such as Thayer-Martin or MTM agar, are used to culture *N. gonorrhoeae* to prevent its overgrowth by other saprophytic organisms present in the specimen. Some strains will fail to grow on these media, and thus specimens from relatively sterile sites (such as cerebrospinal fluid, blood, joints) should be plated on chocolate media that do not contain antibiotics. Special transport media are necessary when a laboratory is not immediately available. Because the organism is extremely sensitive to drying, temperature, and the level of carbon dioxide, cultures can be falsely negative if the specimen is not processed rapidly and correctly.

Several rapid diagnostic techniques have emerged over the years. The direct immunofluorescence and indirect enzyme immunoassays were some of the earlier tests developed. They are neither more sensitive nor more specific than culture. Sensitivity and specificity of **DNA amplification techniques** range from 85% to 99% in various studies. The specificity of the DNA probe ranges from 94% to 99%. False-positive results may be obtained with these rapid tests, particularly in the assessment of cure. Amplification techniques such as the polymerase chain reaction (PCR) and ligase chain reaction have higher sensitivity and specificity compared with other rapid tests. When cervical specimens are used, sensitivity of the ligase chain reaction for gonorrhea is approximately 95%. Noninvasive specimens such as urine can be assayed, although sensitivity on such specimens is lower. Specificity is 99% for cervical and urethral specimens.

When feasible, culture is the preferred diagnostic technique, as it remains an important means of identifying antibiotic-resistant strains of *N. gonorrhoeae.* The use of newer technologies is preferable to culture when logistical problems prevent obtaining a culture properly.

Choice of Therapy

For decades, penicillin was the drug of choice for the treatment of gonococcal infections. Strains of penicillin-resistant *N. gonorrhoeae* appeared in the United States in the 1970s, with the prevalence of these strains approaching 25% to 35% of strains in certain urban areas. Thus recommended regimens no longer include the use of penicillin. Because 35% to 50% of women infected with *N. gonorrhoeae* also are coinfected with *Chlamydia trachomatis,* any regimen for treating gonorrhea should include empiric treatment for *C. trachomatis.* The regimens noted in Box 22-3 are effective for eradicating infection, with reported cure rates of 92% to 98%.

Preliminary studies have shown that ceftriaxone may be effective in treating incubating syphilis. Thus this regimen would be preferable to the use of the fluoroquinolones, which are not effective in the treatment of incubating syphilis. The fluoroquinolones should not be used during pregnancy, in lactating women, or in patients younger than 18 years old. Quinolone resistance occurs commonly in Asia and the Pacific and has been reported in the United States. In most states, the incidence remains low (0.4%). In some states

---

BOX 22-3
Treatment of Gonorrhea

Uncomplicated Endocervical, Urethral, or Rectal Infection
Ceftriaxone 125 mg IM once or
Cefixime 400 mg PO once (level of antibiotic is not as high as with
    ceftriaxone)
plus
Empiric treatment for *C. trachomatis* with Azithromycin 1 gm PO once or
Doxycycline 100 mg PO bid for 7 days or Erythromycin base 500 mg PO
    qid for 7 days or
Ofloxacin 300 mg po bid for 7 days or
Levofloxacin 500 mg po bid for 7 days
The patient allergic to cephalosporins
Ciprofloxacin* 500 mg PO once or
Norfloxacin* 800 mg PO once or
Ofloxacin* 400 mg PO once or
Levofloxacin* 500 mg PO once
Spectinomycin† 2 g IM or
plus
Empiric treatment for *C. trachomatis*
In pregnancy
Ceftriaxone 125 mg IM
plus
Empiric treatment for chlamydia as recommended for pregnancy

Disseminated Infection
Initial treatment: Recommended
Ceftriaxone 1 g IV daily
Alternatives
Cefotaxime 1 g IV q8h or
Ceftizoxime 1 g IV q8h or
Spectinomycin 2 g IM q12h or
Ofloxacin 400 mg IV q 12 h
After 24 to 48 hr of improvement, therapy may be switched to one of the
    following regimens to complete 7 days of treatment:
Continuing treatment: Recommended
Cefixime 400 mg PO bid
Alternatives
Cefuroxime axetil 500 mg PO bid or
Ciprofloxacin 500 mg PO bid or
Levofloxacin 500 mg PO daily or
Ofloxacin 400 mg PO bid
All regimens should include treatment for *C. trachomatis*

---

* Not adequate in the treatment of pharyngeal infection. Can be used in pregnancy.
† Cannot be used during pregnancy or in patients younger than 18 years old.

---

such as Hawaii, where resistance levels have risen >14%, the use of fluoroquinolones is no longer advisable.

All patients with gonorrhea are at risk for syphilis and should receive appropriate screening. All partners of patients with gonorrhea within the preceding 30 days should be evaluated and treated.

CHLAMYDIA TRACHOMATIS

Infection with Chlamydia trachomatis occurs commonly in the United States, with 3 million new cases each year. It is the cause of one fourth to one half of the cases of PID. It is the most common cause of neonatal conjunctivitis and interstitial pneumonia in infants younger than 6 months old born to an infected mother. The prevalence of chlamydial infection ranges from 3% to 5% of asymptomatic women seen in general medical clinics to 15% to 20% of those seen in STD clinics.

Chlamydia are a special type of bacteria. There are many serotypes of *C. trachomatis*. Serotypes A, B, and C cause trachoma, the most common cause of blindness in the world. Serotypes D through K are sexually transmitted and are responsible for the clinical syndromes described in this section. Serotypes L1 to L3 also are sexually transmitted and are the etiologic agents of lymphogranuloma venereum.

Transmission of chlamydial infection is not uncommon; 60% to 75% of women whose male partners have chlamydial urethritis are infected with *C. trachomatis*. Most women with chlamydial cervicitis are asymptomatic. Thus routine screening of women at risk, as well as notification of female partners of infected men, is of utmost importance in helping to identify most of the women infected with this organism.

Screening

Recommendations for screening both men and women for chlamydia have become more aggressive. Screening asymptomatic women at risk for infection with chlamydia has been shown to be cost-effective in view of the risk of development of PID. Women less than 20 years old should be screened at any pelvic examination and *at least once per year.* Women between 20 and 24 years old should be screened *at least once per year.* Women more than 25 years old should be screened at least once a year if at risk (i.e., inconsistent use of barrier methods; a new, or more than one sexual partner in the last 3 months; a new partner since the last screening test; or infection with another STD).

Clinical Presentation

A large proportion of women with genital chlamydial infection have normal findings on cervical examination. If results of the examination are abnormal, there may be evidence of **mucopurulent cervicitis.** The cervix may be erythematous and edematous with increased friability. The mucopurulent discharge may be evident on visual inspection of the cervical os, or yellowish mucopus may be present on a cotton swab of the os. A Gram stain of a cervical smear that reveals more than 10 to 20 PMNs per oil-immersion field in the presence of cervical mucus that is free of contamination with vaginal secretions has been shown to correlate with the presence of *C. trachomatis*. More recent data, however, suggest a greater correlation when more than 30 PMNs per oil field are seen.

C. trachomatis is one of the etiologic agents of the **acute urethral syndrome** and is a cause of sterile pyuria in the sexually active woman. The symptoms of dysuria and frequency can be misdiagnosed as a bacterial urinary tract infection. Urethritis may occur without cervicitis. A urethral discharge, meatal erythema, or swelling can be present. A Gram-stained smear of the urethral discharge may reveal more than 10 PMNs per oil field. Infection of Bartholin's ducts may result in abscess formation and a **Bartholin's gland abscess** similar to that seen with gonococcal infection.

Fitz-Hugh–Curtis syndrome was initially thought to be caused only by *N. gonorrhoeae*. Evidence now suggests that

C. trachomatis may be a more common pathogen. (See preceding discussion of *N. gonorrhoeae* for clinical signs and symptoms.)

Of the cases of **PID** that occur annually in the United States, 25% to 50% are due to *C. trachomatis*. Women complain of unilateral or bilateral abdominal pain, which may be mild or severe. Other symptoms include a vaginal discharge, dyspareunia, and menorrhagia. Fever sometimes occurs. Abdominal tenderness may be mild, or peritoneal signs may suggest an acute abdominal process. Pelvic examination may reveal a mucopurulent discharge from the cervical os. Cervical motion tenderness, uterine tenderness, or unilateral or bilateral adnexal tenderness can be detected on palpation. Adnexal swelling, if present, indicates a possible tuboovarian abscess, a condition that must be distinguished from an ectopic pregnancy. Laboratory tests may not be helpful in the diagnosis of PID. An elevated ESR and a leukocytosis can be seen; however, a normal ESR or WBC does not rule out the diagnosis. Specimens for cultures or for other diagnostic tests for chlamydia and gonorrhea must be obtained from the cervical os.

A woman with one episode of PID has a 10% to 20% risk of infertility and a sevenfold increased risk of an ectopic pregnancy if she becomes pregnant. In addition, some women subsequently experience chronic lower abdominal pain because of scarring and adhesions. Recent studies have shown the presence of *C. trachomatis* DNA in the fallopian tubes of infertile women who have never had a clinical episode of PID. Thus asymptomatic PID caused by *C. trachomatis* may indeed occur and is responsible for the "silent epidemic" of PID that is occurring.

Inclusion **conjunctivitis** can develop in the sexually active adult as a result of spread from the genital region. It manifests by an acute, copious mucopurulent discharge and inflamed edematous conjunctivae. Symptoms may be mild, however, and can mimic other causes of bacterial or viral conjunctivitis.

Chlamydial infection during pregnancy raises special concerns; 8% to 12% of pregnant women are infected with chlamydia. The prevalence approaches 20% to 30% in unwed teenagers in inner-city regions. An infant passing through an infected birth canal has a 35% to 50% chance of developing chlamydial inclusion conjunctivitis and a 25% risk of developing chlamydial neonatal pneumonia. Because of an increased incidence of chlamydial cervicitis and a decreased incidence of gonorrhea, in many hospitals erythromycin is now instilled into the conjunctival sac of newborn infants instead of 1% silver nitrate. This prevents the development of chlamydial conjunctivitis; however, nasopharyngeal colonization still occurs and infants remain at risk for the development of chlamydial pneumonia.

Lymphogranuloma venereum (LGV), which is due to chlamydial serotypes L1 to L3, is endemic in developing countries in Asia, Africa, and South America. Several hundred cases are reported annually in the United States, although the exact incidence is unknown and is likely to be higher. It is seen more commonly in men than in women in a ratio of 5:1 in as much as women tend to have asymptomatic infection. LGV is a systemic illness that begins 3 days to 3 weeks after exposure. A primary lesion appears on the labia or vagina as a papule, a shallow ulcer, or an erosion. This lesion may go unnoticed. Two to six weeks after exposure the second stage begins with the development of painful, swollen lymph nodes that drain the involved site. One third of lymph nodes become fluctuant (buboes) and go on to suppurate with the development of draining fistulas. Constitutional symptoms may occur. Left untreated, progressive ulceration, fistulae formation, and abnormal lymphatic drainage of the genitals can occur. If the rectum is involved, rectal strictures can develop. In addition to genital ulcerative disease, serotypes L1 to L3 also can cause urethritis, cervicitis, and proctitis.

Treatment of LGV consists of the use of doxycycline, tetracycline, or erythromycin at doses similar to that for other chlamydial infections (see discussion later in this section); however, antibiotics should be taken for 3 to 4 weeks.

Diagnostic Tests

Evaluation of potentially infected sites can be accomplished through a variety of diagnostic tests. Regardless of the technology used, it is of paramount importance that the specimen be obtained in the appropriate manner. *C. trachomatis* is an intracellular host parasite, and thus host cells must be obtained. Swabs must be adequately rotated or the site gently rubbed or scraped to obtain an adequate specimen. Obtaining superficial "pus" will give a false-negative result.

Until recently, **tissue culture** had been the "gold standard" for diagnosing chlamydial infection. Samples for isolation, using swabs that are not toxic to the tissue monolayer, are placed in transport media. Specimens inoculated onto cell monolayers are evaluated in 48 to 72 hours for evidence of the development of chlamydial inclusions. This technique is expensive to perform and requires the expertise of trained laboratory personnel. Sensitivity of culture is highest if specimens are planted immediately after collection, but decreases readily if the specimen is stored before inoculation of the monolayer.

More rapid tests based on newer technologic methods have become available. **Direct monoclonal antibody staining (fluorescent antibody [FA])** is a rapid test that takes 30 to 60 minutes to perform. Samples are placed directly onto a slide, stained with a fluorescein-labeled monoclonal antibody, and evaluated for the presence of fluorescing elementary bodies. The sensitivity rate of this assay can range from 75% to 99% and depends greatly on the skill of the technician reading the slide. Host cells can be seen on the slide, thus confirming the adequacy of the obtained specimen and eliminating one cause of false-negative results.

The **enzyme immunoassay (EIA)** was one of the first automated tests to become available, obviating the need for a highly trained laboratory technician and enabling numerous specimens to be processed at one time. The quality of the specimen is especially important because it cannot be assessed as it can with the FA test. Poorly acquired specimens will give false-negative results. Sensitivity of the EIA is low compared with newer techniques. The DNA probe appears to have a higher sensitivity than the EIA, with a sensitivity of 76% to 94% in various studies. Specificity for the DNA probe is 91% to 98%. The original studies, however, used culture as the "gold standard." Amplification techniques have been shown to have a higher sensitivity than chlamydia culture, raising the possibility that the true sensitivity of the DNA probe may be lower than originally thought.

DNA amplification techniques have become the test of choice in screening both men and women for chlamydia, in view of the high sensitivity and specificity of these tests. The sensitivity of the PCR is approximately 95% to 98%, with a specificity of 96% to 100%. Similarly, detection rates of the ligase chain reaction (LCR) is 97% for specimens from the male urethra, 94% for cervical specimens, and 93% for first-void urine specimens. Specificity of the LCR is 99%. Excessive blood in the specimens may interfere with obtaining an accurate result; however, up to 2% blood may be acceptable.

The diagnosis of LGV is best made by use of **serologic evaluation.** A complement fixation (CF) titer of at least 1:64 or a microimmunofluorescence (micro-IF) titer of at least 1:512 is consistent with a diagnosis of LGV. The organism can be isolated from a suppurative lymph node or primary lesion, although this is not commonly recommended.

Although serologic evaluation is useful in the diagnosis of LGV, it is not particularly helpful in the diagnosis of the sexually transmitted syndromes caused by *C. trachomatis* serotypes D through K. Only 50% of patients will have CF titers greater than 1:16. The micro-IF test, however, is more sensitive than the CF test because it can measure immunoglobulin (Ig)M or IgG to specific serotypes when this information is needed. Few laboratories, however, perform this test.

Practitioners occasionally receive results of Pap smears that show inclusions caused by *C. trachomatis.* The finding of chlamydial inclusions on a Pap smear is highly specific; unfortunately, sensitivity is limited. Chlamydial inclusions also can be seen on Giemsa stain of scrapings of the conjunctivae and are helpful in diagnosing active inclusion conjunctivitis.

Choice of Therapy

C. trachomatis has a long life cycle, and thus therapeutic levels of antibiotics are required at the intracellular site for an extended period. Historically, the tetracyclines and erythromycin have been highly successful in the treatment of chlamydial infections. Because these drugs commonly have side effects, including gastrointestinal disturbance, alternative regimens have been sought.

Azithromycin is an azalide with a low minimal inhibitory concentration (MIC) against *C. trachomatis* and an ability to achieve high intracellular levels. Thus this antibiotic is highly effective in eradicating the organism. Azithromycin's long half-life of 60 hours allows infrequent dosing. Its one-time dosing schedule makes treatment convenient for patients and significantly decreases the problem of patient noncompliance. The cost of azithromycin is higher than that of the tetracyclines or erythromycin. Although azithromycin is taken as a one time dose, it may take up to 7 days to eradicate infection, and patients should be cautioned not to have sex for 7 days after treatment.

The newer fluoroquinolones such as ofloxacin and levofloxacin have been shown to have good activity against *C. trachomatis* in vitro. Their high oral bioavailability, long half-life, and high concentration in tissues make them good treatment candidates. The fluoroquinolones are contraindicated during pregnancy and in those younger than 18 years old.

The drug of choice for the treatment of chlamydial infection during pregnancy is erythromycin. The estolate preparation should be avoided in pregnancy. The fluoroquinolones are contraindicated during pregnancy as are the tetracyclines. Although azithromycin is classified as a category B drug, limited data are available on its use in pregnancy (Box 22-4).

Although some women with PID require hospitalization, many do not. Patients should be hospitalized if the diagnosis is uncertain, if surgical emergencies such as appendicitis or ectopic pregnancy cannot be ruled out, if a tuboovarian abscess is suspected, or if the patient is severely ill, an adolescent, pregnant, HIV-positive, unable to tolerate or comply with an outpatient regimen, or unable or unlikely to return for clinical follow-up within 72 hours. Treatment of PID should consist of an antibiotic regimen adequate to treat gonorrheal as well as chlamydial infection (Box 22-5).

BOX 22-4

Treatment of Uncomplicated Genital Infection Caused by *C. trachomatis*

Azithromycin 1 g PO once or
Doxycycline* 100 mg PO bid for 7 days or
Tetracycline* 500 mg PO qid for 7 days or
Erythromycin base or stearate 500 mg PO qid for 7 days or
Ofloxacin† 300 mg PO bid for 7 days or
Levofloxacin† 500 mg PO daily for 7 days

*Should be avoided in pregnancy.
†Should be avoided in pregnancy and in those younger than 18 years of age.

BOX 22-5

Treatment of Pelvic Inflammatory Disease

Ambulatory Regimen
Ofloxacin 400 mg po bid or Levofloxacin 500 mg po daily for 14 days
  plus consideration of metronidazole 500 mg po bid for 14 days
Alternatives
Cefoxitin 2 g IM plus probenecid, 1 g PO concurrently or
Ceftriaxone 250 mg IM (alternative: ceftizoxime or cefotaxime)
plus
Doxycycline 100 mg PO bid 14 days and consideration of metronidazole 500 mg bid for 14 days

Inpatient Treatment
Cefoxitin 2 g IV q6h or cefotetan IV 2 g q12h
plus
Doxycyline 100 mg IV or PO bid
Continue this combination treatment for 24 hours after clinical improvement, followed by doxycycline 100 mg PO bid to complete 14 days. (Addition of metronidazole should be considered for anaerobic coverage, particularly for tuboovarian abscess).
Alternate Regimen
Clindamycin 900 mg IV q8h *plus* gentamicin 1.5 mg/kg IV q8h for 24 hours after clinical improvement.
Continue clindamycin 450 mg PO qid to complete 14 days. (This regimen has good activity against anaerobes but may be less effective against gonorrheal and chlamydial infection.)

All partners of patients with chlamydial infection or PID should be evaluated and treated.

GENITAL ULCERS

Practitioners in primary care practice frequently evaluate women with genital ulcers. A clinical diagnosis often is based on appearance. When multiple lesions are present, a diagnosis of herpes simplex virus infection frequently is made; a painless singular lesion is diagnosed as syphilis. Generalizations such as these often can be misleading and result in misdiagnosis and mistreatment. Practitioners must be aware of the various causes of genital ulcers, incubation periods, and the clinical presentations, both typical and atypical. A thorough understanding of the diagnostic tests available is necessary.

A full discussion of all causes of genital ulcers is beyond the scope of this text (Box 22-6). Syphilis and genital herpes simplex infection are discussed in detail in the next section.

Genital ulcers are a significant risk factor for the transmission of the HIV. Practitioners should take the time to discuss this concern with their patients and to recommend HIV testing.

BOX 22-6
Approach to the Patient with Genital Ulcers

Causes
Infectious
Treponema pallidum
Herpes simplex virus
Chlamydia trachomatis L1-L3 (lymphogranuloma venereum)
Haemophilus ducreyi (chancroid)
Cytomegalovirus (CMV)
Epstein-Barr virus (EBV)
Human immunodeficiency virus (HIV)
Calymmatobacterium granulomatis (granuloma inguinale)
Noninfectious
Trauma
Fixed drug reactions
Behçet's syndrome
Neoplasm

Evaluation
Syphilis serology*
Tzanck test or direct immunofluorescence for herpes simplex virus (HSV 1 and HSV 2)
Viral culture for HSV
Serology for lymphogranuloma venereum (LGV)
Gram stain for *H. ducreyi*†
Culture for *H. ducreyi* (special culture is needed and should be discussed with the laboratory)

---

*Rapid plasma reagin (RPR), Venereal Disease Research Laboratory (VDRL), or automated reagin test (ART) should be performed initially and, if negative, repeated in 1 and 3 months, if the patient is compliant. Empiric treatment may be considered in the appropriate setting.
†A scraping of the edge of the ulcer is placed on a slide; after staining, the smear is evaluated for "tracking" of small gram-negative rods.

SYPHILIS

One in every 7000 to 10,000 infants born in the United States has congenital syphilis. The increase in incidence of congenital syphilis in the early part of the decade was indicative of an increase in the incidence of primary and secondary syphilis in women of childbearing years and in heterosexual men. This number has declined more recently. It is estimated that 70,000 new cases of syphilis occur annually in the United States.

Transmission of the spirochete, *Treponema pallidum,* the causative agent of syphilis, generally occurs through sexual contact, with an acquisition rate of 30% after one exposure to an infected person. Transmission can occur transplacentally, after contact with mucous membranes (including kissing), by transfusion of infected blood, and possibly by direct inoculation. Patients are most infectious during the initial stages; however, potentially they can transmit the organism by sexual contact for an extended period, up to 4 years after acquisition of the disease.

Clinical Presentation

The incubation period is variable, ranging between 3 and 90 days after an exposure. The primary manifestation is the appearance of the **chancre,** which begins as a macule or papule, progressively erodes, and forms an ulcer. Although the chancre usually is painless and indurated, it can be painful (particularly when secondarily infected), soft, and nonindurated. Although usually thought of as a single lesion, multiple chancres can be present and can be mistaken for herpes simplex infection. Chancres most commonly occur in the genital region but can be found on other parts of the body as well. When they appear on the cervix or rectum, they often go unnoticed and thus undiagnosed; in fact, 15% to 30% of chancres go undetected. Painless regional **lymphadenopathy** sometimes is present. Without treatment, the chancre resolves spontaneously within 5 weeks.

The secondary phase of the infection is due to the hematogenous spread of the organism. The signs of secondary syphilis appear 2 to 8 weeks after the appearance of the chancre and may occur while the chancre is still present. Patients have **nonspecific flulike symptoms** of malaise, fever, arthralgias, headache, and pharyngitis.

The most characteristic finding on physical examination is the **rash** of secondary syphilis, which often appears as an erythematous macular or maculopapular rash on various parts of the body, including the palms and the soles. The appearance of the rash can vary from papular, papulosquamous (scaling), to pustular. Classically, the rash is described as nonpruritic, although cases of pruritic rash have been mistaken for dermatologic conditions such as eczema. The rash must be distinguished from a drug allergy (which also can involve the palms and soles), pityriasis rosea, viral exanthems, and other skin conditions. Other findings can include generalized **lymphadenopathy, hepatosplenomegaly,** and **alopecia.** Mucous patches may be present in the oral cavity. **Condyloma lata** in the genital region needs to be distinguished from genital warts (condyloma accuminatum).

Several complications of disseminated infection can occur, including syphilitic meningitis, which manifests as an aseptic meningitis. Ocular involvement can result in the development of uveitis, and the patient complains of a painful, red eye.

Without treatment, the uncomplicated manifestations of secondary syphilis resolve within 2 to 10 weeks and the infection becomes latent. The finding of seropositive syphilis in the absence of clinical manifestations is consistent with the diagnosis of latent syphilis. Within the first 4 years after infection, clinical relapses may occur, with the appearance of lesions at the site of the initial chancre (chancre redux) or other cutaneous manifestations.

Since the use of penicillin for the treatment of syphilis began, the rate of tertiary syphilis, including **cardiovascular involvement** (coronary disease, aortic aneurysms, aortic insufficiency), gummatous lesions, and neurosyphilis, has been significantly reduced. An increase in the number of cases of **neurosyphilis** had occurred more recently, particularly in patients with HIV infection. The manifestations of neurosyphilis vary. Syphilitic meningitis, which often occurs early after infection, can mimic the symptoms of bacterial meningitis. Meningovascular syphilis most often occurs within the first few years after infection and can result in a cerebrovascular accident, or stroke. The later manifestations of neurosyphilis, such as general paresis (mental status changes) and tabes dorsalis (loss of position and vibration sensation), occur after many years. In addition, asymptomatic involvement of the nervous system can persist for many years.

Diagnostic Tests

T. pallidum is a tightly coiled helical cell that is too small to be visualized by the use of light microscopy. Thus **darkfield microscopy,** an easy and excellent method of diagnosing primary syphilis, is needed. The newer models of office microscopes can be made into a darkfield microscope by changing the condenser. Serous material from the abraded ulcer is placed in a normal saline wet mount and evaluated under the darkfield microscope for the presence of the typical, motile, coiled organisms. Results of a darkfield test will be negative if the patient has applied local antiseptics to the chancre or has recently taken systemic antibiotics. When possible, initial negative results should trigger repeat tests on 2 or 3 consecutive days.

Serologic findings can be used to diagnose primary syphilis, although nontreponemal test results may be negative in up to 40% of patients at the time they seek evaluation for a syphilitic chancre. Thus initial seronegativity should prompt consideration of repeat syphilis testing in 3 to 4 weeks in a patient with a genital ulcer. Often, patients may need to be treated empirically at the time they present, without a diagnosis having been made.

The **nontreponemal serologic tests**—the Venereal Disease Research Laboratory (VDRL, rapid plasma reagin (RPR), and the automated reagin test (ART)—are nonspecific tests used to screen patients for syphilis. They are nonspecific tests because they detect a group of antibodies directed against the cardiolipin antigen found on both *T. pallidum* and host cells, which increases in many inflammatory conditions such as systemic lupus erythematosus and tuberculosis. Thus confirmation of the diagnosis of syphilis must be made by a positive treponemal test result, for example, the fluorescent treponemal antibody absorption test (FTA-ABS)) the microhemagglutination–*Treponema pallidum* assay (MHA-TP), the TPPA test, the *Treponema pallidum* immobilization test (TPI), and the hemagglutina-

tion treponemal test for syphilis (HATTS), which assay for the presence of antibody to the organism *T. pallidum.*

At all stages of infection the **treponemal tests** are more sensitive than the nontreponemal tests. In most patients, the treponemal test results remain positive despite therapy, although 15% to 25% of patients treated during the primary stage may revert to seronegativity after 2 to 3 years. A patient's response to therapy can be determined by following nontreponemal tests, the titer of which should decline after treatment.

The diagnosis of neurosyphilis can be difficult. It is made on the basis of clinical manifestations and a lumbar puncture that reveals one or more of the following findings in the cerebrospinal fluid (CSF): an elevated white cell count (0.4 WBC/mm^3), an elevated protein level, or positive VDRL finding. However, a negative CSF VDRL result has been shown in up to 50% of patients with neurosyphilis, and thus does not rule out the diagnosis of neurosyphilis. New techniques to aid in the diagnosis of neurosyphilis, such as PCR, are being investigated.

Women with any sexually transmitted infection should be screened for syphilis. Pregnant women are in a special category. *All* pregnant women, regardless of their sexual history, should be screened for syphilis early in the first trimester. Women at high risk for acquiring syphilis and those who reside in communities where the prevalence of syphilis is high should be retested during the second and third trimesters and at the time of delivery.

Choice of Therapy

Treatment of syphilis requires the presence of adequate antibiotic levels for an extended period. Thus a penicillin with a long half-life, such as benzathine penicillin, must be used (Box 22-7). Doxycycline has been used as an alternative treatment in the penicillin-allergic patient. Limited data suggest that ceftriaxone may be effective in treating early syphilis and may be a consideration in penicillin-allergic patients who are able to tolerate cephalosporins. In addition, single-dose azithromycin may be effective in the treament of early syphilis, but further studies are warranted.

Pregnant women should be treated with the appropriate dose of penicillin for their stage of syphilis. Erythromycin is no longer recommended to treat syphilis in the penicillin-allergic pregnant female because it fails to eradicate fetal infection. Other treatments have not been adequately studied in pregnant women. Thus, pregnant women with syphilis who have a history of penicillin allergy should undergo skin testing to the major and minor penicillin determinants. If skin testing results are positive, desensitization to penicillin should be considered in consultation with an expert and undertaken in an appropriate intensive care setting. Premature labor and fetal distress can be seen in women treated in the second half of pregnancy. Thus, women should be informed as to the possibility of complications and need to seek obstetric assistance.

All patients with primary or secondary syphilis should receive follow-up with serologic testing every 3 months for at least 2 years after treatment to ensure that the titer of the nontreponemal test falls appropriately. Patients with primary syphilis should show a fourfold decline in the nontreponemal titer within 3 to 6 months, and 97% of treated patients should have a negative nontreponemal test result within

---

BOX 22-7
Treatment of Syphilis

Early Syphilis (Primary, Secondary, or Duration < 1 Year)
Benzathine penicillin G 2.4 million units IM once (CDC recommendation)
Benzathine penicillin G 2.4 million units IM weekly 2 wk (Massachusetts
    State Department of Health)*
***Alternative regimens—nonpregnant penicillin-allergic
patient***
Doxycycline 100 mg PO bid for 2 wk
Tetracycline 500 mg PO qid for 2 wk

Latent Syphilis (Duration > 1 Year or Unknown)
Benzathine penicillin G 2.4 million units IM weekly for 3 wk†
Alternative regimen—nonpregnant penicillin-allergic patient
Doxycycline 100 mg PO bid 30 days†
Tetracycline 500 mg PO qid 30 days†

Treatment of syphilis in the HIV positive patient
See text

Treatment of syphilis in the pregnant patient
Penicillin should be used in all stages of pregnancy. Refer to text

---

*Many experts recommend the longer treatment regimen.
†Neurosyphilis should be evaluated by physical examination.
A lumbar puncture should be performed in any patient with neurologic abnormalities.
Patients treated for latent syphilis with alternative antibiotics such as tetracycline or
doxycycline should undergo a lumbar puncture before treatment.

2 years. The greater the duration of untreated infection, the greater the time needed to achieve seronegativity. Patients with latent syphilis should be tested every 6 months. The possibility of treatment failure should be considered in patients with latent syphilis if there is an increase in the nontreponemal titer or if a fourfold decline does not occur within 12 to 24 months in those patients with a titer of 1:32 or more. Failed treatment of syphilis at any stage requires that the patient be retreated. A lumbar puncture to rule out asymptomatic neurosyphilis must be performed before retreatment.

Pregnant women require closer follow-up monitoring, with monthly serologic testing for syphilis repeated throughout the pregnancy, particularly if they are at risk for reinfection. Retreatment should be considered in a pregnant woman if the appropriate fall in titer for the stage of infection is not seen. Some experts would recommend retreatment if a fourfold decrease in the nontreponemal titer does not occur within 3 months in women with early infection.

All partners of infected patients should be appropriately evaluated and treated when indicated. Partners of patients with primary, secondary, and early latent syphilis who have been exposed within the preceding 90 days should be screened for syphilis but should be treated empirically for possible infection at the time they are seen. Partners of patients with primary, secondary, or early latent syphilis exposed more than 90 days earlier should be screened for syphilis and treated at the time of evaluation if syphilis serology results are not immediately available and follow-up cannot be guaranteed. Partners of patients with syphilis of unknown duration with titers of 1:32 or more should be

screened and treated presumptively for possible infection. Partners of patients with late latent syphilis should be screened for syphilis.

Genital ulcer disease is a risk factor for HIV infection. Because there is an increased incidence of HIV infection in patients with syphilis, and vice versa, all patients with syphilis should be counseled on HIV infection, and HIV testing should be recommended. HIV infection generally does not affect syphilis serology, although occasionally higher than expected nontreponemal titers have been seen in some HIV-positive patients, and nontreponemal titers have been shown to be falsely negative in some patients with HIV. Biopsy specimens of skin rashes and lesions that suggest syphilis should be obtained in HIV-positive patients when initial syphilis serology is negative. Standard regimens for syphilis have been noted to fail in some patients with HIV, and the optimal treatment for syphilis in these patients is unclear. Treatment of HIV patients with standard regimens of benzathine penicillin is generally recommended, although some experts would recommend additional treatment (i.e., 3 weekly injections for treatment of primary, secondary, and early latent syphilis). At present, some authorities believe that examination of the CSF should be considered to rule out asymptomatic neurosyphilis before treating HIV-positive patients with early syphilis. A lumbar puncture should be performed in the HIV-positive patient with syphilis of more than 1 year's duration or when the duration of infection is unknown. After treatment, serologic status should be followed every 3 months. Retreatment should be considered if the nontreponemal titer does not decrease by two dilutions within 6 months, or if a rise in titer occurs.

HERPES SIMPLEX INFECTION

Herpes simplex virus (HSV) is a member of the herpesvirus group, which includes HSV 1, HSV 2, cytomegalovirus, Epstein-Barr virus, varicella-zoster virus, and herpesvirus 6 and 8. These viruses have the ability to establish a latent state within host cells and to cause recurrent disease. Genital *herpes simplex virus* infection is due predominantly to HSV 2, although 5% to 30% of cases can be caused by HSV 1. Serologic studies have shown that approximately 20% of young adults between 14 and 49 years old have antibody to HSV 2. Approximately 1 million new cases of genital herpes occur each year, with 45 million people in the United States infected. Transmission of HSV 1 and 2 occurs through close contact with someone who is shedding the virus in secretions, from skin lesions, or from mucous membranes. The incubation period ranges from 2 to 7 days.

Clinical Presentation

Most patients with primary infection have **nonspecific systemic symptoms,** including fever, chills, malaise, headache, and myalgias and appear to have "the flu." Pain or itching may accompany or precede the appearance of the **herpetic lesions,** which can involve the labia, vagina, cervix, perineum, buttocks, urethra, and bladder. More than 70% of women with genital lesions have cervical involvement as well. Lesions begin as papules or vesicles on an erythematous base that go on to ulcerate and heal spontaneously. Often, vesicles will not be present at the time a woman is examined because vesicles located on the labia become macerated and open to form an ulcer. Lesions may manifest as small linear fissures and can be mistaken for trauma or irritation. Tender **inguinal lymphadenopathy** often is present. Patients may report vaginal discharge and can be misdiagnosed as having vaginitis. With involvement of the urethra and bladder, patients may experience symptoms of **urethritis** or **cystitis.**

Symptoms may last for 2 days or for more than 3 weeks. Symptoms associated with primary infection may be milder in women who have previous antibody to HSV 1. Viral shedding from genital lesions may persist for 12 days. Lesions can take up to 3 weeks to heal. Complications of genital HSV infection include sacral radiculopathy that results in urinary or fecal retention. Aseptic meningitis may occur. HSV proctitis can occur in women who have rectal intercourse.

Symptoms do not develop in all women who acquire genital HSV infection. Serologic studies have shown that 60% of women infected with HSV 2 may not have symptomatic outbreaks and may be unaware of their infection. These patients can remain asymptomatic or manifest their first episode of clinical genital herpes infection later in life.

Recurrent outbreaks occur most frequently during the first year after infection. Some patients never experience a clinical recurrence, whereas others have frequent recurrences, some as often as once or twice each month. Many women have recurrences around the time of menses. The degree of severity of the recurrence varies from patient to patient; 50% of women experience prodromal symptoms, including tingling, itching, or pain at the site of the eruption as early as 30 minutes to 2 days before an outbreak. Recurrences generally are milder and shorter in duration than the primary infection. A clinical "recurrence" may occur without a previous primary outbreak.

Asymptomatic cervical viral shedding can occur in the absence of vulvar lesions. Approximately 20% of women with HSV II infection will shed virus asymptomatically within the first year after a primary infection. Asymptomatic shedding tends to occur more frequently in women with more frequent clinical recurrences than in those without clinical recurrences. Most transmission of virus to uninfected persons occurs from persons shedding virus asymptomatically. Virus can be shed from multiple sites, including the external genitalia, perianal area, and the cervix.

Lesions of genital HSV infection in the immunocompromised patient (those on a regimen of chemotherapy or infected with HIV) may appear as progressively enlarging ulcers, several centimeters in size. They can be present for weeks to months. Reactivation of infection occurs more frequently in these patients. Prolonged treatment with antiviral agents is needed for complete healing to occur.

Issues regarding **neonatal HSV** infection often arise during the counseling of women with herpes. Neonatal infection with HSV can occur when an infant passes through an infected birth canal, resulting in significant neonatal morbidity and mortality. Fortunately, this uncommon event is estimated to occur in 1 in 3000 to 20,000 live births. The greatest risk to the neonate occurs in those women who contract a primary infection around the time of delivery; 10% of pregnant women are at risk of contracting primary HSV 2 infection from their HSV 2-seropositive partners. Women who are seronegative for HSV 1 and HSV 2 should avoid genital exposure to HSV 1 or HSV 2 from their seropositive partners during the third trimester. Infection of the neonate can occur during a recurrent episode, but this is a less frequent event. Particular care needs to be taken at and around the time of delivery for those women with a previous history of HSV infection, a history of exposure to a male partner with HSV, or evidence of active lesions that on examination suggest HSV infection. The use of acyclovir around the time of delivery has been suggested by some obstetricians, although this has not become a standard recommendation to date.

Diagnostic Tests

The diagnosis of genital HSV infection is often missed by practitioners based on clinical grounds alone. Genital HSV infection is often misdiagnosed as folliculitis, yeast infections, irritation, allergic reactions, or urethral syndrome. Thus, diagnostic tests are necessary to assist the clinician in making the correct diagnosis.

Viral culture is the "gold standard" test used to confirm the clinical diagnosis of herpes simplex infection. The fluid from a vesicle or a rubbing of the base of an ulcer can be obtained with a Dacron swab, placed in transport media, and forwarded to the tissue culture laboratory. Cultures may show positivity in 1 to 2 days but may take several days if the inoculum is low. The sensitivity of culture is more than 90% if vesicles are present but falls to 30% when lesions are crusted.

The **Tzanck test,** which can be performed while the patient is in the office, provides rapid results. A scraping taken from the base of an unroofed vesicle or from the base of an ulcer is placed on a slide and then stained with Wright or Giemsa stain. The presence of multinucleated giant cells is diagnostic of a herpetic infection, but this finding does not differentiate between infection with HSV or varicella-zoster. The sensitivity of the Tzanck test ranges from 40% to 80% depending on the skill of the person reading the slide. An alternative to the Tzanck test is the use of direct immunofluorescence (DFA) staining of the prepared slides. DFA can be used to distinguish between HSV 1 and HSV 2 infection.

Serologic testing may be helpful in diagnosing primary infection when there is evidence of conversion from seronegativity to seropositivity. Newer serologic tests that eliminate the problem of cross-reactivity between HSV 1 and HSV 2 have recently become available. The Meridian test is an enzyme-linked immunosorbent assay (ELISA) that tests for glycoprotein G1 or G2 specific for HSV 1 or HSV 2. Sensitivity of this assay has been reported to be 81% to 99%, with a specificity of 94% to 99%. Antibody may not become positive for 3 months after primary infection and will therefore be negative at the time that a patient presents with a primary outbreak. The Microbiology Reference Laboratory (MRL) assay is another ELISA test that can distinguish between HSV 1 and HSV 2. The POCKit HSV 2 is a point of care test that assays only for HSV 2. The test itself can take 6 minutes to perform in the office. Sensitivity has been reported to be 96% to 100%, with a specificity of 97%. Antibody may take up to 3 months to develop after a primary infection. These serologic tests can be used to determine if a patient has been infected with HSV in the past, but are not helpful in the diagnosis of a genital ulcer at the time the patient presents.

Choice of Therapy

At present there is no cure for genital HSV infection. The major thrust of treatment for acute infection is to decrease symptoms, decrease time to healing, and decrease viral shedding. Topical acyclovir can decrease the duration of local symptoms but does not reduce the systemic symptoms often associated with primary infection. It should not be placed intravaginally and thus does not affect cervical lesions and cervical viral shedding (see Box 22-8).

Oral acyclovir, when initiated at the onset of a clinical recurrence, has been shown to decrease time of viral shedding and duration of lesions. It may help in decreasing duration of local symptoms, although this has been less well established. Treatment of recurrent outbreaks with the use of any of the three antiviral agents, acyclovir, famciclovir, or valacyclovir, should be started during the prodrome, or with the onset of lesions. Acyclovir has been used for approximately 20 years and is generally well tolerated. Valacyclovir is a prodrug of acyclovir with a bioavailability three to five times that of acyclovir, which enables it to be administered less often. Famciclovir is well absorbed and is the prodrug of the antiviral agent, pencyclovir. It, too, can be given less often than acyclovir, with twice daily dosing.

When taken daily, oral acyclovir has been shown to be effective in decreasing clinical recurrences by up to 75%. Most patients with recurrent infection do not require ongoing treatment with acyclovir; some benefit from intermittent therapy begun at the onset of an outbreak. Suppressive daily therapy should be reserved for those patients with frequent or severe recurrences, complications of herpetic infection (i.e., urinary retention, aseptic meningitis), or for those patients whose emotional well-being may require a break from their herpetic recurrences. Suppressive therapy has been approved for use with acyclovir for up to 5 years and with valacyclovir and famciclovir for 1 year. Information is being gathered on the safety of longer treatment regimens. Suppressive therapy should be discontinued on an annual basis to determine if the pattern and number of recurrences have decreased with time, as is often the case. Patients should be informed that a severe outbreak is likely to occur immediately after discontinuation of suppressive therapy. Patients should be aware that despite the use of suppressive therapy, both symptomatic outbreaks and asymptomatic viral shedding can still occur.

Despite adequate therapy, some women have an extremely difficult time accepting the diagnosis of genital HSV infection. Patients often feel stigmatized. They may have concerns regarding new relationships and are fearful of being rejected. They may become depressed. In addition to making a diagnosis and prescribing medication, each medical provider is obligated to offer all patients appropriate education and counseling regarding HSV infection, as well as appropriate supportive help to those patients in need.

SAFER SEX PRACTICES

Despite all the public awareness of STD and HIV infection, some patients continue to place themselves at increased risk of infection. What can a practitioner do to help patients decrease the likelihood of acquiring an STD? Women and men must be educated to avoid sex with a casual contact. Numbers of sexual partners must be limited. Patients should know their partners well before entering into a sexual relationship. Frank and explicit discussions should be encouraged between partners regarding previous sexual contacts, history of previous STD, and use of recreational drugs. Couples considering a sexual relationship can be counseled together regarding modes of transmission of STD and incubation periods. Testing of both partners at the same time for STDs should be offered.

The practitioner must stress the need for condoms to be used during each and every sexual encounter. Although condoms may decrease transmission rates, women must understand the correct use of condoms and their limitations. Not all condoms are alike, and different brands have been shown to be more effective in preventing transmission of HIV than others. (A rating list can be obtained from the CDC.) Petroleum-based lubricants can react with latex, causing breakage of the condom. The female condom may be helpful to those women whose male partners refuse to comply with condom use.

Aside from abstinence, there are no totally safe sex practices. Medical providers, however, must play an active role in educating their patients about safer sex practices and in helping their patients decrease their risk for an STD.

BOX 22-8
Treatment of Genital HSV Infection

Primary HSV Infection
Acyclovir 400 mg PO tid for 7-10 days or 200 mg PO five times per day for 7-10 days or
Famciclovir 250 mg PO tid for 7-10 days or
Valacyclovir 1 gram PO bid for 7-10 days

Recurrent HSV Infection
Acyclovir 200 mg PO five times per day for 5 days or 400 mg PO tid for 5 days or 800 mg PO bid for 5 days or
Famciclovir 125 mg PO bid for 5 days or
Valacyclovir 500 mg PO bid for 5 days or 1 gm PO daily for 5 days

Suppression of Recurrences
Acyclovir 200 mg PO tid or 400 mg bid
Famciclovir 250 mg PO bid
Valacyclovir 500 mg PO once daily* or 500 mg PO bid or 1 g PO daily

*May be less effective.

BIBLIOGRAPHY

Ashley RL, Wald A: Genital herpes: review of the epidemic and potential use of type-specific serology, *Clin Microbiol Rev* 12:1, 1998.

Ashley RL, Eagleton Mark, Pfeiffer N: Ability of a rapid serology test to detect seroconversion to herpes simplex virus type 2 glycoprotein G soon after infection, *J Clin Microbiol* 37:1632, 1999.

Bryson YJ et al: Risk of acquisition of genital herpes simplex virus type 2 in sex partners of persons with genital herpes: a prospective couple study, *J Infect Dis* 167:942, 1993.

Buimer M et al: Detection of *Chlamydia trachomatis* and *Neisseria gonorrhoeae* by ligase chain reaction-based assays with clinical specimens from various sties: implications for diagnostic testing and screening, *J Clin Microbiol* 34:2395, 1996.

Campbell LA et al: Detection of *Chlamydia trachomatis* deoxyribonucleic acid in women with tubal infertility, *Fertil Steril* 59:45, 1993.

Centers for Disease Control: 1998 Guidelines for treatment of sexually transmitted diseases *MMWR* 47(RR-1):1, 1998.

Chernesky MA et al: Diagnosis of *Chlamydia trachomatits* urethral infection in symptomatic and asymptomatic men by testing first-void urine in a ligase chain reaction assay, *J Infect Dis* 170:1308, 1994.

Frenkel LM et al: Clinical reactivation of *herpes simplex* virus type 2 infection in seropositive pregnant women with no history of genital herpes, *Ann Intern Med* 118:414, 1993.

Holmes KK et al, editors: *Sexually transmitted diseases,* ed 3, New York, 1999, McGraw-Hill.

Hook EW III, Marra CM: Acquired syphilis in adults, *N Engl J Med* 326:1060, 1992.

Ison CA: Laboratory methods in genitourinary medicine: methods of diagnosing gonorrhea, *Genitourin Med* 66:453, 1990.

Iwen PC, Blar TMH, Woods GI: Comparison of the Gen-Probe PACE 2 system in cervical specimens, *Am J Clin Pathol* 95:578, 1991.

Kostman JR, Stull TL: Molecular techniques in the diagnosis of sexually transmitted diseases, *Curr Opin Infect Dis* 5:5, 1992.

Koumans EH, Johnson RE, Knapp JS: Laboratory testing for *Neisseria gonorrheae* by recently introduced nonculture test: a performance review with clinical and public health consideration, *Clin Infect Dis* 27:1171, 1998.

Koutsky LA et al: Underdiagnosis of genital herpes by current clinical and viral-isolation procedures, *N Engl J Med* 326:1533, 1992.

Martin DH et al: A controlled trial of single dose of azithromycin for the treatment of chlamydial urethritis and cervicitis, *N Engl J Med* 327:921, 1992.

Mertz GJ et al: Risk factors for the sexual transmission of genital herpes, *Ann Intern Med* 116:197, 1992.

Norgard MV: Clinical and diagnostic issues of acquired and congenital syphilis encompassed in the current syphilis epidemic, *Curr Opin Infect Dis* 6:9, 1993.

Romanowski B et al: Serologic response to treatment of infectious syphilis, *Ann Intern Med* 114:1005, 1991.

Stary A et al: Performance of transcription-mediated amplification and ligase chain reaction assays for detection of chlamydial infection in urogenital samples obtained by invasive and noninvasive methods, *J Clin Microbiol* 36:2666, 1998.

Wald A et al: Reactivation of genital *Herpes simplex virus* type 2 infection in asymptomatic seropositive persons, *N Engl J Med* 342:844, 2000.

CHAPTER **23**

Acute Dysuria and Urinary Tract Infections

Anthony L. Komaroff

EPIDEMIOLOGY

One fourth of all adult women experience an episode of acute dysuria each year. It is one of the most common clinical problems seen by clinicians in the developed Western nations. Our knowledge about the causes, diagnosis, and treatment of dysuria has been expanded greatly in the last 20 years.

The classic teaching about women with dysuria without symptoms or signs of acute pyelonephritis has included the following:

1. Such patients have bacterial cystitis.
2. The responsible microorganisms are almost always the gram-negative coliform bacteria.
3. The single most important test is a urine culture.
4. More than 100,000 bacteria/ml (a positive culture) constitute proof of a urinary infection.
5. Patients with positive cultures should receive 7 to 14 days of treatment with any of several relatively benign antimicrobial agents.

Recent evidence seriously challenges these assumptions.

This chapter summarizes this evidence and proposes a scheme for categorizing the condition of women with acute dysuria. The discussion pertains only to the problem of dysuria in an office practice as it is most commonly seen and is not applicable to dysuria in adolescents, dysuria in pregnant women, or nosocomial urinary tract infections. (For a more detailed discussion on urinary tract infection during pregnancy see Chapter 78.) Chronic dysuria is discussed in Chapter 24.

CAUSES OF ACUTE CYSTITIS

The clinical syndrome called acute cystitis is now recognized to consist of at least six different conditions, each of which is managed differently. These conditions are summarized in Table 23-1. Each category has important differences from the rest with respect to diagnostic testing, treatment, and prognosis.

Specific Conditions Included in Acute Cystitis
Lower Urinary Tract Bacterial Infection

Many women with acute dysuria have lower tract bacterial infection—infection of both the bladder (cystitis) and

urethra. That is, they have no clinical or laboratory evidence of acute pyelonephritis but have some degree of bacteriuria. Other symptoms commonly include urinary frequency, urgency, suprapubic pain, and hematuria. The only specific physical examination abnormality seen with any frequency is suprapubic tenderness.

In recent years it has become apparent that in 30% to 50% of women who clinically have cystitis the urine culture is negative by the traditional criteria: either bacterial pathogens are found in concentrations less than 100,000/ml or the urine culture is sterile. In fact, it is preferable to use 10^2 to 10^3 organisms/ml of urine as the threshold for defining significant bacteriuria, in *symptomatic* women. The work of Stamm and colleagues has shown that dysuric women with such low colony counts really are infected: urine obtained by suprapubic aspirate or catheter specimen, and hence free of contamination, contained bacteria—but in concentrations less than 100,000/ml. Not only *Escherichia coli* but also *Staphylococcus saprophyticus* and *Proteus* spp., can produce low-count bacteriuria and real infection. (The threshold of greater than 10^5 organisms/ml of urine is still useful in identifying women with *asymptomatic* bacteriuria, the purpose for which the threshold was originally intended.) Moreover, randomized, controlled trials have shown that patients with low-count bacteriuria benefit from antibacterial therapy.

E. coli accounts for 70% to 90% of community-acquired urinary tract infections (UTIs) in women. In the most recent studies, *S. saprophyticus*—a coagulase-negative, novobiocin-resistant organism that sometimes is identified imprecisely by microbiology laboratories as *S. albus* or *S. epidermidis*—is the second most frequent cause of lower tract infection. Thus *S. saprophyticus* should never be dismissed as a contaminant when it grows in pure culture from a urine specimen. (*S. aureus* is only an occasional urinary pathogen, and hematogenous spread to the urinary tract from some other septic focus should always be considered with *S. aureus* UTIs.) The other gram-negative coliform bacteria, group B streptococci and the enterococci, are the other urinary pathogens that are seen with some frequency in community-acquired UTIs. Diphtheroids, alpha-hemolytic streptococci, and lactobacilli—organisms that often are grown from a clean-voided urine specimen—are rarely if ever true urinary pathogens. Although uncomplicated UTIs in women usually involve one organism, polymicrobial UTIs may occur more often than had been thought.

Subclinical Pyelonephritis

Several studies indicate that women with the presenting complaint of dysuria, without symptoms or signs suggesting acute pyelonephritis, nevertheless have *upper* tract infection, or at least tissue invasion of the urinary tract. Such women account for up to 30% of dysuric patients seen in most office settings and up to 80% of women in emergency rooms serving indigent populations.

Subclinical pyelonephritis may produce minimal symptoms, may smolder for long periods, and may be difficult to eradicate. At present there is no practical way of accurately diagnosing subclinical pyelonephritis at the time of the initial visit. Clinical features can increase the likelihood of this condition, as discussed later, but there are no useful diagnostic tests. For practical purposes, subclinical pyelonephritis is diagnosed after the fact, by the detection of treatment failure on follow-up urine cultures. Although patients with subclinical pyelonephritis usually have a prompt symptomatic response, relapse may occur in 10% to 50% after the traditional 7- to 14-day course of treatment, even when the organism is sensitive to the antimicrobial drug used. The optimal antimicrobial regimen for subclinical pyelonephritis has not been established.

Chlamydial Urethritis

Chlamydia trachomatis urethritis accounts for 5% to 20% of cases of dysuria, and its presence may be especially likely when urine cultures are sterile. Risk factors that increase the likelihood of chlamydial infection include (1) a sexual partner with recent urethritis, (2) a new or recent sexual partner, (3) the stuttering onset of symptoms over a period of days rather than abruptly, and (4) the absence of hematuria.

Gonococcal Urethritis

Gonococcal urethritis may account for up to 10% of cases of dysuria among inner-city women. Pyuria is usually present. Even in the absence of symptoms suggesting pelvic inflammatory disease, there may be purulent discharge from the urethral or cervical os. Risk factors that increase the likelihood of gonococcal urethritis are (1) a history of gonorrhea, (2) a recent sexual partner with urethral discharge, and (3) being an indigent inner-city woman.

Other Urethral Infections

Trichomonas vaginalis, Candida albicans, and *Herpes simplex* virus all can occasionally cause urethritis. Other associated symptoms and signs (e.g., cervicitis or vaginitis, vesicular eruptions) can suggest the diagnosis. Trichomonal urethritis typically produces pyuria, whereas candidal urethritis usually does not. Laboratory testing and standard treatment regimens for these organisms are discussed in Chapter 22.

No Recognized Pathogen

Despite extensive studies, no recognized pathogen can be found in some women with dysuria. These patients also often do not have pyuria and do not respond to antimicrobial treatment. This raises the possibility that they suffer from a urethritis caused by noninfectious factors. Postmenopausal, estrogen-deficient women may develop dysuria secondary to desiccation of the urethral and vaginal mucosa. Therefore the patient with acute dysuria, but without pyuria, ordinarily should not be given immediate treatment with antimicrobial agents.

Vaginitis

Vaginitis is an important and often neglected cause of dysuria and "negative" cultures. A patient with vaginitis may not mention vaginal symptoms as a presenting complaint, stating only that she has dysuria—perhaps because some patients are embarrassed to speak of symptoms affecting the genital organs. Vaginitis may be the most common cause of dysuria in some settings. Associated symptoms can include vaginal discharge or odor, vaginal itch, and dyspareunia. Dysuria caused by vaginitis typically is perceived as an external sharp somatic type of pain, caused by the impact of the stream of

Table 23-1
Categorization of Women with Acute Dysuria

Category	LOCATION			Colony Count[†]	Pyuria[‡]	Effectiveness of Antimicrobial Treatment
	Upper Tract*	Bladder	Urethra			
Acute pyelonephritis	+	+	±	>10,000	+	+
Subclinical pyelonephritis	+	+	±	>10,000	+	+
Lower urinary tract bacterial infection	−	+	+	>1000	+	+
Chlamydial urethritis	−	−	+	0-100	+	+
Gonococcal urethritis	−	−	+	0-100	+	+
Other urethritis	−	−	+	0-100	+	+
No recognized pathogen	−	?	+	0-100	−	−
Vaginitis	−	−	−	0-100	−	+

Modified from Komaroff AL: *N Engl J Med* 310:368, 1984.
* Or tissue-invasive infection.
† Colony count in colonies per milliliter.
‡ Pyuria typically is seen with gonorrheal and trichomonal urethritis but is not typically seen with monilial urethritis.

urine as it hits the irritated labia. In contrast, dysuria associated with urethritis typically is perceived as an internal, burning visceral type of pain. Also, urinary frequency and urgency are very unusual in patients with vaginitis.

Recurrent Dysuria

Some women are prone to recurring episodes of dysuria from repeated UTIs. Recurrent UTIs traditionally have been categorized as either reinfections with a new organism or relapses with the same organism. Reinfections generally indicate lower tract infection and account for most recurrences. Relapsing infection, as determined by DNA fingerprinting, has recently proven to be more common than was previously thought. The kind of relapsing infection that should cause the clinician concern is infection that follows within 14 days of completing a course of therapy; this is an indication of uneradicated infection, possibly because of functional or anatomic urinary tract abnormalities, and usually warrants diagnostic evaluation.

There is one practical problem that frequently arises in distinguishing a reinfection from a relapse. Although a recurrent infection with most bacterial species (e.g., a recurrent infection with enterococcus) indicates a relapse, a recurrent infection with *E. coli* may be either a reinfection with a new strain or a relapse from the old, uneradicated strain of *E. coli*. Relapse with the same strain can be assumed if both the former and the current isolate have an identical antibiogram. Vaginal and periurethral colonization has long been identified as the first step in UTI. From the periurethral "beachhead," organisms can begin their ascending spread up the urethra and into the rest of the urinary tract. Several factors seem to facilitate periurethral colonization. Vaginal colonization is increased when the number of vaginal H_2O_2-producing lactobacilli are reduced, such as often results from spermicide use.

The uroepithelial cells of girls and women prone to recurrent infection have glycolipid receptors that greatly increase the adherence for *E. coli;* these receptors, which are present in greater numbers even when these persons are uninfected, are genetically determined. Women who carry a gene that promotes the display of ABO and Lewis blood group antigens on the surface of epithelial cells are protected against recurrent UTIs, perhaps because these blood group antigens prevent bacteria from binding to the cell-associated receptors.

Certain behavioral factors also influence recurrence. Sexual intercourse transiently increases the concentration of bladder bacteria by as much as 10-fold. Intercourse encourages the retrograde movement of periurethral organisms up the urethra and into the bladder. Young women who have sexual intercourse three times a week have nearly three times the risk of developing a UTI, compared with young women who do not have intercourse. Use of a contraceptive diaphragm more than doubles the risk of developing UTIs. The spermicidal jelly (as well as spermicidal foam and condoms, but not oral contraceptives) dramatically increases vaginal and periurethral colonization, in part by reducing the number of H_2O_2-producing lactobacilli in the vagina (see previously). Oral contraceptive users have an increased frequency of asymptomatic bacteriuria, but it is not clear if this association is independent of sexual activity. Use of antimicrobial drugs for any reason in the last 15 to 28 days has been found to strongly predict recurrent UTI's in a careful prospective study. There is no strong evidence that any of the following

factors affect the risk of recurrent UTI: deferral of urination when the urge arises or after sexual intercourse, the direction of wiping after bowel movements, the type of menstrual protection, douching practices, the frequency with which the perineum is washed, or wearing occlusive underpants.

Sometimes, recurrent dysuria may be caused by chlamydial, gonorrheal, trichomonal, monilial, or herpetic urethritis. The natural history and proper management of these conditions are poorly understood. Interstitial cystitis, a disorder of uncertain cause, diagnosed by cystoscopic examination, occasionally causes recurrent cystitis (see Chapter 24).

⚑ EVALUATION OF ACUTE DYSURIA

How does the clinician approach a woman with acute dysuria (an initial or a recurrent attack) on the basis of the preceding information? Clinical data and easily available laboratory data allow the clinician to categorize the individual patient's condition with reasonable, although imperfect, accuracy.

History and Physical Examination

The clinical history guides the extent of the physical examination and laboratory testing (Table 23-2). The severity and duration of dysuria—urgency and frequency—should first be assessed.

The patient should always be asked about symptoms of vaginal discharge and irritation. Such symptoms strongly suggest vaginal infection; therefore a pelvic examination should be performed.

Risk factors suggestive of subclinical pyelonephritis should be sought: a known underlying functional or anatomic urinary tract abnormality, diabetes mellitus, an immunocompromised state, a history of urinary tract infections in childhood, documented relapsing UTI in the past, recent urinary tract instrumentation, symptoms for 7 to 10 days before seeking care (this also suggests chlamydial urethritis), three or more UTIs in the past year, or acute pyelonephritis in the past year. Subclinical pyelonephritis also may be more likely in indigent, inner-city residents who seek care in emergency departments.

The symptoms and signs of acute pyelonephritis—fever, rigors, flank pain, and costovertebral-angle tenderness, nausea and vomiting—reliably indicate the presence of acute pyelonephritis.

If by history one suspects chlamydial infection (see Chapter 22 for a more detailed discussion on diagnosis of chlamydial infection), a pelvic examination is warranted. Chlamydial urethritis often is seen in combination with

Table 23-2
Key Factors in the History and Physical Examination

History	Physical Examination
Vaginal discharge or pelvic pain or infertility	Pelvic examination
Prior UTIs	Examine for costovertebral angle tenderness
Diabetes	
Immunocompromised	
Symptoms or signs of acute pyelonephritis	

chlamydial cervicitis, an entity characterized by mucopurulent cervical discharge and edematous areas on the ectocervix. Although chlamydial cervicitis is generally responsive to the same therapeutic regimen as chlamydial urethritis, it is theoretically possible that patients with cervicitis are more likely to have indolent chlamydial pelvic infection; these patients might benefit from a careful history relating to infertility and might be counseled explicitly about returning for medical care in the case of symptoms that might suggest pelvic inflammatory disease.

Diagnostic Tests

Urinalysis and Urine Culture

Patients with likely acute or subclinical pyelonephritis should have urinalysis (including Gram stain) and urine culture performed (see box 23-1). If the patient's temperature is greater than 101° F or the patient appears toxic, blood cultures should be obtained.

In preparing to collect a urine specimen, the patient should clean the perineum simply with a gauze pad moistened with tap water or saline. Pads that contain disinfectants are widely used, and can artificially lower the colony count.

A Gram stain of uncentrifuged urine is considered indicative of greater than 100,000 bacteria per milliliter of urine if any organisms are seen, although this finding is more sensitive for bacillary rods than for cocci. Gram stain of sediment may be preferable because even in acute pyelonephritis, there can be fewer than 100,000 organisms per milliliter of urine.

Leukocyte esterase tests (part of urine dipstick testing) have a sensitivity ranging from 75% to 96% and a specificity ranging from 94% to 98%, when compared to either the finding of greater than 10 leukocytes per high power field or a culture with at least 100,000 organisms per milliliter of urine.

If there is no evidence to suggest any of the aforementioned conditions, the "diagnosis by exclusion" is still lower tract bacterial infection—which accounts for 60% to 70% of patients with dysuria. In such patients a urinalysis provides immediately useful information because patients who have pyuria will likely require only single-dose/short-course therapy. A urine culture is of less value in patients with presumptive lower tract bacterial infection, except in those patients with one or two previous symptomatic urinary infections during the past year. In such patients the possibility of relapse (and hence of upper tract infection) needs to be pursued by comparing the results of past urine cultures with a current culture. The best definition of a "positive" urine culture in a woman with dysuria is greater than 1000 bacteria per milliliter of urine, and the best definition in a women with symptoms and signs suggesting acute pyelonephritis is 10,000 bacteria per milliliter of urine. The traditional definition of a positive culture as greater than 100,000 (10^5) organisms has been shown to be insufficiently sensitive, missing as many as 50% of real, treatable lower urinary tract infections and 15% of cases of acute pyelonephritis.

Chlamydial Screening

In patients with the risk factors for chlamydial urethritis (described earlier), chlamydial screening during pelvic examination should be performed. A sensitive urine ligase chain reaction test for the amplified DNA of chlamydial organisms is noninvasive, highly sensitive (at least 90%), and specific (at least 98%); it should effectively replace earlier, much less sensitive, antigen detection tests in the urine.

Screening for Gonorrhea

In patients with risk factors for gonococcal urethritis (described earlier), a urethral culture for gonorrhea should be obtained. When purulent discharge from the urethral (or cervical) os is present, it should always undergo a Gram stain. A positive Gram stain result is a reliable indicator of gonorrhea and should lead to immediate treatment. When urethral or cervical discharge is not present, which can occur in gonococcal urethritis, the urethra should be swabbed. The swab needs to be inserted several millimeters into the urethra. The tip of a regular cotton swab is too large; therefore a calcium-alginate-tip swab should be used. The swab should be plated promptly on an appropriate medium (Thayer-Martin agar, or New York City agar) that has been prewarmed to room temperature. An alternative technique is a urine ligase chain reaction test for the gonococcus, which, like the urine ligase chain reaction test for chlamydia, is noninvasive, highly sensitive, and specific.

MANAGEMENT
Uncomplicated Lower Urinary Tract Bacterial Infection

In women with uncomplicated lower urinary tract bacterial infection, a 3-day course (even a single dose given in the office to a patient in whom compliance is uncertain) of oral therapy is nearly as effective as the traditional 7- to 14-day course in patients with lower tract infection (Table 23-3).

The benefits of short-course therapy are as follows:
1. A lower rate of medication side effects, particularly vaginal candidiasis, rash, and diarrhea
2. A reduced problem with noncompliance
3. A lower rate of emergence of resistant bacteria
4. Lower cost, as summarized elsewhere.

The best 3-day regimens are TMP-SMX, 160 to 800 mg twice a day, or (if allergic to TMP-SMX) ciprofloxacin 250 mg two times a day. Three-day short-course regimens appear slightly more effective than single-dose regimens in eradicating bacteriuria and are still associated with low rates of adverse drug reactions. Courses longer than 3 days offer no demonstrated benefits and cause more frequent adverse effects. The single-dose regimen that appears to be most effective is trimethoprim-sulfamethoxazole (TMP-SMX), 160 to 800 mg (one double-strength tablet) or 320 to 1600 mg (two double-strength tablets) by mouth. In

---

BOX 23-1
Diagnostic Tests

Urinalysis
Urine culture
If indicated (patient toxic, temperature 101° F), obtain blood cultures
Gram stain of uncentrifuged urine: if positive for organisms, indicates urine bacterial colony 100,000/ml
Chlamydial screening if clinically indicated, by culture or urine ligase test
Urethral testing for gonorrhea if clinically indicated

Table 23-3
Treatment for Uncomplicated Urinary Tract Infection

Medication	Dosage
Short-course Treatment	
Trimethoprim-sulfamethoxazole (TMP-SMX)	160 to 800 mg (one double-strength tablet) twice a day for 3 days
Fluoroquinolones*, if TMP-SMX-resistant organisms are common	250 mg twice a day for 3 days
Single-dose Treatment	
Trimethoprim-sulfamethoxazole (TMP-SMX)	160 to 800 mg (one double-strength tablet) or 320 to 1600 mg (two double-strength tablets)
TMP alone	200 mg

* Fluoroquinolones are contraindicated in pregnancy.

patients allergic to sulfonamides, trimethoprim alone (200 mg) is effective. Sulfonamides or ampicillin or amoxicillin, alone, are no longer optimal choices because of widespread resistance.

There is some evidence that short course therapy may be less effective in women over age 50 or in women infected with *Staphylococcus saprophyticus.*

Acute Pyelonephritis

The treatment of acute pyelonephritis is still a controversial area (Table 23-4). When the patient has a community-acquired case of acute pyelonephritis, is younger than 55 years old, is not diabetic, has no known underlying urinary tract abnormality, has no past history of acute pyelonephritis, is not pregnant, and is not very sick (temperature less than 101° F, normotensive, no rigors), outpatient management with oral antimicrobial agents is preferable.

For many years, TMP-SMX has been the antimicrobial of choice. However, in many US communities during the 1990s, an increasing number of bacteria causing UTIs have developed resistance to TMP-SMX; in such communities, fluoroquinolones have become preferred first-line therapy. Recent studies indicate that oral ciprofloxacin, 500 mg twice a day for 7 days, is very effective in premenopausal women with uncomplicated acute pyelonephritis. An alternative is to give one parenteral injection of gentamicin in the office or emergency room followed by oral antimicrobial agents. If the Gram stain result suggests enterococcal infection, ampicillin or amoxicillin is the treatment of choice.

When the patient with community-acquired acute pyelonephritis is more than 55 years old, has a known or suspected urinary tract abnormality, is experiencing a recurrence of acute pyelonephritis, is diabetic or is immunocompromised in some way, or is very sick, she should be hospitalized and started on intravenous therapy. If the patient is having a recurrent UTI, particularly if a prior episode has occurred within the past 6 months, the results of the urine culture and sensitivities from the prior episode (along with the Gram stain of the current urine) should guide therapy. Of the quinolones, ciprofloxacin may be the preferred agent; it provides broad-spectrum coverage against both gram-negative and most

Table 23-4
Treatment Options for Acute Pyelonephritis

Type	Management
Uncomplicated course	**Gram-negative Bacteria** TMP-SMX 160 to 800 mg twice a day for 10 to 14 days If TMP-SMX-resistant organisms common in the community, any of several fluoroquinolones for 10 to 14 days
	Enterococcus Ampicillin 500 mg q8h Amoxicillin 500 mg q8h
Complicated	Hospitalize
Toxic (temperature >101° F, hypotensive or rigors) Diabetic Immunocompromised Older than 55 years Known underlying urinary tract abnormality	**Gram-negative Bacteria** Parenteral fluoroquinolone* or Parenteral aminoglycoside or Parenteral extended-spectrum cephalosporin ***Enterococcus*** Amoxicillin 500 mg IV q8h **Unclear Pathogen or Polymicrobial** Ciprofloxacin 200 to 400 mg IV q12h*
Pregnancy	See Chapter 78

* Fluoroquinolones are contraindicated in pregnancy.

gram-positive organisms, is particularly good in the rare case of community-acquired *Pseudomonas* UTI, has excellent tissue penetration even in patients with renal failure, and has relatively little toxicity. If the patient refuses hospitalization, treatment with oral ciprofloxacin is probably the best option except if the patient is pregnant or considering pregnancy. Careful recent prospective studies have found that it is safe to discharge patients from the hospital promptly after discontinuing intravenous antimicrobial therapy and sending them home on oral agents.

Treatment of pyelonephritis during pregnancy is covered in Chapter 78.

Subclinical Pyelonephritis

For suspected subclinical pyelonephritis, immediate treatment for 10 to 14 days should be initiated before the culture result returns (Box 23-2). Pooled data from several trials indicate that 10 days of therapy with TMP-SMX may be the most effective, having only a 1% failure rate (in contrast, single-dose TMP-SMX had a 16% failure rate). However, in communities with increasing resistance to TMP-SMX, as noted previously, the fluoroquinolones may be preferable. There are no good randomized studies comparing alternative antimicrobial regimens in patients with subclinical pyelonephritis. When the urinalysis indicates gram-positive cocci in chains, indicating the likelihood of enterococcal infection, ampicillin or amoxicillin would be the treatment of choice. Every effort should be made to obtain a follow-up culture 2 to 4 days after the end of therapy,

---

BOX 23-2
Treatment of Subclinical Pyelonephritis

10-14 days of treatment
TMP-SMX for 10 days; fluoroquinolones, if TMP-SMX-resistant organisms are common in the community
If enterococcus, then ampicillin or amoxicillin
Follow-up urine culture

---

because patients with subclinical pyelonephritis may be particularly prone to relapse. In patients with recurrent infection caused by the same organism (relapsing infection), treatment for 6 weeks may be indicated, although this is another poorly studied area. In patients who experience relapse after a 6-week course of therapy, diagnostic studies to look for a cause of the persistent infection (e.g., intravenous pyelogram and retrograde studies) are indicated.

Chlamydial Urethritis

For patients with chlamydial urethritis, as well as those with low-count bacteriuria, the best current treatment is probably azithromycin, 1 g taken orally as a single dose. An alternative is doxycycline, 100 mg twice a day for 10 days (see box 23-3). Less-expensive regimens of tetracycline hydrochloride, 500 mg four times a day for 7 days, or erythromycin, 500 mg four times a day for 7 days, probably would be equally effective. Also, patients with chlamydial urethritis should be counseled to return promptly if dysuria recurs. Partners of these patients need to be treated, and the clinician should counsel the woman to abstain from sexual intercourse until the partner has been treated.

Gonococcal Urethritis

For gonococcal urethritis diagnosed by a positive finding on Gram stain or culture should be treated with ceftriaxone, 250 mg intramuscularly once plus oral doxycycline, 100 mg twice a day for 7 days. Again, partners need to be treated, and the woman needs to abstain from sexual intercourse until completion of the partner's therapy.

Symptomatic Relief

Urinary analgesics such as phenazopyridine, 200 mg taken orally three times a day, can be useful when dysuria is severe, but should be used for no more than 2 days because of the risk of allergic reactions and because proper antimicrobial therapy should itself greatly reduce symptoms within 48 hours.

RECURRENT URINARY TRACT INFECTION
Diagnostic Tests

A single episode of relapsing infection, as previously defined, or three or more infections in the past year with the same organism (persistent infection), can reasonably be pursued with intravenous pyelography (IVP) and cystoscopic examination. However, urologic abnormalities are unusual in people who have responded promptly to antimicrobial therapy.

IVP and cystoscopy are less clearly indicated when patients have three or more infections in the past year with dif-

---

BOX 23-3
Treatment of Chlamydial and Gonococcal Urethritis

Chlamydial Urethritis
Azithromycin, 1 g po × 1
    Alternatives:
    Doxycycline 100 mg PO bid for 10 days
    Tetracycline hydrochloride 500 mg 4 times a day for 7 days
    Erythromycin 500 mg 4 times a day for 7 days
Advise partners to seek treatment
Advise patient to abstain from sexual intercourse until partner is fully treated

Gonococcal Urethritis
Ceftriaxone 250 mg IM once plus
Doxycycline 100 mg PO bid for 7 days for potential associated chlamydial infection
Advise partners to seek treatment
Advise patient to abstain from sexual intercourse until partner is fully treated

---

ferent organisms (reinfections). Three studies of the yield of IVP and cystoscopic examination in women with recurrent UTI have been conducted in recent years, but unfortunately none clearly distinguishes relapse from reinfection in the patients studied. On the basis of other studies, it is likely that most of the patients studied were experiencing reinfections. The three studies found that IVP revealed a surgically correctable lesion in fewer than 1% of patients, although cystoscopic examination revealed a correctable lesion (e.g., urethral diverticulum) in up to 4% of patients. Because these studies suggest a somewhat higher yield from cystoscopic examination, without the radiation exposure and dye risk of IVP, cystoscopy is recommended before IVP, although this may not be a choice because urologists often insist on an IVP before performing cystoscopy. When the patient has experienced three or more reinfections in a year, a referral to a urologist should be considered, although the yield of urologic evaluation still will be low.

Although IVP has been the standard imaging technique for years, contemporary ultrasound is proving to be at least as accurate and avoids both the dye and radiation risks.

✳ MANAGEMENT

Antimicrobial prophylaxis can be recommended in a woman who has had three or more bacterial infections in a year. Antimicrobial prophylaxis greatly reduces the frequency of recurrent infection during the period of prophylaxis and for a few months thereafter. TMP-SMX, one half of a regular-strength tablet (40 to 200 mg) each day, taken for 6 to 12 months, appears to be the most effective regimen (Table 23-5).

In women whose recurrences are clearly related to sexual activity, use of the spermicide nonoxynol-9 should be discontinued and a single dose of an antimicrobial taken at the time of intercourse. Oral TMP-SMX, 40 to 200 mg (half of a single-strength dose), nitrofurantoin, 50 mg, or oral cephalexin, 250 mg, is effective.

Table 23-5
Prophylactic Therapy for Recurrent Urinary Tract Infections

Medication	Dosage
TMP-SMX	One half regular-strength tablet (40-200 mg) PO qd
	If associated with sexual activity, take at time of intercourse
TMP-SMX	One half regular-strength tablet (40-200 mg) or one regular-strength tablet (80-400 mg) PO
Cephalexin	250 mg PO qd

"Self-start therapy" also works well for women with recurrent infections who are not on a daily prophylaxis regimen; the woman keeps an antimicrobial agent in the medicine cabinet. Most women with recurrent UTI can reliably identify symptoms indicating that a recurrent UTI is beginning and can quickly eradicate the infection by the immediate use of antimicrobial agents for a 3-day short course of therapy.

Finally, in postmenopausal women with recurrent UTIs, intravaginal estrogen can dramatically reduce the frequency of infection, probably by increasing vaginal lactobacilli (which compete with urinary pathogens) as well as by lowering the vaginal pH.

BIBLIOGRAPHY

Brunham RC et al: Mucopurulent cervicitis—the ignored counterpart in women of urethritis in men, *N Engl J Med* 311:1, 1984.

Dunn AS et al: The utility of an in-hospital observation period after discontinuing intravenous antibiotics, *Am J Med* 106:6, 1999.

Fihn SD et al: Association between diaphragm use and urinary tract infection, *JAMA* 254:240, 1985.

Fowler JE, Pulaski ET: Excretory urography, cystography, and cystoscopy in the evaluation of women with urinary tract infection: a prospective study, *N Engl J Med* 304:462, 1981.

Gupta K et al: Inverse association of H_2O_2-producing lactobacilli and vaginal *Escherichia coli* colonization in women with recurrent urinary tract infection, *J Infect Dis* 178:446, 1998.

Hooton TM et al: A prospective study of risk factors for symptomatic urinary tract infection in young women, *N Engl J Med* 335:468, 1996.

Hooton TM, Stamm WE: Diagnosis and treatment of uncomplicated urinary tract infection, *Infect Dis Clin North Am* 11:551, 1997.

Johnson JR, Stamm WE: Urinary tract infections in women: diagnosis and treatment, *Ann Intern Med* 111:906, 1989.

Komaroff AL: Acute dysuria in women, *N Engl J Med* 310:368, 1984.

Komaroff AL et al: Management strategies for urinary and vaginal infections, *Arch Intern Med* 138:1069, 1978.

Latham RH, Running K, Stamm WE: Urinary tract infections in young adult women caused by *Staphylococcus saprophyticus*, *JAMA* 250:3063, 1983.

O'Hanley P et al: Gal-Gal binding and hemolysin phenotypes and genotypes associated with uropathogenic *Escherichia coli*, *N Engl J Med* 313:414, 1985.

Raz R, Stamm WE: A controlled trial of intravaginal estriol in postmenopausal women with recurrent urinary tract infections, *N Engl J Med* 329:753, 1993.

Schaeffer AJ, Jones JM, Dunn JK: Association of in vitro *Escherichia coli* adherence to vaginal and buccal epithelial cells with susceptibility of women to recurrent urinary-tract infections, *N Engl J Med* 304:1062, 1981.

Shafer M-A, Pantell RH, Schacter J: Is the routine pelvic examination needed with the advent of urine-based screening for sexually transmitted diseases? *Arch Pediatr Adolesc Med* 153:119, 1999.

Sheinfeld J et al: Association of the Lewis blood-group phenotype with recurrent urinary tract infections in women, *N Engl J Med* 320:773, 1989.

Smith HS et al: Antecedent antimicrobial use increases the risk of uncomplicated cystitis in young women, *Clin Infect Dis* 25:63, 1997.

Spencer J, Lindsell D, Mastorakou I: Ultrasonography compared with intravenous urography in investigation of urinary tract infection in adults, *Br Med J* 301:221, 1990.

Stamm WE, Hooton TM: Management of urinary tract infections in adults, *N Engl J Med* 329:1328, 1993.

Stamm WE et al: Causes of the acute urethral syndrome in women, *N Engl J Med* 303:409, 1980.

Stapleton A et al: Postcoital antimicrobial prophylaxis for recurrent urinary tract infection, *JAMA* 264:703, 1990.

Stapleton A, Stamm WE: Prevention of urinary tract infection. *Infect Dis Clin of N Amer* 11:719, 1997.

Talan DA et al: Comparison of ciprofloxacin (7 days) and trimethoprim-sulfamethoxazole (14 days) for acute uncomplicated pyelonephritis in women. A randomized trial. *JAMA* 283:1583, 2000.

Warren JW et al: Guidelines for antimicrobial treatment of uncomplicated acute bacterial cystitis and acute pyelonephritis in women, *Clin Infect Dis* 29:745, 1999.

Wong ES et al: Management of recurrent urinary tract infections with patient-administered single-dose therapy, *Ann Intern Med* 102:302, 1985.

CHAPTER 24

Chronic Bladder Disorders and Chronic Dysuria

Joseph A. Grocela
Neeraj Rastogi

The pathophysiologic mechanisms of lower urinary tract disorders are varied, encompassing many neurologic, anatomic, hormonal, and infectious causes. Similarly, symptom complexes may vary somewhat for each disorder, although they may overlap among different disorders. Imagining a continuum between purely sensory symptoms (e.g., dysuria, dyspareunia, frequency, urgency) and purely motor symptoms (incontinence) may simplify the initial approach. Most symptom complexes fall somewhere between the two but show a predominance of one symptom type. Loosely, then, urinary tract disorders may be categorized as primarily sensory or primarily motor.

This chapter considers the primarily sensory disorders: those associated with chronic irritative symptoms of dysuria, frequency, urgency, and, occasionally, pelvic pain and dyspareunia. Lower urinary tract bacterial infections and urethritis, which sometimes cause chronic irritative symptoms, are discussed in greater detail in Chapter 23. Evaluation of dysuria in pregnancy is also discussed in Chapter 23. Chapter 54 addresses the predominantly motor disorders (incontinence) and prolapse.

INTERSTITIAL CYSTITIS

Interstitial cystitis (IC) encompasses a major portion of the "painful bladder" disease complex, which includes bladder and/or pelvic pain, chronic irritative voiding symptoms (urgency, frequency, nocturia, dysuria), and negative urine cultures. One problem with defining IC is that the symptoms are allodynic—an exaggeration of normal sensations. With no pathognomonic findings on pathologic examination, IC is truly a diagnosis of exclusion. It may have multiple causes and represent a final common reaction of the bladder to different types of insults.

Epidemiology and Definition

What is known of the epidemiology of IC is based on several case series from specialty clinics. The prevalence of IC per se is unknown, but its ulcerative variant accounts for 5% to 20% of patients. The disorder is diagnosed most frequently in white women. Women with IC have a higher frequency of immunopathologic abnormalities (allergies to medications, allergic rhinitis, asthma, food allergies, and

rheumatoid arthritis) and irritable bowel syndrome than do control subjects. The triad of clinical findings of IC includes:

- Characteristic painful bladder symptoms
- Exclusion of specific diseases (bacterial or tuberculous cystitis, bladder cancer, etc.)
- Petechial bleeding at cystoscopy.

Etiology

The etiology of IC continues to remain elusive. Multiple factors are capable of causing the symptoms of IC, so one cannot look at this syndrome as a single disease. Different initiating insults could result in activation of specific pathogenic pathways that result in the classic symptom complex. Current concepts are summarized below.

It is possible that **infection** could work in concert with other mechanisms, leading to bladder injury or an autoimmune reaction. It is also possible that infection can lead directly to an autoimmune response and subsequent bladder injury.

Mast cells have frequently been reported to be associated with IC. Mast cells contain granules, which secrete many vasoactive and nociceptive molecules. Although it is not pathognomonic of the disease, detrusor mastocytosis does occur in a significant subset of IC patients.

It is hypothesized that in a subset of patients, IC is the result of some **defect in the epithelial permeability barrier** of the bladder surface glycosaminoglycans (GAGs). The GAG layer functions as a permeability and antiadherence barrier. Strong evidence for the role of a mucosal leak was reported by Parsons and Stein. Water or 0.4 mol/L potassium chloride (KCl) was placed intravesically into normal volunteers and IC patients. Water did not provoke symptoms in either group, but KCl provoked symptoms in 5% of normal subjects and 70% of IC patients.

The **urine toxicity** theory of pathogenesis postulates access of a component of urine to the interstices of the bladder wall, resulting in an inflammatory response induced by toxic, allergic, or immunologic means. Perhaps the best circumstantial evidence for urine toxicity in IC relates to the failure of substitution cystoplasty and continent diversions in some patients because of development of pain or contraction of the bowel segment over time, and to histologic findings similar to those of IC found in bowel used to augment the small capacity IC bladder.

Diagnosis

As IC is primarily a diagnosis of exclusion, the evaluation includes a thorough history, physical examination, urodynamic evaluation if needed, appropriate urine cultures, and cytologic examination, and may include cystoscopy under anesthesia with hydrodistention of the bladder as well as bladder biopsy (Table 24-1). Although many dispute the need for the urodynamic studies, urodynamics may not only help to assess bladder compliance and sensation, but also may reproduce the patient's symptoms during bladder filling. In addition, urodynamics may help to rule out bladder instability, keeping in mind that patients with discrete, involuntary bladder contractions do not have IC by exclusion criteria.

Arguably, cystoscopy can be performed under local anesthesia without biopsy if the urine cytology and cultures are negative. However in certain groups of patients, cystoscopy may be therapeutic, in which case it should be performed with the patient under general anesthesia to allow sufficient distention of the bladder. Glomerulations are not specific for IC, and should be viewed as significant only when seen in conjunction with the clinical criteria of frequency, pain, and urgency.

There are no pathognomonic histopathologic features of the disease. The role of histopathology in the diagnosis of IC is primarily one of excluding other possible diagnoses. One must rule out carcinoma, tuberculous cystitis, and eosinophilic cystitis, as well as any other entities with a specific tissue diagnosis. Until then, IC is a diagnosis of exclusion, and excluding other diseases that are pathologically identifiable is now the primary use of bladder biopsy in this group of patients.

Treatment

As long as causative factors are unknown, both patient and physician must understand that there is no sure cure for IC, nor is there likely to be a treatment that is effective in reducing symptoms for every patient. Patient education remains the cornerstone of successful therapy. Many patients, however, can benefit from one treatment or a combination of treatments. Most can be maintained in a stable state, punctuated by exacerbations and remissions.

Initial Approach

Hydrodistention of the bladder with the patient under anesthesia, although technically a surgical treatment, is usually the first therapeutic modality used, often as part of the diagnostic evaluation. One approach is to perform an initial cystoscopic examination, obtain urine for cytologic examination, and distend the bladder for 1 to 2 minutes at a pressure of 80 cm H_2O. The bladder is then refilled to establish the diagnosis. A therapeutic hydraulic distention then follows for another 8 minutes. Biopsy follows the second distention.

Responses are seen in 30% to 40% of cases but are usually temporary. Repeat distention may be performed if needed. Acute hydrodistention does not seem to result in any long-term bladder dysfunction. A bladder capacity with the patient under anesthesia of less than 200 ml suggests that medical therapy is less likely to be successful.

Medical Therapy

Amitriptyline has become a staple of oral treatment for IC, with success rates of 64% to 90% at a range of follow-up time of 2 to 14 months. A dosage of 10 mg at bedtime, increased to 25 mg over 2 weeks, is recommended.

The antihistamine **hydroxyzine** may be used, with 25 mg given before bedtime and increased over 2 weeks (if sedation is not a problem) to 50 mg at night and 25 mg in the morning. Hydroxyzine appears to be most effective in the premenopausal woman with biopsy-documented bladder mastocytosis or mast cell activation and a history of allergies.

Pentosan polysulfate (Elmiron) is an agent that replenishes the GAG layer. Results of treatment with pentosan polysulfate, either alone or in combination, have been variable. The dose is 100 mg three times daily.

Various other oral preparations such as the calcium channel blocker nifedepine, the opiate antagonist nalmefene, antispasmodic agents, L-arginine, and the prostaglandin analog misoprostol have been used with variable success.

Intravesical Therapy

The mainstay of treatment of IC is intravesical instillation of **dimethyl sulfoxide (DMSO),** the only drug therapy approved by the Food and Drug Administration. DMSO can be administered alone or as a part of an intravesical

---

Table 24-1
Exclusion and Inclusion Criteria for the Diagnosis of Interstitial Cystitis

Automatic Exclusion	Automatic Inclusion	Positive Factors (2 are required)
Under 18 years of age		Pain on bladder filling, relieved by emptying
Waking frequency <8 times/day		Pain (suprapubic, urethral, pelvic, vaginal)
Bladder cancer		
Radiation cystitis		
Cyclophosphamide cystitis		
Bacterial cystitis		
Bladder stone		
Lower ureteric stone		
Cystoscopic Findings		
Hunner's ulcer and glomerulations		Glomerulations
Cystometric Findings		
Involuntary bladder contractions		Decreased compliance
Capacity of >350 ml		
Absence of urgency with bladder filled to 150 ml of water		

"cocktail" that can include steroids, heparin, and bicarbonate (the latter may enhance the antiinflammatory actions of the DMSO-steroid combination). Treatment regimens are variable and can include 1 to 2 weekly instillations for 4 to 8 weeks. A mixture of 50 ml of 50% DMSO, 10,000 units of heparin, 10 mg triamcinolone, and 44 mEq bicarbonate, instilled intravesically weekly for 6 weeks, has shown an objective response rate of more than 90%.

An alternative for intravesical therapy is sodium oxychlorosene (Clorpactin WCS 90).

Nerve Stimulation

The primary intention in applying transcutaneous peripheral electric nerve stimulation in IC is to relieve pain by stimulating myelinated afferent fibers in order to activate segmental inhibitory circuits. This modality is in early trial stages at this time.

Surgical Therapy

Surgical therapy for IC has been considered a last resort after all trials of conservative treatments have failed. Many experts argue that surgical therapy has no role in the treatment of IC. Surgery has typically been reserved for patients with extremely severe unresponsive disease, a group that accounts for less than 10% of patients. Many surgical approaches, including transurethral resection, neodymium: YAG laser ablation of Hunner's ulcer, and supratrigonal cystectomy with augmentation, have been tried with variable results. The procedure of choice after all other options have been exhausted for a desperate patient may be simple cystectomy with supravesical diversion.

LOWER URINARY TRACT INFECTIONS

Occasionally, persistent bacterial infections of the lower urinary tract may manifest as chronic dysuria. The vast majority of "chronic infections" are actually **sequential infections** caused by different organisms. Reinfections result from inoculation of bladder urine in the sterile urinary system by enterobacteria from vaginal and fecal flora. They may be occasional or frequent. Susceptibility to frequent reinfections is due to enhanced colonization of the vaginal mucosa by enterobacteria.

Persistent infections as opposed to reinfections are characterized by sequential infections caused by the same organism. These infections usually result from continued inoculation of urine by an infected focus within the urinary system.

Virtually all urinary tract infections begin in the lower tract through bacterial adherence phenomena, creating simple uncomplicated infections in otherwise healthy hosts and sometimes serious, complicated infections in others. The diagnosis is usually straightforward, based on the presence of pyuria and growth of bacterial culture (see Chapter 23).

URETHRAL SYNDROME

The term *urethral syndrome* is used liberally to label the symptoms of frequency and voiding dysfunction commonly seen by the urologist in female patients. There is no known pathology typical to this condition, and the cause is obscure. The symptoms vary greatly from patient to patient, but frequency and urgency are always present. Symptoms may also include burning with urination or dysuria, which often leads to misdiagnosis of a urinary tract infection.

Pain or discomfort in the lower abdomen also tends to be a major component of this condition. Discomfort may be relieved with the passage of urine. This is an important point to elicit in the history, as it implies that relaxation of the urethral sphincter is accompanied by easing of symptoms. Similarly, symptoms such as hesitancy, dribbling, or an intermittent stream also implicate the external urethral sphincter in that they represent a complete or partial failure of sphincteric relaxation. Stress incontinence is not part of the syndrome.

The cause of urethral syndrome is obscure, but the following features are worth noting. Most patients are between 25 and 45 years old, a time when urinary tract infections are common. Indeed symptoms are irritative and it is therefore easy to consider that infection of periurethral glands may initiate a sphincteric irritation, which then becomes chronic. In addition, there may be elements of urethral syndrome related to resting urethral sphincter tension, voiding habits, and psychological components. Infection may not be the primary cause, but a secondary aggravating feature may occur largely because of inefficiencies in the washout of bacteria from the bladder during voiding. Excessive use of Kegel exercises may contribute to the problem by interfering with washout of bacteria from the bladder. Some experts believe poor voiding habits may be as much a factor in the cause of the problems as tissue changes resulting from urinary tract infections, childbirth, age, or minor but repeated trauma.

Diagnosis

Videourodynamic studies are now integral to the understanding and diagnosis of the urethral syndrome. Voiding dysfunction, symptoms of irritation (hypersensitivity), and discomfort in these patients correlate directly with the high pressure or instability or both that can be demonstrated urodynamically in the external sphincter. Typically higher than normal closure pressures in the external sphincter and unstable (spastic) behavior will be apparent in response to bladder filling. During a voiding attempt, dysfunction of the external sphincter will be clearly evident as nonrelaxation, delayed relaxation, or dyssynergic activity.

The site of urgency and hypersensitivity typically overlaps the zone of greatest sphincteric tone and is not difficult to appreciate clinically. Urethral dilation may be met with more resistance and more pain than normal. Even passing a catheter or a cystoscope through the zone of the external sphincter will provoke a sense of tension and discomfort. Distention of the anal sphincter or pressure on the levator muscles that pass along the sidewalls of the anal sphincter may also be associated with pain and discomfort. Such simple techniques immediately implicate the levator muscles and intrinsic musculature of the sphincters as the focal point of discomfort. The degree of tension can then be quantified objectively during urodynamic recordings.

Movement of a catheter in the urethra will usually duplicate the patient's symptoms of urgency and discomfort, being most easily elicited at the level of the external sphincter. During testing, the clinician can clearly demonstrate to the patient inappropriate behavior of the levator and sphincter muscles, which can then help her to relearn proper voiding techniques, namely the conscious suppression of spastic urethral behavior.

One factor common to many patients is the inability to tighten and relax the pelvic floor muscles selectively and voluntarily. This inefficient movement of the perineum suggests a dissociation of conscious control over the proper use of these muscles.

Treatment

Patients demonstrating clear evidence of dysfunctional external sphincter behavior affecting evacuation of the bladder are the most amenable to therapy. The most important therapeutic intervention is to **retrain voiding habits.** The voluntary tightening and relaxation of the pelvic musculature throughout the urodynamic evaluation provides an important baseline assessment of the patient's ability to suppress the spastic behavior or inappropriate tightening of the external sphincter voluntarily. The patient should be able, at the completion of the urodynamic assessment, to appreciate what is required to restore voluntary control over the involuntary, abnormal behavior of the external sphincter. Indeed, this appreciation is the essence of biofeedback.

Medication may assist in this regard, and two common classes used are the alpha blockers and skeletal muscle relaxants (cyclobenzamine or diazepam). The two classes are usually used in combination. The best chance for improvement is through better voiding habits and the use of standard hygienic precautions against urinary tract infections.

Some patients with urodynamically proven evidence of spastic behavior within the external sphincter during voiding can reach a point at which they are crippled by their symptoms and refractory to most forms of therapy. Some of these patients may be treated with **neurostimulation.** The basis for using nerve stimulation as a treatment of the urethral syndrome lies in its ability to fatigue muscle. Neurostimulation is selective in its effect; it will fatigue erratic behavior of the striated muscles (hyperreflexive behavior), but will not affect the normal intrinsic sphincter tone.

URETHRAL DIVERTICULUM

Urethral diverticulum in women is common and usually presents between the third and fifth decades. Most cases in women are acquired, resulting from infection of the periurethral glands with subsequent rupture into the urethral lumen. Other etiologies include urethral injury during childbirth, surgery, or repetitive trauma from catheterization.

The pathognomonic presentation is uncommon and consists of episodic postvoid dribbling, urethral pain (as a result of persistent infection), a tender periurethral mass (resulting from pus, stone, or malignancy within), or expression of pus from the urethra on physical examination. Most patients present episodically with nonspecific, refractory, lower urinary tract symptoms and undergo extensive evaluation and empirical treatments before the correct diagnosis is established. Therefore, clinical awareness and a high index of suspicion are essential in making the definitive diagnosis and formulating a treatment plan.

On physical examination the most common pathognomonic finding is a palpable tender cystic swelling (in about 50% of cases) in the anterior vaginal wall. "Milking" of diverticular contents via the urethral meatus is another pathog-

nomonic finding of urethral diverticulum. Regardless of size or complexity, a diverticulum may or may not be palpable or tender and may arise at any point along the circumference and length of the urethra.

Diagnosis

Most cases present as diagnostic dilemmas and are diagnosed and treated by physicians as stress incontinence, urge incontinence, chronic cystitis, urethral syndrome, vulvovestibulitis, cystocele, sensory urgency, idiopathic chronic pelvic pain, and psychosomatic disorders. Obstetricians should be vigilant regarding the possibility of this condition in pregnant or postpartum women with pain, incontinence, or difficulty voiding.

Initial diagnostic measures for the evaluation of a patient with a suspected urethral diverticulum usually include vaginal examination, cystourethroscopy, voiding cystourethrography, and double-catheter urethrography. Cystourethroscopy may allow direct visualization of the diverticular orifice and occasionally, expression of pus or retained urine by digital compression of the mass. Transvaginal digital compression of the vesical neck at cystoscopy may maximize visualization by distending the urethral mucosal folds.

Voiding cystourethrography is a useful diagnostic tool with a detection rate of 65%. Voiding cystourethrography may also reveal "paradoxical stress incontinence" caused by loss of retained urine in the diverticulum during coughing.

In patients in whom a urethral diverticulum is strongly suspected and voiding cystourethrography is equivocal or nonconfirmatory, ultrasound or magnetic resonance imaging (MRI) may be useful adjuncts, particularly when the neck of the diverticulum is functionally occluded.

Transvaginal ultrasound examination may detect a urethral diverticulum that does not fill with contrast material and may further delineate the size, number, location, content, and wall thickness of a diverticulum. However, other cystic lesions such as a Gartener's cyst, vaginal inclusion cyst, ectopic ureterocele, or endometrioma cannot be differentiated from a urethral diverticulum by ultrasound examination alone. MRI, because of its multiplanar capabilities and excellent tissue contrast, is highly recommended when clinical findings strongly suggest a urethral diverticulum.

There is no need to treat asymptomatic diverticula. Transvaginal diverticulectomy is highly effective treatment for urethral diverticulum.

POSTMENOPAUSAL ATROPHY

The postmenopausal woman is frequently more difficult to treat than the premenopausal woman in terms of recurrent cystitis, because she may have more frequent episodes but recurrences caused by an ever changing variety of bacterial species. These individuals tend to be difficult to suppress because they continue to become reinfected with different organisms or become resistant to the drug most recently used. These problems may occur because the source of infection is the perineal flora. The pH of their vaginal secretions is significantly elevated, usually in the range of 7.0, because of lack of estrogen stimulation. As a result, many different rectal organisms will grow in the vaginal introitus.

This problem can be controlled by eliminating this "abnormal" flora from the vagina and urethra. Estrogen will accomplish this readily, but oral estrogens frequently do not suffice. Half an applicator (1 g) of Premarin vaginal cream applied once or twice per week will rapidly reduce the pH of vaginal secretions to 4.0. Once this occurs, the gram-negative bacteria in the perineum will be reduced or disappear, which allows the urine to remain sterile more often.

BIBLIOGRAPHY

Anderson RU: Management of lower urinary tract infections and cystitis, *Urol Clin North Am* 26:729, 1999.

Batra AK, Hanno PM, Wein AJ: Interstitial cystitis. AUA update series. 1999. Lesson 2. Volume xix.

Blaivas LB et al: Urethral diverticulum in women: diverse presentations resulting in diagnostic delay and management, *J Urol* 164:428, 2000.

Daneshgari F, Zimmern PE, Jacomides L: MRI detection of symptamatic noncommunicating intraurethral wall diverticula in women, *J Urol* 161:1259, 1999.

Fleischmann J: Calcium channel antagonists in the treatment of interstitial cystitis, *Urol Clin North Am* 21:107, 1994.

Fontanna D, Porpiglia F, Morra I: Transvaginal ultrasonography in assessment of organic diseases of the female urethra, *J Ultrasound Med* 18:237, 1999.

Ganabathi K et al: Experience with management of urethral diverticulum in 63 women, *J Urol* 152:1445, 1994.

Hanno PM: Amitriptyline in the treatment of IC, *Urol Clin North Am* 21:89, 1994.

Hanno PM: Diagnosis of interstitial cystitis, *Urol Clin North Am* 21:63, 1994.

Khati, NJ et al: MR imaging diagnosis of a urethral diverticulum, *Radiographics* 18:517, 1998.

Koziol IA: Epidemology of interstitial cystitis, *Urol Clin North Am* 21:7, 1994.

Parsons CL et al: Abnormal sensitivity to intravesical potassium in interstitial cystitis and radiation cystitis, *Neurourol Urodyn* 13:515, 1994.

Sant GR, La Rock DR: Standard intravesical therapies for interstitial cystitis, *Urol Clin North Am* 21:73, 1994.

Sant GR, Theoharides TC: The role of mast cells in interstitial cystitis, *Urol Clin North Am* 21:41, 1994.

Smith SD et al: Improvement in interstitial cystitis symptom scores during treatment with oral l-arginine, *J Urol* 158:703, 1997.

Theoharides TC, Sant GC: Hydroxyzine therapy for interstitial cystitis, *Urology* 49 (5A):108, 1997.

Warren JW: Interstitial cystitis as an infectious disease, *Urol Clin North Am* 21:31, 1994.

Wein AJ, Broderic GA: Interstitial cystitis: current and future approaches to diagnosis and treatment, *Urol Clin North Am* 21:153, 1994.

CHAPTER 25

Renal Insufficiency

Elizabeth S. Ginsburg
Julian Lawrence Seifter
Jennifer Ho

Renal insufficiency can have a tremendous impact on the endocrinologic, reproductive, and sexual function of women. This chapter focuses on the various effects in women of acute and chronic renal insufficiency, dialysis, renal transplantation, as well as the impact of renal disease on pregnancy, and that of pregnancy on the progression of preexisting renal disease.

⌘ APPROACH TO THE PATIENT WITH SUSPECTED RENAL DISEASE

Interpreting Serum Creatinine and Blood Urea Nitrogen in Women

There are no prospective studies that evaluate women with mild elevations in the serum creatinine and blood urea nitrogen (BUN) levels to determine the incidence of clinically significant renal failure. Nor are there established recommendations for routine screening of renal function in the nonpregnant woman.

Many factors can affect the measurement of creatinine and BUN (Box 25-1). When assessing these values, one must keep in mind that women have smaller muscle mass than men, and therefore in the normal state, they have lower serum creatinine levels. Thus for each level of creatinine, there is potentially more compromise of the glomerular filtration rate (GFR) for women than for men, necessitating further evaluation for etiologic factors. Table 25-1 compares the laboratory reference ranges for renal function in women and men.

Gender differences in normal creatinine are also important when considering the use of potentially nephrotoxic medications such as aminoglycosides. A serum creatinine value of 1.5 may be normal in a humans but reflects renal insufficiency in a woman and would be an indicator for adjusting the dose of a nephrotoxic agent.

Once an elevation of creatinine has been established on serial testing (even if mild), an estimate of the GFR should be obtained by ordering a 24-hour urine collection for creatinine clearance. Because little data exist on the natural history of abnormal creatinine levels in women, there are no standard recommendations for follow-up monitoring. Generally, evaluation of the BUN, creatinine, and electrolytes is performed every 3 to 4 months until stable, then annually. Evaluation for potential causes must be pursued when renal

insufficiency is diagnosed because the risk of progression to renal failure is dependent on the etiology. Causes and procedures for evaluation are listed in Box 25-2.

ACUTE RENAL FAILURE
Definition

The definition of acute renal failure (ARF) is a fall in GFR that occurs over a period of hours or days. Strictly speaking, ARF is an increase in serum creatinine levels by 0.5 mg/dl if the baseline is 2.5 to 3.0 mg/dl or less and an increase by 1.0 mg/dl if the baseline is higher. It is associated with substantial morbidity and mortality.

Epidemiology and Etiology

A recent population-based study reported the incidence of ARF to be 172 per 1 million adults, with prostatic disease accounting for the largest proportion of cases. After excluding these cases, men still have been found to be 2.8 times more likely to have ARF than women. The risk increases with age regardless of gender. ARF is associated with a mortality ranging anywhere between 35% and 65% depending on associated medical comorbidities.

There are many causes of ARF, and the cause differs for women and men. The categories of ARF are broadly divided based on etiology in the kidney: prerenal, intrarenal or postrenal. Table 25-2 highlights the causes of ARF more commonly seen in women.

Differentiating Specific Types of ARF

In general, history, physical and serum/urine indices can be helpful in differentiating among the various types of ARF. The urinary findings in ARF help to differentiate among specific types of intrarenal causes (Table 25-3). In addition, several laboratory measurements are useful in differentiating the prerenal from renal tubular etiology (Table 25-4).

Because the intrarenal etiologies of ARF encompass a wide variety of intrinsic renal as well as systemic causes, a detailed discussion is beyond the scope of this chapter. Nevertheless, it is important to remember that the most common cause of ARF in both women and men is acute tubular necrosis from shock. Hemorrhage and septic complications from pregnancy and gynecologic surgery can lead to ARF,

---

BOX 25-1

Factors Affecting Creatinine and BUN Measurement

Creatinine
Increases serum creatinine
Cimetidine
Trimethoprim
Increased muscle mass
Cephalosporins*
Acetoacetate*
Decreases serum creatinine
Muscle wasting

BUN
Protein intake
Corticosteroids
Renal perfusion

Modified from Wyngaarden J, Smith L: *Cecil's textbook of medicine*, ed 19. Philadelphia, 1988, WB Saunders.
*Falsely increases measurement by interfering with assay.

Table 25-1
Laboratory Reference Ranges for Renal Function Tests

	REFERENCE RANGE	
Test	**Female**	**Male**
Serum creatinine (serum or plasma)	0.5-1.1 mg/dl	0.6-1.2 mg/dl
Creatinine clearance (serum or plasma plus urine)	88-128 ml/min/ 1.73 m^2	97-137 ml/min/ 1.73 m^2
Uric acid (serum)	2.6-6.0 mg/dl	3.5-7.2 mg/dl

but are fortunately rare. It appears that if the location of the injury in women is tubular rather than cortical, the prognosis for recovery of renal function is better.

As far as postrenal causes, bilateral ureteral obstruction can be seen in women with malignant tumors of the pelvis, such as advanced cervical or ovarian cancer. Ultrasound is an excellent study to evaluate for dilation of ureters and collecting systems and potential obstructive pathology. Computed tomography (CT) scanning can provide similar information but is a poorer study for evaluating pathologic conditions of the uterus and ovaries. Treatment is directed toward bypassing the obstruction, initially with retrograde stents placed via cystoscopy under fluoroscopic examination. If this is unsuccessful, drainage of the urine proximal to the blockage must be performed percutaneously.

Clinical Presentation

The clinical manifestations of acute renal disease can be organized into four different categories, each highlighting a different aspect of deteriorating kidney function: electrolyte imbalances, volume handling, acid-base disturbances, and toxin accumulation.

BOX 25-2

Causative Factors for Abnormal Creatinine Levels in Women

Causes
- Vascular depletion
- Nephrotoxic agents
- Obstruction
- Sepsis and infection
- Contrast dyes
- Hypertension
- Metabolic

Evaluation Strategies
- Serial serum BUN and creatinine levels every 3 to 4 months
- 24-hour urine collection for creatinine clearance (with simultaneous serum creatinine measurement)
- Serum electrolyte levels if creatinine value is rising

BUN, Blood urea nitrogen.

History and Physical Examination

Symptoms that may indicate ARF include hematuria, cloudy foamy urine, dysuria, edema, uremia, fatigue, malaise, dyspnea, orthopnea, renal colic, and flank pain. Oliguria may be present, although urine volume is often normal in early or mild ARF and thus serves as a poor diagnostic marker. Anuria on the other hand is rare and indicates a renal emergency. Signs of ARF include hypertension, uremia, papilledema, edema, and evidence of congestive heart failure (CHF). Although any of these symptoms may be present, the clinical picture depends on the underlying etiology of ARF. Particular areas to address while performing history taking and physical examination and signs and symptoms of uremia are summarized in Box 25-3.

Diagnostic Tests

The laboratory diagnosis of acute renal failure is much like that for renal insufficiency, with an initial evaluation of BUN, serum creatinine, and electrolytes. A 24-hour urine then allows for determination of creatinine clearance and proteinuria. Urinalysis may reveal hematuria, pyuria, and proteinuria, although the urine sediment is generally more accurate in quantifying cells, as well as identifying casts and crystals in the urine (Box 25-3). It is imperative to obtain a clean catch sample of urine, especially in premenopausal women, because contamination with menstrual blood may yield false urinalysis results. Any other tests are determined by the clinician's suspicion for underlying etiology.

Management

In prerenal states, hypovolemic patients should respond to appropriate volume challenges. Depending on the underlying etiology, maximizing cardiovascular function and discontinuing offending drugs also improves renal function. Patients with acute tubular necrosis (ATN) generally recover with conservative management, including removal of offending agents, as well as supportive fluid, electrolyte, and dietary management. Intrinsic renal disease should be treated as promptly as possible by means of standard medical protocols and are beyond the scope of this chapter.

Table 25-2
Causes of Acute Renal Failure in Women

	General Etiology and Causes	Additional Causes More Common in Women
Prerenal	*Hypovolemia:*	
	Hemorrhage	Severe hyperemesis during pregnancy (see Chapter 64)
	GI losses due to emesis or diarrhea	Placenta previa
	Diuretic abuse	Placental abruption
	Sequestration of fluid into extracellular compartment and reduced renal perfusion:	
	CHF	Ovarian hyperstimulation syndrome
	Cirrhosis	
	Sepsis	
	Cardiovascular:	
	Decreased cardiac output	Peripartum cardiomyopathy
	Hepatorenal syndrome	Severe preeclampsia
	Renal artery stenosis	
	Aortic aneurysm	
	Other:	Fatty liver of pregnancy
Intrarenal	*Vascular diseases:*	
	Thrombotic microangiopathy	
	Malignant hypertension	
	Cholesterol emboli	
	Vasculitis:	
	Scleroderma	Lupus nephritis
	Glomerular:	Preeclampsia
	Acute glomerulonephritis (postinfectious)	
	Nephrotic syndrome (minimal change disease, focal glomerulosclerosis, membranous GN)	
	Tubular (Acute necrosis):	
	Toxin induced: aminoglycosides, antibiotics	Septic abortion
	Ischemia	Hemorrhage from placenta previa, placental abruption, or uterine rupture
	Oxalate/uric acid crystals	Eclampsia/preeclampsia
	Multiple myeloma, hypercalcemia	Pyelonephritis
	Cortical:	Placenta previa, placental abruption
Postrenal	*Extrarenal obstruction:*	
	Prostatic disease	Incarcerated uterus
		Cervical carcinoma
		Ovarian carcinoma
		Uterine fibroids
	Extraureteral obstruction:	
	Bilateral renal calculi (rare)	Cervical carcinoma
		Ovarian carcinoma
		Endometriosus
		Complications from pelvic surgery (e.g., hysterectomy)
	Venous obstruction:	
	Bilateral renal vein thrombosis	

GI, Gastrointestinal; *CHF,* congestive heart failure; *GN,* glomerulonephritis.

Regardless of the etiology of ARF, use of hemodialysis should be guided by careful patient evaluation and never by BUN or serum creatinine values alone. Thus indications for hemodialysis include symptomatic volume overload, any manifestations of uremia such as pericarditis or encephalopathy, and otherwise uncontrolled hyperkalemia.

Prognosis and Outcome
The mortality and prognosis for recovery from ARF depend on associated multisystem disease and severity of insult. Generally speaking, the shorter the time interval of injury, the speedier the recovery. Thus prerenal azotemia usually reverses directly with appropriate treatment. In ATN, full recovery as measured by BUN and serum creatinine occurs

Table 25-3
Urinary Sediment and Intrarenal Causes of Acute Renal Failure

Findings	Differential Diagnosis
Hematuria Red cell casts Proteinuria	Glomerular or vasculitis
Renal tubular cells Tubular granular/ epithelial casts	Acute tubular necrosis
Pyuria White cell casts No/mild proteinuria	Tubular, interstitial disease, or pyelonephritis
Hematuria alone	Glomerular
Pyuria alone	Pyelonephritis

Table 25-4
Laboratory Findings in Acute Renal Failure

	Prerenal	Renal (Acute Tubular Injury)
Serum		
BUN: creatinine	>20	10-15
Urine		
Osmolality	>500	300-350
Sodium	<25	>40
Urinalysis	NL/hyaline casts	Granular "muddy brown" casts with epithelial cells
Fractional Excretion of Sodium (FENa) (U/P Na/ U/P Cr × 100)		
FENa	<1%	>2%

NL, Normal.

BOX 25-3
Evaluation of Woman with Suspected Acute Renal Failure

History
Medical history
Pregnancies past and present
Medications

Physical Examination
Blood pressure and orthostatics
Exclusion of signs for volume overload (peripheral edema, rales on lung examination, pericardial friction rub or new murmur on cardiac examination)

Signs and Symptoms of Uremia
Hyperkalemia
Metabolic acidosis
Hyperuricemia
Evidence for volume overload
Congestive heart failure
Pericarditis
Anorexia, nausea, diarrhea, vomiting
Gastrointestinal bleeding
Weakness
Fatigue

Table 25-5
Female/Male Ratio of Incidence of Treated Causes of End-Stage Renal Disease 1987-1990

	RATIO	
Disease	Female	Male
Collagen vascular diseases	2.9	1
Interstitial nephritis	1.2	1
Diabetes	1.1	1

Modified from the US Renal Data System: *Incidence and causes of treated ESRD,* Bethesda, Md, 1993, National Institutes of Health.

within days to weeks, depending on the severity and type of initial insult. However, if ATN persists for >6 to 8 weeks, one can expect only partial recovery of renal function. The best prognosis has been seen in obstetric cases of ARF (other than cortical necrosis) in which there are no other medical comorbidities, although fetal mortality is increased if associated with hemorrhage or preeclampsia.

Often the only advice that the clinician can offer the patient is to monitor the renal function tests closely and observe for stability and recovery over time. Consultation with a nephrologist if available is strongly advised.

CHRONIC RENAL FAILURE
Epidemiology and Etiology

Chronic renal failure (CRF) occurs with equal frequency in women and men. The most common causes of CRF in the United States are diabetic nephropathy (28%), hypertension (25%), and glomerulonephritis (21%), such as human immunodeficiency virus (HIV)-associated nephropathy. Diabetes has a slight female preponderance. Less common conditions accounting for a greater proportion of CRF in women than in men include lupus nephritis, amyloidosis, and other immunologic vasculitides such as scleroderma (Table 25-5).

End-stage renal disease (ESRD) is defined by the need for dialysis therapy or transplantation, and approximately 50% of patients with ESRD are women. The yearly age-adjusted incidence and prevalence of ESRD are slightly higher in men than in women with exception of the Native-American population, according to data from the 1993 United States Renal Data System. The increased protein intake and higher prevalence of hypertension and dyslipidemias in men versus premenopausal women all contribute to these gender discrepancies; however, they cannot account for all of the differences. This has led to the proposed role of sex hormones in influencing renal function.

Natural History and Pathophysiology

It is thought that initial injury and irreversible loss of nephrons leads to compensatory hyperfiltration and hypertrophy in the remaining nephrons. This increase in single nephron GFR (snGFR) initially enables maintenance of near-normal GFRs; however, the compensatory increase in glomerular pressures at the level of the individual nephron predisposes to further fibrosis and scarring over the long term. It has also been found that lower birth-weight infants with a lesser total number of initial nephrons have a greater incidence of renal disease when monitored over time. Thus secondary injury following the compensation to a primary loss of nephrons is important in the continued progression of chronic renal disease.

CRF patients with 30% to 50% of normal GFR can often maintain a new steady state and be asymptomatic despite continuing injury as a result of hyperfiltration. However, these patients often have little functional reserve and easily become uremic with any additional stressors. Most patients with GFRs <20% of normal are symptomatic.

In one prospective study by Ahlman, the rate of disease progression to end-stage renal failure from a persistent abnormal creatinine value of 5 mg/dl was dependent on the underlying etiology. A review of gender differences revealed that women became uremic in 5.9 months compared with 11.6 months for men, but the difference was not statistically significant. A more recent study showed that when women are on hemodialysis for ESRD, they survive longer, possibly because they receive proportionately more dialysis than do men who have higher muscle mass and therefore more nitrogenous waste to clean.

Clinical Presentation

The clinical signs and symptoms of uremia are caused by four main mechanisms: electrolyte and volume imbalances, toxin accumulation, hormonal disturbances, and compensatory responses. CRF has a major effect on organ system function with the significant clinical manifestations listed in Table 25-6. Effects of ESRD on menstrual and reproductive function, bone metabolism, anemia, and thyroid function are discussed in detail.

Clinical Issues for Women

Menstrual Function

Although amenorrhea, oligomenorrhea (menses occurring less than every 35 days), polymenorrhea (bleeding occurring more frequently than every 21 days), and regular menses have all been reported in women with ESRD, few clinical studies have focused on the reproductive endocrinologic function of women with renal failure. As many as 90% of premenopausal women undergoing chronic hemodialysis may have menstrual irregularities. Although heparin given during dialysis increases the amount and duration of bleeding, it has no influence on the frequency of menstrual flow.

The new onset of menstrual irregularity or amenorrhea in a woman with renal disease often indicates worsening renal function and uremia. In fact, the onset of uremic symptoms correlates with the onset of menstrual irregularity and is typically seen with creatinine clearances of 10 to 15 ml/min, whereas amenorrhea occurs with clearances of less than 4 ml/min. Amenorrhea appears to be a common presentation in ESRD except in women receiving continuous ambulatory peritoneal dialysis who may not be amenorrheic despite elevated serum prolactin levels. It is unclear whether the age of true menopause is different for women in ESRD because diagnosis in amenorrheic women is more difficult and requires a documented elevation in serum follicle-stimulating hormone (FSH) to ascertain menopausal status.

Table 25-6
Clinical Manifestations of End-Stage Renal Failure

System	Clinical Manifestations
Electrolytes	*Na/water retention:* CHF, HTN, ascites, edema, hyponatremia if water > sodium retention
	Hyperkalemia: exacerbated by ACE inhibitors, K-sparing diuretics, beta-blockers, as well as increased K loads (hemolysis, infection, diet, etc.), type 4 RTA
	Metabolic acidosis: decreased excretion of H, decreased production of buffers
	Other abnormalities: Hyperphosphatemia, hypocalcemia, hyperuricemia
Musculoskeletal	*Renal osteodystrophy* (discussion to follow)
Cardiovascular	*Hypertension*
	CHF
	Pericarditis
	Atherosclerosis: accelerated progression due to decreased lipoprotein lipase activity, hyperlipidemia
Neurologic	*Central nervous system:* encephalopathy: decreased concentration and memory, sleep disturbances, asterixis, neuromuscular irritability—hiccups, twitching, muscle cramps, fasciculations
	Peripheral neuropathy: sensory stocking-glove distribution, "restless leg" syndrome
Hematologic	Anemia (discussion to follow)
	Platelet dysfunction: abnormal hemostasis, increased bleeding time
Endocrine	*Sexual dysfunction* (discussion to follow)
	Insulin resistance
Dermatologic	*Pruritus*
Gastrointestinal	*Anorexia*
	Nausea/Vomiting
	Uremic Fetor: degradation of urea to ammonia in saliva

CHF, Congestive heart failure; *HTN,* hypertension; *ACE,* angiotensin-converting enzyme.

Pathophysiology. The menstrual irregularities in patients with ESRD reflect chronic anovulation resulting from abnormalities at various levels in the hypothalamic-ovarian feedback loop (see Chapter 43). Small studies of luteinizing hormone (LH) and FSH pulsatility in premenopausal patients on dialysis have shown anovulatory patterns with no midcycle peaks. Because both LH and FSH are glycoproteins that are not cleared by dialysis, renal failure rather than the dialysis itself is the most likely cause of the abnormal ovulatory cycling. Excessive endorphin activity associated with chronic renal insufficiency may inhibit release of gonadotropin-releasing hormone (GnRH), which in turn results in diminished release of LH and FSH at the level of the hypothalamus and leads to anovulation.

Prolactin. Elevation of serum prolactin levels in renal failure has also been shown to cause hypoestrogenism by inhibiting hypothalamic pulsatile GnRH release, subsequent LH and FSH release, and ovulation. Thus anovulation is associated with low serum estradiol and testosterone levels in premenopausal dialysis patients and low progesterone levels in patients with oligomenorrhea. In contrast, some studies have found that menstruating or irregularly menstruating women on dialysis have normal estradiol levels.

The cause of hyperprolactinemia is multifactorial and seems to correlate with the degree of renal insufficiency and decreased renal clearance. In small studies, prolactin levels normalized in patients on erythropoietin therapy; however, regular menses resulted in only 50% of the study population. In addition, both primary pituitary abnormality and abnormal hypothalamic function owing to decreased prolactin inhibitory factor, thought to be dopamine, have shown secondarily increased prolactin levels. Therefore the combination of decreased clearance, increased secretion, and decreased inhibition leads to elevated prolactin levels in most women on dialysis therapy.

Of interest, in response to the lack of ovarian estradiol secretion in menopause, gonadotropins have been found to be appropriately elevated in postmenopausal dialysis patients or post-oophorectomy patients. This indicates that the negative feedback effects of estradiol on the hypothalamus are intact in patients with ESRD.

Clinical Implications. Although the absence of menses in a population likely to have chronic anemia may appear beneficial, the consequences of chronic anovulation are considerable. Development of endometrial hyperplasia increases the risk of endometrial carcinoma, and it is important that a gynecologist determine whether an endometrial biopsy and interventional therapy are indicated (see index for additional entries).

Although elevated prolactin levels in renal insufficiency are quite common, further workup may be necessary, especially if renal failure has not yet occurred. There are no published studies addressing the prevalence of pituitary microadenoma or macroadenoma in patients with CRF; however, prolactin levels of greater than 100 ng/ml are uncommon and suggest the possibility of malignancy. Thus prolactin levels greater than 100 ng/ml, or lower levels associated with either galactorrhea or visual disturbances merit further evaluation with pituitary imaging to exclude prolactinoma.

Infertility

Infertility is common in women receiving either peritoneal or hemodialysis and is due to anovulation, abnormal endometrial maturation, and uremic toxins that may inhibit implantation of the embryo. Pregnancy occurs in as few as 0.9% of female hemodialysis patients of childbearing age, although one study by Souqiyyeh et al. found a pregnancy rate of 7% in a younger nonhypertensive population with previous pregnancies (27 of 380 women). Therefore young patients without vascular disease may have a better chance of conception.

Sexual Function

Severe chronic renal insufficiency requiring dialysis is associated with decreased sexual desire, frequency of inter-

course, and sexual satisfaction in women as well as in men. Hyperprolactinemic dialysis patients have a significantly lower frequency of sexual intercourse and orgasm than those with normal prolactin levels.

The cause behind this change in sexual function is unclear. Some have suggested that lower estradiol levels in amenorrheic dialysis patients cause vaginal atrophy and dryness, which can lead to dyspareunia. Decreased sexual desire and function may also be due to increased prolactin itself, and small studies have shown improvement of sexual function with bromocriptine in male dialysis patients, although there are no such studies involving female populations. Relevant studies have also found a significant psychologic component to the decreased libido and an association with depression experienced by women on dialysis.

General Clinical Issues

Renal Osteodystrophy

Chronic renal failure impairs the metabolism of vitamin D to the biologically active 1,25-dihydroxy vitamin D_3, resulting in decreased gastrointestinal absorption of calcium and phosphate, as well as decreased inhibition of parathyroid hormone (PTH). Low active vitamin D_3 in combination with renal phosphate retention results in hyperphosphatemia and transient hypocalcemia, causing secondary hyperparathyroidism and osteitis fibrosa. The characteristic findings of this disorder include bone demineralization, resorption of both ends of the clavicles and subperiosteal phalanges, and bone cysts.

Other factors exacerbating bone disease are malnutrition and toxic metabolites that lead to osteomalacia, as well as metabolic acidosis depleting bone buffers resulting in decalcification and osteoporosis.

Excess PTH may also lead to metastatic calcifications in arteries and soft tissues because PTH maintains both a near-normal calcium concentration with a high phosphate concentration owing to inadequate renal excretion. Typically, precipitation occurs when the calcium-phosphate product (mg/dl) exceeds 60.

The overall bone density for postmenopausal women receiving dialysis is lower than that for men, although it is unclear whether this is due to the hypoestrogenemia of menopause. There are no data as to whether amenorrheal premenopausal women have lower bone densities than eumenorrheal women. Nor are there data on the efficacy of estrogen replacement therapy in retarding bone loss in menopausal women with ESRD.

Treatment is aimed at reducing phosphate levels via dialysis, dietary changes, and phosphate-binding calcium salts. Vitamin D analogs also lower bone resorption and PTH secretion, although care should be taken not to lower PTH levels below three times normal levels to avoid adynamic bone disease. In cases unresponsive to medical management, parathyroidectomy may be indicated.

Anemia

Renal erythropoietin production is typically inhibited when the GFR drops below 30% of normal, resulting in a normochromic, normocytic hypoproliferative anemia. Other factors contributing to chronic anemia include possible bone marrow suppression from uremic toxins, hemolysis and blood losses associated with hemodialysis, and folate or iron deficiency.

Replacement therapy with Epoetin (EPO), a recombinant human erythropoietin, has taken the place of repeated transfusion therapy and is much safer owing to decreased risk of hepatitis and HIV exposure. Despite the widespread use of EPO, there are limited data on its effect on the menstrual and ovulatory patterns of dialysis patients. One small study suggested a regularization of the menses; however, no data on ovulation were obtained and definitive conclusions could not be drawn from so small a study.

Thyroid Function and Dialysis Treatment

The diagnosis of hypothyroidism in dialysis patients can be difficult, as many of the typical symptoms are similar to those of uremia. In addition, measurement of thyroid function tests may indicate abnormal results despite clinically euthyroid states. Some studies have suggested that the total triiodothyronine (T3) and total and free thyroxine (T4) are lower in the dialysis population compared with control subjects. One study found that 43% of dialysis patients had T3 levels in the hypothyroid range that were not necessarily associated with clinical symptoms. Furthermore, reverse T3 may be normal, elevated, or low; and the T3 resin uptake has been found to be normal or elevated. These abnormalities may be related to the loss of albumin and transferrin protein, which affects the measurement of thyroid hormones.

Thyroid-stimulating hormone (TSH) has been found to be higher in hemodialysis patients compared with age-matched control subjects (5.2/20.4 mU/ml for study group versus 3.0/20.2 mU/ml for control subjects), although values are still within the upper normal laboratory range. Various studies have shown a higher prevalence of clinically enlarged thyroid or goiter in this group.

✺ MANAGEMENT

Prevention

Women with severe chronic renal failure often do not receive routine health maintenance examinations such as pelvic examinations, Pap smears, and mammograms. There may be a tendency for physicians to focus on the renal disease or to assume that the patient's life span is limited and therefore diagnosing an occult malignant condition will not significantly affect longevity. Data indicate that dialysis patients may be at an increased risk of developing solid tumors and that postrenal transplantation patients are at increased risk for leukemia and lymphoma. Therefore it is important that routine health maintenance be addressed in addition to the daily medical needs of chronic renal failure patients.

CRF can lead to gradual hyperlipidemia, and progression of atherosclerosis in dialysis patients is often accelerated and should be monitored closely.

Impaired renal clearance increases susceptibility to potentially toxic substances, and patients should be aware that dietary supplements may have hazardous effects. For example, vitamin A can accumulate to toxic levels, as can many trace metals such as aluminum, fluoride, and lead.

Therapeutic Interventions

Gynecologic Management

Menstrual Dysfunction. The goal of treatment of menstrual dysfunction is to regulate the menstrual cycle as close to normal as possible to decrease effects of chronic anovu-

lation. After excluding pathologic changes of the endometrium by biopsy, a number of treatment options are available to control irregular bleeding in this population. One option is to use exogenous progesterone therapy such as medroxyprogesterone acetate (10 mg orally for 10 days) given at least four times a year to interrupt the proliferation-hyperplasia-carcinoma progression. Alternatively, combination oral contraceptives could be used, although it is unclear whether these medications increase the incidence of arteriovenous shunt clotting. Low-dose pills (.30 μg of estrogen) are unlikely to have a significant effect. A newer treatment is endometrial ablation, or the destruction of the endometrial lining via electrocautery or laser energy, and is appropriate for patients with significant medical problems. Treatment requires only local anesthesia and diminishes or permanently eliminates uterine bleeding in 80% of cases. Repeat treatment is necessary in the remainder of patients.

Despite the aforementioned interventions, some patients continue to have profuse menstrual bleeding and thus require hysterectomy.

Epoetin (EPO) for Treatment of Anemia. Epoetin (EPO) is routinely prescribed for patients with severe anemia secondary to ESRD and is commonly given intravenously at the time of dialysis. Patients generally note improved quality of life owing to resolution of the anemia, and in about half of treated premenopausal women, regularization of menstruation and possible improved fertility occur as well. It has also been reported to improve libido and sexual performance in men despite unchanged hyperprolactinemia and testosterone, LH, or FSH levels. These parameters have not been completely assessed for women receiving EPO therapy.

Calcium Supplementation. Hypocalcemia in CRF is caused by several factors, including decreased intestinal calcium uptake owing to low 1,25-dihydroxyvitamin D_3 levels and high phosphate levels binding to calcium and further lowering free calcium levels. Thus it is important to provide adequate calcium supplementation with goal levels in the high range of normal (10.5 to 11.0 mg/dl), which will decrease PTH secretion and halt the progression of bone disease.

Phosphate Binders. As mentioned previously, phosphate binders are crucial in treating renal bone disease because hyperphosphatemia seems to be closely linked to hyperparathyroidism itself. The most widely used is calcium carbonate, which binds phosphate in the gastrointestinal tract and prevents its absorption, although potential complication includes hypercalcemia. In the past, aluminum salts were used as phosphate binders, although they are rarely used now owing to intoxication and exacerbation of osteomalacia.

DIALYSIS

Dialysis is generally indicated to prevent otherwise uncontrolled life-threatening hyperkalemia, metabolic acidosis, hypervolemia resulting in pulmonary edema and CHF, and other symptoms of uremia. Hemodialysis and peritoneal dialysis are nearly equally effective, and main differences are in patient comfort and potential complications, including hemodynamic instability in the former, and peritonitis in the latter.

TRANSPLANTATION

Epidemiologic studies indicate that women, especially those in minority groups, are less likely to undergo renal transplantation than are men, with a ratio of 1:1.3. Women undergoing transplantation do as well as men, with excellent long-term graft survival and prognosis. In 60% to 89% of these patients, menstrual function regularizes with improvement of the uremic state and sexual interest and libido often return to pre-CRF levels. Hypertrichosis (excess body hair growth) is a common cosmetic problem after transplantation. Pregnancy is optimal in posttransplant patients, as there are many complications associated with pregnancy during dialysis.

◼ PREGNANCY AND RENAL DYSFUNCTION
Normal Renal Physiology in Pregnancy
Parameters for Renal Function
Various physiologic changes occur during normal gestation of which the clinician needs to be aware. In normal pregnancy, blood volume increases by 45% at term, with the greatest increase occurring during the second trimester. Similarly, the GFR increases by approximately 50% by the beginning of the second trimester and remains elevated until delivery. Despite this increase in GFR from a mean of 96 to 148 ml/min, sodium and water handling remains normal. Increased GFR, however, leads to increased filtration of glucose and inability to effectively reabsorb all of it. Excretion often increases up to a factor of 10 and results in glycosuria in pregnant women (for more details about abnormal glycosuria in pregnancy and the diagnosis of diabetes, see Chapter 71). Renal plasma flow does not increase quite as much as GFR and actually decreases during the third trimester. The supine position, which is associated with decreased urinary flow and sodium excretion, has not been shown to consistently decrease GFR or renal flow. Total body water is increased with a resultant decrease in plasma osmolality seen from the fifth week of gestation until delivery. In addition to contributing compression of the inferior vena cava, this reset osmostat leads to lower extremity edema in 35% to 83% of healthy pregnancies. Uric acid clearance is increased in the first two trimesters, leading to a decrease in plasma uric acid levels to 2.5 to 4, which often return to normal levels by the third trimester.

Anatomic Changes with Pregnancy
Anatomic changes include (1) the dilation of the renal calyces, pelves, and ureters, also known as physiologic hydronephrosis of pregnancy, (2) increase in kidney sizes of 1 cm primarily owing to increased renal blood flow, and (3) a decrease in ureteral peristalsis as a result of uterine and iliac artery pressures on the ureters (right worse than left) and the muscle-relaxing properties of placental progesterone.

Abnormal Renal Physiology During Pregnancy
Proteinuria
Despite increases in GFR and glomerular permeability to proteins and subsequent increased fractional excretion of albumin, normal urinary protein should not exceed 300 mg/day in pregnancy, and higher urinary losses indicate renal dis-

ease. If proteinuria is present with hypertension after week 20 of gestation, the diagnosis of preeclampsia must be strongly considered (see Chapter 69 for a detailed discussion of preeclampsia and eclampsia).

Urine Output
Oliguria is defined as a urine output below the level necessary to maintain nitrogenous waste balance. Because absolute urine volume may not necessarily reflect how much waste is cleared, this is difficult to define numerically. Generally any calculation less than 700 ml/24 hr should be suspect.

Specific Renal Disorders in Pregnancy
Acute Renal Failure
Epidemiology and Etiology. The incidence of ARF in pregnancy has been estimated at less than 0.01% and accounts for 2.8% of all cases of ARF. The incidence peaks between 35 and 40 weeks and is mainly due to preeclampsia and bleeding complications. Before the legalization of abortion, the distribution of ARF was bimodal with an early peak around 16 weeks owing to septic abortions and was a major cause of maternal mortality (see Table 25-1).

Hemorrhage. Bleeding complications that cause ARF include hemorrhage from the uterus as a result of placental abruption, placenta previa, and uterine rupture. The greatest occurrence of these life-threatening conditions is during the third trimester from 24 to 40 weeks of gestation. Postpartum hemorrhage from uterine atony, retained placental fragments preventing uterine contraction around the raw placental bed, lacerations of the cervix or vagina, and rupture can all cause ARF as a result of hypovolemia and ischemia as well.

Incarcerated Uterus. Urinary obstruction that results from an incarcerated uterus occluding the bladder outlet is an uncommon event, but when it does happen it can produce postrenal ARF. Affected women usually have a retroverted uterus and manifest acute urinary retention in the late first or early second trimester, although third trimester cases have been reported. The bladder outlet obstruction occurs as the enlarging retroverted uterus becomes wedged between the sacrum and pubic symphysis. On physical examination the cervix is lodged beneath the pubis and often cannot be seen on speculum examination, the bladder is distended and tender, and the second trimester uterus often appears smaller than expected for dates. In some cases the uterus can be dislodged by exerting pressure vaginally on its posterior aspect, usually with the patient under general anesthesia because of the tenseness and extreme pain experienced by the woman, although occasionally a laparoscopy or laparotomy is necessary. Once the uterus is dislodged from the pelvic bones, it is unlikely to incarcerate again. Much like women who undergo removal of large uterine fibroids, these patients will experience a postobstructive diuresis after relief of the obstruction.

Pyelonephritis. Pyelonephritis is the most common infectious problem of pregnancy, and about 30% of patients with asymptomatic bacteriuria can become symptomatic or develop pyelonephritis during pregnancy. This increase in urinary tract infections is probably related to the physiologic dilation of the renal collecting system in pregnancy and subsequent stasis of urine. Maternal consequences from pyelonephritis include bacteremia, ARF, and sepsis, whereas fetal risks include abortion, increased perinatal mortality, and intrauterine growth restriction (for a more detailed discussion of urinary tract infections and pyelonephritis see Chapters 23 and 78).

Preeclampsia. Any woman with preeclampsia should be closely monitored for renal failure (see Chapter 69).

Ovarian Hyperstimulation Syndrome. Ovarian hyperstimulation syndrome may occur after induced ovulation with human menopausal gonadotropins or purified follicle-stimulating hormone, and rarely after clomiphene citrate when human chorionic gonadotropin is given to induce ovulation. The syndrome is characterized by cystic ovarian enlargement, capillary leakage, ascites, weight gain, pleural effusions, and hyponatremia secondary to increased fluid intake. This decreased intravascular volume leads to prerenal azotemia, which is usually self-limited and treated supportively with intravenous hydration and bed rest.

Prognosis and Outcome. Kennedy et al. reviewed 251 patients with ARF of whom 43 were pregnant. The obstetric group was oliguric for 1 to 28 days with a mean of 11 days, and the average rate of rise of BUN was 41 mg/100 ml. In similar studies by Hawkins et al. and Sibai et al., the researchers found that if obstetric patients survived the ARF, renal function would ultimately return to normal regardless of etiologic factors. In approximately 12% of a study population of 81 evaluated by Stratta et al., permanent renal compromise ensued, most often in association with preeclampsia and eclampsia. Placental abruption and prolonged intrauterine fetal death may increase the likelihood of cortical necrosis and associated maternal mortality can be as high as 100% with increasing age and/or hypertension. Fetal mortality in ARF caused by either hemorrhage or eclampsia is 71% and 76%, respectively. Survival after ARF treatment with dialysis in one dialysis center was 78.8% at 1 year and 72.5% at 5 years including women with cortical necrosis. Excluding the latter, survival rate increased to 85.8% at 1 year and 85% at 5 years.

Chronic Renal Failure in Pregnancy

Management. Pregnancy in women with CRF can be complicated by miscarriage, premature labor and delivery, intrauterine growth retardation, placental abruption, and intrauterine fetal death. Preeclampsia is common as well; however, it poses a difficult diagnosis in women with underlying renal insufficiency and hypertension. The prognosis is better for women who are placed on dialysis therapy after conception than it is for those already on maintenance hemodialysis at time of conception. Hydramnios is seen in women on hemodialysis. The poorer prognosis and morbidity associated with dialysis are not linked to heparin use during filtration, but rather to the greater degree of renal compromise itself. Dialysis in pregnancy is usually started when the serum BUN level is >80 mg/dl with a goal of maintaining BUN <50 mg/dl. The physiologic assumption is that decreased azotemia improves the fetal environment and decreases incidence of hydramnios, thereby improving pregnancy outcome. Late in pregnancy, fetal urea production increases and may necessitate increased dialysis frequency or

duration to maintain the goal maternal BUN. It is crucial to be aware that the use of angiotensin-converting enzyme (ACE) inhibitors and angiotensin-receptor blockers in the medical management of hypertension is contraindicated in pregnancy, and that the mainstay of management should therefore rely on beta-blockers or calcium channel blockers instead.

Therapeutic Abortion. A woman's decision to carry or to terminate her pregnancy may hinge on the long-term impact it will have on her health and survival. The physician who recommends therapeutic abortion because of poor pregnancy prognosis, poor maternal health, or a fear that pregnancy may lead to further deterioration of maternal renal function must bear in mind that termination of the pregnancy does not necessarily halt the progression of the underlying renal disease. It is unknown whether therapeutic abortion prevents sensitization to transplant antigens if end-stage renal disease occurs and renal transplantation is pursued.

Dialysis. In the rare instance that a woman on maintenance dialysis therapy conceives, the prognosis of the pregnancy is bleak. Only 19 of 820 pregnancies were reported as successful in the 1990 European dialysis registry. Most conceptions occur in women who have some residual renal function before dialysis. The literature indicates that 45% of women on dialysis elect therapeutic abortion, 11% to 54% have a miscarriage, and up to 61% have premature deliveries. Hydramnios is common and increases risk of premature labor owing to excess uterine distention. Other reasons for early delivery include worsening fetal or maternal condition leading to cesarean section in up to 46% of cases, as well as premature labor, placental abruption, ruptured membranes, fetal distress, growth retardation, preeclampsia, and worsening maternal hypertension. In one registry report, 42% to 90% of newborn infants had evidence of growth retardation, with an average fetal weight of 1900 g at 33.2 weeks.

Appropriate patient counseling with regard to pregnancy prognosis is hindered by the fact that some series report only live births. Available, although limited, data indicate live birth rates between 19% and 63%, with the highest rate in a series of 8 of 14 women on peritoneal dialysis; however, it is not clear which method of dialysis is safer with respect to both fetal and maternal complications. Hemodialysis may be associated with more severe anemia and hypotensive episodes leading to decreased placental perfusion. Peritoneal dialysis, by contrast, may be complicated by obstruction of the peritoneal catheter and by peritonitis causing premature labor and delivery.

EPO successfully treats the anemia of ESRD in pregnant patients, although the same pregnancy complications occur with or without therapy, and EPO has been documented to exacerbate chronic hypertension.

PROGNOSIS AND OUTCOME. Pregnancy outcome in women with **mild renal insufficiency** as defined as a serum creatinine less than 1.5 mg/dl is approximately 90%. In a study by Katz and colleagues, 89 of 121 pregnant women with biopsy-confirmed diagnoses had mild renal insufficiency and had fetal survival rates of 94%, stillbirth rate of 4.1%, and neonatal death rate of 4.9%—four times that seen in the general

BOX 25-4
Pregnancy and Fetal Outcome in Women with Moderate Renal Insufficiency

BOX 25-4
Pregnancy and Fetal Outcome in Women with Moderate Renal Insufficiency

- Higher cesarean section rates
- Increased rate of premature delivery
- High rate of growth retardation
- Increased risk fetal death
- Decreased fetal survival

population. The preterm birth rate (<36 weeks) was 20% compared with 13% nationally and 5.7% in the local population, and 24% of infants (or fivefold the rate in the general population) were small for gestational age. It is unclear whether fetal and neonatal deaths are increased in women with mild chronic renal disease who have glomerulonephritis because the data included women with more severe renal dysfunction, and the study was conducted at a time when less advanced neonatal care was available.

Pregnancy and fetal outcome are less favorable in patients with **moderate renal insufficiency** (serum creatinine >1.5 mg/dl) (Box 25-4) rather than mild renal insufficiency. Therapeutic abortion rates are higher, ranging from 13% to 24%, and premature deliveries occur in 54% to 63% of cases, with a significant number of deliveries performed early because of worsening renal function, hypertension, placental abruption, and fetal distress. Cesarean section rates range from 47% to 61%, up to 40% of infants demonstrate growth retardation with even higher rates in hypertensive mothers, intrauterine death varies between 3% and 10%, and neonatal deaths are 3% to 13% in this population. In general, hypertension indicates a poorer fetal prognosis. Overall fetal survival is 60% to 92%, with higher rates being reported in more recent series; this improvement has occurred as a result of modern maternal and neonatal care.

Pregnancy outcomes in women with **severe renal insufficiency** are poor, especially for women conceiving while on maintenance dialysis therapy. The knowledge of low fetal viability and a potentially emotionally devastating and medically complicated pregnancy does not deter all women whose desire to bear a child outweighs the risks. In these cases, the support and expertise of the medical staff, as well as the general health of the mother and etiology of her renal disease, all play a significant role in obtaining the best maternal and fetal outcome.

Pregnancy is not uncommon in women who have undergone **renal transplantation,** as they generally are ovulatory. In addition, prognosis is excellent in transplant recipients inasmuch as immunosuppressive agents tend to be well tolerated by the fetus and the risk for complications is much lower than in patients on hemodialysis.

Effect of Pregnancy on Future Renal Function

Interpretation of the literature regarding the effect of pregnancy on long-term renal function is hindered by the grouping of patients into "mild" and "moderate" degrees of renal insufficiency that include overlapping ranges of serum creatinine. In addition, patient numbers are small and no statistical analyses were obtained in any series. Taking into account these limitations, it seems likely that patients with serum creatinine levels of less than 1.5 mg/dl are not at significant risk of harming themselves by conceiving. The data are less clear for higher creatinine levels, with postpregnancy deterioration of renal function reported in 23% to 50% of these cases. Until the effect of pregnancy on renal function after pregnancy is further defined, appropriate counseling of women considering childbearing will not be possible.

BIBLIOGRAPHY

Abu-Romeh SH et al: Recombinant human erythropoietin (rHuEPO) and fertility in women on dialysis, *Nephrol Dial Transplant* 5:834, 1990 (letter).

Ahlmen J: Incidence of chronic renal insufficiency: a study of the incidence and pattern of renal insufficiency in adults during 1966-1971 in Gothenburg, *Acta Med Scand (Suppl)* 582:1, 1975.

Bear RA: Pregnancy in patients with renal disease, *Obstet Gynecol* 48:13, 1976.

Bierman M, Nolan GH: Menstrual function and renal transplantation, *Obstet Gynecol* 49:186, 1977.

Bommer J et al: Improved sexual function during recombinant human erythropoietin therapy, *Nephrol Dial Transplant* 5:204, 1990.

Brandes JC, Fritsche C: Obstructive acute renal failure by a gravid uterus: a case report and review, *Am J Kidney Dis* 18:398, 1991.

Cowden EA et al: Hyperprolactinemia in renal disease, *Clin Endocrinol* 9:241, 1978.

Cunningham FG et al: Chronic renal disease and pregnancy outcome, *Am J Obstet Gynecol* 163:453, 1990.

Davison JM, Dunlop W: Changes in renal hemodynamics and tubular function induced by normal human pregnancy, *Semin Nephrol* 4:198, 1984.

Eika B, Skajaa K: Acute renal failure due to bilateral ureteral obstruction by the pregnancy uterus, *Urol Int* 43:315, 1986.

Eschbach JW et al: Treatment of the anemia of progressive renal failure with recombinant erythropoietin, *N Engl J Med* 321:158, 1989.

Finkelstein FO, Finkelstein SH: Evaluation of sexual dysfunction of the patient with renal failure, *Dial Transplant* 10:921, 1981.

Gadallah MF et al: Pregnancy in patients on chronic ambulatory peritoneal dialysis, *Am J Kidney Dis* 20:407, 1992.

Ginsberg ES, Owen WF: Reproductive endocrinology and pregnancy in women on hemodialysis, *Semin Dial* 6:105, 1993.

Gladziwa U et al: Pregnancy in a dialysis patient under recombinant human erythropoietin, *Clin Nephrol* 37:215, 1992.

Gomez F et al: Endocrine abnormalities in patients undergoing long-term hemodialysis, *Am J Med* 68:522, 1980.

Goodwin NJ et al: Effects of uremia and chronic hemodialysis on the reproductive cycle, *Am J Obstet Gynecol* 100:528, 1968.

Grunfeld J-P, Ganeval D, Bournerias F: Acute renal failure in pregnancy, *Kidney Int* 18:179, 1980.

Hankins GD, Cedars MI: Uterine incarceration associated with uterine leiomyomata: clinical and sonographic presentation, *J Clin Ultrasound* 17:385, 1989.

Hou SH, Grossman SD, Madias NE: Pregnancy in women with renal disease and moderate renal insufficiency, *Am J Med* 78:185, 1985.

Hou SH, Grossman S, Molitch ME: Hyperprolactinemia in patients with renal insufficiency and chronic renal failure requiring hemodialysis or chronic ambulatory peritoneal dialysis, *Am J Kidney Dis* 6:245, 1985.

Howmans DC et al: Acute renal failure caused by a gravid uterus, *JAMA* 246:1230, 1980.

Isselbacher KJ, editor: *Harrison's principles of internal medicine,* ed 13. New York, 1994, McGraw-Hill.

Katz AI, Lindheimer MD: Effect of pregnancy on the natural course of kidney disease, *Semin Nephrol* 4:252, 1984.

Katz AI et al: Pregnancy in women with kidney disease, *Kidney Int* 18:192, 1980.

Kennedy AC et al: Factors affecting the prognosis in acute renal failure, *Q J Med* 42:73, 1973.

Lapata RE, McElin TW, Adelson BH: Ureteral obstruction due to compression by the gravid uterus, *Am J Obstet Gynecol* 106:941, 1970.

Levy NB: Sexual adjustment to maintenance hemodialysis and renal transplantation: national survey by questionnaire preliminary report, *TransAm Soc Artif Organs* 19:138, 1973.

Lim VS et al: Ovarian function in chronic renal failure: evidence suggesting hypothalamic anovulation, *Ann Intern Med* 93:21, 1980.

Maher JF: Modifications of endocrine-metabolic abnormalities of uremia by continuous ambulatory peritoneal dialysis, *Am J Nephrol* 10:19, 1990.

Mastrogiacomo I et al: Hyperprolactinemia and sexual disturbances among uremic women on hemodialysis, *Nephron* 37:195, 1984.

McGregor E et al: Successful use of recombinant human erythropoietin in pregnancy, *Nephrol Dial Transplant* 6:292, 1991.

Meislin HW: Incarceration of the gravid uterus, *Ann Emerg Med* 16:1177, 1987.

Meyers SJ, Lee RV, Munschauer RW: Dilatation and nontraumatic rupture of the urinary tract during pregnancy: a review, *Obstet Gynecol* 66:809, 1985.

Morley JE et al: Menstrual disturbances in chronic renal failure, *Horm Metab Res* 11:68, 1979.

Morrin PAF et al: Acute renal failure in association with fatty liver of pregnancy, *Am J Med* 42:844, 1967.

Munk B, Rasmussen KL: Acute urinary retention caused by incarcerated fibromyoma in the eighth week of pregnancy, *Ugeskr Laeger* 150:1937, 1988.

Nageotte MP, Grundy HO: Pregnancy outcome in women requiring chronic hemodialysis, *Obstet Gynecol* 72:456, 1988.

Nelson MS: Acute urinary retention secondary to an incarcerated gravid uterus, *Am J Emerg Med* 4:231, 1986.

Orme BM et al: The effect of hemodialysis on fetal survival and renal function in pregnancy, *Trans Am Soc Artif Organs* 14:402, 1968.

O'Shaughnessy R, Weprin SA, Zuspan FP: Obstructive renal failure by an overdistended pregnant uterus, *Obstet Gynecol* 55:247, 1980.

Pride SM, James CStJ, Ho Yuen B: The ovarian hyperstimulation syndrome, *Semin Reprod Endocrinol* 8:247, 1990.

Pritchard JA: Changes in the blood volume during pregnancy and delivery, *Anesthesiology* 26:393, 1965.

Registration Committee of the European Dialysis and Transplant Association: Successful pregnancies in women treated by dialysis and kidney transplantation, *Br J Obstet Gynaecol* 87:839, 1980.

Rosenthal T, Insler V, Iaine A: Haemodialysis in acute renal failure following hyperemesis gravidarum, *Aust NZ Obstet Gynaecol* 14:57, 1975.

Schiffer MA, Dunn I: Jaundice with hepatorenal failure associated with pregnancy or gynecologic procedures, *Obstet Gynecol* 39:241, 1972.

Sibai BM, Villar MA, Mabie BC: Acute renal failure in hypertensive disorders of pregnancy: pregnancy outcome and remote prognosis in thirty-one consecutive cases, *Am J Obstet Gynecol* 162:777, 1990.

Slater DN, Hague WM: Renal morphologic changes in idiopathic acute fatty liver of pregnancy, *Histopathology* 8:567, 1984.

Smalbraak I et al: Incarceration of the retroverted gravid uterus: a report of 4 cases, *Eur J Obstet Gynecol Reprod Biol* 39:151, 1991.

Souqiyyeh MZ et al: Pregnancy in chronic hemodialysis in patients in the kingdom of Saudi Arabia, *Am J Kidney Dis* 19:235, 1992.

Stratta P et al: Pregnancy-related acute renal failure, *Clin Nephrol* 32:14, 1989.

Strickler RC et al: Serum gonadotropin patterns in patients with chronic renal failure on hemodialysis, *Gynecol Invest* 5:185, 1974.

Surian M et al: Glomerular disease and pregnancy: a study of 123 pregnancies in patients with primary and secondary glomerular diseases, *Nephron* 36:101, 1984.

Turner JH, Ellis CM, Parsons FM: Obstetric acute renal failure 1956-1987, *Br J Obstet Gynaecol* 96:679, 1989.

US Renal Data System: *Incidence and causes of treated ESRD, USRDS 1993. Annual data report, National Institute of Diabetes and Digestive and Kidney Diseases,* Bethesda, Md, 1993, National Institutes of Health.

US Renal Data System: *Methods of ESRD treatment, USRDS 1993 annual report, National Institute of Diabetes and Digestive and Kidney Diseases,* Bethesda, Md, 1993, National Institutes of Health.

Van Winter JT et al: Uterine incarceration during the third trimester: a rare complication of pregnancy, *Mayo Clin Proc* 66:208, 1991.

Whalley PJ, Cunningham FG, Martin FG: Transient renal dysfunction associated with acute pyelonephritis of pregnancy, *Obstet Gynecol* 46:174, 1975.

Wyngaarden J, Smith L, editors: *Cecil's textbook of medicine,* ed 19. Philadelphia, 1988, WB Saunders.

Zingraff J et al: Pituitary and ovarian dysfunctions in women on haemodialysis, *Nephron* 30:148, 1982.

CHAPTER **26**

Headache Syndromes

Egilius L.H. Spierings

A total of 75% of women of reproductive age experience headaches, and most of them experience headaches more than once a month. In 15%, the headaches are severe enough to affect daily activities; however, up to the age of 30, only 25% of women with headaches have sought medical advice.

In their presentation, headaches in women do not differ significantly from those in men. However, in women they occur more frequently, are more intense, last longer, and are more disabling. The estrogens, both endogenous and exogenous, play an important role; they are among the most potent chemicals that cause headaches in women. Headaches occur especially when estrogen levels change, making women more vulnerable to headache during menstruation and ovulation. It is also during these times of the menstrual cycle that headaches are generally more intense and longer lasting. Headaches that occur with menstruation or ovulation are also often more difficult to treat, both abortively and preventively.

DEFINITION OF HEADACHE SYNDROMES

Four headache syndromes account for the majority of headaches in the general population. These headache syndromes are **episodic and chronic tension-type headache, migraine,** and **tension-type vascular headache** (Table 26-1). Tension-type headache, whether episodic or chronic, is equally common in men and women. Migraine, on the other hand, is two to three times more common in women.

A rare headache condition is *cluster headache,* which mostly affects men. It consists of severe, unilateral headaches that last from $1/2$ hour to 2 hours. They occur daily, once or twice per day, for 2 to 8 weeks with remissions of 6 to 12 months.

Episodic and Chronic Tension-Type Headache

Tension-type headache, formerly called muscle-contraction headache, is the most common headache syndrome. It consists of mild or moderate headaches, diffuse in location, and pressing in quality. The headaches usually lack significant associated symptoms, such as nausea, vomiting, photophobia, and phonophobia, because of their relatively low intensity.

Tension-type headache is divided into episodic and chronic, depending on the frequency of occurrence of the headaches. In **episodic tension-type headache,** the headaches occur up to two or three times a week. They begin during the day, usually in the late afternoon, and last for several hours. In **chronic tension-type headache,** the headaches occur daily or almost daily. They are usually present on awakening in the morning or occur shortly after getting up. The headaches gradually build in intensity as the day progresses and last for most or all of the day.

Migraine

In migraine, the headaches are moderate or severe in intensity, localized, usually to the temple or behind the eye, and throbbing in nature. They are generally associated with other symptoms, such as nausea, vomiting, photophobia, and phonophobia. The headaches occur in attacks that last from 4 to 6 hours to 2 or 3 days. The attacks occur with variable frequency, ranging from once per year to weekly. In women, the migraine attacks often occur once or twice per month, in relation to menstruation and ovulation. The headaches usually begin during the day and build to their maximum intensity within several hours. However, they can also be present on awakening in the morning or awake the patient at night.

Migraine is divided into two forms: migraine with aura and migraine without aura, formerly called classic and common migraine, respectively. Migraine with aura constitutes 5% to 10% of migraine.

In **migraine with aura,** transient focal neurologic symptoms occur before the onset of the headache. The symptoms usually last 10 to 30 minutes and occur within an hour before the onset of the headache. The symptoms are always sensory in nature and are either visual or somatosensory.

Visual symptoms are usually unilateral, affecting both eyes and one visual field. Their typical presentation is the scintillating scotoma, which is schematically shown in Fig. 26-1. It generally begins near the center of vision as a small spot surrounded by bright, often flickering and sometimes colorful, zigzag lines. After slight enlargement, the circle of zigzag lines breaks open on the inside to take the form of a horseshoe. The horseshoe then gradually

Table 26-1
Differentiating Symptoms of the Four Most Common Headache Syndromes

Headache Syndrome	Symptoms
Episodic tension-type headache	Mild or moderate headaches Diffuse in location Pressing in quality Not associated with nausea or vomiting
Migraine	Moderate or severe headaches Localized in the temple or behind the eye Throbbing in quality Associated with nausea and sometimes with vomiting
Chronic tension-type headache	Daily or almost daily headaches Mild or moderate in intensity Present on awakening or coming about during the day Not associated with nausea or vomiting
Tension-type vascular headache	Daily or almost daily headaches Frequently moderate or severe in intensity Regularly waking the patient up out of sleep Associated with nausea and sometimes with vomiting

expands into the periphery of a visual field, where it ultimately fades away.

The somatosensory symptoms typically present themselves in the form of digitolingual paresthesias (Fig. 26-1). These paresthesias consist of a feeling of tingling that starts in the fingers of one hand. They gradually extend upward into the arm, ultimately involving the face, especially the nose and mouth area, on the same side. The paresthesias are always unilateral and have to be differentiated from the bilateral tingling in the hands and around the mouth that occurs with hyperventilation syndrome.

Tension-Type Vascular Headache

Tension-type vascular headache is a headache syndrome in which migraine headaches occur superimposed on chronic tension-type headache. The headaches occur daily or almost daily and with certain regularity, often once or twice weekly, build in intensity to cause migraine headaches, with the features mentioned previously; however, the condition may be presented as intermittent severe headaches and the erroneous diagnosis of migraine may then be made. This diagnosis should be considered when migraine headaches occur frequently, that is, on a weekly basis.

Tension-type vascular headache, like chronic tension-type headache, is often associated with frequent use of analgesics and vasoconstrictors, including caffeine. It has been shown that frequent use of these medications for headache is associated with perpetuation of the headaches and ineffectiveness of preventive treatment. It needs to

be addressed before preventive treatment is initiated and often results, by itself, in improvement of the headaches. A 6-day course of prednisone, 15 mg four times a day for 2 days, 10 mg four times a day for 2 days, and 5 mg four times a day for 2 days, can be helpful in discontinuing the medications and reversing the progression.

PATHOPHYSIOLOGY
Headache Mechanisms

The two most common mechanisms in headache are craniocervical muscle contraction and extracranial arterial vasodilation. Muscle contraction causes pain through the accumulation of waste products in the muscles as a result of the prolonged contraction. The pain caused by prolonged muscle contraction is mild or moderate in intensity and diffuse in location. It is often described as an ache more than a pain and tends to be pressing in nature.

The dilation of the extracranial arteries causes pain by stretching of the nerve fibers that coil around the arteries. In response to being stretched, the nerve fibers become activated and send impulses to the central nervous system. At the same time, the nerve fibers release chemicals into the peripheral tissues, such as substance P and calcitonin gene-related peptide. These chemicals have inflammatory properties and cause so-called neurogenic inflammation. The neurogenic inflammation is associated with further dilation of the arteries and a lowering of the pain threshold. The extracranial arterial vasodilation causes a localized pain, usually in the temple or behind the eye but sometimes in the back of the head. The pain is moderate or severe in intensity and described as throbbing or sharp, steady.

The two peripheral headache mechanisms outlined above interact in two ways. Craniocervical muscle contraction can lead to extracranial arterial vasodilation when the mechanical interference with muscle circulation extends beyond a critical point. Extracranial arterial vasodilation can cause craniocervical muscle contraction through a voluntary and involuntary contraction of the muscles, as a result of the intense pain. A vicious cycle can thus be created that over time leads to a progression of the headaches. The involvement of a muscular mechanism in headache, including migraine, can often be ascertained by inquiring about the state of contraction of the neck and shoulder muscles.

With regard to the two headache mechanisms in the four headache syndromes described, the muscular mechanism is predominantly involved in tension-type headache, the vascular mechanism in migraine, and both are involved in tension-type vascular headache. However, the matching of the headache mechanisms and headache syndromes is far from perfect and the muscular mechanism is often more important in migraine than is generally realized.

Headache Continuum

As a result of the interaction of the peripheral headache mechanisms, the four headache syndromes fall on a continuum that is schematically shown in Fig. 26-2. The episodic form of tension-type headache stands on one side of the continuum and migraine on the other. In between are the chronic headache conditions, chronic tension-type headache and tension-type vascular headache. Patients

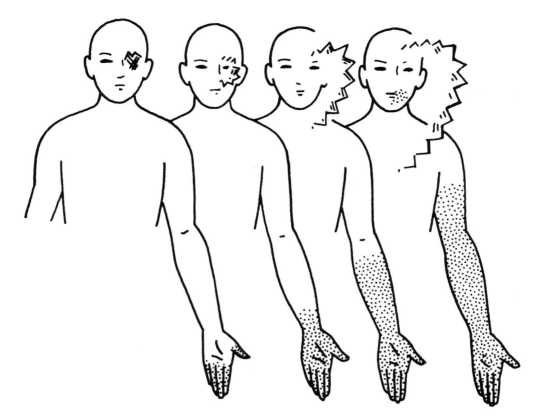

FIG. 26-1 The two most typical aura symptoms of migraine, the scintillating scotoma and digitolingual paresthesias, shown from left to right in their successive stages of development.

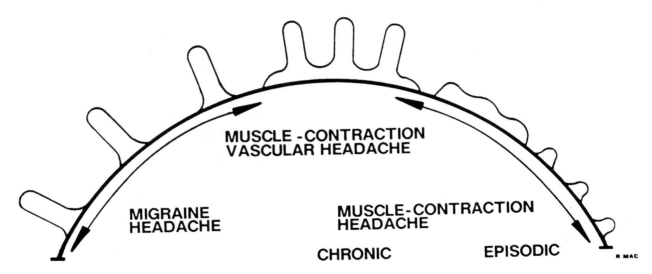

FIG. 26-2 The continuum of tension-type headache, migraine, and tension-type vascular headache.

can experience headaches anywhere on the continuum and can, in the course of time, move along it as indicated by the arrows.

Over time and as a result of a gradual increase in frequency of the headaches, episodic tension-type headache can develop into chronic tension-type headache. The increase in frequency is, in turn, associated with a progressively earlier onset of the headaches during the day, ulti-mately leading to a daily and continuous headache. The most common cause of progression of episodic into chronic tension-type headache is treatment of the headaches with analgesics. Analgesics, whether obtained with or without prescription, address only the symptom of headache but neglect the underlying mechanisms. This neglect of the underlying mechanisms results in the gradual deterioration of the headaches as described.

With further progression of the condition, chronic tension-type headache may develop into tension-type vascular headache. The change in headaches underlying this progression is a gradual increase in intensity resulting in severe headaches. The severe headaches in tension-type vascular headache are similar to those in migraine. This condition, as opposed to migraine, should be considered when the frequency of the severe headaches is high or the onset occurs late in life. Migraine generally has its onset early in life, that is, within the first three decades, with an average age of onset in women of 18.

Tension-type vascular headache, however, may also develop out of migraine as a result of a gradual increase in frequency. The condition is then referred to as *chronic* or *transformed migraine*. An increase in frequency of migraine headaches is generally associated with a progressive interposition of the headaches with tension-type headaches. This ultimately leads to a daily and continuous headache, with a regular increase in intensity to cause severe headaches. Again, treatment of the headaches with analgesics and vasoconstrictors, including caffeine, is often the cause of the progression.

EVALUATION
History

A good history is the key to the diagnosis of the previously described headache syndromes. Patients have a tendency to talk only about their severe headaches, although information regarding their mild headaches is at least as important. Important questions are shown in Box 26-1.

Questions related to the intake of prescription and nonprescription medications are also essential. It is important to know exactly how often a certain medication is taken: how many tablets or capsules per day and how many days per week or month. Of the nonprescription medications, headache and sinus medications are especially important.

Special consideration should always be given to headaches of recent onset, that is, headaches that started within weeks or months before consultation, especially when they have progressed in frequency or intensity. When a patient complains of an acute severe headache, the onset of the headache is important. When did the headache start and how long did it take to build to its maximum intensity? Did the headache build to its maximum intensity in a matter of seconds, minutes, or hours?

Also of special concern are the headaches that are always located on the same side of the head: always on the left or always on the right. This fixed lateralization to one side of the head must be explored. The explanation can sometimes be found in a skeletal asymmetry or ipsilateral tightness of the neck muscles. At other times, an ipsilateral chronic sinusitis is the cause. However, the fixed lateralization can also be due to an intracranial lesion on the side of the headaches. When transient focal neurologic symptoms occur in association with the headaches, it is important that the symptoms alternate sides. If the headaches are fixed to only one side, especially contralateral to fixed transient focal neurologic symptoms, an intracranial lesion is likely.

Physical Examination and Diagnostic Testing

Patients who present with headaches should be given, at the least, a screening neurologic examination. Any abnormality found on the examination is reason for further diagnostic testing, in particular neurodiagnostic imaging. When computed tomography is performed, it should always be conducted with intravenous contrast enhancement, unless the headache is acute and subarachnoid hemorrhage is suspected because of the very acute onset of the headache. Magnetic resonance imaging is an alternative to computed tomography with contrast; however, it is not necessary to perform both.

BOX 26-1
Key Questions in Taking a Headache History

Onset
When did the headaches start?
How often did they occur initially and how long did they last?
Were the headaches severe in intensity, or could they be treated easily with simple analgesics?
Were they initially associated with nausea or vomiting?

Frequency
How often do the headaches, including the mild ones, occur presently?
If the present frequency of the headaches is different from the initial frequency, how did the headaches change over time?
Did the headaches gradually become more frequent and more intense?
Was there a sudden change, and, if so, was it related to any particular event?
Do the headaches come about during the day, or are they present on awakening in the morning?
How often do they wake the patient at night?
How long do the headaches take to build to their maximum intensity?
How often are they severe, and how long do the severe headaches last?

Character
Where are the headaches located?
Do they have a preferential location?
What is the nature of the headaches?
Are the neck and shoulder muscles tight or sore? All the time or only with the headaches?

Associations
Do the severe headaches relate to the menstrual cycle?
How often are they associated with nausea or vomiting?
What makes the headaches worse and what makes them better?
Does physical activity or exertion make them worse?
Do coughing, sneezing, straining, and bending over affect the headaches?
Does lying down make the headaches better?
Does applying a cold pack or heating pad help?
What can bring on a headache?
Does fatigue, lack of sleep, oversleeping, skipping a meal, or physical exertion bring on headache?
When headache is brought on by stress, does it occur during or after the stressful event?
Can a headache be brought on by dietary products, such as chocolate, cheese, or alcohol?

✳ MANAGEMENT
Avoidance of Triggers

Individual headaches are often brought about by endogenous or exogenous factors (Box 26-2). Important and avoidable endogenous trigger factors include fatigue, lack of sleep, oversleeping, and lack of food. Exogenous trigger factors are stress, weather changes, dietary products, and alcoholic beverages. The trigger factors often need each other to bring on headache; therefore one strategy for decreasing headache frequency is to prevent them from compounding.

Caffeine as a dietary ingredient is significant in coffee (50 to 100 mg/8 oz), tea (25 to 50 mg/8 oz), and cola drinks (15 to 25 mg/12 oz). The headache caused by caffeine is probably a withdrawal headache, caused by decreasing of the vasoconstrictor effect of the chemical. Caffeine withdrawal often occurs on weekends partially because of oversleeping, which delays the first cup of coffee. Therefore, it is advisable to limit the total daily caffeine intake to 100 or 200 mg.

Ethanol probably causes headache, directly or indirectly, through its vasodilator effect. However, it also causes the so-called hangover headache in those otherwise not subject to headaches. The hangover headache occurs several hours after the ethanol consumption, usually the next morning, and is not caused by the ethanol itself. Chemicals in alcoholic beverages other than ethanol have been implicated here, the so-called congeners.

The **sympathomimetic amines** that are present in dietary products are tyramine and phenylethylamine. These chemicals are present in aged cheese, red wine, and dark chocolate. They act on the sympathetic nerve fibers to release the neurotransmitters norepinephrine and epinephrine. Once released, the transmitter substances act on their target tissues to produce the sympathetic effects. One of these effects is a constriction of blood vessels. The headache follows as the vasoconstriction wears off and rebound vasodilation of extracranial arteries occurs.

The **food additives** are sodium nitrite, monosodium glutamate, and aspartame. Sodium nitrite is often added to meat to preserve its red color. It is present in cured-meat products, such as frankfurters, bacon, salami, and ham. Monosodium glutamate is a food additive used extensively in the preparation of some Chinese dishes. Aspartame is an artificial sweetener that is present in diet-food products. The mechanism by which the food additives cause headache is not known.

Abortive Treatment

Abortive treatment aims at the individual headaches to decrease their intensity and duration, if possible within 1 or 2 hours. Abortive treatment is generally indicated when the headaches are moderate or severe in intensity.

Tension-Type Headaches

The abortive treatment of tension-type headaches is better accomplished with muscle relaxants than with analgesics. This is not so much because of efficacy, which is higher for the analgesics, but because of the progression of the headaches that occurs with frequent analgesic use. Muscle relaxants that can be used for this purpose are **metaxalone** (Skelaxin) and **carisoprodol** (Soma). Both medications are fast and short acting and therefore suitable for abortive treatment. Metaxalone often has to be given in a dose of 800 mg to be effective, whereas 350 mg of carisoprodol generally suffices. The medications can be taken as needed every 4 hours. Especially carisoprodol can cause drowsiness as an adverse effect.

Migraine Headaches

The treatment of migraine headaches is best accomplished with vasoconstrictors. These medications are the most specific for the condition and, therefore, most effective. When they are taken by mouth, as is often the case, absorption must be considered. It has been shown that oral absorption during migraine headaches is impaired, as a result of dysfunction of the gastrointestinal tract. The dysfunction consists of atony and dilation of the stomach with closure of the pyloric sphincter. It results from activation of the sympathetic nervous system, as it occurs during the migraine headache secondary to the pain.

The gastrointestinal dysfunction characteristic of migraine can be addressed with **metoclopramide** (Reglan), an antinausea medication with gastrokinetic properties. It stimulates the gastrointestinal tract and thereby corrects the impaired absorption of oral medications. It is taken in a dose of 10 mg by mouth but needs to be ingested early, that is, at the onset of the headache and before the headache becomes moderate or severe, to be effectively absorbed. It generally does not cause sedation or any other adverse effects and therefore can be taken early. Medications for treatment of the headache are often more effective when ingested 15 minutes after the metoclopramide, including simple analgesics.

A useful oral medication for the treatment of migraine is a combination of **isometheptene, dichloralphenazone,** and **acetaminophen (Midrin).** Isometheptene is an indirectly acting sympathomimetic with mild vasoconstrictor activity,

---

BOX 26-2
Common Headache Triggers

General
Stress/tension
Fatigue
Lack of sleep
Not eating on time

Foods/Drinks
Caffeine
Tyramine in aged cheese and red wine
Phenylethylamine in dark chocolate

Food Additives
Sodium nitrate
Monosodium glutamate
Aspartame

Alcohol

Menstruation and ovulation

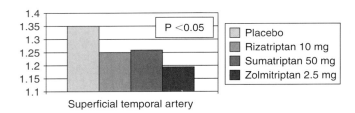

FIG. 26-3 Effect of oral triptans, 1.5 to 2.5 hours after administration, compared with placebo on the diameter of the superficial temporal artery, in millimeters, in migraineurs between attacks (n = 16). (Data obtained from JNJM de Hoon, Migraine and anti-migraine drugs, Thesis, Maastricht University, The Netherlands, 2000.)

Table 26-2
Tablet Strengths, Optimum and Maximum Daily Doses of the Triptans

Name	Tablet Strengths	Optimum Dose	Maximum Daily Dose
Almotriptan (Axert)	6.25 and 12.5 mg	12.5 mg	50 mg
Naratriptan (Amerge)	2.5 mg	2.5 mg	5 mg
Rizatriptan (Maxalt)	5 and 10 mg	10 mg*	30 mg*
Sumatriptan (Imitrex)	25, 50, and 100 mg	50 mg	200 mg
Zolmitriptan (Zomig)	2.5 and 5 mg	2.5 mg	10 mg

*In patients on propranolol, optimal dose is 5 mg and maximal dose is 15 mg of rizatriptan.

and dichloralphenazone is a mild sedative. Midrin is generally well tolerated with few if any adverse effects, of which stomach upset is the most common. It is taken in a dose of two capsules at the onset of the headache, if necessary, followed by one every half hour, with a maximum of six per day. The medication is contraindicated with the concomitant use of a monoamine-oxidase inhibitor.

In the oral abortive treatment of migraine, the **selective serotonin agonists** or **triptans** are a step up in potency from Midrin. The medications cause constriction of the extracranial arteries (Fig. 26-3). They also inhibit the mechanism of neurogenic inflammation, which, together with the vasodilation, causes the migraine headache.

Serotonin agonists attack the migraine cycle of vasodilation and inflammation by inducing vasoconstriction and inhibiting the release of inflammatory factors. The selective serotonin agonists have relatively little effect on the coronary and peripheral vascular beds. Nevertheless, caution is required when they are used in patients with uncontrolled hypertension or coronary artery disease.

All five selective serotonin agonists are available for oral administration (Table 26-2). Naratriptan (Amerge) is slower acting than the others. The concomitant use of propranolol requires a 50% reduction in dose of rizatriptan because of interference with the breakdown of the triptan.

Almotriptan (Axert), rizatriptan (Maxalt), sumatriptan (Imitrex), and zolmitriptan (Zomig) in the doses shown have similar efficacy (Table 26-3). When taken at *mild-to-moderate* headache intensity, they provide full relief of headache in about 70% of patients within 2 hours of treatment. They also have similar recurrence rates of approximately one third, which means that one third of patients experience recurrence of moderate or severe headache within 24 hours of treatment. Naratriptan is somewhat different in that it has a slower onset of action as well as a lower recurrence rate. Hence, it may be particularly useful in those patients with longer lasting but less acute headaches. If necessary, the efficacy of the oral triptans can be enhanced by administration together with a nonsteroidal anti-inflammatory analgesic, for example, 500 to 1000 mg naproxen sodium.

With regard to tolerability, the oral selective serotonin agonists are also very similar. The adverse effects of these medications when given orally are generally mild and brief. The most common are tingling in the fingers and tightness of the throat; sometimes fatigue, light-headedness, or nausea occurs. As mentioned previously, these medications are contraindicated in uncontrolled hypertension and coronary artery disease. Rizatriptan, sumatriptan, and zolmitriptan are also

contraindicated with the concomitant use of a monoamine-oxidase inhibitor.

Nonoral Treatments

When oral medications fail to relieve a migraine headache, it is usually due to impaired absorption. Rather than increasing the strength of the medication, it is generally more effective to alter the route of administration. Administration of a medication by a different route is also more effective once the headache has established itself, for example, when it is present on awakening in the morning or when it wakes the patient up out of sleep at night. An effective way of administering a medication under these circumstances is by nasal spray or rectal suppository.

The **sumatriptan (Imitrex) nasal spray** contains 20 mg sumatriptan administered in one spray. It can be repeated once in 24 hours with a minimum interval of 2 hours. The onset of action of the nasal spray is about twice as fast as that of the tablet. The most common adverse effect of sumatriptan nasal spray is a bad or bitter taste in the mouth.

The dose of **dihydroergotamine (Migranal) nasal spray** is 2 mg, which is administered in four sprays, that is, one in each nostril, repeated after 15 minutes. Its efficacy is slightly less than that of the sumatriptan nasal spray. The most common adverse effect is nasal congestion, followed by a bad taste in the mouth and nausea. The 24-hour headache recurrence rate with dihydroergotamine nasal spray is 15%, considerably lower than what is seen with most selective serotonin agonists (excepting naratriptan). This feature makes dihydroergotamine nasal spray, such as naratriptan, particularly useful in patients with longer lasting headaches. Dihydroergotamine is a potent vasoconstrictor and is contraindicated in uncontrolled hypertension and coronary artery disease.

Indomethacin rectal suppositories provide a potent anti-inflammatory analgesic with mild constrictor effects on the cranial arteries. The dose is 50 mg taken every half hour, up to a maximum of four per day. The most common adverse effect is orthostatic light-headedness, owing to its systemic vasodilator effect. The medication is contraindicated in peptic ulcer disease and bleeding disorders.

Table 26-3
Abortive Medications for Migraine, Categorized by Headache Intensity at Time of Treatment

Intensity	Initial Dose	Maximum Dose	Duration of Action
Mild			
Midrin	2 capsules Can repeat 1 every ½ hr	5 capsules/day 10/week	Short
Naratriptan (Amerge)	2.5 mg Can repeat in 4 hours	5 mg/day	Intermediate
Mild to Moderate			
Almotriptan (Axert)	12.5 mg Can repeat in 2 hours	50 mg/day	Short
Rizatriptan (Maxalt)	10 mg (5 mg with propranolol) Can repeat in 2 hours	30 mg/day (15 mg with propranolol)	Short
Sumatriptan (Imitrex)	50 mg Can repeat in 2 hours	200 mg/day	Short
Zolmatriptan (Zomig)	2.5 mg Can repeat in 2 hours	10 mg/day	Short
Moderate			
Sumatriptan nasal spray (Imitrex)	20 mg Can repeat in 2 hours	20 mg/day	Short
Indomethacin suppository	50 mg Can repeat every ½ hr	100 mg/day	Intermediate
Dihydroergotamine nasal spray (Migranal)	0.5 mg in each nostril Repeat in 15 minutes	2 mg/day	Long
Moderate to Severe			
Cafergot suppository	⅓ suppository Can repeat in ½ to 1 hr	2/day	Long
Severe			
Sumatriptan injection (Imitrex)	6 mg Can repeat in 1 hour	12 mg/day	Short
Dihydroergotamine injection (DHE 45)	1 mg Can repeat in 1 hour	2 mg/day	Long

The **Cafergot suppository** contains 2 mg of ergotamine in combination with 100 mg of caffeine to improve its absorption. Nausea and vomiting are its most common adverse effects. To minimize this problem, patients are advised to take only one third of a suppository at a time and repeat that, if necessary, every ½ to 1 hour, with a maximum of two per day. When taken in this way, the Cafergot suppository often provides effective relief of the migraine headache, without causing significant gastrointestinal adverse effects. However, it can also be combined with an antinausea medication, either orally or rectally.

Parenteral dihydroergotamine (DHE 45) is also available for abortive treatment. The dose of dihydroergotamine is 1 mg, which can be given subcutaneously, intramuscularly, or intravenously. It should *always* be given after an antinausea medication is administered, for example, 10 mg of metoclopramide intramuscularly or intravenously, to prevent the occurrence or worsening of nausea and vomiting.

Parenteral sumatriptan (Imitrex) is available with an autoinjector for easy self-administration by the patient. The injection is given subcutaneously and comes in prefilled syringes that contain 6 mg of the medication. The injection can be repeated, if necessary, after 1 hour, but it has been shown that this does *not* increase the efficacy. Also, administration of sumatriptan by injection during the aura has been shown *not* to affect the ensuing headache; however, administration of the medication during the aura is safe and has no effect on the intensity or duration of the symptoms. The most common adverse effects of sumatriptan when given by injection are a hot, tight, or tingling sensation, generally in the upper chest, anterior neck, and face, and light-headedness.

Preventive Treatment

Preventive treatment aims at decreasing the frequency of occurrence of the headaches. Whether preventive treatment is also indicated depends on the frequency, intensity, and duration of the headaches, as well as on the effectiveness of abortive treatment. It should be considered when moderate or severe headaches occur more often than three or four times a month or when headaches in general occur daily or almost daily.

Tension-Type Headache

The two medications that have been shown to be effective in the preventive treatment of (chronic) tension-type headache are **amitriptyline** and **doxepin**. The doses used are lower than for the treatment of depression and range from 25 to 75 mg/day. It is best to prescribe the medications once daily at bedtime because they often cause sedation. They are particularly helpful in patients who have problems falling asleep or sleeping through the night. Apart from sedation, the medications can cause dry mouth, constipation, and weight gain. They are contraindicated in glaucoma, epilepsy, and cardiac arrhythmias.

If the patient does not tolerate amitriptyline or doxepin because of sedation or weight gain, **imipramine** can be tried. Imipramine has been shown to be effective in the treatment of chronic tension-type headache but in an open study only. Of the selective serotonin reuptake inhibitors, citalopram (Celexa) and paroxetine (Paxil) have been studied in the preventive treatment of chronic tension-type headache and were found to be ineffective.

Physical therapy and relaxation techniques can also be useful for the prevention of tension-type headache. The simplest form of physical therapy is the use of a heating pad on the neck and shoulder muscles. This is an effective way of decreasing the tightness of the neck and shoulder muscles, provided it is applied regularly, preferably daily. Exercises to stretch and strengthen the muscles complement the effect of local heat. More formal physical therapy modalities include massage, ultrasound, and traction. Mobilization or manipulation of the neck can also be helpful in stretching and thereby relaxing the small intervertebral muscles.

Relaxation techniques that can be applied in the treatment of tension-type headache are autogenic and biofeedback training. In autogenic training, suggestions of warmth and heaviness are used to relax successive parts of the body; as an alternative, hypnotherapy can be used with self-hypnosis. **Biofeedback training** is directed at general muscle relaxation or teaching the patient to increase her finger temperature. The latter causes relaxation of the craniocervical muscles. The relaxation therapies, however, are effective only when practiced regularly, preferably daily. In this way, they do not differ from the preventive medications, which also have to be taken daily to be effective.

Migraine

The nonpharmacologic approaches described previously can also be applied in the preventive treatment of migraine. They may be particularly effective when the headaches are associated with considerable tightness and soreness of the neck and shoulder muscles. This is often the case when migraine headaches occur frequently.

Beta-blockers are among the most effective agents for migraine prevention. The beta-blockers that lack partial agonist activity increase peripheral vascular resistance by increasing blood vessel tone, thereby mitigating the process of migrainous vasodilation. **Propranolol** is most commonly used for migraine prevention, generally in doses ranging from 80 to 160 mg/day. When use is made of the long-acting capsule, the medication can be taken once daily. Adverse effects of propranolol are fatigue, depression, insomnia, and sexual dysfunction. The medication is contraindicated in sinus bradycardia, atrioventricular block, congestive heart failure, obstructive pulmonary disease, and diabetes mellitus. **Atenolol, bisoprolol,** or **metoprolol** is preferred over propranolol because they are generally better tolerated, equally effective, and long-acting.

Amitriptyline is a serotonin and norepinephrine uptake inhibitor and has been shown to increase the pain threshold. It is best prescribed once a day at bedtime because it causes sedation. Apart from sedation and dry mouth, amitriptyline can cause constipation and weight gain as adverse effects.

Verapamil is a calcium-entry blocker that also increases the pain threshold. Verapamil is generally well tolerated and constipation is its most common adverse effect. The medication is contraindicated in atrioventricular block and sick-sinus syndrome.

Valproate is a GABA A-receptor agonist and anticonvulsant. It can cause nausea and indigestion and is, therefore, best taken with meals and at bedtime with a snack. The serum level can be determined and should preferably be maintained between 50 and 100 μg/ml. Liver function should be monitored regularly because of a remote risk of hepatotoxicity. Valproate is contraindicated in liver disease.

Of the selective serotonin reuptake inhibitors, fluoxetine (Prozac) and sertraline (Zoloft) have been studied in the preventive treatment of migraine. Fluoxetine was found to be effective in one, but not in another, much larger study. Sertraline was studied in a very small trial and found not to be effective.

A summary of the dosage and efficacy of the preventive antimigraine medications is shown in Table 26-4. The medications are roughly equally effective, with efficacy rates ranging mostly between 50% and 60% in reducing headache frequency. A total of 3 to 4 weeks of treatment are required to assess effectiveness. Verapamil is probably the best tolerated but is not effective unless there is a preponderance of nocturnal headaches. The beta-blockers are next best tolerated and generally more effective in migraine prevention than verapamil. Valproate is less well tolerated, especially because of gastrointestinal adverse effects, and certainly not more effective than verapamil.

The preventive treatment of migraine should always be tried first with a single medication. However, medications can also be combined and a good combination is that of a

Table 26-4
Preventive Medications for Migraine, Categorized on the Basis of Their Efficacy and Tolerability

Medication	Starting Dose	Maximum Dose	Efficacy
First Line			
Atenolol	25 mg/day	100 mg/day	50%
Bisoprolol	2.5 mg/day	5 mg/day	60%
Metoprolol	25 mg/day	200 mg/day	50%
Nadolol	20 mg/day	240 mg/day	70%
Propranol	80 mg/day	160 mg/day	55%
Timolol	10 mg/day	20 mg/day	50%
Second Line			
Amitriptyline	10-25 mg/day	150 mg/day	60%
Third Line			
Verapamil	120 mg/day	480 mg/day	50%
Valproate	500 mg/day	1500 mg/day	55%

beta-blocker with amitriptyline. Special care should be taken when a beta-blocker is combined with verapamil because of bradycardia.

ESTROGENS AND HEADACHE

Headache is one of the most common adverse effects of the oral contraceptive pill (OCP) and is related to the dose of estrogen. Headaches occur in 5% to 10% of women taking low-dose OCPs. OCPs can aggravate preexisting headaches in 40% to 50% of users, whereas improvement in headaches occurs in 10% to 20%. Discontinuing oral contraceptives has been shown to reduce headache frequency by at least 60% in 70% of patients. It is important therefore to inquire about the occurrence of headaches in women who are considering or are taking oral contraceptives. In women with significant headaches, especially when they are related to the menstrual cycle, the potential for aggravation of the headaches should be considered against the potential benefits of using an oral contraceptive.

Postmenopausal hormone replacement therapy (HRT) can also affect headaches, although doses of estrogen are much lower than those in the OCP. For women with preexisting headaches or headaches that develop on HRT, the lowest dose of estrogen possible should be used. Estrogen should be given continuously, with cyclic or continuous progestin as appropriate. It has been shown that decreasing the dose of estrogens by at least half and giving estrogen and progestin continuously can reduce headache frequency by at least 60% in 60% of patients.

PREGNANCY, LACTATION, AND HEADACHE

In general, the use of medications during pregnancy and lactation should be discouraged because of potential effects on the embryo, fetus, or infant. For abortive treatment of migraine, *promethazine* (Phenergan) can be used safely. When prescribed as a rectal suppository of 50 mg, it is often at least somewhat effective. It is generally recommended that patients take one suppository, as needed, every 4 to 6 hours. The medication is also helpful in relieving nausea and vomiting and, in addition, causes drowsiness. The drowsiness makes it easier for the patient to sleep, thereby facilitating the recovery from the headache.

Preventive treatment should be avoided if at all possible. In the presence of tightness of the neck and shoulder muscles, physical therapy or relaxation exercises can be helpful. Fortunately, headaches often improve by themselves once the pregnancy has progressed into the second trimester. In the third trimester, a tricyclic such as amitriptyline or doxepin may be used in low dosages. The beta-blockers should be avoided because they decrease placental blood flow and may cause growth retardation of the fetus.

BIBLIOGRAPHY

Spierings ELH: *Management of migraine,* Boston, 1996, Butterworth-Heinemann.
Spierings ELH: *Headache,* Boston, 1998, Butterworth-Heinemann.
Spierings ELH: *Migraine questions and answers,* ed 2. Carol Springs, Fla, 2001, Merit Publishing International.

CHAPTER 27

Multiple Sclerosis

Tanuja Chitnis
David M. Dawson

▦ EPIDEMIOLOGY AND NATURAL HISTORY

Multiple sclerosis (MS) is a major cause of disability in the adult population in North America. It affects women, compared with men, in a ratio of approximately 2:1. The disease is characterized broadly by an array of neurologic deficits occurring over time and space. Neurologic deficits usually commence during early adulthood and progressively accumulate.

MS is a heterogeneous disease with many variations in disease course, specific neurologic deficits, and responses to treatment in affected individuals. Disease course is now defined in the following categories: relapsing-remitting, primary progressive, secondary progressive, or progressive relapsing. *Relapsing-remitting* is the most common disease type, and one in which the patient experiences episodes of neurologic deficits lasting weeks or months, which then resolve. This may continue for several years. Most of these patients then become *secondary progressive,* in which the relapsing course, after 7 to 10 years on average, changes; and they begin to accumulate progressive and fixed deficits. It is thought that this phase of the illness represents a change in the disease pathophysiology. The primary progressive course is characterized by an accumulation of deficits without periods of improvement.

The median age of clinical onset of MS is 23 to 24 years of age. The onset of neurologic deficits in women is in the early 20s; for men it tends to be 5 years later, in the late 20s. Relapsing-remitting MS has a mean age of onset of 25 to 29 years, with a mean age of conversion of secondary progressive disease at 40 to 44 years. The primary progressive group has a mean onset at 35 to 39 years and tends to affect males more often than females.

MS tends to occur in certain geographic locales. There is a diminishing north to south gradient occurring in the Northern Hemisphere, with an opposite trend in the Southern Hemisphere. However, the prevalence tends to differ between different areas on the same latitude, with a predominance in the Western industrialized nations. Countries with a prevalence of 60/100,000 or more include the northern United States, southern Canada, Europe including Russia, New Zealand, and the southeastern portion of Australia. The high incidence in many of these areas may also reflect migration trends and a predominant European heritage in the more recently settled areas of the world. Low prevalence areas include most of South America, Asia, Mexico, and Africa.

Mortality

Mortality statistics indicate an improvement in life expectancy of MS patients owing to recently improved chronic care. The Department of Health and Human Services reports that of the deaths in the year 1992, MS was a contributing cause of death at a rate of 0.7/100,000 deaths, with a total of 1900 citizens dying of MS in that year. Further analysis indicated that 1187 women (89% white and 10% black) and 713 men (90% white and 10% black) died as a consequence of MS. The mean age of death in all MS patients was calculated to be 58.1 compared with 70.5 years for national average.

ETIOLOGY
Exogenous Factors

Many infectious agents have been proposed as etiologies of the disease; however, none have withstood rigorous scrutiny and testing. Among the proposals have been the canine distemper virus and more recently, chlamydia pneumonia and HHV-6. The evidence in favor of these playing a role in MS is weak.

There has been no association between breastfeeding infants and the subsequent risk of the infant developing MS. No association was found between the use of oral contraceptives and the risk of MS.

Genetics

Genetic studies have indicated a concordance rate of about 27% in monozygotic twins, and 2.4% concordance rate in dizygotic twins of the same sex. The concordance rate in siblings is estimated to be between 2% and 5%, compared with a background risk for the general population of 0.2%. Therefore the risk of a close relative of a patient with MS also developing the disease may be 10-fold higher than the background risk. With families, the highest risk is for siblings, followed by children, aunts, uncles, and cousins. There are no differences in incidence between maternal half-siblings and paternal half-siblings of MS patients, suggesting that transmission is not sex-linked.

PATHOPHYSIOLOGY

MS causes demyelination and axonal damage in the central nervous system (CNS). Strategies to block inflammation have resulted in improvement in disease course.

The immune response in MS has been the central focus of much study. In the animal model of the disease, myelin antigens are injected subcutaneously, which results in a myelin-specific T-cell response, and in some models subsequent CNS infiltration and demyelination. In humans, a myelin-antigen T-cell response has also been observed and is present in both MS patients, as well as controls. However, these cells appear to be in an increased state of activation. The array of cytokines produced by helper T (Th) cells may also play a significant role in disease pathogenesis. There is evidence in both MS and its animal model that Th1 cytokines IFN-gamma and TNF-alpha are harmful in disease, whereas Th2 cytokines IL-4 and IL-10 are protective; however, this is a very general rule, and there are many exceptions.

Many immune-mediated and autoimmune diseases demonstrate a predominance in females, including MS, systemic lupus erythematosus, myasthenia gravis, Graves' disease, and rheumatoid arthritis. This is reflected in the animal model of MS, experimental autoimmune encephalomyelitis, in which female SJL mice are more susceptible to disease induction than males, and the administration of testosterone may protect against disease.

During pregnancy, in the first trimester, estrogen availability is high, which induces secretion of prolactin and growth hormones, which in turn increase the production of T and B cells. In the second half of pregnancy, estrogen levels drop, and progesterone levels rise, with concomitant changes in cellular and humoral immunity, with a shift toward Th2 type immunity. As outlined previously, pregnancy is protective in MS, and this may be due to the concomitant increase in progesterone and corticosteroids, which have the ability to produce a Th2 shift in cytokine production. In addition, during pregnancy several other factors are present in higher concentrations in maternal serum, including TGF-beta and IFN-beta.

CLINICAL PRESENTATION

The deficits in MS vary from patient to patient. Common presenting symptoms are paresthesias, monocular visual loss, and asymmetric eye movements with diplopia. Associated symptoms include weakness, cerebellar ataxia, and sensory disturbances. Many patients experience gait disturbances as a result of one or more of these factors.

One third of patients experience cognitive impairment, usually with abnormalities in conceptualization, recent memory, attention, and speed of information processing. Fatigue is common; however, there is poor correlation between fatigue and overall disease burden or specific lesions.

More than 50% of patients develop bladder dysfunction during the course of the disease, with 45% to 74% reporting

sexual dysfunction. A total of 50% become completely sexually inactive because of the disease, and another 20% become less sexually active. Women usually preserve the ability to experience orgasm, but most men experience erectile dysfunction. The cause of sexual dysfunction is multifactorial and may be attributed to physical challenges, sensory disturbances, as well as changes in psychosocial attitudes of the patient and partner towards sexuality.

APPROACH TO THE PATIENT
History and Physical Examination

Evaluation of a patient with proven or suspected multiple sclerosis should attempt to answer these questions:
1. Is the diagnosis clinically definite, likely, possible, or unlikely?
2. What is the current level of neurologic disability?
3. Is the process active or currently inactive?
4. Are there complicating psychiatric, social, or medical issues?
5. Is the current treatment plan appropriate and sufficient?

The cornerstone of the evaluation remains the clinical examination. Magnetic resonance imaging (MRI) can furnish valuable information, but neither it nor any laboratory test can function as an accurate diagnostic substitute (see Diagnostic Testing). Patients are classified in current practice as clinically definite, clinically probable, and possible MS, with or without laboratory support for the diagnosis. Because MS is a chronic disease, often starting as relapsing-remitting disease, it is not rare for a firm diagnosis to be delayed for several years, even though treatment decisions may be required at an early stage.

Assessment of the level of disability is important and typically involves many neurologic systems. **Cognitive dysfunction,** with memory loss and difficulty in concentration, may occur at any stage of the illness. **Visual loss** is the result of one or more bouts of optic neuritis. In uncomplicated optic neuritis an acute reduction in central vision, loss of color perception, and eye pain lasts for weeks or months, with return of vision to normal. With severe or repeated bouts of neuritis there may be sustained loss of acuity. **Motor disability** may consist of weakness or ataxia. It is most accurately measured by observation of the patient's gait.

Bladder, bowel, and sexual function are often impaired in MS patients. The urinary complaints are usually those of incomplete emptying as a result of sphincter dyssynergy, or recurrent infections, or urgent urination. Constipation is common. In men, impotence and erectile dysfunction are observed; women may have reduced perineal sensation and anorgasmia.

The formal measurement of disability can be scored on a commonly used scale, the Kurtzke Extended Disability Status Score (EDSS). This score is routinely used in experimental or therapeutic studies of MS and is widely quoted in the relevant literature. A score of zero means a diagnosis of MS with no disability; a score of 3.5 is found in a patient with considerable disability in one functional area, a score of 7.0 in a wheelchair patient, and a score of 9.0 in a helpless bedfast patient. The measurement of gait alone (Ambulation Index) is another accurate disability scoring system.

The assessment of disease activity, now that treatment options exist, is of great importance. Clinical evidence of disease activity can be evident as steady progression over months of time, or by relapses. Alternatively, or additionally, MRI may give evidence of activity, even when there are no clinical signs or symptoms of change (see Differential Diagnosis).

Complicating medical and psychiatric issues should always be sought. MS is a chronic lifelong illness, and it is to be assumed that other problems will arise during the lifetime of any patient.

DIFFERENTIAL DIAGNOSIS

The diagnosis of MS is relatively straightforward in a young adult, with relapses and remissions and involvement of the nervous system at several anatomic levels. Difficulties arise when the course is progressive from outset (approximately 15% of cases), in the middle-aged, or when the symptoms are atypical (when a diagnosis of conversion disorder is often considered). Table 27-1 lists some features to support the diagnosis.

DIAGNOSTIC TESTING
Magnetic Resonance Imaging

MRI scanning has greatly changed the managemnt of MS patients. It is the imaging study of choice in the diagnosis of MS. Additional information about disease activity can sometimes be deduced from repeated scans in the established patient.

The lesions of MS are typically seen on T2 and FLAIR sequences and rarely on T1 images (Fig. 27-1). These facts indicate that in large part the scans demonstrate an increased water content in the plaques compared with normal tissue. Fresh lesions also demonstrate enhancement with gadolinium, a paramagnetic contrast agent that can cross the disrupted blood-brain barrier. Lesions are located in the deep white matter of the hemispheres, adjacent to and often radiating from the ventricular surface. Lesions in the cerebellar connections and pons are quite characteristic. Acute optic neuritis can be visualized with special procedures.

The number or size of the lesions, contrary to expectations, is *not* a measurement of disease severity. Some young patients, with low disability scores and a history of only a few relapses, have dozens of visible lesions, whereas the middle-aged person with spinal cord dysfunction may have

only a few, even though wheelchair confined. Change in lesion size or total volume of lesion load can be shown to correlate with disease progression.

Not all T2 bright lesions of the central white matter are as a result of MS. In the older person, small vascular lesions can produce a virtually identical appearance on scan. Granulomatous diseases (especially sarcoidosis, Behçet's disease, and Sjögren's syndrome) may be mistaken for MS. In the proper clinical setting, an MRI scan showing typical lesions can confirm the diagnosis of MS at far earlier stages of the illness than was possible in pre-MRI era. An MRI scan that is normal in a patient with progressive neurologic dysfunction should direct attention toward neuronal degenerative disease rather than demyelination. However in some instances the MRI scan shows only trivial lesion load or is normal in patients with confirmed MS.

Nearly every patient should have at least one MRI to confirm the diagnosis. Repeat scans are sometimes useful to assess disease activity, either by measurement of lesion load or by looking for gadolinium enhancement. In a patient with an isolated single demyelinating episode (for instance, optic neuritis or an incomplete transverse spinal cord syndrome) a head MRI scan can be used to indicate prognosis before it is possible to make an official diagnosis of MS. If the scan is positive with the first episode, the chance of the patient developing clinically definite MS within the next 5 years is more than 50%.

Table 27-1
Clinical Features of Multiple Sclerosis

Features Common in MS	Features Suggesting Another Diagnosis
Onset between ages 15 and 50	Onset before 10, or after 60
Relapses and remissions	Steady progression
Optic neuritis	Early dementia
Lhermitte's sign	Rigidity sustained dystonia
Internuclear ophthalmoplegia	Aphasia, neglect syndrome
Marked fatigue	Deficit developing within minutes
Worsening with elevated body temperature	Fasciculations, muscle atrophy

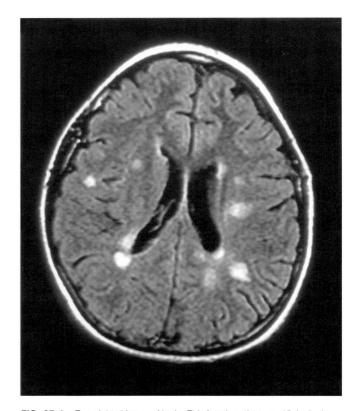

FIG. 27-1 T_2-weighted image of brain. This female patient was 15, had relapsing-remitting multiple sclerosis, and at the time of this scan was asymptomatic. Multiple lesions are seen in periventricular white matter. These lesions have the appearance of acute lesions; in longer term cases many of the lesions are more sharply defined and linear, and radiate outward from the ventricular system.

Recent advances in technology may further enhance the usefulness of MRI. Diffusion weighted imaging, and nuclear magnetic resonance spectroscopy, may give added information. Development of atrophy in the brain of an MS patient is an ominous sign. It implies axon loss, as well as myelin damage and is accompanied by dementia and personality change. Atrophy can be measured on MRI by assessing the volume of white matter tracts, such as the corpus callosum.

Other Diagnostic Tests

In addition to MRI, cerebrospinal fluid (CSF) examination may be helpful diagnostically. In about two thirds of MS patients, the CSF shows evidence of synthesis of immune globulins (Ig) within the CNS. (Synthesis in the nervous system also occurs in viral infections, syphilis, and other infections.) These globulins can be detected by a rise in the total IgG level in the CSF, by calculating a rate of synthesis, or by showing the presence of oligoclonal bands. The total protein is usually normal or nearly so; elevations of protein twice the normal range should be viewed with suspicion.

By means of surface scalp electrodes, one can record evoked electrical potentials after auditory, visual, or other stimuli. With the advent of MRI, this test has become an adjunct to confirm MS but is often not necessary.

A search continues in research laboratories for a marker in peripheral blood of presence or activity of MS. Current interest lies in the ratios of different cytokines, for instance those associated with immune activation (IL-10, IFN-gamma), versus those that appear to reduce immune activity.

As an approximation, MRI is positive in more than 90% of MS cases, whereas CSF IgG levels or presence of oligoclonal bands on electrophoresis is diagnostically useful in 75% of cases. Evoked potentials electrically recorded by scalp electrodes, especially visual evoked potentials, may add information in a few additional patients.

MANAGEMENT

Treatment of Symptoms

Many symptoms of MS can be successfully treated. These include spasticity, bladder dysfunction, depression, pain, fatigue, sexual dysfunction, and some forms of weakness. Medication, physiotherapy, and psychiatric and psychological support are the mainstays of these efforts. Neurologists, rehabilitation specialists, and primary care physicians may be involved; some treatment programs require a specialty MS clinic or tertiary hospital, but many do not. Treatment options are listed in Table 27-2.

Relapses of MS that involve significant dysfunction (e.g., ataxia, weakness, vision less than 20/200) are usually treated with high-dose intravenous steroids. Typical protocols call for methylprednisolone, 1000 g IV repeated daily for 5 to 7 days. It is difficult to achieve this level of steroid dose with oral medication. Because most relapses of MS recover well within 6 to 12 weeks, the purpose of the steroid program is to shorten the period of disability and possibly to limit residual loss of function. Long-term steroids are not useful and lead to many complications of treatment and to steroid dependency.

Within the last decade three medications have been introduced and approved by the Food and Drug Administration for prevention of relapses and limitation of disablement. All three are classified as immunomodulatory drugs. Each of the three appears to reduce the frequency of relapses by about 30%, to limit the number of severe relapses, and to reduce the developing burden of disease as measured by MRI scan. By current practice guidelines, all patients with active relapsing-remitting MS should be under treatment with one of these agents. Details of their administration and their side effects appear in Table 27-3.

A major limitation of the immunomodulatory drugs is the restriction on their use during pregnancy. Two of the three are beta-interferons, and animal studies have shown these to be abortifacient at high dose. *Glatiramer acetate* is in Category C, without either human or animal data relevant to its use in pregnancy. Current practice guidelines dictate that when pregnancy is discovered, any of the three agents should be discontinued until after delivery. If a woman is planning pregnancy, it is reasonable to postpone the use of one of these agents until after the pregnancy. Since none of the three are known to be safe for the infant while breastfeeding, current guidelines indicate that resumption of treatment should await the end of breastfeeding. If there is reason to suspect activity of the MS, discontinuation of breastfeeding is advised.

All three of the approved MS treatments for relapse prevention are injectables. Several orally administered agents are under study. Intravenous high-dose immunoglobulin may be an acceptable alternative. The field is rapidly changing and practice patterns can be expected to change.

The course and rate of progression of MS is highly variable. When patients enter the progressive phase, treatment must be altered, which in most instances involves a shift to a nonspecific immunosuppressive agent, with the expected toxicity of all chemotherapy. Drugs that are currently in use include cyclophosphamide, mitoxantrone, methotrexate, and azathioprine. Continuation of beta-interferon may or may not be indicated; some recent studies have indicated a measurable positive effect on progressive MS. All these treatments are of limited benefit, hence the emphasis in current practice of treating MS early in the hopes of preventing conversion to the progressive phase. Some of these treatment options are listed in Table 27-4.

Table 27-2
Symptomatic Treatments in Multiple Sclerosis

Symptom	Treatment
Spasticity	Physiotherapy Baclofen, 20-80 mg/day Tizanidine, 4-16 mg/day
Depression	Serotonin reuptake inhibitors Tricyclic antidepressants
Fatigue	Amantadine 100-300 mg/day Methylphenidate 10-30 mg/day Pemoline 37.5-65 mg/day
Urinary urgency	Oxybutynin 2.5-10 mg/day Tolterodine 2-4 mg/day Imipramine 50-100 mg/day Self-catheterization
Sexual dysfunction	Counseling Sildenafil 25-100 mg

Table 27-3
Immunomodulatory Drugs for Treatment of Multiple Sclerosis

Generic	Trade	Dose	How Administered	Reduction in Relapse Rate	Side Effects
Interferon B	Ia Avonex	30 μg IM	Weekly	29%	Flu symptoms, headache
Interferon B	Ib Betaseron	250 μg sc	qod	34%	Flu symptoms, site reactions
Glatirimir	Copaxone	20 μg sc	Daily	29%	Rare, angioedema

Table 27-4
Treatment Strategies in Multiple Sclerosis

Course or Stage of MS	Treatment Options
Monosymptomatic attack	IV steroids, 1000 mg × 5-7 days
Relapsing remitting, no disease activity, MRI inactive	No treatment
Relapsing remitting, recent disease activity	"ABC" drugs: Avonex, Betaseron Copaxone, or IV gamma-globulin
Relapse, while under treatment with above agents	IV steroids, 1000 mg × 5-7 days
Relapsing, but after conversion to progressive disablement	Add cyclophosphamide, monthly pulses Mitoxantrone, monthly injection Methotrexate, 7.5-20 mg p.o. weekly Cladribine, IV or sc IV steroids, as monthly pulses

Use of nonspecific immunosuppression with chemotherapeutic agents has many implications for women in their reproductive years. Cyclophosphamide produces ovarian failure and premature menopause, depending on dose, age of the patient, and ovarian reserve. Induction of secondary neoplasm has been rarely observed. Methotrexate is contraindicated at any dose level during pregnancy.

High-dose steroids may be used in pregnancy under certain circumstances. Particularly during the latter months of pregnancy, the risk of steroid use is usually acceptable. As noted previously, relapses are somewhat less common during pregnancy.

■ EFFECT OF PREGNANCY ON MS
Impact on the Course of MS

The largest prospective study of relapsing remitting disease activity found a decreased relapse rate during pregnancy in 256 patients. The greatest protection from relapses occurs in the third trimester, followed by an increase in relapse rate in the first trimester postpartum. Thirteen other studies, most of them retrospective, have observed the same trend. Most of these studies showed a decrease in relapse rate of approximately 33% to 50%. Sequential MRI in two MS patients during pregnancy showed a reduction in active lesions, followed by an increase in MRI activity during the first month postpartum.

Although it is difficult to measure the effect of pregnancy on immediate progression in MS, a review of eight studies that examined the effect of pregnancy on subsequent long-term disability showed either no effect (6/8) or a mild protection (2/8). In addition the period of pregnancy has been associated with a significantly lower risk of onset of MS, again suggesting that pregnancy is protective. There has been no documented adverse effect of breastfeeding by MS patients or receipt of epidural analgesia on long-term disability and course of MS.

Impact on Pregnancy and Childbirth

Two comprehensive reviews found no significant effect of MS on fertility, fetal viability, prematurity, incidence of toxemia, infant mortality, or delivery. Unfortunately, these studies were biased by the fact that most women who attempt childbirth have milder disease, whereas those with severe disease and frequent relapses are more likely to avoid pregnancy. There is an increased rate of childlessness in the MS population, which may relate to physical limitations, as well as psychological concerns of the patient and her partner.

BIBLIOGRAPHY

Bar-or A: The epidemiology of multiple sclerosis. In Batchelor T, Cudowicz M, editors: *Textbook of neuroepidemiology,* Boston 1999, Butterworth Heinemann.

Chancellor MB, Blaivas JG: Urological and sexual problems in multiple sclerosis, *Clin Neurosci* 2:189, 1994.

Chitnis T, Khoury SJ: Cytokines in multiple sclerosis. In Herndon RM, editor: *Multiple sclerosis and other demyelinating diseases,* in press.

Confavreux C et al: Rate of pregnancy-related relapse in multiple sclerosis, *N Engl J Med* 330:285, 1998.

Dalal M, Kim S, Voskuhl RR: Testosterone therapy ameliorates experimental autoimmune encephalomyelits and induces a T helper 2 bias in the autoantigen-specific T lymphocyte response, *J Immunol* 159:3, 1997.

Damek M, Shuster D: Pregnancy and multiple sclerosis, *Mayo Clin Proc* 72:977, 1997.

Hammond S et al: The epidemiology of multiple sclerosis in three Australian cities: Perth, Newcastle, and Hobart, *Brain* 111:1, 1998.

Kurtzke J: Geography in multiple sclerosis, *J Neurol* 215:1, 1977.

Lublin FD, Reingold SC: The National Multiple Sclerosis Society USA Advisory Committee on Clinical Trials of New Agents. Defining the clinical course of multiple sclerosis: results of an international survey, *Neurology* 46:907, 1996.

Olek M, Dawson DM: Multiple sclerosis and other inflammatory demyelinating disease of the nervous system. In Bradley WG et al: *Neurology in clinical practice,* ed 3, Boston 1999, Butterworth Heinemann.

Rao SM et al: Cognitive dysfunction in multiple sclerosis, *Neurology* 41: 685, 1991.

Rudick RA et al: Management of multiple sclerosis, *N Engl J Med* 337:1604, 1997.

Runmarker B, Andersen O: Pregnancy is associated with a lower risk of onset and a better prognosis in multiple sclerosis, *Brain* 118:253, 1995.

Sadovnik A et al: A population based half-sib study of multiple sclerosis. The Canadian Collaborative Group, *Lancet* 347:1728, 1996.

Soldan SS et al: Association of human herpes virus 6 (HHV-6) with multiple sclerosis: increased IgM response to HHV-6 early antigen and detection of serum HHV-6 DNA, *Nat Med* 3:1394, 1997.

Spencely M, Dick G: Breastfeeding and multiple sclerosis, *Neuroepidemiology* 1:216, 1982.

Sriram S et al: *Chlamydia* pneumonia infection of the central nervous system in multiple sclerosis, *Ann Neurol* 46:6, 1999.

Villard-Mackintosh L, Vessey M: Oral contraceptives and reproductive factors in multiple sclerosis incidence, *Contraception* 47:161, 1993.

Weinreb H: Demyelinating and neoplastic diseases in pregnancy, *Neurol Clin* 12:509, 1994.

Wilder R: Hormones, pregnancy, and autoimmune diseases, *Ann NY Acad Sci* 840:45, 1998.

Zhang J et al: Increased frequency of IL-2 responsive T cells specific for myelin basic protein and proteolipid protein in peripheral blood and cerebrospinal fluid of patients with multiple sclerosis, *J Exp Med* 179:973, 1994.

CHAPTER 28

Alzheimer's Disease and Dementia

M. Cornelia Cremens
Olivia I. Okereke

As the elderly population expands in the United States, the incidence of dementia is also on the rise. Because they tend to live longer than men, women are likely to be disproportionately affected by this trend. Thus, the impact of dementia on women is a major public health issue. Knowledge of the epidemiology, diagnosis, and management of dementia, especially as it relates to women, is important for primary care physicians.

Dementia is defined as the development of multiple cognitive deficits, which must include memory loss and one or more of the following: aphasia, apraxia, agnosia, or disturbances of executive function. These domains of cognitive impairment are described in Box 28-1.

▦ EPIDEMIOLOGY

Many etiologies for dementia exist; these include structural, infectious, vascular, hereditary, metabolic, and degenerative central nervous system (CNS) disorders (Box 28-2). Among all causes, Alzheimer's disease (AD) is the most common (accounting for 50% to 70%). Vascular dementia is a relatively distant second; it explains about 15% to 25% of cases. Currently, women outnumber men for AD, and men outnumber women for vascular dementia.

Roughly 4 million Americans are demented. Dementia affects 5% to 7% of individuals over the age of 65 and almost half (47%) of those over the age of 85. The elderly are the fastest-growing segment of the US population; women outnumber men in this cohort (20 million women to 13.9 million men). Because there will be 39.7 million Americans over the age of 65 by the year 2010, many anticipate that dementia will become a public health epidemic in the twenty-first century. Every clinician will need to be cognizant of dementia's growing presence and impact.

Alzheimer's Disease

AD is the leading cause of dementia in this country, accounting for 50% to 70% of all cases of dementia. It is the fourth leading cause of death in adults, creates a major public health problem, fills 50% (or more) of nursing home beds, and costs approximately $100 billion each year.

Alois Alzheimer first described AD in a 1906 case report. The disease is a chronic, progressive neurodegenerative condition. It is identified pathologically by autopsy or biopsy and is characterized by dense beta-amyloid plaques and neurofibrillary tangles.

Not only are women more likely develop AD because of their higher life expectancy, but they are at increased risk compared to men, even after adjusting for longer survival. Such a finding indicates that factors other than age play a role in women's increased AD risk.

On all levels, women are disproportionately affected by AD. Not only are women at increased risk for development of the disease, but caregiver burden is also higher for women. Two thirds of all AD caregivers are women. Among adult children who provide care for their Alzheimer's-afflicted parents, 80% to 90% are women.

Impact of Race and Ethnicity

Studies of incidence and prevalence of AD among different nations and ethnic groups are somewhat confusing (see Ethnic Risk Factors). The incidence of AD is lower in East Asian countries than it is in Europe or the United States. There is an overall lower prevalence among Nigerians compared with African-Americans in Indiana. A major issue, among all ethnic groups in both the United States and in developing nations, is the fact that women's access to education, health care, medication, and other resources affect the risk and expression of AD.

RISK FACTORS FOR ALZHEIMER'S DISEASE
Genetic Risk Factors

Both genetic and environmental factors contribute to the risk of developing AD. Relatives of affected AD patients are at increased risk. Furthermore, female relatives of AD probands show a higher risk of developing AD than their male counterparts. In general, the lifetime risk of first-degree relatives of individuals with AD ranges from 23% to 81%. Nonetheless, the overall risk seems to be less than the 50% we would expect of a gene that is inherited in an autosomal dominant fashion. However, it is important to remember that not all "familial" diseases are necessarily genetic; they may appear as such because of shared environments, shared habits, and other nongenetic risk factors.

BOX 28-1
Domains of Cognitive Impairment

- **Aphasia:** Difficulty finding words, making malapropisms, substituting words (e.g., "the thing" or "whatchamacallit"), losing one's train of thought, or stuttering or repeating words.
- **Apraxia:** Difficulty dressing, bathing, grooming, or feeding *without assistance.*
- **Agnosia:** Difficulty recognizing friends, co-workers, family (late in disease), or familiar objects.
- **Executive dysfunction:** Difficulty following conversations, planning events or activities, operating appliances (e.g., tools, televisions, radios).

Adapted from Steffens DC, Morgenlander JC: *Postgrad Med* 106:72, 1999.

BOX 28-2
Pathology of Dementia

Central nervous system tumor
Head trauma
Subdural hematoma
Infectious diseases: syphilis, HIV/AIDS, Creutzfeld-Jacob Disease (CJD)
Vascular diseases
Congenital/hereditary diseases: Huntington's disease, Down syndrome
Pseudodementia of depression
Seizure disorder
Normal pressure hydrocephalus
Vitamin and nutrient deficiencies (B_{12}, thiamin, folate)
Hypoxia and hypoxemia
Metabolic/endocrine disturbances, e.g., hypothyroidism, hypercalcemia
Neurodegenerative disorders: Alzheimer's disease (AD), Pick's disease, Lewy body disease, Parkinson's disease, progressive supranuclear palsy, Wilson's disease
Demyelinating diseases
Toxins: alcohol, heavy metals, carbon monoxide, medications, radiation

The clear association between the presence of an affected first-degree relative and the likelihood of developing AD has led investigators to pursue genetic risk factors. Interestingly, in early-onset (before age 65) AD families, the presence of AD tends to behave in a Mendelian fashion; this is not the case in late-onset (after age 65) AD families, where the genetic mechanism is more complex. The mechanisms by which genotype may ultimately affect the expression of the phenotype of AD remains unclear, but several AD-associated genes have been identified.

Genes associated with risk can be divided into two categories: causal and susceptibility genes—that is, genes that are known to cause AD and genes that are associated with increased susceptibility to developing AD without proven causal effect. In the causal category, three genes have been located: the mutated amyloid precursor protein (APP) gene on chromosome 21, the presenilin 1 gene on chromosome 14, and the presenilin 2 gene on chromosome 1. These three genes (transmitted in an autosomal dominant manner) account for about 80% of familial early-onset AD but less

than 2% of AD cases overall. Susceptibility genes are likely to play a larger role in most AD cases; these include the genes that encode apolipoprotein E (APOE), and possibly, α1-antichymotrypsin, and the very-low-density lipoprotein receptor.

Apolipoprotein E (APOE)

The APOE genotype deserves special attention in the discussion of AD risk factors. It has emerged as a focus of interest among researchers and of curiosity among the lay public. Many patients and families, especially those who regularly use the Internet, may present to the primary care physician's office with questions about APOE as it relates to the diagnosis and risk of development of AD.

APOE is a plasma protein involved in the transport and metabolism of cholesterol and lipid. The APOE gene is located on chromosome 19, and it is now recognized as the single most important genetic determinant of susceptibility to AD. APOE governs susceptibility for both sporadic and familial late-onset AD. The APOE gene has three alleles, or varieties: ε2, ε3, and ε4; each person has two alleles, in any combination.

APOE genotype appears to mitigate risk of AD; there appears to be a dosage effect of the number of ε4 alleles and the risk of developing AD. In all 34% to 65% of AD patients carry a copy of the ε4 allele, while it is present in only 24% to 31% of the non-AD adult population. APOE ε4 heterozygotes (carriers of a single ε4 allele) have an odds ratio of AD 2.2 to 4.4 times greater than that of ε3/ε3 (ε3 homozygous) individuals; APOE ε4 homozygotes have an increase in the odds ratio from 5.1 to 30.1. It has yet to be established whether ε2 confers a protective effect against AD.

Gender interacts with the degree of risk conferred by APOE genotype: Caucasian females with ε3/ε4 genotype are 1.5 times more likely to develop AD than Caucasian males with the same genotype. Debate exists about the role of APOE among different racial and ethnic groups. Presence of the ε4 allele was not elevated among Swedish samples, and the association is absent altogether in a sample of Nigerians.

Farrer and colleagues studied the impact of ethnicity on the APOE/AD association. The group pooled data on APOE genotype, gender, age of onset, and ethnicity from 5930 patients with probable or definite AD and 8607 control subjects. Results showed that an APOE ε4 association was present but substantially weaker among African-Americans and Hispanics than among Caucasians. Also, there was significant heterogeneity of the odds ratios among African-Americans.

Perhaps, it is equally important to recognize what APOE does not influence. A strong association has not been demonstrated between the APOE ε4 allele and non-Alzheimer's dementias, such as dementia associated with Parkinson's disease, Lewy body disease, or vascular dementia (there is debate about whether the ε4 allele confers susceptibility to Creutzfeldt-Jakob disease (CJD) or Pick's disease). Also, there is a lack of an association between ε4 and the rate of cognitive and functional decline in AD.

Not surprisingly, many patients and their relatives may ask questions in the office about the possibility of APOE genotype tests, hoping to use this information to predict their likelihood of developing the disease or to guide future decisions, such as financial arrangements and family planning. The 1995 consensus report of the American College of Medical Genetics/American Society of Human Genetics speaks to these concerns. While the report's authors recognize the strong association between the APOE ε4 allele and AD, it recommends against genotyping for routine clinical diagnosis or for prediction of AD. Furthermore, the report notes that the presence of the ε4 allele is not required for the expression of AD; and patients with only ε2 or ε3 alleles do develop AD, so these genotypes may be falsely reassuring to some. Also, the value of the notion of predictive testing is questioned: the course of illness cannot be substantially modified using this information; APOE genotype cannot predict the rate of decline; and actual age of onset still cannot be predicted from knowledge of APOE gene status. Despite the important role that APOE plays in the development of AD, the vast majority of cases are clearly governed by multiple factors.

Environmental Risk Factors

Several environmental risk factors for AD have been proposed. Risk-modifying factors can be grouped into *protective* and *negative* categories. Possible protective factors include postmenopausal estrogen replacement therapy, smoking, increased educational level, and chronic use of NSAIDs. Likely negative risk factors include a history of depression, repeated head injury, and thyroid disease. Diminished linguistic ability in early life may be an additional risk factor for dementia in late life; this idea was suggested by results of the longitudinal Nun Study.

Female hormones, especially estrogens, greatly impact women's risk of dementia. Possible positive effects of estrogen include its neurotrophic and antioxidant properties (antioxidants protect against beta-amyloid, which accumulates in the plaques that are diagnostic of AD) and its modulatory role in acetylcholine (ACh) secretion in the hippocampus, a brain structure that plays a critical role in memory. Various psychiatric disorders (e.g., AD, schizophrenia, alcoholism, mood disorders, and anxiety disorders) demonstrate hormone-mediated risks and buffers. Estrogen may protect against neuron degeneration, may enhance growth, and may decrease susceptibility to toxins. On the other hand, cyclic fluctuation of hormones (estrogen and progesterone) may increase a woman's susceptibility to depression and anxiety.

If hormones do in fact create such differences, what is the basis of this action? The human central nervous system is presumed to be most sensitive to the effects of gonadal steroids between 14 and 16 weeks of gestation, when peak testosterone concentrations are found in fetal serum samples. Between this period and puberty, the brain's exposure to hormones is similar in boys and girls. As females become sexually mature, their hormone levels fluctuate cyclically over a much wider range than do those of males. At menopause, ovarian secretion of estrogen drops drastically, while testosterone is produced by the testes throughout the male life cycle. Testosterone is partly converted to estradiol in the brain, albeit at an increasingly slower rate as men age. This may explain why women's neurons begin to degenerate after menopause at a faster pace than men's brain cells.

Estrogen is protective against AD. Possible reasons for the neuroprotective action of estrogen include the role of estrogen in normal brain development, the presence of estrogen receptors in the hippocampus and other brain structures important for memory, estrogen-induced changes in APOE messenger RNA (mRNA) expression, estrogen-related increases in cerebral blood flow, primary neurotrophic effects, estradiol-mediated up-regulation of other neurotrophins, and interactions with the cholinergic basal forebrain system.

Ethnic Risk Factors

The rates of AD in African-American and Hispanic communities are substantially higher than those among Caucasians. However, the reasons for this discrepancy have not been fully elucidated. Tang and co-workers noted that unknown genetic or environmental factors appear to increase the risk for AD for African-Americans and some Hispanics. Even among people without the APOE ε4 allele, African-Americans had a cumulative risk of developing AD before the age of 90 that was four times higher than that of Caucasians. Among Hispanics from the Dominican Republic and elsewhere in the Caribbean, the risk was two times higher than that for Caucasians, again in the absence of the ε4 allele. Studying these ethnic differences and finding their origins could lead to identification of other important AD risk factors. Studies are ongoing in isolated ethnic communities to evaluate the impact of specific factors (e.g. environment, toxins, education, genetics) on AD risk. It is hoped that more researchers will pursue an understanding of ethnic risk factors while investigating possible interactions between gender and ethnicity in the development of AD.

DIFFERENTIAL DIAGNOSIS

The hallmarks of dementia are (1) cognitive decline, especially memory; (2) behavioral disturbance; and (3) impaired daily function. Dementia must be distinguished from other disorders that may present with cognitive and/or behavioral disturbance. In dementia, it is often a patient's family member who reports problems with the patient's memory. **Age-related cognitive decline,** which may prompt concerns voiced by the patient herself, is associated with a decline in acquiring and retrieving new information but not in memory retention. Unlike dementia, the onset of **delirium** is relatively acute; somnolence, fluctuating level of consciousness, and difficulty with attention and concentration may be present. In **depression,** the patient herself is more likely to report memory loss, as well as apathy, hopelessness, or impaired concentration.

Types of Dementia and Dementia Syndromes

Alzheimer's disease (AD), the most common cause of dementia, currently affects about 4 million people in the United States, and by 2040 is expected to attain a high of 9 million. The pathognomonic characteristic of AD is the accumulation of beta-amyloid plaques. The neurotoxic phenomena related to the neural deterioration or degeneration produce a progressive cognitive impairment with widespread neurologic and neuropsychiatric symptoms.

Dementia associated with cerebrovascular disease or **vascular dementia** was referred to as multi-infarct dementia in the past. Prevalence in memory disorder clinics is low, from 5% to 20%. The mixed dementia of both vascular and AD has a higher prevalence.

Lewy body dementia (LBD) presents with both cognitive impairment and extrapyramidal symptoms. The extrapyramidal symptoms can mimic Parkinson's disease, with rigidity, masked facies, resting tremor, shuffling gait, postural instability and at times syncope, hypophonia, and stooped posture. This type of dementia appears less than 10% of the time in patients with dementia. It is often confused with Parkinson's disease in that about one third of patients with Parkinson's disease also develop dementia. Initial symptoms often include prominent hallucinations, delusion misidentification syndromes, and depression, which is more prominent in patients with LBD than AD. An exquisite sensitivity to medications, especially psychotropic agents and the neuroleptics in particular, limit the use of medications to dampen the psychotic symptoms.

The dementia of **Parkinson's disease** may have a mixed picture of Parkinson's disease and AD; conversely patients with AD can develop symptoms of Parkinson's disease late in the course of the dementia. As with LBD, medications must be used with great caution so as not to further impair mobility.

Less common causes of dementia include frontal lobe dementia (including Pick's disease), normal pressure hydrocephalus, central nervous system neoplasms, chronic subdural hematomas, and Creutzfeldt-Jakob disease. Important reversible causes of dementia are those related to medication, alcohol, and metabolic disorders (see Box 28-2).

▣ EVALUATION

The approach to the evaluation of dementia is outlined in Box 28-3. The history, obtained from both patient and family, should include questioning about visual hallucinations, delusions, and depression (to identify possible early Parkinson's disease or LBD), as well as medications that may impair cognition. Formal cognitive testing with an instrument such as the Mini-Mental State Exam (MMSE) is essential for diagnosis, as well as for monitoring the course of disease. Norms for the MMSE that incorporate age, gender, and educational level improve the test's accuracy.

The physical examination includes particular attention to detection of focal neurologic deficits (suggesting possible vascular dementia), signs of Parkinson's disease (rigidity, masked facies, cogwheeling, tremor), and to assessment of gait (normal pressure hydrocephalus should be considered if urinary incontinence and gait disturbance accompany cognitive impairment).

Laboratory testing aims to identify treatable causes of dementia. The yield of such testing and the potential for reversibility has been demonstrated to be quite low. Because neuroimaging has relatively low sensitivity and specificity, there is controversy about its clinical utility in the evaluation of dementia. Clinical factors such as young age, short duration of symptoms, and focal signs should be considered in the decision to obtain neuroimaging with head CT scan or magnetic resonance imaging (MRI).

✳ MANAGEMENT

The goals of treatment of dementia are to demonstrate improvement in behavior and function, or to delay institutionalization.

BOX 28-3
Evaluation of Dementia

History
Memory loss
Disturbance of executive function and/or activities of daily living
Time course of onset
Presence of symptoms suggesting non-Alzheimer dementia
    Visual hallucinations, delusions, depression
Presence of risk factors: family history, head trauma, depression, low educational level
Medical disorders (especially cardiovascular disease, hypertension)
Medications

Cognitive Testing
Mini-Mental State Exam (MMSE)

Physical Examination
Focal neurologic deficits
Signs of Parkinson's disease (tremor, masked facies, cogwheel rigidity)
Gait disturbance

Laboratory Tests
CBC
Electrolytes, calcium, glucose, BUN, Cr
Liver function tests
TSH
Serum B_{12} level
Syphilis serology

Neuroimaging
Cranial CT or MRI

Table 28-1
Available Drugs for Alzheimer's Disease

Medication	Dose	Cost	Adverse Side Effects
Tacrine (Cognex)	10-40 mg po QID	$150	Nausea, vomiting, diarrhea, hepatotoxicity, dyspepsia, myalgias, and anorexia
Donepezil (Aricept)	5 up to 10 mg QD	$135	Diarrhea, nausea, abdominal cramps
Rivastigmine (Exelon)	1.5 to 6 mg BID	$130	Nausea
Galantamine (Reminyl)	4 to 12 mg BID	$130	Nausea, bradycardia

Medications used and approved by the Food and Drug Administration (FDA) in the treatment of AD are tacrine, donepezil, rivastigmine, and galantamine (Table 28-1). Indications for these agents are to slow the progress of the dementia and possibly improve the behavioral problems that accompany these diseases. Cholinesterase inhibitors do not halt the process of neuronal deterioration seen in AD, but slow it and prevent or prolong institutionalization of the individual with dementia. Their efficacy has been established in patients with mild to moderate AD.

Cortical acetylcholinetransferase activity is diminished and acetylcholine neurotransmission is impaired in AD. The central hypothesis underlying the efficacy of anticholinesterase inhibitors is enhancement of central cholinergic function. Evidence now indicates that some AChE inhibitors also may provide neuroprotective effects, perhaps through the activation of nicotinic receptors, and may even enhance neurotrophic regeneration. Other possible actions include the effect of cholinergic agonists on the processing and secretion of the amyloid precursor protein and beta-amyloid.

Tacrine (tetrahydroaminoacridine) is a centrally acting reversible acetylcholinesterase inhibitor that was found to ameliorate some cognitive symptoms in a small number of responders with mild to moderate AD. Tacrine was the first drug on the market and proved to be poorly tolerated and have many side effects, including hepatotoxicity, nausea, and vomiting.

Donepezil, a piperidine-based AChE inhibitor with specificity for AChE, was approved by the FDA subsequently for symptomatic therapy of mild to moderate AD. The bioavailability of donepezil is almost 100%, with peak plasma concentrations occurring between 2 and 4 hours after an oral dose. Food has no significant effect on the drug absorption and mean elimination half-life is 70 hours, allowing once-daily dosing. The usual dose is 5 mg/day, increasing to 10 mg/day after one month.

Rivastigmine is a neuronal selective AChE inhibitor released several years after donepezil. The additional advantage in rivastigmine is that it not only stimulates the AChE but also butyrylcholinesterase (BchE). Patients with AD can tolerate up to 12 mg/day. Adverse effects did not include hepatotoxic effects as with tacrine. The results of the early studies demonstrated significant beneficial effects on measures of cognition using the Alzheimer's Disease Assesment Scale-cognitive subscale (ADAS-Cog), global functioning, and activities of daily living.

Galantamine, a naturally occurring amarylidacea alkaloid, is a long-acting, selective, reversible, and competitive AChE inhibitor. The newest on the market, it is also the least expensive. Galantamine, a selective inhibitor of AChE, also allosterically modulates nicotinic ACh receptors. This dual action is the proposed advantage to galantamine.

Treatment of Behavioral and Cognitive Problems

In addition to memory disturbance, an array of behavioral and cognitive problems manifest in patients with dementia. They include paranoia, delusions, hallucinations, aggression, agitation, anxiety, and mood disturbances. These problems inflict a significant burden on the patient and the caregiver, and when not adequately treated, can lead to placement in a facility. Many novel agents may provide control of aggression and psychotic symptoms but usually do not ameliorate the problems. The typical antipsychotics produce side effects that can precipitate more problems, such as orthostatic hypotension, anticholinergic symptoms, and sedation. Extrapyramidal side effects are particularly common in the elderly, who develop much higher rates of tardive dyskinesia after exposure to typical neuroleptics. The newer atypical antipsychotics are recommended, such

Table 28-2
Atypical Antipsychotics Used in the Treatment of Behaviors and Symptoms Associated with Dementia

Atypical Antipsychotics	Dose	Side Effects	Cost
Olanzapine (Zyprexa)	2.5-15 mg	Weight gain, increased sugars	$122-216
Risperidone (Risperdal)	0.25-3.0 mg	EPS at higher doses	$69-133
Clozapine (Clozaril)	12.5-200 mg	Sedation, hypersalivation requires weekly WBC	$38-95
Quetiapine (Seroquel)	12.5-300 mg	Sedation, mild hypotension	$36-120

EPS, Extrapyramidal symptoms; *WBC,* white blood count.

as **risperidone, quetiapine, olanzapine,** or **clozapine** (Table 28-2). Each has unique side effects, and these can often be used advantageously.

Aggressive treatment of depression and anxiety improves the quality of life in patients who have comorbid illness. Selective serotonin uptake inhibitors (SSRIs) are generally better tolerated in patients with dementia than tricyclic antidepressants because of fewer anticholinergic side effects. Trazodone in low doses (e.g., 25 mg at bedtime) can be useful for nighttime agitation leading to insomnia. Benzodiazepines should be used with great caution and for limited periods.

The progressive nature of dementia mandates frequent reassessment for evaluation of driving ability. An actual on-road driving test is the best determination of the driving capacity of a patient with dementia. Some communities offer such tests, or they may be performed by the department of motor vehicles. Other safety issues including falls, wandering, and injury while cooking should be assessed and managed with appropriate environmental interventions.

Disease Modifying Agents

There is fairly strong evidence that vitamin E 2000 IU daily may help delay the progression of AD. Several recent randomized trials have demonstrated no benefit of estrogen replacement in women with established dementia.

Support of Caregivers

Women have traditionally been the caregivers, and this can be a significant burden for the daughter of a father or mother with dementia. There is a high incidence of depression in caregivers, which can lead to abuse or neglect resulting from an overwhelmed caregiver. Support groups are an important resource for caregivers, providing education and support to people with Alzheimer's disease, their families and caregivers. The Alzheimer's Association has spearheaded the effort for the many support groups that now exist. The Alzheimer's Association web site, www.alz.org, is a good source for information, support and assistance on issues related to Alzheimer's disease. A service of the National Institute on Aging, the web site www.alzheimers.org provides the caregiver with an opportunity to speak with an information specialist to help find answers and get information about the latest research.

BIBLIOGRAPHY

American College of Medical Genetics/American Society of Human Genetics Working Group on ApoE and Alzheimer Disease: Statement on Use of Apolipoprotein E Testing for Alzheimer Disease, *JAMA* 274: 1627, 1995.

Barry PP: Medical evaluation of the demented patient, *Med Clin North Am* 78:779, 1994.

Bidikov I, Meier DE: Clinical decision-making with the woman after menopause, *Geriatrics* 52:28, 1997.

Blessed G, Tomlinson BE, Roth M: The association between quantitative measures of dementia and of senile change in the cerebral gray matter of elderly subjects, *Br J Psychiatry* 114:797, 1968.

Burke JR, Morgenlander JC: Update on Alzheimer's disease: promising advances in detection and treatment, *Postgrad Med* 106:85, 1996.

Callahan CM, Hendrie HC, Tierney WM: Documentation and evaluation of cognitive impairment in elderly primary care patients, *Ann Intern Med* 122:422, 1995.

Cohen D: A primary care checklist for effective family management, *Med Clin North Am* 78:795, 1994.

Cooper JK: Alzheimer's disease: answering questions commonly asked by patients' families, *Geriatrics* 46:38, 1991.

Cummings JL: Cholinesterase inhibitors: a new class of psychotropic compounds, *Am J Psychiatry* 157:4, 2000.

Cummings JL, Vinters HV, Cole GM, Khachaturian ZS: Alzheimer's disease: etiologies, pathophysiology, cognitive reserve, and treatment opportunities, *Neurology* 51(suppl.):S2, 1998.

Cummings JL, Jeste DV: Alzheimer's disease and its management in the year 2010, *Psychiatric Services* 50:1173, 2001.

Dunkin JJ, Anderson-Hanley C: Dementia caregiver burden: a review of the literature and guidelines for assessment and intervention, *Neurology* 51(suppl 1):S53, 1998.

Farrer LA et al: Effects of age, sex, and ethnicity on the association between apolipoprotein E genotype and Alzheimer disease, *JAMA* 278: 1349, 1997.

Farrer LA: Genetics and the dementia patient, *The Neurologist* 3:13, 1997.

Folstein MF, Folstein SA, McHugh PR: Mini-mental state: a practical method for grading the cognitive state of patients for the clinician, *J Psychiatr Res* 12:196, 1975.

Fox GK et al: Alzheimer's disease and driving: prediction and assessment of driving performance, *J Am Geriatr Soc* 45:949, 1997.

Gallo JJ, Lebowitz BD: The epidemiology of common late-life mental disorders in the community: themes for the new century, *Psychiatric Services* 50:1158, 2001.

Gao S, Hendrie HC, Hall KS, Hui S: The relationship between age, sex, and the incidence of dementia and Alzheimer disease: a meta-analysis, *Arch Gen Psychiatry* 55:809, 1998.

Geldmacher DS, Whitehouse PJ: Evaluation of dementia, *N Engl J Med* 335:330, 1996.

Haskell SG, Richardson ED, Horwitz RI: The effect of estrogen replacement therapy on cognitive function in women: a critical review of the literature, *J Clin Epidemiol* 50:1249, 1997.

Henderson VW et al: Estrogen for Alzheimer's disease in women: randomized, double-blinded, placebo-controlled trial, *Neurology* 54:295, 2000.

Inouye SK et al: A multicomponent intervention to prevent delirium in hospitalized older patients, *N Engl J Med* 340:669, 1999.

Johnson J, Sims R, Gottlieb G: Differential diagnosis of dementia, delirium and depression, *Drugs Aging* 5(6):431, 1994.

Jurkowski CL: A multidisciplinary approach to Alzheimer's disease: who should be members of the team? *Am J Med* 104:13S, 1998.

Kalb C: Coping with the darkness, *Newsweek* Jan 31, 2000, 52-54.

Kaye JA: Diagnostic challenges in dementia, *Neurology* 51(suppl):S45, 1998.

Khachaturian ZS: An overview of Alzheimer's disease research, *Am J Med* 104:26, 1998.

Knopman DS: The initial recognition and diagnosis of dementia, *Am J Med* 104(4A):2S, 1998.

Lautenschlager NT et al: Risk of dementia among relatives of Alzheimer's disease patients in the MIRAGE study: what is in store for the oldest old? *Neurology* 46:641, 1996.

Lerner AJ: Women and Alzheimer's disease, *J Clin Endocrinol Metab* 84:1830, 1999.

McKeith I et al: Rivastigmine in the treatment of dementia with Lewy bodies: preliminary findings from an open trial, *Int J Geriatr Psychiatry* 15:387, 2000.

McKhann G et al: Clinical diagnosis of Alzheimer's disease: reports of the NINCDS-ADRDA Work Group under the auspices of the Department of Health and Human Services Task Force on Alzheimer's Disease, *Neurology* 34:939, 1984.

Mittelman MS et al: A family intervention to delay nursing home placement of patients with Alzheimer disease: a randomized controlled trial, *JAMA* 276:1725, 1996.

Mulnard RA et al: Estrogen replacement therapy for treatment of mild to moderate Alzheimer disease: a randomized controlled trial, *JAMA* 283: 1007, 2000.

Overman WH, McCormick WA: Elder law and Alzheimer's disease, *Am J Med* 104:22S, 1998.

Petersen RC et al: Mild cognitive impairment: clinical characterization and outcome, *Arch Neurol* 56:303, 1999.

Reiman EM et al: Preclinical evidence of Alzheimer's disease in persons homozygous for the e4 allele for apolipoprotein E, *N Engl J Med* 334: 752, 1996.

Robinson B: Guideline for initial evaluation of the patient with memory loss, *Geriatrics* 52:30, 1997.

Saunders AM et al: Association of Apolipoprotein E allele with late-onset familial and sporadic Alzheimer's disease, *Neurology* 43:1467, 1993.

Seeman MV: Psychopathology in women and men: focus on female hormones, *Am J Psychiatry* 154:1641, 1997.

Shah Y, Tangalos EG, Peterson RC: Mild cognitive impairment: when is it a precursor of Alzheimer's disease? *Geriatrics* 55:62, 2000.

Small GW: Treatment of Alzheimer's disease: current approaches and promising developments, *Am J Med* 104:32S, 1998.

Steffens DC, Morgenlander JC: Initial evaluation of suspected dementia: asking the right questions, *Postgrad Med* 106:72, 1999.

Tang M et al: Effect of oestrogen during menopause on risk and age at onset of Alzheimer's disease, *Lancet* 348:429, 1996.

Tang M et al: Relative risk of Alzheimer disease and age-at-onset distributions, based on APOE genotypes among elderly African Americans, Caucasians, and Hispanics in New York City, *Am J Hum Genet* 58:574, 1996.

Volicer L, Hurley A: *Hospice care for patients with advanced progressive dementia,* New York, 1998, Springer.

Welsh-Bohmer KA, Morgenlander JC: Determining the cause of memory loss in the elderly: from in-office screening to neuropsychological referral, *Postgrad Med* 106:99, 1999.

Wengel SP, Burke WJ, Roccaforte WH: Donepezil for postoperative delirium associated with Alzheimer's disease, *J Am Geriatr Soc* 47:379, 1999.

Zarate CA et al: Risperidone in the elderly: a pharmacoepidemiologic study, *J Clin Psychiatry* 58:311, 1997.

CHAPTER 29

Chronic Pain Management

May C.M. Pian-Smith

The International Association for the Study of Pain defines pain as an unpleasant sensory and emotional experience associated with actual or potential tissue damage. This definition reinforces the idea that pain is not just a physiologic process mediated by neurotransmitters but also a subjective and emotional process. In fact, without perception and a resultant emotional response, there is not pain but rather a series of complex biochemical mechanisms.

Chronic pain is defined as pain that has not subsided in the expected time of healing after a tissue injury. Generally, pain is considered chronic after it persists for 3 to 6 months. During this time function of the nervous system becomes reorganized (neuroplasticity) and has the potential for spontaneous and atopic nerve excitation. The patient's psychosocial background can further modulate the interpretation of chronic nociceptive signals, and such emotional factors can influence the degree of suffering that is elicited by the pain.

Effective management of chronic pain requires an understanding of the physiologic mechanisms in place, as well as an understanding of the emotional influences that are important in each individual patient. Because pain results from a complex interplay of factors, it is not surprising that it is often best treated with a multidisciplinary approach that fuses conventional and nonconventional methods. This chapter summarizes the physiology, assessment, and treatment of chronic pain. The workup for specific common pain syndromes commonly seen in the primary care of women is illustrated through case discussions.

EVALUATION

The following sections describe the physiologic and anatomic characteristics of different types of pain, namely nociceptive, neuropathic, and psychogenic pain, so that meaningful intervention and pain management can be rendered.

Nociceptive pain occurs when there is activation or sensitization of nerve endings peripherally, which then transduce the noxious stimuli into electrochemical signals. These impulses are then transmitted to the spinal cord and higher rostral areas in the central nervous system. This type of pain is either somatic or visceral. Somatic pain arises from nociceptors in tissue such as bone, periarticular soft tissue, joints, and muscles. Somatic pain is usually well localized anatom-

ically in the area of injury. It is often described as "aching, gnawing, throbbing, or cramping" and can be intermittent or constant and dull. In contrast, visceral pain arises from nociceptors within organs, including those of the cardiovascular, respiratory, gastrointestinal, and genitourinary systems. It is usually more poorly localized and can be referred to other areas. It can be intermittent or constant and is often described as "colicky or squeezing".

Neuropathic pain arises from neural injury within the peripheral or central nervous system. It is usually described as a "hot, burning, or tingling" sensation that occasionally radiates along nerve roots or peripheral nerves. Usually it is not accompanied by motor loss, although motor involvement can be seen. There are three types of neuropathic pain. *Peripherally generated* neuropathic pain includes diabetic neuropathies, cervical or lumbar radiculopathies, spinal nerve lesions, and brachial or lumbosacral plexopathies. *Centrally generated* pain results from injuries to the central nervous system at or above the level of the spinal cord. *Sympathetically maintained* pain can be generated peripherally or centrally and is characterized by localized autonomic dysregulation. Vasomotor or sudomotor changes, edema, sweating, and atrophy can occur in affected areas. This type of pain is sometimes called reflex sympathetic dystrophy, causalgia, or complex regional pain syndrome.

Psychogenic pain describes an entity that occurs when pain cannot be explained on the basis of current medical knowledge. If pain complaints are produced on a voluntary basis, the main distinction is between malingering and factitious disorder. Malingerers obtain secondary gains from their complaints, whereas those with factitious disorder gain only recognition of a sick status. When pain complaints are produced unconsciously, other possible diagnoses include conversion, somatization, hypochondriasis or major depression, or a pain disorder associated with psychological factors.

MANAGEMENT
Drug Therapy

Nonsteroidal antiinflammatory drugs (NSAIDs) produce analgesia peripherally by blocking prostaglandin synthesis. Specifically, these agents block the enzyme cyclooxygenase (COX, prostaglandin synthetase), which converts arachidonic

Table 29-1
Dosing Data for NSAIDS

Drug	Dosage (mg)	Dose Interval (hr)	Maximum Daily Dose (mg/d)	Peak Effect (hr)	Half-Life (hr)
Diclofenac	25-75	6-8	200	2	1-2
Etodolac acid	200-400	6-8	1200	1-2	7
Fenoprofen	200	4-6	3200	1-2	2-3
Flurbiprofen	50-100	6-8	300	1.5-3.0	3-4
Ibuprofen	200-400	6-8	3200	1-2	2
Indomethacin	25-75	6-8	200	0.5-1.0	2-3
Ketoprofen	25-75	6-8	300	1-2	1.5-2.0
Ketorolac*					
Oral	10	6-8	40	0.5-1.0	6
Parenteral	60 load, then 30	6-8	120 (use no longer than 5 d)		
Meclofenamic acid	500 load, then 275	6-8	400		
Mefenamic acid	500 load, then 250	6	1250	2-4	3-4
Nabumetone	1000-2000	12-24	2000	3-5	22-30
Naproxen	500 load, then 250	6-8	1250	2-4	12-15
Naproxen sodium	550 load, then 275	6-8	1375	1-2	13
Oxaprozin	60-1200	Every day	1800	2	3-3.5
Phenylbutazone	100	6-8	400	2	50-100
Piroxicam	40 load, then 20	24	20	2-4	36-45
Sulindac	150-200	12	400	1-2	7-18
Tolmetin	200-400	8	1800	4-6	2

*Use no longer than 5 days.

Table 29-2
Dosing Data for Acetaminophen

Drug	Dosage (mg)	Interval (hr)	Maximum Daily Dosage (mg/d)	Time to Peak (hr)	Half-Life (hr)
Acetaminophen (Tylenol)	325-1000	q4-6	4000	0.5-1.0	2-3

acid to prostaglandins D, E, and F; prostacyclin; and thromboxane. Prostaglandins are algesic mediators that also mediate many components of inflammation including fever, pain, and vasodilatation. New enzyme synthesis overcomes the therapeutic effect.

Pharmacologically, NSAIDs are divided into several groups including salicylates, propionic acids, indoles, and fenamates. They differ in their abilities to affect the different components of the inflammatory response. It has also been theorized that NSAIDs may have a second effect that is central, by facilitating endogenous inhibitory descending pathways.

The side effects of NSAIDs can be divided into those that are prostaglandin-mediated and those that are non-prostaglandin-mediated. Prostaglandin-mediated effects include gastric bleeding or ulceration, disorders of hemostasis, and nephrotoxicity. The nonprostaglandin-mediated effects (idiosyncratic or hypersensitivity reactions) have been attributed to cell-mediated phenomena and include respiratory effects (rhinitis, asthma, nasal polyps) and urticaria, wheals, angioneurotic edema, and hypotension.

The most recently FDA-approved NSAIDs are the **COX II inhibitors.** COX II is expressed in the brain and kidneys but is not found in the gastric mucosa or in platelets where COX I is prevalent. Not surprisingly, there is a lower incidence of gastric complications and platelet inhibition with the COX II inhibitors. Table 29-1 contains dosing data for NSAIDs.

Acetaminophen works centrally to produce analgesia and antipyresis, but its precise mechanism of action is unknown. It does not interact with peripheral COX (it is a poor antiinflammatory agent) and does not have antiplatelet activity. It is metabolized in the liver and excreted renally. It has a very low side-effect profile, but it can cause hepatic and renal toxicity with high doses. Hypersensitivity is rare. Table 29-2 contains dosing data for acetaminophen.

Tramadol (Ultram) is a synthetic analog of codeine and an atypical opioid analgesic. It has very weak μ-opioid receptor affinity and is thought to exert its effect by inhibiting reuptake of norepinephrine and serotonin. It has such minimal opioid side effects that it is not classified as a Schedule II drug.

Tramadol is usually started at doses of 50 to 100 mg and can be given every 4 to 6 hours, not to exceed a 400 mg/day total dose. Side effects, including sedation, nausea, and vomiting, usually occur with the 100-mg dose. Other side effects such as respiratory depression, constipation, or withdrawal signs are minimal.

Table 29-3
Opioid Agonists

	Half-Life	Duration of Action
Weak Opioid Agonists		
Short half-life agents		
Codeine	2 to 4 hours	4 to 6 hours
Hydrocodone	4 hours	4 to 6 hours
Dihydrocodone	4 hours	4 to 6 hours
Long half-life agents		
Propoxyphene	6 to 12 hours	4 to 6 hours
Strong Opioid Agonists		
Short half-life agents		
Morphine	2 hours	2 to 4 hours
Hydromorphine	2 to 3 hours	2 to 4 hours
Meperidine	2 to 3 hours	2 to 4 hours
Oxycodone	2 to 3 hours	3 to 4 hours
Fentanyl	1 to 2 hours	3 to 4 hours
Long half-life agents		
Methadone	15 to 40 hours	4 to 12 hours
Levorphanol	8 to 12 hours	72 hours
Morphine-sustained release*	6 hours	8 to 12 hours
Oxycodone-sustained release*	6 hours	8 to 12 hours

*Behaves like a long half-life opioid.

Table 29-4
Time to Peak Analgesic Effects

	Oral
Short Half-Life	
Morphine	30 to 90 minutes
Hydromorphone	30 to 90 minutes
Meperidine	30 to 120 minutes
Oxycodone	30 to 60 minutes
Hydrocodone	no data
Codeine	60 minutes
Fentanyl	no data
Propoxyphene	120 to 180 minutes
Long Half-Life	
Levorphanol	90 to 120 minutes
Methadone	90 to 120 minutes
Fentanyl (transdermal)	24 to 78 hours
Morphine-sustained release	120 to 180 minutes
Oxycodone	180 minutes

Several surveys of **long-term opioid therapy** for chronic nonmalignant pain have suggested that this class of drugs can be beneficial in a subpopulation of chronic pain patients. For many patients the pain relief is effective (without the "ceiling effect" of other medications, progressive increases in opiates lead to more profound analgesia). It is advised that opiates be given around-the-clock (ATC) rather than on an as-needed basis. In this way a steady plasma opiate level can be maintained. A second, shorter-acting opiate can also be used for transient exacerbations of "break through" pain. The combination of the ATC opiate dose and the supplemental doses offers the best strategy for opiate dosing. See Table 29-3 for weak and strong opioid agonists. Table 29-4 lists the time to peak analgesic effect for commonly used opioid agonists.

Aside from the therapeutic efficacy of the drugs, one must also consider the potential for adverse pharmacologic outcomes and potential risk of opioid addiction and abuse. Long-term opioid use has not been associated with major organ toxicity in large studies of cancer pain patients. Potential side effects such as somnolence, confusion, nausea, and cognitive impairment have not been shown to be of major significance in this group; and side effects are generally reversible. Many times such adverse reactions can be minimized with a switch in opiate type or alteration in the mode of delivery. The most common side effect, constipation, is best treated preemptively with stool softeners or bowel stimulants.

The addiction risk for patients receiving opiates for chronic pain is reassuringly low. The Boston Cooperative Drug Surveillance Study identified only four cases of addiction among 11,882 patients with no history of substance abuse. In a separate survey of 10,000 patients treated for burn pain, no cases of addiction could be identified. It appears that the incidence of iatrogenically induced addiction with protracted use of opioids is less than the prevalence of addiction to alcohol and other drugs within the general population (the rate of alcoholism in the United States is 3% to 16%, and the rate for other forms of substance abuse is estimated to be 5% to 15%).

Drug Therapy for Neuropathic Pain

NSAIDs and opioids can be useful for neuropathic pain, but their effects are nonspecific. Primary pharmacologic management of neuropathic pain includes the use of antidepressants and also membrane-stabilizing agents (anticonvulsants). Neuroleptics (antipsychotic agents) have also been useful in some settings.

Antidepressants can be divided into at least four groups: tricyclics, heterocyclics, serotonin-specific reuptake inhibitors (SSRIs), and monoamine oxidase (MAO) inhibitors. Analgesic and antidepressant effects of the tricyclics and heterocyclics are believed to as a result of the blockade of presynaptic uptake of serotonin and norepinephrine. Serotonin and norepinephrine are known to be involved in the endorphin-mediated pain modulation pathways at the central (descending) and spinal cord levels.

Of the groups, the **tricyclics,** are probably the most clinically useful for analgesia. The tricyclic antidepressants are either tertiary or secondary amines. The tertiary amines (amitriptyline and imipramine) are metabolized to secondary amines (nortriptyline and desipramine). Whereas antidepressant effects occur after 1 to 4 weeks of therapy, analgesic effects can occur immediately.

Therapeutic levels of tricyclics for pain management are not known, so levels are monitored instead to verify compliance or potential toxicity. In general, the secondary amines are associated with fewer side effects than occur with the tertiary amines. Common side effects include anticholinergic effects, antihistaminic effects, alpha-1-adrenergic blockade, and miscellaneous side effects such as jaundice and weight gain.

The choice of drug is based on comparison of the patient's profile with a drug's side-effect profile. It is best to begin with a low dose and to increase the dosing until therapeutic effects or intolerable side effects are obtained.

Table 29-5
Antidepressants

Drug	Dosage (mg)	Usual Daily Dose (mg)	Anticholinergic Activity	Central Action	Hypotension	Sedation
Amitriptyline (Elavil)*	10-300	75-150	Strong	S(N)	Strong	Strong
Amoxapine (Asendin)	50-400	50-200	Minimal	N	Mild	Minimal
Bupropion (Wellbutrin)	50-100	50-300	Minimal	N/A	Minimal	Minimal
Clomipramine (Anafranil)*	25-250	20-150	Moderate	S(N)	Strong	Mild
Desipramine (Norpramin)*	75-300	50-150	Minimal	N	Mild	Minimal
Doxepin (Sinequan)	30-300	30-150	Moderate	S	Strong	Mild
Fluoxetine (Prozac)	5.0-80	20-40	Minimal	S	Minimal	Minimal
Imipramine (Tofranil)*	20-300	20-150	Moderate	N/S	Moderate	Moderate
Isocarboxazid (Marplan)	10.0-40	10.0-40	Minimal	MAOI	Mild	Moderate
Maprotiline (Ludiomil)	75-300	75-150	Mild	N	Mild	Mild
Nortriptyline (Pamelor)*	25-150	50-150	Mild	N/S	Moderate	Mild
Phenelzine (Nardil)	15-90	45-75	Mild	MAOI	Mild	Moderate
Protriptyline (Vivactil)	15-60	15-40	Moderate	N	Minimal	Mild
Sertraline (Zoloft)	50-200	50-100	Mild	S	Minimal	Mild
Tranylcypromine (Parnate)	10.0-45	10.0-20	Minimal	MAOI	Moderate	Mild
Trazodone (Desyrel)	50-600	150-300	Minimal	S	Moderate	Minimal
Trimipramine (Surmontil)	50-200	75-150	Moderate	S(N)	Strong	Mild

S, Serotonergic; *N*, Noradrenergic; *(N)*, weakly noradrenergic; *MAOI*, monoamine oxidase inhibitor.
*Commonly used for neuropathic pain.

SSRIs, although excellent antidepressants, appear to have less utility as analgesics in the management of neuropathic pain. The exception to this generalization may be venlafaxine (Effexor).

MAO inhibitors block monoamine oxidase, an enzyme present in the central nervous system, adrenergic nerve endings, liver, and gastrointestinal tract. Blocking oxidative deamination of synaptic monoamine neurotransmitters results in increased levels of norepinephrine and serotonin in the cytoplasm of the nerve terminals. As with the tricyclic antidepressants, it is unclear how these elevated monoamine levels result in analgesia. The most common side effects include nausea, sedation, weight gain, and dizziness. Orthostatic hypotension may be seen. The interaction of MAO inhibitors with opioids (particularly meperidine) can cause hyperpyrexia and hypermetabolism. Tyramine-containing foods, sympathomimetics, and tricyclic antidepressants can cause a hypertensive crisis (Table 29-5).

Membrane-stabilizing agents (anticonvulsants) seem to benefit patients with neurogenic pain owing to damage or dysfunction of nerves in the central or peripheral nervous systems. Commonly used drugs in this category include **phenytoin** (Dilantin), **carbamazepine** (Tegretol), **valproic acid** (Depakote), **clonazepam** (Klonopin), and **gabapentin** (Neurontin). As with the antidepressants, determining serum levels is not useful in establishing analgesia, but is necessary to monitor potential toxicity (Table 29-6).

The **neuroleptic** and **antipsychotic drugs** are considered second-line adjuvant drugs for chronic pain and are sometimes useful to control adverse effects of opioids such as nausea. There are many mechanisms by which these agents can exert effects. Although these agents exert antipsychotic effects via postsynaptic dopamine blockade, they are also known to block adrenergic, muscarinic, serotonin, and histamine effects. The analgesic effects of these agents are thought to be primarily mediated by interactions with opiate receptors.

There is no evidence to support greater effectiveness of one neuroleptic agent over another. Specific agents are usually chosen based on patient and side-effect profiles. The major side effects of concern include dopaminergic blockade-induced extrapyramidal side effects, sedation, anticholinergic effects, and orthostatic hypotension (Table 29-7).

Nondrug Therapies

Physical therapies are important adjuncts in the management of chronic pain. Drug doses can often be reduced when physical therapies are used. **Superficial heat therapy** (40° to 45° C or 104° to 113° F) can relieve pain of localized inflammation, muscle spasms, and joint stiffness. **Superficial cold therapy** (0° to 5° C or 32° to 42° F) helps muscle spasm and itching. **Massage, vibration therapy,** and **monitored exercise programs** have been helpful for many musculoskeletal problems.

Behavioral and cognitive therapies are part of an integrated approach to pain management. **Behavioral therapies** help patients develop skills to cope with their pain. **Cognitive therapies** focus on thoughts and perceptions that shape patients' interpretations of events and body sensations. The therapies include relaxation and imagery (quiet breathing with pleasant mental images to enhance muscle relaxation and thereby reduce pain), distraction, and reframing (refocusing the patient's attention with an activity such as singing to one's self, and replacing negative thoughts about pain with more positive ones, e.g., "this pain is nothing compared to the way it used to be"), structured support (support groups), and hypnosis.

Many of these techniques can be enhanced through **biofeedback,** with which physiologic responses (many of which the patient is unaware) can be monitored to cue the

Table 29-6
Anticonvulsants

Drug	Half-Life (hr)	Therapeutic Blood Levels, Seizures (ug/ml)	Toxic Concentration (ug/ml)	Maximum Daily Dose (mg/d)
Carbamazepine (Tegretol)	10-20	4.0-12	>8-10	1500
Clonazepam (Klonopin)	18-30	0.02-0.08	>0.06	6
Phenytoin (Dilantin)	6.0-24	10-20	>20	500
Valproic acid (Depakote)	12	50-100	>100-150	1500-2000 (60 mg/kg per day)

Table 29-7
Neuroleptics

Drug	Initial Dose (mg)	Maintenance dose (mg)	ACE	Sedation	Hypotension	EPS
Chlorpromazine (Thorazine)	75-500	25-150	High	High	High	Low
Chlorprothixene (Taractan)	50-200	80-150	High	High	High	Low
Fluphenazine (Prolixin)	1.0-10	1.0-3	Low	Low	Low	High
Haloperidol (Haldol)	0.5-30.0	0.5-10.0	Low	Moderate	Low	High
Methotrimeprazine (Levoprome)*	5-100	10.0-50	High	High	High	Moderate
Perphenazine (Trilafon)	8.0-64	4.0-16	Moderate	Moderate	Moderate	Moderate
Thioridazine (Mellaril)	10-200	25-75	High	High	High	Low

*Available in parenteral form only.
ACE, Anticholinergic effects; EPS, extrapyramidal side effects.

patient to the effects of such responses on body function. Machines used for biofeedback can measure changes in galvanic skin response, body temperature, electromyographic tracings, blood pressure, heart rate, and stomach acidity.

Nerve stimulation therapies include transcutaneous electrical nerve stimulation (TENS), acupuncture, and a subset of acupuncture called percutaneous electrical nerve stimulation (PENS). **TENS** is a form of external peripheral nerve stimulation in which electrode pads are applied to the skin and then stimulated electrically with portable units. This form of counterstimulant therapy is often used for postoperative pain, low back pain, neuropathic pain, headache, intercostal pain, arthritis, phantom limb pain, and cancer pain.

Acupuncture involves the placement of fine needles at distinct points along energy "meridians" on the body surface. The needles are sometimes stimulated with mechanical manipulation, heat, or electrical energy. Traditionally, acupuncture is thought to restore and balance the flow of *qi* vital for good health. In the laboratory setting, it has been shown to stimulate pain-modulating systems involving endorphins, as well as other neurotransmitters such as serotonin and norepinephrine. Recently, controlled and randomized trials have suggested efficacy of acupuncture (and PENS) for diverse conditions including back pain, dysmenorrhea, chemotherapy-induced nausea and vomiting, and dental pain.

Interventional Pain Management

Interventional techniques fall into the territory of a pain specialist, but basic knowledge about the techniques is important for primary care physicians who may need to initiate a referral.

Cryoanalgesia is a process in which nerve fibers are progressively cooled to block conduction and provide a temporary anesthetic block. It is appropriate for pain originating from small, well-localized lesions of peripheral nerves such as neuromas and entrapment neuropathies. It should always be preceded by a diagnostic-prognostic local anesthetic block.

Radiofrequency lesioning uses heat for neural ablation. The radiofrequency voltage on the tip of the radiofrequency probe sets up an electric field that results in heat generated in the tissue rather than in the tip itself. Effects are manipulated by altering tip size and tissue temperature. This type of lesioning is more appropriate for analgesia of deeper structures than is cryoanalgesia; it is used for lumbar and cervical facet rhizotomy, sacroiliac joint rhizotomy, dorsal root ganglionostomy, and lumbar sympathetic chain stereotactic radiofrequency ablation.

Spinal cord stimulation activates many pain-modulating pathways to control pain. Patients are considered for this kind of block when they have evidence of objective pathology underlying their pain (e.g., myelographically demonstrated arachnoiditis) and all conservative therapies have failed. The patients undergo a trial with a temporary electrode before permanent implantation. The percutaneous insertion of a stimulating electrode allows the determination of whether the topography of the pain can be overlapped by a stimulation-induced paresthesia. The trial verifies the efficacy of spinal cord stimulation for each individual, permits exclusion of unsuitable candidates, and is cost-effective. After the temporary lead is placed in an operative setting, a patient is sent home with an external pulse generator for trial screening.

Indications for this kind of trial include lumbar adhesive arachnoiditis, peripheral nerve injury or neuralgia, sympathetically maintained pain, phantom limb pain, medically/surgically optimized peripheral vascular disease with ischemic pain, and spinal cord lesions with well-circumscribed segmental pain. Spinal cord stimulation is most appropriate for neuropathic pain where the pain is relatively stabilized and the distribution of the pain is localized. It is more effective for unilateral extremity pain, although it can be used effectively for bilateral extremity pain. By itself, it is not useful for pain in multiple separate areas of the body.

Implantable drug delivery systems include implanted epidural or subarachnoid catheters and pumps. They are used for cancer pain, treatment of spasticity of both cerebral and spinal cord origin, and intractable nonmalignant pain. Subarachnoid delivery systems allow for more prolonged use, lower drug dosages, and attendant lower incidence of side effects. Trial dosing is carried out before implantation to verify the appropriateness of this therapy. In general, these delivery systems are best for treatment of somatic or nociceptive pain, pain in multiple or diffuse sites in the body, and progressive pain. If necessary, neuropathic pain can also be treated with implantable systems, but it usually requires higher doses of medication.

Case Discussion 1

SOMATIC MYOFASCIAL PAIN SYNDROMES

A 45-year-old concert pianist presented with a 6-month history of bilateral arm pain. She reported that her muscles and elbows were tender, and the pain was affecting the quality of her performance and the degree to which she enjoyed her music. She reported that the problem was causing her to be depressed; it affected her sleep, which in turn exacerbated her fatigue and depression.

■ What is regional myofascial pain syndrome and how is it distinguished from fibromyalgia?

The hallmark characteristics of **regional myofascial pain** are (1) localization within a circumscribed muscle or group of muscles in a specific area of the body and (2) the presence of trigger points. On physical examination, palpation of trigger points elicits an involuntary localized twitch or "jump sign." Trigger points within specific muscles have characteristically described patterns of referred pain, and these patterns often do not follow normal anatomic radiation patterns (i.e., radiation along the course of peripheral nerves or dermatomes).

In contrast, **fibromyalgia** is a diffuse pain syndrome. The American College of Rheumatology has determined that when 11 of 18 tender points elicit pain by palpation (in 9 paired anatomically defined sites) with concomitant widespread muscle aching, a sensitivity of 88% and specificity of 81% is achieved for the diagnosis of fibromyalgia.

Fibromyalgia typically presents without a history of trauma or even an inciting event, whereas regional myofascial pain is the result of repetitive injury or microtrauma to the muscle. Fibromyalgia is characterized by the presence of tender points that are distinct from trigger points; whereas trigger points are in the belly of muscles, tender points can occur at the musculotendon junction. Unlike trigger points, tender points do not radiate.

The presence or absence of other symptoms may also help differentiate between the two syndromes. Fatigue and sleep disturbances are more common with fibromyalgia. There is a nonrestorative sleep pattern, and the patient wakes up unrefreshed. Fibromyalgia can also occur in conjunction with other connective tissue disorders (see Chapter 33).

■ What are the treatment options for regional myofascial pain?

Effective treatment involves medical, invasive, and physical therapeutic modalities. NSAIDs and tricyclic antidepressants (not SSRIs) have been effective. Muscle relaxants seem effective anecdotally but membrane-stabilizing agents are probably not effective. Injection of active trigger points can be helpful. Injectates can include saline, local anesthetics, and corticosteroids. Dry needling has also been used. Physical medicine modalities have also been helpful: Historically vapocoolant spray techniques followed by stretching of affected muscles have been helpful. More recently, specific myofascial release physical therapy techniques have also been successful.

■ Do the same treatments work for fibromyalgia?

The treatment for fibromyalgia requires a multidisciplinary approach. Pharmacologic therapy is best managed with NSAIDs and tricyclic antidepressants. Tender point injections have been disappointing, although acupuncture needling has met with varying success. Physical therapy is essential for the treatment of fibromyalgia, although many patients can be limited because of the painful nature of the disease process and by the depression and anxiety that can accompany the disease. Many patients can benefit from having psychologic intervention as part of an integrated approach.

■ How should a trial of antidepressant medication be done?

If it is decided that a trial of antidepressants should be initiated, a reasonable approach would be as follows: Amitriptyline is started orally at 10 to 25 mg at bedtime and increased every 1 to 3 days until a therapeutic effect is seen or a dose of 150 mg/day is reached. If adverse effects occur, a lower dosage should be continued until a therapeutic effect is noted or 3 weeks have passed. After a 1-week dosage of 150 mg/day, and if no side effects or contraindications have developed, the dose is increased by 25 mg every 1 to 3 days to the maximum dose of 300 mg/day. If there is no therapeutic effect after another 3 weeks, the drug should be tapered. Once a maximal therapeutic effect is achieved for at least 1 month, the dosage can be decreased slowly (by 10 to 25 mg every 1 to 2 weeks). After 3 to 6 months of sustained remission, drug therapy should be slowly tapered in small amounts. If this is not possible, it should be reattempted every 6 months.

■ What treatment options exist if the antidepressant is ineffective?

If the first antidepressant is ineffective, at least five options are available:

1. If the patient is tolerating the drug, check blood levels, and if not toxic, increase dosing.
2. If a drug with a primarily serotonergic effect has failed, substitute with a trial of a drug with a stronger norepinephrine effect.
3. A neuroleptic can be added to the antidepressant, starting with low doses of the neuroleptic. If the combination is successful, the antidepressant can be tapered, since the neuroleptic might be effective alone. If the combination is ineffective, both should be tapered over 7 to 10 days.
4. An anticonvulsant can be added to the antidepressant or antidepressant-neuroleptic combination. Success or failure should be treated as described in (3).
5. The tricyclic should be tapered and an MAO inhibitor instituted, particularly in patients with depressive symptoms. A 2-week washout period between the two regimens prevents drug interactions and adverse effects.

Case Discussion 2

SYMPATHETICALLY MAINTAINED PAIN SYNDROMES

A 35-year-old secretary presented with an exquisitely painful left upper arm. She reported that she received a Benadryl injection there a year ago that was very painful. Since then the pain worsened, and she underwent several surgical procedures to explore the brachial plexus, but nothing helped. Even the lightest touch of her skin in that area produced an exaggerated painful response. She reported the pain as "burning" and the area looked red and swollen.

■ What is the difference between reflex sympathetic dystrophy (RSD) and causalgia?

These terms refer to pain that is dependent on sympathetic efferent innervation of the affected area. **Reflex sympathetic dystrophy** has been used to refer to pain associated with injury to a minor nerve or where the precipitating event is unknown. **Causalgia** refers to pain associated with a similar constellation of autonomic, motor, and trophic changes with known injury to a major nerve trunk.

Recently, these syndromes have been lumped together as **complex regional pain syndromes (CRPS).** These pain syndromes are characterized by (1) pain that is disproportionate to what should be expected after the initiating injury, (2) variably expressed sympathetic dysfunction, (3) dystrophic changes, and (4) a delay in functional recovery. Clinical characteristics can include sustained "burning" pain, allodynia (pain on light touch), hyperalgesia (exaggerated response to a normally painful stimulus), vasomotor and sudomotor disturbances, skeletal muscle hypotonia, and variable onset.

■ Recognizing that the best treatments are multidisciplinary (involving medication, physical therapy, and psychological support), what is a reasonable way to start a patient with sympathetically maintained pain on an anticonvulsant analgesic?

Usually a trial of phenytoin or carbamazepine is tried before initiating a trial of valproic acid or clonazepam:

1. Phenytoin: Initial dosing in adult patients starts at 100 mg three times a day. Blood levels are checked after 3 weeks, with toxic levels over 20 μg/ml. Phenytoin should be taken after meals to avoid gastric irritation, and patients should be monitored for other potential complications, including cerebellar-vestibular dysfunction, allergic reactions, hepatotoxicity, and folic acid deficiency. Often therapy is maintained at initially achieved therapeutic dosages. It should not be discontinued abruptly to avoid withdrawal symptoms.
2. Carbamazepine: Initial dosing starts at 200 mg/day and is increased by 200 mg every 1 to 3 days to a maximum of 1500

mg/day. If side effects are encountered, the dose is decreased to the previous level for several days and then gradually increased. Therapeutic doses usually range from 800 to 1200 mg/day. Carbamazepine may depress hematopoiesis; therefore biweekly complete blood counts (CBCs) are recommended; later monthly CBCs should suffice. It is a gastric irritant that should be taken with food; other potential complications include sedation jaundice, oliguria, hypertension, and rarely acute left ventricular heart failure.

■ What about other pharmacologic approaches?

Alpha-adrenergic receptors may play an important role in the genesis of sympathetically maintained pain. Therefore alpha-adrenergic antagonists such as phenoxybenzamine and prazosin are sometimes used. Intravenous administration of the short-acting alpha-adrenergic blocker phentolamine has been developed as a test for sympathetically maintained pain and is used to determine which patients will respond to sympatholytic therapy (Table 29-8).

Table 29-8
Pharmacologic Treatment of Sympathetically Maintained Pain

Class	Drug	Dose
Oral sympatholytics	Clonidine	0.1 mg tid
	Prazosin	2 mg bid
	Propranolol	80 mg tid
	Phenoxybenzamine	40-120 mg/day
Transdermal sympathectomy	Clonidine patch	0.1 mg every 3 to 7 days
Opioids	Slow release morphine sulfate	15-60 mg bid
	Immediate release or morphine elixir	5-20 mg q3h
Anticonvulsants	Carbamazepine	200 mg tid or qid
	Phenytoin	100 mg tid
	Clonazepam	3-8 mg/day
	Valproate	250 mg tid
Tricyclic antidepressants	Amitriptyline	10-150 mg/day
	Doxepin	10-150 mg/day
	Nortriptyline	25-200 mg/day

BIBLIOGRAPHY

Backonja M et al: Gabapentin for the symptomatic treatment of painful peripheral neuropathy: randomized, controlled trial, *JAMA* 280:1831, 1998.

Borsook D, LeBel AA, McPeek B: *The Massachusetts General Hospital handbook of pain management,* Boston, 1996, Little Brown and Co.

Ferrante FM: Chronic pain management. In American Society of Anesthesiologists Annual Refresher Course Lectures, 1998.

Foley KM: The treatment of cancer pain, *N Engl J Med* 313:84, 1985.

Galer BS: Neuropathic pain of peripheral origin: advances in pharmacologic treatment, *Neurology* 45:S17, 1995.

Merskey H, Bogduk N: *Classification of chronic pain: descriptions of chronic pain syndromes and definitions of pain terms,* Seattle, 1994, IASP Press.

Ness TJ, Gebhart GF: Visceral pain: a review of experimental studies, *Pain* 41:167, 1990.

Nicholas RW, Thompson AR: Orthopaedic management of chronic pain: pain management for the cancer patient. In Price WT, editor: *American Academy of Orthopedic Surgeons Instructional Course Lectures,* Rosemont, Ill, 2000, American Academy of Orthopedic Surgeons.

Portenoy RK: Opioid therapy for chronic non-malignant pain: review of the critical issues, *J Pain Symptom Manage* 11:203, 1996.

Portenoy RK, Kanner RM: *Pain management: theory and practice,* Philadelphia, 1996, FA Davis.

White PF, Phillips J, Proctor TJ, Craig WF: Percutaneous electrical nerve stimulation: a promising alternative medicine approach to pain management, *APS Bulletin* 9:3, 1999.

Willer JC et al: Central analgesic effect of ketoprofen in humans: electrophysiologic evidence for a supraspinal mechanism in a double-blind and cross-over study, *Pain* 38:1, 1989.

CHAPTER **30**

Breast Cancer

Irene Kuter

Carcinoma of the breast is the most common cancer in women, accounting for 31% of female cancers (excluding nonmelanoma cancers of the skin). It is second only to lung cancer as a cause of cancer deaths in women, resulting in an estimated 40,200 deaths in 2001. There has been a great deal of public concern about the high rate of breast cancer, which is heightened by the fact that its cause is unknown. In addition the lack of curative treatments for metastatic disease (1 in 4 women in whom breast cancer develops will die of it) has been alarming.

This chapter provides an overview of the epidemiology and management of breast cancer. Screening for breast cancer is discussed in Chapter 95, and evaluation of breast problems, including suspected cancer, in Chapter 60.

EPIDEMIOLOGY

Carcinoma of the breast, although predominantly a disease affecting women, can also occur in men. In 2001 there will be an estimated 192,200 new cases in women in the United States and 1500 new cases in men. After female gender, age is the most striking risk factor. One in nine women in the United States will develop breast cancer, assuming a life expectancy of 85.

A more useful statistic is the estimated risk of development of breast cancer at different ages (Fig. 30-1, Table 30-1). Despite the apparent "epidemic" of breast cancer it is reassuring that the risk of a diagnosis of breast cancer before age 50 remains relatively small. Nevertheless it has been estimated that 41% of woman-years lost to breast cancer are from women less than 50 years old.

It is well known that there has been a steady rise in breast cancer incidence in the United States since 1940; the incidence now is about two times greater (Fig. 30-2) than in 1940. Although oncologists generally believe that they are seeing an increasing number of cases in young women, this appears to be due to the absolute increase in the number of women less than 50 years old because of the "baby boom." There is, in fact, no significant increase in incidence in women under 50; the slow rise since 1940 is mostly in women above 50 years old.

There are several possible reasons for this increase, which approximates 1% per year. Over this period the mortality rate from many other causes has been declining. Because breast cancer is largely a disease of older women, the number of women surviving to be at risk of development of the disease has therefore increased. It has been estimated that perhaps half the increased incidence over the last five decades is secondary to increased longevity, but as much as half is due to a true increased incidence that is not fully understood. Over this period there have been many lifestyle changes in the US population, such as improved nutrition, resulting in earlier menarche, and increased commitment of women to careers with resulting delay in childbearing. Both of these are known risk factors for breast cancer and may account for some of the increased risk. Oral contraceptive pills do not seem to be responsible for the rise. To what extent environmental exposures can be implicated is not at all clear.

In addition to the gradual rise there has been a sharper increase in incidence since the early 1980s. This is thought to represent the impact of screening mammography with increased detection at an early stage of cancers that would have been discovered clinically at a later time. Consistent with the hypothesis that the accelerated increase in incidence over the last decade is due to increased screening is the observation that the increase has been in early-stage breast cancers, both ductal carcinoma in situ and small infiltrating carcinomas. There has in fact been a decrease in incidence of tumors greater than 2 cm and those associated with positive lymph nodes or metastases.

With the continued widespread use of screening mammography it is predicted that the incidence of new cases will drop as the prevalent cancers are detected and treated. Until recently the mortality rate had remained unchanged; however, beginning in the 1990s, the death rate has begun to decrease (Table 30-2), presumably reflecting the efficacy of screening mammography (which has been used with increased frequency since the early 1980s) and possibly the benefit of adjuvant systemic therapy. The 5-year survival for women diagnosed with breast cancer in this country has improved significantly over the last two and a half decades (Table 30-3).

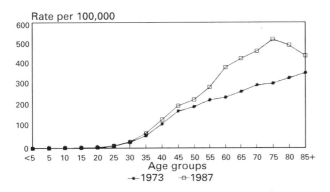

FIG. 30-1 Incidence of breast cancer as a function of age. (From Kessler LG: *Cancer* 69[suppl 7]:1896, 1992.)

Table 30-1
Estimated Risk of Development of Breast Cancer at Different Ages

Current Age	% DIAGNOSED WITH BREAST CANCER BY AGE*			
	+10 yr	+20 yr	+30 yr	Eventually
0	0.00	0.00	0.05	13.24
10	0.00	0.05	0.44	13.34
20	0.05	0.44	1.91	13.38
30	0.40	1.88	4.59	13.40
40	1.50	4.25	7.51	13.16
50	2.84	6.21	9.61	12.04
60	3.62	7.28	9.42	9.89

Modified from Ries LAG et al, editors: *SEER Cancer Statistics Review: 1973-1998,* Bethesda, Md, 2001, National Cancer Institute.
Lifetime Risk of Being Diagnosed with Cancer = 13.24%.
Lifetime Risk of Dying from Cancer = 3.20%.
*Percentage of women diagnosed with breast cancer within 10, 20, or 30 years of their current age, if presently cancer-free.

There is a striking variation in incidence of breast cancer throughout the world. Age-adjusted death rates vary from 5/100,000 to 27.6/100,000, with the highest rates seen in Europe, New Zealand, Canada, the United States, and Israel. The lowest rates are seen in Asian countries and Latin America. Studies of populations have shown that this cannot be accounted for by genetic factors alone. Japanese who move to Hawaii or to the mainland United States experience an increasing risk with each generation, implicating lifestyle factors and environmental exposures as risk factors.

DETERMINING RISK

Although risk factors for breast cancer are much discussed, it should be remembered that 75% of women with breast cancer do not appear to have a high-risk profile. Some risk factors are clearly established, whereas others continue to be quite controversial. The worldwide variation in breast cancer rates suggests that there is hope that we may learn to modify risks by adjusting lifestyle and environment, but whether diet, hormonal profiles related to lifestyle factors, or environmental exposures are most important is still unknown.

When a possible risk factor is tested in a clinical trial, the magnitude of the associated risk is often described in terms of relative risk. This is a numeric measure of the increased likelihood of acquiring breast cancer in the presence of a risk factor compared with the likelihood in the absence of that risk factor. A common misconception is that a relative risk of 2.0 translates into a twofold risk of acquiring breast cancer over that individual's lifetime. It should be noted, however, that the relative risk calculated is in reference to a matched individual at that age, followed over the duration of follow-up observation of that study. Thus, if a 40-year-old woman has a risk factor that is said to carry a relative risk of 1.3 and this was determined in a study that had a follow-up period of 10 years, this woman's risk of breast cancer is not

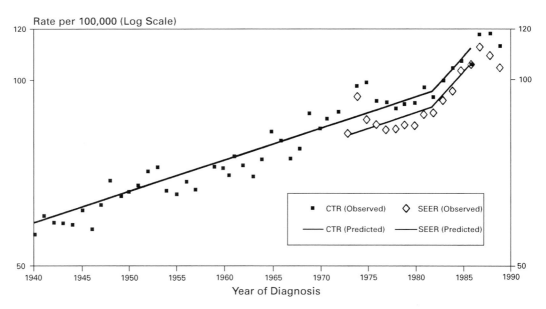

FIG. 30-2 Rising incidence of breast cancer in the United States since 1940. (From Miller BA, Feuer EJ, Hankey BF: *Ca Cancer J Clin* 43:27, 1993.)

Table 30-2
Estimated Number of Cases and Deaths from Breast Cancer in U.S. Women*

	No. New Cases	No. Deaths
1992	180,000	46,000
1994	182,000	46,000
1996	184,300	44,300
1998	178,700	43,500
2000	182,800	40,800

From Greenlee RT: Cancer statistics, 2000, *CA Cancer J Clin* 50:7, 2000.

Table 30-3
Five-Year Survival Rate (%) for Women with Breast Cancer in United States*

	1974-1976	1980-1982	1989-1995
White	75	77	86[†]
Black	63	66	71[†]
All races	75	76	85[†]

*Greenlee RT: Cancer statistics, 2000, *CA Cancer J Clin* 50:7, 2000.
[†]Comparison of 1974-1976 with 1989-1995 statistically significant.

(1 in 9) × 1.3 (equals 1 in 7) but rather (1 in 66) × 1.3 (equals 1 in 48) by age 50.

Risk Factors

In addition to gender, racial/cultural factors, and age, a number of risk factors for breast cancer have been defined. In addition, it should be noted that a prior personal history of breast cancer is a risk factor: a breast cancer patient has approximately a 1% chance per year of developing another breast cancer.

Genetic Susceptibility

Although in a small number of families there is an inherited susceptibility to breast cancer, making genetics the strongest risk factor for this disease, it is estimated that only about 5% of breast cancer is "familial." Familial breast cancer tends to occur in women at a younger age and to be bilateral. When assessing an individual's risk of breast cancer on the basis of family history it is important to focus on first-degree relatives and to determine whether breast cancer in the relatives was unilateral or bilateral, premenopausal or postmenopausal. Breast cancer occurring in a male in the family increases the chance that this family has a susceptibility gene. Table 30-4 gives a rough measure of relative risk to an individual based on characteristics of breast cancer in the family. Women who have a single relative with unilateral, postmenopausal breast cancer can be reassured that their risk is small, but a few women will be at very high risk and deserve special consideration in screening.

At least five **familial syndromes** associated with an increased risk of breast cancer have been described (Table 30-5). The best known of these are bilateral, premenopausal breast cancer and familial breast cancer associated with ovarian cancer, due to an inherited mutation in a gene

Table 30-4
Relative Risk of Breast Cancer According to Family History

Mother or Sister Diagnosed with Breast Cancer	Increased Risk (Fold)
After menopause	
In one breast	1.2
In both breasts	4.0
Before menopause	
In one breast	1.8
In both breasts	8.8

Table 30-5
Familial Syndromes Associated with Breast Cancer

Name of Syndrome	Defective Gene	Other Cancers
Li-Fraumeni (SBLA)	p53	*S*arcoma, *b*rain tumors, *l*eukemia, *a*drenocortical carcinoma
Lynch type II	hMSH2 hMLH1	Colon, gastric, endometrial, genitourinary carcinomas
Bilateral pre-menopausal breast cancer	BRCA1 BRCA2	Ovarian (in some families)
Cowden's disease	PTEN	Thyroid, colon, and other carcinomas
Familial melanoma	CDKN2A	Melanoma

(BRCA1) on chromosome 17q or a second susceptibility gene (BRCA2) on chromosome 13q. Other familial syndromes include Li-Fraumeni syndrome (germline p53 mutation), Lynch syndrome type II (hMSH2, hMLH1 mutations), Cowden's disease (PTEN mutation), and a recently described subset of familial melanoma (CDKN2A mutation). Muir-Torre syndrome was recently shown to be a variant of Lynch syndrome type II.

BRCA1 and **BRCA2 mutations** were initially thought to account for approximately 80% of the families that have a hereditary susceptibility to breast cancer. Subsequently that estimate was called into question, and it is now thought that the role of BRCA1 and BRCA2 may have been overestimated. With either gene, the lifetime risk of breast cancer can be as high as 85% in women who both carry a mutation and have a strong family history of early onset breast cancer. The majority of women develop their breast cancers before age 50 in such families. The risk of a second, contralateral breast cancer in gene carriers who develop early onset breast cancer is approximately 3% per year. Women who develop breast cancer before age 40 have about a 13% to 15% chance of carrying a germline BRCA1 mutation. The overall prevalence of BRCA1 mutations in US breast cancer patients is approximately 3%. BRCA1 mutations are 1.5 to 2 times more common than BRCA2 mutations.

The **magnitude of risk** associated with carrying a mutation may have been overestimated by initial studies, which concentrated on families with many cases of breast cancer. It is known that the carrier rate for BRCA1 and BRCA2 in the Ashkenazi Jewish population is on the order of 1% for each gene. In a study conducted in Washington DC on volunteers from the Ashkenazi Jewish population, mutations in BRCA1 and BRCA2 were sought, and family history was also charted. In this study, it was estimated that the lifetime risk associated with a BRCA1 mutation was 56%, not 85%. This too may actually be an overestimate since the volunteers may have been more likely than average to have a cancer susceptibility in the family. The lifetime risk of breast cancer in a BRCA1 mutation carrier who does not have a family history of breast cancer may be as low as 36%. The lifetime risk of ovarian cancer for a carrier of a BRCA1 or BRCA2 mutation can be as high as 40% in women who also have a strong family history of breast and/or ovarian cancer, and again the risk was much lower, only 16%, in those individuals who were found to carry a mutation but were not selected for study because of a positive family history of cancer. The relative incidence of breast and ovarian cancers in carriers of BRCA1 mutations varies greatly from family to family. There is evidence (still controversial) that the specific site of the mutation in the gene may influence ovarian cancer risk. Male breast cancer is more associated with mutations in BRCA2 than in BRCA1.

Different levels of screening for BRCA1 and BRCA2 mutations are available: whole gene sequencing (which is expensive) and screening for specific mutations (which is significantly less expensive). If a specific gene mutation is identified in an individual with breast cancer in a particular family, other members of that family can be screened for that specific mutation. In women of Ashkenazi Jewish descent with a familial susceptibility, there are certain specific mutations in the BRCA1 and BRCA2 genes (e.g., 185delAG in BRCA1), which are easy to screen for.

Of interest, although breast cancers arising in BRCA1 mutation carriers are more likely to be high grade, with a high proliferation rate and negative estrogen receptors, they have a similar prognosis to sporadic cancers and seem less likely to metastasize than sporadic tumors of the same grade. Recently it was reported that oophorectomy decreased the incidence of breast cancer in BRCA1 carriers by 60%. There are also preliminary data suggesting that tamoxifen may decrease breast cancer incidence in individuals with mutations in the BRCA genes.

Predisposing Benign Breast Condition

It has frequently been quoted that a previous history of biopsies of the breast for benign disease carries with it a risk of future breast cancer. This has caused inordinate anxiety among women. It is now clear that most benign breast disease is not a risk factor for breast cancer. In a classic study by Dupont and Page (Table 30-6) of 10,542 women who had biopsies showing benign breast disease, only the small group of women with atypical hyperplasia were found to be at high risk. If these women also had a positive family history in a first-degree relative, their risk doubled.

Thus most women who have had benign breast disease may be reassured that they are not at high risk of development of breast cancer. Women with atypical hyperplasia or with lobular carcinoma in situ (see later discussion) are counseled that they need careful follow-up observation because of their increased risk. It is reassuring, however, that their risk seems to attenuate with time. If a woman with proliferative disease without atypia has not had breast cancer in

---

Table 30-6
Risk of Breast Cancer in Patients with Benign Breast Disease

Diagnosis	No. of Biopsies	% of Benign Lesions	% of Evaluated Biopsies
Benign Specimens			
Nonproliferative disease	7221	69.7	68.5
Proliferative disease without atypia	2768	26.7	26.2
Atypical hyperplasia	377	3.6	3.6
Total benign	10,366	100	98.3
Total carcinoma in situ	176		1.7
Total evaluated biopsies*	10,542		100

Type of Benign Breast Disease	Relative Risk of Breast Cancer
All patients	1.5
Nonproliferative disease	0.89
Proliferative disease	1.9
Proliferative disease without atypia	1.6
Proliferative disease with atypical hyperplasia	4.4
Proliferative disease with atypical hyperplasia, negative family history	3.5
Proliferative disease with atypical hyperplasia, positive family history	8.9

Data from Dupont WD, Page DL: *New Engl J Med* 312:146, 1985.
*The women who underwent 10,542 consecutive biopsies for a suspicion of breast cancer but who were found to have benign breast disease or carcinoma in situ were monitored for a median period of 17 years. Their relative risk of development of breast cancer as a function of histologic diagnosis of the original biopsy specimen was compared to that of a normal population of case-matched control women. Almost 70% of the women with benign breast disease were at no increased risk. The 4% who had atypical hyperplasia were at significantly increased risk and a positive family history increased that risk considerably.

the first 10 years of follow-up observation, her risk falls to that of a woman without proliferative disease. For a woman who has atypical hyperplasia in whom breast cancer does not develop in the first 10 years of follow-up observation, the risk also falls considerably thereafter.

Reproductive and Hormonal Factors

There is a small (approximately 1.3 times) increased risk of breast cancer associated with early menarche, late menopause, or nulliparity. It is believed that this risk is related to the increased number of ovulatory cycles experienced by these women, with resulting stimulation of the breast epithelium by elevated estrogen levels. There is also a small increased risk associated with delay of first full-term pregnancy until after age 30 and with nulliparity. The longer the interval between menarche and the first full-term pregnancy, the higher the risk of future breast cancer. Most striking, however, is the observation that an early full-term pregnancy is extraordinarily protective. A full-term pregnancy before age 15 results in a decreased relative risk of breast cancer to approximately 0.4 (Fig. 30-3). Lactation after pregnancy confers a small decrease in risk, but this benefit is lost after the menopause. Use of exogenous estrogens can increase a woman's risk of breast cancer, but the risk is small. It is estimated that only prolonged use carries a risk: 15 years of estrogen replacement therapy may elevate a woman's risk to 1.3 over the next 10 years. A small increased risk has also been noted to occur later in life for a woman who took diethylstilbestrol (DES) while pregnant. It was recently reported from the Nurses' Health Study that an elevated endogenous estrogen level is also a risk factor for breast cancer.

Ionizing Radiation Exposure

From experience at Hiroshima, use of therapeutic irradiation of the chest, and use of fluoroscopy in patients with tuberculosis, it has become well established that ionizing radiation can increase the risk of breast cancer. The age of exposure is highly significant, with most of the risk occurring in women irradiated when under 25 years of age. Women who were treated with mantle radiation for Hodgkin's disease before age 25 have a significantly increased risk of breast cancer, and should begin annual mammograms 8 years out from their radiation even if they are less than 40 at that time. It should be noted that the risk of therapeutic radiation used to treat primary breast cancer in conjunction with lumpectomy is associated with an acceptably small increased risk of contralateral breast cancer (relative risk 1.33 at 10 years). The risk of inducing a breast cancer by the use of screening mammography is negligibly small. It is estimated that perhaps less than one case per year per million women screened would be attributable to the radiation exposure, and this is likely to decrease as technology advances: the exposure from digital mammography is even less than from film screen mammography.

Possible Risk Factors

A large number of other endogenous and exogenous risk factors have been proposed, consistent with the fact that we really have little idea of the cause of most breast cancer. There is an intriguing hypothesis that individual variations in endogenous patterns of hormone metabolism, which might be hereditary, could be associated with an increased risk. For example, elevated levels of the enzyme 16-alpha-hydroxylase, which metabolizes estradiol to a more potent estrogen, has been suggested as a risk factor. Levels of breast epithelial growth factors other than estrogen may also play a role; for example, endogenous prolactin levels may be associated with an elevated risk but an association has never been proved. There is some evidence for increased risk associated with elevated insulin-like growth factor-1 levels.

Multiple exogenous factors have been looked at critically. The **high-fat diet** theory emerged on the basis of epidemiologic studies showing a correlation between incidence of breast cancer in various countries and per capita fat consumption. However, it must be cautioned that correlation by no means implies causation. There are no solid data to support the fat hypothesis, and many believe that fat intake per se is irrelevant, but that another correlated factor is responsible.

Alcohol intake has been much in the press over the last few years. There is mounting evidence that daily intake of a moderate quantity of alcohol may be associated with an increased risk. The increased risk mainly affects young women whose baseline risk is already low; thus it is unlikely to be a major risk factor. There are some data to suggest that alcohol may cause increased risk through elevation of endogenous estrogen levels. Recent results from the Nurses' Health Study suggest that adequate intake of folic acid may negate the effect of alcohol.

Oral contraceptive use does not, after decades of study, appear to lead to any significant increase in breast cancer incidence overall; however, recent reanalyses of old studies

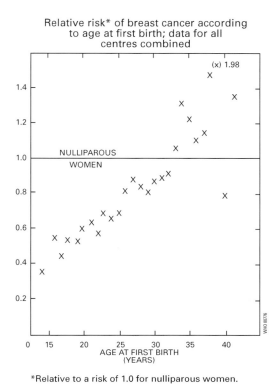

Relative risk* of breast cancer according to age at first birth; data for all centres combined

*Relative to a risk of 1.0 for nulliparous women.

FIG. 30-3   Protective effect of an early full-term pregnancy. (From MacMahon B, et al: *Bull WHO* 43:209, 1970.)

suggest that there may be an increased risk in certain sub-groups. Women who have taken the oral contraceptive pill for prolonged periods (>12 years) or women who took high-estrogen pills in their mid-teens may have an associated increased risk over the next two decades. It has been reported that BRCA2 mutation carriers who take oral contraceptives may develop breast cancer at an even earlier age than carriers who avoid their use, but it would be premature to conclude that in general a positive family history of breast cancer is a contraindication to the use of oral contraceptives. Reassuringly, use for only a few years is extremely unlikely to affect risk significantly in the majority of women. Women using progestins as contraceptives should be studied for any increased risk of breast cancer because, in contrast to their action on the uterus, progestins act on breast tissue as a proliferative stimulus.

Many other putative agents have been examined such as smoking and use of hair dyes, and no definitive link has been proved. Although the risk factors discussed previously are important, we have not yet identified the major etiologic agent of breast cancer. Because genetic alterations in previously normal cells are a key component of carcinogenesis, exposure to chemical carcinogens is an obvious possible causal factor. There is much current interest in evaluating the relationship of environmental exposure to pesticides (which can be detected in body fat) to breast cancer risk, but at this time it is too early to conclude that these toxic agents can be implicated.

CLASSIFICATION OF BREAST CANCER

Figure 30-4 schematizes the subtypes of breast cancer and their frequency. The most common histologic type of breast cancer is "infiltrating ductal carcinoma, not otherwise specified," but there are several identifiable subtypes of infiltrating ductal carcinoma that may have a better or worse prognosis than the common type (e.g., mucinous infiltrating ductal carcinoma or tubular infiltrating ductal carcinoma, both of which have a more favorable prognosis).

Ductal carcinoma in situ (DCIS) is characterized by a proliferation of ductal cells filling the ducts and spreading via the branching ductal network. Microcalcifications are often associated with DCIS within the ducts and can lead to early diagnosis on mammography before the disease spreads extensively through the ductal network or spawns an invasive cancer.

Infiltrating ductal cancer (IDC) is believed to arise by clonal evolution from DCIS and commonly appears as a mass or as a spiculated density on mammography. Small infiltrating ductal carcinomas can be found because of the microcalcifications in the ductal carcinoma in situ from which they arise. With increasing use of screening mammography there has been a gratifying rise in the detection of DCIS as a percentage of all ductal cancers as well as a shift to earlier stages of the invasive cancers that are found. This downstaging is the most important reason for the decrease in mortality rate seen with the use of screening mammography.

Infiltrating lobular carcinoma has distinctive histologic and clinical features. Unlike infiltrating ductal cancer, it does not show up easily on mammograms because it is not associated with microcalcifications and commonly infiltrates insidiously through the breast tissue without forming a

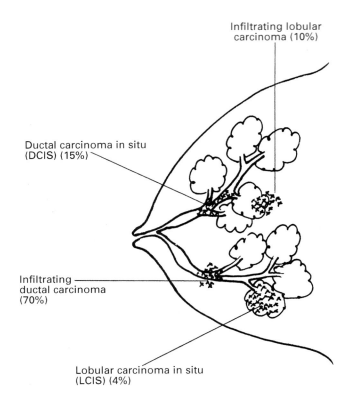

FIG. 30-4 Subtypes of breast cancer. Ductal carcinoma in situ is thought to be a precursor of invasive ductal carcinoma; lobular carcinoma, in contrast, is more akin to atypical hyperplasia and carries a risk of future ductal or invasive lobular carcinoma anywhere in the breast.

discrete mass. It is common for infiltrating lobular carcinoma to appear as a diffusely thickened area of breast tissue.

Lobular carcinoma in situ (LCIS), whose name implies that it has malignant potential, is probably a form of hyperplasia and not a preinvasive neoplasm. Like atypical ductal hyperplasia, LCIS is a risk factor for the future development of DCIS or invasive carcinoma. It is frequently seen in both breasts, and the risk of future cancer is almost the same in the two breasts (approximately 20% to 25% lifetime risk).

MANAGEMENT OF PRIMARY BREAST CANCER

A patient newly diagnosed with breast cancer usually has various treatment options open to her. Because of the complexity of decision making and the need to integrate surgery, radiation therapy, and medical treatment, more and more breast cancer centers are being set up so that multidisciplinary consultations can be offered.

Surgical Options

The rationale behind the Halsted radical mastectomy for primary breast cancer was that cancer was thought to grow like its namesake, the crab, sending out insidious infiltrating projections from the main mass into the surrounding normal tissue. Thus, Halsted reasoned, only a locally extensive surgical procedure had a chance of eradicating all traces of the cancer. Such was the power of Halsted's influence that, from the turn of the century until the mid-1970s, this mutilating surgery, in which the pectoralis major and minor muscles are sacrificed together with the breast and axillary lymph nodes, was standard treatment for breast cancer. Although it was hailed as a major advance in preventing local recurrences (which admittedly can be a major source of morbidity), the radical mastectomy failed to cure the majority of women, who succumbed to distant metastases.

Well-controlled clinical trials over the last several decades have supported a major change in how we use surgery to treat breast cancer. It is clear that the malignant cells in an invasive cancer can gain access to the bloodstream while the primary cancer is still small, and that the cells can also skip lymph nodes and embolize farther down the lymphatic chain. Thus axillary lymph nodes cannot be regarded as "filters" to trap all the cells that have escaped the breast. Axillary lymph node dissection is now regarded less as a therapeutic intervention and more as a staging operation to assess the extent of lymph node involvement by the cancer, which in turn gives an assessment of the likelihood that there has been systemic spread of the cancer cells. Recent studies using monoclonal antibodies have suggested that as many as 30% of women with early stage breast cancer have detectable micrometastases in the bone marrow at the time of initial surgery.

The goal of surgery is now merely to achieve local control of the primary tumor. "Cure" can only be achieved if the cancer is excised before distant metastases have been seeded or if adjuvant medical treatment is successful in eradicating these metastases. Clinical trials documented first that modified radical mastectomy (in which the pectoralis major muscle is spared) is equivalent to radical mastectomy in terms of long-term survival rate and local control, and then that "lumpectomy" with irradiation gives an identical survival rate with an acceptable local recurrence risk in the breast. When amputation of the breast is not performed, there will always be a chance of local recurrence within the breast, but if patients with increased risk of local failure are excluded (see later discussion), this risk should be around 5% and is acceptable to most women. Recurrence within the breast after lumpectomy and radiation therapy with the need for a "salvage" mastectomy has not influenced survival rate.

An NIH consensus report issued in 1990 upheld the position that **lumpectomy with radiation** was preferable to **mastectomy** because it has an equivalent long-term survival rate and spares the breast. Although the majority of women agree with this philosophy, some still choose mastectomy for a variety of reasons, which include an emotional wish to get rid of the cancerous breast, a fear of radiation, or simply a desire to have the treatment over and done with as quickly as possible. In other words most women can choose their surgical option on the basis of the side effects of the treatment with the knowledge that the chance of a cure will be the same, whichever they choose. For mastectomy the major side effect is obvious: physical loss of an appendage with its psychologic toll. Conservative surgery with radiation therapy requires several weeks (usually 5 or 6) of daily radiation treatments, some swelling and erythema of the breast during treatment (and this can sometimes last for months afterward), and the need for more intense surveillance to ensure that the cancer has not recurred in the breast. For some women the fear of finding recurrent disease in the breast is a major stress, but the majority of women are willing and able

to deal with each of these side effects because of a strong motivation to avoid a mastectomy. Recently sentinel lymph node mapping has come into widespread use in an attempt to decrease the morbidity associated with a full axillary dissection (see later).

When it was discovered that the susceptibility genes BRCA1 and BRCA2 were involved in DNA repair, it was feared that women carrying these mutations might not be good candidates for lumpectomy and radiation; however, several studies have indicated that breast cancer patients who are BRCA gene mutation carriers do well with breast conservation. There is, of course, a higher likelihood of a new cancer in the remaining breast tissue (approximately 3% per year, compared with 1% in other breast cancer patients), but the control rate for the cancer treated seems to be similar to what would be expected in a noncarrier.

There are some women for whom breast conservation with radiation therapy is not a good choice. For example, women who have more than one primary cancer in the breast or extensive lymphatic invasion have an unacceptably risk of recurrence. In others, such as those in whom the cancer is centrally located or is large in comparison to the size of the breast, the cosmetic outcome is likely to be poor. Studies are currently ongoing to see whether chemotherapy before surgery (neoadjuvant chemotherapy), which can render large or locally advanced breast cancers more easily operable, will in the long run give acceptable local control rates in the breast (when used with lumpectomy and irradiation). Initial reports are favorable.

Axillary Dissection

Regardless of whether mastectomy or breast conservation is chosen, it has been until recently standard practice to dissect the ipsilateral axilla and remove levels I and II lymph nodes en bloc. The extent of axillary lymph node involvement is the most important prognostic factor currently available, and decisions on adjuvant medical treatment (and eligibility for clinical research protocols) have traditionally been made on the basis of what is found in the axilla. When the treatment will not be affected by these findings (for example, an elderly patient with a large estrogen-receptor-positive cancer will receive tamoxifen whether or not the lymph nodes are positive) or when the morbidity risk of the general anesthesia required is likely to be considerable (for example, in an elderly woman with multiple medical problems), an argument could be made for *not* dissecting the axilla and treating the patient as if the nodes were involved.

Over the last few years, **sentinel lymph node mapping** of the axilla has become popular in an attempt to avoid the morbidity of the full axillary lymph node dissection. Blue dye and/or a radioactive colloid is injected before surgery at the site of the primary tumor (or at the biopsy site). A gamma probe is used at surgery to locate the first lymph node to take up the isotope (the sentinel node). A small incision is made at this site and a blue trail can be visualized leading to the lymph node. This node is removed and subjected to frozen section analysis. Currently, in most centers a complete axillary dissection is done if the sentinel lymph node is involved because decisions regarding both systemic therapy and radiation therapy are frequently based on the number of involved lymph nodes. If the sentinel lymph node is uninvolved, the chance that other lymph nodes are involved is very low, and a full dissection can usually be avoided. The use of sentinel lymph node mapping raises new issues in how to interpret and use the results of axillary staging. More careful analysis of the sentinel node is performed (more cuts, keratin stains) than is normally done on axillary lymph nodes, so that the likelihood of positivity is increased. Whether women with sentinel lymph node involvement detected only by the more rigorous analysis have a poorer prognosis than women with negative lymph nodes is not yet really known, and this question is currently being addressed in a large national trial. Also being studied is whether women with an involved sentinel lymph node (but no gross evidence of residual disease in the axilla) do as well with radiation to the axilla as with a full axillary dissection, and whether the morbidity of this approach is less.

Staging

The international TNM staging system is routinely used for staging breast cancer (Table 30-7). Figure 30-5 shows data from the SEER (*S*urveillance, *E*pidemiology, and *E*nd *R*esults) program of the National Cancer Institute relating survival to stage at diagnosis. It is important to note that the TNM system has been modified over the years, and certain clinical trial data may need to be reinterpreted with this in mind.

The role of radiologic evaluation in the staging of early breast cancer is controversial. One study showed that for clinical stage I disease, the yield of a bone scan was 0% and only 1.5% to 4% of clinical stage II disease had positive scan findings, whereas there was a 16% to 25% positive rate for clinical stage III disease. Another study looking at the role of liver scan results showed that only 5% were positive preoperatively, but only 1% of patients had true positive study results; the others were false-positive results.

Preoperative routine staging therefore should include bilateral mammograms (if not already done) to detect multicentric and bilateral lesions, chest radiographs, and liver function tests, including alkaline phosphatase. Most surgeons still obtain a bone scan, but there is a trend away from obtaining one for clinical stage I or II disease unless the alkaline phosphatase is elevated. Liver scans are no longer done routinely. If abnormal liver function test results are noted, an abdominal computed tomography (CT) is done. Head CT is done only if signs or symptoms of central nervous system involvement are present.

Radiation Therapy

If a mastectomy has been performed as the primary surgery for an invasive breast cancer, radiation therapy has not in the past been given routinely unless the patient was deemed to be at high risk for local recurrence. Local radiation therapy, although effectively decreasing the local recurrence rate, had not convincingly been shown to improve survival rate. This is probably because mortality results from distant metastases and not from local recurrence, and any small benefit from the radiation was negated by its side effects, especially cardiac damage from radiation for left-sided lesions. Patients at high risk for local recurrence include those who have close margins, extensive lymphatic invasion, more than four positive lymph nodes, or locally advanced disease (usually tumors ≤5 cm). These patients are routinely offered chest wall radiation to decrease local recurrence risk.

Table 30-7
TNM Staging System for Breast Cancer

Primary Tumor (T)

Tx	Primary tumor cannot be assessed
T0	No evidence of primary tumor
Tis	Carcinoma in situ
T1	Tumor 2 cm or less in greatest dimension
T2	Tumor between 2 and 5 cm in greatest dimension
T3	Tumor more than 5 cm in greatest dimension
T4	Tumor of any size with any of the following:
	Extension to chest wall
	Edema or ulceration of skin of the breast
	Satellite skin nodules confined to the same breast
	Inflammatory carcinoma

Regional Lymph Nodes (N)

NX	Regional lymph nodes not assessed
N0	No regional lymph node metastasis
N1	Metastasis to movable ipsilateral axillary lymph node(s)
N2	Metastasis to ipsilateral axillary lymph node(s) fixed to one another or to other structures
N3	Metastasis to ipsilateral internal mammary lymph node(s)

Distant Metastases

Mx	Presence of distant metastasis not assessed
M0	No distant metastasis
M1	Distant metastasis (includes metastasis to ipsilateral supraclavicular lymph node[s])

Stage Grouping

Stage 0	Tis	N0	M0
Stage I	T1	N0	M0
Stage IIA	T0	N1	M0
	T1	N1	M0
	T2	N0	M0
Stage IIB	T2	N1	M0
	T3	N0	M0
Stage IIIA	T0	N2	M0
	T1	N2	M0
	T2	N2	M0
	T3	N1	M0
	T3	N2	M0
Stage IIIB	T4	Any N	M0
	Any T	N3	M0
Stage IV	Any T	Any N	M1

From Fleming ID et al: *AJCC cancer staging manual*, ed 5. American Joint Committee on Cancer, Philadelphia, 1997, Lippincott-Raven.

Recent studies have suggested for the first time that **chest wall radiation after mastectomy** may increase *survival*. It is important to note that these women were all premenopausal and all received adjuvant chemotherapy. It has been suggested that when systemic disease is adequately treated with adjuvant chemotherapy, and toxicity of radiation avoided with more modern techniques, a survival benefit may be seen due to a reduction in local recurrence, which in turn can seed systemic metastases. The surgical techniques may not have been comparable to current techniques in this country, because the local recurrence rates were higher than seen here; therefore recommendations regarding

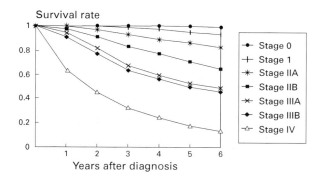

FIG. 30-5 Survival related to stage at diagnosis. (From Beahrs OH, et al, editors: *Manual for staging of cancer,* ed 4, Philadelphia, 1992, Lippincott.)

which patients should actually receive postmastectomy radiation should be made with caution. Women with one to three involved axillary lymph nodes are being asked to participate in a nationwide study in which half the women get radiation to the chest wall and regional lymph nodes and half do not.

Radiation therapy after lumpectomy is required for good local control. It is recommended that clear margins be obtained by lumpectomy, and radiation treatment be delivered in a dose of 4500 to 5000 cGy to the whole breast. If there is a close margin a boost may be necessary. If there is extracapsular invasion from involved axillary lymph nodes or if a large number of nodes are involved, axillary radiation therapy may also be given. It is common for the patient to experience erythema and edema of the breast during and after irradiation. The swelling can last for a number of months and gradually diminishes. There may be a small risk of cancer in the contralateral breast from radiation scatter, but this increase in risk is currently judged to be acceptable (relative risk 1.19, rising to 1.33 at 10 years).

Brachytherapy, which involves placing implants within the breast to deliver localized radiation over only 5 days, has been used successfully in a number of patients with early stage breast cancer. The benefit is a dramatic shortening of the treatment time; the disadvantage is that radiation therapy is less extensive, so that if microscopic disease has spread out of the treated area it might not be adequately treated. This approach remains investigational.

PROGNOSIS

The presence of positive **axillary lymph nodes** and their extent of involvement (number of nodes, level) are the single most important prognostic factors in patients with breast cancer. For example, a woman with a 1.5-cm invasive cancer may have a 10-year disease-free survival rate of 70% after local treatment alone if the lymph nodes are negative but only 50% if two or three axillary lymph nodes are involved.

Other factors that are used to assess prognosis in early-stage breast cancer include tumor size, nuclear grade, histologic subtype, estrogen and progesterone receptor status, and presence of vascular invasion. However, there has been an explosion of information on prognostic factors in recent years. Some, such as ploidy analysis, initially appeared exciting but now do not seem to have independent prognostic value. Others, such as S-phase analysis (one of many assays

that assess mitotic index as a measure of growth rate of the tumor), seem more likely to be useful clinically. The future roles of analyses of oncogene expression, tumor suppressor gene (e.g., p53) expression, neovascularization, growth factor and growth factor receptor expression, and so on, hang in the balance at this time.

In the last few years the **HER2/neu oncogene** has been studied intensively. Approximately 20% to 30% of breast cancers overexpress this oncogene, usually because of gene amplification. The gene codes for a growth factor receptor related to the epidermal growth factor receptor, and the receptor is constitutively active in cells overexpressing it. It is thought that this provides an estrogen-independent growth pathway that causes the breast cancer cell to proliferate. Breast cancers that overexpress HER2 have a worse prognosis, and many oncologists have a much lower threshold for prescribing chemotherapy for women whose tumors overexpress this oncogene.

ADJUVANT SYSTEMIC THERAPY

Breast cancer is a chemotherapy-responsive disease. If the cancer has receptors for estrogen and progesterone, it may also be responsive to hormone therapies. However, chemotherapy and hormonal therapy have not been curative for women who have established metastases. Clinical trials began more than 50 years ago to try to improve the cure rate for breast cancer by giving chemotherapy early in the course of the disease, before distant disease is manifest, on the theory that the micrometastases inferred to be present at the time of the primary treatment might be eradicated and systemic relapse prevented.

The earliest trials included women with positive lymph nodes who were deemed to be at sufficiently high risk of relapse to justify experimental treatment. Perioperative or short postoperative courses, usually with single agents, were given at first. However, it was not until combination chemotherapy (cyclophosphamide, methotrexate, and 5-fluorouracil [CMF] was given for a year or more postoperatively that impressive improvements in disease-free survival and overall survival rates were seen. In the first long-term follow-up evaluation of CMF, Bonadonna and colleagues reported that premenopausal women with positive axillary lymph nodes who were given CMF experienced a 17% improvement in relapse-free survival rate and a 14% improvement in overall survival rate at 10 years compared with untreated control subjects. With other groups reporting similar data, the NIH in 1985 issued a consensus conference report recommending that premenopausal women with positive axillary lymph nodes be given postoperative adjuvant chemotherapy as standard treatment. Postmenopausal women with positive axillary lymph nodes in the Bonadonna study gained only 6% improvement in relapse-free survival rate and 2% improvement in overall survival rate, and this small benefit was considered not significant enough for adjuvant chemotherapy to be offered routinely to this group. It was not clear, however, whether the less favorable results in the older women were due to underdosing with chemotherapy.

In contrast, for postmenopausal women with positive lymph nodes and cancers that were estrogen-receptor-positive (ER+), adjuvant hormonal therapy with tamoxifen was found to produce a remarkable improvement in disease-free survival and overall survival rates, comparable in fact to the effect of chemotherapy in the younger women. Tamoxifen also appeared to benefit postmenopausal women with ER− cancers (although this is no longer thought to be true). Interestingly tamoxifen was much less effective for premenopausal women with ER+ tumors, giving only a small benefit to this group. In 1985 therefore the NIH consensus conference committee recommended adjuvant tamoxifen for postmenopausal women who had ER+ (and even ER−) tumors and positive lymph nodes, but no adjuvant hormonal treatment for premenopausal women (who, as noted, were to have chemotherapy instead). Women with negative lymph nodes were thought to have a sufficiently favorable prognosis so that adjuvant therapy was not advised because of the associated side effects.

Early Breast Cancer Trialists' Collaborative Group Meta-Analysis of Adjuvant Systemic Therapies

Since the 1985 consensus conference report, many new observations have been made with regard to the role of adjuvant medical treatment. Many of these were summarized in a meta-analysis initially published in 1998 and updated in 1992 by the Early Breast Cancer Trialists' Collaborative Group (EBCTCG). This group assembled data from all known trials around the world of adjuvant treatment in breast cancer in which there were both a control and a treatment arm. A total of 133 trials involving 75,000 women were included. Subsequently the EBCTCG reconvened in 1995 and again in 2000 to update their meta-analysis. The main conclusions are summarized next.

Adjuvant Chemotherapy for Women with Positive Lymph Nodes

In the 1992 report the significant benefit of adjuvant chemotherapy in premenopausal women was affirmed with a decrease in the annual recurrence rate of 36% and in the annual mortality rate of 25% compared with those of control subjects. Six months of polychemotherapy (CMF) were shown to be as good as 12 months. Six months of CMF became the "standard" against which all other adjuvant chemotherapy are judged. The survival benefit from chemotherapy was greater at 10 years than at 5 years. In the postmenopausal group as a whole, the benefits were indeed less, but still quite significant in the 50- to 59-year-old group. On the basis of this report chemotherapy was offered more commonly to women in this age range, but hormonal therapy is still the first choice in women above 60 years old if the cancer is hormone-receptor positive. In the update from the 1995 meeting, anthracycline-containing regimens were shown to be marginally superior to CMF. Contrary to popular speculation, dose-intense regimens, including high-dose chemotherapy with stem cell transplantation, have not been shown to be superior to standard regimens in the adjuvant setting.

Adjuvant Hormonal Therapy for Women with Positive Lymph Nodes

In the 1992 meta-analysis report, the substantial benefit of adjuvant tamoxifen in women more than 50 years old (30% decrease in annual recurrence rate, 20% decrease in annual mortality rate) and the relative lack of benefit in

women less than 50 years old (12% decrease in annual recurrence rate, 6% decrease in annual mortality rate) were noted. As is the case with chemotherapy, the survival benefit was greater at 10 years than at 5 years. Comparison between studies showed that 2 years of tamoxifen were better than 1 year, and treatment for more than 2 years was better still. Subsequent studies addressed the optimal duration of adjuvant tamoxifen, and by the time of the update of the meta-analysis from the 1995 meeting, it was clear that 5 years of treatment is better than 2. A few small studies have shown no additional benefit to 10 years of tamoxifen over 5 years (and more complications), so that at the present time the recommendation is for 5 years of tamoxifen in the adjuvant setting pending the outcome of other ongoing trials.

In the earlier meta-analysis, although postmenopausal women with ER+ tumors derived the greatest benefit from tamoxifen (23% decrease in annual mortality rate with 1 to 2 years of adjuvant therapy), there was still a substantial benefit in postmenopausal women with ER− tumors (16% decrease in annual mortality rate). The biologic significance of this was intriguing but not fully understood. There was no benefit to premenopausal women with ER− tumors. Subsequently it has been shown fairly convincingly that neither premenopausal nor postmenopausal women whose tumors are ER− benefit from adjuvant tamoxifen, and the earlier results were probably due to inclusion in the "ER−" group women whose tumors had low levels of ERs. Although premenopausal women with ER+ tumors seemed to benefit little from adjuvant tamoxifen in the 1992 meta-analysis report, the surprising result of the 1995 update was that, with 5 years of therapy, tamoxifen benefited premenopausal and postmenopausal women equally, with about a 50% decrease in recurrence risk in both groups. Tamoxifen therefore is actually superior to chemotherapy in ER+ patients, both premenopausal and postmenopausal, if their tumors are ER+. Current trials are investigating the addition of aromatase inhibitors in the adjuvant setting for postmenopausal women.

Adjuvant Ovarian Ablation

Most of the trials involving oophorectomy in the postoperative setting were conducted at a time when estrogen receptor analyses were not performed. As expected the meta-analysis showed no benefit from ovarian ablation in postmenopausal women, but a surprisingly significant benefit in premenopausal women. In this group the decreases in recurrence and mortality rates resulting from oophorectomy were comparable in magnitude to those seen with chemotherapy. These findings have stimulated a resurgence of interest in adjuvant oophorectomy and ovarian suppression in premenopausal patients. Several small studies have shown that in premenopausal women with ER+ cancers, oophorectomy is as effective an adjuvant therapy as chemotherapy. Ovarian suppression with gonadotropin-releasing hormone (GnRH) agonists is also effective in this group.

Combination Chemotherapy and Hormonal Therapy for Women with Positive Lymph Nodes

In women aged 50 to 69, it was shown in the 1992 meta-analysis report that the combination of chemotherapy and tamoxifen was slightly more effective in decreasing recurrence rate than tamoxifen alone (although there was no effect on overall survival rate). For women younger than 50, tamoxifen is of significant benefit even if chemotherapy has been given. Ongoing trials are addressing which combinations of ovarian suppression, tamoxifen, and chemotherapy provide the optimal benefit in premenopausal women.

Adjuvant Therapy for Women with Invasive Cancer and Negative Lymph Nodes

Since the recommendation in 1985 at the NIH Consensus Conference that women with negative lymph nodes not receive adjuvant systemic therapy, there have been many trials showing that these women do benefit from adjuvant therapy. The meta-analysis by the EBCTCG showed that tamoxifen and chemotherapy use result in the same percentage reduction in recurrence and mortality rates in node-negative as in node-positive women, but because the recurrence and mortality risks are significantly lower in the node-negative women the absolute benefits are also smaller. Thus a treatment that improves 10-year survival rate from 50% to 62% in a node-positive group (12% absolute benefit) might only improve survival from 90% to 92% (2% absolute benefit) in patients with small tumors and negative lymph nodes.

Logically, systemic therapy should be given to those "node-negative" women who are at sufficiently high risk to make the systemic chemotherapy worthwhile in terms of absolute benefit gained. The perfect algorithm that gives appropriate weighting to the various prognostic factors is not yet available. At present, most clinicians recommend adjuvant systemic therapy if the primary tumor is 2 cm or larger and are more likely to recommend chemotherapy for an even smaller tumor if it is ER−, is high-grade, or has a high growth fraction.

Types of Chemotherapy

Six months of chemotherapy with "classic" **CMF,** a well-tolerated regimen with a good track record, is the standard against which other regimens are compared. The original CMF regimen pioneered by Bonadonna gave the cyclophosphamide orally for 14 days in each 28-day cycle, and methotrexate and 5-fluorouracil (5-FU) intravenously on days 1 and 8. With the recognition that Adriamycin (doxorubicin) is a better drug than methotrexate for breast cancer, **CAF,** in which Adriamycin replaces methotrexate, became popular for a number of years. This regimen is more toxic, but is probably slightly more efficacious than CMF. More recently, **CA** (5-FU was dropped and the doses of cyclophosphamide and Adriamycin were increased) given once every 3 weeks for four cycles was shown to be equivalent to 6 monthly cycles of CMF, but the shorter CA regimen (only four treatments done in 3 months) was preferred by the majority of the participants in the study over the longer CMF (12 visits over 6 months). Four cycles of CA is probably now more popular than CMF, although both are widely used. Adriamycin-containing regimens are more commonly used when the patient has four or more axillary lymph nodes involved or when the primary tumor overexpresses the HER2 oncogene because there are data to suggest that Adriamycin is a particularly effective drug for this type of breast cancer.

Recently the CALGB group reported results of a large trial of **paclitaxel (Taxol) plus CA** versus CA alone. Addition of paclitaxel seemed to reduce the systemic recurrence risk by 22% and mortality by 26% in those patients who received it, over and above the benefit seen from CA alone.

Overnight this regimen of CA for 3 months followed by paclitaxel for 3 months became widely adopted for women with involved axillary lymph nodes. It was therefore a shock to hear, late in 2000, that a parallel trial of almost identical design run by the NSABP showed no benefit from the addition of paclitaxel. At the present time long-term results of these and other studies are awaited to define the role of the taxanes in the adjuvant setting.

As noted previously, women whose tumors overexpress the HER2 oncogene have a poor prognosis. Trastuzumab (Herceptin), a monoclonal antibody that targets the HER2 molecule, has been shown to be effective in treating HER2-positive metastatic breast cancer and enhances the effect of chemotherapy. For this reason, trastuzumab is now being tested in the adjuvant setting in randomized trials.

Side Effects of Chemotherapy

The CMF regimen usually causes only mild to moderate nausea in the majority of women, and usually only moderate alopecia and myelosuppression. Other troublesome side effects can include mucositis, conjunctivitis, tearing of the eyes, and unwelcome weight gain. Induction of menopause by chemotherapy is age-related, occurring in only 40% of women less than 40 years old, but in more than 90% of women more than 40 years old. The risk of leukemia secondary to the chemotherapy is estimated to be less than 1%. Anthracycline-containing regimens cause more nausea (although with the advent of Zofran and Kytril the nausea is usually manageable) and more complete alopecia. They also may cause cardiac toxicity at high cumulative doses. With six cycles of Adriamycin at standard doses, the risk of clinically significant congestive heart failure is only about 1%. Taxanes cause little nausea, but can precipitate a significant neuropathy, myalgias, and arthralgias.

Side Effects of Tamoxifen

The only common side effects of tamoxifen are hot flashes and a mucoid vaginal discharge. Sometimes vaginal dryness is exacerbated. Rarely it causes nausea or bloating. With adjuvant therapy currently recommended for 5 years, long-term side effects must be considered. Luckily tamoxifen is not a pure antiestrogen. It is a mixed agonist/antagonist and has proestrogenic effects on several target organs. Its proestrogenic effect on the bones and the cardiovascular system gives some protection against osteoporotic bone loss, decreases cholesterol level, and decreases death of causes other than breast cancer (approximately 12% decrease, mostly attributable to a decrease in vascular events). Because it acts as an estrogen agonist on the endometrium, tamoxifen users experience an increased risk of endometrial cancer, but this small risk (roughly 1.1%, representing a 7.5-fold increase in their baseline risk) is more than counterbalanced in most women by the decreased risk of recurrence of breast cancer. The increased risk of endometrial cancer is seen only in postmenopausal women, as is the slight increase in the risk of thromboembolic disease. There is also a small increase in the risk of cataracts in tamoxifen users.

Neoadjuvant Chemotherapy

Neoadjuvant chemotherapy is defined as chemotherapy given before definitive surgery. It has long been the standard of care for women with inflammatory or locally advanced breast cancer but is now increasingly being used for "operable" breast cancer. Use of neoadjuvant chemotherapy increases the likelihood of breast conservation and improves cosmesis, as surgery is less extensive if the primary tumor is smaller. An additional benefit is the opportunity to assess in vivo the efficacy of chemotherapy. The extent of residual cancer present after neoadjuvant chemotherapy is prognostically significant. Response rates to neoadjuvant chemotherapy are high (75% to 85%) and progression during neoadjuvant chemotherapy is uncommon. The pathologic complete response rate is 10% to 15% in most studies. Some older studies hinted at a survival benefit from neoadjuvant chemotherapy over standard adjuvant therapy. The most recent update from a large NSABP trial suggests equivalence at this time. Perhaps with a longer follow-up period, a benefit from the neoadjuvant therapy will be found. At present, neoadjuvant chemotherapy should be considered if the tumor is large with respect to the size of the breast, the tumor is growing rapidly, or there is clinical evidence of bulky gross regional adenopathy. It is not known with certainty whether sentinel lymph node mapping is accurate after neoadjuvant therapy, whether its use will improve survival, or whether long-term local control will be satisfactory for very large cancers.

MANAGEMENT OF CARCINOMA IN SITU
Ductal Carcinoma in Situ

DCIS is a noninvasive type of breast cancer believed to be a precursor to infiltrating (invasive) ductal carcinoma. Once uncommon, it is being more frequently diagnosed with the advent of screening mammography, because it is detectable on mammograms as microcalcifications even before a mass develops in the breast. Traditionally DCIS has been treated with mastectomy because this will guarantee that this noninvasive cancer will not recur, and historically an unacceptably high rate of recurrence in the breast (between 30% and 75%) has been noted with lumpectomy alone. As lumpectomy and radiation therapy became the accepted treatment for invasive cancer, it was natural to ask whether a similar conservative approach might not be possible for small in situ ductal carcinomas. Recent clinical trials have been encouraging in this regard, and the current trend is to offer excision with radiation to selected women with small in situ tumors. It should be understood, however, that there will always be more risk associated with this approach because there will always be some risk of recurrence in the breast, and a proportion of these recurrences will be invasive. Each individual will therefore need to make a choice of treatment based, on the one hand, on the maximum peace of mind with a mastectomy and, on the other hand, the chance of avoiding a mastectomy but with a moderate risk of a recurrence in the breast that may be invasive and therefore associated with a small risk of life-threatening consequences.

Of the three most important characteristics of DCIS, namely size, grade and margin (the extent of normal tissue around the excised cancer), the width of the margin has emerged as the most important factor influencing local failure. If a 1 cm margin can be obtained, local failure rate is very low. In the NSABP B-24 trial, in which patients with DCIS treated with lumpectomy and radiation were randomized to tamoxifen or placebo for 5 years, there was a significant decrease in recurrence of DCIS (RR 0.82 at 5 years) and invasive breast cancer (RR 0.56) so that tamoxifen is frequently offered now to patients with DCIS who choose conservative treatment.

Lobular Carcinoma in Situ

Lobular carcinoma in situ would be better described as lobular hyperplasia. Its presence signifies that the breast epithelium is abnormal and that the woman has an increased risk in both breasts of a future invasive cancer. The lifetime risk is approximately 20% to 25% in each breast. In the past some surgeons recommended bilateral mastectomy because of this bilateral risk. However, with good screening mammography it is now generally recommended that most women be monitored carefully and surgical intervention offered only when indicated. For some women living with this fear will be unacceptable, whereas for others with mammographically dense breasts the sensitivity of radiography may not be acceptable. For these women bilateral simple mastectomy with or without reconstruction may be preferred. In the NSABP P1 prevention trial (see later) women with LCIS benefited significantly from tamoxifen, with a decrease in breast cancer incidence of 56%. Tamoxifen as a chemopreventive drug should therefore be discussed with women diagnosed with LCIS.

FOLLOW-UP CARE OF THE WOMAN WITH EARLY-STAGE BREAST CANCER

If the primary treatment has been lumpectomy, **serial physical examinations** and **mammograms** of the treated breast are essential to detect a recurrence. Usually the first follow-up mammogram will be obtained at 6 months after completion of irradiation. Physical examination is performed every 3 months in the first year of follow-up observation, every 4 months in the second year, and then every 6 months thereafter. Although chest radiographs and bone scans used to be part of routine follow-up care, clinical studies have shown no benefit in terms of outcome, and their routine use has been largely discontinued. Instead, attention is paid to **symptoms,** such as dry cough, exertional dyspnea, pleuritic chest pain, or bony aches and pains that may signify lung, pleural, or bony involvement. **Blood tests** to screen for bone (alkaline phosphatase) or liver dysfunction (liver function tests) are obtained every 6 months. Many oncologists also monitor tumor markers such as CA27.29 and CEA, elevations in which can be one of the earliest signs of recurrence.

A currently controversial issue is that of **estrogen replacement therapy** in breast cancer survivors. It is widely believed that estrogens must be avoided at all costs in the woman with a history of breast cancer, but recently this has been challenged by a number of experts who point out that the evidence supporting an adverse effect of exogenous estrogens in women with a history of breast cancer is weak. In view of the benefits to the skeletal and cardiovascular systems that postmenopausal women receive from estrogen therapy, many are now calling for prospective randomized trials to assess the actual risk/benefit ratio of estrogen therapy in breast cancer survivors. A small nonrandomized trial in California in which women with a history of breast cancer are prescribed estrogen continues to report no increased incidence of recurrences over what would have been expected. An ECOG trial is currently recruiting women to take estrogen if they are experiencing unacceptable menopausal symptoms on adjuvant tamoxifen. The goal of the trial is to assess the efficacy and safety of adding estrogen to tamoxifen therapy in this group of women.

MANAGEMENT OF METASTATIC DISEASE

Although breast cancer can spread to any part of the body, the common sites for metastases are the bones, lung, liver, and pleura. It is also important to recognize the occasional involvement of the pericardium and intestine and (frequently late) involvement of brain or meninges. Unless recurrent disease is in the breast after a lumpectomy or is locoregional (i.e., in the chest wall or axilla on the side of the original mastectomy), there is little meaningful likelihood of a cure with standard therapy, and the goal of treatment is palliation.

Hormonal Therapy

Unless the patient is in imminent danger of organ compromise from the metastases, hormonal therapy is the treatment of choice for patients whose original cancer was positive for estrogen receptors, because in such cases the likelihood of a response is 60% to 65%. Furthermore hormonal treatments have fewer side effects than chemotherapy. It was first noted by Beatson at the turn of the century that **oophorectomy** in premenopausal patients with breast cancer effected shrinkage of metastatic disease. Oophorectomy is still a valuable therapy for premenopausal women. **GnRH agonists** that lower estrogen levels by turning off ovarian function probably work equally well, but the once-a-month injections are expensive. In postmenopausal women **tamoxifen** is the treatment of choice because it has fewer side effects, although similar response rates can be seen with megestrol acetate. Tamoxifen is as efficacious as oophorectomy in premenopausal women, although a recent study suggested that a combination of tamoxifen and ovarian suppression with a GnRH analog may give superior results. As with many clinical trials, however, the results of this trial may be misleading because the women assigned to single drug therapy instead of the combination did not necessarily get the other drug at the time of progression.

The mean time to response to hormonal therapy is approximately 2 months, with the mean duration of response 1 to 2 years. Responses are more commonly seen in metastases in bone and soft tissue but less commonly in lung, liver, and brain. If a good response is obtained with the first endocrine treatment, it is worth using second-line hormonal therapy at the time of relapse with a likelihood of response of approximately 50%. The **aromatase inhibitors** anastrozole (Arimidex), letrozole (Femara), and exemestane (Aromasin) inhibit the conversion of androgens to estrogen in fat tissue (including breast tissue). Because of equal efficacy and fewer side effects, they have replaced megestrol acetate (Megace) as second-line therapy for postmenopausal patients with hormonally sensitive cancers after tamoxifen fails. They have recently been approved for first-line treatment of metastatic disease. **Megestrol** (Megace), although still a good drug, causes significant weight gain in the ma-

jority of women. It is an excellent choice if a patient also has lost weight or is in need of an appetite stimulant. Antiprogestins such as RU-486 are showing promise in preclinical and early clinical trials and may in the future add to our range of hormonal therapy options.

Chemotherapy

Chemotherapy is the systemic treatment of choice for patients with metastatic disease that is estrogen-receptor-negative (this group has a less than 10% chance of a response to hormonal therapy) or for those whose disease is no longer responding to hormonal manipulation. Even for patients with metastatic disease that is estrogen-receptor-positive, chemotherapy is preferred if they have visceral involvement with imminent symptoms because hormonal therapy gives slow (1 to 2 months) responses compared with chemotherapy, which usually begins to shrink the tumors within a couple of weeks. Patients with hormone-refractory breast cancer can certainly have symptoms palliated by chemotherapy and can live longer with better quality of life. However, it is sobering to discover that, despite response rates that can be greater than 75%, chemotherapy gives only temporary remissions in patients with metastatic breast cancer, and there is little chance of long-term disease-free survival for these patients with standard therapy.

The median duration of response to chemotherapy is 6 to 8 months, and the median survival after institution of chemotherapy is 1.5 to 2 years. There has not been any consistent survival advantage to more aggressive regimens with high response rates, so it is common to use the gentlest, least toxic regimens first (e.g., CMF) and progress to more aggressive regimens (such as those containing anthracyclines such as doxorubicin) later. Paclitaxel (Taxol), an excellent breast cancer drug on its own, is now being tested in combination with other drugs as first-line treatment of metastatic disease with variable results with respect to influence on survival. Because aggressive combination chemotherapy regimens have not been curative, however, the trend is away from aggressive therapy in favor of single agent, sequential therapy.

Trastuzumab (Herciptin), a humanized antibody against the HER2 receptor, is now widely used for HER2-positive breast cancers after the development of metastatic disease. It has been approved by the Food and Drug Administration for use in combination with paclitaxel for first-line treatment of HER2 overexpressing breast cancers. Apart from chills and sometimes rigors with the first infusion, Herciptin is remarkably free from the usual side effects of chemotherapy, although unexpectedly cardiac toxicity can develop in patients treated with this drug. Patients who develop cardiac toxicity have almost always had prior treatment with anthracyclines, and the drop in left ventricular ejection fraction is usually manageable with appropriate medical therapy; however, its occurrence has made many oncologists wary of introducing Herciptin into the adjuvant setting (see previously). Many new drugs including angiogenesis inhibitors and tyrosine kinase inhibitors, as well as a number of vaccines, are currently in clinical trials. For the woman with disease involving the bone, the bisphosphonate pamidronate is now routinely given because clinical trials have shown women who are given it have less bone pain and fewer fractures than those who do not receive it.

Autologous Bone Marrow Transplantation

There is a dose-response relationship in the treatment of breast cancer with chemotherapy. It has been hypothesized that, whereas cure of metastatic disease does not seem possible with standard doses of chemotherapy, increasing the doses many times might be curative if the toxicity of the treatment could be lessened. When drugs such as the alkylating agents, whose dose-limiting toxicity is bone marrow suppression, are chosen a several-fold increase in delivered dose can be obtained if hematopoietic stem cells are harvested before administration of chemotherapy and returned to the patient after metabolism and excretion of the chemotherapy drugs. Autologous bone marrow transplantation (when the stem cells are harvested by marrow aspiration from the iliac bones) and autologous peripheral stem cell transplantation (when the stem cells are harvested from the peripheral blood after mobilization from the bone marrow by chemotherapy or growth factors) provide such a way of overcoming the devastating bone marrow suppression that would otherwise accompany such high-dose chemotherapy.

In the early days of bone marrow transplantation for breast cancer, women who had widely metastatic disease and had been through several types of chemotherapy were recruited, but these women did poorly. Most had relapsed within 6 to 8 months and died within a year or so of transplantation. In subsequent trials, women who had lesser burdens of disease and who had had fewer prior treatments were selected as candidates if they showed a good response to induction chemotherapy before transplantation conditioning. In some series, 15% of such highly selected women were disease-free several years after transplantation. Although these numbers were encouraging, subsequent randomized trials have shown no benefit to high-dose chemotherapy with bone marrow or peripheral stem cell rescue. That some of the transplant recipients in the initial trials did better than expected is thought to be due to selection bias. Currently patients with metastatic breast cancer should not undergo bone marrow or peripheral stem cell transplantation unless they are participating in a clinical trial.

CHEMOPREVENTION

One of the major areas of basic and clinical research in cancer currently is chemoprevention. In breast cancer patients use of adjuvant tamoxifen has been shown to decrease the likelihood of a contralateral new primary breast cancer. A large multi-institutional trial, NSABP-P1, sought to accrue 16,000 women at increased risk of breast cancer for randomization into placebo versus tamoxifen treatment arms to determine the protective potential of tamoxifen. The trial was actually stopped early by the monitoring committee when it became apparent that there was a significant difference between the two arms. Tamoxifen reduced the risk of developing breast cancer by approximately 50% in these high-risk women. Although other European trials have not shown a benefit in this regard for tamoxifen, it is generally agreed that owing to different definitions of "high risk" and other features that differed between the different studies, the negative results from other trials do not negate the results of the carefully done NSABP study.

Women who fall into the high-risk group defined by the Gail model used in the NSABP trial (incidence of breast cancer of 1.66% or above in the next 5 years) should be told of the results of the NSABP prevention trial results and offered tamoxifen. The subgroups of women who benefited most were those with atypical ductal hyperplasia and lobular carcinoma in situ (LCIS). For some women, however, the risk of thromboembolic complications or endometrial carcinoma exceeds the benefit, so clearly not every "high-risk" woman will gain a net benefit from taking this drug. At an NIH conference an attempt was made to define the risk/benefit ratio for different subsets of women in an attempt to assist primary practitioners to decide who should and who should not be given the drug. Preliminary information suggests that tamoxifen is of value as a chemopreventive drug in women with BRCA gene mutations.

In the MORE osteoporosis trial, raloxifene (retrospectively) appeared to decrease the risk of breast cancer to a degree similar to tamoxifen. Because raloxifene does not stimulate the uterus, it is important to know if raloxifene is indeed as efficacious in prevention as tamoxifen, and if so, if it is safer. The NSABP is currently recruiting high-risk women to a study of tamoxifen versus raloxifene in the STAR trial to assess the comparative efficacy for chemoprevention and safety of these two drugs. The study is open only to postmenopausal women.

Fenretinide, a retinoid derivative, is also being tested as a chemopreventive agent for breast cancer in European studies. Another study, at the University of Southern California, is treating women at high risk with GnRH analogs to suppress normal ovulation. These women receive supplementary low-dose estrogen and intermittent pulses of progesterone to minimize the adverse effects of estrogen deprivation and unopposed estrogen, respectively. If chemoprevention and modification of the environment could have a major impact on decreasing the rate of breast cancer, this would be a much more valuable contribution than the discovery of another new drug to treat metastatic disease and will offer women another alternative to surgical ablation (bilateral mastectomy or oophorectomy), which is the only other known way to diminish breast cancer risk.

BIBLIOGRAPHY

Bonadonna G et al: Adjuvant cyclophosphamide, methotrexate, and fluorouracil in node-positive breast cancer: the results of 20 years of follow-up, *N Engl J Med* 332:901, 1995.

Cody HS 3rd: Sentinel lymph node mapping in breast cancer, *Oncology* 13(1):25; discussion 35, 1999.

Cummings SR et al: The effect of raloxifene on risk of breast cancer in postmenopausal women: Results from the MORE randomized trial, *JAMA* 281:2189, 1999.

Early Breast Cancer Trialists' Collaborative Group: Favourable and unfavourable effects on long-term survival of radiotherapy for early breast cancer: an overview of the randomised trials, *Lancet* 355:1757, 2000.

Early Breast Cancer Trialists' Collaborative Group: Polychemotherapy for early breast cancer: an overview of the randomised trials, *Lancet* 352:930, 1998.

Early Breast Cancer Trialists' Collaborative Group: Tamoxifen for early breast cancer: an overview of the randomised trials, *Lancet* 351:1451, 1998.

Early Breast Cancer Trialists' Collaborative Group: Ovarian ablation in early breast cancer: overview of the randomised trials, *Lancet* 348:1189, 1996.

Early Breast Cancer Trialists' Collaborative Group: Systemic treatment of early breast cancer by hormonal, cytotoxic, or immune therapy: (meta-analysis), *Lancet* 339:1-15, 71-85, 1992.

Fentiman IS: Future prospects for the prevention and cure of breast cancer, *Eur J Cancer* 36:1085, 2000.

Fisher B et al: Endometrial cancer in tamoxifen-treated breast cancer patients: findings from the National Surgical Adjuvant Breast and Bowel Project (NSABP) B-14, *J Natl Cancer Inst* 86:527, 1994.

Fisher B et al: Tamoxifen for prevention of breast cancer: report of the National Surgical Adjuvant Breast and Bowel Project P-1 study, *J Natl Cancer Inst* 90:1371, 1998.

Fleming ID et al: *AJCC cancer staging manual,* ed 5, American Joint Committee on Cancer, Philadelphia, 1997, Lippincott-Raven.

Gail M H et al: Weighing the risks and benefits of tamoxifen treatment for preventing breast cancer, *J Natl Cancer Inst* 91:1829, 1999.

Ginsburg ES: Estrogen, alcohol and breast cancer risk, *J Steroid Biochem Mol Biol* 69:299, 1999.

Greenlee RT: Cancer statistics, 2001, *CA Cancer J Clin* 51:15, 2001.

Henderson IC, Patek AJ: The relationship between prognostic and predictive factors in the management of breast cancer, *Breast Cancer Res Treat* 52:261, 1998.

Hudis CA: The current state of adjuvant therapy for breast cancer: focus on paclitaxel, *Semin Oncol* 26(1 Suppl 2):1, 1999.

Martin AM, Weber BL: Genetic and hormonal risk factors in breast cancer, *J Natl Cancer Inst* 92:1126, 2000.

Ollila DW et al: The role of intraoperative lymphatic mapping and sentinel lymphadenectomy in the management of patients with breast cancer, *Adv Surg* 32:349, 1999.

Osborne MP: Chemoprevention of breast cancer, *Surg Clin North Am* 79:1207, 1999.

Overgaard M et al: Postoperative radiotherapy in high-risk premenopausal women with breast cancer who receive adjuvant chemotherapy, *N Engl J Med* 337:949, 1997.

Ries LAG et al, editors: *SEER cancer statistics review, 1973-1998,* Bethesda, Md, 2001, National Cancer Institute.

Scottish Cancer Trials Breast Group and ICRF Breast Unit: Adjuvant ovarian ablation versus CMF chemotherapy in premenopausal women with pathological stage II breast carcinoma: the Scottish trial, *Lancet* 341: 1293, 1993.

Silverstein MJ et al: The influence of margin width on local control of ductal carcinoma in situ of the breast, *N Engl J Med* 340:1455, 1999.

Sledge GW Jr, Miller KD: Metastatic breast cancer: the role of chemotherapy, *Semin Oncol* 26(1 Suppl 2):6, 1999.

Stadtmauer EA et al: Conventional dose chemotherapy compared with high-dose chemotherapy plus autologous hematopoietic stem-cell transplantation for metastatic breast cancer. Philadelphia Bone Marrow Transplant Group, *N Engl J Med* 342:1069, 2000.

Vastag B: Consensus panel recommendations for treatment of early breast cancer, *JAMA* 284:2707, 2000.

Vogel VG: Breast cancer prevention: review of current evidence [see comments], *CA Cancer J Clin* 50:156, 2000.

CHAPTER 31

Gynecologic Cancers

Linda R. Duska

In the year 2000, the three most commonly diagnosed cancers among United States women were cancers of the breast, lung, and colon, in that order. These three sites account for more than half of the cancers diagnosed in women and more than half of cancer deaths, with lung cancer being the leading cause of cancer death.

Gynecologic cancers, although not as significant in number, continue to be a significant health problem for women in the United States. Cancer of the uterine corpus is the fourth most common cancer diagnosed in American women, accounting for 6% of new cancer diagnoses. Ovarian cancer is the fifth most commonly diagnosed cancer, accounting for 4% of new diagnoses and 5% of cancer deaths. Ovarian cancer continues to be a significant health problem because of the high mortality rate. For example, in breast cancer in the year 2000 there were estimated to be 182,800 new diagnoses and 40,800 deaths. In contrast, in ovarian cancer there were estimated to be 23,100 new diagnoses (much fewer than for breast cancer) and 14,000 deaths (much higher proportion of deaths, 22% compared with 61%).

This chapter reviews four gynecologic cancers: cervical, endometrial, ovarian, and vulvar—with emphasis on aspects of diagnosis and management of disease relevant to the primary care clinician. Screening for cervical cancer is discussed in detail in Chapter 96 and screening for ovarian, endometrial, and vulvar cancer in Chapter 97.

CERVICAL CANCER

▦ EPIDEMIOLOGY AND RISK FACTORS

Cervical cancer is the third most common malignant disease of the female genital tract in the United States and is the only genital tract cancer for which an effective screening test has been established. In developing countries, where screening programs are not in place, cervical cancer is the leading cause of death in women. Since the introduction of the Pap smear in 1943 and the widespread institution of screening programs, there has been a decreasing incidence of, and mortality from, invasive cervical cancer. Nevertheless, it was expected that of 12,800 new cases diagnosed,

4600 women would die of cervical cancer in the United States in the year 2000. Many of these deaths are believed to be the result of screening failure.

Risk factors for cervical cancer include early age at first intercourse, multiple sexual partners, cigarette smoking, and low socioeconomic status. The human papillomavirus (HPV) is now thought to be causally related to the development of cervical neoplasia. High-risk subtypes, including types 16 and 18, have been found in more than 90% of preinvasive disease and cervical cancers. HPV is a sexually transmitted virus that is prevalent in the US population. For example, prevalence rates of HPV in women with *normal* cytology range from 25% to 30%. Patients should be counseled that a new diagnosis of dysplasia does not necessarily mean that their partner has given them a new virus; the latent time from infection to development of dysplasia is not known. Condoms are not protective against viral transmission. Currently there is no information to explain what activates the virus, thus causing premalignant change. Women who are immunosuppressed and women who smoke cigarettes are at higher risk for developing genital tract neoplasia and for having recurrent disease.

Treatment of Preinvasive Disease

In 1988 the Bethesda system of Pap smear classification was created to provide more clinically relevant categories of abnormal Pap smears. Table 31-1 details these categories for squamous smears and compares Bethesda system diagnoses with previous diagnostic categories. Abnormal squamous smears are divided into low- and high-grade categories. The low-grade lesions (LGSIL) are often associated with low-risk HPV and have a significant rate of spontaneous regression (as high as 50%). In contrast, the high-grade smears (HGSIL) have an association with high-risk HPV, a lower rate of regression, and a significant rate of malignant transformation. Thus the diagnoses are separated into clinically relevant categories: HGSIL needs to be treated and LGSIL can (usually) safely be monitored. It should be remembered that the Pap smear has a 20% false-negative rate for squamous lesions (possibly as high as 40% for glandular lesions). One of the major causes of the false-negative rate is

Table 31-1
Comparison of Cytology Classification Systems

Bethesda System	Dysplasia/CIN System	Papanicolaou System
Within normal limits	Normal	I
Infection (organism should be specified)	Inflammatory atypia (organism)	II
Reactive and reparative changes		
Squamous cell abnormalities		
Atypical squamous cells of undetermined significance	Squamous atypia	III R
HPV atypia		
Low-grade squamous intraepithelial lesion (LSIL)	Mild dysplasia	CIN 1
High-grade squamous intraepithelial lesion (HSIL)	Moderate dysplasia	CIN 2 III
	Severe dysplasia	CIN 3
Carcinoma in situ	CIS	IV
Squamous cell carcinoma	Squamous cell carcinoma	V

sampling error. Moreover, a diagnosis per se is not made on the basis of cytology (the Pap smear) but rather on histology (cervical biopsy), and treatment planning should be made based on histologic findings.

The Pap smear is a screening test that leads to colposcopy and biopsy as the diagnostic test. Any patient with a high-grade squamous lesion or a glandular lesion of any type (including atypical glandular cells of undetermined significance, AGCUS) on Pap smear should be referred for colposcopy and biopsies. Treatment of preinvasive disease is determined by correlating the Pap smear and biopsy results. Patients who are low risk with an AGCUS or LGSIL smear may have their smear repeated in 3 months or may be referred directly for colposcopy at the discretion of the clinician. If a patient has two or more ASCUS/LGSIL smears, she should be referred for colposcopy. (The ACS definition of high risk includes any woman who began intercourse before the age of 20 or any woman who has had more than two sexual partners during her lifetime.)

Preinvasive disease can often be treated on an outpatient basis with preservation of fertility by use of such techniques as **cryotherapy, carbon dioxide laser,** or **electrosurgical loop excision** (also called LEEP, LOOP, and LLETZ) of the cervical transformation zone. The last involves that portion of the cervix that has undergone squamous metaplasia, which is the area evaluated by colposcopic examination and the site of origin of 80% to 90% of cervical neoplasia. Many clinicians now have the capacity to perform LLETZ in the office using local anesthesia injected directly into the cervical stroma. A LLETZ cone biopsy can also be performed in the office and is appropriate treatment for many preinvasive squamous lesions. Glandular lesions may be managed with LLETZ cone biopsy or cold knife cone biopsy, which must be performed in the operating room.

Clinical Presentation and Diagnostic Evaluation

Early invasive cancer of the cervix can be detected before it is symptomatic by periodic examination and Pap smear. The cervix may appear completely normal to the eye in the presence of a microinvasive cancer.

The most frequent symptom of cervical cancer is abnormal bleeding, either intermenstrual, postmenopausal, or postcoital. Symptoms may also include vaginal discharge, which is often foul smelling. Patients with advanced disease may

Table 31-2
Five-Year Survival Rates by Stage for Gynecologic Cancers

	Stage I	Stage II	Stage III	Stage IV
Cervical cancer	78%	57%	31%	8%
Endometrial cancer	87%	72%	51%	9%
Ovarian cancer	82%	59%	25%	11%
Vulvar cancer	>95%	>90%	50%	10%

Adapted from Pecorelli S et al: *Int J Gynecol Obstet* 65:243, 1999.

complain of back or flank pain (indicating spread of disease to the pelvic sidewall with obstruction of the ureter or involvement of the pelvic nerves).

Physical findings may include a gross tumor on the cervix or palpable groin or supraclavicular nodes. Cervical cancers can be exophytic, with an obvious growth visible on the cervix on speculum examination, or endophytic, where the cervix is expanded by tumor, but no tumor is visible on speculum examination. This last is also called the "barrel" cervix.

Diagnosis is made by biopsy of the cervix. Biopsy of a visible gross lesion can be performed with a long biopsy instrument; biopsy of microinvasive tumors is obtained by excising the entire transformation zone via cone biopsy. The results of cervical cytology may be false negative in 15% to 40% of women with invasive cancer; therefore any clinically suspicious lesion should be biopsied regardless of cytology results.

Histology

Most invasive cancers of the cervix are squamous (80% to 90%), although the proportion of adenocarcinomas has been increasing (10% to 15%). Other rare histologies include clear cell cancer and small cell cancer of the cervix. Small cell cancer of the cervix is a particularly virulent histology, and women often have systemic disease at the time of original presentation.

Staging

Cervical cancer is clinically staged according to the tumor-staging system developed by the International Federation of Gynecology and Obstetrics (FIGO). See Tables 31-2 and 31-3 for survival rates by stage and staging criteria. Patients

Table 31-3
FIGO Staging of Carcinoma of the Cervix Uteri

Preinvasive Carcinoma

Stage 0	Carcinoma *in situ*, intraepithelial carcinoma

Invasive Carcinoma

Stage I		Carcinoma strictly confined to the cervix (extension to the corpus should be disregarded).
	Stage Ia	Preclinical carcinomas of the cervix, that is, those diagnosed only by microscopy.
	Stage Ia1	Minimal microscopically evident stromal invasion.
	Stage Ia2	Lesions detected microscopically that can be measured. The upper limit of the measurement should not show a depth of invasion of more than 5 mm taken from the base of the epithelium, either surface or glandular, from which it originates, and a second dimension, the horizontal spread, must not exceed 7 mm. Larger lesions should be staged as Ib.
	Stage Ib	Lesions of greater dimensions than stage 1a2 whether seen clinically or not. Lesions greater than 4 cm in diameter are classified as stage Ib2.
Stage II		The carcinoma extends beyond the cervix but has not extended on to the wall. The carcinoma involves the vagina, but not the lower third.
	Stage IIa	No obvious parametrial involvement.
	Stage IIb	Obvious parametrial involvement.
Stage III		The carcinoma has extended on to the pelvic wall. On rectal examination, there is no cancer-free space between the tumor and the pelvic wall. The tumor involves the lower third of the vagina. All cases with hydronephrosis or nonfunctioning kidney.
	Stage IIIa	No extension to the pelvic wall.
	Stage IIIb	Extension on to the pelvic wall and/or hydronephrosis or nonfunctioning kidney.
Stage IV		The carcinoma has extended beyond the true pelvis or has clinically involved the mucosa of the bladder or rectum. A bullous edema as such does not permit a case to be allotted to stage IV.
	Stage IVa	Spread of the growth to adjacent organs.
	Stage IVb	Spread to distant organs.

should first undergo a complete history and physical examination. Pelvic examination is performed with the patient under general anesthesia and by multiple examiners including the gynecologic oncologist and radiation oncologist. Cystoscopy and proctoscopy may also be performed to rule out local spread to the bladder or rectum. Other diagnostic tests allowed in the staging system include intravenous pyelogram and barium enema. Many centers in the United States are currently using magnetic resonance imaging to stage patients with cervical cancer, rather than examination under anesthesia (EUA).

✷ MANAGEMENT

Cervical cancer may be treated surgically or with combination radiation and chemotherapy.

Surgery

Surgery is appropriate for early stage cervical cancers, stages I to IIA. In the United States approximately 70% of patients with newly diagnosed cervical cancer have disease limited to the cervix and therefore have primary surgical treatment as an option.

In the United States the Society of Gynecologic Oncologists (SGO) has defined **microinvasive disease (stage Ia1)** as less than 3 mm of invasion into the cervical stroma and less than 7 mm width of tumor without evidence of lymphatic or vascular space invasion. This diagnosis corresponds to FIGO stage Ia, and patients can be treated with simple hysterectomy, performed either abdominally or vaginally, because risk of disease spread to parauterine tissue (parametria) and pelvic lymph nodes is negligible. In the event that a patient wishes to preserve her fertility and is appropriately counseled, cone biopsy alone can be considered treatment for stage Ia1 disease, thus preserving the uterus for future childbearing. These criteria apply only to squamous cancers; management of microinvasive adenocarcinoma is much more controversial.

Stages Ia2, Ib and IIa may be treated either by radical hysterectomy with bilateral pelvic lymph node dissection or by radiation therapy. Recent studies suggest that patients with bulky stage Ib tumors (diameter of tumor greater than 4 cm) and higher stage tumors should ideally be treated with combination cisplatinum and radiation therapy. In very few centers in the United States, patients with stage Ia2 cancer (or very small Ib cancers) may be treated by radical trachelectomy, thus preserving the uterus for childbearing. This operation is *not* considered the standard of care for this disease and should be performed only at qualified institutions, probably with Institutional Review Board approval.

Radical hysterectomy involves resection of the uterus and cervix, their supporting elements (cardinal and uterosacral ligaments), the upper 2 to 3 cm of the vagina, and the regional lymph nodes in the common iliac regions. Radical hysterectomy differs in several ways from the traditional "extrafascial" hysterectomy performed for benign disease. The uterosacral ligaments are ligated closer to the sacrum, the cardinal ligaments are resected to the pelvic floor, and the ureters are unroofed during their course into the trigone of the bladder. These differences result in different postoperative complications. Patients often have neurologic bladder dysfunction and require indwelling catheter for approximately 4 to

6 weeks after radical surgery. Patients often have difficulty with lifelong constipation because the autonomic nerves to the sigmoid colon and rectum travel in the uterosacral ligaments. The surgical approach has the advantage over radiation of preserving ovarian function in the younger patient, and it is associated with less postoperative sexual dysfunction than radiation therapy, which may be associated with vaginal fibrosis and stenosis.

Radiation Therapy

Radiation therapy is the conventional and highly efficacious treatment for patients with more advanced disease or in patients with early-stage disease who are not considered optimal candidates for the surgical approach because of excessive tumor size, coexisting medical illness, or obesity. Radiation therapy in early stage cervical cancer gives equivalent cure rates to surgical therapy. Radiation therapy for cervical cancer involves a combination of external beam therapy delivered to the entire pelvis by linear accelerators, given over the course of 4 to 6 weeks as an outpatient, followed by brachytherapy. Placement of radiation sources directly in the uterus and vagina (brachytherapy) permits safe administration of doses to the cervix and vagina in excess of 10,000 cGy while minimizing the amount of radiation to the more radiation-sensitive adjacent bladder and rectum. As noted previously, it is now considered standard of care to add weekly cisplatin to radiation therapy for improved cure rates.

Chemotherapy

In the past, chemotherapy was reserved for patients with metastatic or recurrent disease. However, low-dose weekly cisplatin in combination with radiation therapy is now the standard of care for many cervical cancer patients. For patients with metastatic or recurrent disease, active agents include cisplatin, bleomycin, vincristine, 5-fluorouracil (5-FU), and ifosfamide. Gemcitabene is a new agent with activity against cervical cancer and is now being tested in clinical trials. Although response rates ranging from 50% to 80% are routinely reported with combination therapy, durations of response are short, with survival benefits of 1 year or less for patients who respond to treatment. Other newer options for patients with advanced or recurrent cervical cancer include clinical trials looking at new chemotherapy combinations and HPV vaccine. Patients with recurrent disease who have already had radiation therapy may also be treated and sometimes cured with a radical surgical procedure called pelvic exenteration. Pelvic exenteration may be total, anterior, or posterior and involves removal of the pelvic organs, including the bladder and the rectum, with creation of ostomies.

Prognosis and Follow-up Monitoring

Stage and tumor size are the most important clinical prognostic factors. Within each stage category, after correction for lesion volume, nodal status takes precedence as the most important prognostic factor. In stages IB and IIA disease, survival of patients without involvement of the pelvic nodes is in excess of 85% at 5 years in contrast to 50% in patients with disease metastatic to these regional nodes. Survival rates for cervical carcinoma in the United States in 1990 to 1992 are as follows: stage I, 78%; stage II, 57%; stage III, 31%; and stage IV, 8%.

Patients usually are seen at 3-month intervals the first year after treatment, every 4 months the second year, at 6-month intervals to the 5-year mark, and thereafter at annual examinations. The most common site of recurrence is the pelvis, although other sites are also at risk, including bone, lung, brain, upper portion of the abdomen, and the paraaortic lymph nodes. Risk of recurrence is directly related to stage of disease.

Follow-up visits should include examinations of the supraclavicular and nodal regions of the groin, abdomen, and pelvis. A Pap smear is obtained at each visit. For all patients, radiologic studies should include a computed tomography (CT) scan of the abdomen and pelvis and a chest radiograph at the 1-year mark. Further radiologic testing may be performed at the discretion of the treating clinician, usually involving annual CT scanning and chest radiographs for an additional 1 to 5 years.

New developments in the field of cervical cancer include the HPV vaccine. HPV vaccine clinical trials are currently open for women with metastatic or recurrent disease. Ideally in the future, HPV vaccines will be developed that will completely eradicate cervical cancer.

ENDOMETRIAL CANCER

EPIDEMIOLOGY AND RISK FACTORS

In the United States, endometrial cancer is the most common malignant disease of the female genital tract. It is estimated that 36,000 new cases of endometrial cancer will be diagnosed in 2000, with 6500 deaths. A woman's lifetime risk of developing endometrial cancer is 2% to 3%.

Endometrial cancer occurs most often in the postmenopause, with an average age of onset of 60 years. Risk factors include obesity, nulliparity, late menopause, diabetes, hypertension, and unopposed estrogen. The pathophysiology of these epidemiologic factors is related to chronic unopposed estrogen stimulation of the endometrium that may result from increased production (estrogen-secreting tumors or obesity via increased peripheral conversion of androstenedione to estrone by the aromatase reaction in adipose cells), decreased degradation (liver disease), or exogenous sources. The risk of developing endometrial cancer triples for those women who are 21 to 50 pounds overweight and is 10 times higher for those who are more than 50 pounds overweight. Conditions associated with anovulation such as polycystic ovarian disease (PCO) also favor an estrogenic environment and so increase risk. In contrast, the oral contraceptive pill decreases risk, particularly in those women who are at increased risk because of anovulation.

Patients on tamoxifen have been shown to be at increased risk for developing endometrial cancer. There is currently no role for routine screening of these patients and yearly vaginal ultrasounds or endometrial biopsies in the asymptomatic woman on tamoxifen should not be performed. Any patient with abnormal uterine bleeding while on tamoxifen needs to undergo histologic evaluation.

Clinical Presentation and Diagnostic Evaluation

The most common presenting symptom of endometrial cancer is postmenopausal bleeding. Other signs and symptoms of advanced disease may include pelvic pressure, abdominal distention, or ascites.

Any abnormal uterine bleeding should be assessed by **endometrial biopsy,** either via the Pipelle sampler or formal dilatation and curettage (D&C). Endometrial biopsy with a Pipelle instrument can be performed easily in the office, in most cases with minimal discomfort to the patient. In the case of cervical stenosis dilatation can also be performed in the office with the aid of a paracervical block if necessary. D&C generally is reserved for patients in whom a biopsy cannot be obtained adequately in the office or in whom symptoms persist after negative biopsy results. Risks associated with either of these techniques include infection, uterine perforation, and patient discomfort.

Pelvic ultrasound should not be substituted for histologic sampling in the presence of symptoms. Although an endometrial stripe of less than 5 mm has been shown statistically to be unlikely to have carcinoma, if the patient is symptomatic most gynecologic oncologists recommend that a histologic diagnosis should still be made. In contrast, an endometrial stripe greater than 5 mm in a postmenopausal patient does not necessarily mean that patient has cancer of the endometrium. Other histologic abnormalities can account for a thickened stripe, including endometrial polyps, which most often are benign, or endometrial hyperplasia.

Sonohistography is a new technique that can help to diagnose endometrial abnormalities. In this technique a tiny catheter is used to inject saline into the endometrial cavity, thereby aiding the ultrasonographer to view endometrial anatomy. This technique is particularly useful in patients on tamoxifen. In these patients the endometrial stripe may look falsely thick on routine ultrasound because of subendometrial cystic change in the myometrium. Sonohistography can resolve this diagnostic problem via better delineation of the endometrial stripe and may therefore allow a patient to forego endometrial sampling.

Histology

A total of 80% of endometrial cancers are endometrioid adenocarcinomas. These tumors are graded 1, 2, and 3, with grade 1 tumors having the best prognosis. Rare histologies include papillary serous adenocarcinoma of the endometrium and clear cell carcinoma. Both of these histologies carry poor prognosis and patients are more likely to present with advanced disease.

Staging

Endometrial cancer is a surgically staged disease. See Table 31-4 for FIGO staging criteria. Stage I disease is confined to uterine corpus. In the United States, more than 80% of endometrial cancers are diagnosed as stage I. In stage II disease, there is extension to the cervix. Stage III incorporates disease that has spread to the tubes and ovaries, to the vagina, or to the retroperitoneal lymph nodes. Positive peritoneal cytology is also included with stage III. Stage IV indicates spread to the bladder or rectum, or distant disease (essentially, out of the pelvis).

To perform surgical staging, exploratory laparotomy is undertaken. Washings of the pelvis are sent and full exploration of the peritoneal cavity is performed. An extrafascial (not radical) hysterectomy and bilateral salpingo-oophorectomy (BSO) is performed. Pelvic and para-aortic lymph node sampling is performed if appropriate. If advanced disease is encountered, all gross disease should be removed if pos-

Table 31-4
1988 FIGO Surgical Staging for Endometrial Carcinoma

Stage Ia	Tumor limited to endometrium
Stage Ib	Invasion to less than half the myometrium
Stage Ic	Invasion to more than half the myometrium
Stage IIa	Endocervical glandular involvement only
Stage IIb	Cervical stromal invasion
Stage IIIa	Tumor invades serosa and/or adnexa, and/or positive peritoneal cytology
Stage IIIb	Vaginal metastases
Stage IIIc	Metastases to pelvic and/or para-aortic lymph nodes
Stage IVa	Tumor invasion of bladder and/or bowel mucosa
Stage IVb	Distant metastases including intra-abdominal and/or inguinal lymph nodes

sible. Endometrial cancer is then staged based on pathologic evaluation of the specimens sent from the operating room. Rarely a patient will not be a candidate for this operation, usually for medical reasons, and so will be staged clinically.

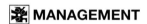 **MANAGEMENT**

In some cases, **stage I disease** will be completely treated by surgery alone. The decision to administer postoperative radiation therapy is based on tumor grade and depth of myometrial invasion. Patients with low-grade disease or minimal myometrium invasion, or both, are at low risk for recurrence and require no adjuvant therapy. Patients with higher grade disease or more extensive involvement of the myometrium receive whole-pelvis radiation therapy, which has been shown to decrease the risk of pelvic recurrence but has not demonstrated a clear survival advantage. Patients who fall into an intermediate risk category may receive postoperative vaginal radium or cesium therapy, which minimizes dose to the bladder and rectum, thus virtually eliminating side effects and, at the same time, minimizing the risk of vaginal apex recurrence.

Patients with **stage II disease** (spread to the cervix) are considered to be at high risk (30% to 40%) for pelvic nodal involvement and pelvic recurrence. In general these patients are treated with postoperative pelvic radiation therapy. Alternatively, they can be primarily treated with radical hysterectomy, BSO, and retroperitoneal node dissection without adjuvant radiation therapy, assuming involvement of the cervix can be diagnosed preoperatively.

Patients with **stage III or IV disease** are generally treated with postoperative radiation therapy tailored to the sites of known disease and areas believed to be at high risk for recurrence. Patients with pelvic or para-aortic nodal spread are treated with pelvic or extended field radiation therapy, respectively. Patients with evidence of peritoneal involvement may be considered candidates for whole abdominal radiation therapy, combination chemotherapy and radiation, or chemotherapy alone.

Patients with advanced disease or with disease that cannot be resected or radiated require systemic therapy.

Progestational agents, which reverse estrogen's trophic effects on the endometrium, have been used with response rates ranging from 10% to 30%. Higher response rates have been associated with increased differentiation and the presence of progesterone receptors. Poorly differentiated tumors in general do not respond to hormonal manipulation and require cytotoxic chemotherapy. Active agents include cisplatin, doxorubicin (Adriamycin), cyclophosphamide, paclitaxel (Taxol), and 5-FU. Reported response rates for combined therapy range from 25% to 60%, with only modest impact on survival because of relatively short durations of response.

Prognosis and Follow-up Monitoring

The 5-year survival rates that have been reported based on the FIGO surgical staging system of 1988 are 87% for stage I, 72% for stage II, 51% for stage III, and 9% for stage IV. In patients with endometrioid histology, between 80% and 90% have stage I disease. Thus the overall survival for endometrial cancer is excellent. Early diagnosis is likely secondary to early symptoms of this disease.

Posttreatment follow-up monitoring of patients depends on the extent of disease noted initially. In general, all patients are seen at 3- to 4-month intervals the first year. Patients at low risk (stage I, well- or moderately well-differentiated tumors, minimal invasion) may then be seen at 3- to 6-month intervals until the 5-year mark is reached and annually thereafter. Patients at higher risk (deep invasion, poorly differentiated, advanced-stage disease) usually are seen at 3- to 4-month intervals for several years, then at 6-month intervals to the 5-year mark. In general, patients fitting into this last category are seen by the operating clinician or primary care provider and by a radiation oncologist.

Follow-up visits should include examinations of the supraclavicular and groin node regions, the abdomen, and pelvis. The utility of Pap smear for diagnosing early vaginal recurrence has not been studied. Major sites of recurrence include the pelvis, bone, brain, upper portion of the abdomen, and the lung, with the last representing the most common extrapelvic site. Again, radiologic testing should be based on risk. The patient at high risk, as already defined, should undergo CT scanning and chest radiography annually to the 5-year mark. Patients at low risk for recurrence may have scans less frequently at the discretion of the treating physicians.

CA-125 has been used as a serum marker in women with advanced endometrial disease to follow progress in therapy and to diagnose early recurrence. It is particularly useful in women with the unusual papillary serous subtype.

Hormone Replacement Therapy After Treatment for Endometrial Cancer

There are currently no prospective data with regard to the safety of hormone replacement therapy (HRT) in patients treated for endometrial cancer. Several retrospective reviews suggest that women with good prognosis disease may benefit from HRT if appropriately counseled. The Gynecologic Oncology Group is currently conducting a national randomized prospective trial for women with early stage endometrial cancer comparing estrogen replacement with placebo. Patients with endometrial cancer who wish to use HRT should be encouraged to participate in this trial.

OVARIAN CANCER

▦ EPIDEMIOLOGY AND RISK FACTORS

Cancer of the ovary is the second most common gynecologic malignant disease after cancer of the endometrium; however, it accounts for more deaths than all other gynecologic cancers combined. Overall, 1 in 70 women in the United States will develop ovarian cancer during their lifetime; 23,100 new cases were expected in 2000 and 14,000 deaths. The incidence of ovarian cancer increases with age, with a peak incidence at age 59 years. This disease is more commonly seen in the industrialized and developed countries, and it is more common in Caucasian than in African-American women.

The molecular etiology of ovarian cancer is unknown; however, there are some well-defined epidemiologic risk factors. These include nulliparity, infertility, early age of menarche with late age of menopause (all associated with the "incessant ovulation" theory), the use of talcum powder on the perineum, and possibly a diet high in animal fat. Multiparity and the use of oral contraceptives appear to have a protective effect. A study from the Centers for Disease Control concluded that the use of the pill may decrease the lifetime risk of ovarian cancer by as much as 50% and that this effect increases with duration of use and persists for several years after discontinuance.

Women who are at high risk of ovarian cancer by family history can be treated with oral contraceptive pills to decrease risk.

Most cases of ovarian cancer are not familial but sporadic; in fact, it is estimated that only between 1% and 5% of patients with ovarian cancer will be part of a hereditary syndrome. However, family history plays an important role in identifying those patients who may be at increased risk on a genetic basis. Patients with one second-degree or one first-degree relative are believed to be at approximately two or four times the risk, respectively, of patients without a family history. Women with multiple affected relatives are at substantially greater risk, as high as 50%, of developing ovarian cancer in their lifetime, with a tendency for the disease to occur at a much earlier age. As a result of this increased risk, prophylactic oophorectomy has been advocated in patients with more than one first-degree relative affected. This usually is performed at completion of childbearing—optimally by age 35 years given the nature of familial ovarian cancer to occur at an early age. With the discovery of the genes BRCA1 and BRCA2, patients with significant family histories should be encouraged to undergo genetic counseling, followed by genetic testing only if desired and appropriate.

Clinical Presentation and Diagnostic Evaluation

In 80% of cases, patients with ovarian cancer present with advanced disease. This is because, unlike endometrial cancer, symptoms are vague, nonspecific, and often not present until disease is advanced. Typically the patient first consults a health care provider (frequently an internist or a family practitioner) complaining of vague abdominal pain or pressure, early satiety, anorexia, or dyspepsia, usually of about 4 to 6 weeks' duration. Nausea, vomiting, constipation, or increasing abdominal girth also may be described. With this constellation of findings the diagnosis of ovarian cancer must be considered, as well as primary gastrointestinal disease. Often the patient with ovarian cancer will try multiple remedies for her gastrointestinal complaints with no relief. *It is the patient with persistent symptoms even after what would normally be considered appropriate therapies for whom the diagnosis of ovarian cancer should be considered.* Pelvic examination should be part of the primary evaluation of these women; it is inexpensive and often reveals a pelvic mass. Rectovaginal examination may be necessary to appreciate cul-de-sac involvement or a cul-de-sac mass. It is not unusual for a patient to have had a normal pelvic examination within 12 months and be asymptomatic until 2 to 3 weeks before presentation, with rapidly progressing symptoms.

Preoperative evaluation should include a full history and pelvic examination, including stool guaiac examination. Preoperative studies should include a baseline CA-125 in addition to usual preoperative testing. CA-125 is used primarily to follow response to chemotherapy. CT scan of the abdomen and pelvis may be useful to identify ascites, omental mass, retroperitoneal adenopathy, or liver metastases but is not necessary preoperatively. Barium studies of the upper or lower gastrointestinal tracts, or both, may be performed for evaluation of severe symptoms arising from these areas. Generally they are not required inasmuch as formal bowel preparation is a procedural element in virtually all patients with a tentative diagnosis of ovarian cancer, thereby permitting resection of the gastrointestinal tract if so required at exploration.

Histology

Epithelial ovarian cancers are classified as borderline or frankly malignant. In contrast to the malignant epithelial tumors, **borderline tumors** (also called low malignant potential tumors), although capable of metastases, do not behave in a fulminant manner. Surgical resection is all that is required in treatment and chemotherapy is not necessary.

Epithelial ovarian tumors account for 70% of all ovarian tumors and 90% of the cancers; they arise from the ovarian capsular epithelium, which is derived from the coelomic epithelium. Epithelial ovarian cancers mimic the normal cells of the female reproductive tract. Histologic subtypes are serous papillary, mucinous, endometrioid, clear cell, transitional, or undifferentiated.

The ovary is also capable of producing **germ cell** and **stromal cell tumors.** These tumors are unusual and often do not present as advanced disease as do epithelial tumors. Malignant germ cell tumors occur most commonly in girls and young women, and many produce specific biologic markers including hCG and AFP. Stromal tumors account for 7% of ovarian malignancies, most are of low malignant potential, and in general they have a good prognosis.

Staging

Ovarian cancer is a surgically staged disease. See Table 31-5 for FIGO stages. Simply put, stages I and II are confined to the pelvis, with stage I disease confined to the ovaries and stage II disease outside of the ovary but still confined to the pelvis. Approximately 75% to 85% of patients have stage III or IV disease. In stage III disease, the cancer has spread outside of the pelvis to involve the peritoneal surfaces of the abdomen, the omentum, or the retroperitoneal lymph nodes. Stage IV disease is outside of the peritoneal cavity or parenchymal liver metastases.

✖ MANAGEMENT

Primary management of ovarian cancer is via surgical cytoreduction, also called debulking. Patients undergo preoperative mechanical and antibiotic bowel preparation the day before surgery, usually as an outpatient. Exploration of the

---

Table 31-5
FIGO Staging for Primary Carcinoma of the Ovary

Stage I	Growth limited to the ovaries.	
	Stage Ia	Growth limited to one ovary; no ascites containing malignant cells. No tumor on the external surface; capsule intact.
	Stage Ib	Growth limited to both ovaries; no ascites containing malignant cells. No tumor on the external surfaces; capsules intact.
	Stage Ic	Tumor either stage 1a or 1b but with tumor on the surface of one or both ovaries; or with capsule ruptured; or with ascites present containing malignant cells or with positive peritoneal washings.
Stage II	Growth involving one or both ovaries with pelvic extension.	
	Stage IIa	Extension and/or metastases to the uterus and/or tubes.
	Stage IIb	Extension to other pelvic tissues.
	Stage IIc	Tumor either stage IIa or IIb but with tumor on the surface of one or both ovaries; or with capsules(s) ruptured; or with ascites present containing malignant cells or with positive peritoneal washings.
Stage III	Tumor involving one or both ovaries with peritoneal implants outside the pelvis and/or positive retroperitoneal or inguinal nodes. Superficial liver metastasis equals stage III. Tumor is limited to the true pelvis, but with histologically proven malignant extension to small bowel or omentum.	
	Stage IIIa	Tumor grossly limited to the true pelvis with negative nodes but with histolologically confirmed microscopic seeding of abdominal peritoneal surfaces.
	Stage IIIb	Tumor of one or both ovaries with histologically confirmed implants of abdominal peritoneal surfaces, none exceeding 2 cm in diameter. Nodes negative.
	Stage IIIc	Abdominal implants > 2 cm in diameter and/or positive retroperitoneal or inguinal nodes.
Stage IV	Growth involving one or both ovaries with distant metastasis. If pleural effusion is present, there must be positive cytologic test results to allot a case to stage IV. Parenchymal liver metastasis equals stage IV.	

abdomen and pelvis is performed through a vertical incision. Pelvic washings are sent and hysterectomy and BSO are performed. Disease must be "debulked" to less than 2 cm for optimal outcome; this debulking may include bowel resection. The omentum is removed. If the disease is grossly confined to the ovary, a full staging procedure is performed, including multiple peritoneal biopsies and retroperitoneal node dissection.

After surgery, patients with ovarian cancer that is stage IC or greater should be treated with chemotherapy. The combination of carboplatin and paclitaxel (Taxol) administered for six cycles currently is the standard regimen in most centers. In most cases this chemotherapy can be given in the outpatient setting without need for hospitalization.

With cytoreductive surgery and platinum-based chemotherapy, 70% to 80% of patients will achieve clinical remission. Unfortunately, most of these patients will eventually present with recurrent disease. Only 20% of patients with optimally cytoreduced disease achieve long-term survival (more than 5 years). Patients who have stage IV disease or bulky residual disease after primary cytoreduction have a poor prognosis and few are cured. Chemotherapy and/or surgery may be used for patients with recurrent disease, but is often unsuccessful in achieving cure.

Because primary therapy is often unsuccessful, patients with ovarian cancer, either primary or recurrent, should consider being treated at tertiary centers where they may participate in clinical trials. These clinical trials include new chemotherapy combinations, as well as novel treatments such as genetic therapy, monoclonal antibody conjugated intraperitoneal therapy, and vaccine trials.

Prognosis and Follow-Up Monitoring

The prognosis for stages III and IV ovarian cancer is similar to that of the same stages of endometrial cancer. The difference in mortality rates for the two disease arises in the proportion of cases diagnosed in late stages; whereas most endometrial cancers are diagnosed at stage I, the majority of ovarian cancers are diagnosed as stage III and IV. Survival rates have improved slightly over the last 5 years, likely secondary to the use of the platinum-based chemotherapy. Five-year survival for stages I, II, III, and IV in 1990 to 1992 were 82%, 59%, 25%, and 11%, respectively.

Patients with ovarian cancer are considered at high risk for recurrence and generally are monitored closely after completion of therapy. Office visits at 2- to 3-month intervals for 2 years is fairly standard, with CA-125 testing performed at least this frequently. Thereafter office visits may be scheduled less frequently at 3- to 6-month intervals to the 5-year mark. Less frequent visits may be recommended for the patient at low risk (stage I) at the discretion of the treating clinician. The abdominal cavity remains the site at greatest risk for the development of recurrent disease. CT scanning at 6-month intervals for 2 to 3 years is commonly used in the management of these women. Annual scans to the 5-year mark may be considered in the patient at high risk.

Hormone Replacement Therapy After Ovarian Cancer

There have been no prospective trials evaluating HRT in patients with ovarian cancer. Retrospective studies suggest that HRT in most histologic subtypes does not increase risk of recurrence (endometrioid histologies being the exception).

VULVAR CANCER

▦ EPIDEMIOLOGY AND RISK FACTORS

Cancer of the vulva is unusual, accounting for 3% to 5% of gynecologic malignancies. Although vulvar cancer arises on a visible portion of the body, there is often up to a 12-month delay between symptoms and diagnosis. In the year 2000 in the United States, there were an estimated 3400 new cases of vulvar cancer resulting in 800 deaths.

The incidence of vulvar cancer increases with age, with a peak occurring at age 70 to 79. Preinvasive disease is seen predominantly in younger women, whereas invasive carcinoma is predominantly a disease of the postmenopausal woman. Approximately 10% of patients with vulvar neoplasia, either invasive or in situ disease, have a synchronous primary neoplasm elsewhere, usually involving the lower genital tract, specifically the cervix. Patients with immunosuppression, diabetes, hypertension, and chronic vulvar dystrophies appear to be at increased risk for developing vulvar cancer. In the young woman with preinvasive disease, smoking is a risk factor both for development of preinvasive disease and for recurrence after local therapy.

Treatment of Preinvasive Disease

Most patients with either preinvasive or invasive disease are symptomatic. Symptoms include vulvar itching and discomfort.

Preinvasive disease of the vulva appears in many forms. Any suspicious lesion of the vulva should be biopsied promptly to make a diagnosis. Lesions are often multifocal but can be unifocal. Lesions may be raised or flat and may be pink, white, brown, or black. What appears to be an obvious condylomata to the eye may be VIN III on biopsy. Office biopsy is easily performed using local infiltration of lidocaine and a punch biopsy instrument. This procedure can be tolerated well in the office in most cases.

The pathophysiologic basis of vulvar dysplasia is not clear, but may be related to HPV infection (similar to the cervical counterpart). Although invasive vulvar carcinoma is primarily a disease of older patients, VIN is being diagnosed more frequently in younger age groups. This increased frequency appears to coincide with an increase in the frequency of such genital infections as HPV and herpes simplex virus type 2. Younger patients with vulvar neoplasia frequently have lesions that exhibit the histologic changes associated with HPV and have a history of, or current infection with, condyloma, whereas patients more than 50 years old rarely demonstrate these associations. Instead, VIN can occur in older patients with lichen sclerosus, although lichen sclerosus itself is not considered to be a premalignant lesion. In a patient being treated chronically for lichen sclerosus, any new change in symptoms or in the appearance of the lesion should be biopsied.

Preinvasive disease can be treated via a variety of modalities. Surgical modalities include wide local excision (in the office or in the operating room) and laser ablation. The benefit of local excision is the procurement of a specimen for histology. The benefit of laser ablation is often an improved cosmetic result, with excellent healing. If laser ablation is considered, multiple biopsies should be performed preoperatively to rule out invasive disease. Recurrent vulvar dysplasia can be treated medically with 5-FU cream. This cream can be irritating to the vulva and vagina and should be used with caution by experienced clinicians.

Patients with vulvar dysplasia may also have preinvasive disease elsewhere in the genital tract. Careful examination of the vagina and cervix with Pap smear of the cervix should therefore be performed in these patients.

Clinical Presentation and Diagnostic Evaluation

Most women with vulvar cancer present with pruritis and a recognizable lesion. Careful examination of the vulva with the naked eye is often sufficient to identify carcinoma, which may appear as a raised lesion, a flat plaque, or an ulcer. Biopsy is necessary for diagnosis. Many elderly women are embarrassed about vulvar symptoms and reluctant to mention them to their doctor, believing them to be related to poor hygiene. These patients may present with advanced disease and symptoms of local pain, bleeding, and drainage. Women with advanced disease may also be symptomatic from enlarged inguinal nodes.

Histology

Most vulvar cancers are squamous. Approximately 60% of squamous cancers have associated VIN, and lichen sclerosus can be found in association with cancer in 15% to 40% of cases. The second most frequent primary vulvar cancer is melanoma, accounting for 10% of vulvar cancers.

Other unusual histologies include basal cell carcinoma, adenocarcinomas of the Bartholin's gland, sarcoma, and Paget's disease. Paget's disease of the vulva is not carcinoma per se, but is associated with an underlying vulvar carcinoma in 10% to 15% of cases. Paget's disease presents as a red, eczematous, weepy lesion on the vulva that is often extensive. Extensive surgical removal is usually necessary.

Staging

Vulvar cancer is a surgically staged disease. Important prognostic factors include tumor size and presence of lymph node metastases. See Table 31-6 for FIGO staging of vulvar cancer.

✳ MANAGEMENT

Stages I to III vulvar cancer are usually treated surgically. The appropriate surgical treatment for lesions with greater than 1 mm invasion is radical vulvectomy with inguinal node dissection. Unilateral lesions can be treated with radical hemivulvectomy and ipsilateral node dissection. Midline lesions have the propensity to metastasize to either groin; therefore bilateral node dissection needs to be performed.

The morbidity from radical surgery can be significant, particularly in the elderly woman with comorbid medical problems. Common problems for these patients in the immediately postoperative period include wound breakdown, groin seroma or infection, and pulmonary embolus. Late complications include lower extremity lymphedema. Complications are decreased by tailoring the surgical procedure to the individual lesion, performing unilateral groin node dissections when appropriate and dissecting superficial nodes only if appropriate.

Subsequent therapy is based on surgical stage. The most important prognostic factor for vulvar cancer is groin node status. If there are positive groin nodes the patient should be treated with adjuvant radiation.

Table 31-6
FIGO Staging of Vulvar Cancer

FIGO	StageTNM	Clinical Findings
Stage 0		Carcinoma in situ, e.g., VIN 3, noninvasive Paget's disease
Stage 1	$T_1N_0M_0$ $T_1N_1M_0$	Tumor confined to the vulva, 2 cm or less in largest diameter, and no suspicious groin nodes
Stage II	$T_2N_0M_0$ $T_2N_1M_0$	Tumor confined to the vulva more than 2 cm in diameter, and no suspicious groin nodes
Stage III	$T_3N_0M_0$ $T_3N_1M_0$ $T_3N_2M_0$ $T_1N_2M_0$ $T_2N_2M_0$	Tumor of any size: (1) adjacent spread to the urethra and/or the vagina, the perineum, and/or (2) clinically suspicious lymph nodes in either groin
Stage IV	$T_xN_3M_0$ $T_4N_0M_0$ $T_4N_1M_0$ $T_4N_2M_0$ $T_xN_xM_{1a}$ $T_xN_xM_{1b}$	Tumor of any size: (1) infiltrating the bladder mucosa, or the rectal mucosa, or both, including the upper part of the urethral mucosa, and/or (2) fixed to the bone and/or (3) other distant metastases

Patients with more advanced disease (exceptionally large tumors or involvement of adjacent organs) not amenable to surgical excision—or in cases in which resection would require rectal or bladder resection with diversion—may undergo a combined modality approach with preoperative radiotherapy and/or chemotherapy to achieve tumor shrinkage and permit more conservative resection.

The prognosis of patients with early diagnosis and tailored therapy is excellent, with survival rates in excess of 80% or 90% in stage I and II disease, respectively. Prognosis clearly is related to lesion size and the status of the regional lymph nodes. The cure rate in early-stage disease in which nodes are not affected exceeds 95% in some series. Survival in stage III disease may fall to 50% and to 10% with stage IV disease.

Most patients with vulvar cancer are diagnosed with early-stage disease, obviating the need for extensive radiologic testing in the follow-up period. Most recurrences are noted on the vulva and in the inguinal regions. Thus these areas are carefully examined at all visits, which are recommended at 3-month intervals the first year and then at 3- to 6-month intervals to 5 years; the frequency is based on the extent of the initial lesion. Patients are carefully instructed to observe the vulva monthly, using palpation and hand mirrors, and to report any changes such as discolorations and lumps. They also are instructed to report any new or recurrent symptoms such as itching, burning, bleeding, or discharge. Radiologic screening, chest radiograph, and CT scan of the abdomen and pelvis usually are reserved for patients at high risk for recurrence (groin node involvement or extensive central disease).

BIBLIOGRAPHY

Bast RC Jr et al: CA 125: the past and the future, *Int J Biol Markers* 13:179, 1998.

Bauer HM et al: Genital human papilloma virus infection in female university students as determined by PCR-based method, *JAMA* 265:472, 1991.

Berchuk A, Schildkraut JM, Marks JR, Futreal PA: Managing hereditary ovarian cancer risk, *Cancer* 86:1697, 1999.

The Bethesda system for reporting cervical/vaginal cytologic diagnoses, *JAMA* 267:1892, 1992.

Centers for Disease Control and Steroid Hormone Study: Oral contraceptives and the risk of ovarian cancer, *JAMA* 249:1596, 1983.

Chu CS et al: Primary peritoneal carcinoma: a review of the literature, *Obstet Gynecol Surv* 54:323, 1999.

Creasman WT et al: Estrogen replacement therapy in the patient treated for endometrial cancer, *Obstet Gynecol* 67:326, 1986.

Eelles RA et al: Hormone replacement therapy and survival after surgery for ovarian cancer, *Br Med J* 302:259, 1991.

Fisher B et al: Endometrial cancer in tamoxifen-treated breast cancer patients: findings from the National Surgical Adjuvant Breast and Bowel Project (NSABP) B-14, *J Natl Cancer Inst* 86:527, 1994.

Goldstein SR, Nachtigall M, Snyder JR, Nachtigall L: Endometrial assessment by vaginal ultrasonography before endometrial sampling in patients with postmenopausal bleeding, *Am J Obstet Gynecol* 163:119, 1990.

Greenlee RT, Murray T, Bolden S, Wingo PA: Cancer statistics, 2000, *CA Cancer J Clin* 50:7, 2000.

Keys HM et al: Cisplatin, radiation and adjuvant hysterectomy compared radiation and adjuvant hysterectomy for bulky stage IB cervical carcinoma, *N Engl J Med* 40:1154, 1999.

Landoni F et al: Randomised study of radical surgery versus radiotherapy for stage Ib-Iia cervical cancer, *Lancet* 350:535, 1997.

Lee RB, Burke TW, Park RC: Estrogen replacement therapy following treatment for stage I endometrial carcinoma, *Gynecol Oncol* 36:189, 1990.

McGuire WP et al: Comparison of combination therapy with paclitaxel and cisplatin versus cyclophosphamide and cisplatin in patients with suboptimal stage III and stage IV ovarian cancer: a Gynecologic Oncology Group study, *Semin Oncol* 24:S2, 1997.

McGuire WP, Ozols RF: Chemotherapy of advanced ovarian cancer, *Semin Oncol* 25:340, 1998.

Morris M et al: Pelvic radiation with concurrent chemotherapy compared with pelvic and para-aortic radiation for high-risk cervical cancer, *N Engl J Med* 340:1137, 1999.

Pearce KF, Haeffner HK, Sarwar SF, Nolan TE: Cytopathological findings on vaginal Papanicolaou smears after hysterectomy for benign gynecologic disease, *N Engl J Med* 335:1559, 1996.

Pecorelli S, Benedet JL, Creasman WT, Shepherd JH: FIGO staging of gynecologic cancer. 1994–1997 FIGO Committee on Gynecologic Oncology. International Federation of Gynecology and Obstetrics, *Int J Gynecol Obstet* 65:243, 1999.

Rose PG et al: Concurrent cisplatin-based radiotherapy and chemotherapy for locally advanced cervical cancer, *N Engl J Med* 340:1144, 1999.

Smith-Bindman R et al: Endovaginal ultrasound to exclude endometrial cancer and other endometrial abnormalities, *JAMA* 280:1510,1998.

Suh-Burgmann EJ, Goodman A: Surveillance for endometrial cancer in women receiving tamoxifen, *Ann Intern Med* 131:127, 1999.

CHAPTER 32

Approach to the Woman with Rheumatic Disease

Margaret Seton

Rheumatic diseases are common. Estimates of prevalence in the United States based on radiographic evidence, self-report of illness, or clinical documentation of disease suggest an overall prevalence of rheumatic disease of 15% in the general population. Pain, impairment of function, and disability all increase with age. Impaired mobility is compounded in many postmenopausal women by obesity, physical deconditioning resulting from lack of exercise, and cardiovascular disease.

This chapter describes the general approach to the woman with rheumatic disease or musculoskeletal complaints in the primary care setting. The reader is referred to Chapters 33 through 39 for detailed information on management of specific conditions.

▦ EPIDEMIOLOGY

Projections are that by the year 2020, as our population ages, almost 60 million Americans (18%) will have limitation in their activity owing to arthritis. This approximation does not encompass the numbers of women injured by violence or those with impairment resulting from osteoporotic fractures. These women, too, present with chronic musculoskeletal complaints and loss of independence. Table 32-1 summarizes the frequency of some of these rheumatic diseases in the United States, with comments about ascertainment or disease patterns.

Environmental factors, race, gender, and ethnicity undoubtedly play a role in disease expression; these along with psychosocial status also affect outcome. The increased prevalence of systemic lupus erythematosus (SLE) in African-American women in the United States, as opposed to native Africans, has focused on the environment in which genes are expressed—the microscopic environment at the cellular level of gene transcription and the macroscopic environment of the neighborhoods that support these lives. Classically, studies in women with SLE have highlighted poor outcomes in women of color, correlating these with issues of race and socioeconomic status. On closer inspection, however, outcomes may have as much to do with activity of disease at presentation as level of education, access to health care and compliance with medical regimens, genetics, and neighborhoods. To date, no consensus has been reached on these issues.

Understanding the interplay of psychosocial factors with biologic and ethnic variations in the clinical expression of rheumatic disease is equally important in disorders marked by chronic pain. Osteoarthritis, fibromyalgia, tendonitis, low back pain, and the fractures of osteoporosis represent some of these disorders that present with sustained pain, early disability, and loss of independence. What contributes to the loss of functional status associated with these chronic pain syndromes? Jordan, in her review on the effect of race and ethnicity on outcomes in arthritis, emphasized how disruptive chronic pain and dysfunction can be within a family. Arthritis may affect a woman's perceived sexuality and her role in the family, school, or church; this may lead to depression, loss of competence in the workplace, and loss of self-esteem. Further, Jordan writes that "pain intensity, higher rates of chronic pain, and lower pain threshold have been reported in areas with highly traditional ethnic identification, high migration rates, and high proportions of individuals of foreign background." To provide effective care for all populations of women with rheumatic disease, the norms with which one measures the cause and experience of illness will have to be reevaluated to enable these women to live healthy, fruitful lives.

▦ APPROACH TO THE WOMAN WITH MUSCULOSKELETAL COMPLAINTS

History and Physical Examination

Despite the widespread prevalence of arthritis, the etiology of most rheumatic maladies is unknown. For this reason, rheumatic illness is most often characterized by clinical phenotype, and a detailed history and physical examination is the most useful approach to a woman with musculoskeletal complaints. To address functional status, the history should also include living conditions, number of children, issues of work, support, and domestic violence. The manifestations in any given woman at presentation and the spectrum of disease over time are variable, colored by these psychosocial issues and the fluctuation in disease activity.

A practical way to assess a patient with rheumatic disease is to attend to the **age** of the woman. For example, sexually transmitted arthritides are more common in young women of reproductive age, SLE and the arthralgias of hypothyroidism

Table 32-1
Prevalence and Gender Differences in Rheumatic Disorders in the United States

Rheumatic Condition	Female/Male Ratio	Prevalence Estimates	Comments
Rheumatoid arthritis	2-3:1	0.5-1%	The prevalence increases with age Some recent reports suggest a decreasing incidence of RA An excess mortality from all causes seen in these women
Systemic lupus erythematosus	5-9:1	40-50 per 100,000 persons	Incidence/outcomes are modified by race, gender, ethnicity, environment and socioeconomic status Prevalence estimates include definite plus suspected cases
Osteoarthritis (OA)	With aging, increase in female/male ratio of those with symptoms	12.1% Americans > 25, with clinical signs and symptoms	Prevalence estimates vary on whether one is looking at the knee vs. hip vs. hands No standard definition of OA; some studies use histology, others radiographic evidence, others presence of symptoms Virtually everyone has changes of osteoarthritis with aging
Scleroderma	7-12:1	Between 4 and 253 persons per million	Rare disease, occurring in reproductive years, peaking age 40-50 years
Gout	1:2-7	8.4 per 1000 persons	Prevalence affected by race and menopause in women Prevalence reflects self-reported incidence in United States Hyperuricemia is more common occurrence than gout
Sjögren's	Studied in women	1 in 1250 women	Estimates vary depending on self-report of symptoms vs. serologic or tissue diagnosis Recent estimates in UK suggest 3%-4% general population Association with rheumatic disease, HIV and hepatitis C
Polymyalgia rheumatica	2:1	700 per 100,000 persons over age 50	Occurs most frequently after age 50, increasing in prevalence with age, peaking in women age 70-79 Association with giant cell arteritis
Fibromyalgia	9:1	Overall estimates 2%, increasing with age	Most commonly reported by women, with prevalence affected by race and socioeconomic factors Increased frequency in men reported after the Gulf War Historically, epidemics of regional pain syndromes reported in workplace; stress, domestic violence and depression may play role in reported symptoms
Spondyloarthropathy	1:2 Often more symptomatic in men	2.1 per 1000 persons	Associated with HLA-B27 Spectrum of disease including psoriatic arthritis, inflammatory bowel disease, ankylosing spondylitis and Reiter's Historically, gastrointestinal and genitourinary tract infections may be associated with onset of disease

HIV, Human immunodeficiency virus.

or depression may be associated with the early postpartum period, and polymyalgia rheumatica is more common in the elderly woman.

The second practical question to ask is **how many joints are involved?** If one, was there antecedent trauma? Or is there a risk factor for infection, such as intravenous drug use, a prosthetic joint, or underlying rheumatoid arthritis? If many joints are involved, is there a pattern? Symmetric, small joints of the hands and feet are often seen in rheumatoid arthritis. Osteoarthritis may be seen in the hands (Heberden's nodes), knees, or hips of middle-aged, often obese women. Reiter's disease may affect one knee and/or the Achilles tendon. Ankylosing spondylitis may spare peripheral joints and present with low back pain, which is protracted on rising and eased with activity. These simple observations in the context of a competent medical history help to determine whether the woman is likely to be suffering from an inflammatory or noninflammatory condition. Further elucidation of the patterns of rheumatic disease are outlined in more detail in subsequent chapters.

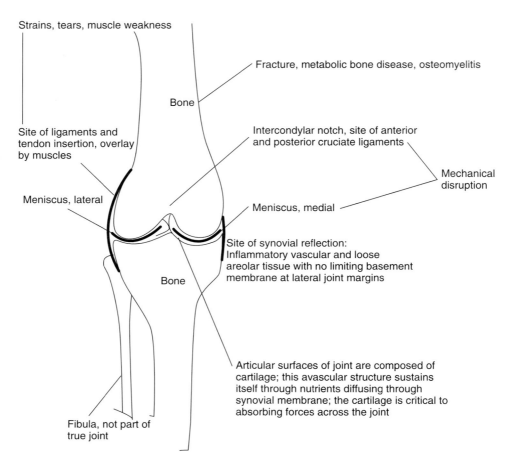

Strains, tears, muscle weakness

Fracture, metabolic bone disease, osteomyelitis

Bone

Site of ligaments and tendon insertion, overlay by muscles

Intercondylar notch, site of anterior and posterior cruciate ligaments

Mechanical disruption

Meniscus, lateral

Meniscus, medial

Site of synovial reflection: Inflammatory vascular and loose areolar tissue with no limiting basement membrane at lateral joint margins

Bone

Articular surfaces of joint are composed of cartilage; this avascular structure sustains itself through nutrients diffusing through synovial membrane; the cartilage is critical to absorbing forces across the joint

Fibula, not part of true joint

R Knee, sketch of femur & tibia

FIG. 32-1 Anatomy of the knee joint and correlation with disease processes.

It is important to remember that inflammation has anatomic correlates that should be sought based on an understanding of the disease process and the anatomy of the joint (Fig. 32-1). Clues that suggest an inflammatory origin are the systemic nature of the illness (fever, weight loss, malaise, loss of function across joint(s), visual disturbance, bloody diarrhea) in the context of true findings on physical examination (synovitis, hair loss, rashes/skin lesions, thickened skin, ulcers, dry eyes or mouth, pleural or pericardial rub). Sometimes, what is not evident on first inspection becomes evident over time. This may be as a result of a stuttering onset of the manifestations of illness or a subtlety of findings. During this time of diagnostic ambiguity, careful observation is indicated and early treatment with nonsteroidal antiinflammatory drugs (NSAIDs) may be helpful.

Diagnostic Testing

A routine complete blood count with differential and platelets, urinalysis, creatinine, liver function tests, and a thyroid-stimulating hormone are useful screening tools in this setting to exclude early involvement of any internal organ. Blood cultures, an antinuclear antibody (ANA), rheumatoid factor, erythrocyte sedimentation rate, antineutrophil cytoplasmic antibody, or Lyme titer may also be indicated based on the history and findings. In cases of monoarticular arthritis or pauciarticular arthritis, arthrocentesis with synovial fluid analysis for cell count, differential and crystals, as well as culture for microorganisms may be indicated. Patients with polyarthritis secondary to bacteremia, vasculitis, or diffuse vasculopathy tend to appear toxic, have frank physical findings, and often require hospital admission to better define the illness. Polyarthritis caused by viral illnesses or reactions to vaccines or drugs is usually self-limited, resolving over days to weeks. Polyarthritis of inflammatory rheumatic diseases tends to persist for 6 weeks or more, and this duration alone suggests an evolving autoimmune process. A physician is often anxious to provide a working diagnosis for a patient in distress, but it is important to remember that overdiagnosis of a rheumatic disease such as SLE or rheumatoid arthritis may be as deleterious to outcome in a young person's life as underdiagnosis of these conditions. Diagnostic uncertainty is an important indication for referral to a rheumatologist.

The approach to a patient with rheumatic disease can be less categorical when the concern of a progressive erosive arthritis, inflammatory disease with internal organ involvement, or untreated infection has been allayed. Here, the woman's misery and poor quality of life may be as real as in the woman suffering from an inflammatory process, but the objective findings of impairment will be few.

Goldenberg wrote in his update on fibromyalgia that "between 10% and 12% of the general population has chronic widespread pain." The prevalence is higher in women and increases with age. Fibromyalgia and other regional pain syndromes, uneased by medication or other therapeutic intervention, are difficult for many physicians to manage. It is difficult as well for the patient and her family; they experience this identity in family relationships and use it to shape their expectations and their choices in their day-to-day lives. Psychosocial issues including depression and domestic violence, comorbid disease such as SLE or posttraumatic stress disorder, and job dissatisfaction involving workers compensation and litigation all contribute to perpetuate the fatigue, pain, and misery of women with fibromyalgia.

The cause of this diffuse, symmetric pain remains unknown. There are no diagnostic findings in the laboratory or in the physical examination that convey more legitimacy to the diagnosis than the subtle findings of pressure points. However, new insights into the laying down of pain fibers in infancy and into the affective management of pain in the brain may clarify the experience of patients with chronic pain and bring more effective therapies to the treatment of fibromyalgia (see Chapter 33).

The absence of true anatomic correlates for pain and the absence of progressive deformity do not equal the absence of pain, but they do suggest an alternative approach to treatment. The expectations of the patient must be clear; a pill is not going to make this go away. More tests have not been shown to improve outcome. This is a syndrome in which pain does not herald worsening disfigurement, progressive impairment of joints, or destruction of the underlying tissue. The woman's involvement in understanding the limits of the diagnosis, participating in psychotherapy, and pursuing exercise may have a greater role to play than formal medical therapy. Except in cases of malingering and in cases in which distress is exaggerated by litigation or the promise of compensation by money or drugs, validating the woman's experience and giving it a context are often helpful. In a woman suffering from domestic violence or depression, chronic pain may be the symptom of pain that allows her to seek help in a medical setting. Diminishing this pain without identifying its roots excludes her from the help she needs. It is important to remember that facilitating the impairment, such as filing for disability or advocating the use of handicapped license plates, has not proven therapeutic. In the absence of understanding the pathophysiology of widespread pain, treatment should be supportive, and aimed toward living life.

Treatment

In all rheumatic disease, treatment is eventually successful for many, although cures are few enough. Realistic hopes should be fostered, and a practical approach to treatment of the disease should be outlined. This includes the importance of exercise and physical therapy to protect joints, weight loss to ease the work of tender joints, and psychotherapy to facilitate coping with the implications of the disease. In arthritis, the experience of illness often occurs within a woman's reproductive years, affecting her sexuality, self-esteem, and ability to work. Without understanding the measures of well-being in this fuller context, medicine will fail to ease her distress and promote, in a larger sense, her health.

Alternative therapies have moved into the world of medicine, perhaps reflecting a need to choose safer drugs or "natural remedies." Copper bracelets, raisins soaked in rum, herbal teas and incantations, voodoo, and cathartics continue to show up in the arthritis clinic as women from all over the world immigrate into our communities. Acupuncture, massage, and yoga are useful modalities for easing pain and improving a sense of well being. Glucosamine, chondroitin, and keratan sulfate supplements seem benign in trials to date and perhaps are effective for some patients with osteoarthritis. Other agents seem less benign, some ineffective, and many costly. A comprehensive well-referenced database on natural remedies with information regarding drug/nutrient interactions is now available in print and on the web.

Literature by women including their novels and memoirs, arthritis organizations and the resources on the web, and spiritual healing through the church and family are all important systems of support. Although one does not have to subscribe to all practices or promote those with no scientific basis, one can use the art of healing, defined by compassion and listening to the voice of the patient, to support those choices that promote well-being and do no harm. One can still think rigorously about the cause of a woman's distress in medical and scientific terms and yet opt for alternative care as a treatment more apt to produce health than an invasive procedure or new drug.

Nonsteroidal antiinflammatory drugs remain a mainstay in the treatment of pain and inflammation of arthritis. The selective cox-2 inhibitors celecoxib (Celebrex) and rofecoxib (Vioxx) are an advance in this class of drugs in the treatment of arthritis in the elderly, in those with intractable gastritis or ulcer disease, in those on anticoagulation therapy, and those on concurrent high-dose prednisone therapy. These medications are no better in easing pain than the traditional nonsteroidal drugs, but may be less harmful and better tolerated in terms of gastrointestinal disease. As a rule, celecoxib and rofecoxib are no safer for patients with renal insufficiency or liver disease than other NSAIDs; both are contraindicated in patients with an allergy to aspirin and other NSAIDs; and both are more costly than traditional NSAIDs.

In the systemic inflammatory rheumatic diseases, new medications have been designed that seem more potent and/or less toxic than those formerly available. These include **antimetabolites,** more selective **immunosuppressives,** and **antiinflammatory drugs.** Primary care physicians once saw patients with rheumatoid arthritis routinely on gold therapy in their clinics. This treatment has become increasingly rare. New drugs, etanercept and infliximab, have been designed that bind tumor necrosis factor-α, a potent cytokine in the proinflammatory pathways of erosive arthritis. These new drugs are startling in their efficacy and well tolerated, with few side effects reported to date. However, their long-term safety as defined by the incidence of infections or malignancies has yet to be determined. The medications are potent modulators of the immune response, and as such, may alter the environment of genes and the expression of autoimmunity. Women on these drugs may become ANA-positive, and there are rare reports now of pancytopenia and other autoimmune phenomena that bear watching.

The antimetabolites leflunomide and methotrexate are effective in the treatment of inflammatory rheumatic disease and are often used in combination with other drugs such as hydroxychloroquine and Azulfidine in the treatment of patients with rheumatoid arthritis. Prednisone remains a cornerstone in treatment regimens at some point in those with progressive, inflammatory disease; ideally, it should be prescribed at doses equal to or lower than 10 mg/day. In the treatment of lupus nephritis, mycophenolate mofetil has been shown to have comparable efficacy to cyclophosphamide, with a suggestion of far less morbidity. Other experimental medications, including interleukin-1 antagonists, intravenous gamma globulin, and gamma interferon, are being tested in the treatment of rheumatic disease.

Another breakthrough in the care of patients with inflammatory rheumatic disease has been the development of the **bisphosphonates** for prevention of osteoporosis resulting from corticosteroids and for the treatment of existent osteoporosis. Women with rheumatoid arthritis and SLE are particularly vulnerable to osteoporosis and subsequent fracture, both because of the inflammatory disease state and the drugs used to treat them. The bisphosphonates, alendronate, risedronate, and to a lesser extent cyclical etidronate are potent inhibitors of bone resorption and protect these women from progressive bone loss. They are not approved for use in women of reproductive age, since their safety in pregnancy has not been tested. An alternative for young women at high risk of fracture may be calcitonin. Raloxifene also has a role in prevention of vertebral fractures in postmenopausal women, but it has many of the side effects of estrogen, and its safety in women with SLE and/or vasculopathy is questionable. The use of estrogens for treatment of osteoporosis has become more controversial. These issues are addressed in more detail in Chapter 12.

Finally, **exercise** is essential for the health of women and particularly for women with rheumatic disorders. Cardiovascular fitness, weight loss, and improved functional status are the goals. In women with limited resources, this may mean a walking program, weightlifting at home or in the school gymnasium after hours, or bicycling when the weather permits. In women with access to a fitness center, exercise may mean an aquatics program, use of a treadmill, or classes of low-impact aerobics, yoga, or spinning. In senior citizen centers, *tai chi* may be taught to improve balance and well-being. And for some elderly women at home, the use of simple weights made by filling a sock with beans and draping it over the ankle may strengthen the quadriceps, improve balance, and reduce falls (Fig. 32-2). Home physical therapy visits to perform an "elderly checklist" intended to prevent falls and injuries is a useful intervention for many families, especially with elders following hip or knee replacement surgery and those with prior falls or early dementia and instability of gait. Whatever is prescribed should be thoughtful and tailored to the patient in a way that respects the constraints in her life.

The approach to a patient with rheumatic disease is an important concept as one undertakes the lifelong care of an individual woman. Details that clarify this approach are outlined in the ensuing chapters.

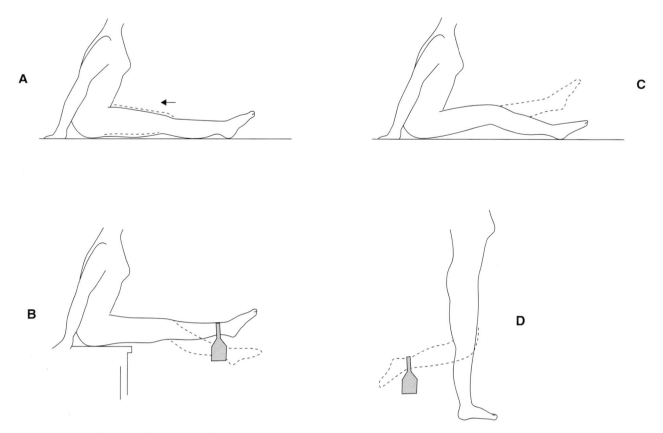

FIG. 32-2   Knee exercises. **A,** Isometric quadsetting. The muscle is tightened and the knee stiffened and relaxed several times. **B** and **C,** Isotonic short-arc knee extension. The knee is straightened through the last 30 degrees (to prevent peripatellar pain). **D,** Isotonic knee curls for hamstring strengthening. All exercises are performed as five sets of ten lifts each. (Modified from Mercier: *Practical orthopedics,* ed 5, St Louis, 2000, Mosby.)

BIBLIOGRAPHY

Alarcon GS et al: Systemic lupus erythematosus in three ethnic groups. V. Acculturation, health-related attitudes and behaviors and disease activity in Hispanic patients from the LUMINA cohort, *Arthritis Care Res* 12:267, 1999.

Bae SC, Fraser P, Liang MH: The epidemiology of systemic lupus erythematosus in populations of African ancestry: a critical review of the "prevalence gradient hypothesis," *Arthritis Rheum* 41:2091, 1998.

Barthon JM et al: A comparison of etanercept and methotrexate in patients with early rheumatoid arthritis, *N Engl J Med* 343:1586, 2000.

Cappell MS, Schein JR: Diagnosis and treatment of nonsteroidal anti-inflammatory drug-associated upper gastrointestinal toxicity, *Gastroenterol Clin North Am* 29:97, 2000.

DaCosta D et al: Determinants of health status in fibromyalgia: a comparative study with systemic lupus erythematosus, *J Rheumatol* 27:365, 2000.

Feldman M, McMahon AT: Do coclooxygenase-2 inhibitors provide benefits similar to those of traditional nonsteroidal anti-inflammatory drugs, with less gastrointestinal toxicity? *Ann Intern Med* 132:134, 2000.

Goldenberg DL: Fibromyalgia syndrome a decade later: what have we learned? *Arch Intern Med* 159:777, 1999.

Identification of racial and socioeconomic influences, *Arch Intern Med* 150:849, 1990.

Jellin JM: How to select between Celebrex, Vioxx and the other NSAIDs, *Prescriber's Letter* 7:55, 2000.

Jordan JM: Effect of race and ethnicity on outcomes in arthritis and rheumatic conditions, *Curr Opin Rheumatol* 11:98, 1999.

Karlson EW et al: The relationship of socioeconomic status, race, and modifiable risk factors to outcomes in patients with systemic lupus erythematosus, *Arthritis Rheum* 40:47, 1997.

Lawrence RC et al: Estimates of the prevalence of arthritis and selected musculoskeletal disorders in the United States, *Arthritis Rheum* 41:778, 1998.

Leventhal LJ: Management of fibromyalgia, *Ann Intern Med* 131:850, 1999.

Liang MH et al: Strategies for reducing excess morbidity and mortality in blacks with systemic lupus erythematosus, *Arthritis Rheum* 34:1187, 1991.

McAlindon TE et al: Glucosamine and chondroitin for treatment of osteoarthritis: a systematic quality assessment and meta-analysis, *JAMA* 283;1469, 2000.

Price DD: Psychological and neural mechanisms of the affective dimension of pain, *Science* 288:1769, 2000.

Reveille JD, Bartolucci A, Alarcon GS: Prognosis in systemic lupus erythematosus. Negative impact of increasing age at onset, black race, and thrombocytopenia, as well as causes of death, *Arthritis Rheum* 33:37, 1990.

Reveille JD et al: Systemic lupus erythematosus in three ethnic groups. I. The effects of HLA class II, C4, and CR1 alleles, socioeconomic factors, and ethnicity at disease onset, *Arthritis Rheum* 41:1161, 1998.

Ruda MA et al: Altered nociceptive neuronal circuits after neonatal peripheral inflammation, *Science* 289:628, 2000.

Walker EA et al: Psychosocial factors in fibromyalgia compared with rheumatoid arthritis. I. Psychiatric diagnoses and functional disability, *Psychosom Med* 59:565, 1997.

Walker EA et al: Psychosocial factors in fibromyalgia compared with rheumatoid arthritis. II. Sexual, physical, and emotional abuse and neglect, *Psychosom Med* 59:572, 1997.

Wallace DJ, Shapiro S, Panush RS: Update on fibromyalgia syndrome, *Bull Rheum Dis* 48:1, 1999.

Ward SM, Studenski S: Clinical manifestations of systemic lupus erythematosus.

Weinnblatt ME et al: A trial of etanercept, a recombinant tumor necrosis factor receptor: Fc fusion protein, in patients with rheumatoid arthritis receiving methotrexate, *N Engl J Med* 340:253, 1999.

Woolf CJ, Salter MW: Neuronal plasticity: increasing the gain in pain, *Science* 288:1765, 2000.

CHAPTER 33

Arthralgias, Fibromyalgia, and Raynaud's Syndrome

Robert H. Shmerling
Matthew H. Liang

▦ EPIDEMIOLOGY

Approximately one of every seven visits to the primary care physician is for musculoskeletal symptoms. In women, most visits are probably for aches and pains or low back pain, the so-called nonarticular rheumatic syndromes. Diffuse connective tissue disease as a cause of arthritis is infrequent in the general population, but the syndromes are more common in women than in men (Table 33-1). For example, in the United States 1% of the population is afflicted with rheumatoid arthritis (RA), which is two to three times more common in women than in men. The differences are even greater for systemic lupus erythematosus (SLE). In contrast, many forms of spondyloarthropathy (including ankylosing spondylitis and Reiter's disease) and gout are less common in women. Why the diffuse connective tissue diseases that are considered to be immune-mediated occur more frequently in women is unknown, but it is suspected that sex hormones (estrogen, progesterone, testosterone) may be important.

▦ APPROACH TO THE PATIENT WITH RHEUMATOLOGIC COMPLAINTS

The goals of evaluating patients with musculoskeletal complaints irrespective of gender are to exclude treatable illness, to identify which patients need more extensive diagnostic tests and follow-up evaluation, and to prevent disability. Laboratory tests are rarely diagnostic in rheumatic disease but serve as adjuncts to a detailed history and physical examination. Similarly, x-ray studies are rarely diagnostic at initial presentation. Laboratory tests may be deferred at the initial visit except when a morbid condition such as malignancy or infection is suspected, or when a systemic rheumatic condition is suspected, in which case it is prudent to screen for multisystem involvement. Radiographs early in disease are most likely to be helpful only in select situations (Box 33-1).

History

The history should determine the location of pain (by having the patient point) and whether the pain is likely to be articular, inflammatory, or part of a systemic illness. How and when the pain started, what makes the pain worse or better,

its temporal pattern, and the presence of constitutional symptoms (such as fever or weight loss) are important details.

Pain originating from joint structures should be improved by resting the joint and made worse by stretching the joint or by weight bearing. **Stiffness after prolonged immobility ("gelling")** suggests inflammatory joint disease or synovitis. This symptom probably results from altered viscosity of inflammatory joint fluid but is also experienced by older patients, as well as by patients with hypothyroidism, fibromyalgia, Parkinson's disease, and disorders with only a minor inflammatory component such as osteoarthritis. Clinically significant gelling lasts at least 15 to 30 minutes. In inflammatory disease the length of gelling may be proportional to the severity of the inflammatory process and may shorten as the patient's condition improves. The physician, in ascertaining morning stiffness, should ask about the usual time of awakening and the time when the patient is as limber as she will be during the day. The time elapsed is probably the most reliable way of eliciting this symptom.

Night pain may be a clue to a diagnosis and is also a major factor in impairing sleep, an important component of quality of life. Pain that awakens the patient may be infectious, neurogenic, vascular, or crystal-induced (e.g., gout or pseudogout) or may result from movement of a joint with severe structural damage during sleep. Tendinitis and bursitis also may awaken a patient. Synovitis without structural damage rarely causes night pain.

Neurogenic pain is often described in vague terms ("I can't describe it") or as numbness, an extremity falling asleep, shooting or burning pain, or pins and needles. Pain from vascular insufficiency is brought on by use and is relieved with rest within a few seconds. In neuroclaudication or spinal stenosis, use-related pain usually is bilateral, does not radiate below the knee, and improves slowly with sitting or bending forward.

A complaint of **locking of a joint** suggests a mechanical derangement of the fingers, knees, and occasionally the hip or shoulder. It may occur without warning when caused by ligamentous disruption or muscle weakness, or with pain when caused by a meniscal tear or loose bodies within the joint. Locking is the inability to move a joint smoothly through its complete range of motion because of an internal derangement (loose body, torn cartilage, or meniscus) or an

Table 33-1
Diffuse Connective Tissue Diseases

Disease	Estimated Prevalence (%)	Female: Male
Rheumatoid arthritis	1	2-3:1
Systemic lupus erythematosus	0.054	3-8:1
Systemic sclerosis	0.014	12:01
Polymyositis/dermatomyositis	0.006	2:01
Ankylosing spondylitis	0.13	1:03
Gout	1.6	1:07

BOX 33-1

Indications for Radiographic Evaluation of Musculoskeletal Complaints

No antecedent history, with abnormal joint examination
Significant trauma (especially near joint in prepubertal patient)
Age younger than 15 years
Progressive symptoms and failing conservative management
Symptoms not relieved by rest of involved area
Symptoms in patient with weight loss, prior malignant disease, fever, immune dysfunction
Recurrent acute monoarthritis

BOX 33-2

Functional Assessment

Screening
Which activity is most difficult for you?
Are you worse, better, or the same as before?
What can't you do now that you could do before?
What can't you do but need to or want to do?
How do you sleep? Can you sleep through the night?

Specific Activities of Daily Living: Ask About Difficulties With
Childrearing responsibilities
Ambulation
Dressing
Eating
Personal hygiene
Transfers
Sexual activity

---

extra-articular soft tissue block such as a tendon nodule, the cause of trigger finger.

Review of Systems

A brief review of systems should be undertaken to determine whether the musculoskeletal symptoms might be related to a systemic illness or a systemic rheumatic illness. This can be done simply by asking the following questions: "If you didn't have this [complaint], would you be feeling well?" "Do you have any other medical problems?" "Do you have any other joints involved?"

Functional Assessment

Inability to function is the final common pathway of all rheumatic illness; dysfunction and pain are the issues that most concern patients. The clinician should always assess how the symptoms affect the person in childrearing responsibilities, work, home activities, and sexual function. The presence of functional impairment may point the physician toward different or more aggressive treatment. In the patient with polyarthritis, for example, a joint that is symptomatically out of proportion to the others may indicate advanced structural damage or possibly even infection. Screening for functional problems can be accomplished quickly with five questions, and a more detailed inventory can be used to complete the assessment (Box 33-2). For patients with cognitive difficulties or multiple disabilities, direct observation of essential activities usually is needed to identify specific deficits.

When self-reported function is compared with observed ability to perform certain tasks, women report more disability than do men for the same level of musculoskeletal impairment. This also appears to be true for pain reporting. Studies of decompression laminectomy for lumbar spinal stenosis and total joint arthroplasty show that although the outcomes of the surgery for pain relief and functional improvement are the same, women tend to have more severe symptoms at the time they decide to proceed with surgery.

Physical Examination

The history, physical examination, and duration of symptoms are the three most important and useful "tests" in the diagnosis and management of rheumatic disorders. The goal of the examination is to locate the anatomic site, to identify whether the symptoms come from inside the joint or an extra-articular source, and to determine whether the problem is inflammatory or noninflammatory. The cardinal signs of true joint inflammation (**synovitis**) are effusion (fluid), warmth, palpable swelling over the joint line, diminished range of motion in all directions of the joint, and pain over all palpable areas of the joint capsule.

Point tenderness over anatomic sites of bursa is **bursitis** or a tear in a muscle or tendon. **Tendinitis,** on the other hand, is suggested by linear swelling, warmth, tenderness over the course of tendon, and occasionally an audible rub. Stretch of the tendon should reproduce the pain, although active motion is typically more painful than passive motion in tendinitis. In the examination the patient is asked to imitate the examiner taking the major joints through an active range of motion. If the active range of motion is limited, the examiner should note whether it is limited by pain, weakness, or mechanical block. The joint should then be taken through a passive range of motion. If the passive range is normal and active range is limited, disease of soft tissue such as tendinitis, myopathy, torn ligament or muscle, or peripheral neuropathy should be suspected. If the active and passive ranges of motion are equally limited, a soft tissue block such as in a frozen shoulder or synovitis should be considered.

Women tend to have more spine and joint mobility than do men until about the fourth or fifth decade. It is also a clinical impression that rheumatoid synovitis in women leads to more deformity and dysfunction than in men, perhaps because of the relatively smaller-sized joints and thinner bone structure in women.

Diagnostic Tests

Laboratory Tests

Acute-phase reactants are a heterogeneous group of proteins synthesized in the liver whose levels appear to reflect inflammation or tissue necrosis. The most commonly used of these is the **erythrocyte sedimentation rate (ESR).** The ESR can be high or low in the absence of a pathologic condition, it increases with age and anemia, and it is higher in women than in men. A rough rule of thumb is that an ESR's age-adjusted upper limit of normal for men is the age divided by 2; for women, it is the age plus 10 divided by 2.

The ESR is important in the diagnosis and monitoring of giant cell arteritis (GCA) and polymyalgia rheumatica (PMR) inasmuch as it is part of the criteria for the clinical diagnosis of these disorders. However, up to 20% of patients with GCA/PMR may have a normal ESR. The ESR generally is elevated in systemic vasculitis but is often normal in certain vasculitides such as primary central nervous system (CNS) angiitis or Henoch-Schönlein purpura.

Autoantibodies—immunoglobulins directed against autologous intracellular, cell surface, and extracellular antigens—are seen in a number of rheumatic illnesses. The intracellular antigens include nuclear components (antinuclear antibody [ANA]) and cytoplasmic components (e.g., antineutrophilic cytoplasmic antibodies [ANCA]).

Antibodies to cell-surface antigens react with a variety of antigens, including human leukocyte antigen (HLA) molecules. Other antibodies may react with plasma components such as coagulation factors (e.g., lupus anticoagulant). Low titers of autoantibodies are present in a small proportion of the normal population; therefore a diagnosis of rheumatic disease should not be based solely on the presence of an autoantibody.

Testing for **antinuclear antibodies (ANA)** is helpful in the evaluation of suspected SLE inasmuch as the test is highly sensitive (95% to 99%) in this disease. Certain ANA types—for example, Sm and dsDNA—are highly specific

for SLE. The ANA's predictive value is highest when the titer and pattern of the ANA are considered in the context of the clinical presentation. The pattern of the ANA (diffuse, peripheral, speckled, or nucleolar) correlates with the antigen against which the antibody is targeted (Table 33-2). For example, anti-dsDNA antibody generally produces a peripheral staining in ANA, whereas anti-Ro antibody produces a speckled ANA. Although some of these precipitins add to the specificity of the test, they possess variable and limited sensitivity. When SLE is highly suspected and the ANA is negative, an anti-Ro antibody and a hemolytic complement (CH_{50}) assay should be obtained because some SLE patients with a negative ANA will have a positive anti-Ro antibody and others may be complement-deficient.

Although anti-Sm and anti-dsDNA antibodies are highly specific (but not highly sensitive) for SLE, the ANA's most important limitation is its lack of specificity. Rheumatic disorders such as systemic sclerosis, Sjögren's disease, and rheumatoid arthritis also are associated with ANA positivity, although the sensitivity of the test in these diseases is much lower than in SLE. Patients without rheumatic disease, including healthy elders, patients with infectious illness (e.g., mononucleosis, acquired immunodeficiency syndrome), or those taking certain medications (e.g., procainamide, hydralazine, phenytoin), also may be seropositive for ANA. Although false-positive ANA results tend to be in low titer, a proportion will be of medium to high titer. The ANA titers of patients with SLE also may be low. Thus the ANA test is most helpful when ordered in settings of moderate pretest probability. (For a more detailed discussion on ANA and SLE see Chapter 38.)

The detection of **anticytoplasmic antibodies (ANCA)** is extremely valuable in the diagnosis of suspected Wegener's granulomatosis (sensitivity is up to 95% in the context of active diffuse disease) and crescentic glomerulonephritis. These antibodies may also have a pathogenic role. The most frequently used method for detecting ANCA

Table 33-2
Antinuclear Antibodies in Rheumatic Disease

| Disease | ANTINUCLEAR ANTIBODY | | | PRECIPITIN PANEL | | | | |
	ANA (%)	Pattern*	Titer	Anti-dsDNA (%)	Anti-Sm (%)	Anti-RNP (%)	Anti-Ro (%)	Anti-La (%)
SLE	95-99	P,D,S,N	50% > 1:640	20-30	30	30-50	30	15
Sjögren's	75	D,S	Low	5	0	15	50	25
RA	15-35	D	10% > 1:640	<5	0	10	10	5
Scleroderma	50-90	S,N,D	Often high	0	0	30	5	1
DILE	100	D,S	May be high	0	<5	<5	<5	0
MCTD	95-99	S,D	May be high	0	0	95	<5	5
Normal	<5	D	Rarely > 1:80	0	0	<5	<5	Rare

From Schumacher HR, ed: *Primer on the rheumatic diseases,* Atlanta, 1997, Arthritis Foundation.
*P, Peripheral; D, diffuse; S, speckled; N, nucleolar. Presented in order of decreasing frequency.
SLE, Systemic lupus erythematosus; *RA,* rheumatoid arthritis; *DILE,* drug-induced lupus erythematosus; *MCTD,* mixed connective tissue disease.

is indirect immunofluoresence microscopy in which two fluorescence patterns are observed: cytoplasmic (C-ANCA) and perinuclear (P-ANCA). ANCA also may be detected by enzyme-linked immunosorbent assay, which detects the antigens proteinase-3 (PR-3) and myeloperoxidase (MPO) that frequently are responsible for the immunofluorescent patterns, C-ANCA or P-ANCA, respectively. Patients who demonstrate C-ANCA with PR-3 specificity are likely to have active Wegener's granulomatosis, whereas P-ANCA directed against MPO suggests pauciimmune glomerulonephritis or other systemic vasculitis. P-ANCA may be positive because of antibodies directed against antigens other than MPO in a variety of disorders, including inflammatory bowel disease and other inflammatory disorders.

Rheumatoid factors (RF) are antibodies directed against serum gammaglobulins. These autoantibodies appear to be synthesized in response to immunoglobulin that has been conformationally altered after reaction with an antigen. The most commonly found rheumatoid factor is an IgM antibody to IgG.

The RF is one of the most frequently ordered tests in the evaluation of patients with suspected rheumatic disease, but its clinical utility is limited. The estimated sensitivity of the test among patients with RA is 75% to 90%, but such estimates are derived from highly selected populations in whom the prevalence of RA is relatively high. Other rheumatic diseases may be accompanied by the presence of RF, but the sensitivity in most of these conditions is even lower. The assay technique and titer of the RF may alter the sensitivity, but use of a more sensitive assay or using a lower titer as a cutoff for a positive test result will produce lower specificity.

Results of RF testing exhibit low specificity and low positive predictive value in a primary care practice. A variety of nonrheumatic diseases are associated with the presence of RF. Rheumatic diseases such as Sjögren's, SLE, and cryoglobulinemia may have clinical features in common with RA and may manifest RF. The test's usefulness is largely determined by the prevalence of RA and the prevalence of diseases associated with a false-positive test in the population for whom the test is ordered. For patients older than 75 years of age, the reported incidence of false-positive RF reactions is 2% to 25%. Given the modest sensitivity and specificity of the RF test, it should be ordered only for patients with a moderate likelihood of RA.

Serum **complement** represents a series of more than 20 biologically active proteins and inhibitors produced in the liver and accounts for 2% to 3% of the total plasma protein concentration. The best screening test for a complement abnormality is the CH_{50}, which is a functional assay of the entire classic pathway. A low level would suggest either consumption of complement or a deficiency of one or more components. Complement activation and consumption generally are triggered by exposure of the host to a foreign protein, especially when bound to host antibody (immune-complex disease).

Conditions with immune-complex formation are those in which measurement of complement may be useful, including SLE (especially with nephritis), cryoglobulinemia, chronic infections that cause glomerulonephritis (GN) or vasculitis (e.g., endocarditis or hepatitis B), generalized vasculitis (e.g., rheumatoid vasculitis or active polyarteritis no-

dosa [PAN]), and serum sickness. In SLE nephritis, serial measurement of complement may prove useful in monitoring patients inasmuch as complement levels may decrease just before or concomitant with disease flare and return to normal over weeks to months when disease activity diminishes. The correlation of lupus nonrenal disease activity with complement is variable, however, and thus complement should be considered in the context of the clinical picture.

The association between the **HLA-B27** allele and the spondyloarthropathies makes this genetic marker a potentially useful test in evaluating patients with possible spondyloarthropathy. The diagnostic sensitivity of this test is approximately 95% in ankylosing spondylitis, 80% in Reiter's disease, 70% in patients with the spondylitis of psoriatic arthritis, and 50% in symptomatic spondylitis associated with inflammatory bowel disease. Moreover, patients without rheumatic symptoms but with HLA-B27 positivity have an increased relative risk (although low absolute risk) for the development of these spondylitides compared with those who are seronegative to HLA-B27. The background prevalence of this genetic marker (approximately 6% to 10% in white populations) and the fact that only a small number of persons who are seropositive to HLA-B27 will ever develop a spondyloarthropathy limit the utility of the test. In general, because spondyloarthropathies are uncommon in women, HLA-B27 testing should not be ordered unless there is at least a moderate pretest probability.

Assessment of Organ Damage or Involvement

In patients with systemic rheumatic disorders, extra-articular involvement is often the rule even in the absence of signs or symptoms. In addition, agents used in their treatment may have systemic toxicity. Such involvement can be deduced by appropriate laboratory testing, such as renal or liver function tests, blood counts, muscle enzyme values, or urinalysis. For selected patients, more elaborate testing may be indicated, such as a 24-hour urine collection for protein and creatinine clearance, imaging studies (e.g., brain magnetic resonance imaging [MRI]), or lumbar puncture, depending on the suspicion of specific organ systems involved and diagnosis under consideration.

Synovial fluid analysis can differentiate infection, crystal-induced disease, or hemarthrosis and characterizes the process as inflammatory or noninflammatory (Table 33-3). In all cases, joint fluid should be handled using universal precautions.

| Table 33-3 |
| **Rapid Joint Fluid Examination** |

Method	Noninflammatory	Inflammatory
Gross appearance	Clear Can read print through joint fluid	Cloudy Print difficult to read through joint fluid
String test	Strings 1-2 inches	Drips like water from syringe
Wet preparation unspun joint fluid	Less than 2 WBC/hpf ($\leq$2000/mm^3)	Greater than 2 WBC/hpf (>2000/mm^3)

WBC/hpf, White blood cell count per high-power field.

The routine joint fluid analysis should include a white blood cell count and differential, Gram stain, and culture and crystal examination by polarizing microscopy. The mucin clot, complement, and sugar and protein determinations on joint fluid have little or no usefulness. If gonococcal or tuberculosis infection is suspected, appropriate culture media should be used, and other sites should be cultured (e.g., genitourinary system, blood or sputum).

Normal or noninflammatory joint fluid has the consistency and color of egg white and is clear; inflammatory fluid tends to be cloudy. The string sign is elicited after the fluid has been withdrawn by pressing slowly on the plunger with the syringe held parallel to the floor until a drop appears at the end of the needle and falls. Normally the fluid should string for about 2 to 3 inches. The more inflammatory the fluid, the more waterlike the consistency and the fluid will fall in drops. Inspecting the fluid for cells and crystals can be accomplished quickly by placing a drop of fluid on a slide with a cover glass and examining it at low and higher power (wet preparation). White blood cell counts greater than 2 per high-power field suggests inflammation, and this can be confirmed by the formal cell count, in which fluids with more than 2000 cells or more than 75% polymorphonuclear leukocytes are considered inflammatory.

A search for crystals requires careful scrutiny of fresh synovial fluid. Crystals may be seen without a polarizing microscope. The light source should be reduced by closing the diaphragm of the light source and lowering the condenser. In most fluids that contain urate crystals, pine needle-shaped crystals in and outside of white blood cells will be seen; under polarizing microscopy, they will be yellow when parallel to the axis of the polarizer. Pseudogout crystals are scanty, less brightly bi-refringent, and pleomorphic in appearance; blunt-ended rhomboids are most typically seen. They are blue when parallel to a polarizing lens.

In contrast to arthrocentesis, radiographs for a new joint complaint are rarely helpful, and, accordingly, the indications are limited (Box 33-1). Plain radiographs show changes in bone best and in soft tissue less well. Soft tissue findings usually confirm the physical examination. The changes in bone include erosions, joint space narrowing, osteophytes, fractures, and primary or metastatic bone tumors. Because it takes 4 to 6 months of inflammation for chronic synovitis to cause erosions that are radiographically evident, a film taken before this is rarely helpful. One exception is the patient who has had recurrent attacks of acute arthritis in a joint. A radiograph may demonstrate an erosion typical of gout. X-ray films of septic joints show abnormal findings 10 days to 2 weeks into the course. The process should have been detected by arthrocentesis well before radiographic changes are evident.

Ultrasound of joints by an experienced operator may be useful in identifying a joint effusion in sites where fluid or other abnormalities may be difficult to detect by examination; a Baker's cyst, torn rotator cuff, and ankle effusion are examples of such abnormalites. **MRI** of bone and joints are increasingly performed, but its role in diagnosis and treatment is uncertain. MRI provides detailed resolution of the bones and soft tissues such as in spinal stenosis or mechanical joint derangement, but it is not clear how much it adds to clinical assessment. Guidelines for ordering these tests may improve their utility while reducing costs.

CLINICAL PATTERNS OF ARTHRITIS
Monarthritis

A woman reporting pain or stiffness of a single joint may have an extra-articular problem, systemic rheumatic disease such as monarticular rheumatoid arthritis, a crystal-induced disease, or an infection. The differential diagnosis in approximate order of frequency in a primary care setting is noted in Box 33-3.

The patient's age is key in interpreting the history. Monarticular complaints in prepubertal patients require careful evaluation for traumatic conditions and congenital defects such as a slipped capital epiphysis and hip dysplasia. A sexually active woman may have gonococcal or reactive arthritis. Crystal-induced arthritis is rare in premenopausal women. In postmenopausal women, gout may be related to use of diuretics.

The degree of pain and the circumstances with which joint symptoms occur are helpful clues to diagnosis. Severe pain, especially during rest, narrows the differential diagnosis but is infection until proved otherwise. Mild to moderate pain is seen in inflammatory monarthritides but also in many other conditions such as hemarthrosis and ligamentous strains. The duration of the complaint may provide a clue. Pain that has been present for weeks is unlikely to be a bacterial arthritis but could be mycobacterial or fungal infection.

If there is a moderate or larger effusion, the joint should be aspirated. Only arthrocentesis for culture can definitively rule out infection, the only disorder in which prompt identification is crucial. A single episode of bleeding in the joint (hemarthrosis) should clear within several days to 1 week and may be seen in association with trauma or pseudogout. Persistent blood in the joint after this point implies rebleeding; a coagulopathy or a joint tumor (e.g., pigmented villonodular synovitis) should be considered.

Polyarthritis

Polyarthritis is synovitis of three or more joints and is distinct from polyarthralgia in which joint complaints are not associated with actual inflammation. Acute polyarthritis is a diagnostic dilemma that may be a feature of almost any systemic rheumatic disease, including some associated with high morbidity. Acute polyarthritis of less than 6 weeks' duration often cannot be diagnosed with any certainty and could be benign. A complete history, physical examination, and diagnostic evaluation are always necessary (Table 33-4).

The elements of the history particularly helpful in sorting out this presentation are the pattern of joint involvement, the

---

BOX 33-3
Differential Diagnosis of Monarthritis

Infection
Crystalline synovitis (rare in premenopausal women) (particularly first metatarsophalangeal joint)
Systemic rheumatic illness (knee in rheumatoid arthritis)
Hemarthrosis

temporal sequence, the course, the presence or absence of extra-articular symptoms or signs, and the functional consequences of the articular involvement.

The sequence of symptoms generally follows three major patterns: additive, migratory, and intermittent. In **additive arthritis,** new joints are added to previously involved joints. In **migratory arthritis,** an inflamed joint subsides as new ones become involved. In **intermittent arthritis,** inflammation is episodic with virtually no signs or symptoms between flare-ups.

When one pattern dominates the clinical presentation, a diagnosis may be suggested. For instance, an additive pattern is seen in patients with rheumatoid arthritis, SLE, and Still's disease; migratory arthralgia and arthritis occur typi-

Table 33-4
Selected Differential Diagnosis Suggestive History, and Findings in Common Rheumatic Conditions

Joint Disease	Suggestive History	Most Diagnostic
Traumatic		
Fracture	Acute onset after significant trauma	Radiographs and fat in joint fluid
Internal derangement (e.g., meniscal tear, loose body)	Acute onset, locking, giving way, often after trauma	MRI or arthroscopy
Tendinitis/bursitis	Localized pain, nighttime pain, worse with use, following overuse	Active motion more painful and limited than passive motion
Hemarthrosis	After trauma or with history of coagulopathy	Tests of coagulation, synovial fluid analysis
Inflammatory		
Rheumatoid arthritis	Chronic, symmetric polyarthralgia	Chronic symmetric polyarthritis
Systemic lupus erythematosus	Multisymptom inflammatory disease, especially skin and joints	Rash, oral ulcers, arthritis, pericardial or pleural rub, blood count/differential, antibodies to dsDNA, Sm, ANA, urinalysis
Spondyloarthropathies		
Inflammatory bowel disease	Oligoarthraligia, back pain, chronic or episodic diarrhea	Oligoarthritis, sacroiliitis by x-ray film; endoscopic evidence for inflammatory bowel disease
Psoriatic arthritis	Oligoarthralgia, skin plaques, nail pitting	Oligoarthritis, especially of the DIPs, sacroiliitis by x-ray film, psoriasis, nail pitting
Ankylosing spondylitis	Oligoarthralgia, back pain that improves with exercise	Oligoarthritis, sacroiliitis by x-ray film
Reiter's disease	Oligoarthralgia, eye symptoms, dysuria, rash, history of chlamydia or dysentery	Oligoarthritis, conjuctivitis, sterile urethritis, rash, sacroiliitis by x-ray film
Crystal-induced arthritis	Acute, episodic monarthritis	Synovial fluid analysis with polarizing microscopy; erosions or chondro-calcinosis on x-ray film
Infection		
Bacterial (nongonococcal)	Abrupt onset arthralgia, fever, systemic symptoms	Fever, CBC, synovial fluid analysis with Gram stain, culture
Gonococcal	Abrupt onset migratory arthralgia in sexually active patient; vaginal or urethral discharge; rash	Fever, tenosynovitis, rash, urethral or cervical discharge, Gram stain, culture (oral, rectal, genital)
Viral	Abrupt onset polyarthralgia of small joints; self-limited	Serology, liver function tests
Lyme disease	Tick bite or exposure, rash, polyarthralgia followed by monarthralgia	Expanding rash, serologic testing, synovial fluid testing (to rule out other causes of inflammatory monoarthritis)
Noninflammatory		
Osteoarthritis	No morning stiffness, use-related pain, night pain	Lack of inflammatory findings (e.g., no effusion), x-ray films
Avascular necrosis	Abrupt onset, predisposition (e.g., alcohol or steroid exposure)	X-ray films, MRI, or bone scan
Tumor	Chronic, unrelenting pain, history of malignant disease	X-ray films, bone scan

ANA, Antinuclear antibody; *CBC,* complete blood count; *DIP,* distal interphalangeals; *MRI,* magnetic resonance imaging; *dsDNA,* double-stranded DNA; *Sm,* Smith antigen.

cally in patients with disseminated gonococcal infection, acute rheumatic fever, and the arthritis associated with bacterial endocarditis and hepatitis. Intermittent arthritis is typically seen in crystal-induced disease and palindromic rheumatism (a variant of RA).

The specific joints involved and the pattern can narrow the diagnostic possibilities. For instance, RA would be the most likely diagnosis in the patient with a symmetric synovitis of the small joints of the hands, wrists (excluding the distal interphalangeal [DIP] joints), elbows, knees, ankles, and feet. DIP involvement without synovitis usually is due to osteoarthritis. Asymmetric synovitis of knees and ankles with backache suggests a spondyloarthropathy such as ankylosing spondylitis, Reiter's syndrome, psoriatic arthritis, or arthritis associated with inflammatory bowel disease.

DIFFUSE ACHES AND PAINS

Polyarthralgia is a common but nonspecific complaint in women, with an extensive differential diagnosis (Box 33-4). Such complaints can be evaluated through the history, physical examination, and limited laboratory tests, particularly an ESR in patients older than 60 years of age. Gelling or morning stiffness longer than 30 minutes suggests inflammatory rheumatic diseases such as polymyalgia rheumatica, rheumatoid arthritis, or SLE. When symptoms are less than 6 weeks in duration, postviral arthralgias/myalgias are common diagnoses.

Myalgias—muscle pain and aching—often occur with arthralgias. This sensation differs from other sources of pain by being less intense, and it usually does not awaken the patient from sleep or prevent function. Common causes of myalgia include bacterial or viral infections and unusual or prolonged exertion. Weakness, malaise, and fatigue are nonspecific symptoms and are frequently used interchangeably. True weakness implies loss of power or endurance. Such patients have difficulty initiating and maintaining a functional activity that requires strength. A patient with weakness or decreased endurance of one extremity may have a myopathy, a neurologic lesion, muscle atrophy, or a disrupted musculoskeletal unit such as a torn tendon (e.g., rotator cuff tear) or torn muscle.

Some patients mention weakness when they have decreased stamina. This can be a symptom of any chronic disease probably related to deconditioning, toxic-metabolic effects (uremia, severe anemia), or myopathies such as polymyositis, myasthenia gravis, or a variety of muscle-enzyme disorders. Patients frequently use the term *weakness* for malaise, asthenia, or nonspecific loss of well-being.

Patients without functional impairment and with normal findings on physical examination and laboratory evaluation usually have benign arthralgias that wax and wane; synovitis or impaired function rarely develops in such patients. Most of these patients are women, but no systematic study has been made of the epidemiology, course, or pathogenesis of the condition. The clinical impression is that its peak prevalence is in women of childbearing age and that its prevalence is more common and seems worse during the second part of the ovulatory cycle and postpartum. It may be a part of premenstrual syndrome. No specific treatment is reliably effective, but it is important to take the symptoms seriously and to legitimize the condition as real but benign.

BOX 33-4
Differential Diagnosis of Polyarthralgia

Viral infection
Idiopathic benign arthralgia
Early rheumatic disease (e.g., rheumatoid arthritis, systemic lupus erythematosus [SLE])
Lyme disease
Medications
   Accutane
   Fluoride
   Drug-induced SLE (especially procainamide, hydralazine)
   Enalapril
Steroid withdrawal
Fibromyalgia
Hypothyroidism
Hyperparathyroidism
Subacute bacterial endocarditis
Sarcoidosis
Metabolic bone disease (e.g., osteomalacia)

Antiinflammatory drugs seem to have an inconsistent effect; exogenous hormones have not been studied formally.

Arthritis has long been considered a condition that often begins at the time of menopause. One study reported the onset of RA at the time of menopause in 9.7% of approximately 250 cases. Diffuse aches, pains, and stiffness in the muscles and joints in the first 2 years after cessation of menstruation, without objective signs of synovitis or increase in acute-phase reactants, have been termed **menopausal arthralgias.** The same profile has been said to follow oophorectomy in women of childbearing age, with the symptoms controlled by estrogens. There are no epidemiologically valid studies to show that menopause is an etiologic factor or that hormonal replacement is specifically effective in putative menopausal arthralgias or arthritis. The best population-based evidence, in fact, suggests that joint pain is reported with about the same frequency in the following groups: approximately 20% in unselected premenopausal women, 12% in postmenopausal women before final menses, and 17% in postmenopausal women after final menses.

Fibromyalgia

When the patient has diffuse aches without a definable systemic rheumatic, infectious, or endocrine disease, and the findings of laboratory evaluation are negative, fibrositis or fibromyalgia should be considered. Fibromyalgia is a distinct syndrome characterized by diffuse aches and pains that do not seem to correspond to specific anatomic structures and that lack physical findings other than characteristic tender points (Fig. 33-1). Sleep disturbance, fatigue, and depression are common, but its cause is not well understood. Deprivation of non-rapid eye movement (REM) sleep in healthy persons can result in generalized aching. A number of metabolic disturbances involving estrogens, endorphins, and enkephalins have been suggested but not proved. Muscle biopsy specimens of tender points compared with those taken from nontender points in patients and healthy control subjects show reduced high-energy phosphate compounds.

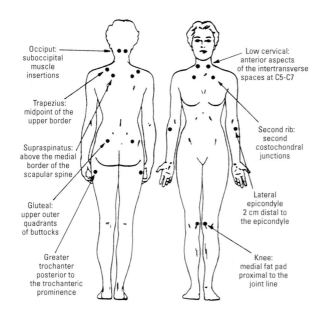

FIG. 33-1 Characteristic tender points in fibromyalgia. (From Schumacher HR, editor: *Primer on the rheumatic diseases,* Atlanta, 1993, Arthritis Foundation.)

As with many unexplained illnesses, psychosomatic factors have been implicated.

The patient with fibromyalgia needs support and reassurance that nothing life-threatening exists. Often the issue for such patients is not a dreaded illness but validation of their symptoms. To provide reassurance, the clinician needs to be attentive to and concerned about the patient's complaints, provide information about the illness and the theories about its cause, what to expect, and a treatment strategy. In controlled trials, aerobic exercise and tricyclic antidepressants for sleep disturbance (such as amitriptyline, 25 to 50 mg) help improve symptoms, but long-term benefit may not always result. Some patients with fibromyalgia, as in patients with chronic fatigue syndrome (a potentially related condition), may be very sensitive to low doses of amitriptyline (e.g., 10 to 12.5 mg/day) that would not normally be expected to be therapeutic for depression. Cyclobenzaprine (Flexeril), 5 to 10 mg orally at night, is a muscle relaxant chemically related to the tricyclic antidepressants and is an alternative first-line option. Nonsteroidal antiinflammatory drugs and corticosteroid therapy rarely help.

In summary, a woman with polyarthralgias should be questioned about antecedent illness, prior episodes, arthritis, medications that can cause arthralgias/myalgias (Box 33-4) symptoms from other organ systems, functional limitations, and mood. If these are normal and the examination shows no tender points, synovitis, or other abnormalities, benign arthralgia is the most likely diagnosis. If tender points can be identified, fibromyalgia is the diagnosis.

Raynaud's Syndrome

Pain in the digits may be caused by Raynaud's phenomenon, a reversible pallor caused by vasospasm of the vessels in the fingers and toes that is precipitated by cold or emotion. The reaction is episodic and may be accompanied by numbness or pain; it occurs only rarely in the nose, earlobe,

---

BOX 33-5

Conditions Associated with Raynaud's Phenomenon (Secondary Raynaud's Phenomenon)

Small Vessel Disease
Idiopathic
Systemic sclerosis (scleroderma)
Systemic lupus erythematosus
Rheumatoid arthritis
Dermatomyositis/polymyositis
Vasculitis
Vibration, chronic (e.g., jackhammers, chain saw)
Cold injury
Primary pulmonary hypertension

Large Vessel Disease
Arteriosclerosis
Thoracic outlet syndromes
Thromboangiitis obliterans

Intravascular (Cyanosis Without Blanching)
Cryoglobulinemia
Cold agglutinins
Polycythemia

Drug or Toxin Associated
Beta blockers
Ergots
Bleomycin
Cisplatin
Vincristine/vinblastine
Nicotine
Pseudoephedrine
Polyvinylchloride
Cocaine

Hormonal
Hypothyroidism
Estrogen/progesterone
Pheochromocytoma

---

or even tongue. It is classically described as a triphasic response with blanching white color, usually clearly demarcated from the rest of the digit, followed by cyanosis and then rubor as reperfusion takes place. Many patients, however, report only the initial vasospastic component associated with digital pallor. Occasionally, edema accompanies reperfusion; in long-standing disease, sclerodactyly may develop. This disorder is much more common in women, affecting up to 18% of the female population in some studies. A distinction is made between Raynaud's phenomenon, which occurs with or is an early manifestation of a connective tissue disease or another condition (secondary Raynaud's), and Raynaud's disease, which occurs as an isolated condition. The diagnosis must be made clinically, primarily based on the history, although cold challenge (e.g., running cool water over the hands) may be useful in select cases. The episodic nature of symptoms and the development of sharply demarcated pallor are the most specific historical features.

> **BOX 33-6**
> **Referral Criteria**
>
> Undiagnosed synovitis
> Failing function
> Multisystem disease
> Consideration of immunosuppressive, steroid, or disease-modifying agent, or intravenous colchicines
> Diagnostic arthrocentesis/biopsy
> Unresolved symptoms more than 6 weeks, especially if unresponsive to symptomatic or supportive therapy
> Progressive symptoms or signs
> Pregnancy in systemic lupus erythematosus, progressive systemic sclerosis

Even in a referral practice rheumatic disease develops in only 5% of patients with Raynaud's phenomenon. Many rheumatic diseases may be associated with Raynaud's phenomenon (systemic sclerosis, limited scleroderma, SLE, mixed connective tissue disease, dermatomyositis, or RA), but the most important are scleroderma and related disorders.

The principal task for the primary care physician in evaluating Raynaud's phenomenon is to determine whether it is isolated (primary) or associated with other diseases or exposures. Box 33-5 displays the diagnoses associated with secondary Raynaud's phenomenon. Most patients with the disease can be evaluated quite simply, and the pace of further evaluation depends on associated features (Table 33-4). If Raynaud's phenomenon is present for several years without the development of another rheumatic disease, it is likely to remain an isolated problem.

Treatment of Raynaud's phenomenon begins with advice to avoid cigarettes, cold, and beta-blockers and to wear a hat, gloves or mittens, and a vest in the cold weather. Waving the involved arm can be helpful. Biofeedback if available may be beneficial. Calcium channel blockers, including nifedipine and diltiazem, have been used with success. A recent study by Dziadzio and colleagues also found benefit in patients treated with losartan; thus blockade of the angiotensin II receptor may be a useful approach.

Patients with sclerodactyly or who are ill should have laboratory measurement of renal function, ANA, ESR, and complete blood count, as well as a urinalysis.

Any patient with Raynaud's phenomenon who has other organ involvement could have secondary Raynaud's phenomenon and should be referred to a rheumatologist. Raynaud's phenomenon with ischemic manifestations requires urgent referral and possible hospitalization (see Chapter 6).

INDICATIONS FOR REFERRAL TO A RHEUMATOLOGIST

Most musculoskeletal problems a primary care physician sees can be effectively diagnosed and managed initially in the office. Exceptions are situations in which greater experience and specialized knowledge are needed to ensure optimal outcome (Box 33-6). The primary care physician should refer these problems for another opinion, but in most cases is still the best person to integrate and execute advice from the specialist.

BIBLIOGRAPHY

American College of Rheumatology Ad Hoc Committee on Clinical Guidelines: Guidelines for the initial evaluation of the adult patient with acute musculoskeletal Symptoms, *Arthritis Rheum* 39:1, 1996.

Arnett FC et al: The American Rheumatism Association 1987 revised criteria for the classification of rheumatoid arthritis, *Arthritis Rheum* 31:315, 1988.

Baker DG, Schumacher HR Jr: Acute monoarthritis, *N Engl J Med* 329:1013, 1993.

Clayburne G, Baker DG, Schumacher HR Jr: Estimated synovial fluid leukocyte numbers on wet drop preparations as a potential substitute for actual counts, *J Rheum* 19:60, 1992.

Coope J, Thomson JM, Poller L: Effects of "natural oestrogen" replacement therapy on menopausal symptoms and blood clotting, *Br Med J* 4:139, 1975.

Dziadzio M et al: Losartan therapy for Raynaud's phenomenon and scleroderma, *Arthritis Rheum* 42:2646, 1999.

Fitzgerald O et al: Prospective study of the evolution of Raynaud's phenomenon, *Am J Med* 84:718, 1988.

Fletcher E: *Medical disorders of the locomotive system including the rheumatoid diseases,* Baltimore, 1947, Williams & Wilkins.

Gerbarcht DD et al: Evolution of primary Raynaud's phenomenon (Raynaud's disease) to connective tissue disease, *Arthritis Rheum* 28:87, 1985.

Hawkins BR et al: Use of the B27 test in the diagnosis of ankylosing spondylitis: a statistical evaluation, *Arthritis Rheum* 24:743, 1981.

Hebert LA, Cosio FG, Neff JC: Diagnostic significance of hypocomplementemia, *Kidney Int* 39:811, 1991.

Hoppenfeld S: *Physical examination of the spine and extremities,* New York, 1976, Appleton-Century-Crofts.

Jennette JC, Falk RJ: Antineutrophil cytoplasmic autoantibodies associated disease: a review, *Am J Kidney Dis* 15:517, 1990.

Juby A, Johnston C, Davis P: Specificity, sensitivity and diagnostic predictive value of selected laboratory generated autoantibody profiles in patients with connective tissue diseases, *J Rheumatol* 18:354, 1991.

Katz JN et al: Differences between men and women undergoing major orthopaedic surgery for degenerative arthritis, *Arthritis Rheum* 37:687, 1994.

Lichtenstein MJ, Pincus T: Rheumatoid arthritis identified in population based cross-sectional studies: low prevalence of rheumatoid factor, *J Rheum* 18:989, 1991.

Litwin SD, Singer JM: Studies of the incidence and significance of antigamma globulin factors in the aging, *Arthritis Rheum* 8:538, 1965.

Maddison PJ, Provost TT, Reichlin M: Serologic findings in patients with "ANA-negative" systemic lupus erythematosus, *Medicine* 60:87, 1981.

McCarty GA: Autoantibodies and their relation to rheumatic diseases, *Med Clin North Am* 70:237, 1986.

Pinals RS: Polyarthritis and fever, *N Engl J Med* 330:769, 1994.

Polley HF, Hunder GG: *Rheumatological interviewing and physical examination of the joints,* ed 2, Philadelphia, 1978, WB Saunders.

Richardson B, Epstein WV: Utility of the fluorescent antinuclear antibody test in a single patient, *Ann Intern Med* 95:333, 1981.

Schur PH: Inherited complement component abnormalities, *Annu Rev Med* 37:333, 1986.

Shmerling RH, Delbanco TL: The rheumatoid factor: an analysis of clinical utility, *Am J Med* 91:528, 1991.

Shmerling RH, Delbanco TL: How useful is the rheumatoid factor? Analysis of sensitivity, specificity, and predictive value, *Arch Intern Med* 152:2417, 1992.

Shmerling RH, Liang MH: Evaluation of the patient: laboratory assessment. In Schumacher HR, editor: *Primer on the rheumatic diseases,* Atlanta, 1997, Arthritis Foundation.

Sox HC Jr, Liang MH: The erythrocyte sedimentation rate: guidelines for rational use, *Ann Intern Med* 104:515, 1986.

Thompson B, Hart SA, Durno D: Menopausal age and symptomatology in a general practice, *Johns Hopkins Biosoc Sci* 5:71, 1973.

Wolfe F, Cathey MA, Roberts FK: The latex test revisited: rheumatoid factor testing in 8,287 rheumatic disease patients, *Arthritis Rheum* 34:951, 1991.

Wood C: Menopausal myths, *Med J Austr* 1:496, 1979.

CHAPTER 34

Osteoarthritis

Ronald J. Anderson

EPIDEMIOLOGY AND RISK FACTORS

Osteoarthritis is the one of the leading causes of morbidity in the female population. Although the disease clearly affects both sexes, the incidence of osteoarthritis of the knee in women is twice that seen in men. In the Framingham study the prevalence of knee osteoarthritis was 30% between ages 65 and 74 years. In addition to pain and loss of independence, osteoarthritis was responsible for 68 million work-loss days each year and nearly 4 million hospitalizations. Most of these hospitalizations were related to the performance of total joint arthroplasties. Various risk factors exist for the development of osteoarthritis, including obesity, repetitive trauma, female gender, several metabolic defects of cartilage metabolism, and genetic factors. This chapter deals with the diagnosis of osteoarthritis and addresses some of the key issues in treatment and rehabilitation.

PHYSIOLOGY

Critical to the understanding of osteoarthritis is the appreciation of several key points concerning the normal physiology and anatomy of the diarthrodial joint, its clinical and radiographic implications, and the pathophysiology of the disease process itself (Box 34-1).

Hyaline Cartilage

Hyaline cartilage, which forms the articular surface of all diarthrodial joints, has an understructure consisting of arcades of collagen fibers encased in a matrix of proteoglycan. This understructure provides an elastic, resilient surface that is nearly free of friction. Cartilage does not normally deteriorate with age, and degenerative joint disease should not be viewed as a normal accompaniment of aging. Unlike bone, however, cartilage lacks the ability, at least on a macroscopic level, to repair and reconstruct itself. Thus one should regard any lesion of cartilage on a clinical level as a permanent and irreversible step.

When cartilage loss does occur, it tends to develop initially in the region of the articular cartilage most exposed to weight bearing and stress. The subchondral and periarticular bone adjacent to areas of cartilage loss tends to buttress this region by local proliferation, resulting in the formation of subchondral and periarticular osteophytes.

PATHOPHYSIOLOGY AND DEFINITION OF OSTEOARTHRITIS

The term *osteoarthritis* is misleading because the suffix "itis" implies an inflammatory process. Most of the data suggest a degenerative rather than an inflammatory process. Pathologic examination, however, rarely demonstrates synovial inflammation, and the synovial fluid is characteristically free of inflammatory exudate. A leukocytosis of greater than 1000 cells/ml is seldom seen in the synovial fluid, and inflammatory mediators are found in low concentrations. Antiinflammatory agents are relatively ineffective in relieving symptoms and have not been shown to reverse the process. Although the precise mechanism responsible for producing pain in osteoarthritis is unclear, it appears that the symptoms are related to the mechanical opposition of two imperfect surfaces on each other. The term *degenerative joint disease* or *osteoarthrosis* is often used as a synonym for osteoarthritis, implying the noninflammatory and degenerative nature of the process.

Cartilage loss in osteoarthritis is related either to localized trauma and mechanical stress or to these factors operating on cartilage that has an underlying metabolic or structural abnormality. The abnormalities can be divided into those associated with collagen structure and those related to an underlying biochemical abnormality of the cartilage matrix. Although various kindreds may be identified with an apparent propensity for the development of osteoarthritis, only recently has a specific abnormality of collagen formation been identified and genetically defined. Other abnormalities of collagen structure undoubtedly will be defined in the future, but the incidence of these syndromes would seem to be rare. Metabolic abnormalities of cartilage, which include acromegaly, hemachromatosis, Wilson's disease, and ochronosis, predispose the patient to premature degeneration of the cartilage. These conditions also are associated with the radiographic appearance of **chondrocalcinosis,** a clinically useful marker for abnormal cartilage and the resultant development of osteoarthritis. Chondrocalcinosis is associated with acute inflammatory attacks of **pseudo-gout,** in which calcium pyrophosphate crystals existing within lacunae in the articular cartilage enter the synovial fluid by an unknown mechanism and provoke an inflammatory response that clinically has the appearance of gout.

Only a small proportion of patients with osteoarthritis have a defined metabolic abnormality or genetic predisposition to arthritis. Most patients suffer cartilage loss related to "trauma" occurring in an "anatomically disadvantaged joint." Therefore the joints affected are those involved with major weight bearing and stress, such as the metacarpocarpal joint at the base of the thumb, the hip, the knee, and the metacarpophalangeal (MCP) joint of the great toe. Prior injury to the cartilage of any joint such as occurs in congenital dislocation of the hip, slipped femoral epiphysis, avascular necrosis, intraarticular fracture, or any subtle asymmetry of the joint also creates a predisposition to mechanical wear and cartilage deterioration.

Osteophytes and Osteoarthritis

Although x-ray study is the usual technique by which a diagnosis of osteoarthritis is made, it is helpful to remember that plain radiographs basically show only bone and not cartilage. Alterations in cartilage can be detected only by the rather insensitive method of demonstrating that bone margins are closer together. The radiographs will not pick up subtle changes in the articular surface. Radiologists also use the presence of osteophytes as a criterion for the diagnosis of osteoarthritis. The presence of osteophytes does not automatically follow the deterioration of cartilage, and it is absent in cartilage loss related to the destruction of cartilage by synovitis. In addition, the degree of osteophyte formation does not correlate well with the extent of cartilage loss in degenerative joint disease but is useful as a radiographic marker that the cartilage loss is not inflammatory in nature. Moreover, there are several clinical syndromes, such as **Heberden's nodes** and **diffuse idiopathic skeletal hyperostosis (DISH)** in which osteophyte formation is the dominant lesion and not directly related to the extent of primary cartilage loss.

DEGENERATIVE JOINT DISORDERS WITH A PREDILECTION FOR WOMEN

Heberden's Nodes

Heberden's nodes is a hereditary disorder with a predilection for women in which a secondary spurt of bone growth occurs during the middle years of life and is localized to the distal interphalangeal joints of the hands. The condition is unrelated to osteoarthritis in other joints and is not an apparent risk factor for any other disorder. The symptoms are correlated with the phase of bone growth that usually persists for 1 to 2 years. Once the osteophyte is formed, the stiffness usually improves significantly, although the rigidity and protuberance of bone persist. **Bouchard's nodes** is the term applied to the identical process when it occurs in the proximal interphalangeal joints.

Metacarpocarpal Joint Degeneration of the Thumb

Metacarpocarpal (MCC) joint degeneration of the thumb is related to the hypermobility and resultant shear forces associated with ligamentous instability in the MCC joint of the thumb. Symptoms related to the degeneration of the MCC articulation of the thumb usually occur between the ages of 50 and 70 years. On physical examination, pain is produced by stressing the base of the metacarpal on the triquetral bone. Often a high-pitched crepitus characteristic of cartilage loss may occur. X-ray films show cartilage loss when symptoms arise, and osteophytes will develop over the next few years. The natural course of the condition is symptomatic improvement as the development of osteophytes stabilizes the joint and reduces motion and therefore the pain associated with it. The syndrome needs to be distinguished from **de Quervain's tendinitis** in which pain is produced by forced flexion at the MCP and ulnar deviation of the wrist, which causes tenderness and pain along the abductor pollicis longus (Finkelstein's test). (For more details on this syndrome see Chapter 35.)

Patellofemoral Osteoarthritis

The same instability and mobility that occur in the MCC joint also occur in the female patellofemoral joint. This is related to an increased angle of the patellar groove of the female femur. This syndrome commonly occurs in younger women aged 15 to 35 years and is rare in middle-aged or elderly women, although knee radiographs in this older age group frequently show degenerative changes in the patellofemoral joint. The symptoms do not correlate well with radiographic findings, which often are negative in the younger age group. The pain is most often felt anteriorly and bilaterally. It is accentuated by use, particularly by walking downstairs. Pain that interferes with sleep is common and related to pivoting on the patella while switching from a prone to a supine position. On physical examination the pain can be reproduced by grinding the patella on the femur. Also, the maximal pain during range of motion occurs during the last 30 degrees of extension. The management of the syndrome is controversial, and surgical therapy is aimed at stabilizing the patella. Clinical observation has revealed, however, that the majority of patients will experience relief of symptoms over a period of several months to few years. The interventions for these patients include maintenance of strength and the use of benign analgesic and nonsteroidal antiinflammatory agents (NSAIDs).

DIFFERENTIAL DIAGNOSIS

A physician's first concern on the presentation of probable osteoarthritis is to attempt to make another diagnosis. Pragmatically, osteoarthritis should be a diagnosis of exclusion. Once again, the radiographic evidence of osteoarthritis should never be accepted as adequate evidence for the diagnosis. The clinical picture needs to be consistent with the diagnosis of osteoarthritis, and other readily treatable conditions need to be excluded. Frequently another condition, such as inflammatory arthritis, is superimposed on underlying osteoarthritis and is sufficient to precipitate symptoms in the affected joint. Another example is the generalized stiffness associated with Parkinson's disease and myxedema. These diseases, particularly in the elderly population, can be confused with osteoarthritis.

Local inflammatory disorders, **tendonitis** and **bursitis,** are prone to develop adjacent to joints whose leverage and anatomy are altered by degenerative changes. The most common syndrome is anserine bursitis, an inflammation of the anserine bursa located inferior and medial to the knee joint. The classic picture of this syndrome is the abrupt accentuation of knee pain, frequently with nocturnal pain, occurring in a patient with medial compartment osteoarthritis of the knee with its resultant bowlegged deformity. Exquisite tenderness over the anserine bursa is evident on physical examination. Erythema or swelling is seldom seen. The pain should respond to the local injection of 1 or 2 ml of 1% lidocaine (Xylocaine) mixed with 1 ml of a long-acting steroid such as methylprednisolone (Depo-Medrol), 40 mg/ml. Whenever doubt exists regarding the diagnosis, it is advisable to inject the tender area; the complications are minimal and the benefits may be significant and long-lasting.

The coexistent development of an inflammatory condition, most commonly **rheumatoid arthritis, gout, pseudogout,** and **polymyalgia rheumatica,** should always be excluded, at least on clinical grounds. Patients with these diseases often manifest mechanical symptoms but also have associated systemic malaise, physical findings of joint inflammation, a dramatic response to antiinflammatory therapy, and symptoms and deformities that occur in non–weight-bearing joints such as the elbow, wrist, or MCP joint.

CLINICAL PRESENTATION

To reiterate, the diagnosis of osteoarthritis as the cause of the patient's symptoms should never be based solely on the radiologic demonstration of cartilage loss with associated osteophyte formation. Although radiographic evidence is required for the diagnosis of osteoarthritis, its presence should never be sufficient in itself to make the diagnosis. The physician should rely on other clinical criteria to ensure that the patient's symptoms are truly related to osteoarthritis. The criteria are as follows (Box 34-2).

History and Symptom Presentation

Mechanical Symptoms

The cause of pain in osteoarthritis seems to evolve from the abrasive grinding of two imperfect surfaces, and symptoms therefore occur only when weight-bearing or similar mechanical stress occurs. In contrast, although an accentuation of symptoms occurs with use in patients with

---

> **BOX 34-2**
> **Summary of Clinical Presentation of Osteoarthritis**
>
> Mechanical symptoms
> Gradual and progressive deteriorating course
> Lack of inflammatory features
> Failure to respond to antiinflammatory therapy
> Involvement of mechanically stressed joints only
> High-pitched crepitus on physical examination
> Radiographic or arthroscopic evidence of cartilage loss

---

inflammatory joint disease, they also experience rest pain and stiffness. Rest pain and particularly nocturnal pain, defined as pain sufficient to interfere with sleep, is uncommon in osteoarthritis and seen only in the most advanced stages of the process when failure to consciously splint the joint during sleep allows surfaces totally devoid of cartilage to rub on each other and produce pain. The typical patient with degenerative joint disease of the knee has pain on walking and is asymptomatic at rest.

Gradual and Progressive Deteriorating Course

Cartilage loss is irreversible, with a gradual rate of change that becomes obvious only over months or years and not days or weeks. The latter pattern is more suggestive of inflammatory arthritis. An occasional exception to this rule occurs in osteoarthritis of the hip, which may infrequently follow an aggressively severe and rapid course of accentuated symptoms despite only gradual changes when monitored radiographically or by physical examination. The reason for this presentation is unknown and seems more related to the observation that early osteoarthritis of the hip is often asymptomatic except for a characteristic difficulty in putting on shoes or socks. Because the pathologic changes of osteoarthritis are permanent, the clinical occurrence of a remission or significant improvement almost excludes degenerative joint disease as the diagnosis.

Failure to Respond to Antiinflammatory Therapy

Because osteoarthritis is essentially a noninflammatory condition, its symptoms do not usually respond dramatically to the use of nonsteroidal and other antiinflammatory agents. Often acetaminophen is as effective. This may not be true, however, for degenerative joint disease of the hip in which some patients will experience significant symptomatic relief from the use of NSAIDs. The mechanism behind this unique situation is unknown. There is no evidence, however, that antiinflammatory therapy either reverses or prevents the progression of the changes to osteoarthritis.

Lack of Inflammatory Features

Joints involved with osteoarthritis do not exhibit significant synovitis or pannus formation. The presence of a large synovial effusion is rare, and the synovial fluid white cell count is low—in the range of under 1000 cells/ml. Symptomatic patterns of prolonged (more than 2 hours) morning stiffness, easy fatiguability, and generalized malaise, which are characteristic of systemic rheumatic diseases, are absent in osteoarthritis; their presence should lead the clinician to reassess the working diagnosis of osteoarthritis.

Patients with underlying osteoarthritis and articular chondrocalcinosis are prone to episodic attacks of inflammation related to pseudogout. (Joint aspiration and the diagnosis of pseudogout are detailed in the next section.)

Involvement Only of Mechanically Stressed Joints

In the absence of a unique trauma or injury such as intra-articular fracture, osteoarthritis develops only in weight-bearing or mechanically stressed joints, namely the MCC joint of the thumb (a fulcrum joint), the hip, the knee, and the MTP joint of the great toe. Presumably because of the spring-like action of the tibiofibular-talar joint and the added resilience of the subtalar and intratarsal joints, osteoarthritis of the ankle is extremely rare and usually seen only after intraarticular fractures of the ankle or in persons with metabolic defects of the cartilage metabolism. Symptoms related to or the appearance of a deformity in a non–weight-bearing joint such as the elbow, wrist, or MCP joint are characteristic of an inflammatory joint disease in which any joint may be involved.

Physical Examination

In addition to a complete physical examination, a thorough joint examination should be completed. Pertinent physical findings for the diagnosis of osteoarthritis are as follows.

High-Pitched Crepitus

The findings of high-pitched crepitus can be of help in the diagnosis. When a high-pitched palpable or audible crepitus is present on manipulating the joint during the physical examination, it is specific for the absence of cartilage covering the articular surface and is indicative of bone grinding on bone. It is not specific for osteoarthritis, as any process that destroys cartilage may be associated with this characteristic physical finding.

Quadriceps Muscle Weakness

Often degenerative changes of the knee joint are associated with profound quadriceps muscle weakness. Two physical findings are indicative of quadriceps muscle weakness. The first is instability on lateral stress. This can be demonstrated by having the patient hold the knee in full extension while the examiner applies lateral stress to the calf with the thigh held stable. Normally the tibia should not move on the femur. The other finding is the presence of an extensor lag that is demonstrated by asking the patient to extend the knee fully. The examiner then attempts to further extend the knee by passive motion. Additional motion would be abnormal and indicative of weakness of the quadriceps, a condition that can be reversed by quadriceps strengthening exercises.

Diagnostic Tests

Joint Aspiration

As mentioned before, generally the joint fluid in osteoarthritis either is not detectable on physical examination or is benign, with lack of inflammatory cells or crystals. Intra-articular calcium pyrophosphate crystals are identifiable within polymorphonuclear leukocytes in the synovial fluid aspirated from an affected joint of a patient with pseudogout. These crystals are difficult to identify by means of polarized light microscopy compared with the readily apparent urate crystals seen in attacks of gout; a period of 10 to 15 minutes of careful observation is required under polarized light until the examiner can say with certainty that calcium pyrophosphate crystals are not present.

Radiographic and Arthroscopic Evidence of Cartilage Loss

Although **x-ray examination** is the usual technique by which a diagnosis of osteoarthritis is made, it is helpful to remember that plain radiographs basically show only bone and not cartilage and will not detect subtle alterations of the cartilage surface. Any joint that has deteriorated structurally to the point of producing symptoms should have at least some of the characteristic features of osteoarthritis on an x-ray film, especially joint space narrowing, which reflects cartilage loss and adjacent osteophyte formation. However, the radiographic appearance of osteoarthritis should never be accepted as adequate evidence that the patient's symptoms are related to osteoarthritis.

In recent years **magnetic resonance imaging (MRI)** has developed an increasingly larger role in the diagnosis of musculoskeletal disorders. Its major role has been in the more precise definition of lesions that are not apparent on plain films. This includes lesions such as meniscal derangements, soft-tissue lesions such as synovial proliferation or neoplasms, and the early osseous changes associated with avascular necrosis. This later condition may have clinical manifestations for several weeks before the plain films show abnormal findings. Although all of these conditions may cause a predisposition to cartilage degeneration, by the time symptoms related to degenerative joint disease develop, the plain films will show characteristic changes.

Arthroscopic examination, particularly of the knee, may be an even more sensitive technique for the early diagnosis of osteoarthritis, albeit not the most cost-effective. Several studies have compared arthroscopy with MRI or arthrography in defining early structural changes of the knee and meniscal derangements and have suggested increased sensitivity with the use of arthroscopy. However, in view of the paucity of significant therapeutic interventions currently available, arthroscopy cannot be recommended as a routine early diagnostic procedure for this condition.

❋ MANAGEMENT

Goals of Management

The guiding principles in the management of osteoarthritis are as follows:

1. There is no evidence that either medical or surgical therapy can reverse the course of the disorder.
2. The pathologic process appears to be irreversible, at least on a macroscopic level, and the lesion at best will remain stable but more likely will progress over the ensuing months to years.
3. Advances in orthopedic surgery over the past 25 years have provided patients with procedures for the reconstruction of damaged joints that not only relieve pain but also restore meaningful function. These procedures, although in a state of technical evolution, have been highly successful and have dramatically improved the quality of life for persons with these conditions.

4. The role of the nonorthopedist in the management of osteoarthritis is to initially and accurately diagnose the disorder, develop a program aimed at obtaining symptomatic relief and maintaining function, and, when indicated, orchestrate appropriate orthopedic intervention.

Choice of Therapy

Pharmacologic Therapy

The optimal pharmacologic agent for the treatment of osteoarthritis would be a substance that induces cartilage to regrow and repair itself. Such an agent does not exist. Acromegaly is the only condition in which cartilage is seen to increase quantitatively, but the cartilage formed is of poor quality and premature osteoarthritis develops.

NSAIDs are marketed for the treatment of both inflammatory arthritis and osteoarthritis. A study by Bradley et al comparing acetaminophen with high- and low-dose ibuprofen in the treatment of osteoarthritis of the knee showed benefit from all agents but no significant difference among the three regimens. This result would be expected given the usual noninflammatory nature of knee osteoarthritis, and it is consistent with clinical experience. On the other hand, hip osteoarthritis for reasons that are unclear may be symptomatically more responsive to the use of NSAIDs, particularly indomethacin, and a trial of these agents is worthwhile. There is no evidence, however, that NSAIDs alter the pathologic process or course of the disease. Therefore if complications from the use of nonsteroidal agents occur, such as gastritis or renal dysfunction, it seems best to avoid these medications and use acetaminophen for pain or consider other options. The recent development of the inhibitors of cyclooxygenase-2, Celebrex and Vioxx, presumably will reduce the risk of gastrointestinal bleeding associated with the use of nonsteroidals. These agents do not offer any improvement in efficacy or pain relief, however, when compared to the "traditional nonsteroidals." Because of the chronic nature of the pain, narcotic analgesics should be avoided.

Viscosupplementation

In recent years the use of intraarticular viscosupplements (Hyalgan and Synvisc) has been advocated in the management of osteoarthritis of the knee. These agents were developed to serve as a "synthetic synovial fluid" and are given as a series of several injections over a period of a few weeks. The efficacy of this therapy is open to debate. Early studies sponsored by the manufacturer showed efficacy comparable to the use of nonsteroidals, and only slightly better than placebo. There is little evidence that the symptoms of osteoarthritis are related to an abnormality in synovial fluid and intraarticular therapy has an obvious placebo effect. On the other hand, the treatment seems to have little in the way of complications.

Chondroitin Sulfate and Glucosamine

The use of these two agents in combination has developed via the health food stores and a great deal of publicity in the lay press. Although there is no evidence that a dietary deficiency of these agents or any dietary substance predisposes to osteoarthritis, the popularity of this supplement has snowballed. Presumably chondroitin sulfate is degraded in the gastrointestinal tract to simple amino acids and never reaches the joint in its original form. Glucosamine is commonly found in many food substances. A recent meta-analysis of published trials of these agents by McAlindon et al demonstrated positive effects of this combination in the development of osteoarthritis of the knee, both radiographically and symptomatically. There were several methodological flaws in the trials analyzed in addition to a potential bias related to sponsorship of the studies. It has been suggested that any benefit shown could be related to a possible analgesic effect of the compounds. The strongest evidence for efficacy demonstrates a benefit in the prevention of osteoarthritis, which is apparent only after several months to years of use. Currently the combination is being used in aches and pains of diverse etiologies with an anticipation of immediate relief. This seems unrealistic. At this time a randomized control trial comparing a combination of glucosamine and chondroitin versus placebo versus glucosamine alone versus chondroitin alone versus a nonsteroidal agent is being instituted by the National Institute of Arthritis and Musculoskeletal Diseases in conjunction with the National Center for Complementary and Alternative Medicine. In the meantime these agents are being used by a significant number of patients with both minor musculoskeletal complaints and destructive arthritis of varying etiologies. The substances seem safe and vary tremendously in price to the consumer. The strongest evidence for efficacy involves glucosamine in a dose of 1.5 g/day.

Weight Reduction

Obesity has been shown to be a risk factor in the development of osteoarthritis of the knee, and weight reduction in the asymptomatic obese woman does reduce the risk of developing symptomatic knee osteoarthritis. Whether weight reduction should be used as a universal therapy for osteoarthritis is controversial. In general the rate and degree of symptomatic relief achieved by weight reduction in the obese patient with osteoarthritis are equal to or exceeded by the rate of worsening caused by the natural progression of cartilage deterioration during the time period taken to lose the weight. Thus patients seldom perceive any symptomatic benefit from the tremendous effort involved in weight reduction, often feel frustrated and misled, and frequently respond inappropriately by rapidly regaining the lost weight. On the other hand, weight reduction significantly decreases the morbidity associated with reconstructive surgery and presumably will defer or delay the development of symptomatic osteoarthritis in currently unaffected joints. A reasonable practice would be to explain the benefits and options to the patient and strongly encourage weight reduction.

Weight Bearing and Exercise

Because osteoarthritis is a disease of weight-bearing joints, patients adjust their activities to remain comfortable. A patient should not be advised to avoid activity in hopes of "saving" the joints. Patients should maintain their present level of activity, including the optimal level of employment, aerobic exercise, and social and personal activities. If these activities become difficult to do, the patient might want to consider surgical options.

Use of External Braces

The use of external braces is ineffective in most situations. Any brace rigid enough to provide stabilization of a weight-bearing joint will compress the soft tissue in a way that is detrimental to the patient. Soft elastic braces do not provide any real stability and create venous occlusion. In non–weight-bearing joints such as the MCC joint at the base of the thumb, splinting may provide symptomatic relief.

Physical Therapy and Rehabilitation

The obvious tendency is to avoid using a painful joint. Immobility will lead to both muscle atrophy and restricted motion related to soft-tissue contracture. Motion also may be lost in osteoarthritis as a result of the stabilizing effect of periarticular osteophyte formation creating a "bony blockade." In certain joints such as the MCC joint at the base of the thumb, this immobility is beneficial, and with time much of the pain and disability disappear. In other joints such as the knee, immobility is deleterious. For a person to climb stairs and arise from a low chair, the knee should be able to move from 0 to 110 degrees. In addition, the muscular strength of the quadriceps lends stability to the knee, particularly in the flexed position.

The techniques of physical therapy are primarily of value when the goal is to add muscle strength or range of motion. Range of motion can be added either passively or actively. Restoring muscle strength requires active effort on the part of the patient.

The findings of quadriceps muscle weakness are an indication for an aggressive program of muscle strengthening, usually by means of quadriceps-setting exercise. Because at least some degree of thigh-muscle weakness exists in almost every patient with knee arthritis, these exercises may be routinely prescribed. Muscle strengthening can be achieved only by the patient's individual efforts. The therapist's role in obtaining this goal is that of an educator, and frequent visits to the therapist are not required after the patient has mastered the exercise routine. In the beginning of the process, the therapist may need to take an active role inasmuch as passive range of motion exercises may be needed. The use of other modalities such as local heat, massage, whirlpool, and ultrasound may be of preliminary value in manipulating the patient to increase passive range of motion. They have little role otherwise in the management of osteoarthritis.

Orthopedic Interventions

Few prophylactic procedures will affect the development of osteoarthritis. **Arthroscopic débridement** of loose bodies may provide symptomatic relief from symptoms of internal derangement, but the clinical indications for the procedure are still unclear. Prior meniscectomy promotes the development of osteoarthritis in that specific knee. However, it is highly probable that the presence of a torn meniscus provides an intraarticular nidus and thus may accelerate the development of degenerative changes in that joint.

Over the last decade several groups have advocated the use of periodic **intraarticular lavage** of the knee with saline, often under arthroscopic guidance. Recent studies seem to negate its value and currently the popularity of this treatment is declining. At best it may provide temporary palliation of symptoms.

Tibial osteotomy should be considered for patients with unicompartmental knee symptoms and a varus (bowlegged) or valgus (knock-kneed) deformity. Unicompartmental knee osteoarthritis is a "self-fulfilling prophecy" in that the more

the cartilage deteriorates in the medial compartment, the greater the bowlegged deformity and thus the greater the stress on that compartment, leading to a more rapid cartilage deterioration. In this situation, a tibial osteotomy consisting of the surgical removal of a triangular wedge of bone from the lateral aspect of the lateral upper tibia would correct the varus deformity and create a valgus deformity so that the patient will bear weight primarily on the healthy normal cartilage covering the lateral compartment of the knee. This procedure is indicated in relatively young persons (younger than 50 years old) who are physically active and wish to defer the more definitive procedure involved in a total joint replacement. The major disadvantage of the procedure is the need to use crutches for several months. Given that this procedure is performed in patients with "mild" disease, this group may be less eager to accept the long period on crutches.

Fusion of osteoarthritic joints is seldom done. Although considered a low-risk procedure, joint fusion requires a long period of immobility, and the resulting "long lever arm" produced by the fusion increases the stress on the adjacent joint and facilitates the development of osteoarthritis in that joint. It is the procedure of choice in unstable, painful interphalangeal joints of the hand and occasionally in the MCC joint of the thumb or the MTP joint of the great toe.

Repair of cartilage defects with explants is currently an experimental procedure. Patients with a localized cartilage defect in the knee, as might occur secondary to avascular necrosis of bone, have a sample of their own cartilage removed arthroscopically from a non–weight-bearing site in the same knee. This explant is cultured ex vivo and, at a later date, implanted surgically into the defect. This procedure is:

1. Currently experimental
2. Used only in localized cartilage defects ("divots")
3. Requires several months of partial weight-bearing after the implant
4. Not covered by health insurance and is anticipated to cost more than $30,000

However the procedure does offer significant hope to younger individuals with an isolated defect in an otherwise normal joint. It is not anticipated that this procedure will have a future role in the treatment of diffuse cartilage loss, which is a hallmark of advanced osteoarthritis.

The definitive treatment for any destroyed joint is a **total joint replacement.** This is a surface replacement arthroplasty in which the destroyed articular surface is removed and replaced by a metallic prosthesis on one side and a plastic prosthesis on the other. The prosthesis is sometimes cemented to the bone.

General experience with joint replacement has been positive. The major complication has been infection in the prosthetic site, and the risk increases with each operation. It also should be assumed that the life expectancy of a total joint replacement is 5 to 15 years.

Once the clinician is certain that the symptoms arise from the mechanical lesion of osteoarthritis, the indication for an operation is based solely on the patient's symptoms of pain and dysfunction, surgical risk, and the anticipated result. There is no reason to assume that an operation performed early is more successful than delayed surgery.

Pain is difficult to measure but may be defined as being severe enough to interfere with sleep. Function can be defined more quantitatively. Except in rare situations, pain sufficient to interfere with sleep in a major way is an indication for surgery irrespective of other problems. In considering an operation aimed at achieving a functional gain, it is critical to determine whether there is another factor such as angina, vascular or pulmonary insufficiency, or another marginal joint that is currently asymptomatic only because the patient is unable to stress herself past the limits set by the severity of symptoms arising from the one worst joint.

Finally, once convinced that osteoarthritis is the cause of the patient's symptoms, the clinician should never defer surgery with the expectation that the situation will spontaneously improve. If the diagnosis is correct, the symptoms will only increase in severity. The current critical issue in reconstructive joint surgery focuses on the longevity of the implants, with further research in progress.

BIBLIOGRAPHY

Adams ME et al: The role of viscosupplementation with SYNVISC in the treatment of OA of the knee, *Osteoarthritis Cartilage* 3:213, 1995.

American College of Rheumatology Subcommittee on Osteoarthritis Guidelines: Recommendations for the medical management of osteoarthritis of the hip and knee: 2000 update, *Arthritis Rheum* 43:1916, 2000.

Bradley JD et al: Comparison of an anti-inflammatory dose of ibuprofen, and analgesic dose of ibuprofen and acetaminophen in the treatment of patients with osteoarthritis of the knee, *N Engl J Med* 325:87, 1991.

Brittberg M et al: Treatment of deep cartilage defects in the knee with autologous chondrocyte transplantation, *N Engl J Med* 331:889, 1994.

Felson DT et al: Obesity and knee osteoarthritis: the Framingham study, *Ann Intern Med* 109:18, 1988.

Felson DT et al: Weight loss reduces the risk for symptomatic knee osteoarthritis in women: the Framingham study, *Ann Intern Med* 116:535, 1992.

Fischer SP et al: Accuracy of diagnoses from magnetic resonance imaging of the knee: a multicenter analysis of one thousand and fourteen patients, *J Bone Joint Surg (Am)* 73:2, 1991.

Gillies H, Seligson D: Precision in the diagnosis of meniscal lesions: a comparison of clinical evaluation, arthrography, and arthroscopy, *J Bone Joint Surg (Am)* 61:343, 1979.

Hochberg MC et al: Guidelines for the medical management of osteoarthritis. Part 1. Hip, Part 2. Knee, *Arthritis Rheum* 38:1535, 1995.

Harris WH, Sledge CB: Total hip and total knee replacement, *N Engl J Med* 323:725, 1990.

Klippel JH, editor: *Primer on the rheumatic diseases,* ed 11, Atlanta, 1997, Arthritis Foundation.

McAlindon TE et al: Glucosamine and chondroitin for treatment of osteoarthritis: a systematic quality assessment and meta-analysis, *JAMA* 283:1469, 2000.

CHAPTER 35

Regional Musculoskeletal Diseases

Karen H. Costenbader
Jeffrey N. Katz

Regional musculoskeletal disorders are common and disabling, yet often underrecognized and inappropriately managed by clinicians because they fall between the cracks of rheumatology, orthopedics, neurology, and physical medicine. Box 35-1 lists a variety of regional musculoskeletal disorders by anatomic region and pathophysiologic mechanism. This chapter focuses on the most common of these disorders and particularly those frequently seen in women.

DISORDERS OF THE SHOULDERS AND ELBOWS
Epidemiology and Pathophysiology
Shoulder Syndromes

Frequently encountered shoulder syndromes include **impingement syndromes, rotator cuff tears,** and **adhesive capsulitis.** An understanding of the basic anatomy of the shoulder is important in evaluating shoulder pain. The rotator cuff muscles originate along the scapula and insert on the humerus. These muscles hold the humeral head in the glenoid fossa and assist in the motion of the shoulder. Pain can occur with impingement of an inflamed subacromial bursa, biceps tendon, or rotator cuff tendon on the acromion, coracoacromial ligament, acromioclavicular joint, or coracoid process. Inflammation of any one or all of these structures, typically due to acute or chronic repetitive motion injury, can give rise to an impingement syndrome.

Calcific tendinitis of the shoulder is a relatively common cause of shoulder pain in which calcium deposits crystallize in the tendons of the rotator cuff, producing pain, decreased range of motion, and occasionally swelling. The calcium deposits typically resorb over time. The prevalence of impingement syndromes increases after age 45 and is associated with physical demand and repetitive motion.

Rotator cuff tears typically occur as a result of weakening or chronic damage, poor blood supply, or chronic impingement secondary to inflammation. Young patients most often suffer rotator cuff tears as the result of acute trauma or sports activities. The incidence of nontraumatic rotator cuff tears in women has been found to be two to ten times that in men and increases with age over 80 years, and other debilitating systemic conditions such as chronic renal failure necessitating hemodialysis, use of systemic corticosteroids, and infections.

Adhesive capsulitis (frozen shoulder) can complicate any inflammatory process or injury of the shoulder, which causes restriction of mobility and the formation of contracted, fibrous adhesions within the joint capsule. Women ages 40 to 65 years; patients with trauma, diabetes, depression, hypothyroidism, recent stroke or neurosurgery, Parkinson's disease or other chronic, debilitating illnesses are at highest risk for the development of a frozen shoulder.

Elbow Syndromes

Lateral epicondylitis, or tennis elbow, affects 1% to 2% of the population at some point in time, with peak incidence between ages 40 and 60 years. Inflammation at the origins of the wrist and finger extensors at the lateral humeral epicondyle give rise to the symptoms and are most often caused by chronic, repetitive injuries from work or sports activities.

Medial epicondylitis, or golfer's elbow, is five to eight times less prevalent than lateral epicondylitis and similarly results from inflammation of the flexors at the medial epicondyle. In both medial and lateral epicondylitis, repeated forceful contraction of these muscle groups is proposed to cause small tears of the tendons followed by an inflammatory response.

Olecranon bursitis is seen commonly in diabetics, in athletes who play contact sports, and in persons who repeatedly traumatize the elbows leading to pressure over the bursa or skin breakdown. Inflammation of the bursa with overlying erythema and warmth can arise from infection (usually *Staphylococcus* or *Streptococcus* spp.), gout, rheumatoid arthritis, or trauma alone.

Clinical Presentation
Shoulder Syndromes

Patients with **impingement syndromes** of the shoulder present with the gradual onset of anterior and lateral shoulder pain, typically radiating to the deltoid area. Night pain and difficulty sleeping on the affected side are common. After symptoms have been present for several months, localized atrophy over the superior and posterior aspects of the shoulder may appear. On examination, the patient experiences pain with overhead abduction and with internal rotation of the shoulder; often there is a sensation of the shoulder "catching" during this motion. Prolonged shoulder pain,

BOX 35-1

Chronic Regional Musculoskeletal Disorders Commonly Seen in Office Practice

Shoulder
Impingement syndrome
Calcific tendinitis
Rotator cuff tear
Adhesive capsulitis (frozen shoulder)

Elbow
Olecranon bursitis (gout, trauma, or infection)
Lateral epicondylitis
Medial epicondylitis
Elbow joint inflammatory arthritis
Ulnar nerve entrapment

Wrist and Hand
Carpal tunnel syndrome
De Quervain's tenosynovitis
Carpometacarpal osteoarthritis
Scaphoid fracture
Colles' fracture

Neck and Upper Back
Cervical radiculopathy

Lower Back and Pelvis
Mechanical low back pain
Herniated intervertebral disk
Lumbar spinal stenosis
Vertebral compression fracture
Metastatic tumor to the spine
Epidural abscess

Knee
Anterior (patellofemoral) pain
Osteoarthritis
Anserine bursitis
Meniscal tear
Anterior cruciate ligament tear
Crystalline arthritis (gout and pseudogout)
Septic arthritis
Rheumatoid arthritis

night pain, and difficulty sleeping are also characteristic complaints in patients with **rotator cuff tears.** On examination, atrophy may be seen over the superior and posterior aspects of the shoulder. Passive range of motion is normal, while active range of motion is limited by pain and weakness. With large tears, patients are not able to hold the arm elevated at 90 degrees against resistance. The classic presentation of **adhesive capsulitis** is the insidious onset of pain with decreased passive and active range of motion, in particular after a known injury to the shoulder. Examination reveals marked reduction in range of motion in all planes.

Elbow Syndromes

Patients with **lateral epicondylitis** report pain over the lateral elbow and forearm with activities involving the wrist extensor muscles, classically the tennis backhand swing, but also in power grip activities such as lifting a heavy frying pan.

Examination reveals point tenderness over the lateral epicondyle, increased with resisted wrist extension. In **medial epicondylitis,** the point tenderness is located on the medial side of the elbow and patients have pain with activities involving wrist flexors, such as a golf swing, or lifting with the palms up. In both conditions, there is no limitation of range of motion at the elbow joint itself, nor any intraarticular elbow effusion. Erythema, warmth, swelling, and variable pain over the tip of the elbow are reported by patients with **olecranon bursitis.** Symptoms can develop gradually or acutely in infection or trauma. The inflamed extensor structures result in painful active extension; passive motion is usually preserved.

Differential Diagnosis and Diagnostic Testing

Shoulder Syndromes

Plain radiographs of the shoulder (axillary and anteroposterior views) should be obtained to exclude occult fractures, dislocation, arthritis, or neoplasm. Occasionally, a subacromial bone spur or calcification of the rotator cuff tendons adjacent to the greater tuberosity of the humerus is seen, suggesting the etiology. In large rotator cuff tears, a high-riding humeral head relative to the glenoid may be seen. In patients at risk for joint sepsis (for example, recent infections, diabetes or human immunodeficiency virus [HIV]) or, if the shoulder is warm, swollen, or erythematous, the joint may need to be aspirated to exclude infection. Magnetic resonance imaging (MRI) can confirm a rotator cuff tear and determine the size and extent of the injury. Since 20% of asymptomatic older persons have rotator cuff tears, however, the MRI should be used judiciously.

Elbow Syndromes

Plain radiographs of the elbow may be necessary to exclude an underlying arthritis, loose body, or occult fracture. A joint effusion indicates elbow joint involvement. In olecranon bursitis, examination reveals a warm, tender swelling over the tip of the elbow. Often there is an intense overlying erythema; associated cellulitis of the forearm must be considered and worked up appropriately with blood cultures. If the olecranon bursitis is secondary to gout, tophi (subcutaneous collections of urate crystals) may be appreciated within the bursa. If there is a collection of fluid in the bursa, it must be aspirated sterilely and the fluid sent for Gram stain and culture, as well as crystal analysis. Gouty olecranon bursitis and infection may coexist.

Management

Shoulder Syndromes

The use of oral nonsteroidal antiinflammatory medications (NSAIDs) for 1 to 2 weeks with rest of the shoulder is usually effective for impingement syndromes. These interventions are later combined with exercises to gently stretch the shoulder capsule and thus prevent the development of adhesive capsulitis. Corticosteroid injections into the subacromial bursa can often decrease local inflammation and provide long-lasting relief. Ultrasound therapy has been found to lead to short-term improvement in calcific shoulder tendinitis and may help reduce local soft tissue inflammation. Complete rotator cuff tears usually require surgery, and acute tears have been shown to do better if they undergo operative repair within 6 weeks of injury of the start of symptoms. Conservative treatment for partial thickness tears

Table 35-1
Prevalence and Key Clinical Findings in Select Upper Extremity Regional Disorders

Disorder	Prevalence	% Female	Clinical Findings
Carpal tunnel syndrome	0.1%	>60%	See Table 35-2
De Quervain's tenosynovitis	NA	77%-91%	Finkelstein maneuver; tenderness at radial styloid
Osteoarthritis	30% in patients >65 years old	66%	Tender joint line; pain with loading; radiographic changes
Lateral epicondylitis	1%	60%-70%	Tenderness at lateral epicondyle; pain with wrist extension

NA, Not available.

includes NSAIDs, physical therapy with gentle stretching, and strengthening exercises. The recommended treatment for adhesive capsulitis involves NSAIDs and pain medications, physical therapy with warm packs, and frequent, gentle range of motion exercises. In severe cases, arthroscopy to excise adhesions or manipulation of the shoulder with the patient under anesthesia may be necessary.

Elbow Syndromes

Modification of activities and antiinflammatory medicines are the initial interventions for epicondylitis. Corticosteroid injections for lateral epicondylitis have up to 90% short-term success but frequent relapse. Medial epicondyle injections, although effective, carry the risk of iatrogenic injury to the ulnar nerve. Commercially available forearm straps may be used to absorb force across the extensor tendons. Lateral release of the extensor aponeurosis is performed rarely. Septic olecranon bursitis is treated with drainage, often repeated, and a prolonged course of antibiotics. Applying a compression bandage to the bursa and keeping the arm extended and elevated may help prevent the reaccumulation of fluid in the bursa.

DISORDERS OF THE WRISTS AND HANDS
Epidemiology and Pathophysiology

The wrists and hands are prone to repetitive strain injuries. Carpal tunnel syndrome, de Quervain's tenosynovitis, and carpometacarpal osteoarthritis commonly present to primary care providers.

Carpal tunnel syndrome has an annual incidence of 0.1% in the general population, with highest incidence in women in the sixth and seventh decade. In workers, there is no female predominance and the peak decade of onset is the 30s. Carpal tunnel syndrome is caused by compression of the median nerve in the carpal tunnel, bounded posteriorly by the carpal bones and anteriorly by the transverse carpal ligament. Any process that increases pressure within the carpal tunnel can lead to median nerve compression and the symptoms of carpal tunnel syndrome, including inflammatory tenosynovitis (e.g., rheumatoid arthritis), infiltrative disorders, and generalized swelling as occurs in pregnancy or with use of birth control pills. Repeated forceful movements of the fingers, especially with the wrist in flexion or extension, produces a low-grade tenosynovitis within the carpal canal leading to carpal tunnel syndrome. Risk factors include medical conditions such as diabetes, amyloidosis, hypothyroidism, inflammatory arthritis, and corticosteroid use, as well as forceful repetitive occupational hand movements.

The incidence of **de Quervain's tenosynovitis** has not been studied. In major clinical series, over three fourths of patients with de Quervain's are female. De Quervain's tenosynovitis arises from inflammation of the abductor pollicus longus or extensor pollicus brevis. These tendons share a passage through a thick fibrous sheath at the distal radius. Inflammation generally results from repeated forceful thumb extension. Activities that involve resisted extension of the thumb, excessive pinch, and excessive ulnar deviation of the wrist predispose to de Quervain's tenosynovitis. The problem is seen commonly among parents who lift their babies by the axillae.

The carpometacarpal (CMC) joint is one of the most common sites of osteoarthritis, with reported prevalence of 20% in males and 40% in females more than 65 years old. **Carpometacarpal osteoarthritis** arises from excessive load at the carpometacarpal joint. Joint space narrowing occurs along with osteophyte formation and decreased motion.

Work-related upper extremity disorders are the fastest-growing source of disability in the American workplace, yet fewer than half of patients with these disorders fit neatly into any of the entities listed in Box 35-1 and Table 35-1. The incidence of repetitive strain injuries in females is greater than that in males. While manufacturing, assembly work, and food processing, all of which involve forceful repetitive motion, pose the highest risk, epidemiologic data show that computer work for more than 4 hours a day is also a risk factor.

Clinical Presentation

Carpal tunnel syndrome is typically accompanied by numbness, tingling, and nocturnal symptoms involving the first three fingers. Percussion of the median nerve at the wrist *(Tinel's sign)* and prolonged wrist flexion *(Phalen's sign)* may produce paresthesias in the median nerve distribution. In advanced cases, the physical examination may reveal sensory loss in the first three fingers and wasting of the thenar eminence. The sensitivity and specificity of these historical and physical findings are listed in Table 35-2.

Patients with **de Quervain's tenosynovitis** complain of pain along the radial styloid exacerbated by movements of the thumb, particularly extension against resistance. Physical examination reveals marked tenderness over the radial styloid, as well as a positive *Finkelstein sign,* elicited by having the patient fold the thumb into the palm, curl the fingers around the thumb, and then deviate the wrist toward the ulnar side.

Table 35-2
Diagnostic Value of Clinical Findings in Carpal Tunnel Syndrome

Finding	Sensitivity	Specificity	POSITIVE PREDICTIVE VALUE WITH POPULATION PREVALENCE =	
			0.15	0.01
Nocturnal symptoms	0.77	0.28	0.16	0.87
Tinel's sign	0.60	0.67	0.25	0.91
Phalen's sign	0.75	0.47	0.20	0.91
Sensory loss	0.32	0.81	0.23	0.87
Hand symptom diagram	0.61	0.71	0.27	0.91
Neurologist's assessment	0.84	0.72	0.34	0.96

Carpometacarpal osteoarthritis, like other forms of osteoarthritis, is generally worse with use and better with rest. The joint margin is tender and "squaring" of the first carpometacarpal joint may be seen. Resisted flexion and extension of the thumb reproduce pain at the base of the thumb, often with crepitation.

Differential Diagnosis and Diagnostic Tests

The "gold standard" for the diagnosis of **carpal tunnel syndrome** is nerve conduction testing that has a sensitivity of 90% to 92% and unknown specificity. The opinion of an experienced neurologist is more valuable than any of the diagnostic tests. The aching pain, weakness, and paresthesias of carpal tunnel syndrome can be mimicked by lower **cervical radiculopathy** or an **ulnar neuropathy,** secondary to entrapment of the ulnar nerve at the elbow or, less commonly, at the wrist. Cervical radiculopathy is usually accompanied by back pain and reduction in the deep tendon reflexes of the brachioradialis (C6-7) or biceps (C7-8). If there is compression of the ulnar nerve, paresthesias involve the fourth and fifth fingers. Nerve conduction studies help to distinguish among these entities.

In **carpometacarpal arthritis,** radiographs reveal joint space narrowing and osteophyte formation, whereas in **de Quervain's tenosynovitis,** plain films are generally normal. If the patient reports trauma, classically a fall on an outstretched hand and wrist, it is important to exclude a fracture, typically of the scaphoid. **Scaphoid fractures** are often complicated by osteonecrosis. Patients report pain on the radial aspect of the wrist, and are tender to palpation in the "anatomical snuffbox" and directly over the scaphoid. Plain radiographs of the wrist initially may not reveal a scaphoid fracture; often repeat films and occasionally a bone scan are necessary. In addition, **fractures of the distal radius (Colles' fractures)** and **fractures of the thumb** can be detected on plain radiographs. A Colles' fracture should be a red flag to caregivers to suspect osteoporosis in menopausal or postmenopausal women.

Management

Patients with **carpal tunnel syndrome** should be offered neutral wrist splints that can be worn at night and during the day unless they interfere with work activity. Underlying disorders such as inflammatory arthritis, diabetes mellitus, or hypothyroidism should be sought and treated. Antiinflammatory medicines are typically of marginal value. Modification of work and recreational activities is critical. Corticosteroid injection into the carpal tunnel is safe and usually effective in patients with intermittent symptoms and no evidence of sensory dysfunction.

For patients unresponsive to conservative measures, carpal tunnel surgery is generally safe and effective in 80% to 90% of patients. The transverse carpal ligament is incised under direct visualization. Endoscopic carpal tunnel release has been found to be a reliable and effective alternative to open surgery, with success and complication rates comparable to that of open surgery in most studies. In cases with long-standing nerve compression, sensory and motor function may not return completely.

The most important goal in the management of **de Quervain's tenosynovitis** is modification of activities that provoke symptoms. Antiinflammatory medications are useful, as is immobilizing the thumb with a splint. Injection of corticosteroids/lidocaine into the first dorsal compartment over the radial styloid is effective in 60% to 90% of cases. In over half of cases unresponsive to injections, an aberrant separate sheath for the extensor pollicus brevis tendon is noted. Surgical release of the extensor tendon sheath is highly successful and can be done under local anesthesia.

Carpometacarpal osteoarthritis is generally treated by reducing load across the joint with activity modification and a splint that immobilizes the CMC joint. Injection of corticosteroids is also effective. Both arthroplasty (joint replacement) and arthrodesis (joint fusion) can be performed in refractory cases. More details on management can be found in Chapter 23 on osteoarthritis.

LOW BACK PAIN
Epidemiology and Pathophysiology

Back pain affects more than 80% of Americans at some point in their lives, and its direct and indirect costs exceed $50 billion annually. Low back pain can be categorized into (1) **mechanical back pain syndromes,** which involve injury to musculoligamentous structure without nerve root involvement; (2) **herniated disk syndromes** with sciatica; and (3) **lumbar spinal stenosis.** Compression fractures (covered elsewhere in this text), tumors, infections, inflammatory arthritis, and a few other diagnoses account for the remainder.

Mechanical low back pain is the most common and peaks in incidence in the third or fourth decade. Risk factors include smoking, lower socioeconomic status, and occupational activities that involve lifting or exposure to vibration. Myofascial pain is a frequent concomitant. Mechanical back pain is also a common complication of the late months of pregnancy, presumably because the added weight and lordosis impose increased demand on the paraspinal muscles. Unfortunately, low back pain in pregnancy appears to be associated with a higher risk of low back pain later in life.

Documented **herniated disk syndrome** occurs in 1% or 2% of Americans, with peak incidence in the fourth and fifth decades. There does not appear to be any male or female predominance. Lumbar disk herniation appears to result from repeated torsional and compressive stresses on the

Table 35-3
Prevalence and Key Clinical Findings in Low Back Syndromes

Syndrome	Prevalence %	Female	Clinical Findings
Mechanical LBP	>80%	50%	Use related; no neurologic deficits
Herniated disk	1%-2%	50%	Sciatica (dermatomal) root tension signs; dermatomal neurologic deficits
Degenerative spinal stenosis	NA	60%	Dermatomal and nondermatomal pain; pseudoclaudication; pain with extension; polyradicular neurologic deficits

lumbar disks, resulting in weakening of the annular fibers and protrusion of the disk material into the spinal canal, impinging on the exiting nerve root.

The incidence and prevalence of degenerative **lumbar spinal stenosis** are not known. Lumbar spinal stenosis is more common in women, who account for about 60% of most series. Degenerative lumbar spinal stenosis arises from compression of the cauda equina or nerve roots within the spinal canal. Repeated loading of the spine leads to disk degeneration, loss of disk height, apophyseal joint osteoarthrosis with osteophyte formation, and attendant ligamentum flavum hypertrophy. The osteophytes, ligamentum flavum, and protruding disks all narrow the space available for the cauda equina and exiting nerve roots, resulting in a nerve compressive lesion.

Clinical Presentation

The differential diagnosis of **low back pain** syndromes requires a careful history and physical examination. Table 35-3 lists some of the key clinical findings. **Mechanical back pain** is usually of a deep aching quality, generally perceived in the lower lumbar spine, and may radiate to the buttock and thighs. Paralumbar muscle spasm is frequent. Straight leg raising and the neurologic examination in the lower extremities are negative. Radiographs are of little value. **Herniated disk syndromes** characteristically produce sciatica, a lancinating pain radiating from the back to the buttock and along the posterior thigh and calf, usually into the foot. In more than 90% of cases, the vertebral levels involved are L4-5 or L5-S1. Numbness and paresthesia are also commonly perceived in a dermatomal pattern. On physical examination, a positive straight leg-raising test produces pain and/or paresthesia radiating down the leg. The sensitivity of the straight leg-raising test is more than 90%, with specificity of about 40%. The neuromuscular examination (sensory, strength, reflexes) is less sensitive and more specific than the straight leg raise.

Patients with **spinal stenosis** generally have insidious onset of aching pain, exacerbated with lumbar extension and improved with flexion, causing patients to stoop. Pain worsens with continued walking and improves with rest, often suggesting a diagnosis of vascular claudication. The pain is often bilateral; radiates into the thighs, legs, and feet; involves more than one dermatome; and is accompanied by paresthesias and numbness. The physical examination generally reveals normal straight leg raising. Pain with lumbar extension is probably the most useful diagnostic clue to spinal stenosis. Vibratory sensation is lost early in the course of the disease, followed by pinprick sensation and motor loss in a polyradicular distribution.

Differential Diagnosis and Diagnostic Tests

Approximately 0.7% of patients in primary care settings presenting with low back pain have **malignant spinal neoplasms.** These are generally metastatic, and in women the most common tumor is breast carcinoma. Factors that raise the likelihood of cancer include age greater than 50, previous history of cancer, unexplained weight loss, and back pain that is unrelieved by bed rest and unimproved after a month of therapy. Unexplained weight loss and previous history of cancer should prompt aggressive investigation for carcinoma. Patients with **spinal infections** also fail to improve with conservative therapy and generally, but not always, have systemic features.

Imaging tests should be performed in two circumstances: first, to exclude tumor, infection, or other ominous lesions; or second, if an intervention requiring visualization of the anatomy is contemplated, such as epidural steroid injection or surgery. Up to 20% to 25% of asymptomatic individuals have **disk herniations** or **spinal stenosis** on computed tomography (CT) or magnetic resonance imaging (MRI). Hence, these studies must be used judiciously. MRI has superior sensitivity in detecting abnormalities of soft tissues including disks and neural structures, whereas CT has better resolution of bony structures.

Management

Management of **low back pain** syndromes requires an understanding of the natural history. More than 90% of patients with mechanical back pain improve after 1 month. Similarly, more than 90% of patients with sciatica are improved after 6 months. Spinal stenosis, on the other hand, worsens insidiously as the underlying degenerative disease in the spine progresses.

The management of **mechanical back pain and sciatica** includes explanation of the excellent prognosis along with nontoxic interventions to accelerate the healing process and prevent future episodes. Acetaminophen, antiinflammatory medicines, and muscle relaxants may be useful. It is critically important that patients maintain as many of their usual daily and work activities as possible, to avoid deconditioning, social isolation, and depression. A randomized trial of physical therapy versus chiropractic manipulation versus an educational booklet alone for low back pain found no difference in symptoms between the three groups at 12 weeks, in days of work lost, or rates of recurrent back pain. Patient satisfaction, however, was greater in the two active groups. Transelectrical nerve stimulation for chronic low back pain has been found to be no better than placebo. Alternative therapies such as massage, acupuncture, and meditation are used commonly. Traction has been used in sciatica but without scientific support.

Epidural steroid injections provide transient (weeks to months) relief of leg pain in many patients with herniated disks and nerve root compression, with no influence on long-term function. Invasive interventions and antiinflammatory drugs are relatively (though not absolutely) contraindicated in pregnant women; thus postural education, acetaminophen, physical medicine modalities, and alternative therapies assume a more prominent role in management. In a controlled trial, the implementation of an educational program for workers at high risk of back injury did not prevent subsequent back pain episodes.

More than 300,000 diskectomies are performed in the United States annually. Surgery is typically elective. **Cauda equina syndrome,** which occurs in less than 2% of disk prolapses, is an absolute indication for surgery. Rapid progression of muscle weakness is also a rare but important indication for surgery. In a randomized trial involving patients without absolute indications for surgery, 70% of operated patients, compared with 33% of unoperated patients, were completely satisfied with their status after 1 year. Ten years after diskectomy, 63% of operated patients were satisfied compared with 55% of unoperated patients. Women accounted for 40% of patients in this study and had similar outcomes to men. Thus the long-term outlook is little changed, but surgery has a striking short-term benefit.

Conservative therapy for degenerative **lumbar spinal stenosis** is much less effective than in mechanical or disk syndromes because of the poor natural history of disease. Antiinflammatory medicines may be useful, lumbar corsets are valuable although inconvenient, and exercises to increase abdominal strengthening are rational but have not been studied critically. Epidural steroid injections may offer pain relief. Laminectomy appears to be successful in the short-term in approximately 70% of patients. However, up to 20% of patients may ultimately require a second operation. Women undergoing laminectomy appear to be more functionally limited preoperatively than men, suggesting they are operated on at a more advanced stage in the course of the disease. It is unclear if this reflects women's preferences for avoiding surgery, or lack of access.

KNEE PAIN

Epidemiology and Pathophysiology

Knee pain is a common complaint, particularly in women. Four of the most frequently encountered entities are covered in this section including **anterior** or **patellofemoral knee pain, osteoarthritis, anserine bursitis,** and **meniscal tears.** Unfortunately, prevalence data are not available for any of these conditions except osteoarthritis.

Anterior knee pain is probably the most common cause of knee disability in patients under 40 years old. Women are affected much more frequently than men. Patients with patellofemoral disorders generally have lateral deviation of the patella with respect to the distal femur, as a result of excessive tension in the lateral supporting structures, particularly the lateral retinaculum. Continued tension on the patella from a tight lateral retinaculum ultimately damages the patellofemoral joint producing cartilage damage. This is a late finding, however, generally occurring after patients have been symptomatic for years.

Osteoarthritis (OA) of the knee is a leading cause of pain and disability in patients over 50 years old. Risk factors for OA of the knee include older age, female gender, obesity, occupations involving repeated trauma to the knee, previous knee injury, and smoking. Postmenopausal hormone replacement therapy in women over age 50 has been found to slightly increase the relative risk of osteoarthritis of the knee in some series. Mechanical load from acute trauma or repetitive injury is the primary insult. Morphologic changes in the articular cartilage include fragmentation with pitting, clefts, and ultimately ulceration of cartilage down to bone. Bony proliferation, in the form of osteophytes, accompanies the cartilage destruction. Although men are more likely to develop a bow-leg deformity *(genu varum)* causing greater medial than lateral compartment degeneration, women, as a result of the geometry of the pelvis, are more likely to develop a knock-knee *(genu valgum)* deformity, giving rise to accelerated lateral knee compartment osteoarthritis. Radiographic OA is present in 27% of women 65 to 69 years old and 53% over age 80 years. Symptomatic OA occurs in 8% of women 60 to 70 years old and 16% of those over 80 years. Men have slightly lower rates of OA. (More information can be found in Chapter 23.)

Meniscal tears generally arise from trauma in younger patients, with males affected more frequently. Degenerative meniscal tears often occur in older patients with degenerative arthritis of the knee and therefore are more common in females. The menisci provide stability against rotational forces and cushion load applied across the joint. The medial two thirds of the meniscus is sparsely vascularized and heals poorly, whereas the outer third may heal spontaneously. Mechanical symptoms arise from the free flap of meniscus moving about the joint.

Another lesion that often arises in association with degenerative arthritis of the knee is **pes anserine bursitis,** inflammation of the insertion of the medial hamstrings onto the tibia. This lesion is seen considerably more frequently in females than in males. The pes anserinus bursa surrounds the medial hamstring tendons and allows them to glide smoothly over the bony prominence of the superior tibia. These tendons may become inflamed acutely from athletic activities or chronically from valgus stress, as often occurs in women with osteoarthritis.

Clinical Presentation

Anterior knee pain is perceived just behind the patella and is exacerbated by forceful knee flexion as occurs in kneeling or squatting. Patients often complain of onset of pain after periods of inactivity, such as sitting in the theater or a long car trip. The physical examination often shows lateral tilting of the patella, tenderness at the insertion of the lateral retinaculum insertion onto the patella, and pain with compression of the patellofemoral joint (Table 35-4).

In **OA,** dull aching pain is perceived deep within the knee and increases with activity. In advanced cases, pain occurs at night. The physical examination may show quadriceps atrophy and usually reveals joint line tenderness. Range of motion is normal until late in the disease, when bony crepitus may also be noted.

Table 35-4
Key Clinical Findings in Select Regional Disorders of the Knee

Disorder %	Female	Clinical Findings
Anterior knee pain	80%	Pain with stairs, squat tender lateral retinaculum patellar tilt patellofemoral compression tenderness
Osteoarthritis	60%	Use-related pain joint line tenderness radiograph: cartilage loss, osteophytes, sclerosis
Meniscal tears	40%	Mechanical symptoms joint line tenderness MacMurray's maneuver
Anserine bursitis	80%	Tenderness at anserine bursa

Prevalence unknown except for osteoarthritis; see text.

This work was supported in part by grant PO1 AR36 308 from the National Institutes of Health to the Robert B. Brigham Multipurpose Arthritis and Musculoskeletal Diseases Center, and grants from the Arthritis Foundation.

The signs and symptoms of **meniscal tears** are locking, giving way, joint line tenderness, a joint effusion and a positive McMurray's sign. The McMurray's sign involves flexion of the knee and concomitant internal or external rotation of the tibia. A positive response is a painful and palpable click as the knee goes through the arc of flexion.

Patients with **pes anserinus bursitis** complain of pain along the medial aspect of the knee inferior to the medial joint line. The physical examination reveals exquisite tenderness at the pes anserinus bursa, located about four finger breadths below the medial joint line. Radiographs are unnecessary.

Differential Diagnosis and Diagnostic Tests

The differential diagnosis of knee pain includes a variety of noninflammatory, inflammatory, and systemic conditions that can affect the knee, including **OA, meniscal, bursal** or **tendinous disorders, crystalline arthritis (gout** and **pseudogout), rheumatoid arthritis** (RA), and **infectious arthritis,** such as **bacterial infection, Lyme disease, tuberculosis,** and others. Radiographs, including a patellar view, can assess damage to the retropatellar cartilage and alignment of the patellofemoral joint in anterior knee pain. In OA, radiographs will reveal sclerosis of the bony endplates, followed by a narrowing of the joint space, formation of osteophytes, and subchondral cysts. Chondrocalcinosis, calcification along the meniscal cartilage of the knee, is seen in pseudogout, and reflects deposition of calcium pyrophosphate dihydrate within these tissues. Joint erosions and periarticular osteopenia may be found on plain radiographs in RA. If a joint effusion and signs of inflammation (warmth, erythema, and swelling) are present, a sterile arthrocentesis should usually be performed to exclude infectious, crystalline, or other inflammatory arthritis.

If instability of the knee is found on examination and an internal derangement is suspected, MRI is the best noninvasive method, with sensitivity over 90% for medial meniscal tears and 80% for lateral meniscal tears. MRI is an excellent imaging modality for the other soft tissues of the knee and can be used to evaluate the **cruciate ligaments,** the **collateral ligaments,** and the **patellar tendon,** all of which can be torn or damaged in trauma to the knee. Arthroscopy, the "gold standard" for the diagnosis of meniscal tears, has specificity of about 95% for lateral meniscal tears and 90% for medial meniscal tears.

Management

More than 80% of patients with significant **anterior knee pain** can be managed successfully with conservative therapy. The treatment program should consist initially of eliminating or modifying activities that produce symptoms, then progressive resistance exercises to strengthen the medial knee extensors, counterbalancing the tight lateral structures. Next, a graduated running or other exercise protocol is instituted. A maintenance program of quadricep strengthening should be continued indefinitely. Adjunctive measures such as knee pads, patellar braces, and shoe orthotics can be used if appropriate. Patients unresponsive to the preceding measures who desire a high level of functional activity may be candidates for release of the lateral retinaculum.

Treatment of **OA** of the knee begins with modification of activities. A cane can relieve up to 30% of the load off the affected joint. Acetaminophen is as efficacious as antiinflammatory doses of ibuprofen. Newer Cyclooxygenase-2 (COX-2)-specific NSAIDs, Celecoxib, and Rofecoxib have been shown to be as effective as traditional nonspecific NSAIDs in the treatment of osteoarthritis, with a lower incidence of gastric ulceration in endoscopic studies. Studies of intraarticularly injected purified hyaluronan, a glycosaminoglycan produced by normal chondrocytes and synoviocytes, have shown only a small benefit over placebo for relief of pain in OA of the knee with no serious side effects. Small trials examining the effect of oral glucosamine on the pain and stiffness of OA have demonstrated a minimal benefit versus placebo, whereas larger, longer term randomized trials are ongoing. Intraarticular injections of steroids are effective in some patients, suggesting an inflammatory component (see Chapter 34).

In severe cases of OA of the knee, total knee arthroplasty is remarkably effective. Approximately 300,000 are performed annually in the United States at a direct cost of about $30,000 per case. Medical complications occur in 1% to 2% of patients. Prostheses ultimately loosen and require revision, seldom before about 15 years. In view of the need for revisions, other procedures such as osteotomy should be attempted in younger patients. As mentioned regarding laminectomy for spinal stenosis, women have been noted to undergo knee arthroplasty for OA at a more advanced point in the course of functional decline than men.

In patients with OA of the knee, it is important to diagnose and treat associated lesions that may be more amenable to therapy. Chief among these is **pes anserine bursitis,** which is relieved predictably with a local injection of corticosteroid mixed with 1% lidocaine.

Meniscal tears are managed with decreased activity, antiinflammatory therapy, and simple observation. Arthroscopic partial meniscectomy is indicated for meniscal tears that have not responded to several months of conservative therapy. The torn flap of meniscus is removed, preserving as much meniscal tissue as possible. Arthroscopic partial menisectomy is successful in up to 85% of patients, but may be a risk factor for subsequent OA.

BIBLIOGRAPHY

Ahlgren BD, Garfin SR: Cervical Radiculopathy, *Orthop Clin North Am* 27:253, 1996.

Altman RD et al: Intra-articular sodium hyaluronate (hyalgan) in the treatment of patients with osteoarthritis of the knee: a randomized clinical trial, *J Rheumatol* 25:2203, 1998.

Bensen WG et al: Treatment of osteoarthritis with Celecoxib, a cyclooxygenase-2 inhibitor: a randomized controlled trial, *Mayo Clin Proc* 74:1095, 1999.

Bernard BP, editor: *Musculoskeletal disorders and workplace factors. National Institute for Occupational Safety and Health. DHHS (NIOSH)*, publication no. 97-141, Cincinnati, 1997.

Bradley JD et al: Comparison of an anti-inflammatory dose of ibuprofen, an analgesic dose of ibuprofen, and acetaminophen in the treatment of patients with osteoarthritis of the knee, *N Engl J Med* 325:87, 1991.

Bradshaw DY, Shefner JM: Ulnar neuropathy at the elbow, *Neurol Clin* 17:447, 1999.

Cherkin DC et al: A comparison of physical therapy, chiropractic manipulation and provision of an educational booklet for the treatment of patients with low back pain, *N Engl J Med* 339:1021, 1998.

Cohen RB, Williams GR: Impingement syndrome and rotator cuff diseases as repetitive motion disorders, *Clin Orthop* 351:95, 1998.

Daltroy L et al: A controlled trial of an educational program to prevent low back injuries, *N Engl J Med* 337:322, 1997.

Daigneault J, Cooney LM: Shoulder pain in older people, *J Am Geriatrics Soc* 46:1144, 1998.

Deyo RA, Rainesville J, Kent DL: What can the history and physical examination tell us about low back pain? *JAMA* 268:760, 1992.

Dieppe P et al: Knee replacement surgery for osteoarthritis: effectiveness, practice variations, indications and possible determination of utilization, *Rheumatology* 38:73, 1999.

Ebenbichler GR et al: Ultrasound therapy for calcific tendinitis of the shoulder, *N Engl J Med* 340:1533, 1999.

Fadale PD, Noerdlinger MA: Sports injuries of the knee, *Curr Opin Rheumatol* 11:144, 1999.

Gabel GT: Acute and chronic tendinopathies at the elbow, *Curr Opin Rheumatol* 11:138, 1999.

Hart DA et al: Gender and neurogenic variables in tendon biology and repetitive motion disorders, *Clin Orthop* 351:44, 1998.

Herno A et al: Long-term clinical and magnetic resonance imaging follow-up assessment of patients with lumbar spinal stenosis after laminectomy, *Spine* 24:1533, 1999.

Houpt HB et al: Effect of glucosamine hydrochloride in the treatment of pain of osteoarthritis of the knee, *J Rheumatol* 26:2423, 1999.

Hulstyn MJ, Weiss AP: Adhesive capsulitis of the shoulder, *Orthop Rev* 22:425, 1993.

Jensen K et al: Rotator cuff arthropathy, *J Bone Joint Surg* 81A:1312, 1999.

Jensen MC et al: Magnetic resonance imaging of the lumbar spine in people without back pain, *N Engl J Med* 331:69, 1994.

Jimenez DF, Gibbs SR, Clapper AT: Endoscopic treatment of carpal tunnel syndrome: a critical review, *J Neurosurg* 88:817, 1998.

Katz JN: The assessment and management of low back pain: a critical review, *Arthritis Care Res* 6:104, 1993.

Katz JN et al: The carpal tunnel syndrome: diagnostic utility of the history and physical examination findings, *Ann Intern Med* 11:321, 1990.

Katz JN et al: Maine carpal tunnel study: outcomes of operative and nonoperative therapy for carpal tunnel syndrome in a community-based cohort, *J Hand Surg* 23:697, 1998.

Katz JN et al: Predictors of surgical outcome in degenerative lumbar spinal stenosis, *Spine* 24:2229, 1999.

Katz JN et al: Differences in functional status between men and women undergoing major orthopedic surgery for osteoarthritis, *Arthritis Rheum* 37:687, 1994.

Lawrence RC et al: Estimates of the prevalence of arthritis and selected musculoskeletal disorders in the United States, *Arthritis Rheum* 41:778, 1998.

Malanga GA, Nadler SF: Nonoperative treatment of low back pain, *Mayo Clin Proc* 74:1135, 1999.

Morrison DS, Fragmeni A, Woodworth P: Non-operative treatment of subacromial impingement syndrome, *J Bone Joint Surg* 79A:732, 1997.

Mueller T, Nikolic A, Vecsei V: Recommendations for the diagnosis of traumatic meniscal injuries in athletes, *Sports Med* 27:337, 1999.

Oliveria SA et al: Body weight, body mass index, and incident osteoarthritis of the hand, hip and knee, *Epidemiology* 10:161, 1999.

Rettig AC: Elbow, forearm and wrist injuries in the athlete, *Sports Med* 25:115, 1998.

Rivest C et al: Effects of epidural steroid injection on pain due to lumbar spinal stenosis or herniated disks: a prospective study, *Arthritis Care Res* 11:291, 1998.

Sanchis-Alfonso V et al: Pathogenesis of anterior knee pain syndrome and functional patellofemoral instability in the active young, *Am J Knee Surg* 12:29, 1999.

Sandmark H et al: Osteoarthrosis of the knee in men and women in association with overweight, smoking and hormone therapy, *Ann Rheum Dis* 58:151, 1999.

Solomon DH et al: Nonoccupational risk factors for carpal tunnel syndrome, *J Gen Intern Med* 14:310, 1999.

Steinfeld R, ValenteRM, Stuart MJ: A commonsense approach to shoulder problems, *Mayo Clin Proc* 74:785, 1999.

Towheed TE, Anastassiades TP: Glucosamine therapy in osteoarthritis, *J Rheumatol* 26:2294, 1999.

Towheed TE, Hochberg MC: A systematic review of randomized controlled trials of pharmacological therapy in osteoarthritis of the knee, with an emphasis on trial methodology, *Semin Arthritis Rheum* 26:755, 1997.

Van der Hoogen HJ et al: On the course of low back pain in general practice: a one year follow up study, *Ann Rheum Dis* 57:13, 1998.

Wainner RS, Hasz M: Management of calcific tendinitis of the shoulder, *J Orthop Sports Phys Ther* 27:231, 1998.

Weiss AP, Akelman E, Tabatabai M: Treatment of de Quervain's disease, *J Hand Surg* 19A:595, 1994.

CHAPTER 36

Rheumatoid Arthritis

Bonnie L. Bermas

EPIDEMIOLOGY AND RISK FACTORS

Rheumatoid arthritis (RA) is a chronic systemic inflammatory disease that affects the musculoskeletal system and other organ systems. The worldwide prevalence of rheumatoid arthritis is estimated to be between 1% and 2%. Two to three times as many women as men have this disease. Although rheumatoid arthritis can occur at any age, the peak onset is in the fourth to sixth decade of life. In women over the age of 65, the prevalence of RA is about 4%.

The HLA haplotypes, HLA-DR 4 and DR, are found in greater frequency in patients with rheumatoid arthritis. In RA patients, these haplotypes contain an area of DNA sequence that is similar and is called a shared epitope. The penetrance in patients who contain this epitope is incomplete as manifested by the rheumatoid arthritis concordance rate of 30% in monozygotic twins. First-degree relatives of patients with rheumatoid arthritis have a 3% to 5% risk of developing the disease.

PATHOPHYSIOLOGY

The etiology of rheumatoid arthritis is unclear. Many researchers believe that infectious or environmental triggers may precipitate rheumatoid arthritis in genetically predisposed individuals. These triggers probably activate the T lymphocytes that in turn causes the secretion of inflammatory mediators such as cytokines. These cytokines stimulate the proliferation of synovial cells. The growing synovium can then destroy cartilage and underlying bone.

Relationship of Estrogens to Rheumatoid Arthritis

During pregnancy, a high estrogen state, rheumatoid arthritis improves in 70% to 80% of patients. The incidence of rheumatoid arthritis in women increases after menopause. These observations have led researchers to hypothesize that rheumatoid arthritis may improve with estrogen-containing therapy. However, studies in patients with RA who have received oral contraceptives and estrogen replacement therapy have failed to demonstrate any disease improvement.

CLINICAL PRESENTATION

The diagnosis of rheumatoid arthritis is based on a careful history, physical examination, and laboratory testing. The ACR criteria (Table 36-1) are still used to confirm the diagnosis. Rheumatoid arthritis should be considered as a diagnosis in patients who present with several weeks of pain and joint swelling. However, other inflammatory conditions should also be investigated (see section on differential diagnosis).

Patients with rheumatoid arthritis typically present to their health care provider with a several week history of joint pain, stiffness, and swelling. Occasionally patients may present for evaluation after only a few days of severe polyarticular joint pain and swelling. Almost any joint can be involved, but the most commonly affected joints are the proximal interphalangeal (PIP) and MCP (metacarpal phalangeal) joints of the hand, the wrist joints, the elbows, the shoulders, the upper cervical spine, the jaw, the hips, the knees, the ankles, and the feet. Often, patients will require several hours to loosen up their joints in the morning, a symptom commonly referred to as morning stiffness. The clinician can assess for morning stiffness by asking patients how long it takes them to feel their best during the day. Greater than 1 hour of morning stiffness is considered significant for active disease. Some patients, after sitting for any prolonged period, will also experience stiffness and will have to reloosen up their joints. This latter phenomenon is called "gelling." Other symptoms include fevers, fatigue, weight loss, and generalized achiness.

On examination, the patient's joints may appear red or feel warm. The joints can be swollen and the range of motion can be decreased. Patients may have squeeze tenderness or pain with movement of the joint (Boxes 36-1 and 36-2). They may also have muscle weakness and atrophy in the muscles surrounding the affected joint. If the inflammation continues unchecked, joint deformities, secondary osteoarthritis, tendon damage, and tendon ruptures can occur. These changes generally do not occur until the patient has had disease for more than a year (Box 36-3).

Major Joint Involvement

Most patients with rheumatoid arthritis will have involvement in their **hands and wrists.** Swelling and pain are common in the proximal interphalangeal (PIP) and metacarpal phalangeal (MCP) joints. The wrist joints are also involved, especially in patients who present with adult onset Still's disease.

Table 36-1
The American Rheumatism Association 1987 Revised Criteria for the Classification of Rheumatoid Arthritis

Criterion*	Definition
Morning stiffness	Morning stiffness in and around the joints, lasting at least 1 hour before maximal improvement
Arthritis of three or more joint areas	At least three joint areas simultaneously have had soft tissue swelling or fluid (not bony overgrowth alone) observed by a physician. The 14 possible areas are right or left PIP, MCP, wrist, elbow, knee, ankle, and MTP joints
Arthritis of hand joints	At least one area swollen (as defined above) in a wrist, MCP, or PIP joint
Symmetric arthritis	Simultaneous involvement of the same joint areas (as defined in 2) on both sides of the body (bilateral involvement of PIPs, MCPs, or MTPs is acceptable without absolute symmetry)
Rheumatoid nodules	Subcutaneous nodules, over bony prominences, or extensor surfaces, or in juxta-articular regions, observed by a physician
Serum rheumatoid factor	Demonstration of abnormal amounts of serum rheumatoid factor by any method for which the result has been positive in <5% of normal control subjects
Radiographic changes	Radiographic changes typical in rheumatoid arthritis on posterior hand and wrist radiographs, which must include erosions or unequivocal bony decalcification localized in or most marked adjacent to the involved joints (osteoarthritis changes alone do not qualify)

*For classification purposes, a patient shall be said to have rheumatoid arthritis if he/she has satisfied at least 4 of these 7 criteria. Criteria 1 through 4 must have been present for at least 6 weeks. Patients with 2 clinical diagnoses are not excluded. Designation as classic, definite, or probable rheumatoid arthritis is *not* to be made.

BOX 36-1
Key Features of the History

Morning stiffness
Persistent pain and swelling of joints:
  PIP and MCP joints of hands and wrists
  Elbows, shoulders, knees, ankles, feet
Pain and stiffness of cervical spine

BOX 36-2
Key Findings on Physical Examination

Joint swelling and pain
  PIP, MCP of wrist joints
  Symmetric swelling
Swelling of periarticular soft tissue, synovial thickening, and/or joint effusions
Deformities (generally in long-standing disease):
  Ulnar deviation of fingers MCP joints
  Extensor subluxation of metacarpals at MCP joints
  Swan-neck deformities
  Boutonniere deformities
  Ankylosing of wrist and ankle
  Hallux valgus
  Subluxation of metatarsophalangeal joints
  Flexion deformities of toes

BOX 36-3
Chronic Joint Changes Seen in Rheumatoid Arthritis

Ulnar deviation of the MCP joints
Swan-neck deformities
Boutonniere deformities
Volar subluxation of the hands or the wrists
Fusions of the wrists and ankles
Hallus valgus
Flexion deformities of toes
Subluxation of metatarsophalangeal joints

The **elbows** can be involved in rheumatoid arthritis. Patients will often hold their elbows in fixed flexion with joint inflammation.

The **shoulder** can be involved in rheumatoid arthritis. Reaching, lifting, and activities of daily living such as combing one's hair can be limited in patients with shoulder disease. Shoulder involvement can be difficult to distinguish from other disorders, in particular, rotator cuff tendinitis and frozen shoulders, as well as polymyalgia rheumatica (PMR).

The upper **cervical spine,** mainly C1 and C2, can be affected by rheumatoid arthritis. When the involvement is severe, instability myelopathy and neurologic symptoms can occur. Patients with rheumatoid arthritis who complain of neck pain should have a careful neurologic examination and often require radiographic evaluation.

The **hip** is commonly involved in RA. In early disease, the findings can be subtle. Often patients will complain of difficulty getting out of a chair, crossing legs, and putting on their shoes and socks. On physical examination, loss of internal rotation of the hip is one of the earliest findings.

The **knees** are often involved in rheumatoid arthritis. Effusions, synovial thickening, and reduced range of motion can be readily detected.

As in the hands, the **feet** are commonly involved in rheumatoid arthritis. Joint swelling, pain, and stiffness are common. Hammer toes and other deformities can occur.

Extraarticular Manifestations of Rheumatoid Arthritis (Box 36-4)

Rheumatoid **nodules** are subcutaneous nodules that generally appear on the extensor surfaces of the joints. The hands, elbows and the Achilles tendon are all common locations

---

BOX 36-4
Extraarticular Manifestations

Rheumatoid nodules
Rheumatoid vasculitis
Pleural disease
Pericardial effusion/pericarditis
Neurologic
    Entrapment neuropathies
    Carpal tunnel syndrome
    Tarsal tunnel syndrome
    Cervical cord compression
    Mononeuritis multiplex
Eye
    Xerophthalmia
    Keratoconjunctivitis sicca
    Episcleritis
    Scleritis
Anemia
Felty's syndrome
Still's disease

---

for these nodules. They are seen in 30% of patients with rheumatoid arthritis, and most patients with nodules will have a positive rheumatoid factor. Occasionally they can get superinfected. They can also be seen in the lung and in the eye (sclera). When they occur in the lung, Caplan's syndrome, they need to be differentiated from other pulmonary nodules.

Bone thinning can occur in rheumatoid arthritis both from the disease process itself and some of the medications that are used to treat rheumatoid arthritis. Periarticular bone thinning is one of the first abnormalities seen on radiographic examination.

Muscle inflammation or **myositis** is occasionally seen in patients with rheumatoid arthritis. Proximal muscle weakness can occur after prolonged corticosteroid use.

Pleuritic chest pain and pleural inflammation are the most common **pulmonary manifestations** of RA. Patients can get an interstitial pneumonitis and fibrosis. Smokers and patients with pneumoconiosis are particularly at risk. Rheumatoid nodules can occur in the lung and can be difficult to distinguish from other lesions. Bronchiolitis obliterans and organizing pneumonia (BOOP) and pulmonary fibrosis can also occur.

The most common **cardiac manifestation** of rheumatoid arthritis is pericarditis. Myocarditis can rarely occur.

Renal involvement in rheumatoid arthritis is rare and is most likely secondary to treatment in particular nonsteroidal antiinflammatory drugs (NSAIDs), gold, and cyclosporine therapy.

Patients with rheumatoid arthritis can develop a small or medium vessel **vasculitis.** In the small vessel vasculitis, purpura, splinter hemorrhages, and small ulcerations can occur. Some patients may have associated cryoglobulinemia. In the medium vessel vasculitis, mononeuritis multiplex can occur. The most common clinical presentation of mononeuritis multiplex is a foot drop. These patients may require high-dose immunosuppressive therapy or even cyclophosphamide therapy.

Ocular involvement most commonly manifests as episcleritis, which causes mild pain and redness, lasting only a few weeks. Scleritis, which is much rarer, can cause severe pain and ulcerations that can result in permanent damage to the eye. Occasionally rheumatoid nodules appear in the sclera.

Sjögren's syndrome or keratoconjunctivitis sicca can be seen in patients with rheumatoid arthritis. Patients complain of dry irritated eyes with associated itchiness. In severe cases abrasions and infections can happen. Patients may also have decreased saliva production. This can lead to dry mouth and dental caries.

Carpal tunnel syndrome can occur in patients with RA. Inflammation within the carpal tunnel with concomitant compression of the medial nerve lead to the finding. Symptoms include burning and numbness of the thumb, index finger, middle finger, and radial portion of the fourth finger. Many patients will complain of diffuse hand numbness. Symptoms tend to be worse at night and can awaken the patient from sleep. Patients may also complain of weakness and pain in their hands, forearms, and upper arms. Similar symptoms can occur in the feet if the tarsal tunnel becomes compressed.

DIAGNOSTIC TESTS

In all 70% to 80% of patients with rheumatoid arthritis will have a positive rheumatoid factor. The rheumatoid factor is an immunoglobulin (Ig)M directed against the Fc portion of IgG. It is detected by a latex-fixed agglutination technique. Nearly all patients who form rheumatoid nodules will have a positive rheumatoid nodule. The diagnosis of rheumatoid arthritis can be made in the absence of a rheumatoid factor. Conversely, having a rheumatoid factor that is positive does not make the diagnosis of rheumatoid arthritis, as roughly 3% to 5% of the population will have a positive rheumatoid factor. Rheumatoid factors are more common after an infection, in patients with cancer, as patients get older, or with other medical conditions (Box 36-5).

Many patients with rheumatoid arthritis will have an elevated erythrocyte sedimentation rate (ESR) or C-reactive protein (CRP) during periods of disease activity. For some of these patients, these laboratory tests can be a useful way of monitoring how a patient is responding to therapy.

Patients with rheumatoid arthritis can have an anemia of chronic disease. This normocytic anemia usually will improve with disease treatment. Occasionally, patients with rheumatoid arthritis will have low complement levels.

Synovial fluid analysis of an involved joint will show an inflammatory fluid, white blood cell count >2000/mm^2. The protein tends to be high and the glucose is low to normal.

OTHER PRESENTATIONS OF RHEUMATOID ARTHRITIS

Rheumatoid arthritis can sometimes present as a disorder characterized by high fevers, a skin rash that comes and goes, and joint swelling. Hepatosplenomegaly and elevated white blood cell counts can be seen. This condition is called **Still's disease.** Although this disorder is much more common in the pediatric population, it should be considered in the patient who present with fevers of unknown origin.

Felty's syndrome is a disorder where patients have neutropenia in the setting of rheumatoid arthritis. Constitutional

BOX 36-5
Conditions in Which a Positive Rheumatoid Factor Is Frequently Present

Rheumatologic Diseases
Rheumatoid arthritis
Systemic lupus erythematosus
Sjögren's syndrome
Scleroderma
Polymyositis/dermatomyositis
Mixed cryoglobulinemia

Infectious Diseases
Bacterial endocarditis
Tuberculosis
Syphilis
Viral hepatitis
Schistosomiasis
Leprosy
Kala azar

Noninfectious Conditions
Healthy elderly persons
Chronic active hepatitis and cirrhosis of the liver
Diffuse interstitial pulmonary fibrosis and silicosis
Intravenous drug abuse
Sarcoidosis
Waldenström's macroglobulinemia

Modified from Zvaifler NJ. In Schumacher HR Jr, Klippel JH, Robinson DR, editors: *Primer on the rheumatic diseases,* ed 9, Atlanta, 1988, The Arthritis Foundation.

BOX 36-6
Differential Diagnosis

Polymyalgia rheumatica (PMR)
Systemic lupus erythematosus (SLE)
Psoriatic arthritis (PA)
Inflammatory bowel disease (IBD) associated arthritis
Reiter's syndrome
Sarcoidosis (Lofgren's syndrome)
Lyme arthritis
Septic arthritis
Viral arthropathy
Crystal induced arthropathy including polyarticular gout and pseudogout
Osteoarthritis
Tendinitis
Fibromyalgia

symptom, splenomegaly, lymphadenopathy, leg ulcers, and thrombocytopenia can occur.

Palindromic rheumatism is an associated disorder in which patients get episodes of migratory joint pain and inflammation that can occur for a few days or a few weeks. Some patients will have only one episode; others will have several episodes but no long-term joint destruction or involvement. Finally, others will develop into full-blown rheumatoid arthritis.

Differential Diagnosis

Rheumatoid arthritis can be difficult to distinguish from other inflammatory joint conditions including systemic lupus erythematosus (SLE), psoriatic arthritis, inflammatory bowel disease associated arthritis, polyarticular gout, polyarticular septic arthritis, rheumatic fever, viral arthritis, and fibromyalgia (Box 36-6).

One of the key features of rheumatoid arthritis is the radiographic changes that are seen in the joints. Cartilage erosion and symmetric joint space narrow, periarticular osteopenia, are some of the abnormalities seen on radiographs. Magnetic resonance imaging (MRI) can demonstrate synovial thickening and pannus formation, as well as early cartilage destruction.

Polymyalgia rheumatica (PMR) can be particularly difficult to distinguish from rheumatoid arthritis in the elderly population. Patients with PMR are over 50 years old, have achiness and stiffness in their shoulders and hips, and have an elevated erythrocyte sedimentation rate (ESR). Some rheumatologists believe that patients with PMR can have in-

volvement of their wrists and hands. These latter patients can be difficult to distinguish from patients with RA. A rheumatoid factor can be helpful in making the correct diagnosis.

In the younger female patient, SLE can be confused with rheumatoid arthritis. Patients with SLE generally have more skin findings and systemic findings and less joint swelling than is found in rheumatoid arthritis. In all, 95% of patients with SLE will have a positive antinuclear antibody test. Some patients have features of both rheumatoid arthritis and SLE and may be called "rhupus."

Patients with psoriatic arthritis, Reiter's syndrome, and inflammatory bowel disease associated arthritis tend to have fewer joints involved and less symmetric involvement. They are more likely to have PIP and DIP swelling and will rarely have MCP swelling. They tend to get joint involvement in a ray (the MCP, PIP, and DIP joint of the same digit) rather than joint involvement across all of the MCP or PIP joints.

✱ MANAGEMENT

Some patients will have a mild intermittent course, which requires minimal pharmacologic intervention. Most patients will have a chronic course that will progress and lead to joint damage without medications.

The treatment of rheumatoid arthritis involves a multidisciplinary approach. Education, medications, physical therapy, occupational therapy, and orthopedic intervention all play a role. Alternative therapy such as nutritional supplementation, acupuncture, and behavioral modification may be beneficial as well. When considering pharmacologic therapy, consultation or co-management with a rheumatologist is appropriate.

Pharmacologic Therapy (Table 36-2)

Many medications are available for the treatment of rheumatoid arthritis. The original treatment paradigm for rheumatoid arthritis was to start patients on aspirin and nonsteroidals after diagnosis. If these medications did not work, then corticosteroids were added. If corticosteroids did not work or were used for a long period, a second-line agent was added. This approach was referred to as the treatment pyramid. During the last decade, this approach has fallen out of favor. In general, when a patient is diagnosed with rheumatoid

Table 36-2
Drugs for the Treatment of Rheumatoid Arthritis

	Hydroxychloroquine	Gold Compounds	Sulfasalazine	Methotrexate	Penicillamine	Azathioprine
Indications	Disease unresponsive to NSAIDs and physical medicine; seronegative or less aggressive disease than for gold or methotrexate as the first SAARD	Disease unresponsive or progressive on hydroxychloroquine regimen or disease responsive to NSAIDs and relatively more aggressive disease	Disease unresponsive or progressive on hydroxychloroquine regimen or disease unresponsive to NSAIDs and relatively more aggressive disease	Disease unresponsive or progressive on hydroxychloroquine regimen or disease unresponsive to NSAIDs and relatively more agressive disease	Failure of gold and methotrexate	Failure of gold, methotrexate, and penicillamine
Relative contraindications	Preexisting macular disease	Proteinuria, renal disease	Allergy to sulfa antibiotics, sensitivity to salicylates; porphyria	Alcohol consumption; liver or renal disease	Proteinuria, renal disease	Renal or liver disease
Usual dosage	200-400 mg qd	10-mg test dose; week 2 start 50 mg IM q/wk, tapering to 50 mg q/mo, starting after 0.5-1 g auranofin 3 mg bid 50 mg q/wk	2-4 divided tid to qid	7.5-15 mg once weekly; can be in divided doses over 1 day	125-750 mg daily; start with 125 daily and advance by 125 mg/mo	50-150 mg/day; start with 50 mg qd and raise dose by 25 mg every other week
Maximal dosage	400 mg qd or 200 mg bid		1 g qid	25 mg q/wk	750 mg daily	200 mg qd
Major and common toxicities	Gastrointestinal upset, pigmented macular degeneration and rashes	Rashes, oral ulcers, rare exfoliation, membranous glomerular nephritis, bone marrow suppression	Rashes (may rarely be severe), hepatitis, bone marrow suppression, renal toxicity	Rashes, oral ulcers; rarely pulmonary or hepatic fibrosis, or cirrhosis; bone marrow suppression	Rashes, oral ulcers, membranous glomerular nephritis, bone marrow, suppression, and rarely autoimmune diseases	Gastrointestinal upset, rashes, and bone marrow suppression
Suggested monitoring	Ophthalmologic examinations at baseline and q6mo, including Amsler grids, color vision testing, and retinal examinations	CBC, differential and platelet count; urine dipstick before each injection	CBC, differential, and platelet count, BUN, creatinine and liver function tests every 4-6 wk	CBC, differential, and platelet count' BUN, creatinine and liver function tests every 4-6 wk	CBC, differential, and platelet count; urine dipstick for protein every 2 wk; may lengthen interval to monthly at 6 mo	CBC, differential, and platelet count, before adjusting dosage and every month; liver function tests every month
Length of typical trial	3-6 mo	6 mo	6 mo	3 mo	7-9 mo	3 mo
FDA category for pregnancy	No official category; not recommended in pregnancy	Category C	Category B	Category X	No official category; not recommended in pregnancy	Category D

Modified from Ruddy S, Roberts WN: In Kassirer JP, editor: *Current therapy in internal medicine*, ed 3 Philadelphia, 1991, BC Decker.
NSAIDs, Nonsteriodal antiinflammatory agents; *SAARD*, slow-acting antirheumatic drugs; *CBC*, complete blood count; *BUN*, blood urea nitrogen.

arthritis, NSAIDs and corticosteroids may be used at the outset for symptom relief. However, clinicians are more aggressive about starting a second-line agent shortly after diagnosis. Some clinicians prefer using less toxic second-line agents such as antimalarials, gold, and azathioprine; but many clinicians are using more potent and toxic therapy such as methotrexate early after disease diagnosis. More recently, the use of combination therapy, two or more second-line agents, has been advocated as the best approach to active rheumatoid arthritis. Methotrexate is considered the cornerstone of therapy unless a patient cannot tolerate this drug. The use of the newer agents such as a TNF-alpha blocker and leflunomide before initiation or more standard therapy is unclear.

Aspirin and NSAIDs are among the more commonly used medications in the treatment of rheumatoid arthritis. These medications block the production of prostaglandins, substances that mediate joint inflammation. The nonsteroidals are effective medications in reducing pain and inflammation. They are often used in early disease or in combination with other medications. They have no effect on disease course and are used for symptom relief. The major side effect of NSAIDs is the gastrointestinal toxicity particularly seen in older patients. Gastric erosions and sometimes ulcers can occur. Patients need to be monitored for these symptoms. Patients need to have their renal and liver function monitored with prolonged NSAID use, as these medications can be toxic to the kidneys and the liver. Other side effects include dyspepsia, nausea, headaches, and confusion. These medications can interfere with the metabolism of warfarin (Coumadin) and should not be used in patients on this medication. In addition, aspirin and NSAIDs can interfere with platelet function and need to be discontinued before surgery.

Recently, newer nonsteroidal type medications have been developed. These medications are selective **Cox-2 inhibitors.** Because the gastrointestinal tract has Cox-1 inhibitors, this new class of medications was developed to avoid gastrointestinal toxicity. Although, the Cox-2 inhibitors dramatically reduce the risk of gastrointestinal toxicity, they do not eradicate the risk of this toxicity and should still be used cautiously if at all in individuals with a history of ulcer disease. Because these medications do not act on platelets, their use can be continued up to surgery. Furthermore, these medications theoretically do not interact with warfarin and can be used in patients on these medications. Patients on warfarin should have their prothrombin time monitored carefully at the initiation of therapy with Cox-2 inhibitors to ensure that no interaction is occurring.

Corticosteroids can be used to treat the inflammation and pain of rheumatoid arthritis. These medications have the advantage of quick onset of action and the majority of patients will respond. However, the many side effects of glucocorticoids, both short-term (glucose intolerance, hypertension) and long-term (Cushingoid appearance, osteoporosis, weight gain, stria, avascular necrosis, adrenal suppression), make this medications less than ideal. Intraarticular steroids are sometimes used for immediate relief from joint inflammation.

Second-line agents (also called SSARDs and DMARDs) are medications that theoretically modify the underlying process of rheumatoid arthritis. These medications can take from a few weeks to a few months to start to work. Almost all of these medications have toxicities that require the monitoring of organ system.

The **antimalarial medications** hydroxychloroquine and chloroquine have been used for many years in the treatment of rheumatoid arthritis. The antimalarials take 4 to 12 weeks to start to work. These medications are well tolerated and are effective against mild rheumatoid arthritis. The major side effect is retinal toxicity that tends to occur in older patients. Regular ophthalmologic examinations (every 6 months) should be done in patients on these medications to prevent ocular damage. Some patients may develop a rash to hydroxychloroquine and rarely bone marrow toxicities can be seen.

Gold salts have been used in the treatment of rheumatoid arthritis for many years. They can be used in an injectable form or taken orally. However, the oral preparations have not been shown to be as effective as the injectable forms in studies. This medication takes 6 to 12 weeks to work. Patients can get skin rashes, oral ulcers, and occasionally hair loss. The major toxicities include proteinuria and hematologic abnormalities, so the renal and hematologic organ systems need to be monitored on a regular basis.

Penicillamine has been used to treat rheumatoid arthritis for many years. This medication has many side effects and is rarely used.

Azathioprine is an immunosuppressive medication that is predominantly used for the immunosuppression of organ transplant recipients. Although not one of the more commonly utilized medications, it can be used in RA patients who have not responded to other second-line agents.

Cyclosporine is also an immunosuppressive agent that has been used in patients who have received transplants. This medication can be used for the treatment of rheumatoid arthritis alone or in combination with other medications.

Although **sulfasalazine** is better known for its treatment of inflammatory bowel disease, this medication was originally developed to treat rheumatoid arthritis. It was rarely used in the United States until the late 1980s. This medication has some hepatotoxicity and bone marrow suppression, so these organ systems need to be monitored. In general, it has a fast onset of action, 2 to 3 weeks, and is well tolerated. It is less toxic than methotrexate and may be a viable alternative for patients with moderate disease.

Methotrexate is a folic acid antagonist that has been used as a chemotherapeutic agent. In the early 1980s, it was shown to be an effective agent for the treatment of rheumatoid arthritis and is now the cornerstone of any RA treatment regimen. This medication is highly effective and has a quick onset of action. Side effects include oral ulcers and hair loss. The major toxicities are hepatotoxicities and hematologic toxicities. For the former, patients should avoid alcohol intake and use of hepatotoxic medications. For the latter, patients should be given either folic acid or folinic acid to avoid toxicity. There is a hypothetical risk of non-Hodgkin's lymphoma with methotrexate that goes away on drug removal.

The **cytotoxic agents** such as cyclophosphamide are reserved for patients with complicated systemic features of RA or patients who have been refractory to other second-line agents.

More recently there have been several biologic agents approved that are **antibodies directed against TNF-alpha,** an inflammatory cytokine that is thought to be important in the mediation of the inflammation and joint destruction seen in RA. These medications are either given in biweekly injections or by monthly infusions. These medications are contraindicated in debilitated individuals who have comorbidity that can predispose them to infection or in patients who have had cancer. These are extremely costly medications and should probably be prescribed only after consultation with a rheumatologist.

Leflunomide is related to thalidomide. This medication has recently been approved for use in rheumatoid arthritis and is effective either alone or in combination with methotrexate. This medication is extremely teratogenic and should be used cautiously in patients of child-bearing potential. Reliable contraception and careful counseling are required in patients who are of child-bearing age who use this medication.

There have been several studies that have shown that **antibiotics** such as minocycline can be effective in the treatment of mild rheumatoid arthritis. This treatment is not commonly used.

Other Treatments

Data on the use of **nutritional supplements** in rheumatoid arthritis have been equivocal at best. Some studies have shown that diets extremely high in fish oils can cause modest improvement in the symptoms of rheumatoid arthritis. However, the amount of fish oils that patients had to ingest led to multiple side effects. Although the newer cartilage supplements such as chondroitin sulfate and hyaluronic acid have been shown in limited studies to be beneficial for the treatment of osteoarthritis, there have been no studies demonstrating their effectiveness in the treatment of rheumatoid arthritis.

Physical and occupational therapy are crucial in the treatment of rheumatoid arthritis. The physical therapist can help with the rehabilitation of joints post surgery or can strengthen an improve range of motion. The occupational therapist can help patients with splinting or adaptive devices to make the activities of daily living more tenable.

Joint replacement surgery has revolutionized the treatment of chronic long-standing RA. The techniques have improved over the last 10 years, and the outcomes are significantly better. Joint replacement therapy can make a dramatic improvement in the quality of life of patients with rheumatoid arthritis.

Many patients with RA use **complementary therapy.** One study found that 90% of RA patients had used some form of complementary therapy defined as herbal remedies, chiropractic manipulations, high-dose vitamins, and elimination diets. Although few studies have explored the efficacy of these treatments, they probably play a role as adjunctive therapy in patients with RA.

PREGNANCY AND RHEUMATOID ARTHRITIS

Patients with rheumatoid arthritis have no reduction in fertility or increased risk of miscarriage. In general, patients do well, with about 70% to 80% of patients going into remission when pregnant. Unfortunately, many of these patients will flare again in the postpartum period. Some medications such as glucocorticoids, azathioprine, cyclosporine, and sulfasalazine may be used cautiously during pregnancy. Glucocorticoids slightly increase the risk of cleft palate. Glucocorticoids, azathioprine, and cyclosporine predispose for premature rupture of the membranes, intrauterine growth retardation, and small-for-gestational-age infants and should be used cautiously. Penicillamine, cyclophosphamide, methotrexate, and leflunomide are all absolutely contraindicated for use during pregnancy. A high-risk obstetrician or a rheumatologist with expertise in this area can help with the decision of what treatments are appropriate during pregnancy.

BIBLIOGRAPHY

Bermas BL, Hill JA: Immunosuppressive drugs during pregnancy, *Arthritis Rheum* 38:1722, 1995.

Gregerson PK, Silver J, Winchester RJ: The shared epitome hypotheses: an approach to understanding the molecular genetics of susceptibility to rheumatoid arthritis, *Arthritis Rheum* 34:43, 1991.

Harris ED: Pathogenesis of rheumatoid arthritis, *Up To Date* 2000.

Lanza FL et al: A pilot endoscopic study of the gastroduodenal effects of SC-58635 as COX-2 inhibitor, *Arthritis Rheum* 40:S93, 1997.

Liang MH, Karlson EW: Female hormone therapy and the risk of developing of exacerbating systemic lupus erythematosus or rheumatoid arthritis, *Proc Assoc Am Physicians* 108:25, 1996.

Moreland LW et al: Treatment of rheumatoid arthritis with a recombinant human tumor necrosis factor receptor (p75)-Fc fusion protein, *N Engl J Med* 337:141, 1997.

Pincus T, O'Dell JR, Kremer JM: Combination therapy with multiple disease modifying anti-rheumatic drugs in rheumatoid arthritis: a preventive strategy, *Ann Intern Med* 131:768, 1999.

Rao JK et al: Use of complementary therapies for arthritis among patients of rheumatologists, *Ann Intern Med* 131:409, 1999.

Shmerling RH, Delbanco TL: The rheumatoid factor: an analysis of clinical utility, *Am J Med* 91:528, 1991.

Smolen JS et al: Efficacy and safety of leflunomide compared with placebo and sulphasalazine in active rheumatoid arthritis: a double blind, randomised, multicentre trial, *Lancet* 353:259, 1999.

Spector TD: Rheumatoid arthritis, *Rhem Dis Clin North Am* 16:513, 1990.

Stein CM et al: Combination treatment of severe RA with cyclosporine and methotrexate for forty-eight weeks, *Arthritis Rheum* 40:1843, 1997.

Wolfe F et al: Use of second line "disease modifying" anti-rheumatic drugs (DMARDs) within 5 months of disease onset by 64% of 750 rheumatoid arthritis patients under care of 142 US rheumatologists: an inception cohort study, *Arthritis Rheum* 40:S218, 1997.

CHAPTER **37**

Antiphospholipid Antibody Syndrome

Kristine Phillips
Bonnie L. Bermas

The antiphospholipid antibody syndrome (APS) is a disorder in which patients produce specific antibodies directed against phospholipids in the setting of recurrent venous or arterial thrombotic events or recurrent fetal losses. Other associated features include migraines, Raynaud's disease, thrombocytopenia, hemolytic anemia, and renal disease.

EPIDEMIOLOGY

Primary APS is found in patients with no clinical evidence of any other autoimmune conditions. When this disorder is found in patients with other autoimmune conditions, it is called secondary APS. Secondary APS has been reported in patients with systemic lupus erythematosus (SLE), as well as other rheumatic diseases such as rheumatoid arthritis or scleroderma; after some infectious diseases; and after the administration of certain medications. Although women are more frequently diagnosed with the condition, the actual prevalence of the syndrome is unknown. About 1% to 2% of the healthy adult population produces antiphospholipid antibodies. The significance of these antibodies in the healthy adult population is unclear.

CLINICAL PRESENTATION AND EVALUATION

In evaluating a patient for the presence of the APS, a complete history and physical examination should be performed.

Antiphospholipid antibodies can precipitate the formation of a clot. Thus patients with the APS may develop **venous** or **arterial thrombi.** Clots can occur in any of a number of places, and the symptoms may be different at each site. Patients who have venous events tend to have recurrent venous events, and patients who have arterial events tend to have recurrent arterial events.

Many of the associated symptoms result from these blood clots. For example, if blood clots have occurred in the lungs, **pulmonary hypertension** can develop. If a clot occurs in an artery that supplies bone, **avascular necrosis** can result. Antiphospholipid antibodies have been implicated in 20% of individuals under age 40 years who present with a **stroke** or **heart attack** with no other risk factors. *Sneddon's syndrome,* stroke in young women who have livedo reticularis, has been attributed to APS. Other neurologic symptoms in-

clude seizures, myelopathy, and chorea. Heart valve abnormalities, although rare, do occur and may be demonstrated by echocardiogram. Small heart valve vegetations, which are thought to be microthrombi, are called *Leibman-Sacks endocarditis.* Renal involvement is unusual but can occur with resultant renal failure in some cases. Biopsy reveals microthrombi but no autoimmune deposit. A rare complication is sudden multisystem occlusive disease, where multiple clots occur at once. This rare life-threatening condition can be difficult to treat.

Many patients will develop a fine lacy rash over the legs known as livedo reticularis. This is common in young women, particularly after cold exposure. Migraine headaches or Raynaud's phenomenon are also seen in patients with the APS.

DIAGNOSTIC TESTS

Thrombocytopenia is one of the most common findings in the APS. For most, the number is only mildly decreased and no specific therapy is required. Clinically significant thrombocytopenia can be treated with steroids, danazol, intravenous immune globulin (IVIG), and splenectomy (see Management). A large proportion of patients with Evan's syndrome (hemolytic anemia and thrombocytopenia) has antiphospholipid antibodies.

Blood testing should be done for the presence of antiphospholipid antibodies. Three types of blood tests can be performed.

Anticardiolipin Antibody

Many different types of antiphospholipid antibodies are used; however, the immunoglobulin (Ig)G and IgM anticardiolipin antibodies are the only approved tests to make the diagnosis of the APS. The newer β2 glycoprotein I may also be tested. Testing is most valid in laboratories that have been standardized using an internationally accepted standardization.

Lupus Anticoagulant

Although patients with APS are thrombotic, standard testing for clotting—activated partial thromboplastin time, kaolin clotting time, platelet neutralizing, and Russell viper venom time can all be prolonged. This paradoxical prolongation is called a lupus anticoagulant. Some laboratories have developed specialized coagulation testing to evaluate for the presence of a lupus anticoagulant.

False-Positive VDRL

Patients with APS may have a false-positive VDRL but negative fluorescent treponemal antibody absorption (test) (FTA-ABS). This test is of low sensitivity and specificity and should not be sent as a screening tool.

Diagnosis of the syndrome is based on one clinical finding and one abnormal laboratory finding during the course of the disease. The abnormal antibody test must be positive on at least two occasions more than 3 months apart. If the clinician is suspicious that the patient has the disorder, both the anticardiolipin antibody and lupus anticoagulant should be tested, since some patients will have only one test that is positive (Box 37-1).

DIFFERENTIAL DIAGNOSIS

The presence of an antiphospholipid antibody in individuals with no symptoms does not imply that they will develop a blood clot in the future, but they are at higher risk for this complication. Before making a diagnosis of APS, the doctor must first exclude other disease states that may present in a similar fashion. Thromboses may be caused by other clotting disorders, and patients should be screened appropriately (e.g., Protein S, Protein C, antithrombin III, Factor V Leiden, prothrombin mutation 20210). The presence of more than one disorder may increase the risk of thrombosis.

✳ MANAGEMENT

Although smoking is never a good idea, it is particularly important that patients with APS discontinue smoking.

Patients who have experienced thrombosis should be treated with lifelong anticoagulation. Several studies have suggested that the INR be maintained at 3 to 3.5 to avoid further clots. If patients continue to suffer from repeated blood clots despite the use of adequate anticoagulation, high-dose steroids, and immunosuppression may be recommended. Plasmapheresis to remove the antibody has also been used on occasion. This procedure only temporarily removes the antibody from the blood and is only indicated for life-threatening situations. Patients with pregnancy complications should be treated with low-dose aspirin and heparin during the pregnancy. Occasionally IVIG is used. For patients with no history of blood clots but high levels of IgG anticardiolipin antibody or lupus anticoagulant, low-dose aspirin (81 mg) may be recommended for prophylaxis of blood clots, although there are no data to support this treatment's efficacy.

◼ PREGNANCY

Antiphospholipid antibodies can be associated with recurrent pregnancy losses. These generally occur in the late first trimester (after 10 weeks when the embryo becomes a fetus). This coincides with the dependence of the fetus on the placenta. Second trimester miscarriage and stillbirths can also occur. Other pregnancy complications include intrauterine growth retardation and preeclampsia. Postpartum

clotting events may be seen as well. Pathologic evaluation of the placenta reveals a small placenta that is filled with clots and thrombi.

Evaluation of the patient with recurrent miscarriages should include antiphospholipid antibody testing.

BOX 37-1

Preliminary Criteria for the Classification of the Antiphospholipid Syndrome

1. **Vascular Thrombosis**

   One or more clinical episodes of arterial, venous, or small vessel thrombosis, in any tissue or organ. Thrombosis must be confirmed by imaging or Doppler studies or histopathology, with the exception of superficial venous thrombosis. For histopathologic confirmation, thrombosis should be present without significant evidence of inflammation in the vessel wall.

2. **Pregnancy Morbidity**

   (a) One or more unexplained deaths of a morphologically normal fetus at or beyond the 10th week of gestation, with normal fetal morphology documented by ultrasound or by direct examination of the fetus, or

   (b) One or more premature births of a morphologically normal neonate at or before the 34th week of gestation because of severe preeclampsia or eclampsia, or severe placental insufficiency, or

   (c) Three or more unexplained consecutive spontaneous abortions before the 10th week of gestation, with maternal anatomic or hormonal abnormalities and paternal and maternal chromosomal causes excluded.

   In studies of populations of patients who have more than one type of pregnancy morbidity, investigators are strongly encouraged to stratify groups of subjects according to a, b, or c above.

Laboratory Criteria

1. Anticardiolipin antibody of IgG and/or IgM isotype in blood, present in medium or high titer, on two or more occasions, at least 6 weeks apart, measured by a standardized enzyme-linked immunosorbent assay for β2-glycoprotein I-dependent anticardiolipin antibodies.

2. Lupus anticoagulant present in plasma, on two or more occasions at least 6 weeks apart, detected according to the guidelines of the International Society on Thrombosis and Hemostasis (Scientific Subcommittee on Lupus Anticoagulants/Phospholipid-Dependent Antibodies), in the following steps:

   (a) Prolonged phospholipid-dependent coagulation demonstrated on a screening test (e.g., activated partial thromboplastin time, kaolin) clotting time, dilute Russell's viper venom time, dilute prothrombin time, Textarin time.

   (b) Failure to correct the prolonged coagulation time on the screening test by mixing with normal platelet-poor plasma.

   (c) Shortening or correction of the prolonged coagulation time on the screening test by the addition of excess phospholipid.

   (d) Exclusion of other coagulopathies (e.g., factor VIII inhibitor or heparin, as appropriate).

Definite antiphospholipid antibody syndrome is considered to be present if at least one of the clinical criteria and one of the laboratory criteria are met.

From Wilson WA et al: *Arthritis Rheum* 42:1309, 1999.

BIBLIOGRAPHY

Ames PR, Khamashta MA, Hughes GR: Clinical and therapeutic aspects of the antiphospholipid syndrome, *Lupus* 4(Suppl 1): p. S23, 1995.

Arnout JP, Meijer, Vermylen J: Lupus anticoagulant testing in Europe: an analysis of results from the first European Concerted Action on Thrombophilia (ECAT) survey using plasmas spiked with monoclonal antibodies against human beta2-glycoprotein I, *Thromb Haemost* 81:929, 1999.

Branch DW: Antiphospholipid antibodies and reproductive outcome: the current state of affairs, *J Reprod Immunol* 38:75, 1998.

Branch DW, Scott JR, Kochenour NK, Hershgold E: Obstetric complications associated with the lupus anticoagulant, *N Engl J Med* 313:1322, 1985.

Cuadrado MJ et al: Can neurologic manifestations of Hughes (antiphospholipid) syndrome be distinguished from multiple sclerosis? Analysis of 27 patients and review of the literature, *Medicine (Baltimore)* 79:57, 2000.

D'Agati V, Kunis C, Williams G, Appel GB: Anticardiolipin antibody and renal disease: a report of three cases, *J Am Soc Nephrol* 1:777, 1990.

Finazzi G: The Italian registry of antiphospholipid antibodies, *Haematologica* 82:101, 1997.

Finazzi LB et al: Natural history and risk factors for thrombosis in 360 patients with antiphospholipid antibodies: a four year prospective study from the Italian registry, *Am J Med* 100:530, 1996.

Harris EN et al: Anticardiolipin antibodies in autoimmune thrombocytopenic purpura, *Br J Haematol* 59:231, 1985.

Harris EN, Pierangeli, SS: Utilization of intravenous immunoglobulin therapy to treat recurrent pregnancy loss in the antiphospholipid syndrome: a review, *Scand J Rheumatol Suppl* 107:97, 1998.

Infante-Rivard C et al: Lupus anticoagulants, anticardiolipin antibodies, and fetal loss, *N Engl J Med* 325:1063, 1991.

Khamashta MA et al: The management of thrombosis in the antiphospholipid-antibody syndrome, *N Engl J Med* 332:993, 1995.

Love PE, Sanlon SA: Anticardiolipin and the lupus anticoagulant in systemic lupus erythematosus (SLE) and non-SLE disorders, *Ann Intern Med* 112:682, 1990.

Nesher G et al: Thrombotic microangiopathic hemolytic anemia in systemic lupus erythematosus, *Semin Arthritis Rheum* 24:165, 1994.

Petri M: 1998 update on antiphospholipid antibodies, *Curr Opin Rheumatol* 10:426, 1998.

Rand JH et al: Pregnancy loss in the antiphospholipid-antibody syndrome—a possible thrombogenic mechanism [published erratum appears in *N Engl J Med* 1997 Oct 30;337(18):1327]. *N Engl J Med* 337:154, 1997.

Rosove MH, Brewer PM: Antiphospholipid thrombosis: clinical course after the first thrombotic event in 70 patients, *Ann Intern Med* 117:303, 1992.

Vianna JL et al: Comparison of the primary and secondary antiphospholipid syndrome: a European Multicenter Study of 114 patients, *Am J Med* 96:3, 1994.

Wilson WA et al: International consensus statement on preliminary classification criteria for definite antiphospholipid syndrome, *Arthritis Rheum* 42:1309, 1999.

CHAPTER 38

Systemic Lupus Erythematosus

Patricia A. Fraser

EPIDEMIOLOGY

Systemic lupus erythematosus (SLE, lupus) is an auto-immune systemic rheumatic disease of unknown etiology that preferentially afflicts women. Lupus is found world-wide and the prevalence varies among population groups. This is best exemplified by lupus statistics in the United States, where a several-fold variation in the prevalence of SLE exists, ranging from 140/100,000 in white women, 280/100,000 among Native Americans in Alaska, to 410/100,000 in African-American women. These differences in lupus prevalence may be due to an interaction between genetic and environmental factors that modulate the differential risk of lupus observed in US racial and ethnic groups. Disease expression, prognosis, and survival for SLE also vary in the United States, where we see significantly greater disease severity, ethnicity-dependent autoantibody profiles, and poorer survival in African Americans and Hispanic individuals with SLE compared with whites. Socioeconomic factors are the most important predictors of prognosis.

PATHOPHYSIOLOGY

Most symptoms of SLE are due to immune complex formation in or adjacent to venules, arterioles, and capillary beds. The exact etiologies of the small vessel vasculitis commonly seen in lupus are unknown. Exposure to microorganisms such as herpes viruses may initiate the disease process through the induction of T and B lymphocyte dysfunction in genetically susceptible persons. Alternatively, exposure to genotoxic compounds that damage DNA may also trigger lupus. Antibodies to double stranded DNA (anti-dsDNA) cause renal injury through the formation of immune complexes. Similarly, the deposition of immune complexes containing anti-Ro antibodies in the fetal myocardium is the presumed mechanism for complete congenital heart block in neonatal lupus. Cutaneous lupus lesions, lupus arthritis, serositis, and central and peripheral nervous system dysfunction in SLE are all consistent with the sequelae of small vessel vasculitis. Proinflammatory cytokines such as tumor necrosis factor-alpha and CD40-CD40 ligand-mediated interactions between CD4 T cells and B cells may also contribute to the perpetuation of the chronic inflammatory state in SLE.

CLINICAL PRESENTATION
Criteria for Classification

Criteria for the classification of SLE underwent major revisions in 1982 and 1997. The purpose of these criteria of SLE is to facilitate the design of and comparisons between epidemiologic studies of SLE (Box 38-1). Clinical and laboratory manifestations are combined to define the spectrum of common signs and symptoms associated with SLE. These criteria permit comparisons between clinical studies in which patient selection is limited to those who have at least 4 of 11 criteria. It is important for clinicians to appreciate that the clinical diagnosis of SLE does not depend on the number of criteria met. Rather, the diagnosis of SLE is framed by the clinical impression of the practitioner and the specific clinical manifestations.

History and Symptom Presentation

Fever (temperature greater than 100° F) often accompanies lupus flares. Lupus patients who are receiving systemic corticosteroids or immunosuppressive agents such as azathioprine (Imuran) and cyclophosphamide (Cytoxan) are immuno-compromised and at risk for opportunistic infections, as well as for serious sequelae of routine bacterial infections. Even if a lupus flare is present, the febrile lupus patient should be evaluated and treated for infection. In addition to fevers, lupus patients often report severe, disabling **fatigue.**

Transient **menstrual abnormalities** in SLE most often are due to acute severe illness or rapid weight loss and systemic corticosteroid use. It is not known whether menarche is significantly delayed in childhood-onset SLE. Secondary amenorrhea and premature ovarian failure may occur with daily or pulse (monthly intravenous) cyclophosphamide therapy (see Chapter 43 for discussion on amenorrhea and premature ovarian failure).

Cutaneous Manifestations

Disease-specific cutaneous symptoms of SLE may be acute, subacute, or chronic.

The common acute cutaneous lupus eruptions include **malar erythema,** the so-called butterfly rash, and generalized facial and truncal erythema. Rarely, focal or diffuse acute bullous lesions develop in the setting of SLE.

Chronic cutaneous lesions comprise the majority of the cutaneous symptoms in patients with SLE. **Discoid lupus erythematosus** (DLE) is more common in men but frequently occurs in women. It may be localized to either the face or scalp, limited to the head, or generalized. The scarring hypopigmentation and/or hyperpigmentation and permanent alopecia associated with DLE may pose a major cosmetic problem. **Lupus profundus** or **lupus panniculitis** appears as painful, hyperesthetic, indurated truncal lesions. Oral and nasal ulcerations, urticaria, psoriasis-like eruptions, and chilblains are also seen in SLE.

Alopecia is a troublesome symptom for lupus patients because it dramatically affects body image. As stated before, DLE lesions often are accompanied by scarring and the alopecia associated with DLE is frequently permanent. Transient alopecia also occurs with SLE. Patchy alopecia (**alopecia areata**) occurs in up to 10% of SLE patients, whereas diffuse alopecia is even more common, with more than 50% of patients affected. Alopecia correlates with disease activity (see also Chapter 8 for discussion of alopecia).

Ultraviolet light (UVB and UVA) exposure is an important exacerbating factor for both acute and chronic cutaneous lupus symptoms in patients with **photosensitivity.** Symptoms of photosensitivity may include rash (urticarial, vesicular or petechial) on sun-exposed areas, nausea, headache, arthralgias/arthritis, and fever. Photosensitivity is more common among SLE patients who have anti-Ro autoantibodies and also among those who are homozygous for the glutathione-S-transferase M1 (GSTM1) null genotype.

Lupus arthritis is a **symmetric peripheral arthritis** that usually affects (in order of decreasing frequency) the small joints of the hands, knees, and small joints of the feet. Cricoarytenoid arthritis also occurs and can manifest as persistent or intermittent sore throat, hoarseness, or even episodic stridor. Characteristic inflammatory signs are seen with laryngoscopy.

The arthritis of SLE is classically described as nondeforming. Because SLE patients with arthritis rarely develop erosive joint disease but frequently develop deformities, it may be more appropriate to characterize lupus arthritis as nonerosive. In fact, chronic lupus arthritis may lead to joint deformities that are indistinguishable from those seen in rheumatoid arthritis, such as swan neck, boutonniere deformities, and ulnar drift (ulnar deviation of the metacarpophalangeal joints). Reconstructive surgery is effective in reducing these deformities.

Recurrent tendon ruptures occur more commonly in SLE than in other systemic rheumatic diseases. The cause of this tendon disorder is unclear, but chronic steroid therapy has been implicated as one predisposing factor.

Acute monarticular arthritis in SLE requires urgent evaluation. The chronic lymphopenic state associated with SLE results in decreased natural immunity to microbial agents, which is compounded by corticosteroid and other immunosuppressive therapies. Arthrocentesis of the affected joint (and simultaneous fluoroscopic examination for hip joint involvement), synovial fluid analysis (cell count, differential, Gram stain, and polarized microscopic examination for crystals), and culture should be performed when the patient manifests acute monarticular arthritis even in the absence of fever (see Chapter 33 for a more detailed discussion). In the febrile patient, parenteral antibiotic therapy that includes coverage for *Staphylococcus aureus* should be continued until the joint fluid culture is negative for the organism.

Pleuropulmonary Disease

Pleurisy is the most common pulmonary symptom of SLE. At least 50% of the patients will have either unilateral or bilateral pleural involvement at some time during the course of their disease. Frequently an afebrile patient reports pleuritic pain, but a pleural rub is inaudible and a chest film shows no effusion. It is important to consider other causes of the pleuritic chest pain such as pulmonary embolism. If there is no obvious cause, the practitioner generally treats the symptoms (see Management) and then, if unsuccessful, the radiograph should be repeated. Often a pleural effusion will develop later in the course of disease. In the febrile patient with effusion and pulmonary infiltrate, diagnostic thoracentesis should be considered to exclude infection.

Parenchymal involvement is less common in SLE but may take the form of diffuse interstitial pneumonitis or acute focal, migratory infiltrates. Infectious processes must always be considered in this setting, even if the patient is afebrile. It may be necessary to consider bronchoscopy, bronchoalveolar lavage, and transbronchial or open lung biopsy to confirm the diagnosis. Diffuse interstitial pneumonitis often progresses to diffuse pulmonary fibrosis, with restrictive lung disease, pulmonary hypertension, and cor pulmonale even after appropriate treatment.

The **"shrinking lungs syndrome"** in SLE is distinct from diffuse interstitial pneumonitis. This syndrome is characterized by severe progressive dyspnea, restrictive lung disease, and an elevated diaphragm. There is uncertainty about the pathogenetic mechanisms leading to the shrinking lungs syndrome. Popular theories include alveolar microatelectasis and diaphragmatic weakness secondary to fibrosis.

Pulmonary hemorrhage also may complicate SLE. The prominent features of this presentation are variable amounts of hemoptysis, profound hypoxemia and acute respiratory distress, diffuse pulmonary infiltrates, and a sudden drop in hematocrit.

Cardiovascular Disease

Pericarditis is the most common cardiac manifestation of SLE. Massive pericardial effusions may occur and can be associated with echocardiographic evidence of impending cardiac tamponade. Serial echocardiographic imaging is an essential part of management. Management issues are discussed later in the chapter.

Accelerated atherosclerosis affects 6% to 12% of SLE patients. This lupus complication, along with **coronary artery disease,** contributes significantly to early lupus mortality. Multiple predisposing factors for these complications include obesity, steroid therapy, hypertension, hyperlipidemia, and antiphospholipid antibodies.

SLE may be complicated by **myocardial dysfunction** (including hypertrophic cardiomyopathy) and **valvulitis.**

Serositis and Other Causes of Abdominal Pain

Frequently encountered causes of abdominal pain in SLE are listed in Box 38-2. Abdominal pain associated with **lupus serositis** is nonspecific and may even suggest an acute abdominal condition. Patients with lupus serositis are often febrile, with diffuse abdominal pain. Abdominal ultrasound examination may demonstrate a localized fluid collection consistent with lupus serositis. Because lupus serositis is a diagnosis of exclusion, it is often necessary to exclude acute abdominal and pelvic conditions by exploratory laparotomy, or laparascopy. If other causes for the symptoms have been excluded, treatment with steroids (equivalent to prednisone, 40 mg/day) may be considered.

Another cause of abdominal pain in SLE is **acute pancreatitis.** The mechanisms proposed for its occurrence in SLE include pancreatic vasculitis and corticosteroids. Recurrent bouts of pancreatitis may develop and are treated with standard pancreatitis management.

Less common causes of abdominal pain in SLE include **mesenteric vasculitis** and **colonic perforation.** Mesenteric vasculitis may be associated with intermittent, sharp, or crampy abdominal pain and hematochezia. The symptoms of colonic perforation are nonspecific and intermittent. The cause of perforation is unclear but also may be vasculitic in origin.

Lupus Nephritis

Predisposition to renal involvement in SLE varies among different ethnic groups. The risk of lupus nephritis is highest among African-American SLE patients who carry FC gamma RIIA alleles. Renal disease is an important cause of morbidity and mortality in SLE. More than 70% of all SLE patients will have renal involvement sometime during the course of their illness. Ideally, potential therapies used early in the course of renal involvement may prevent or minimize permanent renal damage. It is important to assess whether the renal dysfunction (usually manifested by elevated creatinine levels and a spectrum of abnormalities of the urinary sediment) is active or inactive before considering invasive studies or cytotoxic therapy. Renal biopsy should be considered if there is either an active urinary sediment (red blood cells and/or cellular casts) or significant proteinuria (0.1 g/24 hr). Other indications for biopsy are abnormal renal function (abnormal serum creatinine level or creatinine clearance) of unknown duration and decrements in renal function observed by the practitioner in association with an active urinary sediment or proteinuria or consideration of cytotoxic drug therapy.

Neurologic Syndromes

Headache is one of the most common neurologic symptoms in SLE. Some patients have classic migraine, especially those with antiphospholipid antibodies. Many lupus patients with chronic recurrent headaches may not have symptoms that suggest a vascular component to the headache. Chronic headache is well tolerated and is not a major cause of disability.

Depression may be the most common neuropsychiatric manifestation of SLE and is usually multifactorial in origin. The chronic and acute symptoms of systemic illness such as SLE may induce reactive depression. Reactive depression also may result from disability caused by SLE. Alteration in physical appearance because of SLE (e.g., hyperpigmentation/hypopigmentation and the scarring DLE, alopecia, and malar rash) or side effects of medications used to treat SLE (moon facies and generalized weight gain from systemic steroids) all may cause reactive depression.

It is difficult to distinguish between steroid-induced depression and that caused by central nervous system (CNS) SLE. Magnetic resonance imaging (MRI)-angiography can be used to identify vasculitic lesions in the CNS.

Cognitive impairment in SLE may manifest as attention deficit and memory disorders that interfere with activities of daily living. For example, work capacity, shopping, banking, driving, and housekeeping may be impaired. Frequently, depressive symptoms are superimposed. Psychometric testing is helpful in identifying the contribution of depression to cognitive impairment. Imaging techniques such as single photon emission computed tomography (I-123 SPECT) scan may be useful in the evaluation of cognitive disorders in SLE.

Coma, seizure disorder, cranial and peripheral neuropathies, myelopathy, stroke, movement disorders, and aseptic meningitis may occur in patients with SLE. The mechanisms for manifestations are unclear, but microangiopathy from immune complex disease or vascular thrombosis resulting from antiphospholipid antibodies is suspected. Variable success in localizing pathologic lesions has been obtained by use of diagnostic techniques, such as electroencephalography, MRI, and lumbar puncture.

BOX 38-2
Causes of Abdominal Pain in Systemic Lupus Erythematosus

Serositis
Acute pancreatitis
Mesenteric vasculitis
Colonic perforation

DIAGNOSTIC TESTS
Laboratory Tests

Although many of the **antinuclear antibody** (ANA) patterns are highly specific for lupus, others are not. The spectrum of the pattern of ANA is important in differentiating the various connective tissue disorders but is always supplemental to the history, symptoms, and physical examination.

The fluorescent antinuclear antibody test is the screening test of choice for SLE. ANA findings are positive in more than 90% of persons with SLE. Positive test reactions for ANA may show one of several different patterns of immunofluorescence, which assist the practitioner in choosing the necessary additional diagnostic studies to distinguish among the various systemic rheumatic diseases. Homogeneous and peripheral patterns correlate with antibodies to DNA and are most specific for SLE. A speckled pattern indicates antibodies directed toward extractable nuclear antigen (ENA). Antibodies to ENA may be further subdivided into four antibody types. Anti-Sm is commonly found in SLE. Anti-RNP also is commonly found in SLE but is seen in mixed connective tissue disease (MCTD) as well. Anti-Ro (SSA) and anti-La (SSB) are positive in SLE, Sjögren's syndrome, and rheumatoid arthritis. These two antibodies, especially anti-Ro, are important risk factors for neonatal lupus syndrome and should be measured in every pregnant lupus patient (pregnancy and lupus are discussed in greater length at the end of this chapter). The nucleolar and centromeric staining patterns suggest systemic sclerosis and related syndromes. Cytoplasmic staining, which occurs rarely in SLE, may be seen in primary biliary cirrhosis and autoimmune thyroiditis. The diagnostic tests and diagnoses that the patterns of ANA suggest are summarized in Fig. 38-1.

A **complete blood count** (CBC) should be obtained in any patient for whom the diagnosis of SLE is considered. Anemia in lupus may be multifactorial. Hemolysis (positive Coombs' test reaction), iron deficiency (exacerbated by menses, poor iron intake, and chronic gastrointestinal bleeding from nonsteroidal antiinflammatory medications), pernicious anemia, and anemia of chronic disease may all contribute to the anemia of SLE. Thrombocytopenia and leukopenia/lymphopenia seen in SLE may be on an autoimmune basis, although specific antibodies may not be detected.

Renal disease occurs in up to 70% of SLE patients and is an important cause of morbidity and mortality. Screening tests of renal function should include a serum **creatinine** and **urinalysis** specifically to ascertain the presence of hematuria, cellular casts, and proteinuria.

Other Diagnostic Tests

Serositis, specifically pleurisy, pericarditis, and peritonitis, may complicate early SLE. Chest pain should be evaluated with a chest film to exclude pleural or pericardial effusions. Abdominal ultrasound examination is useful in assessing focal peritoneal fluid collections caused by SLE.

The presence of IgG **antiphospholipid antibodies** (APL) is often associated with a coagulopathy that may occur independently of SLE. APL is a risk factor for peripheral arterial and venous thromboses, CNS thrombotic events, migraine, transverse myelopathy, recurrent spontaneous abortion, and fetal demise in the second and third trimesters. Screening nonpregnant lupus patients for these

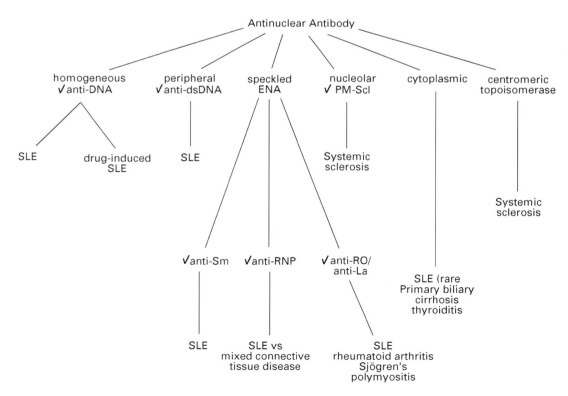

FIG. 38-1 Diagnostic tests and diagnoses to consider from antinuclear antibody pattern.

antibodies should be limited to individuals with a history of thromboses or associated clinical manifestations. All pregnant lupus patients should be screened for APL because this may require specific management. Screening should include a serologic test for syphilis, anticardiolipin antibody, a Russel Viper venom test, and an activated partial thromboplastin time. A summary of the initial laboratory workup for probable SLE is shown in Table 38-1. A different panel of tests is needed to evaluate definite, active, inactive, and pregnant SLE patients.

DIFFERENTIAL DIAGNOSIS

Several clinical and laboratory features of SLE also occur in other rheumatic conditions. For this reason, it is sometimes difficult to distinguish SLE from other systemic rheumatic diseases (Box 38-3).

Rheumatoid Arthritis

Symmetric, peripheral polyarthritis is a frequent initial presentation of SLE and may be indistinguishable from the arthritic manifestations of early rheumatoid arthritis (RA). Rheumatoid factor is present in most RA patients (more than 75%) and is uncommon in SLE. In contrast, ANA is present in more than 90% of persons with SLE but also may occur in up to 30% of those with RA. When present, anti-dsDNA antibodies are specific for active SLE. Similarly, hypocomplementemia is highly suggestive of active SLE but also can occur in RA in the setting of cutaneous or systemic vasculitis. Subcutaneous nodules are commonly found in rheumatoid factor–positive (seropositive) RA but are seen infrequently in SLE. Hand films, with posteroanterior, lateral, and oblique views of both wrists and both hands, provide a useful comparison. Although periarticular osteopenia is present with RA and SLE polyarthritis, marginal erosions are specific for RA (see Chapter 36).

Dermatomyositis

The proximal muscle weakness associated with early dermatomyositis may be subtle and overshadowed by the patient's more prominent complaints of symmetric, poly-

arthralgias, polyarthritis, and severe myalgias. The heliotrope rash of dermatomyositis affects the periorbital and malar areas, may be exacerbated by sun exposure, and can be confused with the butterfly rash of SLE. ANA is present in dermatomyositis and SLE. The speckled pattern of ANA is more common in dermatomyositis, whereas homogeneous (diffuse) and peripheral ANA patterns are seen almost exclusively in SLE.

Systemic Sclerosis (Scleroderma) and Mixed Connective Tissue Disease

Raynaud's phenomenon (see Chapters 6 and 33) is a prominent feature of systemic sclerosis (SS) and MCTD but also occurs in SLE. ANA is present in all of these conditions. Speckled, centromeric and nucleolar ANA are more likely to occur in SS and MCTD. In some ethnic groups the pattern of antibodies to nuclear precipitins may help to distinguish SLE from MCTD. For example, anti-RNP is more common in MCTD, whereas anti-Sm is specific for SLE in whites. In contrast, both anti-SM and anti-RNP occur more commonly in African Americans, and distinction between SLE and MCTD may not be possible solely on the basis of autoantibody profile in this ethnic group.

✳ MANAGEMENT

Goals

Because there is currently no cure for SLE, therapeutic interventions focus on reducing the symptoms and organ dysfunction that affect lupus-related morbidity and mortality. Lupus disease activity may vary spontaneously, even with optimal therapy. Prophylactic measures for maintaining lupus remissions are limited but for certain patients may include sun avoidance or protection (suncreens) and hydroxychloroquine therapy.

Choice of Therapy by Organ System Manifestation
Cutaneous Manifestations

Malar rash may respond to topical corticosteroid creams or ointments. If possible, treatment with fluorinated corticosteroid preparations for facial lesions should be prescribed for a limited period to minimize the complications of fluorinated corticosteroid creams, namely atrophy, hypopigmentation/hyperpigmentation, and telangiectasias. Once the acute lesions respond to the fluorinated preparations, attempts should be made to switch to hydrocortisone cream. Steroid- and antimalarial-unresponsive bullous lesions that have neutrophils on biopsy may respond to dapsone. The use of dapsone is contraindicated in glucose-6-phosphate dehydrogenase (G6PD) deficiency. Starting dose is 25 to 50 mg/day. Weekly laboratory testing should include CBC,

---

Table 38-1
Initial Laboratory Workup for Probable Systemic Lupus Erythematosus

Test	Probable SLE	Definite SLE	Active SLE	Inactive SLE	Pregnant SLE
ANA	Yes	No	No	No	No
CBC	Yes	Yes	Yes	Yes	Yes
Anti-DNA	No	Yes	Yes	Yes	Yes
Serum creatinine	Yes	Yes	Yes	Yes	Yes
Urinalysis	Yes	Yes	Yes	Yes	Yes
Ro/La	No*	No	No	No	Yes
Anticardiolipin	No	No	No	No	Yes
CH$_{50}$	No	Yes	Yes	Yes	Yes

ANA, Antinuclear antibody; *CBC*, complete blood count.
*Ro/La testing would not be performed at the initial visit but might be undertaken subsequently if ANA results are negative and there is strong suspicion of SLE.

BOX 38-3
Differential Diagnosis of Systemic Lupus Erythematosus

Rheumatoid arthritis
Mixed connective tissue disease
Polymyositis/dermatomyositis
Systemic sclerosis

reticulocyte count, and lactic dehydrogenase measurement. If laboratory parameters remain stable, the dose may be increased to 100 to 200 mg/day.

Combinations of therapies usually are required to treat chronic cutaneous symptoms. Regimens include hydroxychloroquine (Plaquenil) (400 mg/day) and/or topical and intradermal injections of corticosteroids into the active lesions. Hydroxychloroquine deposits in the retina and occasionally is associated with retinopathy and permanent visual disturbance. For this reason, baseline and serial (every 6 to 12 months) ophthalmologic evaluation is necessary. If there are baseline retinal abnormalities, the use of fluorescein angiography may be required. Refractory skin lesions can be treated with combination antimalarial therapy (hydroxychloroquine and quinacrine [Atabrine]). Atabrine does not cause retinopathy but does cause yellow-orange skin discoloration. There is limited data on the efficacy of thalidomide and low-dose weekly methotrexate (10 to 25 mg) in refractory discoid lupus.

Lupus profundus may be refractory to conventional treatments. Combinations of therapies usually are required to treat these cutaneous symptoms. Dapsone or cyclophosphamide may be effective when the conventional regimens of combination antimalarial therapy (hydroxychloroquine and quinacrine) and topical and intralesional corticosteroids fail.

Alopecia often responds to systemic steroids as the other disease manifestations improve. Systemic steroids should not be used routinely to treat alopecia unless the alopecia is associated with some other manifestation of SLE that requires systemic therapy.

Sun avoidance and topical sunscreens are the best treatments for the associated photosensitivity. Sunscreens of skin protection factor (SPF) 2 to 15 protect against UVA, whereas those with an SPF greater than 15 provide protection from UVB.

Lupus Fatigue

Chronic fatigue that is severe enough to interfere with activities of daily living is common in SLE and may improve with a low-impact aerobic exercise program. (For a more detailed discussion on management of fatigue, see Chapter 86.)

Polyarthritis

Aspirin and nonsteroidal anti-inflammatory drugs (NSAIDs) provide the first line of therapy. Hydroxychloroquine, 200 mg twice a day, is used in combination with ASA or NSAIDs. As mentioned before, patients who are treated with hydroxychloroquine need baseline and semiannual ophthalmologic examinations to monitor potential retinal toxicity from this medication. Short courses of low-dose prednisone (5 to 10 mg orally every morning) provide transient relief of joint complaints. Resting wrist and hand splints reduce inflammatory symptoms. Maintenance physical therapy exercises help to maintain range of motion of inflamed joints.

Pleuropulmonary Disease

For those patients with pleurisy but no evidence of pleural effusion or pulmonary embolism, a brief course of steroids (prednisone 10 to 20 mg orally for 7 to 10 days) generally controls pleuritic symptoms. Sometimes combination therapy with NSAIDs (in particular, indomethacin

50 mg orally three times daily if tolerated) and transient narcotic analgesic use (codeine preparations for the first 3 days of symptoms) becomes necessary. For pleurisy that the clinician believes is caused by the lupus rather than infection, higher doses of steroids (prednisone 30 mg orally every morning) often are needed for 4 to 6 weeks.

For parenchymal involvement, high-dose corticosteroids (prednisone 40 to 60 mg daily) are used in this setting with variable efficacy.

Uncontrolled studies on the shrinking lung syndrome suggest that treatment with prednisone 40 mg/day may be beneficial.

For pulmonary hemorrhage, treatment includes maintenance of respiratory function, reversal of coagulopathy if present, and the administration of parenteral steroids and cyclophosphamide.

Cardiac Disease

For pericardial effusion with impending tamponade, the decision about invasive versus noninvasive treatment—that is, whether to rapidly decompress the pericardial sac by pericardiocentesis or pericardial window to prevent progression to tamponade or whether to treat with steroids—is a difficult one. High-dose steroids have been shown to improve symptoms and reduce fluid volumes within 48 to 72 hours. Clinically, however, if the patient's cardiac status is unstable, a more invasive approach may be required.

Myocarditis requires the use of steroids in combination with standard therapies. Valvulitis and vegetations in the SLE patient may be due to acute or subacute bacterial endocarditis.

Pancreatitis

During an episode of pancreatitis, there is no known therapeutic benefit of adjusting the dose of steroids.

Lupus Nephritis

Randomized control trials in severe lupus nephritis suggest that combinations of cyclophosphamide and corticosteroids may be efficacious for the treatment of renal lesions within World Health Organization (WHO) guidelines. This regimen is limited to WHO classification grades III, IV, and V disease (segmental, proliferative, and diffuse proliferative and membranous nephritis with either segmental or proliferative features, respectively) that show some degree of active inflammation (fibrinoid necrosis, crescent formation, hyaline thrombi, or subendothelial deposits). The "pulse" (intravenous monthly) cyclophosphamide regimen is more popular because it is better tolerated and equally effective as daily dosing schedules. A randomized control trial of plasmapheresis plus cyclophosphamide and prednisone showed no additional benefit attributable to plasmapheresis.

Neurologic Syndromes

Depression may respond to combination treatment with antidepressants and long-term psychotherapy, informal group counseling, or support group participation. (See Chapter 81 for discussion of treatment for depression.)

For CNS vasculitis, high-dose steroids (orally or intravenously administered) are used most often alone or in combination with cytotoxic drugs, although their benefit is unknown. Aseptic meningitis in SLE occasionally is associated with NSAID use (ibuprofen and other NSAIDs). Pleiocytosis and meningeal signs rapidly improve with cessation of medication.

Corticosteroid Use

Steroid preparations are used to treat almost all manifestations of SLE. The most serious side effects of corticosteroids are increased susceptibility to opportunistic infections and predisposition to osteoporosis and aseptic necrosis. Other side effects are associated diabetes, hypertension, and cataract formation. Prolonged use of systemic corticosteroids is unavoidable in the treatment of renal and CNS SLE. The goal is to relieve symptoms related to SLE and to decrease long-term morbidity.

Daily prednisone dosages as low as 5 mg orally may alter mood and sleeping patterns. Emotional lability and insomnia develop within several days of initiating oral corticosteroid therapy and usually improve in 7 to 10 days. Severe depression and psychosis are more likely to occur at higher doses and may develop at any time during the course of steroid use. Acne, moon facies, and weight gain resolve when steroids are tapered or discontinued, but cataracts and purple striae are permanent sequelae. Calcium supplementation (1000 to 1500 mg elemental calcium on a daily basis), vitamin D (calcitriol 0.25 μg/day), and calcitonin nasal spray (miacalcin) are administered to minimize steroid-induced osteoporosis. Serial determinations of serum and 24-hour urinary calcium excretion are necessary on this regimen.

Hydroxychloroquine

Hydroxychloroquine (Plaquenil) affects disease activity. The mechanisms are unknown and do not appear to be only organ-specific. Generally the therapy is used when any of the symptoms of lupus appear with a twice-daily oral dose of 200 mg. Cessation of this medication may result in lupus flare. As mentioned before, the side effects include retinopathy; thus close ophthalmologic follow-up monitoring is necessary.

Immunization and Chemoprophylaxis

Immunization with pneumococcal and *Haemophilus B* vaccine is an essential component of the management of the SLE patient who has undergone splenectomy. Similarly, pneumococcal vaccine is recommended in lupus patients with leukopenia and also in those receiving corticosteroid and other immunosuppressive therapies. Isoniazid is not routinely used in SLE patients who receive long-term steroids, but close screening for tuberculosis exposure is important.

Monitoring Disease Activity

Accurate assessment of disease activity is essential for appropriate decision making in caring for SLE patients. The activity indexes SLAM and SLEDAI have been developed to facilitate epidemiologic studies and clinical trials. These standardized measures are valuable research tools but remain too time-consuming for use by most busy practitioners. Serial sedimentation rates are useful for monitoring disease activity in most lupus patients, whereas CH_{50} and anti-DNA antibody factors assist in monitoring many forms of lupus nephritis and some patients with pleuropericardial disease. CNS disease activity is difficult to assess and often requires serial cognitive and imaging studies.

▪ PREGNANCY AND LUPUS

Overview

Outcomes of interest for SLE patients considering pregnancy are fertility, the influence of pregnancy on SLE, lupus effects on pregnancy, and the possible adverse fetal effects of maternal SLE (Box 38-4).

With the exception of the subset of SLE patients who experience severe lupus nephritis with chronic renal failure or who require cytotoxic drugs such as cyclophosphamide, fertility studies of SLE show no direct effects of the disease and no overall reduction in fertility.

Cohort analyses indicate that pregnancy causes mild exacerbations in SLE. Patients with SLE require clinical and laboratory monitoring of disease parameters (anti-DNA, CH_{50}, platelet count) on a biweekly to monthly basis during their pregnancies.

Preeclamptic toxemia (PET) is three times more common in SLE than in women with normal pregnancies. PET is more common in patients with any renal dysfunction and may explain the higher prevalence of this condition in SLE. The manifestations of preeclampsia may be indistinguishable from active lupus nephritis (Table 38-2), and simultaneous treatment for both lupus nephritis and preeclampsia often is necessary.

Fetal wastage (early and late fetal loss) is more common in SLE pregnancy. Fetal distress and late fetal loss are associated with antibodies to phospholipids (APL), which occur in 6.7% to 25% of SLE patients. APL can be detected by a biologically false-positive test for syphilis, by prolongation of the activated partial thromboplastin time (APTT), by tests of the lupus anticoagulant (LAC) (Russell viper venom), or by assays for IgG antibodies to cardiolipin (ACL). Pregnant

Table 38-2
Manifestations of Lupus Nephritis and Preeclamptic Toxemia

| | SYSTEMIC LUPUS | |
	Erythematosus	Preeclampsia
Hypertension	+	+
Proteinuria	+++	+
Edema	+/−	+/−
Oliguria	+/−	+/−
Thrombocytopenia	+	+
Uric acid	Normal to elevated	Elevated
Active sediment	+	−
Complement (CH_{50})	Low	Low
	Normal	Normal
	High	High

BOX 38-4
Pregnancy and the Lupus Patient

Fertility in SLE
Impact of pregnancy on lupus
SLE effects on pregnancy
Fetal effects of SLE

SLE patients with ACL require close fetal observation (biophysical profiles weekly) throughout the third trimester. Preterm delivery is also more common in lupus pregnancies. Estimates of the frequencies of intrauterine growth retardation and low birth weight that are adjusted for known risk factors are not available for SLE, so we cannot determine whether there is SLE-specific predisposition to these adverse pregnancy outcomes.

Neonatal lupus erythematosus (NLE) is a rare condition with transient cutaneous or hematologic manifestations or permanent congenital complete heart block (CCHB) (Box 38-5). The presence of maternal anti-Ro (SSA) or La (SSB) antibodies is a risk factor for NLE. There are no preventive therapies with proved efficacy, nor are there any known therapies to reverse CCHB.

SLE patients should have testing for antibodies Ro (SSA), antibodies La (SSB), anticardiolipin antibodies (IgG and IgM ACL), and APTT in early pregnancy. CCHB can occur as early as week 20. If anti-Ro or anti-La antibodies are present, fetal heart auscultation after week 20 may detect the regular bradycardia of CCHB. If ACL or an abnormal APTT is detected, nonstress testing should be performed. SLE monitoring should include serial measurements of serum complement (CH_{50}) and platelet counts (Box 38-6). Serum complement rises to supernormal levels in pregnancy. Normal, low, or decreasing levels during pregnancy suggest active or flaring disease but are not conclusive because normal or low-normal complement levels also may be associated with PET.

Drug Therapy

During Pregnancy

The most commonly used drugs in SLE include aspirin and NSAIDs, corticosteroids, antimalarial agents, and cyclophosphamide. If the patient can tolerate dose adjustment, NSAIDs are reduced or discontinued in early pregnancy to minimize maternal and fetal bleeding tendencies associated with the drugs and also to reduce the risks of delayed labor in the mother and premature closure of the ductus arteriosus in the fetus. Prednisone is the most commonly used corticosteroid preparation. Because it is metabolized by the placenta, only very small amounts are present in the fetal circulation and minimal—if any—fetal adrenal suppression is associated with it. The dose of prednisone often is adjusted to compensate for the withdrawal or reduction of NSAIDs. Prophylactic use of prednisone is not recommended for patients with inactive lupus because no evidence exists of its benefit. In addition, prednisone causes fluid retention and hypertension, and these effects may increase the risk of pregnancy-induced hypertension, which is more common in SLE. Maintenance therapy with antimalarial agents sustains a stable course or remission in SLE. This clinical observation must be balanced against the finding in experimental animals of hydroxychloroquine deposition in fetal retinal tissue. The options are to discontinue hydroxychloroquine as soon as pregnancy is confirmed and to observe for possible flare of symptoms, or to maintain the medication throughout pregnancy if the patient is informed of the experimental data and the lack of known adverse effects on the fetus and she can accept this uncertainty. Cyclophosphamide should not be used in the first trimester because of its teratogenic potential.

During Lactation

Most of the literature on drug use in lactation stems from case reports. Thus the absence of a case report of adverse effect on a nursing infant may reflect the low frequency of side effects or a truly "safe" drug. Aspirin and indomethacin should not be used. Ibuprofen (Motrin, Advil) and piroxicam (Feldene) have no reported side effects. Although hydroxychloroquine has no reported adverse effects, it may precipitate hemolysis in a G6PD-deficient infant and should be avoided during lactation. Prednisone has no reported adverse effects in nursing infants.

PROGNOSIS AND OUTCOME

Longitudinal studies suggest that at least 4% of SLE patients will experience serologic and clinical remission. Survival in SLE is influenced by age of onset, race, socioeconomic status, duration of disease, pattern of organ involvement, and the presence of IgM anticardiolipin antibodies. Cardiopulmonary, renal (especially the histology of the renal lesion) and CNS symptoms are all important predictors of survival. In whites with SLE, prognosis continues to improve, as is demonstrated by survival rates at 5 and 10 years of 90% and 80%, respectively. In contrast, survival in African Americans with SLE continues to decline, especially if lupus nephritis is present.

BOX 38-5

Features of the Neonatal Lupus Syndrome

Skin lesions
Thrombocytopenia and/or hemolytic anemia
Congenital complete heart block (CCHB)

BOX 38-6

Laboratory Tests in the Pregnant Lupus Patient

Anti-Ro (SSA)
Anti-La (SSB)
  If positive, monitor fetal heart rate
Anticardiolipin (IgG/IgM)
  If positive, monitor fetal biophysical profile
Activated partial thromboplastin time
  If abnormal, monitor fetal biophysical profile
Baseline and serial complement (CH_{50}) levels
  Normal to low CH_{50} suggests active SLE, follow-up 2/mo
  Sudden decrease suggests SLE flare and/or preeclamptic toxemia, treat specific symptoms
Baseline and serial platelet counts

BIBLIOGRAPHY

Alarcon GS et al: Systemic lupus erythematosus in three ethnic groups: II. Features predictive of disease activity early in its course. LUMINA Study Group. Lupus in minority populations, nature versus nurture. *Arthritis Rheum* 41:1173, 1998.

Amigo MC, Khamashta MA: Antiphospholipid (Hughes) syndrome in systemic lupus erythematosus, *Rheum Dis Clin North Am* 26:331, 2000.

Austin HA 3rd, Boumpas DT, Vaughan EM, Balow JE: High-risk features of lupus nephritis: importance of race and clinical and histological factors in 166 patients. *Nephrol Dial Transplant* 10:1620, 1995.

Bae A-C, Bae PA, Fraser DP, Liang: The epidemiology of systemic lupus erythematosus in populations of African ancestry: a critical review of the "prevalence gradient hypothesis." *Arthritis Rheum* 41:2091, 1998.

Bakir AA, Levy PS, Dunea G: The prognosis of lupus nephritis in African-Americans: a retrospective analysis, *Am J Kidney Dis* 24:159, 1994.

Boehm IB, Boehm GA, Bauer R: Management of cutaneous lupus erythematosus with low-dose methotrexate: indication for modulation of inflammatory mechanisms, *Rheumatol Int* 18:59, 1998.

Bush TM, Shlotzhauer TL, Grove W: Serum complements: inappropriate use in patients with suspected rheumatic disease, *Arch Intern Med* 153: 2363, 1993.

Callen JP. Management of skin disease in lupus, *Bull Rheum Dis* 46:4, 1997.

Cooper GS et al: Hormonal environmental, and infectious risk factors for developing systemic lupus erythematosus, *Arthritis Rheum* 41:1714, 1998.

Ginzler EM: Clinical features and complications of systemic lupus erythematosus, and assessment of disease activity, *Curr Opin Rheumatol* 2:703, 1990.

Ginzler EM et al: Hypertension increases the risk of renal deterioration in systemic lupus erythematosus, *J Rheumatol* 20:1694, 1993.

Hochberg MC: Systemic lupus erythematosus, *Rheum Dis Clin North Am* 16:617, 1990.

Hochberg MC: Updating the American College of Rheumatology revised criteria for the classification of systemic lupus erythematosus, *Arthritis Rheum* 40:1725, 1997.

Jacobs L et al: Central nervous system lupus erythematosus: the value of magnetic resonance imaging, *J Rheumatol* 15:601, 1988.

Lawrence RC et al: Estimates of the prevalence of selected arthritic and musculoskeletal disease in the United States, *J Rheumatol* 16:427, 1989.

Lewis EJ et al (Lupus Nephritis Collaborative Study Group): A controlled trial of plasmapheresis therapy in severe lupus nephritis, *N Engl J Med* 326:1373, 1992.

Liang MH et al: Reliability and validity of six systems for the clinical assessment of disease activity in systemic lupus erythematosus, *Arthritis Rheum* 32:1107, 1989.

Lockshin MD et al: Neonatal lupus risk to newborns of mothers with systemic lupus erythematosus, *Arthritis Rheum* 31:697, 1988.

Millard TP, Hawk JL, McGregor JM: Photosensitivity in lupus, *Lupus* 9:3, 2000.

Molina JF et al: Ethnic differences in the clinical expression of systemic lupus erythematosus: a comparative study between African-Americans and Latin Americans, *Lupus* 6:63, 1997.

Ortman RA, Klippel JH: Update on cyclophosphamide for systemic lupus erythematosus, *Rheum Dis Clin North Am* 26:363, 2000.

Perez-Gutthann S, Petri M, Hochberg MC: Comparison of different methods of classifying patients with systemic lupus erythematosus, *J Rheumatol* 18:117, 1991.

Petri M, Howard D, Repke J: The frequency of lupus flare in pregnancy, *Arthritis Rheum* 34:1538, 1991.

Petri M: Detection of coronary artery disease and the role of traditional risk factors in the Hopkins Lupus Cohort, *Lupus* 9:170, 2000.

Robb-Nicholson C et al: Effects of aerobic conditioning in lupus fatigue: a pilot study, *Br J Rheumatol* 28:500, 1989.

Salmon JE et al: Fc gamma RIIA alleles are heritable risk factors for lupus nephritis in African Americans, *J Clin Invest* 97:1348, 1996.

Studenski S, Ward MM: Systemic lupus erythematosus in men: a multivariate analysis gender differences in clinical manifestations, *J Rheumatol* 17: 220, 1990.

Tan EM et al: The 1982 revised criteria for the classification of systemic lupus erythematosus, *Arthritis Rheum* 25:1271, 1982.

Tebbe B, Orfanos CE: Epidemiology and socioeconomic impact of skin disease in lupus erythematosus, *Lupus* 6:96, 1997.

Urowitz MB, Gladman DD: Accelerated atheroma in lupus—background, *Lupus* 9:161, 2000.

Walz-Leblanc BAE et al: The "shrinking lungs syndrome" in systemic lupus erythematosus—improvement with corticosteroid therapy, *J Rheumatol* 19:1970, 1992.

Ward MM, Studenski S: Clinical manifestations of systemic lupus erythematosus: identification of racial and socioeconomic influences, *Arch Intern Med* 150:849, 1990.

Yell JA, Mbuagbaw J, Burge SM: Cutaneous manifestations of systemic lupus erythematosus, *Br J Dermatol* 135:355, 1996.

Zonana-Nacach A, Barr SG, Magder LS, Petri M: Damage in systemic lupus erythematosus and its association with corticosteroids, *Arthritis Rheum* 43:1801, 2000.

CHAPTER 39

Sports Injuries

Sheila Ann Dugan

Passage of Title IX of the 1972 Education Amendments Act marked an important triumph for proponents of women's sports. It prohibits discrimination by gender in providing educational programs and activities for all secondary and post-secondary institutions receiving federal funding. Over the succeeding three decades, women's sports participation and performance have grown. Today, girls and women are able to benefit from the enriching environment of sports participation. This participation occurs across a wide spectrum, from intercollegiate play to weekend road races.

We can expect to care for a growing number of women who have been active in sports over their lifetimes. There are also many women who embark on exercise later in life, in some cases, following in the footsteps of their daughters! Life cycle issues and changes must be considered when evaluating a female athlete. In adolescence, hypermobility and laxity place some girls at risk of injury. Women who remain active with exercise during pregnancy present with unique biomechanical issues. Postpartum pelvic floor weakness can lead to lumbar pain, pelvic pain, and urinary incontinence. Middle-aged women may be at increased risk of overuse injuries in sports as a result of hormonally induced soft-tissue atrophy and bone density loss. Master athletes have degenerative changes of the spine and extremities that may limit joint mobility, leading to altered movement patterns and injury.

Although the health benefits of regular exercise are innumerable, vigorous exercise can put some women at risk for significant health consequences. Women have an increased susceptibility to particular injuries owing to biomechanical, hormonal, and training issues. The term *female athlete triad* was coined by the American College of Sports Medicine (ACSM) to draw attention to the interrelatedness of menstrual irregularities, disordered eating, and premature osteoporosis. It has been shown that women with this triad have an increased incidence of musculoskeletal injuries.

Studies of the epidemiology of injury in female athletes reveal that many of these injuries are similar to male athletes in the same sport. These injuries can be considered sports related rather than gender specific. Contact sports by their very nature put the participant at risk for injury related to the transfer of force to the tissues of the body. Overuse injuries are common owing to the repetitive nature of practice and competition.

This chapter addresses selected musculoskeletal injuries that occur in female athletes. Individuals managing sports-related injuries must recognize the individuality of the patient; there is no "typical woman athlete" just as there is no "typical woman." Returning the athlete to participation or competition as soon as possible, without risking ongoing injury, is our challenge.

Table 39-1 provides a regional overview of injuries in women who participate in sports. The ankle is the most common site of injury. National Collegiate Athletic Association (NCAA) data reveal that the sports in which women are most commonly injured are, in order, gymnastics, soccer, basketball, field hockey, volleyball, lacrosse, and softball.

Functional sports medicine rehabilitation management strategies are shown in Table 39-2, as described by Kibler and colleagues, and provide the framework for how individual injuries are managed. Sports rehabilitation requires a team approach. It is most successful when the lines of communication are open and respect is given for the unique knowledge and skill set each of the team members provides, whether physician, physician assistant, nurse practitioner, nurse, physical therapist, occupational therapist, chiropractor, trainer, or complementary medicine practitioner.

HEAD INJURY

Concussion should be considered a minor head injury, as it causes a decreased level of consciousness. The highest rates of concussion in college women's sports are seen in softball, soccer, and lacrosse. Concussion requires the same medical approach as any brain injury. Sideline evaluation of neurologic status must be thorough yet efficient. In the setting of loss of consciousness or change in level of alertness, the athlete is closely monitored serially. Consensus statements on the management of sports-related concussion recommend a period of exertion in conjunction with mental status testing to tax the blood supply to the brain and uncover any subtle abnormalities before consideration for return to play. There is some controversy on return-to-play guidelines when a player has her "bell rung" but does not lose consciousness,

Table 39-1
Injuries in Women Athletes

Site of Injury	Type of Injury
Head	Concussion/mild brain injury
	Second impact syndrome
Cervical spine	Burners or stinger syndrome (cervical root or upper trunk of brachial plexus stretch or compression injury)
Thoracic spine	Compression fracture
Lumbar spine	Spondylolysis/spondylolisthesis
	Mechanical low back pain
	Internal disk disruption
	Radiculopathy
Shoulder	Impingement syndrome
	Rotator cuff tear
	Instability/dislocation
	Scapulothoracic joint dysfunction
Elbow	Lateral epicondylitis
	Medial epicondylitis
Wrist and hand	Mallet finger (tear of the extensor mechanism of digit)
	Fracture of scaphoid
	Scapholunate dissociation
Pelvis and sacrum	Stress fracture (ilium, sacrum, pubis)
	Sacroiliac joint dysfunction
	Piriformis syndrome
Hip	Femoral stress fracture (neck, greater trochanter)
	Acetabular labrum tears
	Iliotibial band syndrome
	Greater trochanteric bursitis
	Snapping hip syndrome
Knee	ACL tears
	Meniscal tears
	Patellofemoral syndrome
Leg, foot, and ankle	Inversion ankle sprain
	Medial tibial stress syndrome/stress fracture
	Compartment syndrome
	Stress fracture (metatarsal, navicular)

with the more conservative guidelines recommending removal for the duration of the contest.

There has been some concern that repetitive minor head impacts via "heading" the ball in soccer can lead, at least, to acute neuropsychologic changes and, at worse, to cumulative traumatic encephalopathy. The majority of research in this area has been done on male athletes and methodologic issues have been raised in some studies. Newer studies are underway including female soccer players.

SPINE
Cervical Spine Injury

Burners or **stingers** are terms given to temporary burning or stinging pain that travels down an arm after a traction or compression injury to the cervical nerve root or upper trunk of the brachial plexus. The symptoms are generally self-limiting but occasionally can recur and progress; when this occurs, the symptoms must be recognized and managed aggressively. A force that distracts the shoulder from the head and neck can lead to compression on the contralateral side or distraction on the ipsilateral side (Fig. 39-1). The neurologic and musculoskeletal examination, if positive, directs any need for radiographic testing such as bony pain requiring plain films or neurologic deficit requiring magnetic resonance imaging (MRI) or electromyography (EMG) testing. The rehabilitation focus is twofold: to address both the biomechanical factors leading to the injury and the deficits associated with the injury. Although men's football is the sport with the greatest incidence of burners and stingers, they also occur in wrestling and hockey; all are sports in which women's participation is growing.

Thoracic Spine Injury

Compression fractures of the thoracic spine are reported infrequently in woman athletes. Cheerleading and other sports, in which excessive loads are placed on a flexed spine, especially with landing from a height, are associated with this injury. Attention to the underlying bone health of the injured athlete is mandatory. The history must include menstrual history, nutritional status, including questioning about eating disorders, and previous history of bone injury, including stress fracture. Management of compression fractures is largely symptom based and may require an orthosis set in extension. Rehabilitation stresses maintenance of trunk and hip range of motion, posture, and spine stabilization.

Lumbar Spine Injury

Spondylolysis is a relatively common radiographic finding, more so in the athletic population. Studies of adolescent female gymnasts demonstrate a rate of spondylolysis that is five times the rate for nonathletic females. It involves a defect in the pars interarticularis of the vertebral arch, usually involving the fifth lumbar vertebrae. The pars defect is most likely a fatigue fracture from repetitive loading of a congenitally weaker bony structure.

Spondylolisthesis refers to an anterior displacement of the vertebral body on the one below, coincident with spondylolysis in roughly 25% of cases. There is controversy in the literature regarding the optimal treatment regimen. When spondylolisthesis is associated with low back pain, healing and symptom control are achieved via bracing or at a minimum, activity restriction. Some type of radiographic study is used serially to document the extent of initial injury and healing, including single proton emission computed tomography, computed tomography (CT), or MRI. Surgical intervention is required when conservative managed has not led to pain control, when there is a progressive slip, or when neurologic deficits are identified.

Women athletes are also susceptible to low back pain arising from conditions that affect the general population, including **mechanical low back pain, internal disk derangement,** and **disk herniation with or without nerve root impingement.** It is unclear from the scientific literature whether athletes are at a higher risk for developing lumbar spine injuries. Athletes are at risk for internal disk derangement because of the repetitive loads placed, with both compressive and torsional forces, on the spine. The physical examination rules out any ominous findings related to

Table 39-2
Functional Sports Medicine Rehabilitation Management Strategy

Rehabilitation Phase/Target	Treatment Focus	Goals/Criteria to Advance
Acute Phase Target: Control symptoms and facilitate local tissue healing	Medications Rest/immobilization Modalities Manual therapy Range of motion +/− assist based on pain Isometric strengthening Pain-free cross training	Pain control Edema management Tissue healing Normalize range of motion Minimize deconditioning
Recovery Phase Target: Restore tissue, muscle and joint flexibility and restore normal movement patterns	Flexibility Proprioception and balance Strengthening with limited joint stress, (i.e., straight leg raises, closed kinetic chain exercises) Trunk stabilization	Full pain free range-of-motion Adequate flexibility Strength involved side 75% of uninvolved

Functional Phase
Target: Address biomechanical issues, restore advanced movement patterns without abnormal compensatory patterns to prevent recurrence
	Power and endurance
	Advance strengthening:
	  High reps/low resistance for endurance and
	  Low reps/high resistance for power
	  Neuromuscular re-education
	  Agility drills and pylometrics
	  Sports-specific activity
		Full flexibility
		Pain-free sports activity with normal mechanics
		Normal strength and cardiovascular fitness

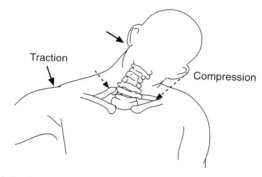

FIG. 39-1 Burners or stingers are caused by a blow to the shoulder or neck. As the neck is forced into lateral flexion, the brachial plexus may be stretched via traction on the ipsilateral side or compressed via loading on the contralateral side. (From Feinberg JH, Nadler SF, Krivickas LS: *Sports Med* 24[6]:385, 1997.)

fracture or nerve root impingement and evaluates the length and strength of muscles, being alert for abnormal movement patterns. Radiographic testing is seldom required initially as low back pain generally resolves spontaneously over several weeks. Pain management includes the use of medications, primarily nonsteroidal anti-inflammatory drugs (NSAIDs), modalities, and physical therapy. In the setting of nerve root impingement or radiculopathy, consideration is given for epidural steroid injections when other pain management strategies fail. Emergent referral for surgical evaluation is mandatory in the setting of cauda equina syndrome or progressive neurologic decline. Diskectomy is performed in less than 2% of individuals who present with low back pain.

UPPER EXTREMITY
Shoulder Injury

Shoulder injuries in female athletes occur for a variety of reasons. Longitudinal studies of strength differences between men and women demonstrate greater differences in upper body than lower body strength. This difference is virtually eliminated when strength is expressed relative to fat-free weight. Women have shorter arm length and shorter body length and thus require more strokes for swimming the same distance compared with men. Women historically have poorer conditioning than men do. This conditioning gap should narrow as girls become involved in sports at a younger age. Some authors argue that increased joint laxity, more common in women, may equate to increase injury risk. Finally, women may be at an increased injury risk owing to use of resistance training equipment designed for the male body.

The most common shoulder injuries seen in athletes include impingement syndrome, rotator cuff tendinitis or tendinopathy, and instability. Swimming, racquet sports, and sports requiring throwing are associated with **impingement syndromes.** In the setting of ongoing pain, maladaptive movement patterns can develop and evaluation of the scapulothoracic joint is included on physical examination. Physical examination maneuvers such as Hawkin's and Neer's tests, in which the examiner passively abducts or flexes the arm and narrows the subacromial space, are painful with impingement.

Rotator cuff tendinitis is a common overuse injury and can present with localized pain or with a pain referral pattern to the lateral arm. Scaption testing, in which the patient performs resisted shoulder abduction with the arm positioned in the plane of the scapula at 90 degrees of abduction, is done to assess for integrity and pain in the supraspinatus.

Instability is usually due to capsular laxity. Anterior instability is the most common clinical scenario. In the setting of mild laxity, symptoms occur only with repetitive overhead activities. Moderate laxity presents with recurrent subluxations. Severe laxity presents with recurrent dislocations. MRI testing may be pursued in the setting of rotator cuff tear or labral injury to plan for possible invasive procedures such as arthroscopy.

Treatment of shoulder injuries begins with pain control and restoration of normal joint kinematics, including not only the glenohumeral joint, but also the scapulothoracic, acromioclavicular, and sternoclavicular joints. Strength training of the shoulder girdle is added to the rehabilitation program as soon as possible. Despite inequity in upper body strength, men and women experience similar relative strength gains with training. Biceps and rotator cuff strengthening contribute to the stiffness and rigidity of the glenohumeral ligaments, decreasing instability. Restoration of normal movement patterns and strength of the scapular stabilizers avoids recurrent injury. Maintaining full range of motion, especially of the hip and neck in throwing athletes, allows for appropriate force generation and dissipation. As in all sports injuries, sports-specific training precedes return to play.

Elbow Injury

Overuse injuries of the wrist extensor and flexor muscles and their attachment sites at the lateral and medial elbow occur in sports requiring repetitive arm and hand movements. It is clinically relevant to describe these injuries anatomically (lateral epicondylitis) rather than athletically (tennis elbow). Sports associated with **epicondylitis** include tennis, golf, rowing, and softball. The differential diagnosis of elbow pain includes cervical radiculopathy or disk herniation with referred somatic pain, internal derangement of the elbow, and referral from the joints above and below the elbow (shoulder and wrist). Management includes local pain control, restoration of normal range of motion, and strengthening along the entire kinetic chain. A tennis-elbow brace worn 2.5 cm below the epicondyle may help relieve the strain. Equipment modification, such as increased racquet grip size, can decrease the tendency for overuse.

Wrist, Hand, and Finger Injury

Although primary care physicians are familiar with common causes of hand and finger pain such as carpal tunnel syndrome, injuries not to be missed in the female athlete include scaphoid fracture, scapholunate dissociation, and mallet finger. **Scaphoid fracture** is the most common carpal fracture in athletes, typically resulting from a fall on an outstretched hand. Tenderness can be elicited by palpating the scaphoid at the base of the anatomic snuffbox. One can also apply a load to the scaphoid, while assessing for pain, by axial compression of the thumb toward the radius or by loading the wrist in radial deviation. X-ray studies in the setting of fracture can be negative initially and if the suspicion for fracture is high, one can consider casting and repeating the x-ray study in 2 weeks. There is a high risk of nonunion and surgically treatment may be indicated.

Scapholunate dissociation, from scapholunate ligament tear, is another cause of radial wrist pain that can be evaluated using Watson's test. The examiner applies pressure to the scaphoid while passively radially deviating the wrist. If the athlete feels pain dorsally (at the scapholunate ligament) or the examiner feels the scaphoid move dorsally, the test is positive. Plain x-ray films taken while the patient makes a clenched fist assess for a gap greater than 3 mm between the scaphoid and lunate. Operative treatment may be necessary.

Mallet finger results from avulsion of the extensor mechanism at the distal interphalangeal (DIP) joint. It commonly occurs from a ball striking the end of an outstretched finger, forcing finger flexion while the extensor mechanism is activated (catching a pass in basketball). On examination, the athlete is unable to extend the DIP joint actively. Once x-ray studies exclude an avulsion fracture, treatment includes splinting the DIP joint in slight hyperextension continuously for 8 weeks to avoid a permanent loss of terminal extension.

LOWER EXTREMITY

Stress Fractures

Stress fractures occur more commonly in female athletes. Stress fractures are complete or partial bone fractures caused by the accumulation of microtrauma. If the normal bone remodeling system does not keep pace with the force applied, stress reaction (microfractures) and finally stress fracture can result. Malalignment and poor flexibility of the lower extremities (intrinsic factors) and inadequate footwear, changes in training surface, and increases in training intensity and duration without an adequate ramp-up period (extrinsic factors) can lead to stress fractures. Stress fractures in female athletes are most common in the lower extremities, including the tibia, metatarsals, and fibula. They affect runners and dancers most commonly (Fig. 39-2). Patients may report a recent increase in training or activity level preceding the onset of symptoms. In general, pain improves with rest.

On physical examination, there is a local area of exquisite, well-localized tenderness, warmth, and edema over the affected region of the bone. Placing a vibrating tuning fork over the fracture site intensifies the pain. In the pelvis, the inferior pubic rami, near the symphysis pubis, is the most common location for stress fractures. In the tibia, stress fractures primarily occur along the medial border. In the fibula, they usually present one hand's breadth proximal to the lateral malleolus. Tarsal or metatarsal stress fractures present with localized foot tenderness. Weight-bearing activity such as a one legged-hop test can provoke the pain by increasing the ground reaction forces. For a presumed femoral stress fracture, the examiner can provoke pain by applying a downward force on the distal femur while the affected individual is seated with the distal femur extending beyond the edge of the seat. Examination of the lumbar spine and lower limbs evaluates for any biomechanical abnormalities. For example, an individual with rigid supinated feet or weak foot intrinsic muscles may transmit more ground reaction forces to the tibia.

Plain films may take as long as 6 weeks to show fracture. Technetium-99m diphosphonate bone scanning will yield the earliest confirmatory data for stress fractures, showing a "hot spot" in 1 to 4 days. The fracture site may not return to normal on a bone scan for 5 months or longer. CT may be necessary for differentiating stress fractures of the sacrum and pelvis. MRI provides soft tissue definition, which can be helpful in the setting of stress reaction. One should

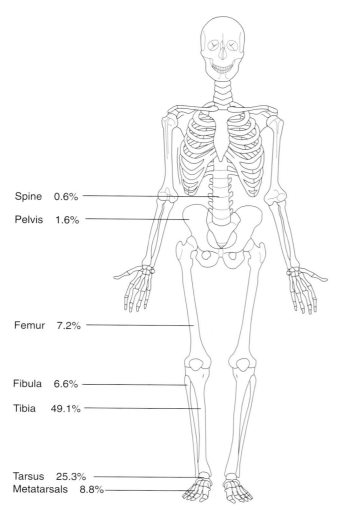

Spine   0.6%

Pelvis   1.6%

Femur   7.2%

Fibula   6.6%

Tibia   49.1%

Tarsus   25.3%
Metatarsals   8.8%

FIG. 39-2   Common sites of stress fractures in athletes. (From Matheson GO et al: *Am J Sports Med* 15[1]:46,1987.)

consider bone density testing in a female with a history of amenorrhea.

The mainstay of stress fracture treatment is activity modification. Pain resolution is used as the clinical guide to progression of activity. Pneumatic leg braces are thought to stabilize the fracture site and limit force transduction. Orthotics can provide shock absorption and reduce foot deformities such as hyperpronation. Conservative management successfully treats lower extremity stress fractures, with a few exceptions. Femoral neck stress fractures on the tensile (superior) aspect may require pinning if they do not heal after a course of non-weight bearing. Midshaft tibial fractures are at risk of nonunion and must be immobilized and followed closely; an open bone grafting procedure may be indicated in the setting of nonunion.

Compartment syndrome can mimic stress reaction or stress fracture of the leg. It can involve the anterior, superficial posterior, or deep posterior muscles, with anterior or posterior lower leg pain, respectively; pain increases with exercise and is associated with a feeling of tightness. There may be associated distal neurologic symptoms indicative of local nerve compression. Compartment pressure testing is the definitive test, with normal pressure between 0 and

10 mm Hg. If conservative treatment with rest, local superficial and deep soft tissue release, and correction of biomechanical abnormalities fails, fasciotomy may be indicated.

Pelvis and Sacrum Injury

In addition to the stress fractures noted in the preceding section, other injuries in the pelvis and sacrum can present a diagnostic dilemma. As in other areas of the body, muscle strains, bursitis, and tendonitis, often associated with muscle imbalances, are common. The piriformis muscle is prone to overuse and can be stretched and activated by the examiner as one attempts to define a specific pain generator. The sciatic nerve travels in close proximity, through the piriformis in a small percentage of the population, and may be involved. One should evaluate distal neurologic function of both the peroneal and tibial portions of the sciatic nerve.

The examiner must be adept at evaluating the joints of the pelvis, including the pubic symphysis and sacroiliac (SI) joint. Leg length discrepancy has been identified as an instigator of pain and dysfunction in the spine and pelvis. The SI joint can be painful in women who exercise; sports that require asymmetric movement of the lower extremities, such as skating, golfing, and gymnastics, are associated with SI joint pain. Stair steppers and elliptic trainers may exacerbate the pain. Pregnant women are more susceptible to SI joint pain owing to ligamentous laxity reducing the force closure component of SI joint competence. Diagnostic testing rarely defines the pathology. Treatment must address the muscle imbalances in addition to bony alignment issues to be successful.

Hip Injury

Snapping hip is a symptom complex sometimes reported by exercising women. The source of the snapping sensation can typically be discovered on examination, including intra-articular hip joint pathology, tendon issues, such as the iliopsoas muscle snapping over the iliopectineal eminence, or pubic symphysis instability. Intra-articular concerns may require further diagnostic testing to rule out acetabular labral tear, loose body, or other bony lesions; the decision to pursue further testing is based on the complete history and physical examination findings.

Greater trochanteric bursitis and **gluteus medius tendinitis** often occur together and are seen in long-distance runners. If acute rehabilitation strategies (relative rest, NSAIDS, stretching) are unsuccessful, corticosteroid injection may be required. Strengthening of the hip and lumbopelvic area is mandatory.

Iliotibial band syndrome can also cause hip pain. The iliotibial band is tight commonly and can cause pain anywhere along its course from its origin at the tensor fascia lata muscle to its attachment at Gerdy's tubercle just distal to the lateral knee joint line. It responds well to local treatment and stretching.

Conditions not to be missed in the hip region include stress fracture and referred pain. **Femoral stress fractures** occur primarily in long distance runners and must be included in the differential for any female presenting with recalcitrant hip or groin pain. Stress fracture management is based on the location and intensity of symptoms, as noted previously. Neurogenic causes of hip pain must always be considered, such as **referred pain** from lower lumbar disk disease. Visceral structures, such as the ovary, can also be the source of hip and pelvic pain. The woman should be questioned about association of the pain with the menstrual cycle, abnormal bleeding, or other pelvic symptoms.

Knee Injury

Retrospective and prospective studies of female athletes at all levels of play have shown an increased risk for **anterior cruciate ligament (ACL) injuries** of the knee vis-a-vis men in comparable sports. Factors contributing to increased ACL injuries in women include both extrinsic and intrinsic factors (Table 39-3). Historical clues to ACL tears include a weight bearing, rotatory mechanism of injury and acute knee effusion. Specific ACL physical examination techniques are the Lachman's maneuver and anterior drawer test. In these tests, the femur is stabilized while the examiner passively glides the tibia anteriorly. Prevention strategies for ACL injuries include sports participation at early age, improved preseason conditioning, and strength training with a hamstring focus versus quadriceps focus. These hamstring-focused strengthening techniques are integrated into the rehabilitation program. The gastrocnemius can also be strengthened for dynamic knee stabilization. Plyometric, or weight-bearing eccentric, training of the lower limbs is necessary before the athlete returns to play. Coaching should include modified jumping and cutting movement patterns. Depending on the level of the athlete, surgical repair may be pursued. Recreational athletes can be managed successfully without surgical repair of the ACL.

The **patellofemoral pain syndrome** is another common cause of anterior knee pain in women athletes; it is thought to be related to the "miserable malalignment syndrome" (pronation of the feet, increased femoral anteversion, and increased genu valgus) observed in women more often than men (Fig. 39-3). It occurs after direct macrotrauma (volleyball) or repetitive microtrauma (running, especially hills) with recurrent flexion and extension of the weight-bearing knee joint. A short period of immobilization from days to weeks is indicated, depending on the severity of symptoms and instability. Local imbalance of muscle length and strength about the knee joint must be recognized and remedied for pain control and prevention of recurrent injury. Beyond the usual pain and edema management noted in Table 39-2, taping or bracing may provide increased proprioceptive feedback and improve tracking of the patella.

Meniscal tears and **other ligamentous knee injuries** including the medial collateral ligament, lateral collateral ligament, and posterior cruciate ligament do occur; but the female athlete does not appear to be at greater risk than her male counterpart participating in the same sport. Meniscal tears present with joint line tenderness with variable amounts of swelling. The athlete should be questioned about locking of the knee joint. Squatting and walking in a crouched position can provoke meniscal pain. McMurray's test, in which the menisci are loaded with passive knee flexion and rotation with the athlete supine, can elicit meniscal pain. Apley's compression test is done prone with the examiner applying a load to the meniscus through the long axis of the tibia with the knee flexed at 90 degrees. Rehabilitation includes the principles of acute pain and edema management followed by progressive, controlled flexibility and strength training of the lower extremities, with introduction of plyometric and sports specific training before return to play.

Table 39-3
Proposed Etiology of ACL Injuries in Women

Extrinsic Causes	Intrinsic Causes
Conditioning	Gender differences in hamstring and
Body movement	quad strength
Jump landing	Knee muscle recruitment pattern
Planting and cutting	Females use quadriceps to stabilize
Ankle bracing	knee
	Female knee muscles with longer time
	to peak force production
	Female knee more ligament dominant
	Joint laxity greater in women
	Hormonal effect
	Variability during menstrual cycle
	Biomechanical differences between
	genders
	Wider pelvis
	Genu recurvatum
	Increased femoral anteversion
	Static postures
	Increased subtalar pronation and
	navicular drop
	Notch width/Notch Width Index
	smaller in women

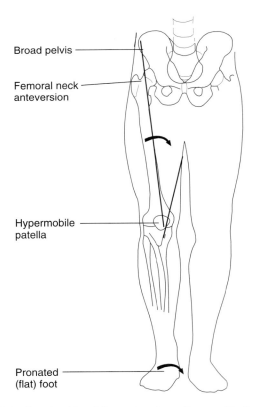

FIG. 39-3 The miserable malalignment syndrome. These combinations of biomechanical factors express a phenotypic difference in females that cause a propensity toward knee pain. (From Ciullo JV: Lower extremity injuries. In Pearl AJ, editor: *The athletic female*, Champaign, 1993, Human Kinetics.)

Broad pelvis

Femoral neck anteversion

Hypermobile patella

Pronated (flat) foot

Ankle and Foot Injury

As noted at the beginning of the chapter, the ankle is the most common anatomic area of injury according to NCAA data. **Inversion ankle sprain** is by far the most common ankle injury suffered, with the three lateral ligaments being torn, in order, depending on the severity of the injury as follows: anterior talofibular ligament (ATFL), calcaneofibular ligament (CFL), and posterior talofibular ligament. The anterior drawer test in which the examiner stabilizes the tibia and fibula and glides the foot anteriorly, assesses the integrity of the ATFL. The talar tilt test, in which the examiner stabilizes the tibia and fibula and passively moves the foot medially and laterally, assesses the integrity of the CFL. Beyond initial pain and edema management, training for restoration of normal proprioception of the ankle joint must be provided. Many athletes with chronic ankle sprains use taping or bracing for sporting events.

BREAST INJURY

Women who exercise complain of breast discomfort, particularly if they are large breasted or during the premenstrual phase of the menstrual cycle. Sports bras with strong back construction and nonstretch straps give support from all sides and can reduce discomfort. Breast trauma with associated contusion occurs infrequently and is managed like contusion in other areas, with ice, analgesics, and support. Padding can be added to sports bras for contact sports to protect the breasts from injury.

Nipple injury such as "runner's nipples," in which the nipples are irritated and abraded by clothing during prolonged activity, is more common in males. Prevention is brought about by local use of petroleum jelly or tape, use of a bra with a seamless cup, and using a wind-breaking material over the chest for exercise in cold weather.

FEMALE ATHLETE TRIAD

No review of sports injuries in women would be complete without mentioning the female athlete triad. The triad includes three interrelated conditions, namely disordered eating, amenorrhea, and osteoporosis. The triad is associated with decreased fertility and increased injury, especially stress fractures. Disordered eating can lead to menstrual disturbance, most likely related to negative calorie balance and hypothalamic dysfunction. Menstrual disorders can lead to reduced fertility owing to anovulatory cycles or amenorrhea. Premature osteoporosis occurs as a result of estrogen deficiency and not only increases the immediate risk of fracture but has long-term implications for bone health. Some studies have shown that reduction in bone density persists despite resumption of normal menses or use of hormone replacement.

Strategies on preventing the female athlete triad are key in minimizing its impact. Ideally, these strategies are aimed at preventing all three components of the triad. Identifying and treating disordered eating can prevent the associated menstrual and bone metabolism disorders. Similarly, identifying exercise-induced amenorrhea and providing treatment before the occurrence of stress fracture is important not only for athletic performance but for long-term musculoskeletal health. Providing an open, self-empowered, and caring environment for athletes enhances their willingness to discuss personal matters, especially as pertains to disordered eating, such as dissatisfaction with body shape or family dysfunction. Educational material is available from the ACSM and NCAA and should be prominently displayed in locker rooms and training areas. Principles of proper hydration and nutrition should be presented in required team meetings and reinforced during practice, competition, and team meals. Coaches and parents of younger athletes should be team members in our goal of preventing the female athlete triad and its sequelae.

BIBLIOGRAPHY

Arendt EA: Orthopedic issues for active and athletic women, in Agostini R, editor: The athletic woman, *Clin Sports Med* 13:483, 1994.

Arendt E, Dick R: Knee injury patterns among men and women in collegiate basketball and soccer. NCAA data and review of the literature, *Am J Sports Med* 23:694, 1995.

Barrow G, Saha S: Menstrual irregularity and stress fracture in collegiate female distance runners, *Am J Sports Med* 16:209, 1988.

Bennell KL, Brukner PD: Epidemiology and site specificity of stress fractures, *Clin Sports Med* 16:179, 1997.

Brody DM: Techniques in the evaluation and treatment of the injured runner, *Orthop Clin North Am* 13:541, 1982.

DeHaven KE, Lintner DM: Athletic injuries: comparison by age, sport, and gender, *Am J Sports Med* 14:218, 1986.

Feinberg JH: Burners and stingers, *Phys Med Rehabil Clin North Am* 11(4):771, 2000.

Hewett TE, Stroupe AL, Nance TA, Noyes FR: Plyometric training in female athletes: decreased impact forces and increased hamstring torques, *Am J Sports Med* 24:765, 1996.

Huston LJ, Wojtys EM: Neuromuscular performance characteristics in elite female athletes, *Am J Sports Med* 24:427, 1996.

Hutchinson MR, Ireland ML: Knee injuries in female athletes, *Am J Sports Med* 19:288, 1995.

Kibler WB: Rehabilitation of the shoulder. In Kibler WB, Herring SA, Press JM, editors: *Functional rehabilitation of sports and musculoskeletal injuries,* Gaithersburg, Md, 1998, Aspen Publishers.

Kibler WB, Chandler TJ, Pace BK: Principles of rehabilitation after chronic injuries, *Clin Sports Med* 11:668, 1992.

Leblanc KE: The female athlete. *Comp Ther* 24:256-264, 1998.

Lewis DA, Kamon E, Hodgson JL: Physiological differences between genders: implications for sports conditioning, *Sports Med* 3:357, 1986.

Marcus R et al: Menstrual function and bone mass in elite women distance runners: endocrine and metabolic factors, *Ann Intern Med* 102:158, 1985.

Myburgh KH et al: Low bone density is an etiologic factor for stress fracture in athletes, *Ann Intern Med* 113:754, 1990.

O'Brien SJ: Developmental anatomy of the shoulder in throwing, swimming, gymnastics, and tennis, *Clin Sports Med* 2:247, 1983.

Prather H: Pelvis and sacral dysfunction in sports and exercise, *Phys Med Rehabil Clin North Am* 11(4):805, 2000.

Richards DB, Kibler WB: Rehabilitation of knee injuries. In Kibler WB, Herring SA, Press JM, editors: *Functional rehabilitation of sports and musculoskeletal injuries,* Gaithersburg, Md, 1998, Aspen Publishers.

Standaert CJ, Herring SA, Halpern B, King O: Spondylolysis, *Phys Med Rehabil Clin North Am* 11(4):785, 2000.

Traina SM, Bromberg DF: ACL injury patterns in women, *Orthopedics* 20:545, 1997.

Young JL, Press JM: Rehabilitation of running injuries. In Buschbacher R, Braddom R, editors: *Sports medicine and rehabilitation: a sports specific approach,* Philadelphia, 1994, Hanley and Belfus.

CHAPTER **40**

Sleep Disorders

Joyce A. Walsleben
David M. Rapoport

Throughout their lifetime women suffer more sleep difficulty than men. This is true despite the fact that biologically women tend to have more delta (slow wave sleep) and rapid-eye-movement (REM) sleep than men. Recent research suggests this implies "better" sleep.

Research studies and surveys all show that women complain of more insomnia and more pain and stress-related interference of sleep than men. In addition, women's cyclic sex hormones and changing life stages such as menarche, pregnancy and lactation, and menopause affect sleep. Sleep problems among women typically emerge during the childbearing years, when many are trying to juggle work and home life and tend to careers, marriages, and children. Some must work the night shift. Most work "the second shift" of home and family. There are just so many hours in the day and something has to give. That something is usually sleep.

This chapter briefly presents normal sleep, discusses the impact of women's issues on sleep, and explores the more common sleep disorders for women.

NORMAL SLEEP

Typically sleep is divided into two states of consciousness: nonrapid eye movement (NREM) and REM, which cycle every 70 to 90 minutes across the night. NREM sleep is divided into four stages denoting depth based on one's ability to arouse. The lightest, transitional stage is 1, which occurs about 5% to 7% of the night. Next in depth is stage 2, occupying 45% to 50% of the night. Stages 3 and 4, also called delta or slow wave sleep, are the deepest stages, occurring most frequently during the first third of the night and thought to be the most restorative stages of sleep. REM sleep, sometimes referred to as dream sleep, occurs about 20% of the night in adults. Sleep onset is regulated by both the circadian pacemaker and the homeostatic drive mechanisms, which respond to the total amount of prior wake time. The average adult needs about 7 to 8 hours of sleep, but few accomplish that goal. Sleep loss, even on a small scale, accumulates over time and can lead to significant symptoms of irritability, memory loss, and even injury, since short bursts of unattended micro sleeps can occur.

Sex Hormones

Although we recognize the potential impact on sleep of cyclic estrogen and progesterone across a woman's life, few studies have systematically evaluated the effect of cyclic hormones on sleep. Only the original work on sleep of normal subjects has controlled for the hormonal changes by studying women only in the follicular phase of the menstrual cycle. Worse, most animal work has studied male rats as models. Unfortunately, the studies that have examined sleep in women are small and have not even systematically considered the phase of the menstrual cycle or even described the cycle in the same terms. This is true despite the fact that the cycling of estrogen and progesterone varies both within and among women.

We do know that in humans, contrary to animals, **estrogen** appears to enhance REM sleep by decreasing the latency to onset and increasing the total amount of REM sleep captured. Similarly, estrogen replacement appears to increase slow wave sleep after menopause, lessening the age-related decline of that sleep stage. Estrogen also regulates the flow of other key hormones that are secreted during sleep, among them growth hormone, prolactin, cortisol, and melatonin. Melatonin, known as the "hormone of darkness," because it is produced by the pineal gland during the dark cycle, is thought to have a role in regulating sleep. This effect on sleep may come through its action of lowering body temperature. (We are more likely to fall asleep when our body temperature is falling and wake as it rises.) A number of drugs may suppress melatonin secretion, among them aspirin and ibuprofen, as well as beta blockers, alcohol, nicotine, and caffeine.

Progesterone seems to have a hypnotic and anxiolytic effect that is dose dependent. Its action is similar to that of the benzodiazepines. In studies administering progesterone, there is a reduction in the amount of time it takes to get to sleep and the number of episodes of wakefulness after sleep onset and increase NREM stage 2 sleep.

Testosterone, excreted by the adrenals in women and converted into estrogen in the brain, has variable effects on sleep. In men testosterone decreases REM sleep. For women as estrogen is waning, the ratio of estrogen to testosterone changes. Women sensitive to the effects of androgens will feel symptoms of irritability, sleeplessness, and depression similar to that of estrogen loss.

Menstrual Cycles

In studies of sleep, the menstrual cycle has been divided into two to eight phases. If two phases are studied, they are the follicular (preovulation) and luteal (postovulation). If more than two, authors separate each phase into parts, early or late. They may also include menstruation and ovulation as phases.

In the follicular phase, as increased estrogen is triggered by follicle-stimulating hormone, many women experience an increased depth of sleep if not actual increased sleep time and increased slow wave sleep and total sleep time. At midcycle, after ovulation, the corpus luteum produces progesterone. This increase in progesterone acts to increase body temperature and blunt circadian rhythm. Over the course of the next 14 days, there is increased wakefulness and increased sleep disturbance. Because of the blunting in melatonin rhythm, women tend to get sleepy earlier and wake up early. The metabolic rate increases as well. Researchers see a decrease in the depth of sleep and an increase in time to fall asleep.

Additional estrogen is secreted in the early luteal phase perhaps modulating these changes. In the late luteal phase, when estrogen and progesterone fall, studies indicate that women have more nighttime awakenings and a greater percentage of NREM sleep. There is a significant decrease in slow wave sleep premenstrually, decreased sleep efficiency, an increase in the time it takes to fall asleep, and decreased sleep quality. A total of 68% of menstruating women surveyed felt sleepiest during the week before or the first few days of their periods, compared with the rest of the month.

During menstruation, female hormone secretion lessens as does metabolic rate. As a result, many women experience excessive daytime sleepiness. In rare cases, women can suffer debilitating hypersomnia, excessive daytime sleepiness that begins premenstrually and clears up after a menses begins. This may be as a result of sensitivity to progesterone's sedating effects.

Women who experience premenstrual syndrome (PMS) may experience these symptoms to a greater degree. PMS varies from woman to woman. Clinically, PMS symptoms arise in the period between ovulation and menstruation. There may also be daytime sleepiness and increased sleep disturbances. Some researchers have likened PMS to jet lag. Both are temporary conditions involving nighttime sleep disturbance and daytime sleepiness, with mood changes and difficulty concentrating. Both also involve shifts in the secretion of melatonin. Melatonin has been found to be higher premenstrually and during menstruation. Low serotonin may also contribute to PMS-related mood swings, depression, and anxiety.

For women who suffer premenstrual dysphoric disorder (PMDD), sleep problems are common. Despite these general findings, it is important to note the vast individuality of responses among women.

Pregnancy and the Postpartum Period

Being pregnant and caring for an infant also affects sleep. Owing to the rapid rise of progesterone during the first trimester, many women are unable to stay awake during the day. Progesterone also inhibits smooth muscle contraction and may be responsible for their frequent trips to the bathroom during the night. By 11 weeks of pregnancy, sleep becomes disrupted with increased awakenings, a shorter time to fall asleep, and less efficient sleep. Some studies show a slight decline in REM and slow wave sleep, perhaps as a result of more awakenings. REM sleep returns to almost normal levels during the last month of pregnancy. Some women may also be bothered at night by nausea (which is hormonally related) and by backaches.

By the second trimester sleep is the most consistent. However, women are bothered by fetal movements and the emergence of pregnancy-related heartburn. Restless leg activity may also start during the second trimester and may be caused by an imbalance of ferritin in the brain. Despite the normal serum level, brain ferritin may be low. Additional iron in supplement form is frequently helpful.

During the third trimester, there is increasing sleep difficulty, in part because of the physical girth of the body and the inability to be comfortable and in part because of changing hormones before delivery. Sleep deprivation and fatigue are major issues late in the third trimester. Women also suffer from shortness of breath, frequent urination, cramps, itching, and frequent nightmares. Heartburn increases along with the size of the belly. Additionally, the growing uterus also can press on the sciatic nerve causing pain. Each of these problems interferes with sleep continuity.

In addition to the hormonal aspects of pregnancy and childbirth, there are the physical stresses of pregnancy and the demands of taking care of a newborn who needs to be fed on a schedule (day or night). In striving to do their best, parents often put their own sleep needs on the back burner. Postpartum depression or anxiety may be overlooked as a cause of sleep problems because we expect disrupted sleep at this time of life.

On the other hand, sleep loss is a major culprit in mood problems and in the memory loss of new mothers (which may also be hormonally related). First-time mothers show a significant decrease in sleep efficiency and increase in fatigue compared with women with other children. Furthermore, the sleep systems of women with a history of depression may be more sensitive to the psychobiological changes of childbearing. Those women may have an earlier onset or more severe sleep disruption.

Perimenopause and Menopause

During the perimenopausal years, physical and psychological symptoms such as hot flashes and depression can also take their toll on sleep, but in differing ways. Menopausal symptoms caused by hormones keep some women from a good night's sleep. Stress also plays a role. A recent study evaluated the sleep, physical symptoms, and stress of perimenopausal women 40 to 59 years old and found that those who complained of poor sleep frequently showed good sleep when measured objectively in the sleep laboratory. However, these women also reported more stress and body symptoms, such as muscle pain, than women with no sleep complaints. The women who did have objectively documented poor sleep reported menopausal-related physical symptoms such as hot flashes. The hot flash of menopause is a global excitation of central as well as peripheral sympathetic activity. The increase in norepinephrine acts to alert and arouse the sleeping brain. Daytime sleepiness and memory deficits occur as a result of frequent awakenings with subsequent difficulty falling back to sleep.

SLEEP DISORDERS
Insomnia

Insomnia, generally thought to be a symptom rather than its own entity, is the complaint of a significant inability to fall asleep or stay asleep, which ultimately interferes with day time functioning through the progression of sleep deprivation. Most surveys recognize 30% to 35% of adults (two to three times more women than men) will suffer this phenomenon during their lifetime. For many it will be fleeting, perhaps linked to sudden life changes or illness. For others, however, the symptoms appear to be unrelenting. Short-term insomnia is that which lasts less than 1 week and is generally related to a significant self-contained life stress. Transient (more than 1 and less than 3 months) and chronic insomnia (longer than 3 months) may have begun with a stressful event but are now the combination of anxiety, poor reactive habits and lifestyle, and continuing stress.

Pathophysiology

The pathophysiology of insomnia is multifactorial. Physical, physiologic, psychological, psychiatric, and pharmacologic causes exist, and each deserves exploration for its impact on sleep. Physical factors that interfere with sleep include noises, illness, and pain. Physiologic interference includes jet lag, shift work, and hormonal changes. Psychological factors include stress, anger, and a perceived lack of safety. Psychiatric illnesses frequently note insomnia as part of their symptom list. It is often difficult to assess the impact of subtle disease such as clinical depression. Recent work has suggested that insomnia may precede relapse of known depression. Similarly, pharmacologic interactions exist between drugs and the modulation of sleep. Medication used to treat other conditions (e.g., hypertension) may foster or impede sleep. The administration time may need to be altered to minimize side effects or even to take advantage of these incidental physiologic effects. Further subdivisions of insomnia are described in the International Classification of Sleep Disorders (ICSD). They include psychophysiologic insomnia, sleep state misperception, idiopathic insomnia, fatal familiar insomnia, food allergy insomnia, and menstrual-related sleep disorders.

Diagnosis

Both the ICSD and the *Diagnostic and Statistical Manual of Mental Disorders,* Fourth Edition (DSM-IV) urge a complete evaluation of insomnia including a complete review of systems, physical examination, and blood chemistries to rule out other obvious causes such as anemia, thyroid disorder, fever, or pain. Both diagnostic systems have practical use for clinicians. In addition, a review of current medication, as well as over-the-counter drugs such as herbal products, should be included in the evaluation. It is important to learn when the disorder began and what the initial situation was. Frequently, the patient can tell you about the onset of the symptoms as they relate to a stress or life change that may be very current or years old. In addition, detailed information regarding sleep/wake schedules and daily habits is

essential. When is the sleep period? How regular is it? What are the bedtime habits, daytime stressors, typical interference? What remedies have been tried and how did they work? It is helpful to have the patient graph her sleep/wake activity including hours of meals, physical activity, medications, alcohol, and tobacco use for the 2 weeks before the evaluation. This may help her spot a trend or recognize that she is getting more sleep than she thinks.

Treatment

Treatment of insomnia is also multifactorial. Correction of any underlying cause is essential. Treatment should always include the teaching of good sleep habits (see later discussion). Short-term insomnia may be well treated with short-acting sedative/hypnotics. There are many choices, depending on the form of insomnia. When considering the choice, it is important to consider the symptoms (onset or maintenance insomnia), the patient's health status, other medications, social support, and responsibilities, as well as age. Short half-life drugs such as zolpidem or zaleplon are good choices for sleep-onset difficulties. Zaleplon is a safe choice for maintenance insomnia as well because its half-life is 1 hour, and it can be taken again during the night or late in the night without morning hangover effects. Zaleplon has also been well tolerated in elderly people. Drugs useful for sleep maintenance difficulties include longer half-life preparations such as temazepam or triazolam. In this case it is important to warn the patient who made need to rise suddenly in the night that the drug effect may still be active and care should be taken regarding decision making and physical activity such as driving. Over-the-counter preparations for sleep generally contain diphenhydramine, which carries the possibility of long drug effect and hangover, as well as side effects of dryness that could affect respiratory and renal systems. Similarly, no studies of the efficacy of sedating antidepressants as hypnotics have been carried out, yet they are frequently prescribed for insomnia.

The treatment of long-term insomnia may require specialized skill found in sleep centers. Medications may be used initially along with structured routines. Good sleep habits/hygiene need to be taught (Box 40-1). In this case, teaching good investigatory skills is also helpful. Logs of sleep and wake activity over several weeks help the patient see what life practices influence sleep. They also become reinforcing as sleep improves and serve as a more objective measure in a very subjective arena.

Many techniques have been developed to refocus and retrain the patient. One such method is *sleep restriction.* This method acts to restrict the hours in bed to the number of average hours slept per night over the previous week. Once the allowed time in bed has been at least 90% filled with sleep for most of a week, the patient is allowed to increase the time in bed by 15 minutes. These increases can continue until the patient reaches the desired amount of sleep (7 to 8 hours). *Stimulus control* is another technique developed to reduce the impact of negative cognitions. In this technique, the patient uses the bedroom for sleep and sex. If the patients is not asleep in 30 minutes, she gets up and leaves the bedroom until she is sleepy again. Box 40-1 presents suggestions for good sleep hygiene.

Even when obvious causes such as other illnesses or medication changes have been resolved, the patient with

---

BOX 40-1
Good Sleep Hygiene

Set a regular wake time.
Limit time in bed to the number of hours usually slept.
Keep the bedroom quiet, safe, and dark.
Separate the bedroom from active living space and use it only for sleep.
Limit alcohol and tobacco.
Establish a worry book and worry well during the early afternoon.
Investigate stress-reducing routines to be used before bedtime.

BOX 40-2
Factors Related to Apnea

Increasing age
Obesity
Position
Alcohol and sedatives
Hypothyroidism
Facial abnormalities
Excessive airway tissue

---

long-term insomnia may continue on with learned behaviors/reactions that are damaging to good sleep. Studies show good symptomatic relief with the combination of behavioral approaches and medication. In addition, the use of estrogen replacement therapy has been shown to improve the sleep of postmenopausal women and may be an added benefit for those using this treatment option.

Apnea

Apnea refers to the cessation of airflow, usually as a result of complete closure of the airway. In obstructive sleep apnea, the closure is brief, lasting 10 or more seconds, but may be repeated every minute across the night. Incomplete closures also occur. These may be labeled hypopnea or increased upper airway resistance depending on the amount and consequence of the closure. Each of these episodes may result in oxygen desaturations and short, unrecognized arousals. The consequence over time is cardiovascular morbidity, excessive daytime sleepiness, and neurocognitive deficits. Estimated prevalence of sleep-disordered breathing, which is defined as an apnea-hypopnea score over 5 per hour of sleep, is 9% of adult women. Two percent will have the apnea-hypopnea syndrome, which includes daytime sleepiness.

Pathophysiology

The pathophysiology of obstructive apnea is multifactorial, reflecting a combination of anatomic and neuromuscular factors. Small pharyngeal airway size, nasal obstruction, inadequate muscle tone in the upper airway, the effect of sleep and position on airway tone, and obesity are all factors that interact to cause respiratory disturbance in sleep. In rare cases, other diseases may influence the onset of apnea. These include hypothyroidism, muscular dystrophies, and lung disease. Sleep deprivation, sedatives, and alcohol worsen the disorder by dampening the arousal mechanism that acts to end each event.

Diagnosis

Symptoms of obstructive apnea in both men *and* women include dramatic snoring (although many women do not know if they snore), gasping during sleep, restlessness, and daytime sleepiness. Unfortunately, despite giving the classic symptoms of apnea to their health care provider, many women are not diagnosed. It is not clear whether this results from a bias of the health care worker or the concurrent reporting of psychologically oriented symptoms, which attract more attention in women. In addition to a good physical workup, a thorough evaluation may include a nocturnal polysomnogram (PSG) to assess the form and severity of the respiratory event.

Obesity tends to be a large factor in the development of obstructive apnea. However, the placement of weight is also important. In women, weight tends to be more evenly distributed across the hips and chest than in men. For equal degrees of obesity, a man would probably experience more sleep apnea than the woman, perhaps because of the placement of male fat in the mid torso area. Women who have very large and heavy breasts may seem to be at risk, but research has not shown that the added weight of breast tissue affects her ability to move her rib cage and breathe. However, women who are severely overweight are in jeopardy at any age. They may not have apnea from airway obstruction but may suffer hypoventilation, a decreased effort to breathe particularly in REM, allowing significant hypoxia to develop. Box 40-2 lists factors related to apnea.

Treatment

Several forms of treatment exist depending on severity of the respiratory disorder and anatomic factors. Weight loss is helpful as are changes in sleeping position when appropriate. Others may use a variety of surgical techniques such as uvulopalatopharyngoplasty (UPPP), laser assisted-UPPP, and a radiofrequency method of trimming excess tissue to alter airway anatomy. Still others may be helped with dental devices that move the mandible forward. CPAP (continuous positive airway pressure) frequently is used in symptomatic obstructive sleep apnea. It is the most uniformly physiologically successful treatment, but it is tolerated by only about 70% to 80% of subjects. This treatment consists of the fitting of a tight mask to be worn over the nose during sleep, to which is connected a source of pressurized air from a quiet blower. This arrangement maintains pressure in the upper airway at a level that usually prevents or significantly reduces the occurrence of airway occlusions. A similar device can also provide assisted ventilation if needed.

PREGNANCY AND APNEA

Women can develop a temporary form of sleep apnea during pregnancy. In fact, a recent study of 500 Swedish women found that habitual snoring was a sign of pregnancy-induced high blood pressure (preeclampsia) and was associated with lower birth weights and lower Apgar scores (an evaluation of a newborn's heart rate, respiratory effort, muscle tone, response to stimulation, and skin color). The study also noted that women started to snore before any sign of hypertension appeared and that snoring was related to sleep apnea. Although it may seem reasonable to suppose that the increased abdominal girth of pregnancy (with or without excessive weight gain) underlies the increase in apnea, there is little evidence to support this. A more likely explanation is that the frequent nasal congestion experienced by pregnant women predisposes to upper airway collapse owing to the large negative pressure in the airway needed to overcome nasal obstruction.

Central Apnea/Cheyne-Stokes Respiration

A different form of apnea, known variously as central apnea or Cheyne-Stoke respiration, occurs without clear airway obstruction. This is due to a failure of breathing efforts and may also contribute to sleep disruption and daytime symptoms. Cheyne-Stokes respiration (waxing and waning breaths with or without apnea) occurs predominantly in the elderly and in those with a low cardiac output. It may also occur in certain neurologic diseases. It is rarely associated with retention of CO_2 or cardiorespiratory failure and is generally thought to be more of a marker of the underlying disease than a primary process. The most important therapeutic effort should be to treat the underlying disease. However, oxygen and respiratory stimulants have been used. A recent intriguing development has been the proposal that CPAP, by overcoming any small upper airway obstruction and by the pressure's effect on improving cardiac function, may play an important role in the treatment of congestive heart failure when associated with Cheyne-Stokes respiration.

BIBLIOGRAPHY

American Psychiatric Association: *Diagnostic and statistical manual of mental disorders,* ed 4, Washington DC, 1994, American Psychiatric Association.

Bootzin RR, Epstein D, Wood JM: Stimulus control instructions. In Hauri P, editor: *Case studies in insomnia,* New York, 1991, Plenum Publishing.

Coble PA et al: Childbearing in women with and without a history of affective disorder. II. Electroencephalographic sleep, *Compr Psychiatry* 35: 215, 1994.

Driver HS et al: Sleep and the sleep electroencephalogram across the menstrual cycle in young healthy women, *J Clin Endocrinol Metab* 81:728, 1996.

Driver HS, Baker FC: Review article: Menstrual factors in sleep, *Sleep Med Rev* 2:213, 1998.

Ehlers CL, Kupfer DJ: Slow-wave sleep: do young adult men and women age differently? *J Sleep Res* 6:211, 1997.

Giampiero P et al: HRT as a first step treatment of insomnia in post menopausal women, *Eur Menopause J* 4:145, 1997.

Guilleminault C, Hold J, Mitler MM: Clinical overview of the sleep apnea syndromes. In Guilleminault C, Dement WC, editors: *Sleep apnea syndromes,* New York, 1978, Alan R Liss.

Guilleminault C et al: Upper airway sleep-disordered breathing in women, *Ann Intern Med* 122:493, 1995.

Kryger MH, Roth T, Dement WC, editors: *Principles and practice of sleep medicine,* ed 3, Philadelphia, 1999, WB Saunders.

Lee KA: Alterations in sleep during pregnancy and postpartum: a review of 30 years of research, *Sleep Med Rev* 2:231, 1998.

Lee KA, DeJoseph JF: Sleep disturbance, vitality and fatigue among a select group of employed childbearing women, *Birth* 19(4):208, 1992.

Manber R, Armitage R: Sex, steroids and sleep: a review, *Sleep* 22:540, 1999.

Morin CM et al: Behavioral and pharmacological therapies for late life insomnia: a randomized controlled study, *JAMA* 281:991, 1999.

Morin CM et al: Nonpharmacological treatment of chronic insomnia, *Sleep* 22:1134, 1999.

O'Connor C, Thornley KS, Hanly PJ: Gender differences in the polysomnographic features of obstructive sleep apnea, *Am J Respir Crit Care Med* 161:1465, 2000.

Rapoport DM: Treatment of sleep apnea syndromes, *Mount Sinai J Med* 61:123, 1994.

Sin DD et al: Effects of continuous positive airway pressure on cardiovascular outcomes in heart failure patients with and without Cheyne-Stokes respiration, *Circulation* 102:61, 2000.

Spielman AJ, Saskin P, Thorpy MJ: Treatment of chronic insomnia by restriction of time in bed, *Sleep* 10:45, 1987.

Thorpy MJ, editor: Diagnostic classification steering committee. *The International classification of sleep disorders diagnostic and coding manual,* Rochester, MN, 1990, American Sleep Disorders Association.

Van Cauter E, Leproult R, Plat L: Age-related changes in slow wave sleep and REM sleep and relationship with growth hormone and cortisol levels in healthy men, *JAMA* 284:879, 2000.

Walsleben JA, Baron Faust R: *A woman's guide to sleep,* Crowne Books, 2000, New York.

Williams RL, Karacan J, Hursch CJ: *Electroencephalography of human sleep: clinical applications,* New York, 1974, Wiley.

Woodward S, Freedman RR: The thermoregulatory effects of menopausal HF on sleep, *Sleep* 4:497, 1994.

Young TB et al: The occurrence of sleep-disordered breathing among middle-aged adults, *N Engl J Med* 328:1230, 1993.

Young T et al: The gender bias in sleep apnea diagnosis, *Arch Intern Med* 156:2445, 1996.

CHAPTER 41

Chronic Cough

Barbara Ann Cockrill

Cough is one of the most common reasons for patients to seek medical care. This chapter describes the normal physiology of cough, some of the frequent syndromes causing cough with a normal chest x-ray study, with an emphasis on aspects particular to women, and nonspecific cough suppressant therapies. An important essential point is that, even in a referral practice, causes of cough are common. Using a systematic approach the cause of cough is almost always identified, and more than 90% of the time one (or more) of a few common etiologies is found. Treatment failures usually reflect failure to recognize one of these common causes of cough or failure to treat it with sufficient intensity.

Cough accounts for more than 30 million visits per year to primary care physicians in the United States. It can be a distressing symptom. Cough can cause sleep disturbance, headache, musculoskeletal pain, vomiting, rib fracture, and syncope. A common complaint in women is that of cough-induced stress incontinence. The social consequences of cough may be debilitating and are often underestimated. Patients may stop participating in activities such as going to church or attending social gatherings because of embarrassment resulting from a chronic cough. This can result in isolation and depression.

PHYSIOLOGY

Cough is a vital protective mechanism, and the consequences of not being able to cough are recurrent chest infection and lung damage. Four discrete steps are involved in a normal cough. The first is an inspiratory gasp, accomplished by a functioning diaphragm. The increase in lung volume stimulates pulmonary stretch receptors that augment the cough stimulus via the Hering-Breuer reflex. This step is impaired—and cough is weak—in patients with inspiratory muscle weakness. Examples include patients with diaphragmatic weakness or more commonly in patients with thoracic hyperexpansion and a flat diaphragm resulting from chronic obstructive pulmonary disease. Step two is a Valsalva maneuver: forced exhalation against apposed vocal cords. Patients with an open tracheostomy or paralyzed vocal cords have impaired cough because of their inability to raise intrathoracic pressure against a closed glottis.

The third step is the expiratory blast, since the vocal cords suddenly abduct. Expiratory muscle function is crucial for this step; expiratory muscle weakness (e.g., patients with spinal cord injuries above T6) causes ineffective cough. Finally, in step four there is a post-tussive prolonged inspiration.

Some of the neural pathways involved in the normal cough mechanism are shown in Fig. 41-1. The cough center is located in the medulla and pons. Cough receptors in the nose are thought to be innervated by the trigeminal nerve. The vocal cords receive innervation from the superior laryngeal nerve. Below the vocal cords, other branches of the vagus nerve carry signals from cough receptors. There are also cough receptors in the ear, pericardium, diaphragm, esophagus, and stomach. The efferent signal generated in the medulla travels via the vagus, phrenic, and spinal nerves. Mechanical receptors, which respond to stretching and displacement, are more prevalent in the upper respiratory tract. Chemical receptors, which respond to noxious small particles and gases, are more prevalent in the lower respiratory tract. The total density of cough receptors decreases progressively from the proximal to the distal airways to the point that there are no cough receptors in the alveoli.

It appears that women have a more sensitive cough reflex mechanism than men. The mechanism for this is uncertain, but may involve a heightened sensitivity in women of the sensory receptors within the respiratory tract.

EVALUATION

For research purposes, chronic cough is usually defined as a cough lasting more than 3 weeks. In practice, many patients will have been coughing for months or years. In most series, the most frequent causes of chronic cough are postnasal drip, asthma, and gastroesophageal reflux disease (GERD). As an example, Irwin and colleagues reported their experience evaluating patients referred for chronic cough of at least 3 weeks' duration. Patients were approached in a systematic fashion. Workup included history, physical examination, and chest x-ray studies in all patients, with further testing as indicated. Postnasal drip accounted for 41%, asthma 24%, and GERD 21%. Other common causes included chronic bronchitis and bronchiectasis. More unusual

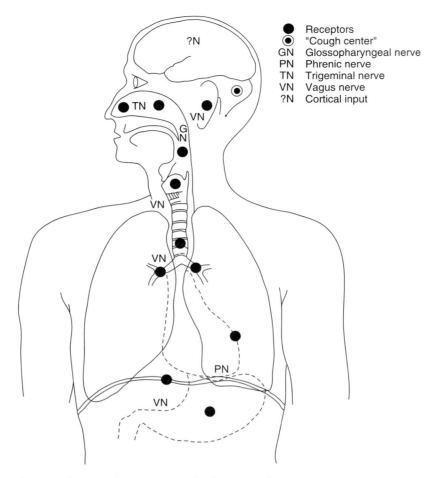

FIG. 41-1   The afferent limb of the cough reflex. (From Irwin RS et al: *Arch Intern Med* 137:1189, 1977.)

causes were occasionally discovered, including broncho-genic cancer, sarcoidosis, congestive heart failure, and esophageal diverticulum (Fig. 41-2).

Many patients with prolonged cough are found to have more than one cause of cough. In one study, a quarter of patients were found to have more than one cause. In a referral-based pulmonary practice, patients have often been diagnosed and treated for more than one cause of cough sequentially. However, if for example both asthma and GERD are present, it is essential that both problems be aggressively treated *simultaneously* before the cough will abate.

A systematic approach to chronic cough, derived from the work of Irwin and colleagues, is shown in Fig. 41-3. **History and physical examination** may indicate a diagnosis, such as the onset of cough following a respiratory tract infection (postinfectious cough). Nocturnal cough suggests possible asthma, esophageal reflux, or congestive heart failure. Cough related to meals may indicate aspiration or regurgitation. An early morning productive cough is typical of chronic bronchitis and bronchiectasis. Seasonal cough or exercise-induced cough points to a diagnosis of asthma. Cough with hoarseness raises the possibility of laryngeal disease or esophageal reflux. Among medications causing cough, angiotensin-converting enzyme (ACE) inhibitors are the most common. One study, however, indicated that a

careful history is not very helpful in diagnosing the cause of a chronic cough.

When no diagnosis is evident from patient interview and examination, a **chest x-ray** and **spirometry** should be obtained. A radiographic or spirometric abnormality will direct further workup. If the chest x-ray and spirometry are normal, consider a **methacholine challenge** (to evaluate for bronchial hyperresponsiveness), **esophageal pH probe** (for GERD), and/or a full set of **pulmonary function tests with lung volumes** (to detect unsuspected restrictive pulmonary disease).

Bronchoscopy has a relatively low yield among patients with chronic cough and a normal chest x-ray film. In a retrospective review by Poe and colleagues, only one bronchoscopy proved diagnostic out of 51 procedures performed among 109 patients referred for evaluation of chronic cough. Nonetheless, bronchoscopy may occasionally be indicated. For example, in one series 17 of 46 patients with carcinoid tumors presented with chronic cough and clear chest radiographs. In another case series six patients with postoperative retained suture material had cough and unremarkable chest films. We tend to perform bronchoscopy after diagnostic testing or treatment trials have excluded all of the more common causes of cough, especially if there is a history of smoking.

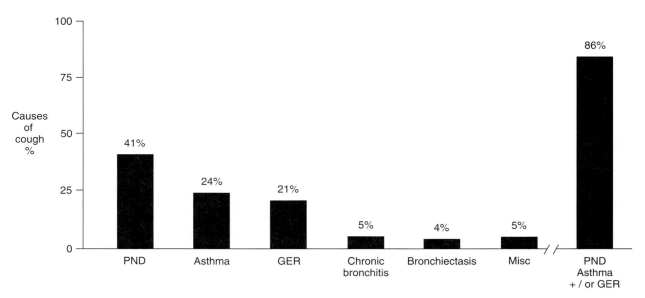

FIG. 41-2   Causes of chronic cough found in a referral population with cough for more than 3 weeks. Note that postnasal drip and asthma with or without gastroesophageal reflux disease account for the large majority and often occur together. *PND,* Post-nasal drip; *GER,* gastroesophagical reflux. (From Irwin RS et al: *Am Rev Respir Dis* 141:640, 1990.)

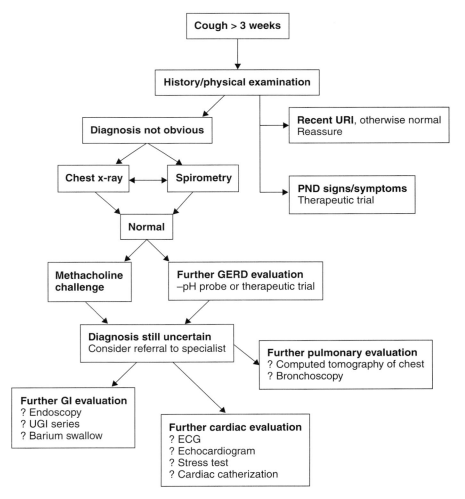

FIG. 41-3   Diagnostic approach to chronic cough.

SPECIFIC COUGH SYNDROMES

Post-nasal drip (PND) is probably the most common cause of chronic cough. Patients generally experience a sensation of mucus dripping or a tickle in the back of their throats. On physical examination one finds "cobblestoning" of the mucosa of the posterior pharynx, representing mucous gland hyperplasia. Treatment depends on the cause of the rhinorrhea. Nasal steroids are the treatment of choice for allergic postnasal drip. Other options include antihistamines (including the older antihistamines with greater anticholinergic effects), decongestants, and nasal ipratropium.

Postnasal drip may be a sign of **chronic sinusitis.** Patients with chronic sinusitis may have a paucity of symptoms—sometimes only cough and PND. When PND symptoms do not respond to treatment, further evaluation of the sinuses should be considered. In our institution, computed tomography of the sinuses is the first step because it is sensitive and similar in cost to plain films. Some authorities recommend four-view sinus films as a starting point. In one study, radiography of the sinuses was the most useful test in patients with chronic cough who required further testing. It is important to note that chronic sinusitis requires prolonged treatment with antibiotics (4 to 8 weeks), and the patient may not have complete resolution until sinus surgery is undertaken.

An important consideration in women is the **rhinitis of pregnancy.** As a result of estrogen effects on mucous membranes, some pregnant patients notice marked nasal congestion. The symptom can be extremely aggravating and make it more difficult to sleep. Rhinitis of pregnancy does not respond to nasal steroids, but will go away shortly after delivery. In selected patients, short-term use of decongestant nasal sprays or pseudoephedrine may be indicated.

Asthma, either typical or cough-variant, is a frequent cause of cough. It is said that as many as 25% of persons with asthma may present with cough as their sole symptom ("cough-variant asthma"). Spirometry by definition is normal. The diagnosis can be made by identifying bronchial hyperresponsiveness on bronchoprovocation challenge (methacholine challenge test) *or* by resolution of the cough with treatment for asthma. It has been hypothesized, but not confirmed with endobronchial biopsies, that cough-variant asthma is a manifestation of more proximal airway inflammation, whereas more typical asthma with wheezing involves peripheral airways. This follows from the observation that cough receptors are more prevalent in the proximal than in the distal airways.

Approximately one third of women with asthma note an increase in symptoms, including cough, during the premenstrual period. Although the increase in symptoms has been documented repeatedly, the mechanism for this is not certain. Increased asthma symptoms do not appear to be related to a change in airways hyperresponsiveness or to progesterone level. The effects of the menstrual cycle on cough-variant asthma have not been studied directly; it is likely, however, that findings would be similar.

Treatment of cough-variant asthma is the same as treatment of typical asthma. A stepped approach according to current NIH guidelines is recommended.

Cough related to **gastroesophageal reflux disease** (GERD) may be caused by two different mechanisms: by gastric acid irritation of the larynx and proximal trachea or by a cholinergically mediated reflex initiated by stimulation of nerve endings in the distal esophagus. The first mechanism is easy to understand: gastric acid stimulates irritant cough receptors. What about patients who have GERD but do not reflux to the level that might lead to aspiration or irritation of the larynx? One study indicated a lower cough threshold in patients with GERD even in the absence of cough related to GERD. Subjects with GERD were compared with normal subjects in their cough-sensitivity to inhaled capsaicin (the chemical that makes hot peppers "hot"). Patients with GERD required a much lower dose of capsaicin to induce coughing than normal subjects. Airway responsiveness to methacholine was normal in both groups.

In a study further investigating the mechanism by which GERD might cause cough, Ing and colleagues instilled hydrochloric acid onto the distal esophagus in persons with GERD and cough and in normal control subjects. Acid instillation caused more cough among persons with GERD. This coughing could be attenuated by pretreatment with the general anesthetic, lidocaine, instilled onto the esophagus and by the anticholinergic agent, ipratropium, inhaled onto the airways, but *not* by ipratropium installation onto the esophagus. This study suggests a reflex mechanism involving afferent neural pathways in the esophagus and efferent cholinergic pathways in the trachea or more distal airways.

It has been reported that as many as 75% of patients with cough owing to GERD will not have symptoms of acid reflux or "heartburn." In an analysis of various testing procedures to establish a diagnosis of GERD, esophageal pH monitoring was found to be more sensitive than barium swallow or endoscopy. An alternative approach utilizes a therapeutic trial of treatment for asthma or GERD. The relative risks and benefits of these two approaches have not been fully evaluated. In one study, only 6 of 17 patients with esophageal reflux documented by pH-probe testing and cough responded to high-dose omeprazole. These authors recommend going directly to an empiric trial rather than to pH probe testing. An approach used in our institution is to institute a therapeutic trial with omeprazole (or other proton-pump agent). If the patient does not respond with a decrease in cough and GERD is still suspected, the clinician can obtain a pH probe while medication is continued to confirm that the acid has been suppressed.

Treatment of GERD should begin with conservative measures such as elevating the head of the bed and dietary adjustments. Bed elevation is essential because reflux is common in the supine position. Proton pump inhibitors such as omeprazole or lansoprazole are the most effective medical therapies. Relatively high doses of the proton pump inhibitors (e.g., omeprazole, 20 to 40 mg twice a day) are needed for treatment of GERD-induced cough. Motility agents such as metoclopramide are also effective and may provide additive benefit to the proton pump inhibitors, but the side effects usually outweigh the benefit. Surgery represents a final option. Surgical approaches include fundoplication and, among patients with delayed gastric emptying, pyloroplasty. It is essential that the surgeon be experienced in these techniques.

Post-infectious cough typically follows certain viral or bacterial upper respiratory tract infections and may be present for up to 8 weeks. More than one mechanism may be involved. Postnasal drip is common. Increased irritant cough-receptor sensitivity is also present. This may be due to injury to the proximal airway epithelium with exposure of afferent nerves that are present just below the surface of tight junctions between epithelial cells. Many patients may have a component of bronchoconstriction and will show evidence for airway hyperresponsiveness on methacholine challenge testing. Treatment with bronchodilators and inhaled corticosteroids is often effective in relieving the cough, although most patients will respond to the tincture of time. As Voltaire said, "The art of medicine is amusing the patient while nature cures the disease."

A special instance of postinfectious cough is **pertussis** or "whooping cough," caused by the bacteria *Bordetella pertussis* or *B. parapertussis.* The name "whooping cough" is based on the presence of a loud "whoop" that occurs during the post-tussive inspiration and occurs only in small children owing to the smaller size of the upper airway. Vaccination programs greatly reduce the incidence of pertussis in children. Most infants in the United States are vaccinated against pertussis, but immunity wanes after about 12 years. Safe, acellular vaccines are now available. Although reasonable, especially for patients with severe lung disease, revaccination of adults has not been recommended for routine practice. Pertussis begins with a runny nose, watery eyes, and cough, as with an ordinary "head cold." It progresses, however, to a phase of severe paroxysmal coughing that can last for 8 to 12 weeks or longer.

The diagnosis is suggested by the severe paroxysmal nature of the coughing, and by the presence of a known outbreak of pertussis. Adults do not typically have the loud "whoop" heard on the post-tussive inspiration because of the larger upper airway. Many patients simply notice a "bad cold." For example, in one study, 21% of 75 adults presenting with a chronic cough had serologic evidence of recent pertussis infection. If obtained within 2 weeks of the onset of cough, nasal culture, using special nasal swab and culture medium, may grow the bacteria. After 2 weeks, acute and convalescent serologies are needed to confirm the diagnosis. Treatment with macrolide antibiotics reduces infectivity but has no effect on the cough. The cough is best treated with cough suppressants and possibly inhaled steroids. The value in making a specific diagnosis of pertussis is mainly in excluding alternative diagnoses and eliminating the need to test for them, as well as reassuring the patient. Also, prophylactic treatment with macrolide antibiotics is recommended for persons with serious lung disease who have been exposed to a known case of pertussis.

Cough related to ACE inhibitors is distinctly more common in women than in men. The cough is likely related to an increase in bradykinin stimulation of pulmonary c-fibers. Bradykinin is normally metabolized by ACE, and inhibition of the enzyme by ACE inhibitors leads to a build up. In susceptible patients, cough usually appears within 1 week of starting the medication, although it can be delayed by up to 6 months. The cough will recur if another ACE inhibitor is started, but cough does not appear to be associated with the newer angiotensin II receptor antagonists. The only curative treatment is withdrawal of the medication.

UNUSUAL CAUSES OF COUGH

Although the common causes of cough predominate, the more unusual and potentially dangerous causes of cough in persons with a normal chest x-ray film must be kept in mind. These include **lung cancer, interstitial lung disease, pulmonary hypertension, pulmonary embolism, thyroiditis,** and **foreign body aspiration** (especially in children and the mentally retarded). A rare cause of cough specific to women is **pulmonary endometriosis,** which will present with menstrual hemoptysis. Finally, **cerumen impaction** in the auditory canal can trigger cough by irritating sensory receptors of Arnold's nerve, a branch of the vagus nerve.

COUGH SUPPRESSANTS

Treatment of cough should be aimed at the underlying etiology. However, some patients may require the addition of a nonspecific cough suppressants, especially early in the course of treatment.

Cough suppressants can be divided into two types: those that act centrally at the level of the cough center in the brainstem and those that act on peripheral neural pathways. The two most commonly used centrally acting agents are **codeine (and its derivatives)** and **dextromethorphan.** One trial compared 30 mg of codeine with 60 mg of dextromethorphan in awake adults and found no difference in the antitussive effects. Codeine and its derivatives are narcotics and may be more effective for overnight cough suppression because of their greater sedative effect. A word of caution: given in sufficient quantities any narcotic can cause respiratory depression. For patients with persistent cough who are already taking narcotic analgesics (e.g., for pain control in metastatic cancer), addition of dextromethorphan may prove helpful because its effect is mediated through nonopioid receptors in the brain. Inhaled morphine has been tried for cough suppression but found to be only minimally effective. There are no opioid receptors in the lungs of humans, so that the observed cough suppression is probably due to systemic absorption of morphine after inhalation.

Peripherally acting cough suppressants include **inhaled lidocaine** and **oral benzonatate.** Inhaled lidocaine can be given by nebulizer (2.5 ml of a 4% solution) up to four times a day. In my experience, results with inhaled lidocaine have been mixed. Benzonatate acts by anesthetizing stretch receptors in the airways, pulmonary parenchyma, and pleura. It has no effect on respiratory drive. For the persistent cough, one can consider the simultaneous use of a centrally and peripherally active agent.

BIBLIOGRAPHY

Allen CJ, Anvari M: Gastro-esophageal reflux related cough and its response to laparoscopic fundoplication, *Thorax* 53:963, 1998.

Aylward M et al: Dextromethorphan and codeine: comparison of plasma kinetics and antitussive effects, *Eur J Respir Dis* 65:283, 1984.

Birkebaek NH et al: Bordetella pertussis and chronic cough in adults, *Clin Infect Dis* 29:1239, 1999.

Cheriyan S, Greenberger PA, Patterson R: Outcome of cough variant asthma treated with inhaled steroids, *Ann Allergy* 73:478, 1994.

Corrao WM, Braman SS, Irwin RS: Chronic cough as the sole presenting manifestation of bronchial asthma, *N Engl J Med* 300:633, 1979.

Curley FJ et al: Cough and the common cold, *Am Rev Respir Dis* 138:305, 1988.

Dicpinigaitis PV, Rauf K: The influence of gender on cough reflex sensitivity, *Chest* 113:1319, 1998.

Fouad YM, Katz PO, Hatlebakk JG, Castell DO: Ineffective esophageal motility: the most common motility abnormality in patients with GERD-associated respiratory symptoms, *Am J Gastroenterol* 94:1464, 1999.

Ing AJ, Ngu MC, Breslin AB: Pathogenesis of chronic persistent cough associated with gastroesophageal reflux, *Am J Respir Crit Care Med* 149:160, 1994.

Irwin RS, Curley FJ, French CL: Chronic cough: the spectrum and frequency of causes, key components of the diagnostic evaluation, and outcome of specific therapy, *Am Rev Respir Dis* 141:640, 1990.

Irwin RS, Curley FJ, Bennett FM: Appropriate use of antitussives and protussives. A practical review, *Drugs* 46:80, 1993.

Irwin RS et al: Chronic cough due to gastroesophageal reflux. Clinical, diagnostic, and pathogenetic aspects, *Chest* 104:1511, 1993.

Irwin RS et al: Managing cough as a defense mechanism and as a symptom. A consensus panel report of the American College of Chest Physicians, *Chest* 114:133S, 1998.

Matthys H, Bleicher B, Bleicher U: Dextromethorphan and codeine: objective assessment of antitussive activity in patients with chronic cough, *J Intern Med Res* 11:92, 1983.

Ours TM, Kavuru MS, Schilz RJ, Richter JE: A prospective evaluation of esophageal testing and a double-blind, randomized study of omeprazole in a diagnostic and therapeutic algorithm for chronic cough, *Am J Gastroenterol* 94:3131, 1999.

Pratter MR, Bartter T, Lotano R: The role of sinus imaging in the treatment of chronic cough in adults, *Chest* 116:1287, 1999.

Smyrnios NA, Irwin RS, Curley FJ, French CL: From a prospective study of chronic cough: diagnostic and therapeutic aspects in older adults, *Arch Intern Med* 158:1222, 1998.

Trochtenberg S: Nebulized lidocaine in the treatment of refractory cough, *Chest* 105:1592, 1994.

PART II
Gynecology and Obstetrics

CHAPTER **42**

Normal Gynecologic Examination and Common Findings

Erin E. Tracy

For many women, annual pelvic examinations are faced with much reluctance and trepidation. Pelvic examinations, however, remain an integral, important part of health maintenance. In recognition of the significant decrease in cervical cancer in countries with available routine cytologic screening, the American College of Obstetricians and Gynecologists recommends annual screening for all women who have reached age 18 or who have been sexually active for at least 3 consecutive years. Pelvic examinations encompass much more than simple cervical cytologic assessment and essential components are highlighted here. It is important in approaching each patient to always bear in mind the reticence she may feel in having this particular examination and to be particularly sensitive to her concerns.

Certain techniques may be used. The presence of a chaperone may put the woman at ease and, incidentally, be helpful from a liability perspective. Some patients benefit from a clear explanation of what the examination entails. Efforts to make the environment more comfortable may be considered, such as having covers on the stirrup feet, artwork on the ceiling, and a private setting. Specific details in the history should be considered in doing the examination, including a history of sexual activity, previous pelvic examinations, gravidae and parity, and sexual assault. A conscious effort should be made to avoid sudden unexpected movements, to use warm instruments, and to be gentle. Taking the history while the patient is fully dressed may enable the patient to feel less vulnerable and to help establish trust. Similarly, once the patient is in dorsal lithotomy position, the patient will relax more if she is notified as to when and where she will be touched. A common error is to manually try to separate her legs to facilitate the examination. This will only result in causing further anxiety and having her tighten her abdominal and leg muscles, thereby impeding the process.

INSPECTION

At the beginning of the examination, the pubic region should be inspected for the presence of lice (pediculosis) or other dermatologic lesions. In adolescent women, Tanner staging can be assessed (Fig. 42-1). The presence or absence of inguinal lymphadenopathy should be determined. The external genitalia should be inspected (Fig. 42-2). The clitoris should be evaluated; it may be enlarged in conditions of hyperandrogenism. The urethra should be evaluated for the presence of a urethra caruncle or urethrocele. A red urethra may be indicative of a urinary tract infection, a caruncle, or a carcinoma. If the patient has had urinary symptoms, inflamed Skene's glands may be the etiology, and purulent material can be expressed from the urethra. Urethral diverticula, present in up to 5% of women, should be suspected in the presence of a palpable, tender suburethral mass in the posterior mid-portion of the urethra.

A detailed examination of the vulva should be undertaken. Specific details of vulvar diseases are highlighted in Chapter 44. The vulva should be inspected for macular, papular, or ulcerative lesions. Inflammatory changes may result in edematous vulvar epithelium, obscuring the typically visible capillary network underlying normal vulvar epithelium. Discharge visible on the perineum should generally be considered pathologic in nature. Hyperpigmented lesions must be evaluated. A general rule regarding specific identifiable lesions is, "when in doubt, biopsy." Approximately 2% to 5% of all melanomas are vulvar in origin. As vulvar malignancies may also present as hypopigmented or ulcerative lesions, careful visual inspection of the vulva and selective biopsies are essential. Empiric treatment with steroid therapy without a clear diagnosis is generally not appropriate. The extensive differential diagnosis of vulvar lesions includes lichen sclerosus, squamous cell hyperplasia, psoriasis, lichen simplex chronicus, lichen planus, and vulvar intraepithelial neoplasia, in addition to infectious etiologies (e.g., condyloma acuminatum, syphilis, chancroid, herpes simplex virus, lymphogranuloma venereum).

Bartholin's glands, which open into the vestibule at the 5 and 7 o'clock positions, may be inspected and palpated. These glands are often not appreciated on routine examinations. Patients may have a blockage of the Bartholin duct on either side, resulting in a Bartholin's cyst. Although often asymptomatic, they can become secondarily infected, causing significant discomfort. Even asymptomatic Bartholin cysts should be evaluated in the postmenopausal woman to rule out a primary, albeit rare, Bartholin's gland carcinoma.

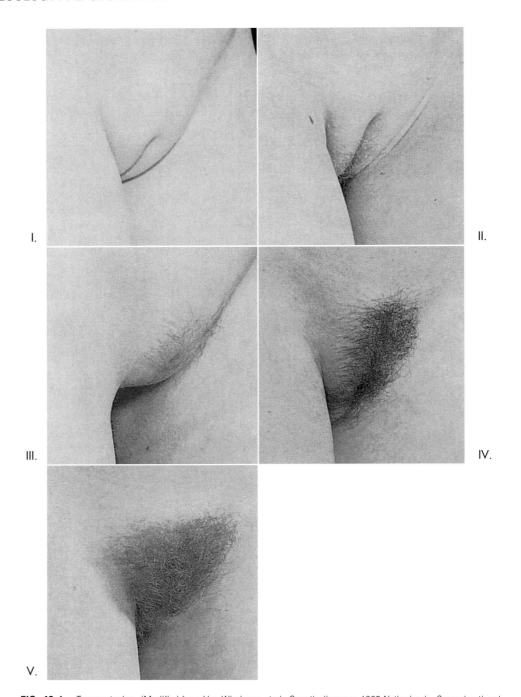

FIG. 42-1 Tanner staging. (Modified from Van Wieringen et al: *Growth diagrams 1965 Netherlands. Second national survey on 0-24-year-olds.* Netherlands, 1971, Wolters-Noordhoff.)

The vulva should also be carefully inspected for evidence of sexual abuse. Lacerations and ecchymosis should be noted, and the patient should be asked specific questions regarding the etiology of these findings (see Chapter 88).

The hymenal ring should be evaluated. An intact hymen is generally found only in a virginal patient; after coitus, the hymen is usually recognized as the carunculae myrtiformes, a semicircular arrangement of small membranous elevations. It may be difficult to identify hymenal remnants in patients who have had many children. In general, there are several types of hymens, as seen in Fig. 42-3. If the hymen is cribriform or septate, menstrual flow may occur normally. Patients with imperforate hymens may present with hematocolpos, requiring surgical correction. It is estimated that imperforate hymens occur in approximately 1 in 1000 women, with patients commonly presenting with abdominal pain, delayed menarche/amenorrhea, and a bulging hymenal mass. This must be differentiated from other congenital conditions such as vaginal agenesis or a transverse vaginal septum.

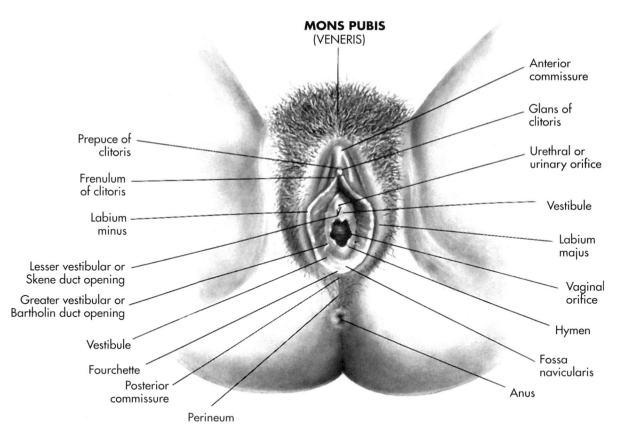

MONS PUBIS
(VENERIS)

Anterior
commissure

Glans of
clitoris

Prepuce of
clitoris

Urethral or
urinary orifice

Frenulum
of clitoris

Vestibule

Labium
minus

Labium
majus

Lesser vestibular or
Skene duct opening

Vaginal
orifice

Greater vestibular or
Bartholin duct opening

Hymen

Vestibule

Fossa
navicularis

Fourchette

Anus

Posterior
commissure

Perineum

FIG. 42-2   External female genitalia. (From Lowdermilk DL, Perry SE, Bobak IM: *Maternity and women's health care,* ed 6, St Louis, 1997, Mosby.)

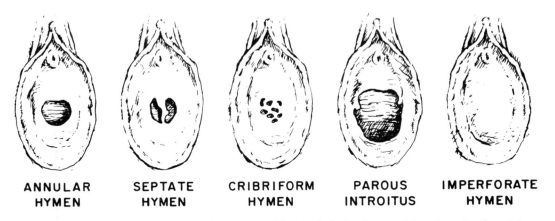

ANNULAR HYMEN   **SEPTATE HYMEN**   **CRIBRIFORM HYMEN**   **PAROUS INTROITUS**   **IMPERFORATE HYMEN**

FIG. 42-3   Various types of hymens. (From Kaufman RH, Paro S: *Benign diseases of the vulva and vagina,* ed 4, St Louis, 1994, Mosby.)

SPECULUM EXAMINATION

The speculum examination is an important component of the pelvic examination. Although the Talmud refers to a similar tubular instrument, the earliest known speculums were discovered among the ruins of Pompeii, destroyed in the year 79 AD. Currently, when evaluating a patient, the proper speculum should be chosen, taking into consideration her obstetric history, age, body habitus, and menopausal status. Although nulliparous, thin, virginal women would benefit from the more narrow Pederson speculum, multiparous, sex-

ually active women would be better evaluated using the larger Graves speculum. A Sims vaginal retractor is helpful to visualize specific areas of pelvic relaxation. Some examining tables have warmers for the speculum drawer; a heating pad may be utilized as well. The speculum should be nonetheless heated with warm water before insertion. Lubrication may be used instead if Papanicolaou screening is not planned. With the fingers of the nondominant hand separating the labia, the speculum should be inserted gently, in a closed position, at a 45-degree angle downward. If the perineum is poorly supported or if the walls of the vagina are redundant, it may be helpful to use the index and middle fingers of the nondominant hand to exert downward pressure on the perineal body to permit entrance of the speculum into the vagina. It is helpful to keep the speculum tilted, so the maximum diameter is at a 45-degree angle relative to the horizontal axis of the perineal body. Care must be taken to avoid pulling the pubic hair or closing the blades on the vulvar or vaginal tissue. Once the speculum blades have entered the vagina, one can feel it "give," as it advances over the muscular support of the levator ani into the posterior vaginal fourchette. Once this is appreciated, the speculum can be rotated into the horizontal position, and the blades gently opened with the thumb of the dominant hand. The cervix should be fully visualized. If it is not seen, carefully close the speculum, withdraw it a short distance, and redirect the speculum posteriorly before reopening it. If the uterus is retroverted, the cervix will be more anteriorly displaced, and the speculum should be redirected accordingly. Once the cervix is seen in its entirety within the speculum blades, the screw on the speculum should be tightened, being careful not to pinch the vulvar skin.

The vagina should be closely inspected. The estrogen status of the patient may affect the quality of the vaginal tissue. Postmenopausal women may exhibit signs of atrophy, including thinning of the vaginal tissue, loss of rugae, and generalized pallor. These women may particularly benefit from the previously mentioned lubrication or warming of instruments. Excoriations or ulcers should be noted. Historical factors such as douching practices and sexual history should be considered. The vagina should be inspected for the presence of foreign bodies and for lesions such as polyps and condyloma. In the pediatric population, such vaginal polyps must be differentiated from the highly malignant sarcoma botryoides. Vaginal lesions should be inspected, and consideration given to cytologic or histologic sampling, especially to rule out squamous intraepithelial lesions or adenosis. Patients who report a history of diethylstilbestrol (DES) exposure in utero should be meticulously evaluated, given their increased risk of vaginal adenosis, vaginal clear cell adenocarcinoma, and intraepithelial neoplasia. Clear cystic structures (e.g., Gartner's duct cysts or müllerian remnants) should be recognized. Sometimes inclusion cysts on the lines of previous scars or episiotomy incisions may be encountered. These are often asymptomatic, requiring no further therapy.

A vaginal discharge that is present at the introitus should be considered pathologic in nature and investigated with a wet preparation. A swab is rubbed against the vaginal mucosa, and the resulting discharge smeared thinly on two slides. On one slide, a drop of KOH (10% potassium hydroxide) should be placed and on the other slide, a drop of normal saline (NS). Cover slips are placed. The "whiff test" is positive when the KOH is applied and a "fishy odor" results, secondary to the presence of anaerobic bacteria. The NS slide is reviewed for the presence of clue cells, trichomonads, leukocytes, and sperm. The KOH slide is helpful in diagnosing monilial vaginitis, characteristically with budding hyphae. The vaginal pH, normally 3.8 to 4.2, may be abnormal in the setting of vaginitis as well. To assess this, pH paper is placed in the lateral vaginal wall or immersed in a sample of vaginal discharge. A pH greater than 4.5 is con-

sistent with a predominance of gram-negative facultative anaerobes in addition to gram-positive and gram-negative obligate anaerobic bacteria. A pH greater than 4.5 is seen in the presence of bacterial vaginosis, as well as with *Trichomonas vaginalis*. For additional details regarding vaginitis, see Chapter 51.

The cervix should now be evaluated. Usually, the cervix appears pink, smooth, and shiny. If the patient is nulliparous, the external cervical os should appear as a small round "fish-mouth" shape. A multiparous patient's cervix, on the other hand, may have more of a slitlike appearance. If she has had prior cervical lacerations, the cervix may have healed in a stellate manner. The cervix may be difficult to visualize in a postmenopausal patient. In these women, it is sometimes helpful to do a bimanual examination first, to identify where the cervix is located, and recognize its general contour. If this is done first, and cytologic screening is planned subsequently, warm water should be used on the glove, instead of a vaginal lubricant. Recording the cervical location in the patient's chart may facilitate future examinations.

Nabothian cysts are commonly visualized. These are benign inclusion cysts that develop as squamous epithelium covers columnar epithelium. The transformation zone, which is the region where the squamous epithelium from the external cervix meets the endocervical columnar epithelium, should be identified. Grossly, squamous epithelium appears more shiny, smooth, and light pink, whereas the columnar epithelium is more irregular in appearance and commonly more red in color. As squamous metaplasia occurs, a non-neoplastic process, the squamous epithelium, covers the columnar epithelium (hence the name, *transformation zone*). Thus columnar epithelium is usually difficult, if not impossible, to visualize in older women, and prominent in younger patients. Postpartum patients can exhibit another normal finding, an ectropion. This occurs when the irregularly shaped external os of the cervix is everted in certain areas, resulting in some columnar epithelium being visible more distally.

Any suspicious cervical lesions should be biopsied, regardless of cytologic results. Colposcopy is invaluable in the setting of cytologic abnormalities or visible lesions (see Chapter 96). Some infectious conditions may manifest themselves on the cervical examination. Ulcerative lesions may indicate herpes simplex virus, whereas flat lesions may represent condyloma acuminatum, caused by human papillomavirus. A mucopurulent cervicitis is most commonly caused by *Chlamydia trachomatis*, but the majority of chlamydia or gonorrhea infections do not exhibit this finding. Mucopurulent cervicitis can be diagnosed by visualizing a yellow material on a cervical swab, or by seeing more than 10 polymorphonuclear leukocytes per microscopic field (with $1000\times$ magnification) on a Gram stain of the endocervical discharge. Similarly, cervical friability, hyperemia, and ulcerations are consistent with this diagnosis. When suspected, cervical cultures should be obtained from the endocervical canal.

Cervical polyps are often visualized during the speculum examination. These typically appear as smooth and soft, varying in color from pink to bright red. The cervix is sometimes friable, and the polyp can usually be easily grasped by its stalk and removed in the office. It is important to rule out concurrent endometrial pathology, which has been reported in asymptomatic patients at a rate of 5%.

PAPANICOLAOU SCREENING

The importance of regular Pap smears has been previously stated in this chapter. Since the introduction of vaginal and cervical cytology screening by Papanicolaou and Trout in 1943, the incidence of invasive cervical cancer has decreased by approximately 50%. The cervix should be clearly visualized, and the endocervical canal should be sampled, in addition to the ectocervix. Several studies have shown that using an endocervical brush is preferable to a simple swab technique. Whether the newer liquid-based technology is utilized, or the traditional cervical smear, the preparation should be immediately fixed to avoid air drying artifact. The entire transformation zone should be included in the sample. If the patient has had a previous hysterectomy, and a vaginal Pap is being done, it is important to sample the posterior vaginal surface, in the superior one third of the vagina, since that is where the majority of vaginal cancers arise. To adequately screen this area, the speculum must be gently turned perpendicularly, as this procedure is explained to the patient. If any suspicious visible lesions are identified, they should be biopsied and consideration should be given to a follow-up colposcopic examination.

BIMANUAL EXAMINATION

After the speculum is removed, the examiner uses his or her dominant hand, putting lubrication on the index and middle fingers, and gently places them in the vaginal canal. The cervix can usually be easily palpated as a round cylindrical structure measuring approximately 3 to 4 cm in diameter. The consistency is typically uniformly firm. The external os is generally closed in nulliparous women, and may be slightly dilated in multiparous patients. Nabothian cysts, polyps, or other neoplasias can be often be palpated. The cervix should be compressed between the two fingers, which exert pressure medially on the cervix. An unduly firm cervix may signify the presence of cervical fibroids or a malignancy. The cervix should be moved laterally right and left. This will cause the broad ligament to move, which may result in cervical motion tenderness in patients with peritonitis. This should be done before placing the other hand on the abdomen to try to decrease the false-positive rate. Similarly, the motion should be a lateral one, because an anterior/posterior direction may signify peritonitis of the anterior abdominal wall or posterior cul de sac, instead of localizing movement to the pelvic ligaments. If the cervical movement is restricted, one should suspect pelvic adhesions, neoplasia, or scarring resulting from inflammation (i.e., prior pelvic inflammatory disease or endometriosis.)

The uterus should then be evaluated. In the majority of women it is anteverted, although a retroverted uterus does not ordinarily signify pelvic pathology. Some conditions that result in scarring in the cul de sac of Douglas or involve the uterosacral ligaments may cause the uterus to be retroverted, but uterine motility in these cases should be restricted. Several features of the uterus should be described, including its position, consistency, size (often expressed in comparison to the uterine size at specific gestational ages, in weeks), and shape. Adenomyosis should be suspected in a uterus that is globally enlarged, without specifically palpable tumors or irregularities. Leiomyoma may present as an enlarged irregularly shaped uterus, or specific fibroids may be palpable as

distinct pelvic masses. Rarely, submucous fibroids may prolapse through the endocervical canal. Pedunculated fibroids may actually be mobile and difficult to distinguish on examination from masses of ovarian origin. Although the uterus is not ordinarily tender on direct palpation, it may be tender in cases of endomyometritis, degenerating fibroids, and septic abortions. The mobility of the uterus should be assessed, including any degree of prolapse (to be further described later). Congenital uterine anomalies are usually difficult to diagnose based on history and physical examination alone.

The vaginal fingers should then be moved to the right lateral vaginal fornix, adjacent to the cervix, to assist in adnexal evaluation. The nondominant hand can be used to make a sweeping downward motion in the right lower quadrant, trying to gently push the ovary into the waiting vaginal fingers, to assess ovarian size and mobility. Ovaries, like male testicles, are tender when directly compressed, but inordinate tenderness should be noted. Ovaries may be especially difficult to palpate in obese or postmenopausal women. Pelvic ultrasound serves as a useful adjunctive tool when the diagnosis is uncertain or further assessment is warranted. Adnexal masses that are irregular in shape, fixed in position, or enlarged on palpation merit further workup. Normal fallopian tubes are usually approximately 7 mm in diameter and difficult to palpate. They may be enlarged in benign conditions (e.g., hydrosalpinx, cysts of Morgagni) or malignancy, although the latter is very rare. The left adnexae should be evaluated in a manner mirroring the right.

RECTOVAGINAL EXAMINATION

The rectovaginal examination is an essential part of a full pelvic examination, especially important in postmenopausal women, or anyone with symptoms of pelvic fullness or incontinence. The examiner should change his or her glove, and after being properly lubricated, the middle finger of the dominant hand is gently placed in the rectum, while the index finger is reintroduced into the vagina (Fig. 42-4). Hem-

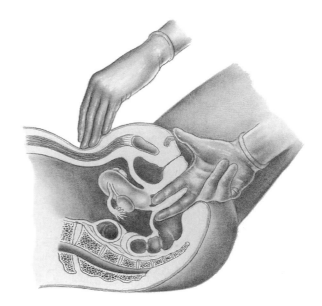

FIG. 42-4 Rectovaginal palpation. (From Seidel HM et al: *Mosby's guide to physical examination,* ed 4, St Louis, 1999, Mosby.)

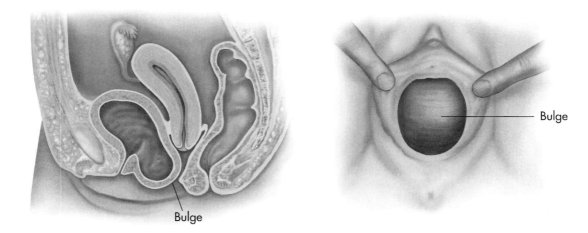

FIG. 42-5 Side and direct views of cystocele. (From Seidel HM et al: *Mosby's guide to physical examination*, ed 4, St Louis, 1999, Mosby.)

orrhoids may be noted. The rectal finger, less frequently, may palpate sigmoid polyps or lesions. The uterosacral ligaments can be palpated as thickened or with recognizable nodularity in cases of significant endometriosis or malignancy. The perineal body can be assessed between the vaginal and rectal fingers, evaluating the strength and muscular tone. Once again, the abdomen should be evaluated with the nondominant hand, using the added depth offered by the vaginal and the rectal fingers in assessing the uterus and adnexal structures. When the cervix is elevated toward the anterior abdominal wall, the uterosacral ligaments are put under tension. Although this procedure is ordinarily not painful, it may be in cases of endometriosis, in which the uterosacral ligaments are involved.

PELVIC RELAXATION

As previously alluded to, in postmenopausal women, or in any patient who complains of urinary or fecal incontinence or pelvic fullness, the status of the pelvic floor must be assessed. This can be done with the aid of a Sims vaginal retractor, with a speculum, and during the bimanual examination. The perineal body should be visualized. If this is weakened, it is possible to visualize a significant proportion of the anterior vaginal wall without separating the labia. Advancing age and parity contribute to scarred or torn perineal fascial supports and muscular atrophy.

A cystocele can be appreciated visually by seeing a bulge downward of the vaginal mucosa from the anterior vaginal wall. This can be accentuated by asking the patient to cough or bear down (Fig. 42-5). When the patient does the Valsalva maneuver, urinary incontinence may be demonstrated in cases of genuine stress incontinence or urethral sphincter deficiency. The cystocele may be reduced by upward displacement of the bladder with the examining fingers. Similarly, a rectocele can be diagnosed by visual inspection, seeing a bulge upward from the posterior vaginal wall. This should be confirmed on rectovaginal examination, appreciating the fascial defect and ruling out fecal impaction as the etiology for the visible protuberance on inspection. Enterocoele or herniation of the small bowel

through a vaginal fascial defect can be more difficult to diagnose in the office setting, but should be suspected in cases of general pelvic relaxation, which worsens when the patient bears down.

Relaxation of the cardinal and uterosacral ligaments can similarly result in uterine prolapse. The degree of prolapse can be described, based on the amount of uterine descent. A mobile uterus can be further evaluated by placing a tenaculum on the cervix, to see how much descent occurs with pressure, which may be predictive of the potential for worsening prolapse. Some authors recommend describing a minimal descent of the cervix into the vagina as stage I, with stage III being complete prolapse of the cervix through the introitus. Similarly, cystoceles, enteroceles, and rectoceles should be graded as 1+ (minimal) up to 4+ (bulging through the introitus). This grading enables the examiner to better communicate his or her findings and to follow a given patient over time more objectively.

BIBLIOGRAPHY

The American College of Obstetricians and Gynecologists: *Recommendations on Frequency of Pap Test Screening,* Committee Opinion 152, Washington, DC, 1995, ACOG.

The American College of Obstetricians and Gynecologists: *Pediatric gynecologic disorders,* Technical Bulletin 201, Washington, DC, 1995, ACOG.

The American College of Obstetricians and Gynecologists: *Vaginitis,* Technical Bulletin 226, Washington, DC, 1996, ACOG.

The American College of Obstetricians and Gynecologists: *Vulvar nonneoplastic epithelial disorders,* Educational Bulletin 241, Washington, DC, 1997, ACOG.

The American College of Obstetricians and Gynecologists: *Routine cancer screening,* Committee Opinion 185, Washington, DC, 1997, ACOG.

Black MM, McKay M, Braude P: *Obstetric and gynecologic dermatology,* St Louis, 1995, Mosby.

Chalvardjian A, De Marchi WG, Bell V, Nishikawa R: Improved endocervical sampling with the cytobrush, *Can Med Assoc J* 144, 1991.

Decherney A, Pernoll M: *Obstetrics and gynecologic diagnosis and treatment,* East Norwalk, CT, 1994, Appleton & Lange.

Disai PJ, Creasman WT: *Clinical gynecologic oncology,* ed 4, St Louis, 1993, Mosby.

Farber M, Noumoff J, Freedman M, Oberkotter L: Understanding and correcting genital anomalies, *Contemp Ob Gyn* 113, 1984.

Julian TM: Simple examination techniques to aid in the diagnosis of urethral diverticulum, *Obstet Gynecol* 76:5, 1990.

Kaufman R, Paro S: *Benign diseases of the vulva and vagina,* ed 4, St Louis, 1994, Mosby.

Koonings PP et al: A randomized clinical trial comparing the Cytobrush and cotton swab for Papanicolaou smears, *Obstet Gynecol* 80:1, 1992.

Mishell DR, Stenchever MA, Droegemueller W, Herbst AL: *Comprehensive gynecology,* ed 3, St Louis, 1997, Mosby.

Pradhan S, Chenoy R: Dilatation and curettage in patients with cervical polyps: a retrospective analysis, *Br J Obstet Gynecol* 102:415, 1995.

Quint E, Elkins T: Cervical cytology in women with mental retardation, *Obstet Gynecol* 89:1, 1997.

Roman LD et al: Pelvic examination, tumor marker level and gray-scale and Doppler sonography in the prediction of pelvic cancer, *Obstet Gynecol* 89:4, 1997.

Rock JA, Thompson JD: *Te Linde's operative gynecology,* ed 8, Philadelphia, 1997, Lippincott-Raven.

Speert H: *Obstetrics and gynecology,* ed 2, San Francisco, 1994, Norman Publishing.

CHAPTER 43

Amenorrhea

Janet Elizabeth Hall

Normal menstrual cycles occur monthly, with the exception of pregnancy, from their onset in adolescence until the time of menopause, which occurs between the ages of 45 and 55 years. Studies of the duration of the menstrual cycle during the reproductive years in a large cohort of American women indicate that the median menstrual cycle length is 28 days, with a range between 25 and 35 days considered normal. Menstrual-cycle disturbances occur relatively infrequently, with estimates of amenorrhea ranging from 2% to 8% in large studies. However, both the delayed onset of menstrual function and subsequent menstrual-cycle abnormalities represent an important biologic marker of potential disease. A framework for the diagnosis and therapy of these disorders can best be constructed by combining a functional and anatomic approach using gonadotropin measurements to help locate the site of the primary abnormality. Key to this framework is an understanding of the physiology of normal reproductive cycles.

PHYSIOLOGY OF THE NORMAL MENSTRUAL CYCLE

The normal menstrual cycle requires precise integration of hormonal events involving the hypothalamus, pituitary gland, and ovaries, with the uterus acting as an end organ for ovarian steroid effects (Fig. 43-1). The reproductive system functions in a classic endocrine mode with hypothalamic stimulation of the pituitary via the releasing hormone, gonadotropin-releasing hormone (GnRH), which is also known as luteinizing hormone-releasing hormone (LHRH), resulting in pituitary secretion of the gonadotropins, luteinizing hormone (LH) and follicle-stimulating hormone (FSH). LH and FSH, in turn, stimulate ovarian follicular development and hormone secretion. Ovarian secretion of estradiol, progesterone, and probably inhibin restrains the secretion of LH and FSH through actions at both the hypothalamus through control of GnRH secretion and directly at the pituitary level. In addition to these negative feedback controls, the menstrual cycle is uniquely dependent on positive feedback to produce the preovulatory LH surge.

The normal menstrual cycle is generally divided into the follicular or preovulatory phase, which begins on the first day of menses, and the luteal phase, which begins with ovulation (Fig. 43-2). During the early follicular phase, FSH is responsible for recruitment of a cohort of follicles, one of which will achieve dominance and eventually ovulate. The increases in estrogen produced by the emerging follicles inhibit further FSH secretion to ensure that a single egg is ovulated each month. The dramatic rise in estrogen secretion that occurs late in the follicular phase stimulates the LH surge required for ovulation. In addition, estrogen has a proliferative effect on the lining of the uterus, resulting in thickening of the endometrium that can be monitored by ultrasound.

The luteal or postovulatory phase begins immediately after ovulation and is characterized by secretion of progesterone and estrogen by the corpus luteum. These hormones produce the secretory changes of the endometrium that are necessary for implantation. Progesterone is also responsible for the postovulatory rise in basal body temperature that can be used clinically as an indicator of ovulatory cycles. The luteal phase ends with menses, which results from removal of the hormonal support of the endometrium that accompanies the natural regression of the corpus luteum. If a pregnancy has been established, human chorionic gonadotropin (hCG), which is produced by the placenta, can prolong the function of the corpus luteum until placental production of progesterone and estrogen is adequate to sustain the pregnancy.

The length of the luteal phase is fairly constant among women (12 to 16 days) and therefore the major variability in cycle length is in follicular-phase duration. With age, both follicular-phase length and total cycle length decrease somewhat. At both ends of reproductive life, adolescence and perimenopause, there is an increased incidence of anovulatory cycles and erratic bleeding patterns.

DEFINITIONS

Amenorrhea refers to the absence of menses. It is termed *primary* in an adolescent or woman who has never menstruated. Normal menarche (the first menstrual period) occurs relatively late in the series of pubertal milestones that mark the onset of reproductive function. The appearance of pubic hair (adrenarche), breast development (thelarche), and the growth spurt all precede the first menstrual period, which occurs at 12.7 years on average, with the ages between 11

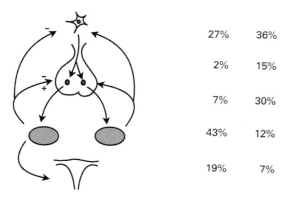

27%	36%
2%	15%
7%	30%
43%	12%
19%	7%

FIG. 43-1 Integration of the hypothalamic-pituitary-ovarian axis with the uterus as an end organ for estradiol and progesterone action. This schema is key to the evaluation of amenorrhea. The prevalence of a given cause of amenorrhea depends on whether amenorrhea is primary or secondary. *FSH*, follicle-stimulating hormone; *LH*, luteinizing hormone; *GnRH*, gonadotropin-releasing hormone; *PCOS*, polycystic ovary syndrome. (Modified from Hall JE, Crowley WF Jr. In DeGroot LJ, editor: *Endocrinology*, ed 3, Philadelphia, 1994, WB Saunders. Prevalence figures are derived from Reindollar [1981; 1986]).

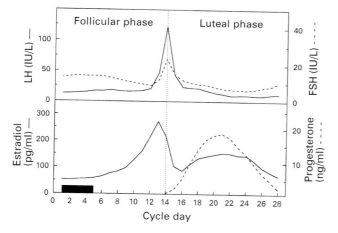

FIG. 43-2 Dynamic changes in mean LH, FSH, estradiol, and progesterone levels throughout the normal menstrual cycle based on daily blood samples in more than 100 normal cycles emphasize the importance of anchoring a sample drawn for clinical indications to preceding and subsequent menses. Menses is indicated by the *solid box*. The *dotted line* indicates ovulation, which separates the follicular and luteal phases.

and 15 years constituting the 95% confidence limits. Amenorrhea is termed *secondary* in a woman who previously has had at least one episode of menstrual bleeding. *Oligomenorrhea* refers to infrequent or irregular menstrual bleeding, with cycle lengths generally in excess of 35 to 40 days.

DIFFERENTIAL DIAGNOSIS (Table 43-1)

The distinction between primary and secondary amenorrhea is an important one because primary amenorrhea encompasses a more extensive differential diagnosis that includes congenital and genetic abnormalities. In addition, the relative frequency of presentation of disorders at each level of consideration is influenced by whether amenorrhea is pri-

mary or secondary (Fig. 43-1). However, it is also important to remember that most processes commonly thought of in association with secondary amenorrhea also can produce primary amenorrhea. Oligomenorrhea is a manifestation of disordered ovulation; therefore the pathophysiologic considerations in the following discussion are the same for oligomenorrhea as for secondary amenorrhea.

Primary Amenorrhea
Uterine and Outflow Tract Disorders

Abnormalities at the level of the uterus or outflow tract account are particularly important in the diagnosis of primary amenorrhea (Fig. 43-1). Most patients with anatomic causes of primary amenorrhea have **müllerian agenesis** (congenital absence of the vagina and/or uterus), also known as Mayer-Rokitansky-Küster-Hauser syndrome. Less commonly, patients manifest other **outflow tract anomalies** such as a transvaginal septum or an imperforate hymen, although they have otherwise normal pubertal developmental and normal levels of sex steroids and gonadotropins. Depending on the level of the anatomic obstruction, they may have cyclic abdominal pain and distention from blood within the obstructed uterus.

Some of these patients are difficult to distinguish from the much smaller proportion of patients with primary amenorrhea who have androgen resistance, an X-linked dominant syndrome also known as **androgen resistance syndrome** or testicular feminization. These patients are genotypic males with one of a number of defects in the androgen receptor that leads to its inability to respond to testosterone. As such, there is failure to develop normal male external genitalia, a testosterone-dependent process, and thus normal female external genitalia develop. However, because the testes of these persons produce müllerian-inhibiting substance (MIS), the müllerian system regresses and they do not have a uterus or the proximal two thirds of the vagina. Therefore the clinical presentation is primary amenorrhea in the presence of minimal body hair, good breast development, an absent uterus and a blind vagina. FSH levels are normal, but levels of LH, estradiol, and testosterone are elevated. A karyotype confirms the diagnosis. Because of the potential for malignant change, gonadectomy is recommended in these patients.

Ovulatory Disorders

A much larger proportion of patients with primary amenorrhea have ovulatory disorders. Measurement of gonadotropin levels is key to the further subdivision of these patients into those with ovarian failure (hypergonadotropic), abnormalities of the hypothalamus or pituitary (hypogonadotropic), or polycystic ovary syndrome (elevated LH to FSH ratio).

Primary amenorrhea rarely can be associated with **ovarian agenesis,** but the most common cause of primary amenorrhea and the most common genetic cause of ovarian failure is **Turner's syndrome** (45,X gonadal dysgenesis), in which primary amenorrhea is associated with the characteristic somatic features of short stature, webbed neck, shield chest, cubitus valgus, and multiple nevi, as well as cardiac and renal malformations and a predisposition to hypothyroidism. In these patients the ovarian failure results from a process of rapid atresia both in utero and after birth, and

Table 43-1
Differential Diagnosis of Amenorrhea

Site of Abnormal Function	Disorder	Primary or Secondary Amenorrhea	Gonadotropin	Estradiol Levels	Clinical Findings	Confirmatory Tests
Uterus or Outflow Tract	Müllerian anomalies or agenesis	Primary	LH, FSH normal	Normal	May have cyclic pelvic pain	
	Testicular feminization	Primary	LH increased, FSH normal	Increased	Minimal body hair, good breast development, blind vagina	Elevated testosterone, karyotype
	Uterine synechiae (Asherman's syndrome)	Secondary	LH, FSH normal	Normal	History of instrumentation or infection	Hysteroscopy or hysterosalpingogram
Ovary	Turner's syndrome (or mosaic)	Primary; sometimes secondary in mosaic form	FSH increased	Decreased	Short stature, webbed neck, shield chest, cardiac abnormalities and hypothyroidism (mosaics may be atypical)	Karyotype
	Premature ovarian failure	Secondary	FSH increased	Decreased	May have history of autoimmune disorder	
	Resistant ovary syndrome	Primary	FSH increased	Decreased		
Pituitary Gland	Prolactinoma	Secondary	FSH, LH decreased or normal	Decreased	May have galactorrhea	Prolactin, cranial imaging
	Other tumors	Secondary	FSH, LH decreased or normal	Decreased	Signs of Cushing's syndrome or acromegaly	Urine free cortisol, growth hormone, cranial imaging
	Pituitary infarction	Secondary	FSH, LH decreased or normal	Decreased	Usually occurs postpartum	
Hypothalamus	Hypothalamic amenorrhea	Primary or secondary	FSH, LH decreased or normal	Decreased	Sometimes associated with stress, exercise, weight loss, chronic illness	
	Pituitary tumors	Primary or secondary	FSH, LH decreased or normal	Decreased	May manifest headache, visual symptoms	Cranial imaging
	Traumatic: head injury or irradiation	Secondary	FSH, LH decreased or normal	Decreased	History of head trauma or cranial irradiation	
Other	Polycystic ovarian syndrome	Secondary	Increased LH:FSH ratio	Decreased or normal	Signs of androgen excess	Testosterone, dehydroepiandrosterone sulfate, ultrasound

LH, Luteinizing hormone; *FSH,* follicle-stimulating hormone.

studies have documented a normal complement of germ cells early in gestation, suggesting that the second X chromosome is vital to the protection of the germ cells from accelerated atresia.

It is likely that autoimmune mechanisms are responsible for some of the reported cases of **resistant ovary syndrome** in which amenorrhea and elevated FSH levels occur in the presence of a large complement of ovarian follicles. Evidence exists for the presence of both antibodies to the ovarian FSH receptor and substances that compete for binding of FSH to its receptor. In addition, this syndrome could result from defects in the FSH receptor or defects in the FSH molecule as has been reported for LH.

Pituitary and Hypothalamic Disorders

In patients with hypogonadotropic hypogonadism, the absence of cyclic gonadal function may be associated with gonadotropin levels that often are normal or only slightly decreased in comparison with those of normal women in the follicular phase.

The most common group of patients in whom low levels of gonadotropins accompany low levels of estrogen is that in whom a structural neuroanatomic lesion cannot be found. The diagnosis given to such patients is **hypothalamic amenorrhea.** In some situations an antecedent cause can be found, but in most of such patients the pathophysiology is not understood. Studies in which the patterns of pulsatile secretion of LH have been compared with those of normal women matched for sex steroid levels have revealed an underlying spectrum of defects of pulsatile GnRH levels (Fig. 43-3). The most severe form of this GnRH abnormality is characterized by a complete lack of pulsatile secretion of GnRH, which manifests by extremely low levels of LH but FSH levels that are often within the normal range. This pattern is seen in patients with a **congenital defect in GnRH secretion,** often in the presence of anosmia (Kallmann's syndrome). A similar pattern is seen in **anorexia nervosa** (see further discussion of anorexia nervosa and other causes of hypothalamic amenorrhea below).

In a small subset of patients, structural lesions of the pituitary or hypothalamus interfere with the normal pattern of GnRH secretion and stimulation of gonadotropin secretion, resulting in hypogonadotropic amenorrhea. In most of such patients, a careful history provides specific clues that suggest a neuroanatomic lesion. **Craniopharyngiomas** are the most common of these abnormalities and usually occur with growth retardation, visual impairment, or headache. Other midline **central nervous system** (CNS) **tumors** such as germinomas, gliomas, meningiomas, and endodermal sinus tumors, as well as rare metastatic tumors, dermoid cysts, or teratomas, are found rarely and often are associated with headache and visual symptoms. **Histiocytosis X** and **infiltrative disorders** such as sarcoidosis, hemochromatosis, and tuberculosis generally manifest with diabetes insipidus. **Head injuries** are a rare cause of hypogonadotropic hypogonadism. **Cranial irradiation** for CNS and head and neck tumors frequently is associated with abnormalities in gonadotropin secretion but normal pituitary responsiveness. The hypothalamus generally is more radiosensitive than is the pituitary, and therefore many of these patients have intact pituitary responsiveness to the hypothalamic-releasing factors.

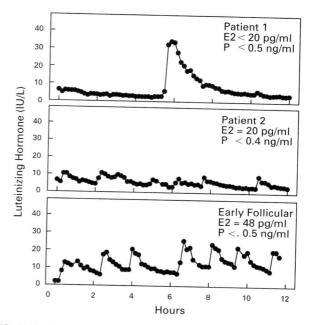

FIG. 43-3   Three representative patterns of pulsatile LH secretion in women with hypothalamic amenorrhea compared with the pattern seen in normal women in the early follicular phase *(lower panel)* emphasizing the range of values that are compatible with this diagnosis on single samples. (Modified from Crowley WF et al: *Rec Prog Horm Res* 41:473, 1985.)

Other Disorders

Polycystic ovary syndrome (PCOS) may occasionally present as primary amenorrhea. An increased ratio of LH/FSH typically is seen in patients with PCOS (see later and Chapter 14).

Secondary Amenorrhea

Uterine Disorders

In patients with a history of uterine instrumentation, particularly in the setting of infection or pregnancy, **Asherman's syndrome** (uterine synechiae or scarring) may account for amenorrhea. These patients have normal levels of all reproductive hormones, absence of a normal endometrial stripe on pelvic ultrasonography, and absence of withdrawal bleeding after a trial of estrogen and progestin replacement. Asherman's syndrome accounts for approximately 7% of all cases of secondary amenorrhea.

Ovulatory Disorders

Females begin life at birth with approximately 2 million primary oocytes. However, as a result of a natural process of atresia, only 400,000 oocytes remain at the time of puberty, and despite ovulation of only 400 oocytes during the period of normal reproductive capability, **ovarian failure** occurs between the ages of 45 and 55 years. Factors that can advance the time of ovarian failure may be genetic (decreased initial complement of germ cells or accelerated atresia) or acquired (destruction of oocytes). An elevation of FSH greater than 2 SD above the normal follicular-phase range in a patient with amenorrhea and low levels of estrogen is virtually pathognomonic of ovarian failure. Levels of LH may be elevated, but FSH is a more sensitive marker of ovarian failure than is LH because of its greater sensitivity to estrogen negative feedback. FSH also is more sensitive to the negative feedback effects of inhibin. Although the physiology of inhibin is still being elucidated, it is likely that a deficiency of inhibin plays a role in the selective rise in FSH with ovarian failure. The clinical history often reveals the finding of hot flashes that cause nighttime wakening. It is important to bear in mind that the course of ovarian failure may be one of waxing and waning, with reciprocal changes in estradiol and FSH levels occurring over several years.

Premature ovarian failure is defined as menopause before the age of 40 years. Autoimmune mechanisms are likely to be involved in a large subset of patients with premature ovarian failure. Premature ovarian failure has been associated with a number of autoimmune disorders, including the polyglandular failure syndromes in which autoimmune destruction is responsible for failure of a number of endocrine organs, for example, the adrenal gland, pancreas, parathyroid glands, and thyroid. Other autoimmune associations include pernicious anemia, rheumatoid arthritis, systemic lupus, myasthenia gravis, vitiligo, and premature gray hair. Follicular destruction is the mechanism behind the ovarian failure associated with chemotherapy, radiation therapy, viral factors such as mumps, oophoritis, and galactosemia.

Although patients with **Turner's syndrome** generally are of short stature and have primary amenorrhea, they may be of normal height or have secondary amenorrhea, or both. Many of these exceptions to the typical presentation of Turner's syndrome have been documented to be mosaics. Because some patients may have an XO/XY mosaic pattern, with a high potential for development of malignant changes in the gonad, it is important to obtain a karyotype on all patients with ovarian failure who are younger than 30 years old.

Hypothalamic and Pituitary Disorders

Approximately 15% of cases of secondary amenorrhea result from defects at the pituitary level, with most of these being **prolactinomas.** Amenorrhea is often the earliest symptom of a prolactin-secreting microadenoma, and up to one third may manifest with galactorrhea. Other patients have infertility associated with a luteal-phase deficiency. The gonadotropin profile of these patients is identical to patients with hypothalamic amenorrhea; however, the prolactin level will be consistently elevated. Although the anatomic defect is clearly at the level of the pituitary in these patients, the cause of gonadotropin deficiency is not the inability of the pituitary to secrete gonadotropins but rather the increase in dopamine turnover as a result of increased prolactin secretion that, in turn, inhibits GnRH secretion. Cranial imaging is important to determine whether the prolactin-secreting tumor is a microadenoma or a macroadenoma and to rule out the rare occurrence of a large pituitary mass in which relatively mild degrees of hyperprolactinemia may result from stalk compression and interference with the normal inhibitory control of prolactin secretion by dopamine. Hyperprolactinemia is discussed in detail in Chapter 15.

Other **pituitary tumors** such as those secreting growth hormone, adrenocorticotropic hormone (ACTH), or gonadotropin subunits or those considered nonfunctional are rare causes of hypogonadotropic hypogonadism and generally are associated with other clinical or biochemical features that help to localize the site of the defect to the pituitary. **Pituitary infarction** has been associated with postpartum hemorrhage (Sheehan's syndrome) and occasionally occurs spontaneously in the perimenopausal age-groups. The degree of hypopituitarism in such patients is highly variable, as is the potential for recovery. **Lymphocytic hypophysitis,** an inflammatory infiltrate of the pituitary of unknown etiology, also has been reported in association with isolated gonadotropin deficiency, again primarily in the postpartum period. **Pituitary irradiation** and extensive **pituitary surgery** are uncommon causes of amenorrhea.

Hypothalamic amenorrhea is associated with disordered pulsatile GnRH secretion caused by stress, strenuous exercise, or weight loss. Occasionally no precipitating cause for hypothalamic amenorrhea can be found. Hypothalamic amenorrhea accounts for over one third of cases of secondary amenorrhea.

Anorexia nervosa often is associated with the most profound suppression of gonadotropin and estrogen levels. Other endocrine abnormalities associated with anorexia nervosa include hypersecretion and decreased metabolism of cortisol, decreased adrenal androgen secretion, partial diabetes insipidus that is usually asymptomatic, elevated growth hormone levels with very low levels of somatomedin C, and thyroid function abnormalities compatible with the euthyroid sick syndrome. Of importance is that both the resumption of a normal weight and the amelioration of psychologic and behavioral traits are required for resumption of normal menses in these patients. (Eating disorders are discussed further in Chapter 84.)

Other abnormalities of pulsatile GnRH secretion in patients with a hypothalamic cause of their menstrual cycle disturbance include patterns of low amplitude, slow frequency, and nighttime augmentation (Fig. 43-3), all of which are inadequate to sustain orderly folliculogenesis and ovulation. Patients in whom amenorrhea is clinically associated with **strenuous exercise, weight loss, stress,** and acute or chronic **intercurrent illness** (including other endocrine disorders such as hypothyroidism and hyperthyroidism, Cushing's syndrome, and diabetes) attest to the clinical consequences of environmental factors on control of hypothalamic coordination of the reproductive axis. Exercise usually is associated with amenorrhea only when there is significant weight loss (weight less than 10% of ideal body weight) or a marked decrease in the percentage of body fat. The recent recognition of both the frequency of **bulimia** in young women of reproductive age and its association with a similar spectrum of hypogonadotropic menstrual cycle disorders indicates that this is a diagnosis that must be specifically excluded in women with amenorrhea.

Other Disorders

The clinical presentation of **polycystic ovary syndrome** usually is oligomenorrhea beginning around the time of puberty in association with clinical or biochemical evidence of hyperandrogenism. However, patients may have amenorrhea or dysfunctional bleeding, and infertility is common. The diagnosis is made on clinical grounds (oligomenorrhea/amenorrhea plus signs of androgen excess), assuming that other causes of hyperandrogenism have been ruled out. Differentiation of patients with PCOS from those with hypothalamic amenorrhea is important because the management issues may be somewhat different. (PCOS is discussed further in Chapter 46.)

EVALUATION

The patient with primary amenorrhea should be evaluated if neither menarche nor breast development has occurred by age 14 years or in the absence of menarche by age 16 years, even in the presence of normal breast development. In addition, the girl with primary amenorrhea should be evaluated if menarche has not occurred within 3 years of the onset of breast development or if she also is under the third percentile for height by age 14 years.

Once menses have been established, it is not uncommon for normal women to skip an occasional menstrual period. Even this should prompt the clinician to rule out pregnancy in the patient who is sexually active, but a more thorough evaluation of amenorrhea should be reserved for those who have had 3 to 6 months of irregular or absent menses.

History and Physical Examination

A careful and directed clinical history can provide many clues to the underlying cause of the patient's menstrual cycle disorder (Box 43-1). Specific questions should focus on the developmental history, previous menstrual history, and elicitation of relevant localizing symptoms. From a developmental perspective, the pattern of growth and pubertal development is key, as well as parental height and a family history of pubertal delay, anosmia, or androgen-resistance syndromes. Menstrual history should include the age and weight at menarche, the characteristics of early and most recent cycles—including regularity and duration of menstrual interval and menstrual flow—the presence or absence of symptoms associated with ovulation (breast tenderness, mood changes, food cravings), and the date of the last menstrual period. The manner of onset of amenorrhea and associations with other events such as illness, stress, weight changes, exercise patterns, medications, pregnancy, and uterine instrumentation should be delineated. In addition, it is critical to determine whether the patient is sexually active and to discuss contraceptive practices. Relevant localizing symptoms include hot flashes, anorectic behaviors or attitudes, galactorrhea, headache or visual disturbances, significant weight changes, acne, hirsutism or oily skin, symptoms of other endocrine dysfunction, systemic illness, and depression.

Physical examination may include height, weight, arm span, secondary sexual characteristics, evaluation for the stigmata of Turner's syndrome already noted, visual field defects, galactorrhea, signs of androgen excess, and clues to the presence of anorexia nervosa (such as lanugo hair or carotenemia). A pelvic examination is performed to determine the presence of normal external and internal genitalia.

Diagnostic Tests

Initial evaluation of the amenorrheic patient includes a pregnancy test to rule out the most common cause of amenorrhea in women of reproductive age, an FSH level to rule out ovarian failure, and a prolactin level to help to determine whether further investigation for a neuroanatomic cause of hypogonadotropic hypogonadism is required (Box 43-2).

BOX 43-1
History and Physical Examination

History
Developmental history
Growth, pubertal development
Previous menstrual history
Last menstrual period
Sexual activity, use of contraception
Age, weight at menarche
Characteristics of previous cycles (regularity, duration, molimina)
Other events or illnesses
Stress, weight changes, anorectic behavior, medications, pregnancy, instrumentation
Exercise patterns
Other symptoms
Androgenic symptoms (acne, oily skin, hirsutism)
Nausea, breast tenderness, weight gain
Galactorrhea or visual symptoms
Significant weight loss or gain
Hot flashes

Physical Examination
General
Height, weight
Stigmata of Turner's syndrome
Skin
Axillary and public hair development
Acne, hirsutism, oiliness, acanthosis nigricans
Signs of weight loss, lanugo hair, carotenemia
Stigmata of Cushing's syndrome
Visual fields
Breasts
Breast development
Galactorrhea
Pelvic examination
Presence of normal external and internal genitalia
Vaginal atrophy
Ovarian and uterine enlargement

Administration of medroxyprogesterone acetate (Provera) (10 mg for 5 days) provides an assessment of overall estrogen status. Any amount of bleeding within 10 days of stopping the medication is considered a positive result. Alternatively an estradiol level can be measured, and basal body temperature charting or a progesterone level can help determine the ovulatory status of the patient.

Further evaluation is based on the history and physical examination findings and may include thyroid function tests, androgen levels, pelvic ultrasound, karyotype, and cranial imaging. Measurement of bone density may help to determine the course of treatment.

Cranial imaging may be performed by use of computed tomography (CT) or magnetic resonance imaging (MRI), with attention to the hypothalamic-pituitary area, and should be undertaken in any patient with a persistently elevated prolactin level, even if the elevation is only modest. In addition, cranial imaging should be used for any patient with hypogonadotropic primary amenorrhea, as already outlined, and in patients with amenorrhea and headache, visual field defects, neurologic symptoms, diabetes insipidus, or evidence of pituitary hypofunction such as growth abnormalities.

MANAGEMENT

Therapy for amenorrhea depends on both the diagnosis and goals of the patient, in particular whether pregnancy is desired. In addition, long-term follow-up is important to evaluate the results of therapy if instituted, as well as to respond to the changing concerns of the patient. Although ongoing management of these patients is often complex and is best managed by a specialized endocrinologist or gynecologist, the primary care physician should be aware of the options available to the patients and the general therapeutic issues that are unique to each group of patients.

Uterine or Outflow Tract Disorders

Surgical correction may be possible in some patients with congenital müllerian abnormalities, whereas most patients with Asherman's syndrome will be successfully cured with hysteroscopic lysis of synechiae and administration of estrogen. In patients with androgen-resistance syndromes, removal of the gonads is important because of risk of testicular malignant disease. The timing of removal of the gonads is controversial, with some investigators suggesting that this should be performed as soon as the diagnosis is made (often in conjunction with surgery for bilateral hernias) and others suggesting that there is some advantage in terms of normal breast development if removal is delayed until secondary sexual development is complete. Thereafter, estrogen replacement therapy is required for protection from osteoporosis, vaginal dryness, and possibly cardiovascular disease. Progestin replacement is not indicated in these patients.

Ovulatory Disorders

In patients with ovarian failure, pregnancy is often not possible other than with the use of ovum donation, the results of which are extremely promising. Hormonal replacement with estrogen and a progestin are required for long-term management of symptoms (hot flashes and vaginal dryness) and for prevention of osteoporosis and possibly cardiovascular disease. Hormone-replacement therapy is discussed in detail in Chapter 48.

Pituitary and Hypothalamic Disorders

Dopamine agonists (bromocriptine or cabergoline) are the treatment of choice for patients with a microprolactinoma and generally will restore normal ovulatory cycles. Transsphenoidal surgery and radiation also have been used but usually are reserved for those patients with larger tumors. In patients who are interested in fertility, the ovulation-induction agents detailed in the next section for use in patients with hypothalamic amenorrhea also are appropriate if the patient remains infertile or anovulatory despite the use of dopamine agonists. Management of prolactinomas is discussed in detail in Chapter 15.

In the patient with hypothalamic amenorrhea who is not interested in fertility, the major concerns are the long-term consequences of hypoestrogenism. There is ample evidence that many of these women have bone-density measurements that are below the normal range for their age, placing them at increased risk for osteoporotic fractures with age, and that even young amenorrheic athletes and ballet dancers have a high incidence of stress fractures. These same women are also at risk for inadequate calcium intake and should receive supplementation to a total intake of 1500 mg of elemental calcium per day, including that from dietary sources.

As a rule, estrogen replacement should be seriously considered in any patient who has been amenorrheic for more than 6 months, and it must be administered in association with a progestin. Oral contraceptives are often the most convenient form of estrogen replacement and also address the issue of contraception for any patient who is sexually active. In the patient who is resistant to consideration of estrogen replacement or in whom estrogen replacement is contraindicated, bone-density measurements may help to ensure that the appropriate decisions are made. Specific interventions and appropriate referral are required for patients with eating disorders.

For patients who are interested in fertility, lifestyle changes with weight and exercise modification may be all that are necessary to restore ovulatory cycles. If these interventions are not successful, ovulation induction is generally highly successful. Before proceeding, however, it is necessary to rule out a significant male factor by performing a semen analysis. The simplest form of ovulation induction is oral therapy with clomiphene citrate, an estrogen antagonist. Although clomiphene citrate is often unsuccessful in this group of patients because of their inherently low estrogen level, a limited trial is generally worthwhile inasmuch as this form of therapy has relatively low risk and is convenient for the patient compared with other ovulation-induction methods. Pulsatile GnRH is the therapy of choice for those who fail to respond to clomiphene citrate, since the risk for hyperstimulation and multiple gestation with this form of therapy is relatively low compared with exogenous gonadotropins. However, the availability of pulsatile GnRH is limited in the United States. Exogenous gonadotropin therapy is also highly successful but must be used conservatively in this population of patients. These forms of ovulation induction generally are managed in specialized endocrine or gynecology practices.

Polycystic Ovary Syndrome

In all patients with infertility who are overweight, weight loss is likely to be beneficial whether or not they are currently interested in fertility. For the patient with PCOS who is not interested in fertility, the main concerns are endometrial protection, management of androgenic effects, and contraception. Treatment of oligomenorrhea or amenorrhea in women with PCOS is discussed in Chapter 46.

In patients who are interested in fertility, estrogen-antagonist treatment (clomiphene citrate) is the therapy of first choice; it is successful in induction of ovulation in approximately 60% of patients. Recent studies indicate that insulin sensitizing agents may be of benefit for ovulation induction either alone or in combination with clomiphene citrate. Exogenous gonadotropins also are highly successful, although they present an increased risk of hyperstimulation and multiple gestation. In addition, pulsatile GnRH has been found to be effective in some patients, although not all patients ovulate in response to this form of therapy. Overall, women with PCOS have a slightly increased rate of pregnancy loss with all forms of therapy compared with other anovulatory patients.

BIBLIOGRAPHY

Broome JD, Vancaillie TG: Fluoroscopically guided hysteroscopic division of adhesions in severe Asherman syndrome, *Obstet Gynecol* 93:1041, 1999.

Crowley WF et al: The physiology of gonadotropin-releasing hormone (GnRH) secretion in men and women, *Recent Prog Horm Res* 41:473, 1985.

Dunaif A et al: *Current issues in endocrinology and metabolism—polycystic ovary syndrome,* Boston, 1992, Blackwell Scientific Publications.

Hall JE: Polycystic ovarian disease as a neuroendocrine disorder of the female reproductive axis, *Endocrinol Metab Clin North Am* 22:75, 1993.

Laufer MR et al: Hormone testing in women with adult-onset amenorrhea, *Gynecol Obstet Invest* 40:2000, 1995.

Martin K et al: Comparison of exogenous gonadotropins and pulsatile GnRH for induction of ovulation in hypogonadotropic amenorrhea, *J Clin Endocrinol Metab* 77:125, 1993.

Reindollar RH, Byrd JR, McDonough PG: Delayed sexual development: a study of 252 patients, *Am J Obstet Gynecol* 140:371, 1981.

Reindollar RH et al: Adult-onset amenorrhea: a study of 262 patients, *Am J Obstet Gynecol* 155:531, 1986.

Saenger P: Current concepts: Turner's syndrome, *N Engl J Med* 335:1749, 1996.

Sanborn CF, Martin BJ, Wagner WW: Is athletic amenorrhea specific to runners? *Am J Obstet Gynecol* 143:859, 1982.

Schlaff WD, Hurst BS: Preoperative sonographic measurement of endometrial pattern predicts outcome of surgical repair in patients with severe Asherman syndrome, *Fertil Steril* 63:410, 1995.

Soules MR: Adolescent amenorrhea, *Pediatr Clin North Am* 34:1083, 1987.

Suh BY et al: Hypercortisolism in patients with functional hypothalamic amenorrhea, *J Clin Endocrinol Metab* 66:733, 1988.

Taylor AE et al: Ovarian failure, resistance and activation. In Adashi EY, Leung PCK, editors: *The ovary,* New York, 1993, Raven Press.

Villaneuva AL et al: Increased cortisol production in women runners, *J Clin Endocrinol Metab* 633:133, 1986.

Warren MP et al: Functional hypothalamic amenorrhea: hypoleptinemia and disordered eating, *J Clin Endocrinol Metab* 84:873, 1999.

Yen SSC, Jaffe RB: *Reproductive endocrinology,* Philadelphia, 1991, WB Saunders.

CHAPTER 44

Benign Vulvar Disorders

Harold Michlewitz

With the control of common gynecologic cancers, the field of gynecology has refocused attention on the vulva. Primary care physicians have assumed greater responsibility for identifying vulvar complaints. This chapter is designed to expand their familiarity with common benign vulvar disorders. Diagnosis and management of vulvovaginitis are discussed in Chapter 51 and herpes genitalis in Chapter 22.

Vulvar disorders can be categorized according to their predominant presenting characteristics (Table 44-1). These include vulvar masses, pruritus, and pain or irritation. A high index of suspicion for preinvasive carcinoma of the vulva is necessary whenever a vulvar complaint is evaluated. The clinical presentation of a preinvasive vulvar lesion may be a reddened or whitish, flattened, or slightly raised patch, often with hyperkeratosis. Biopsy is the only way to establish a diagnosis of benign disease. If any lesion is treated with topical agents without biopsy, it is important that the patient be reevaluated in 3 to 4 weeks and a biopsy performed if signs and symptoms have not remitted.

BENIGN VULVAR MASSES

Epidermal Inclusion Cyst

The most common subcutaneous vulvar lesion, the epidermal inclusion cyst, is a smooth, yellowish cyst that generally measures 5 to 15 mm in diameter. It usually is nontender and slow-growing. Multiple lesions may occur.

Differential Diagnosis

Subcutaneous labial cystic masses must be distinguished from **inguinal hernias.** Rarely a **cyst of Nuck's canal** (a vestigial peritoneal sac passing through the inguinal canal) can manifest as a large, nontender, cystic vulvar mass.

✳ MANAGEMENT

Asymptomatic cysts can be managed by observation alone. If significant enlargement takes place under observation, or if the cyst causes discomfort, excision is needed. Aspiration of fluid should be avoided because of the likelihood of inoculating the cyst with bacteria, leading to abscess formation.

Bartholin's Gland Cysts

Bartholin's gland cysts are common vulvar lesions that arise in the labia minora in the greater vestibular gland, that is, Bartholin's gland. The swelling encountered is in the posterior labia minora and deep to the perineal body. A noninfected cyst usually is compressible and not tender. Secondary bacterial infection may occur in an obstructed Bartholin's gland duct, usually with mixed flora. Infection produces a fluctuant, extremely tender mass at the inferior margin of the labia minora. Swelling may extend superiorly under the labia majora. An abscess that ruptures subcutaneously will track superiorly toward the mons pubis or deep toward the ischiorectal fossa. In severe cases, necrotizing fasciitis may occur.

Differential Diagnosis

Rarely, a **cutaneous fistula** from **Crohn's disease** may resemble a Bartholin's duct abscess. In a postmenopausal woman, a mass at the site of Bartholin's gland may arise from a **benign** or **malignant neoplasm.**

✳ MANAGEMENT

When a Bartholin's gland abscess points and ruptures spontaneously, sitz baths and analgesia are the only treatments needed. However, incision and drainage usually are required. This can be performed under no or local anesthesia (ethyl chloride spray or lidocaine injection). Maintaining drainage and disruption of septations are essential for satisfactory resolution. Broad-spectrum antibiotic coverage (for example, with ceftriaxone or cefixime plus clindamycin) is recommended at the time of drainage, unless culture results identify a specific organism. Bartholin's gland abscesses are generally polymicrobial, involving aerobic and anaerobic bacteria, but may result from sexually transmitted organisms such as *Chlamydia trachomatis* and *Neisseria gonorrhoeae.*

Chronic or recurrent Bartholin's gland abscess is best treated with marsupialization.

Folliculitis

Subcutaneous masses of the labia majora can represent infection at the base of the hair follicle. These tender lesions

Table 44-1
Typical Presentations of Benign Vulvar Disorders

Predominant Symptom	CAUSES	
	More Common	Less Common
Mass		
Cystic	Epidermal inclusion cyst	Inguinal hernia
	Bartholin's gland cyst	Pilonidal cyst
	Follicular cyst	Cysts of embryonic origin
		Hidradenoma
		Urethral diverticulum
Solid	Condyloma acuminatum	Seborrheic keratosis
	Acrochordon (skin tag)	Nevi
		Fibromas and lipomas
		Urethral caruncle
		Endometriosis
Pruritus	Infectious vulvitis (Candida, Trichomonas)	
	Contact dermatitis	
	Bacterial vaginosis	
	Squamous hyperplasia	
	Lichen sclerosus	
	Human papillomavirus	
Pain	Herpes genitalis	Dysesthetic vulvodynia
	Human papillomavirus	Pudendal neuralgia
	Lichen planus	
	Vulvar vestibulitis	

may vary from 5 mm up to several centimeters. These lesions or small abscesses may respond to warm compresses or sitz baths. When large, they require incision and drainage.

Condyloma Acuminatum

Condyloma acuminatum (an anogenital wart) is a benign growth caused by human papillomavirus (HPV). Spread can occur through sexual contact and, less frequently, through inadvertent touching of the genitals with wart-infested hands or during delivery. Condylomata often proliferate during pregnancy; rarely, significant bleeding or obstruction of the birth canal may require cesarean section. Laryngeal papilloma may be transmitted to the neonate.

An association between vulvar intraepithelial neoplasia and vulvar condylomata has been observed. The malignancy potential of HPV is discussed in detail in Chapter 97.

The moist vulvar environment, concomitant vaginal infections, pregnancy, and an immunocompromised state influence the quantity and location of genital warts. Inspection of the genitals by the naked eye—even careful inspection—may miss numerous condylomata. A magnifying glass or colposcope allows for more comprehensive detection of warts. The warts may be minute or grow to 8 to 10 cm, interfering with the ability to sit or walk.

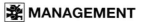 **MANAGEMENT**

Local treatment with topical agents such as trichloroacetic acid (TCA) or podophyllum is the initial therapy for small lesions (<2 cm). TCA (50% to 80% solution) is a caustic agent applied directly to the lesions, which typically blanch within a few hours and slough within 2 to 4 days. Temporary intense burning usually occurs, but a local reaction of the surrounding skin is less common than with podophyllum.

Podophyllum (20% solution or 25% ointment) is applied similarly, but it must be washed off after 4 to 6 hours. A 0.5% podofilox cream, applied twice daily by the patient for 3 consecutive days each week, for up to 3 weeks, also has been effective. Topical podophyllum occasionally is associated with a severe local reaction and, rarely, with severe systemic toxicity. Podophyllum should not be used during pregnancy.

After ablative topical therapy, complete healing usually occurs in 1 week. The patient should then be reexamined for persistent or new lesions requiring further applications. Regrowth of lesions may reflect inadequate treatment or resistance. Resistance demands histologic clarification of potential cancer before a long-term plan of local therapy is initiated.

Imiquimod (Aldara) is an immune modulating agent that can be applied by the patient. It is available as a 5% cream, which is applied three times a week until resolution. As with other topical agents, local irritation can occur.

For lesions greater than 2 cm, the patient should be referred for laser treatment or loop electrode excision. Laser treatment of extensive areas of warts is not without complications. Occasional residual perineal pain may be incapacitating and can lead to vulvar vestibulitis (see next section). The presence of micropapillations or areas that blanch with acetic acid application is insufficient cause to initiate laser therapy.

For persistent or recurrent warts, intralesional interferon injection may be effective, with a complete response rate of up to 60%. Intramuscularly administered interferon-alpha is a successful and less painful therapy.

Examination and treatment of the sexual partner are advised to help stop the spread of infection in the general population. However, recurrence rates in women are similar regardless of whether the male partner is examined and treated.

VULVAR DERMATITIS

Vulvar dermatitis is one of the most frequent vulvar disorders seen in primary care practice. Contact dermatitis, by far the most common form, may be caused by external irritants (Box 44-1) or by an immunologically mediated allergic reaction. Irritation and burning, rather than pruritus, are characteristic of contact dermatitis. The intrinsic susceptibility of vulvar tissue to irritants, coupled with the frequency of certain personal hygiene practices among women, accounts for the predominance of the irritant form of dermatitis. In one study of women seen in a specialty clinic for vulvar disorders, 60% reported personal care habits that were likely to aggravate their condition.

Classic eczema, or atopic dermatitis, may also manifest vulvar involvement, although the frequency of true atopic dermatitis of the vulva is debated.

Differential Diagnosis

A careful history of personal hygiene practices and self-treatment for vulvar complaints is important. The patient should also be asked about a history of eczema or other atopic conditions. Physical examination can reveal a spectrum of findings, ranging from mild erythema to severe fissuring, excoriations, serous oozing, and secondary bacterial or yeast infection. Chronic irritations and scratching can lead to development of papillae, a sign of chronic inflammation, and to the histologic changes of squamous hyperplasia (see later discussion).

Laboratory testing may be necessary to rule out infection. If fissuring or open lesions are present, culture for herpes simplex should be done to rule out genital herpes. A wet mount with potassium hydroxide of vaginal and vulvar secretions may identify yeast vulvitis if hyphae are present; culture for yeast will definitively rule out fungal infection if the wet mount is negative. A vulvar biopsy may be necessary if the diagnosis is uncertain.

❖ MANAGEMENT

Elimination of any external irritants is a crucial first step in management of vulvar dermatitis. For treatment of contact or eczematous dermatitis, low to intermediate potency topical corticosteroids twice a day for 1 to 4 weeks, then twice a week, can be used safely for an indefinite period. High-potency topical corticosteroids required for severe cases, such as clobetasol, may be used for up to 12 weeks without adverse effects. Reexamination after 3 months is important to be certain that any persistent lesion warranting biopsy is detected.

Adjunct measures include treatment of any associated yeast vulvitis, best done with oral fluconazole because of the potentially irritating effects of topical treatments. Warm water soaks and oral antihistamines are helpful for itching.

VULVAR DYSTROPHIES

The vulvar dystrophies are nonneoplastic epithelial disorders of the vulvar skin and mucosa. Clinically they often appear as thickened or thinned white vulvar lesions. Biopsy is essential for diagnosis and determination of any malignancy potential.

Squamous Hyperplasia

The cause of squamous hyperplastic lesions is unknown. They typically manifest with pruritus. On examination, the appearance is highly variable, ranging from a dusky-red vulva in mild cases to well-defined white patches, often with lichenification, fissures, and excoriations. The histopathologic findings are hyperkeratosis and epithelial thickening.

Lichen Sclerosus

Lichen sclerosus is one of the most prominent of the white vulvar lesions. It usually appears in postmenopausal women, although it can occur at any age. The lesion also can be seen in locations outside the vulva. Although the skin appears atrophic, that appearance belies a truly active epithelium. There is increased cell turnover, epithelial thinning, and subjacent dermal inflammation. An autoimmune mechanism is postulated.

Pruritus is a common symptom of lichen sclerosus. The typical lesion is white and initially can occur in an isolated area, evolving to encompass the entire vulva. The skin appears atrophic and glistening, and focal areas may be thickened or eroded. Focal ecchymosis also may be seen. The atrophic appearance is accompanied by progressive loss of the labia majora, labia minora, and fusion of the clitoral hood, which appears as marked introital narrowing (kraurosis).

Biopsy is required for diagnosis. Lichen sclerosus, which is associated with vulvar carcinomas, is present in the epithelium in about 10% of such cancers. A recent cohort study calculated a 15% cumulative risk of invasive squamous cell cancer in women with lichen sclerosus followed prospectively after treatment, compared to a risk of less than 1% in the general population.

Differential Diagnosis

Vulvar lesions appear in a variety of forms; thus their pathologic characteristics cannot be distinguished solely by visual inspection. One must be ready to sample tissue by means of excisional or incisional biopsy to make the proper diagnosis. A biopsy specimen should be obtained from any white, ulcerated, nodular, fissured, or abnormal raised pigmented area.

Local anesthesia is achieved with use of lidocaine 1% or 2% by injection (with a 27- or 30-gauge needle), ethyl chloride spray, or topical anesthetic ointments. The lesion can be excised with either a scissors or scalpel. A Keyes punch biopsy also allows a core of tissue to be readily retrieved with use of forceps and a scissors to free the base of the tissue core. The biopsy specimen from an area of erosion or ulcer should include adjacent noneroded tissue to help make the diagnosis. Control of bleeding can be achieved with either Monsel's solution (a paste of ferrous subsulfate) or silver nitrate sticks. Larger biopsy sites may require sutures. In general, the wound will heal in 7 to 10 days and will require some local anesthetic application if significant pain is encountered.

The incidence of vulvar carcinoma is low, but this should not discourage biopsy when an undiagnosed lesion is encountered. Early identification of its pathology, even if benign, will allow for proper treatment.

❖ MANAGEMENT

After diagnosis by biopsy, squamous hyperplasia is treated with topical steroids. A regimen of high-potency or medium-potency steroids (such as 0.01% triamcinolone acetonide or 0.025% to 0.01% fluocinolone acetonide), applied two or three times a day for 4 to 6 weeks, generally is effective.

For lichen sclerosus, superpotent steroids such as clobetasol 0.05% ointment have been shown to be effective for both treatment and maintenance. A typical regimen is clobetasol ointment daily for 6 to 12 weeks, followed by maintenance therapy with application one to three times a week. Maintenance therapy has not been associated with complications such as systemic steroid effects or local epidermal atrophy.

Recurrence of lichen sclerosus is common. For this reason, and because of the increased risk for vulvar carcinoma, it is optimal for affected women to be monitored by physicians with a special interest in this condition.

OTHER VULVAR CONDITIONS

This section considers other common vulvar conditions that often are accompanied by pain or irritation.

Lichen Planus

Lichen planus affects the mucosal surfaces of the vulva, especially the vestibule. The cause of this condition is unknown. There is thickening of all layers of the epithelium, as well as hyperkeratosis and a subepithelial lymphocytic infiltrate. Vulvar involvement occurs in half of women with extravulvar evidence of lichen planus, which typically appears on the skin as shiny, flat, violaceous papules with white striae.

Clinically, painful erosive areas may be present on the vulva and adhesions of opposite mucosal surfaces can cause marked stenosis of the introitus and vagina. Bleeding on contact and severe dyspareunia are characteristic of the lesion.

On physical examination, lichen planus appears as a white, raised lesion with a reticular, lacy pattern. The erosive variant has the appearance of a desquamation bordered by reticular white epithelium. The external labia may have the appearance of lichen sclerosus (see previous discussion), but the mucosal changes are quite characteristic. The condition can be associated with changes in other mucosal surfaces such as the vagina and particularly the gingivobuccal mucosa.

✴ MANAGEMENT

Whereas dermal lichen planus typically resolves spontaneously, vulvar and other mucosal lesions tend to be persistent. High-potency topical steroids may control the condition. To reestablish the vaginal canal in severe cases of scarring, systemic steroids or reconstructive surgery may be required. Referral to a clinician with a special interest in vulvar disorders is recommended.

Vulvar Pain Syndromes

Women with vulvar pain syndrome (vulvodynia) experience varying levels of vulvar discomfort manifested as either burning, stinging, pain, dryness, irritation, or rawness. Pruritus is absent. Vulvodynia may have an organic cause, or it can occur with no apparent predisposing condition (dysesthetic or "essential" vulvodynia).

Common organic causes of vulvodynia include irritant and contact dermatitis, infection with yeast or trichomonal organisms, HPV, and herpes genitalis. Vulvar vestibulitis (see next section) represents a subset of vulvodynia.

In dysesthetic vulvodynia, constant vulvar burning, not localized to a specific focus, is a typical symptom. There is no pain related solely to touch or introital sexual intercourse. The pain does not radiate as it might in a pudendal neuralgia. It is also distinct from vulvar pain associated with sexual arousal (occlusion of the Bartholin's gland duct must be suspected in this circumstance). The pain pattern is reminiscent of a cutaneous distribution as seen in postherpetic neuralgia.

✴ MANAGEMENT

Treatment with low-dose antidepressants has been fairly effective for this condition, as for other neuropathic pain syndromes. A starting dosage of amitriptyline, 10 mg twice a day, can be increased every 2 to 3 weeks until pain is relieved. In McKay's series of patients with essential vulvodynia, the average dose required was 60 mg/day, and the average length of treatment was 7 months. For pain that is refractory to antidepressants, a computed tomography scan or magnetic resonance imaging to exclude sacral tumors or nerve root cysts is advisable.

Women with essential vulvodynia may have histories of pain that date back decades. The disruption in their lives is significant enough to produce psychologic difficulties that need recognition.

Vulvar Vestibulitis

The hallmarks of vulvar vestibulitis are (1) severe pain with touch or attempted vaginal entry, (2) focal areas of tenderness to light touch localized within the vulvar vestibule (the portion of the vulva that extends from the clitoris to the fourchette, visible on separating the labia minora), and (3) physical findings limited to vestibular erythema.

The etiology of vulvar vestibulitis has not been established. Mann's study of the variables associated with this condition found that recurrent candidiasis and previous condyloma acuminatum were more common in women with vulvar vestibulitis than in control subjects. Some investigators have theorized that a candidal or HPV infection may elicit an autoimmune response, leading to local inflammation. The histopathologic examination reveals a chronic inflammatory response without evidence of allergic phenomena or a hypersensitivity reaction.

Symptoms associated with vulvar vestibulitis include superficial dyspareunia, pain with any vulvar pressure, and persistent burning. Occasionally dysuria and frequency are present, and an association with interstitial cystitis has been observed by some investigators.

Patients in many instances have received therapy or have self-treated for "vaginitis" without the establishment of a proper diagnosis. The acute phase of common vaginitides will result in a vulvitis, but with appropriate treatment the condition is limited. Other inciting causes (irritants, topical therapeutic agents) may be identified. Only when symptoms persist for 6 months or more is the patient said to have chronic vulvar vestibulitis.

On physical examination the external vulva appears normal except for erythema of the vestibule. Rarely, shallow ulcers may be seen adjacent to the hymenal ring. The classic finding of vulvar vestibulitis is the elicitation of typical burning pain with gentle pressure from a cotton-tipped applicator on specific foci within the vestibule.

✹ MANAGEMENT

Lack of understanding of the etiology of vulvar vestibulitis has hampered efforts to find effective treatment for this disorder. Most reported studies are case series, and there are few clinical trials. Topical or injectable steroids, estrogen, antibiotics, antifungal agents, and retinoid compounds appear to have no significant effect. Local destruction of tissue with either topical acids, cryotherapy, or laser treatment has had limited, if any, benefit; and concern has arisen that overzealous treatment with these modalities may lead to residual vulvar vestibulitis.

Solomons and colleagues reported an association between excessive urinary oxalate excretion and vulvar vestibulitis. A low-oxalate diet, coupled with calcium citrate tablets (200 mg calcium/950 mg citrate, two tablets three times a day) has been recommended. This regimen, which inhibits calcium oxalate-crystal formation, needs further study but appears to have little potential toxicity.

Recombinant interferon-alpha 2b, approved by the Food and Drug Administration for treatment of condyloma acuminatum, has been effective for reducing or relieving symptoms in 50% to 80% of patients with vulvar vestibulitis. Recombinant interferon is administered by injection beneath the vulvar mucosa (0.5 mg to a single site, repeated every 2 to 3 days at different locations around the vestibule for a total of approximately 12 injections). Local pain and mild flulike symptoms may occur.

The most successful treatment for vulvar vestibulitis has been surgical excision of the vestibule and hymen, with significant improvement reported in 60% to 80% of women. The healing process can sometimes be slow and require several weeks for complete recovery. Sexual function has been reported to be restored to normal in more than 75% of patients.

Studies of the psychosexual aspects of vulvar vestibulitis suggest that the syndrome may result from an interaction of physiologic and psychologic factors. Psychiatric treatment as the sole modality is not appropriate until full evaluation by a physician knowledgeable in the area of vulvar vestibulitis is completed.

BIBLIOGRAPHY

Borenstein J: Clobetasol dipropionate 0.05% versus testosterone propionate 2% topical application for severe vulvar lichen sclerosus, *Am J Obstet Gynecol* 178:80, 1998.

Carli P et al: Squamous cell carcinoma arising in vulval lichen sclerosus: a longitudinal cohort study, *Eur J Cancer Prev* 4:491, 1995.

Fischer G, Spurrett B, Fischer A: The chronically symptomatic vulva: aetiology and management, *Br J Obstet Gynaecol* 102:773, 1995.

Kaufman RH, Faro S: *Benign diseases of the vulva and vagina,* ed 4, St Louis, 1994, Mosby.

Krebs HB, Helmkamp BF: Treatment failure of genital condylomata acuminata in women: role of the male sexual partner, *Am J Obstet Gynecol* 165:337, 1991.

Lorenz B, Kaufman RH, Kutzner SK: Lichen sclerosus. Therapy with clobetasol propionate, *J Reprod Med* 43:790, 1998.

Mann MS et al: Vulvar vestibulitis: significant variables and treatment outcome, *Obstet Gynecol* 79:122, 1992.

Marin M, King R, Sfameni S, Dennerstein GJ: Adverse behavioral and sexual factors in chronic vulvar disease, *Am J Obstet Gynecol* 183:34, 2000.

Marinoff SC, Turner MLC: Vulvar vestibulitis syndrome: an overview, *Am J Obstet Gynecol* 165:1228, 1991.

McKay M: Dysesthetic ("essential") vulvodynia, *J Reprod Med* 38:9, 1993.

Powell JJ, Wojnarowska F: Lichen sclerosus, *Lancet* 353:1777, 1999.

Solomons CC, Melmed MH, Heitler SM: Calcium citrate for vulvar vestibulitis, *J Reprod Med* 36:879, 1991.

Von Krogh G, Hellberg D: Self-treatment using a 0.5% podophyllotoxin cream of external genital condylomata acuminata in women, *Sex Transm Dis* 19:170, 1992.

CHAPTER 45

Endometriosis

Toufic I. Nakad
Keith B. Isaacson

Endometriosis is defined as the presence of endometrial glands and stroma outside the endometrial cavity and uterine musculature. Because it is such a common condition, the primary care clinician must be familiar with the clinical manifestations, spectrum of treatment options, and prognosis of endometriosis. These topics are reviewed in this chapter. Chapter 55 discusses the differential diagnosis of pelvic pain, which includes consideration of endometriosis.

EPIDEMIOLOGY

The prevalence of a disease is defined as the number of known cases at any given time. Because endometriosis is a disease that can be diagnosed only by direct visualization or biopsy, the reported prevalence of the disease is biased by the indication for surgical exploration. The prevalence of endometriosis has been reported to be 1% to 50% depending on the indication for surgery. Fertile patients undergoing tubal ligation will have the lowest prevalence, and as may be expected, the highest prevalence (nearly 50%) is reported in women with pelvic pain and infertility. In Wheeler's series of 858 hysterectomies performed for indications other than those in which endometriosis was suspected, 8% had histologically confirmed endometriosis. However, nearly 40% of women undergoing laparoscopy for infertility have endometriosis.

The median age for the diagnosis of endometriosis is 29 years. Most endometriosis patients are in the reproductive age group, although a small population is postmenopausal. Endometriosis is diagnosed in similar proportions of white, African-American, Israeli, Afghani, Iranian, and Japanese women. Endometriosis crosses all socioeconomic barriers. The early data suggesting that the disease was more prevalent in women of higher socioeconomic status were flawed by not correcting for access to technologically advanced medical care.

Certain reproductive factors affect the likelihood of developing endometriosis. Cyclic oral contraceptives appear to reduce the risk of endometriosis. This protective effect persists for up to a year after discontinuation. Early and frequent pregnancies also confer some reduction in risk.

HISTOGENESIS

The exact histogenesis of endometriosis is unknown. The most accepted theories include transplantation, lymphatic/vascular metastasis, coelomic metaplasia, and the embryonic rests theory.

The *transplantation theory,* or Sampson's theory, was proposed in 1927 and suggests that viable endometrial tissue is refluxed through the fallopian tubes at the time of menses and that this endometrial tissue is capable of implanting on surfaces within the peritoneum. This theory is supported by recent data from Halme et al demonstrating that up to 90% of women have bloody peritoneal fluid at the time of menses and by others who have shown that endometrial cells within the menstrual effluent are capable of glandular formation. Critical to Sampson's theory is the viability of the sloughed endometrium, and its ability to implant at ectopic sites. Viability in culture was demonstrated by Keetel and Stein in 1951, who demonstrated that endometrial epithelial cells and stroma could be maintained in culture more than 2 days. Supporting data were also provided by Ridley and Edwards, who were able to implant collected menstrual effluent in the subcutaneous abdominal fat of women and prove histologically that these implants had viable endometrial glands and stroma after 90 to 180 days. The major problem in Sampson's theory is that although more than 90% of women have retrograde menstruation, only 10% to 15% of menstruating women develop endometriosis.

The transplantation theory for endometriosis is supported by the fact that endometriotic lesions do occur in the scars from cesarean sections and episiotomies. Furthermore, "natural experiments" from humans also favor that theory, since patients with müllerian anomalies or outflow tract obstruction were found to have an increased risk of endometriosis. Finally, animal models demonstrated that endometrium can be surgically transplanted and that the transplanted material behaves similarly to spontaneous endometriosis.

At the turn of the century, Von Recklinghausen and Russell suggested that endometriosis results from stimulated cell rests of müllerian origin. In support of what was later coined as the *embryonic cell rests theory,* Russell reported the presence of scattered foci of "uterine glands and inter-glandular connective tissue" in histologic sections of normal ovary. However, there is still no evidence that these remnants could develop into endometriosis.

The presence of extrapelvic endometriosis in the lung, brain, and lower extremities was taken as a proof of the *hematogenous and lymphatic spread theory.* Furthermore, experimental demonstration that intravenous injection of homogenized endometrium results in pulmonary endometriosis in the rabbit also supports this concept.

The *coelomic metaplasia theory,* proposed initially by Iwanoff and Meyer, states that endometriosis arises from metaplasia of totipotential mesothelial cells within the peritoneum. This concept implies that in the presence of certain stimuli—for example, infection, hormones, or menstrual effluent—these cells will differentiate into endometriotic cells. The reports of endometriosis in men and in women with Rokitansky-Kuster-Hauser syndrome often were used as a proof of this theory. However, in these reported male cases all the patients were taking estrogen therapy, and the location of endometriosis could not exclude the possibility that it resulted from stimulated müllerian rests. So conclusive evidence that peritoneal epithelium can undergo spontaneous or induced metaplasia is still lacking.

Recently, genetic studies have shown that first-degree female relatives of women with endometriosis have a sevenfold-increased risk of developing the disease. Analysis of available data suggests a polygenic/multifactorial mode of inheritance; however, a dominant gene of low penetrance still cannot be ruled out.

In conclusion, there seems to be little doubt that more than one factor plays a role in the development of endometriosis. It is logical that a disease with such protean manifestations may originate through several mechanisms, and that no single theory can explain every case of endometriosis. There are convincing data to suggest that retrograde menstruation and implantation of endometrial fragments is a primary mode of developing endometriosis in the peritoneal cavity. Because retrograde menstruation is a universal phenomenon occurring in menstruating women with patent tubes, recent work has focused mainly on the mechanisms behind implantation or clearance of viable endometrium from the pelvic cavity.

PATHOPHYSIOLOGY

There have been many well-described immune and non-immune pathologic changes identified in women with endometriosis. These include increased peritoneal fluid volume, increased concentration of peritoneal macrophages, activation of macrophages with subsequent increase in cytokine release into the peritoneal fluid, and decreased NK (natural killer) cell cytotoxicity. However, it remains uncertain whether these changes antecede the development of endometriosis or are a result of the disease. It is also unknown how these changes contribute to the process of implantation and proliferation of endometriosis. One possibility involves an inherent alteration in the macrophages of patients with endometriosis that may be responsible for the immunologic changes, as well as the implantation and proliferation of ectopic endometrium. However, women with endometriosis do not appear to have greater susceptibility to other immuno-logically related diseases when compared to the general population.

A second theory to explain how the presence of ectopic endometrium may yield the pathophysiologic changes seen in endometriosis hypothesizes that the active endometriotic glands and stroma may synthesize and secrete proteins that create these changes. Endometrial tissue produces prostaglandins and complement component–3 (C3). This may be an important factor in the pathophysiology of endometriosis because C3, the most abundant protein in the complement system, plays an integral role in the classic and alternate complement cascade. Directly or indirectly, C3 can increase capillary permeability, stimulate fibroblasts leading to the formation of pelvic adhesions, and attract and activate peritoneal macrophages that then deposit monokines into the peritoneal environment.

Through a different line of thinking, many studies looked at the "hormonal milieu" that surrounds endometriotic implants. Bulum recently reported that endometriotic tissues over express aromatase (the enzyme that converts androstenedione to estrogen) while they under express 17-β hydroxysteroid dehydrogenase (responsible for inactivation of 17-β estradiol), thus favoring a high estrogen milieu in endometriotic tissue compared to eutopic endometrium. This high estrogen can stimulate more production of prostaglandin (PG)E$_2$, which in turn stimulates aromatase activity. Whether such a cycle could be responsible for maintaining endometriotic implants awaits further elucidation.

It is estimated that up to 50% of infertile women have endometriosis and that 30% to 50% of women with endometriosis are infertile. In support of this, data suggest a lower fecundity rate in women with laparoscopically proven endometriosis undergoing donor insemination compared with those without endometriosis. Furthermore, in the prospective randomized Canadian Endocan study, Marcoux and Maheux showed a higher fecundity rate in surgically treated infertile patients with mild or minimal endometriosis, compared with expectant management alone. Proposed mechanisms for endometriosis-associated infertility include pelvic adhesions and tubal obstruction, anovulation, luteal phase defects, luteinized unruptured follicle syndrome, spontaneous abortion, and embryo toxic effects from prostaglandins and peritoneal macrophages. Of these proposed mechanisms, only the presence of significant pelvic adhesions, which rarely lead to tubal blockage but may alter the tube's ability to capture an oocyte, has been clearly demonstrated to play a major role in endometriosis-related infertility.

Just as primary dysmenorrhea has been linked to elevated prostaglandin production from the myometrium, severe dysmenorrhea in patients with endometriosis may result from local prostaglandin production by the ectopic endometrium. Vernon et al suggested that endometriotic lesions could be characterized by their prostaglandin production, which may explain why some patients with minimal disease experience intense pelvic pain, whereas others with severe disease remain asymptomatic.

In conclusion, other than mechanical factors from pelvic adhesions contributing to infertility, and the elevated prostaglandin production causing dysmenorrhea, there are only limited in vivo data to explain the relationship of the various immunologic changes to symptomatology.

CLINICAL PRESENTATION
History and Physical Examination

It is well known that the amount of endometriosis does not correlate with the degree of symptoms. These symptoms are varied and often depend on the organs involved (Box 45-1). The most common symptoms include dysmenorrhea, pelvic pain, dyspareunia, premenstrual spotting, and infertility. This is not surprising since endometriotic lesions are found most commonly on the peritoneal surfaces of the cul-de-sac, the uterosacral ligaments, and the ovaries. When the bowel or bladder is deeply involved, cyclic dyschezia or hematuria may be the first presenting complaint. Patients rarely have catamenial hemoptysis, pleuritic chest pain, pneumothorax, incisional masses, footdrop, posthysterectomy vaginal bleeding, irritable bowel symptoms, and bowel obstruction. Endometriosis has been found in 10% to 40% of women with infertility, in up to 65% of women with chronic pelvic pain, and in more than half of women who have undergone laparoscopy for cyclic pain and dysmenorrhea.

Unfortunately, just as there is no specific symptom complex to aid in the diagnosis of endometriosis, there are no specific physical signs of the disease. Many patients with endometriosis have no abnormal findings on physical examination. However, certain findings should create suspicion that endometriosis may be present. These findings include uterosacral and cul-de-sac nodularity and tenderness, adnexal mass or ovarian enlargement, rectovaginal septal mass, and a retroflexed uterus with limited mobility (Box 45-2). Pigmented lesions in any site that either enlarge or become symptomatic at the time of menses also may represent endometriosis.

Diagnostic Tests

The diagnosis of endometriosis, unlike most other neoplasms, is made mostly by visual identification of endometriotic lesions at the time of surgery. Although many patients have various signs and symptoms that may raise the clinician's suspicions about the presence of the disease, the diagnosis can be made with certainty only at the time of surgery. Because endometriosis is a benign disease and is usually not considered premalignant (although it has been suggested that 5% of ovarian endometrioid cancers may arise from prior endometriotic lesions), it is not necessary to perform surgery to diagnose it unless the patient's complaints (pelvic pain or infertility) require surgical or medical intervention and therapy. In fact, based on a study he conducted to evaluate the efficacy of gonadotropin hormone releasing agonist (GnRHa), Ling suggested that in patients with moderate to severe pelvic pain of at least 6 months and who had a negative workup, a GnRHa treatment trial can be helpful in making the diagnosis of endometriosis. The problem with this approach is that other organ systems such as bowel may respond to GnRHa therapy. Therefore a patient with pain who responds to treatment does not necessarily have endometriosis.

Endometriotic lesions have classically been characterized as "powder-burn lesions." These lesions do not require histologic confirmation for the diagnosis. Today, however, we understand that many endometriotic lesions have an atypical appearance, including peritoneal implants that are white, red, brown, yellow, or clear and whose configuration may be polypoid, flat, or raised (Box 45-3). When atypical lesions are seen at surgery a biopsy specimen should be obtained for histologic confirmation of the diagnosis. Other lesions seen at surgery that suggest the presence of endometriosis include peritoneal pockets and adhesions, as well as subovarian adhesions. Because more than 50% of endometriotic lesions are clear or atypical, endometriosis remains an underdiagnosed condition even with the tremendous increase in the use of laparoscopy.

Imaging modalities such as ultrasound, computed tomography (CT), and magnetic resonance imaging (MRI) can provide information about the likelihood of endometriosis but have limited value in the diagnosis of the disease. The

---

BOX 45-1
Symptoms of Endometriosis

More Common
Dysmenorrhea
Dyspareunia
Infertility
Premenstrual spotting
Pelvic pain

Less Common
Cyclic hematochezia or dyschezia
Cyclic hematuria or dysuria
Cyclic hemoptysis or pleuritic chest pain
Constipation, bowel obstruction, or irritable bowel symptoms
Posthysterectomy vaginal bleeding
Incisional masses
Footdrop or sciatic pain

BOX 45-2
Physical Examination Findings

Uterosacral and cul-de-sac nodularity and tenderness
Adnexal mass or ovarian enlargement
Rectovaginal septal mass
Retroflexed uterus with limited mobility

BOX 45-3
Visual Appearance of Endometriosis

Typical Lesions
Black "powder-burn" lesions

Atypical Lesions
White opacification
Red, brown, yellow, and clear vesicular lesions
Glandular excrescences
Petechial peritoneum
Circular peritoneal defects

main role of ultrasound is defining whether an adnexal mass is cystic, solid, or mixed. Endometriotic cysts are homogeneous; their echogenic pattern is increased, and their appearance is similar to corpora lutea, dermoid cysts, or borderline ovarian carcinomas. CT and MRI scanning also detect cystic lesions, as well as fibrous lesions that may be present in the rectosigmoid wall, rectovaginal septum, and retroperitoneal space. Rarely does this additional information justify the added expense of the CT and MRI over a pelvic ultrasound examination.

It would be helpful if a serum test were available to aid in the diagnosis of endometriosis. Three substances currently being investigated include CA-125, placental protein 14 (PP-14), and antiendometrial antibodies. Assays for antiendometrial antibodies and PP-14 are available only in research laboratories and their clinical usefulness has not been determined. The CA-125 assay is commercially available. A great deal of work has been done by Pittaway et al who have demonstrated that the sensitivity of the serum CA-125 assay ranges from 100% in women with endometriomata greater than 4 cm to 33% in women with dysmenorrhea. CA-125 levels correlate with the stage of endometriosis, and they are most useful when elevated levels are detected preoperatively with Stage III and Stage IV disease. After medical or surgical therapy or both, the CA-125 levels likely will fall, and serial levels correlate well with the status of the disease.

MANAGEMENT

Treatment for endometriosis can include surgical or medical intervention, a combination of these two therapies, or expectant management. Because endometriosis generally is considered neither a premalignant nor a progressive disease, it should be treated only because of symptoms that are not tolerated by the patient. The course of endometriosis is unpredictable. The probability of progression to moderate or severe disease in a woman with early-stage endometriosis is 25% to 40%. Unfortunately, the inability to predict in which patients the disease will progress makes it imprudent to treat asymptomatic endometriosis for the purpose of preventing or delaying future sequelae. The clinician should not subject a patient to medical or surgical therapy if the patient's only concern is fertility in the distant future.

Finally, endometriosis may persist during the entire reproductive life of a woman. Thus it is essential that the physician and the patient develop a long-term management plan combining and alternating different treatment modalities from medical therapy to surgery, or even both, taking into consideration the age of the patient, her desire of fertility, her quality of life, and her work obligations.

CHOICE OF THERAPY FOR PELVIC PAIN

Medical Therapy

Nonsteroidal Antiinflammatory Drugs

Since prostaglandins are correlated with the pelvic pain and dysmenorrhea in patients with endometriosis, nonsteroidal anti-inflammatory drugs (NSAIDs), which inhibit prostaglandin biosynthesis, can be helpful for these symptoms. They are fairly well tolerated and inexpensive and are recommended as first-line treatment for pain in patients with mild disease.

Hormonal Therapy

The rationale behind hormonal therapy is supported by the fact that steroid hormones (mainly estrogen) are the major regulators of growth and function of endometriotic tissue. This theory has been supported by the clinical observation that endometriosis is rare before menarche, after menopause, and in amenorrheic women. Furthermore, endometriosis improves during pregnancy. Early and frequent pregnancies protect against the disease. Thus the current strategy for hormonal therapy for endometriosis is to create an acyclic, hypoestrogenic environment with or without increased serum androgens. Low estrogen levels create atrophy of the endometriotic lesions, whereas the acyclic environment minimizes the chance of miniature menstruation within the implants and prevents reseeding via retrograde menstruation. High androgens and synthetic progestins also induce endometrial atrophy and interfere with follicular development, thereby lowering estrogen levels.

The currently available hormonal therapies for endometriosis include continuous oral contraceptive regimens, progestins (e.g., gestrinone, medroxyprogesterone acetate, norethendrone acetate), danazol, antiprogestins (RU486), and gonadotropin-releasing hormone agonists and antagonists. Some of these drugs have been approved by the Food and Drug Administration (Table 45-1), whereas others are still under trials. Systematic reviews of published evidence have found that 6 months of continuous ovarian suppression using oral contraceptives, danazol, gestrinone, depot medroxyprogesterone acetate, or gonadotropin-releasing hormone (GnRH) agonists are equally effective for reducing moderate and severe pain. There is no evidence that hormonal therapy improves fertility.

Continuous oral contraceptive regimens produce a pseudodecidualized endometrium that contains inactive glandular epithelia with little potential for growth. The use of continuous oral contraceptives without a monthly withdrawal period is approximately 80% effective in relieving pelvic pain and dysmenorrhea. Any low-dose oral contraceptive can be used if administered continuously for 15 weeks followed by 1 week of withdrawal. The progestins within the birth control pill have sufficient androgenic and progestational activity to block the activity of the coadministered estrogen that is present to minimize breakthrough uterine bleeding. This treatment is associated with minimal side effects and can be taken for extended periods. It is for these reasons that this regimen is recommended in patients with early symptomatic disease who are not attempting conception.

No data are available to indicate a role for cyclic oral contraceptives in the management of endometriosis.

The most common progestogen therapy for endometriosis is orally administered **medroxyprogesterone acetate** (MPA) (Provera), 30 mg daily for 3 to 6 months. MPA also can be given intramuscularly in its depot form at a dose of 100 to 300 mg every 3 months. At this dose MPA will inhibit luteinizing hormone (LH) and follicle-stimulating hormone (FSH) secretion and lead to suppression of follicular activity and the creation of a hypoestrogenic acyclic environment. MPA also may have direct effects on endometriotic tissue via binding to androgen and progestin receptors. This medication has been found to be 80% to 90% effective in relieving pelvic pain. It is not used more commonly because of the

Table 45-1
Hormonal Therapy for Endometriosis

Treatment	Dosage	Side Effects
Pseudopregnancy	Any 21-day low-dose OCP continuously, with 1 wk withdrawal every 15 wk	Breakthrough bleeding
Medroxyprogesterone acetate	30 mg qd for 3-6 mo	Weight gain, breast pain, bleeding, mood changes
Danazol	200-400 mg bid	Acne, hirsutism, weight gain, hot flashes, fatigue
Gonadotropin-releasing factor (GnRH) agonists	Leuprolide acetate 1 mg SC qd or depot form 3.75 IM monthly Nafarelin acetate 1 spray bid Goserelin acetate implant every 28 days	Hot flashes, irregular headaches, depression, vaginal dryness, weight loss, insomnia

OCP, Oral contraceptive pill; *SC,* Subcutaneous; *IM,* intramuscularly.

high rate of unacceptable side effects. More than 80% of women experience a 5- to 30-pound weight gain, and a high percentage suffer from breast tenderness, breakthrough bleeding, irritability, and depression.

Gestrinone is a 19-nor-testosterone derivative manufactured in France. It was originally developed in the 1970s as a once-a-week contraceptive with an efficacy rate equivalent to established oral contraceptives. Its development was abandoned because of the high costs of phase 2 trials. This medication is similar to danazol in its binding to estrogen receptors, progestin receptors, and androgen receptors, as well as its effect on steroid-binding proteins. It does not, however, block steroidogenic enzymes or prostaglandin synthesis. Gestrinone does not eliminate endometriotic implants but arrests glandular proliferation, thus producing a cellular progesterone withdrawal effect. Gestrinone generally is well tolerated at doses of less than 5 mg (twice weekly) or 2.5 mg (three times weekly); 95% of patients are asymptomatic on a regimen of 5 mg twice weekly, and all are amenorrheic at the completion of 2 months of therapy. A multicenter randomized double blind study conducted in Italy in 1996 compared the efficacy of gestrinone vs. leuprolide in pain management of endometriosis. Oral gestrinone was as effective as leuprolide with no effect on bone density. Only 5% to 15% of patients discontinue therapy because of unwanted side effects. The most frequent side effects are increased appetite, acne, and vaginal discharge.

Danazol was the first medication approved by the US Food and Drug Administration for the treatment of endometriosis. It is an isoxazole derivative of 17-α-ethinyl testosterone. The usual oral dosage is 400 to 800 mg daily in divided doses. Danazol acts on endometriosis via many mechanisms, including pituitary suppression of gonadotropin secretion, binding to steroid receptors in endometriotic implants, inhibition of ovarian and adrenal steroidogenesis, and alterations in steroid-binding proteins. Normally approximately 40% of testosterone is loosely bound to albumin, and 1% is free. In patients taking danazol, 80% of testosterone is bound to albumin and 2% is free as a result of the reduction in testosterone-binding globulin. Although this phenomenon is responsible for the 80% reduction in pelvic pain related to endometriosis, it also is responsible for the common side effects associated with danazol use.

Studies have shown that more than 80% of women on a regimen of danazol complain of one or more of the following side effects: weight gain, edema, acne, breast atrophy, oily skin, hot flashes, muscle cramps, libido changes, and fatigue. Danazol also lowers the levels of high-density lipoprotein (HDL) cholesterol and raises those of low-density lipoprotein (LDL) cholesterol. It has no detrimental effect on bone density. Because danazol has been associated with the development in utero of female pseudohermaphroditism, it should be used only in conjunction with effective contraception.

Although many antiprogestins are being evaluated by pharmaceutical companies for various therapeutic purposes, only one **mifepristone** has been used widely. Preliminary studies on its use in endometriosis showed that a dose as low as 50 mg daily of mifepristone achieved a condition of ovarian acyclicity while decreasing the pain and extent of pelvic endometriosis. Side effects of this drug include atypical flushes, anorexia, and fatigue. No decrease in bone mineral density of the lumbar spine and the hip has been reported. Mifepristone may provide a safe and well-tolerated alternative for the medical management of endometriosis if these results are confirmed by larger clinical studies.

Gonadotropin-releasing hormone (GnRH) agonist administration is now the treatment of choice if the pain fails to respond to surgery, recurs after surgery, or does not respond to continuous oral contraceptives. The administration of a GnRH agonist produces a paradoxic fall in the pituitary secretion of bioactive LH and FSH, resulting in a hypogonadal state. The serum estradiol concentrations are similar to those seen in women after menopause. Unlike menopause, however, this hypogonadal state is reversible.

Currently, three GnRH agonist formulations have been approved by the FDA for gynecologic conditions: leuprolide acetate (Lupron), nafarelin acetate (Synarel), and goserelin acetate (Zoladex). Lupron may be given by daily subcutaneous injection or in a depot form requiring monthly intramuscular injections. Synarel is administered by nasal spray twice daily, and Zoladex is a 3.6-mg subdermal implant placed within the upper abdominal wall every 28 days.

While taking these medications, 95% of patients will experience hot flashes, 20% to 40% irregular bleeding, and 5% to 15% headache, depression, insomnia, vaginal dryness, weight loss or gain, hair loss, or edema. There have been rare reports of vaginal hemorrhage and allergic reactions. Of patients with pelvic pain from endometriosis 90% to 95% will experience pain relief from GnRH agonist therapy. However, pelvic pain returns to pretreatment levels in most patients 6 months after cessation of therapy.

Because of the risk of bone loss created by the hypoestrogenic state (which has been reported to be as great as 15% after 6 months of therapy when the lumbar vertebrae are measured by quantitative CT), GnRH agonist therapy is only FDA-approved for one 6-month treatment cycle. As noted, however, the recurrence of pelvic pain is quite high after the discontinuation of therapy, and thus many clinicians currently are prescribing longer term therapy in conjunction with estrogen and/or progestin "add-back" therapy. The goal of add-back therapy is to titrate the estrogen to a level that provides protection from trabecular bone loss but ensures that the endometriosis will not be stimulated.

Other drugs such as tibolone, alendronate, and raloxifene have been evaluated in add-back therapy. Tibolone is a synthetic steroid that exhibits estrogenic, progestogenic, and androgenic activity. It has been shown to prevent bone loss and symptomatic side effects associated with GnRH agonist treatment of endometriosis without affecting its efficacy. Patients on add-back therapy should have bone density measurements every 6 months. If bone density decreases, the add-back regimen should be changed or the treatment discontinued.

Surgery

During surgery, the goal for the relief of pelvic pain is the same as for the treatment of infertility: the destruction or excision of all endometriotic disease. This may be accomplished by means of laparoscopy or laparotomy. In refractory cases, hysterectomy with bilateral salpingo-oophorectomy may be performed to reduce formation of new lesions in women who do not wish to preserve fertility.

Pelvic pain resulting from endometriosis is correlated with the amount of deeply penetrating disease. Consequently, treatment of pain from endometriosis should consist of excision of as much of the lesion as possible to a depth where normal underlying tissue is reached. Excision can be performed equally well with laser, electrosurgery, and sharp dissection. Sharp dissection has the added advantage of providing the pathologist with a specimen without thermal damage; however, hemostasis is easier to achieve with electrosurgical or laser excision.

In 12 studies that examined the effect of hysterectomy with bilateral salpingo-oophorectomy for relief of pain related to endometriosis, 345/390 (88%) of patients reported improvement, and 84% experienced pain relief with the removal of only one affected ovary. In studies of ablative techniques, approximately two thirds of patients experienced relief with electrocautery and 80% reported relief after laser therapy. A success rate of more than 85% also has been reported with excisional techniques; however, there are no controlled studies to validate these reports.

Using life-table analysis, Redwine evaluated the recurrence rate after laparoscopic excision and found it to be comparable to excision via laparotomy: approximately 20% within the first 5 years. If a patient has been diagnosed and surgically treated for pain related to endometriosis, and sim-

ilar pain remains or recurs, a trial of medical therapy should then be offered.

Combined Medical and Surgical Treatment

Because medical therapy cannot eradicate the disease and surgical therapy is associated with a high recurrence, it is logical to try to combine both modalities. Potential advantages of preoperative treatment, which remain to be proven in randomized controlled studies, include reduced volume of endometriotic tissue that facilitates surgery and decreased risk of some of complications such as ureteral injury, blood loss, and bowel injury.

The data on postoperative hormonal treatment of women with endometriosis is conflicting. Although there are very few published placebo-controlled trials of hormonal therapy after surgical ablation, the preliminary results indicate that combined treatment is at least as effective as surgical excision, and may carry a lower recurrence rate.

CHOICE OF THERAPY FOR INFERTILITY
Medical Therapy

There are no controlled data that demonstrate improvement in fertility rates with hormonal therapy.

Surgical Treatment

The objective of surgery for endometriosis-related infertility is to destroy or resect as much disease as possible without creating new adhesions that may affect ovum capture. The available methods include electrocautery, endocoagulation, laser vaporization, and excision. Unfortunately, almost all reports on the treatment of endometriosis-related infertility utilize crude pregnancy rates obtained by dividing the number of pregnancies by the number of patients treated. Obviously, the longer the follow-up period, the higher the pregnancy rate. A more useful statistic now used is the monthly fecundity rate, defined as the rate of achieving pregnancy per ovulatory cycle.

The crude pregnancy rates for the treatment of minimal, mild, and moderate endometriosis with electrocautery are approximately 65%, 50%, and 35%, respectively. The pregnancy rate for severe endometriosis has been reported at 50% in a small number of patients. Overall, approximately 75% of patients who achieved pregnancy did so within the first 6 months. Murphy et al, using life-table analysis, studied 72 patients with stages I and II endometriosis who underwent electrocoagulation and noted a 10% and 8% fecundity rate, respectively.

Overall, the use of the laser therapy has not improved the crude pregnancy rates over other methods of ablation. The overall crude pregnancy rates in the literature for stages I, II, III, and IV are 59%, 58%, 58%, and 64%, respectively. As with electrocoagulation, most of the pregnancies occurred within the first 6 months. In a large retrospective study, the monthly fecundity rates of stages I and II endometriosis treated with laser were comparable with those found with expectant management, danazol treatment, and conservative surgery. With stage III endometriosis the fecundity rate was 5% with laser treatment and 2% after danazol therapy.

In an overview of controlled trials in endometriosis-associated infertility, Hughes et al concluded that no medical therapy for endometriosis provided benefit for infertility. There was a treatment benefit in all laparoscopic surgery, including laser and electrosurgery, with an odds ratio (OR) of 2.67 (95% confidence interval [CI] 2.08–3.45), as well as with conservative laparotomy (OR of 1.67, 95% [CI] 1.27–2.10). In particular, the Endocan study showed that laparoscopic treatment (resection or ablation) of minimal and mild endometriosis increased the cumulative probability of a pregnancy that lasted more than 20 weeks by 73% (31% compared with 18% for diagnostic laparoscopy alone). Finally, there appears to be no benefit in adding danazol therapy to either laparoscopic surgery or conservative surgery via laparotomy.

Assisted Reproductive Techniques

Endometriosis is the second most common cause of referrals to assisted reproductive techniques (ART) clinics. In general, it is recommended in women who fail other treatment modalities (medical, surgical, ovulation induction). Controlled ovarian hyperstimulation with intrauterine insemination (COH/IUI) is usually the first line of treatment for a number of causes of endometriosis associated infertility. Tummon et al reported a higher live birth rate (11% versus 2%) in patients with mild and minimal endometriosis who had COH/IUI versus patients who had expectant management. This study and others address the outcome in stages I and II disease, but no similar studies have been conducted so far in higher stages of the disease.

Recently, many trials have focused on the effect of endometriosis and its manifestations on the outcome of ART. Preliminary results show no evidence that endometriosis decreases the success rate of either in vivo fertilization or intracytoplasmic sperm injection (ICSI) as practiced today. Only a higher early pregnancy loss has been reported in patients with endometriosis compared to controls.

PROGNOSIS

As with many problems associated with chronic pelvic pain and infertility, there is an absence of data from randomized controlled clinical trials to guide the therapy of endometriosis-related symptoms. There is little published evidence describing the natural history of endometriosis. In one trial in which laparoscopy was repeated in the placebo-treated group, after 1 year endometriosis resolved in one fourth, worsened in nearly half, and was unchanged in the rest.

However, as a result of improved training and the development of innovative surgical techniques and technology, physicians are making great strides in providing maximum therapeutic benefit while minimizing patient morbidity through operative laparoscopy. On average, patients will obtain between 18 and 24 months of pain relief from surgery or suppressive hormonal therapy (i.e., danazol or GnRH agonist). Because of the risks and side effects of both forms of therapy, alternating medical and surgical therapy often is advised. With this approach, the patient will undergo laparoscopic examination to evaluate the pelvis and treat the disease about every 4 years and will be exposed to the side effects of the medical therapy every 4 years until menopause. The immediate goal is to significantly lengthen these treatment intervals with improved laparoscopic excisional techniques and innovative medical therapy.

BIBLIOGRAPHY

Bulum SE et al: Estrogen production in endometriosis and use of aromatase inhibitors to treat endometriosis, *Endocrine-Related Cancer* 6:293, 1999.

Cook AS, Rock JA: The role of laparoscopy in the treatment of endometriosis, *Fertil Steril* 55:663, 1991.

Dicker D et al: The impact of long-term gonadotropin-releasing hormone analogue treatment on preclinical abortions in patients with severe endometriosis undergoing in vitro fertilization-embryo transfer, *Fert Steril* 57:597, 1994.

Farquhar C: Endometriosis, *Clinical Evidence* 4:1058, 2000.

Franssen AMHW et al: Endometriosis: treatment with gonadotropin-releasing hormone agonist buserelin, *Fert Steril* 51:401, 1989.

Friedman AJ, Hornstein MD: Gonadotropin-releasing hormone agonist plus estrogen-progestin "add-back" therapy for endometriosis-related pelvic pain, *Fert Steril* 60:236, 1993.

Gestrinone Italian Study Group: Gestrinone versus a gonadotropin-releasing hormone agonist for the treatment of pelvic pain associated with endometriosis: a randomized, double blind study, *Fert Steril* 66:911, 1996.

Halme J et al: Retrograde menstruation in healthy women and in patients with endometriosis, *Obstet Gynecol* 64:151, 1984.

Hughes EG, Fedorkow DM, Collins JA: A quantitative overview of controlled trials in endometriosis-associated infertility, *Fert Steril* 59:963, 1993.

Isaacson KB et al: Production and secretion of complement component 3 by endometriotic tissue, *J Clin Endocrinol Metab* 69:1003, 1989.

Koninckx PR et al: Suggestive evidence that pelvic endometriosis is a progressive disease whereas deeply infiltrating endometriosis is associated with pelvic pain, *Fert Steril* 55:759, 1991.

Ling F et al: Randomized controlled trial of depot Leuprolide in patients with chronic pelvic pain and clinically suspected endometriosis, *Obstet Gynecol* 93:51, 1999.

Marcoux S et al: Laparoscopic surgery in infertile women with minimal or mild endometriosis, *N Engl J Med* 337:217, 1997.

Marcus SF, Edwards RG: High rates of pregnancy after long-term down regulation of women with severe endometriosis, *Am J Obstet Gynecol* 171:812, 1994.

Murphy AA et al: Laparoscopic cautery in the treatment of endometriosis-related infertility, *Fert Steril* 55:246, 1991.

Olive DL, Henderson DY: Endometriosis and müllerian anomalies, *Obstet Gynecol* 69:412, 1987.

Olive DL, Martin DC: Treatment of endometriosis-associated infertility with CO_2 laser laparoscopy: the use of one- and two-parameter exponential models, *Fert Steril* 48:18, 1987.

Pittaway DE: CA-125 in women with endometriosis, *Obstet Gynecol Clin North Am* 16:227, 1989.

Redwine DB: Conservative laparoscopic excision of endometriosis by sharp dissection: life table analysis of reoperation and persistent or recurrent disease, *Fert Steril* 56:628, 1991.

Tummon IS et al: Randomized controlled trial of superovulation and insemination for infertility associated with minimal and mild endometriosis, *Fert Steril* 68:8, 1997.

Vernon MW et al: Classification of endometriotic implants by morphologic appearance and capacity to synthesize prostaglandin F, *Fert Steril* 46:801, 1986.

Wheeler JM: Epidemiology of endometriosis-associated infertility, *J Reprod Med* 34:41, 1989.

CHAPTER 46

Polycystic Ovary Syndrome

Ann E. Taylor

Polycystic ovary syndrome (PCOS) is one of the most common conditions in women of reproductive age, affecting 4% to 6% of women. This complex syndrome affects many organ systems and has several important long-term health implications. Although PCOS has historically been considered a condition associated with cosmetic changes and infertility, recent data have emphasized the long-term health consequences of PCOS, including obesity, endometrial hyperplasia and cancer, insulin resistance, and an increased prevalence of diabetes mellitus.

DEFINITION

Although the condition was originally diagnosed based on the appearance of the ovaries at laparotomy, and the ovarian appearance remains part of the name, in the last decade the definition has shifted away from ovarian morphology to a functional description of the patient. Currently, the most widely accepted diagnosis of PCOS requires the presence of:

- Any hyperandrogenism (symptoms of acne, hirsutism, or androgenic alopecia; and/or an elevated serum androgen level) **plus**
- Menstrual dysfunction (often defined by fewer than 6 to 9 menses per year)
- In premenopausal women in whom other conditions are excluded

Thus PCOS is now a diagnosis of exclusion for women with hyperandrogenic symptoms combined with menstrual abnormalities. The conditions to be excluded are those in the differential diagnosis of menstrual dysfunction and hyperandrogenic symptoms, including pregnancy, thyroid dysfunction, hyperprolactinemia, ovarian failure, androgen-secreting tumors (including Cushing's syndrome), late onset congenital adrenal hyperplasia, and severe insulin resistance syndromes. (See Evaluation for the recommended evaluation to exclude these conditions.)

▦ EPIDEMIOLOGY

Three recent population-based studies that have assessed the prevalence of PCOS in the United States, Spain, and Greece have consistently found that between 4% and 7%

of reproductive-age women are affected. Of those women, 10% (Spain) to 38% (United States) had significant obesity, with a body mass index greater than 30 kg/m². This compares with the most recent data from the United States NHANES III study, which found that 15% of women aged 20 to 29 years old and 26% of women aged 30 to 39 years old had a body mass index greater than 30. Thus, PCOS appears to be associated with an increased prevalence of obesity, but less than half of all women with PCOS are obese.

ETIOLOGY

Despite years of investigations, the underlying mechanism of PCOS remains enigmatic. There is growing evidence that PCOS has a genetic basis, although the genetics of the syndrome appear to be complex. Up to 50% of siblings of PCOS patients have evidence of hyperandrogenism, but typical pedigrees do not consistently show a dominant pattern of inheritance. Although several candidate genes have been associated with PCOS, no gene has yet been proven to be the cause. Most investigators predict that more than one gene will be involved in the phenotypic expression of the syndrome.

Several logical hypotheses have been promoted to explain the pathophysiology of PCOS, and none have yet been confirmed or disproven. Obesity seems to worsen the phenotypic features, and weight loss can improve the frequency of menses. Whether a tendency to weight gain is part of the underlying defect, or whether weight gain can bring out and expose the defect remains to be determined. Obesity is linked with several of the phenotypic features, including insulin resistance and impaired glucose tolerance. However, the gonadotropin defects typically observed in women with PCOS in fact tend to be less marked in the heaviest patients.

Other potential theories to explain PCOS include primary defects of insulin sensitivity or insulin secretion (with hyperinsulinemia contributing to exaggerated ovarian androgen secretion), of gonadotropin secretion (with elevated luteinizing hormone levels contributing to excess ovarian androgen secretion), and of ovarian androgen synthesis (presumably associated with the distinctive ovarian morphology). To date, it remains unclear whether subsets of women with PCOS have unique underlying etiologies, or whether all of these reported findings are somehow related to each other.

CLINICAL PRESENTATION

The clinical presentation of women with PCOS is extremely diverse and can vary with the subject's age, weight, personal expectations, and place in the life cycle. Younger women tend to present more with cosmetic symptoms, including **hirsutism, acne,** and **androgenic alopecia.** In women, androgenic alopecia is more likely to present with general hair thinning, rather than temporal recession. Mid-life women may be more likely to present with weight problems, infertility, or menstrual dysfunction.

The **menstrual dysfunction** of PCOS ranges from complete **amenorrhea,** to **oligomenorrhea,** to heavy and frequent **dysfunctional uterine bleeding.** It is believed that the menstrual pattern depends somewhat on the serum hormone levels. Women with higher serum androgens may have amenorrhea owing to endometrial atrophy effects of androgens, whereas obese women may have excess bleeding due to increased aromatization of androgens to estrogens in peripheral fat tissue. Unopposed estrogen exposure without the progesterone produced after ovulation can result in endometrial proliferation, erratic and sometimes very heavy menstrual bleeding, even leading to **endometrial hyperplasia** and **endometrial carcinoma** in young women. Although many women with PCOS do occasionally ovulate, their ovulatory rate is reduced, leading to absolute or relative **infertility,** such that it takes longer to spontaneously conceive a child, or ovulation-inducing medications are required.

Other clinical features of PCOS include **acanthosis nigricans,** a thickening and darkening of the rugal folds of the skin most commonly seen at the nape of the neck, the axillae, and the knuckles, knees, and elbows; a tendency to **central body fat accumulation;** a tendency to **preserved bone density** in spite of amenorrhea; and a classic ovarian morphology that is seen on pelvic ultrasonography or laparoscopy.

SIGNIFICANCE OF POLYCYSTIC OVARIAN MORPHOLOGY

The classic polycystic ovarian morphology is characterized by the presence of multiple small ovarian cystic structures in a peripheral array around the ovary, often called the "string of pearls" sign. By definition, there must be at least 8 or 10 cysts observed in a single plane, and they must each be between 4 and 10 mm in diameter (less than half an inch). Ovaries are also usually enlarged. However, the small ovarian cysts are typically asymptomatic, and PCOS is *not* a condition of large painful ovarian cysts (Fig. 46-1).

Although the syndrome of PCOS has been named by the classic ovarian histologic or ultrasonographic appearance of the ovaries, it is now clear that the morphology alone is insufficient to establish the diagnosis of the syndrome. Several series have demonstrated that 20% to 25% of regularly ovulating, otherwise normal women have this classic ovarian morphology. Thus the demonstration of polycystic ovarian morphology is *not* sufficient to make the diagnosis of PCOS. In addition, women who have androgen excess for other reasons, such as congenital adrenal hyperplasia or female-

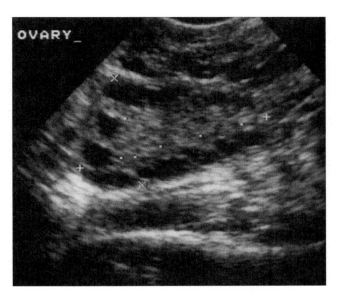

FIG. 46-1 A typical polycystic ovary on transvaginal ultrasonography. The markers represent centimeters. Note the peripheral ring of many follicles less than 1 cm in diameter. Despite the name, PCOS rarely causes growth of large cysts. (Courtesy of Ms. J. Adams.)

to-male transsexuals, also frequently have this morphology. There is a growing body of evidence that the average ovulatory woman with polycystic ovarian morphology may have slightly higher (but normal) serum androgen levels, a mild metabolic defect, and exaggerated ovarian responses to gonadotropin stimulation for ovulation induction, compared with women with normal-appearing ovaries. The clinical significance of these findings remains unclear.

ASSOCIATED METABOLIC ABNORMALITIES

The most important metabolic abnormality associated with PCOS is a strikingly elevated prevalence of **type 2 diabetes mellitus** and **impaired glucose tolerance** (IGT). Two independent series demonstrated remarkable agreement that 7% to 10% of obese women with PCOS had frank diabetes, and another 30% had impaired glucose tolerance, with a high rate of progression to diabetes each year. The rates of diabetes and IGT in lean women with PCOS are significantly less, but still well above the background rate expected for young women. Unfortunately, the current fasting criteria for the diagnosis of IGT and diabetes (fasting glucose greater than 110 and 126 mg/dl respectively) fail to identify a significant percentage of PCOS subjects who have abnormal oral glucose tolerance tests (2 hr glucose greater than 140 and 200 mg/dl, respectively).

Women with PCOS as a group also have **insulin resistance,** which can be observed independent of obesity. Insulin resistance means that their serum insulin levels fasting or after a meal are higher than expected for age and weight. However, there are no clearly established normative data on normal insulin levels, nor are there established insulin levels above which significant morbidity is known to occur at increased prevalence, or above which therapy should be initiated. Thus screening for insulin resistance per se independent of abnormalities of glucose intolerance currently cannot be recommended.

Insulin resistance in some populations is associated with several other defects, including hypertension and lipid abnormalities. Most evidence suggests that women with PCOS are not any more likely to be hypertensive than would be expected for their weight. The prevalence of **lipid abnormalities** is controversial in women with PCOS. Some studies suggest that younger and leaner PCOS patients are more likely to have higher total cholesterol and triglyceride levels, and lower HDL levels, than weight-matched control subjects, whereas older and heavier women with PCOS may have similar lipid levels as weight-matched control subjects.

Because of an increased prevalence of diabetes, insulin resistance, obesity, and perhaps lipid abnormalities, it is reasonable to expect that women with PCOS are at increased risk for cardiovascular disease. If so, screening for PCOS would be a simple way to identify younger women at risk, in whom more rigorous risk factor modification could be initiated. At least two studies of women undergoing cardiac catheterization suggest that women with coronary lesions are more likely to have clinical features suggestive of PCOS. Another study suggests that women with PCOS have greater carotid artery intimal thickness than normal women. However, only one study to date has looked at cardiovascular endpoints, and it has not identified any increased cardiovascular mortality or events in women with a history of PCOS. Because these patients had been diagnosed up to 30 years earlier, when diagnostic criteria varied, and almost all received a potential disease-modulating therapy (wedge resection of the ovaries), further study is necessary to determine if women with PCOS have adverse long-term cardiovascular outcomes.

Finally, it must be acknowledged that a growing body of new literature raises the possibility that these adverse metabolic abnormalities may be observed in all hyperandrogenic women, not just those who meet strict criteria for PCOS. Such findings are under active investigation and need further confirmation.

✻ MANAGEMENT
Goals

The management of PCOS, like the management of hirsutism and acne, has four phases:

- Determining the patient's primary current concerns
- Ruling out other pathologic causes of menstrual dysfunction and hyperandrogenism
- Evaluating the patient for the metabolic consequences of PCOS
- Choosing a therapy that protects the patient from long-term consequences of PCOS and meets the woman's immediate needs

The first priority in managing a women with PCOS is determining her primary concerns, since the choice of therapy and the potential evaluation to be completed will vary dramatically depending on whether she is seeking cosmetic control, menstrual control, or fertility.

Evaluation

At initial presentation, a minimal evaluation must be done to make sure that no other treatable conditions are missed. The most important part of the clinical evaluation is the history and physical examination. Specific points to emphasize are the following:

- The **timing of onset of symptoms:** a peripubertal onset suggests benign PCOS, whereas a recent onset or rapid progression is more consistent with tumors.
- **Other associated symptoms:** mood changes or depression, bruising, or weakness suggest Cushing's syndrome, an increase in libido and other evidence of virilization suggests a tumor, symptoms of hyperthyroidism or hypothyroidism, symptoms of pituitary tumor (visual changes, galactorrhea), symptoms of early menopause (hot flushes, sleep disturbances, urogenital symptoms).
- **Medication history:** some medications cause hypertrichosis; others are androgen analogs. Some medications, such as oral contraceptive pills, may have treated previous signs of PCOS and masked the diagnosis until they were stopped.
- **Family history:** a strong family history of hirsutism suggests a benign condition; a history of early childhood death or other affected members may suggest congenital adrenal hyperplasia.

A laboratory evaluation may not be necessary in a woman who has regular menstrual cycles with evidence of ovulation, but most women with irregular menses will need a minimal evaluation including **human chorionic gonadotrophin, prolactin, thyroid-stimulating hormone,** and **follicle-stimulating hormone.** The following additional testing may be considered:

- A serum testosterone and dehydroepiandrosterone sulfate (DHEAS) level is indicated *if* there is clinical suspicion of an androgen-secreting tumor. A total testosterone level greater than 150 ng/dl or a DHEAS level greater than 800 ug/dl have been validated to suggest an increased risk of androgen producing tumor, whereas levels lower than these are rarely associated with pathologic causes.
- A 24-hour urine sample for volume, creatinine, free cortisol, and 17-keto steroids is indicated if there is concern about Cushing's syndrome.
- A serum progesterone level 7 days before expected menses may be helpful to determine if the patient is ovulating.
- A morning, follicular phase 17-OH progesterone *may* be indicated if there is reason to suspect late-onset congenital adrenal hyperplasia and the patient plans conception with a possible carrier of the defect.

If all tests are normal, (allowing for mildly elevated serum androgens if they are measured), and the patient has irregular menses, the diagnosis is PCOS.

Women with PCOS need an initial evaluation for metabolic risk factors. At this time, we recommend measuring **body weight, blood pressure,** and **fasting lipids.**

Obese women with PCOS should also be screened for impaired glucose tolerance and diabetes with a **2-hour glucose tolerance test** (serum glucose level 2 hours after a 75 g oral glucose load).

At this time, population normative data for insulin levels, either fasting or after a glucose load, are not available, and there are no data to suggest a number above which one should consider treatment. In addition, the efficacy of insulin-reducing drugs in women with PCOS does not appear dependent on specific insulin levels. Thus the measurement of insulin levels in routine clinical practice cannot yet be recommended.

Choice of Therapy

There are two major decision points before choosing therapy. First, does the patient desire pregnancy at this time? Second, does the patient have diabetes mellitus (a glucose level greater than 200 two hours after an oral glucose load or on random testing)?

Patients desiring pregnancy should not be treated with oral contraceptive pills or antiandrogens and are likely to need referral to an endocrinologist or gynecologist if they are not ovulating frequently. They also need additional evaluation for other causes of infertility, including a semen analysis on the male partner, cervical cultures for infections, and possibly evaluation of fallopian tube patency. Women with PCOS who achieve pregnancy will need extra monitoring for signs of gestational diabetes because of the increased risk.

PCOS patients with diabetes should attempt to achieve the same goals as do all patients with diabetes mellitus. Weight loss and increased exercise remain first-line therapy. Because PCOS is associated with insulin resistance, it makes sense for these patients to initiate therapy with a drug that improves insulin action, either metformin or a thiazolidinedione, if lifestyle changes are inadequate. Diabetic PCOS patients who do not desire conception need to be warned that menstrual frequency, and possibly fertility, may be improved with these therapies. Although the first-generation thiazolidinedione troglitazone (now removed from the market because of concerns about liver toxicity) reduced serum levels of oral contraceptive pills and may have reduced their efficacy, there is no evidence that pioglitazone or rosiglitazone have similar effects. Thus, oral contraceptives may be useful in conjunction with insulin-lowering medications in diabetic women with PCOS. Diabetic PCOS patients who do desire pregnancy should be preferentially treated with metformin to avoid the theoretic teratogenicity of the thiazolidinediones.

The optimal therapy for **PCOS patients with impaired glucose tolerance** remains unknown and awaits the results of the Diabetes Prevention Trial, expected in 2003, which is sponsored by the National Institutes of Health. However, it makes sense to advocate weight loss and exercise in these patients, since they have been shown to decrease the risk of progression to diabetes. Women with documented IGT should probably be screened annually for the development of frank diabetes mellitus, since the rate of progression to diabetes is relatively high. Without outcomes data suggesting that pharmacologic treatment of IGT or hyperinsulinemia is beneficial, the use of insulin-lowering drugs for these indications alone cannot yet be recommended. However, these medications may be considered for possible efficacy in improving menstrual function and hyperandrogenism.

PCOS patients with hypertension or lipid abnormalities should also be treated as would any patient with hypertension or dyslipidemia. Some lipid abnormalities associated with PCOS, especially elevated triglyceride levels, may respond well to insulin-lowering medications such as metformin or a thiazolidinedione, but the average patient with elevated low-density lipoprotein cholesterol (>160 without risk factors, >130 with other risk factors, or >100 with known coronary disease) should be treated with an HMG-CoA inhibitor.

PCOS patients without evidence of a metabolic disorder and not desiring pregnancy can be treated with any of the options available to women with **hyperandrogenic symptoms,** such as oral contraceptive pills and/or antiandrogens (see Chapter 14). It is important to ensure that withdrawal menstrual bleeding occurs regularly to prevent endometrial hyperplasia. For many newly diagnosed patients, a pelvic ultrasound after a progestin-induced withdrawal bleeding provides reassuring evidence that the endometrium is homogeneous and thin (<5 to 8 mm) and unlikely to harbor hyperplasia.

An insulin-lowering medication such as metformin, which has been shown to be safe in long-term use, may be indicated in those patients with PCOS who cannot tolerate oral contraceptives or antiandrogens. However, it must be acknowledged that such therapy is currently unapproved by the Food and Drug Administration, and that the largest series to date suggests that only about half of women with PCOS treated with metformin respond with improvement in menstrual function. Of those with improved menses, at least some of them continue to have anovulatory bleeding episodes, which may not protect against endometrial hyperplasia. At this time, currently available thiazolidinediones (pioglitazone or rosiglitazone) cannot be recommended for the treatment of PCOS without diabetes owing to the lack of proven efficacy and concerns about hepatotoxicity and potential teratogenicity.

BIBLIOGRAPHY

Adams J, Polson DW, Franks S: Prevalence of polycystic ovaries in women with anovulation and idiopathic hirsutism, *Br Med J* 293:355, 1986.

Dahlgren E et al: Women with polycystic ovary syndrome wedge resected in 1956 to 1965: a long-term follow-up focusing on natural history and circulating hormones, *Fertil Steril* 57:505, 1992.

Dunaif A et al: Profound peripheral insulin resistance, independent of obesity in polycystic ovary syndrome, *Diabetes* 38:1165, 1989.

Guzick DS et al: Carotid atherosclerosis in women with polycystic ovary syndrome: initial results from a case-control study, *Am J Obstet Gynecol* 174:1224, 1996.

Knochenhauer ES et al: Prevalence of the polycystic ovary syndrome in unselected black and white women of the southeastern United States: a prospective study, *J Clin Endocrinol Metab* 83:3078, 1998.

Pasquali R et al: Clinical and hormonal characteristics of obese amenorrheic hyperandrogenic women before and after weight loss, *J Clin Endocrinol Metab* 68:173, 1989.

Polson DW et al: Polycystic ovaries—a common finding in normal women, *Lancet* 1:870, 1988.

Stuart CA et al: Insulin resistance with acanthosis nigricans: the roles of obesity and androgen excess, *Metabolism* 35:197, 1986.

Taylor AE: Polycystic ovary syndrome. In Burger H, McLachlan R, editors: Gonadal disorders, *Endocrinol Metab Clin North Am* 27:877, 1998.

Taylor AE: Insulin lowering medications in polycystic ovary syndrome. In Penzias A, editor: *Obstet Gynecol Clin North Am* 27:583, 2000.

Wild RA, Bartholomew MJ: The influence of body weight on lipoprotein lipids in patients with polycystic ovary syndrome, *Am J Obstet Gynecol* 159:423, 1988.

Wild S, Pierpoint T, McKeigue P, Jacobs H: Cardiovascular disease in women with polycystic ovary syndrome at long-term follow-up: a retrospective cohort study, *Clin Endocrinol* 52:595, 2000.

Zawadzki JK, Dunaif A: Diagnostic criteria for polycystic ovary syndrome: towards a rational approach. In Dunaif A et al, editors: *Polycystic ovary syndrome,* Boston, 1992, Blackwell Scientific.

CHAPTER 47

Infertility

Jan L. Shifren

Infertility is generally defined as the inability to conceive after 1 year of intercourse without contraception. Normally fertile couples have a monthly conception rate of approximately 15% to 20% per cycle; therefore by the end of 12 months the majority of fertile couples will have conceived. An infertility evaluation therefore is indicated after 1 year without pregnancy, although certain factors may suggest an earlier evaluation. A prompt evaluation is indicated if a woman's cycles are very irregular, or if either partner received radiation or chemotherapy or had significant prior pelvic or genitourinary tract surgery or infection. As one of the critical factors determining a couple's fertility is the age of the female partner and associated egg quality, it may be advisable to evaluate a couple before 1 year if the female partner is 38 years or older; both spontaneous and treatment-associated pregnancy rates decline at this time, and a more aggressive approach is indicated.

CAUSES OF INFERTILITY

Infertility may be due to specific male or female factors, although often the cause is multifactorial or remains unexplained. As infertility is just as likely to be secondary to male as to female factors, both members of the couple should be encouraged to participate fully in the fertility evaluation.

Female Factors

Oocyte Quality

Decreased oocyte quality with increasing age is currently a major cause of infertility, likely owing to a trend for women to marry later and delay childbearing while they establish their careers. Observational studies document a clear decrease in fertility rates with advancing age (Fig. 47-1). This decline in ovarian reserve appears to be a genetically programmed event minimally affected by environmental factors, as reflected in the stable age at menopause over the last 200 years despite extraordinary increases in women's health and longevity. Environmental factors that do reduce oocyte quality include cigarette smoking, pelvic radiation, and some forms of chemotherapy. Not only are cycle fecundity rates decreased in older women, but rates of miscarriage and

chromosomal abnormalities increase, additional consequences of ovarian aging. Studies of pregnancy rates in older women undergoing in vitro fertilization (IVF) using oocytes donated from younger women confirm that reduced oocyte quality is the primary cause of reduced fertility rates and poorer pregnancy outcome in older women. Premature ovarian failure, or menopause occurring before the age of 35, is a rare cause of infertility. Premature ovarian failure may be idiopathic or secondary to genetic or chromosomal abnormalities, autoimmune disease, or environmental factors such as those noted previously.

Anovulation

A woman who is not ovulating regularly will have reduced fertility, despite normal oocyte quality. **Polycystic ovary syndrome,** or chronic anovulation with hyperandrogenism, is an important cause of anovulation. The etiology is likely multifactorial, including obesity, hyperinsulinemia, ovarian hyperandrogenism, and dysregulation of the hypothalamic-pituitary axis. Anovulation secondary to disruption of normal hypothalamic-pituitary signaling also may be due to **thyroid disease** or **hyperprolactinemia; a low percent body fat** associated with an eating disorder, restricted eating, and/or an intense exercise program; **extreme stress;** or rarely a **central tumor. Recent use of long-acting contraceptives,** such as Depo-Provera, may be associated with delayed return of ovulation; in contrast, ovulatory cycles should commence rapidly after cessation of oral contraceptives.

Although anovulation clearly is a cause of infertility, more subtle hormonal changes in the menstrual cycle may or may not be important. **Luteal phase deficiency** describes the finding of an endometrium histologically out of phase with a woman's menstrual cycle. This is thought to be caused by abnormal ovarian estrogen or progesterone production, or the inability of the endometrium to properly respond to normal steroid production; theoretically, an embryo arriving in the uterus would then be unable to implant properly. Although basic research and clinical experience in IVF confirm a narrow window of implantation, luteal phase deficiency is unlikely to be a major fertility factor in ovulatory women.

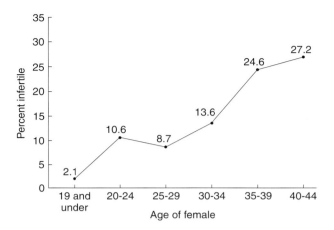

FIG. 47-1 Infertility related to age in the female. (From Mosher WD: *AM Demographics* 9:42, 1987.)

Pelvic Factors

Pelvic **adhesions,** particularly those affecting the fallopian tubes or anatomic relationship between the tube and ovary, are a major cause of infertility. Adhesions may be secondary to a prior infection, surgery, or endometriosis. Gonorrhea, chlamydial infection, or polymicrobial pelvic inflammatory disease often result in pelvic adhesions and dilated, distorted, and poorly functioning fallopian tubes, known as hydrosalpinges. Infertility and ectopic pregnancy are both consequences of these sexually transmitted diseases. Unfortunately, particularly with chlamydia, women may be relatively asymptomatic at the time of acute infection and receive delayed or no treatment. Appendicitis may cause pelvic adhesions, especially if treatment is delayed. In addition, pelvic adhesions may be associated with any prior pelvic surgery, including ovarian cystectomies, myomectomies, and rarely cesarean deliveries. **Endometriosis** also is associated with infertility. In advanced stages of the disease, infertility is likely secondary to distorted pelvic anatomy, but the etiology of reduced fertility in women with minimal or mild disease is unclear. Occasionally women who have had **prior tubal sterilization** desire a return of fertility.

Cervical and Uterine Factors

Cervical or uterine factors rarely are a sole cause of infertility. Normal, midcycle **cervical mucus** is critical for extended sperm viability and transport in the female reproductive tract and should be adequate in the absence of active infection or extensive prior cervical surgery that might destroy the mucus-producing glands, such as a large cone biopsy or cryosurgery. An abnormal uterine cavity may be associated with infertility or recurrent miscarriage. **Congenital uterine abnormalities** include a uterine septum, or one (unicornuate) or two uterine horns (bicornuate or didelphys); rarely the uterus is absent (Rokitansky-Kuster-Hauser syndrome). Occasionally, the endometrium may be severely scarred (**Asherman's syndrome**), typically following curettage of a recently pregnant uterus in the setting of infection. **Exposure to DES in utero** may cause structural abnormalities of the cervix and uterus, associated with increased rates of infertility and miscarriage. **Fibroids,** both intramural and

submucous, also may distort the uterus and contribute to infertility or miscarriage.

Male Factors

Major male infertility factors include **erectile or ejaculatory dysfunction** and **abnormal sperm number, motility, or morphology.** The causes of male sexual dysfunction include neurologic or psychologic problems, medications, or structural abnormalities including hypospadias. Causes of abnormal semen parameters may be hormonal or structural. Normal spermatogenesis will not occur if there is **central disruption of the hypothalamic-pituitary axis** without appropriate secretion of luteinizing hormone (LH), follicle-stimulating hormone (FSH), and testosterone. Even with normal hormonal signals, there may be **testicular failure,** either idiopathic or associated with prior surgery, trauma, radiation, chemotherapy, Klinefelter's syndrome, or infections such as postpubertal mumps. Normal spermatogenesis may occur, but **obstruction** (secondary to trauma or infection) or **congenital absence of the epididymis or vas deferens** may prevent sperm from entering the ejaculate.

A **varicocele,** dilated veins in the pampiniform plexus, may cause decreased sperm parameters, possibly resulting from a slight increase in testicular temperatures. Occasionally, abnormal spermatogenesis may result from **chronic elevation of testicular temperatures** secondary to job or recreational exposures, such as long distance truck driving or frequent use of hot tubs. High concentrations of **antisperm antibodies** bound to sperm may impair sperm function and fertilization; this is a rare occurrence, usually in the setting of disruption of the blood-testis barrier after surgery or trauma. Occasionally men with a prior vasectomy desire a return of fertility.

EVALUATION OF INFERTILITY
Patient Education

The first infertility visit is an ideal time to review the basic steps required for pregnancy, including the deposition of sperm in the vagina and cervical mucus, tubal transport of sperm and later the developing embryo, the functions of the ovary including cyclic hormone production and ovulation, and the role of the uterus in implantation and fetal growth. An understanding of normal fertility is critical for a couple to understand possible causes of infertility, the infertility evaluation, and fertility therapies.

Couples should be educated as to the optimal time to have intercourse and to avoid any lubricant use during midcycle activity, as most are spermicidal. Ovulation occurs approximately 14 days before the first day of menses, therefore a women's fertile period is calculated based on her typical cycle interval. The couple is instructed to have intercourse every other day starting approximately 4 days before ovulation, on the day of presumed ovulation, and 2 days after. Daily intercourse for more than several days consecutively may result in decreased sperm concentration. As sperm survive approximately 72 hours in the female reproductive tract, whereas the oocyte likely survives only 12 to 24 hours, couples should be encouraged to have intercourse before and on the presumed day of ovulation. For example, if a women's typical cycle interval is 30 days, she most likely ovulates on cycle day 16 and optimal timing would include cycle days 12, 14, 16, and 18. Of note, cycle day 1 is defined as the first day of menstrual bleeding heavy enough to require the use of a pad or tampon. As high estradiol levels before ovulation lead to clear, copious cervical mucus, women should be encouraged to notice midcycle mucus changes to assist them in timing intercourse.

Preconception counseling also should be part of the initial infertility visit. Women who smoke, drink excess alcohol, or use illicit drugs should be informed of the significant risks of these behaviors to their developing child and provided with appropriate support services. Women should begin a multivitamin or prenatal vitamin daily that contains at least 400 μg of folate to reduce the risk of neural tube defects. Obese women and women with polycystic ovarian syndrome are often insulin resistant and should be screened for diabetes before conceiving, as poor glucose control in the first trimester of pregnancy is associated with an increased risk of fetal malformations. Women who are rubella or varicella nonimmune should be vaccinated to prevent infection during pregnancy; testing for the human immunodeficiency virus (HIV) should be offered. Couples whose racial or ethnic background or family history suggests an increased risk of a specific genetic disease, such as Tay-Sachs, cystic fibrosis, or sickle cell anemia, should be offered genetic counseling and screening.

History

A thorough history is an important part of the infertility evaluation (Box 47-1). Couples should be asked **how long they have been trying to conceive,** including types and dates of use of previous contraception. **Frequency** and **timing of intercourse** should be discussed, as well as the use of **lubricants** or any **difficulties with sexual relations.** A general, open question about sexual difficulties should be part of the basic fertility history, as it allows couples to discuss possible erectile or ejaculatory dysfunction or the stress of timed intercourse. Any **history of sexually transmitted diseases,** as well as **pregnancies with current or past partners,** should be reviewed. Smoking, alcohol, illicit drug use, and other **toxic exposures,** including prior radiation or chemotherapy, should be discussed. For both partners, it is important to ask about **major medical problems, current medications, prior surgical procedures,** and a **family history** of infertility or genetic diseases or birth defects.

For the **male partner,** the history should include specific questions about genitourinary infections, surgery, or trauma. For the **female partner,** a careful menstrual history is important, as well as a review of pelvic infections and surgery. In addition, women should be asked specifically about vaginal discharge, dysmenorrhea, dyspareunia, headaches, visual changes, heat or cold intolerance, nipple discharge, eating disorders, exercise frequency, and significant stresses.

Physical Examination

For the woman, a thorough general physical examination will identify any major medical problems requiring evaluation and treatment before pregnancy can occur. The presence of hirsutism, acne, galactorrhea, or thyroid enlargement suggest specific diagnoses. During the pelvic examination, care should be taken to identify any abnormalities of uterine size or contour, adnexal masses, signs of infection including discharge or pelvic tenderness, and signs of endometriosis including a fixed retroverted uterus or uterosacral nodularity.

BOX 47-1
The History in the Evaluation of Infertility

Nature and duration of infertility
How long couple has been trying to conceive
Any previous children for either partner
Any prior infertility evaluation
General medical history for both partners
Past surgical history for both partners
Pelvic or abdominal surgery in female
Past gynecologic history
Menstrual history: age of menarche, cycle interval, duration, flow
Presence of molimina, pelvic pain, abnormal bleeding
Past birth control methods
History of pelvic inflammatory disease
History of abnormal Papanicolaou test results and any treatment
DES exposure in utero
Other gynecologic problems (e.g., fibroids, endometriosis)
Coital history (frequency, use of lubricants, sexual difficulties)
Past obstetric history
Social history of both partners
Alcohol, tobacco, and drug use
Occupational exposures
Stress
Eating disorders
Exercise patterns and frequency
Family history
Endocrine disorders
Endocrine review of systems
Hirsutism, acne
Galactorrhea
Weight loss and gain
Tiredness, weakness
Medication use by both partners

DES, Diethylstilbestrol

Diagnostic Tests

The basic infertility evaluation is quite straightforward and includes confirmation of ovulation, assessment of ovarian reserve, evaluation of tubal status and uterine contour, and a semen analysis.

Confirmation of Ovulation

The majority of women with regular menses occurring every 26 to 34 days are ovulatory, but ovulation should be confirmed as part of the fertility evaluation. Basal body temperature (BBT) charting for 1 month will document ovulation, as a slight sustained rise in temperature occurs in the luteal phase. It is important to note that BBT charts do not assist couples in timing intercourse, as the temperature rise occurs after ovulation has occurred. Monthly charting is not needed, as this may be stressful for couples and unlikely to improve pregnancy rates.

Home monitoring of urinary LH surges will predict day of ovulation and aid in timing intercourse, but the kits are costly and unnecessary for most couples. A mid-luteal progesterone level on approximately cycle day 21 will confirm ovulation; conception cycles often are associated with values ≥10 ng/ml.

Assessment of Ovarian Reserve

Fertility is dependent on oocyte quality; therefore a test of ovarian reserve is an important part of a complete infertility evaluation. FSH concentrations clearly increase with age and elevated values reflect follicular depletion. An FSH level drawn on cycle day 3 (when estradiol levels are low) reflects oocyte quality and, interestingly, is an excellent predictor of success in IVF cycles. Although there is much variability among laboratories, a cycle day 3 FSH level >10 IU/L may reflect reduced ovarian reserve.

Hysterosalpingogram

Patency of the fallopian tubes and contour of the uterine cavity are both assessed by hysterosalpingogram (HSG). This study is performed by injecting radiopaque dye through the cervix and monitoring its flow under fluoroscopy through the uterus and fallopian tubes into the peritoneal cavity. Uterine anomalies including septa, adhesions, and submucous myomas are easily identified by HSG, as are abnormalities of the fallopian tubes including hydrosalpinges and peritubal adhesions. One limitation of HSG is that significant pelvic adhesions may be present in the setting of a normal HSG if the tubal lumen or distal fallopian tube is unaffected. This study should be scheduled after menses, but before ovulation, as it should not be performed during pregnancy. Pelvic infection is a risk of HSG, occurring in <1% of all studies, but in 3% of cases when tubal disease is present. Antibiotic prophylaxis may be prescribed for high-risk patients. Discomfort is decreased by treatment with a nonsteroidal antiinflammatory agent approximately 1 hour before the study.

Semen Analysis

Semen analysis assesses the volume, concentration, motility, and morphology of a semen sample and should be performed as an initial study in all fertility evaluations. The specimen is produced by masturbation into a clean container and should be brought to the laboratory, at body temperature, within 1 hour of collection. Couples should abstain from intercourse for approximately 2 to 3 days before collection, as frequent ejaculation may reduce the sperm count. Normal semen parameters are listed in Table 47-1. Any abnormal semen analysis should be repeated, as there may be significant variability between specimens. As the sperm maturation cycle is approximately 70 days, repeat collections should be delayed 6 to 10 weeks to allow for resolution of the effects of an acute event, such as a febrile illness.

Couples often are concerned that the woman is "rejecting" the sperm, or that somehow the couple is reproductively "incompatible." There are no good data to support this misconception, and couples should be reassured. The testing of cervical mucus and serum samples for antisperm antibodies fuels these concerns and is of no proven utility in establishing a specific diagnosis or treating infertility.

Additional Tests

Additional tests may be indicated based on the history and physical examination. Prolactin and thyroid-stimulating hor-

Table 47-1
World Health Organization (WHO) Criteria Used for Semen Evaluation

Volume	≥2 ml
pH	7.2-7.8
Sperm concentration	20×10^6 spermatozoa/ml or more
Total sperm count	40×10^6 spermatozoa or more
Motility	50% or more with forward progression or 25% or more with rapid linear progression within 60 min after collection
Morphologic characteristics	50% or more with normal morphologic features

Modified from *WHO laboratory manual for the examination of human semen and semen-cervical mucus interation*, New York, 1987, Cambridge University Press.

mone levels should be checked in any woman with menstrual irregularities. Cervical cultures for gonorrhea and chlamydia should be performed in couples at increased risk; the utility of *Ureaplasma* cultures remains controversial.

Tests with Limited Utility

Several traditional fertility tests are of limited utility in establishing a diagnosis or leading to a specific therapy proven to increase pregnancy rates.

Postcoital Test

A postcoital test (PCT) involves assessing cervical mucus under the microscope 2 to 12 hours after intercourse for periovulatory characteristics (such as clarity, spinnbarkeit, and ferning) and the presence of motile sperm. This test is considered intrusive and stressful for most couples and has extremely poor sensitivity and predictive value with respect to any specific fertility diagnosis. The most common reason for an abnormal test is inappropriate timing, distant from ovulation, yet couples are very discouraged by a poor result. The PCT is never a substitute for a semen analysis, as significant information regarding semen parameters is unavailable.

Endometrial Biopsy

Although traditionally part of the infertility evaluation, a postovulatory endometrial biopsy to establish a diagnosis of luteal phase deficiency may be of limited clinical utility. To establish the diagnosis, two endometrial biopsies more than 2 days out-of-phase with a woman's calculated cycle day are required, as a high percentage of fertile women will have an out-of-phase biopsy, and there is significant variability in endometrial dating. As discussed previously, luteal phase deficiency is unlikely to be a sole cause of infertility for the majority of couples and should this truly be a factor, it would be corrected by treatments otherwise recommended for idiopathic infertility.

Procedures

Laparoscopy and Hysteroscopy

Laparoscopy is part of a complete fertility evaluation, as it is the only way to confirm a diagnosis of pelvic adhesions or endometriosis and may effectively treat the problem at the same time. As laparoscopy is a procedure with both anesthetic and operative risk, it should be performed when initial testing has not identified a cause, or when indicated by findings at history, physical examination, or a previous test, such as an abnormal HSG. Hysteroscopy is used both to diagnose and treat intrauterine lesions that may reduce fertility. This procedure is indicated primarily when the HSG suggests a uterine abnormality.

TREATMENT OF INFERTILITY

Although couples with bilaterally blocked fallopian tubes, ovarian failure, or azoospermia are unable to conceive, the majority of couples have reduced fertility, or decreased cycle pregnancy rates, and ultimately may conceive on their own. The goal of fertility therapy for these couples is to increase the monthly chance of conception. The diagnosis and treatments for infertility may be enormously stressful. Couples should be provided with resources and support including referrals to therapists and local groups, such as the national fertility education and support network, RESOLVE.

Infertility Secondary to Female Factors

Anovulation

Anovulatory infertility is quite amenable to medical therapy. In women with polycystic ovarian syndrome or other forms of anovulation when endogenous estrogen is present, treatment with **clomiphene citrate** results in ovulatory cycles in 70% to 90% of women. After using a short course of progestins to initiate a withdrawal bleed, clomiphene citrate (50 mg) is given on cycle days 5 to 9, and the couple is instructed to have regular intercourse. Ovulation should be confirmed by BBTs or a luteal phase progesterone level, although the occurrence of menses by cycle day 34 is indirect evidence of ovulation. The dose of clomiphene may be increased up to 150 mg/day if ovulation does not occur. Couples who do not conceive after three ovulatory cycles on clomiphene, or women who do not ovulate with these doses of clomiphene, should be referred to a fertility specialist. Risks of clomiphene therapy include multiple pregnancies and rarely ovarian hyperstimulation syndrome; side effects include hot flashes, vision changes, headaches, and mood changes.

Anovulation secondary to hyperprolactinemia should be treated with the dopamine agonist, bromocriptine, after central imaging has ruled out a significant mass lesion. Anovulation associated with abnormal thyroid function should respond to treatment of the underlying thyroid disease. Hypothalamic amenorrhea, or anovulation associated with low endogenous estrogen production, may not respond to clomiphene therapy and women may need to be referred to a fertility specialist for ovulation induction with a GnRH pump or injectable gonadotropins. Clearly lifestyle modifications including weight gain, limiting exercise, and stress reduction should be encouraged first and may result in resumption of ovulatory cycles.

Pelvic Factors

Infertility associated with significant pelvic adhesions, tubal disease, or endometriosis should be treated at laparoscopy. Women who fail to conceive after surgical treatment of pelvic disease, or whose disease is so significant that surgery is unlikely to result in pregnancy, are excellent candidates for IVF. Prior tubal sterilization procedures may be reversed surgically or pregnancies achieved with IVF. Women with pelvic adhesions and tubal disease are at high risk for ectopic pregnancy and should be monitored closely in early pregnancy with serial quantitative β-human chorionic gonadotropin levels (hCG) levels and ultrasound.

Cervical and Uterine Factors

Cervical factors are unlikely to be a major or sole cause of infertility. Absent or abnormal periovulatory cervical mucus may be treated by bypassing the cervix with intrauterine insemination of the partner's sperm. Although uterine factors such as fibroids, congenital abnormalities, and the effects of DES exposure may be associated with infertility, surgical treatment rarely has been proven to improve fertility rates. Effective surgical therapies include hysteroscopic resection of uterine septa, submucous fibroids, endometrial polyps, and intrauterine adhesions; these procedures may improve pregnancy rates and decrease the risk of miscarriage, especially in women with a history of recurrent pregnancy loss.

Infertility Secondary to Male Factors

Treatment of male factor infertility depends on the specific diagnosis. Men who use tobacco, marijuana, cocaine, excess alcohol, or anabolic steroids should be advised to stop. Alternatives to medications such as cimetidine and certain antidepressants should be sought, as they may affect semen parameters or sexual function. Men exposed to high temperatures at work or during recreation should modify their activities. If a varicocele is present, repair may improve semen parameters and increase the likelihood of pregnancy. Obstruction, including that from elective vasectomy, may be treated surgically or, as in congenital absence of the vas deferens, sperm may be aspirated from the genitourinary tract and used in IVF. Hyperprolactinemia and thyroid disease should be treated, and some men with central hypogonadism may respond to gonadotropin therapy. Primary testicular failure associated with elevated gonadotropin levels rarely is associated with successful pregnancy. Even after a complete urologic evaluation, many cases of male infertility remain unexplained. Treatment in these situations may include ovarian hyperstimulation with intrauterine insemination (IUI), IVF, or donor insemination, depending on semen parameters and preferences of the couple.

Assisted Reproductive Technologies

Gonadotropin-IUI Cycles

Ovarian hyperstimulation combined with intrauterine insemination is effective therapy for unexplained infertility and for infertility associated with endometriosis, mild male factor, and an age-related decline in oocyte quality. Injectable gonadotropins (FSH and LH) or occasionally clomiphene citrate are used to recruit multiple ovarian follicles per cycle, with frequent ultrasound monitoring. When follicles reach a size consistent with oocyte maturity, ovulation is triggered with an hCG injection and an intrauterine insemination is performed 36 hours later. Several randomized, controlled trials have demonstrated that this therapy results in pregnancy rates of approximately 15% per cycle (near normal fecundity) in couples whose chance of conceiving spontaneously is 3% to 5% per cycle. This therapy is costly, time-consuming, and stressful for couples; risks include multiple pregnancy and rarely ovarian hyperstimulation syndrome.

In Vitro Fertilization (IVF)

In vitro fertilization is effective therapy for couples with the above diagnoses who fail to conceive after three to six cycles of ovarian hyperstimulation and IUI, and for those with significant pelvic disease or male factor infertility. Injectable gonadotropins are used to recruit multiple ovarian follicles, and mature oocytes are retrieved transvaginally under ultrasound guidance. Fertilization occurs in the laboratory and embryos are transferred through the cervix into the uterus several days later. In cases of severe male factor infertility, fertilization may not occur with conventional IVF, and a form of micromanipulation involving intracytoplasmic sperm injection may be required. Pregnancy rates approximate 30% per cycle of IVF, but are dependent on a woman's age and oocyte quality. Risks include multiple pregnancy and rarely ovarian hyperstimulation syndrome or surgical complications such as bleeding or infection. There appears to be no increased risk of birth defects in children conceived through assisted reproductive technologies.

Donor Insemination

Donor insemination is an option in cases of severe male factor infertility. Although many couples elect to use an anonymous donor with the privacy this decision affords, some couples choose a donor related to the male partner to establish a genetic link between the child and both parents. Donor insemination also is an option for women without male partners who desire to be single parents or for women with female partners. Anyone using donor insemination should be encouraged to use cryopreserved sperm that has been quarantined for 6 months to allow for interval HIV testing of the donor and detection of latent infection. Cryobanks carefully screen donors for both genetic and sexually transmitted diseases and typically offer a wide selection of donors with varying ethnic origins and physical characteristics. If no other fertility factors are present, pregnancy rates approximate 10% per cycle.

IVF with Donor Oocytes

In vitro fertilization using oocytes from a known or anonymous donor is an option for women with premature ovarian failure or for women with significantly decreased ovarian reserve who are unlikely to conceive using their own oocytes.

BIBLIOGRAPHY

Cedars M: Controlled ovarian hyperstimulation as therapy for unexplained infertility, *Infertil Reprod Med Clinics North Am* 8:649, 1997.

Griffith C, Grimes D: The validity of the postcoital test, *Am J Obstet Gynecol* 162:615, 1990.

Guzick D et al: Efficacy of superovulation and intrauterine insemination in the treatment of infertility, *N Engl J Med* 340:177, 1999.

Hull M et al: The value of a single serum progesterone measurement in the mid-luteal phase as a criterion of a potentially fertile cycle derived from treated and untreated conception cycles, *Fertil Steril* 37:355, 1982.

Menken J, Trussell J, Larsen U: Age and infertility, *Science* 233:1389, 1986.

Sharara F, Scott R, Seifer D: The detection of diminished ovarian reserve in infertile women, *Am J Obstet Gynecol* 179:804, 1998.

Stumpf P, March C: Febrile morbidity following hysterosalpingography: identification of risk factors and recommendations for prophylaxis, *Fertil Steril* 33:487, 1980.

Wentz A, Kossoy L, Parker R: The impact of luteal phase inadequacy in an infertile population, *Am J Obstet Gynecol* 162:937, 1990.

CHAPTER 48

Menopause

Kathryn A. Martin

Menopause is an important time of transition in a woman's life. Life expectancy for women has gradually increased and is now estimated to be approximately 78 years. Therefore for most women up to one third of their total life span occurs after the menopause. This observation highlights the importance of understanding the impact of hormone replacement therapy on this growing segment of the population.

Because of the explosion of information about menopause now available to women, many women discuss questions and concerns about menopause with their primary physicians. Others will experience symptoms related to menopause. Although estrogen replacement was initially used short term to treat symptoms of the menopause, the emphasis for the past two decades has been on long-term use of estrogen to prevent osteoporosis and possibly coronary heart disease (CHD). Although epidemiologic data had demonstrated a dramatic reduction in CHD risk, recent clinical trials investigating hormone replacement therapy (HRT) for the secondary prevention of CHD have not supported these epidemiologic observations. Thus definitive recommendations for long-term HRT use are unclear pending further clinical trial data, in particular on primary CHD prevention.

EPIDEMIOLOGY

The average age of menopause in epidemiologic studies is approximately 51, although the range considered to be normal is quite wide, since menopause can occur in normal women anytime between the ages of 42 and 58. Two factors appear to be associated with earlier menopause: cigarette smoking and a history of short intermenstrual interval. As an example, women who are smokers have menopause, on average, two years earlier than nonsmokers.

PHYSIOLOGY

Although menopause is defined clinically as permanent cessation of menses, the neuroendocrine and ovarian changes leading up to the menopause occur over a 5- to 10-year period referred to as the perimenopausal transition. The groundwork for menopause begins in utero, and by the sixth month of fetal life the human ovary contains approximately 6 to 7 million oocytes. However, after this peak a degenerative process known as follicular atresia occurs until there are no remaining oocytes at the time of menopause. Less than 1% of oocytes are lost via ovulation; the remainder are lost via atresia, a process that is poorly understood.

Endocrine changes seen during menopause include changes in ovarian sex steroid biosynthesis and pituitary gonadotropin secretion. The premenopausal ovary contains three functioning compartments: the stroma, follicle, and corpus luteum. After menopause, however, the only remaining functional compartment is the stroma, the site of androgen production. Although testosterone production rates and levels do not change significantly after menopause, androstenedione levels decrease by approximately 50%. The postmenopausal ovary appears to make little or no estrogen, and circulating estrogen in postmenopausal women is derived primarily from peripheral conversion of androstenedione to estrone.

The earliest endocrine finding during the perimenopausal transition is a selective rise in serum follicle-stimulating hormone (FSH), which is often seen in women over 40 with ovulatory cycles. This rise in FSH occurs despite preservation of estradiol secretion, suggesting that a fall in ovarian inhibin (a hormone that normally suppresses FSH) may be one of the earliest endocrine events in perimenopause.

CLINICAL PRESENTATION

The earliest clinical finding during the perimenopausal transition is a **decrease in cycle length.** It has been demonstrated that ovulatory women over 40 have a mean cycle length of 25 days compared with 30 days in 18- to 30-year-old control subjects, whereas 45-year-old women have a mean cycle length of only 23 days. Although most women initially experience these short cycles, many then have long, anovulatory cycles that may be interspersed with shorter, ovulatory cycles. The reasons for this waxing and waning of ovarian activity are unclear but may reflect a difference in the responsiveness of the remaining oocytes, or a difference in the types of FSH the pituitary secretes during the perimenopausal transition.

The **vasomotor flush** is the most common clinical finding of the menopause. Approximately 75% of women having a natural menopause, and as many as 90% of women who have surgical menopause experience vasomotor flushes. There are two components to a flush. The hot flash describes the subjective feeling of warmth that precedes any physiologically measurable change. The hot flush is the physiologically measurable change and is characterized by visible redness in the chest, neck, and face, usually followed by sweating in the same distribution. Nocturnal hot flushes are more common than daytime hot flushes, and sleep deprivation is a common result. Studies have demonstrated nocturnal flushes with corresponding waking episodes, using skin temperature and electroencephalographic (EEG) recordings. This is clinically relevant since many of these women experience insomnia-related symptoms such as fatigue, irritability, and depression. It has been demonstrated that estrogen treatment of these symptomatic women results in improved sleep latency and an increased percentage of rapid eye movement (REM) sleep.

Genitourinary atrophy is another common phenomenon, since the vagina and the outer third of the urethra are estrogen-responsive tissues. Therefore patients often experience vaginal dryness, dyspareunia, and urinary symptoms that mimic urinary tract infection. All of these symptoms are responsive to estrogen.

In addition to these immediate consequences, menopause affects a woman's risk for other chronic diseases, chiefly **osteoporosis** and **coronary heart disease.** The increased risk of osteoporosis is related to accelerated decrease in bone mass per unit volume during the years following menopause. The effect of menopause on coronary risk is less straightforward. When age and smoking are taken into account, there is no difference in heart disease risk between naturally premenopausal and postmenopausal women. However, bilateral oophorectomy in premenopausal women does increase the risk of heart disease, even though natural menopause does not. By age 60, the risk of CHD in women is identical to that in men.

APPROACH TO THE WOMAN AT MENOPAUSE

Counseling

The proliferation of information in recent years has helped many women become more knowledgeable about menopause. However, the negative tone of much of this information, coupled with cultural stereotypes, has fostered fears and worries about menopause in some women. It is important for the primary care physician to be able to counsel patients about what to expect at menopause. Some perimenopausal women with concerns may be reluctant to voice their worries. Counseling about what to expect as a woman approaches menopause should be part of routine primary care for women in their 40s.

The primary care clinician can provide information about the epidemiologic and physiologic characteristics of menopause and guidelines for what is normal and when symptoms should prompt medical attention (Box 48-1). It is important to acknowledge the cultural emphasis on negative aspects of menopause and provide a more balanced view of the positive physical, emotional, and social aspects. The au-

---

BOX 48-1

Counseling the Perimenopausal Woman

Epidemiology of Menopause
Average age is 51; 1-2 years earlier in smokers
Typical changes in cycles before menopause
    Shortening cycle length
    Skipped menstrual periods
    Occasional heavy menstrual periods

What to Expect at Menopause
Symptoms related to menopause significant for a *minority* of women
Great variation among individual women in the experience of menopause

When to Seek Medical Attention
Vaginal bleeding more frequently than every 21 days
Heavy bleeding or bleeding lasting more than 7 days
Bothersome hot flashes, insomnia, or other symptoms
After 6 to 12 months of amenorrhea

---

thority of the clinician's role can be helpful in countering negative expectations, which may influence a woman's experience of menopause.

Menopause is a convenient time for examining health maintenance and prevention measures. Fluctuations in the rate of change in serum cholesterol levels around menopause may make more frequent screening desirable. Nutrition should be reviewed to ensure that a woman is receiving 1000 to 1500 mg of calcium daily. A regular weight-bearing exercise program is important for women at midlife, both for osteoporosis prevention and for maintenance of appropriate body weight.

A discussion of HRT should generally be initiated with every menopausal woman. Because of the widespread interest in HRT, the clinician can anticipate that a perimenopausal woman will have questions about its use for symptom relief or prevention of disease, even if its use is not appropriate in her case.

Hormone Replacement Therapy
Pharmacology

The relative potency of estrogens in HRT is much less than in the oral contraceptive pill. Most low-dose oral contraceptives currently contain 35 μg of ethinyl estradiol, a dose equivalent to approximately seven times what is used for menopausal replacement. In contrast, estrogen replacement doses are more physiologic and in general restore follicular phase levels of estrogen. Therefore, when considering the risks and benefits of HRT, one cannot necessarily extrapolate from the oral contraceptive literature because of the large difference in estrogen dose.

The exogenous estrogens that are used clinically have striking variability in potency. All oral preparations are metabolized in the liver, with potential effects on liver protein synthesis, including renin substrate, clotting factors, and hepatic lipase. In contrast, transdermal preparations avoid this first-pass hepatic metabolism. With regard to potency, the synthetic estrogens (ethinyl estradiol) are the most potent estrogens available. Conjugated estrogens are the next most potent, and natural estrogens such as estradiol are the least potent.

Progestins are synthetic compounds with progesterone-like activity, most of which have mild androgenic properties. Medroxyprogesterone acetate is the progestin used most commonly after menopause. An oral, micronized preparation of natural progesterone is now approved by the Food and Drug Administration (FDA) and commercially available. Natural progesterone is less potent than the synthetic progestins, but it has some metabolic advantages (more favorable impact on lipoprotein profiles). New combination HRT formulations have included progestins derived from testosterone (19-nor-testosterones), such as norethindrone.

Risks and Benefits

When making a risk/benefit analysis of HRT, the risk of CHD is the most important factor, since death of CHD is four to five times more common than death of breast and endometrial cancer combined. Therefore a very small change in risk could result in a profound change in morbidity and mortality rates.

The increased risk of **endometrial hyperplasia** and **carcinoma** with estrogen use has been well documented (Box 48-2). Endometrial cancer risk has been studied in users versus nonusers of estrogen. It has been found that short-term users (less than 1 year of use) appear to have no increased risk in cancer, whereas long-term users have a fivefold increase in risk. Similar results have been confirmed in many other studies as well.

It is known that addition of a progestin dramatically reduces the risk of endometrial cancer. Although dose and type of progestin are obviously important, there are data suggesting that the duration of progestin exposure is equally important. The incidence of hyperplasia with unopposed estrogen is 20% to 40%, with a decrease to 3% to 4% if a progestin is added for 7 days, and a further reduction to <1% for 12 to 13 days of progestin. The current trend in clinical practice is to give a low dose of medroxyprogesterone acetate (5 mg) or natural micronized progesterone 200 mg for 12 to 14 days, or if using a continuous combined regimen, 2.5 mg daily. Continuous administration of natural progesterone has not been studied.

The risk of **breast cancer** secondary to estrogen replacement has been controversial. Individual observational studies and meta-analyses have reported conflicting results, with many reporting no increase in breast cancer risk, while some

---

BOX 48-2
Risks of Hormone Replacement Therapy

Estrogen
Gallbladder disease
Endometrial hyperplasia and cancer
Breast cancer (risk unresolved)

Progestins
Adverse effect on serum lipid levels
Effect on breast cancer unknown
Effect on coronary artery disease unknown

---

report an increased breast cancer risk after many years of use. To help resolve this controversy, the Collaborative Group on Hormonal Factors in Breast Cancer reanalyzed approximately 90% of the available epidemiologic evidence and concluded that the relative risk of developing breast cancer increased by a factor of 1.023 for each year of HRT use after menopause. This increase is the same as that seen for the effect of delaying menopause by 1 year. Five or more years of HRT use was associated with a relative risk (RR) of breast cancer of 1.35 (1.21 to 1.49).

Although estrogen given for 5 or more years does appear to increase breast cancer risk, both the media and patients often misinterpret relative risk estimates. It is more useful for physicians and their patients to understand the attributable risk (the absolute risk of breast cancer that can be attributed to estrogen), since it is quite low. Using the Collaborative Group's relative risk estimates, attributable risks of breast cancer owing to estrogen were calculated based on duration of use. Using this model, a 50-year-old woman's attributable risk of breast cancer if she uses estrogen for 2 years or less (i.e., for symptomatic relief) is 0.02 per 100 women. For 10 years of estrogen use in the same age group, 0.58 in 100 women would be expected to develop breast cancer that they would not have developed had they not taken estrogen.

Recent data suggest that progestins may further increase breast cancer risk. Two observational studies report an increased risk of breast cancer in combined estrogen-progestin users versus unopposed estrogen users. In the follow-up study of a cohort of women from the Breast Cancer Detection Demonstration Project, combined HRT was associated with a relative risk of breast cancer of 1.4 (Confidence Interval [CI] 1.1 to 1.8) versus that seen in the unopposed estrogen group (RR 1.2; CI 1.0 to 1.4). The increase in risk was seen only in women with a body mass index (BMI) less than 24.4 kg/m^2. Similar results were seen in the National Cancer Institute's case-control study, where the relative risks for combined HRT versus unopposed estrogen were 1.24 (1.07 to 1.45) and 1.06 (0.97 to 1.15), respectively. In this study, risk appeared higher with cyclic versus continuous HRT use, although this was not significant.

Data from the Collaborative Group also suggests that treatment with estrogen plus progestin is associated with a higher risk of breast cancer than unopposed estrogen (relative risk 1.53 and 1.34, respectively), although this difference was not statistically significant. It is anticipated that this group will readdress this issue, in particular the impact of BMI and cyclic versus continuous progestin use.

It is possible that the breast cancers that develop in the setting of postmenopausal estrogen use are associated with a better prognosis, although data have been somewhat conflicting. The Iowa Women's Health study recently examined the association of HRT use with histologic types of invasive breast carcinoma in a population-based study. They observed no overall increase in the risk of invasive lobular or ductal cancers, or DCIS, in estrogen users (these types account for 95% of all breast cancer cases). However, estrogen use was associated with an increased risk of invasive breast cancer with a favorable prognosis. Further data are needed to confirm these observations.

Several conclusions can be drawn from the current breast cancer literature: (1) There is no evidence that short-term use of replacement estrogen (up to 3 years) is associated with an increase in breast cancer risk (the recent 3 year PEPI [Postmenopausal Estrogen/Progestin Intervention Trial] would support this notion); (2) an increase in breast cancer risk is likely with long-term use, although the attributable risk is quite low; (3) the impact of progestins on breast cancer is of concern, but warrants further study; and (4) breast cancers that develop in the setting of postmenopausal estrogen use may have a more favorable prognosis. Further data from the Collaborative Group on Hormonal Factors in Breast Cancer and the Women's Health Initiative (a large, randomized clinical trial) are needed to resolve these issues.

Postmenopausal estrogens have been shown to be effective for both prevention and treatment of **osteoporosis.** It has been thought that conjugated estrogen, 0.625 mg or its equivalent, was the minimally effective dose. However, there has been recent interest in using even lower doses of estrogen for bone protection. Many women prefer lower doses of estrogen to avoid side effects and to theoretically lower their risk of both endometrial and breast cancer. Several studies have demonstrated that conjugated or esterified estrogens (0.3 mg) given with calcium have similar effects on bone density as 0.625 mg. Further data are needed before recommending these lower dose estrogen regimens routinely.

Within 2 years after menopause, changes in **lipid profiles** are seen in most women with a fall in high-density lipoprotein (HDL) and increase in low-density lipoprotein (LDL). The impact of HRT on lipid profiles has been extensively studied, and in general, conjugated estrogen 0.625 mg or its equivalent causes a decrease in LDL concentrations, increase in triglycerides, and an increase in HDL concentrations by approximately 12%. Similar improvements are not seen with transdermal estrogens because of first-pass hepatic metabolism. Synthetic progestins, but not natural progesterone, negate some of this beneficial effect. Use of a natural progesterone preparation is a reasonable option in patients with hypercholesterolemia. While there had been concern that use of synthetic progestins would negate cardiovascular benefit, epidemiologic data suggest that combined estrogen-progestin users have the same reduction in coronary disease risk as unopposed estrogen users.

Although there are no published clinical trials investigating the role of HRT in the **primary prevention of CHD,** there is an abundance of epidemiologic studies that suggest that estrogen is cardioprotective. A meta-analysis has demonstrated that the relative risk of CHD in any user of estrogen versus nonusers is approximately 0.56 (i.e., there is a 44% decrease in risk). The Women's Health Initiative (WHI), a large clinical trial, is expected to provide more definitive data in this area. The WHI recently released information on an interim analysis showing a small increase of cardiovascular events in years 1 and 2. Participants were notified, but a decision was made to continue the study. A similar trial in Europe, the WISDOM study, will be completed in the year 2010.

The role of estrogen in **secondary prevention of CHD,** suggested by many observational studies, has been challenged by the findings of several randomized trials of estrogen replacement in women with established heart disease. Data from a clinical trial known as the HERS study (Heart and Estrogen/progestin Replacement Study) suggests that estrogen might, at least initially, be harmful for women with established CHD. In this prospective trial of 2763 women on placebo or combined continuous HRT, no overall reduction in risk of CHD events was seen (nonfatal myocardial infarc-

tion or sudden coronary death). In a time-table analysis, the risk of CHD events in year 1 was higher in women taking HRT versus placebo. However, there was then a trend toward a protective effect by year 4. A possible explanation for these observations is that the prothrombotic effect of estrogen dominates during early therapy, but that later lipid effects result in a reduction of CHD risk. This time lag would be consistent with many of the lipid-lowering agent studies, where a reduction in CHD risk is not seen for the first 1 or 2 years. Based on the findings of the HERS study, it seems reasonable to continue HRT in those women who are already receiving therapy. However, initiating HRT in women with newly established CHD might increase risk in the first year of therapy.

A more recent study further supports the findings of the HERS study. In the ERA (Estrogen Replacement and Atherosclerosis) trial, postmenopausal women with established CHD were randomized to unopposed estrogen, estrogen plus medroxyprogesterone acetate, or placebo. Quantitative coronary angiography was performed before and after 3 years of treatment. Although both HRT regimens had beneficial effects on lipid profiles, neither affected the progression of coronary atherosclerosis.

Estrogen's effects on the **coagulation system** include an increase in clotting factors and thromboembolic events when high doses of estrogen are used. For example, there is an increased risk of deep venous thrombosis, pulmonary embolism, and myocardial infarction in patients on high-dose oral contraceptives who are over 35 years and who smoke. Although many studies have shown that replacement doses of estrogen do not affect clotting factors, estrogen preparations increase C-reactive protein, a factor known to predict vascular disease.

Recent reports from several observational studies suggest that there is a significant increase in the relative risk of deep venous thrombosis and pulmonary embolism in postmenopausal estrogen users versus nonusers (although the absolute risk remains very small; 1 in 3000 to 5000 women per year). In one study, the increased risk occurred only in the first year of use. Results from the Postmenopausal Estrogen/Progestin Interventions (PEPI) trial suggest that women who had a thromboembolic event on HRT had significantly lower fibrinogen levels before treatment.

In addition, the HERS study demonstrated a higher risk of venous thromboembolic events in postmenopausal women with established CHD who took HRT versus placebo (RR 2.7 over 4 years of follow-up). The risk was particularly high in women who had other risk factors, such as immobilization (lower extremity fracture, surgery, or nonsurgical hospitalization) or cancer. In contrast, risk was decreased in women who also took daily aspirin or a statin (RR 0.5 for both). Underlying activated protein C resistance is another risk factor for venous thrombosis embolism in postmenopausal women on HRT.

Thus it appears that there is a small but significant increase in risk of venous thromboembolic events with current HRT. For healthy postmenopausal women, the absolute risk is extremely low. However, for women with other known risk factors such as immobilization, cancer, or activated protein C resistance, the risk is significant.

Other Possible Benefits of Estrogen
There are data to suggest that estrogen is associated with a decreased risk of colon cancer and Alzheimer disease.

However, neither benefit is firmly established. It is also possible that estrogen improves cognitive function, but this too is not well established. It has been shown that the use of estrogen in women with established Alzheimer's dementia has no beneficial effect on cognitive function.

CHOICE OF THERAPY

Menopause is a time when many women can benefit from examining their health habits and considering the available interventions for prevention of chronic disease. Although some women seek medical attention for symptoms related to menopause, the majority adapt well to this transition. The clinician should counsel all premenopausal women about what to expect at menopause and should review preventive measures, including the use of HRT. Indications for HRT are summarized in Table 48-1.

Almost all postmenopausal women (with the exception of those who have had breast cancer) are candidates for short-term HRT for up to 5 years to treat symptoms. Long-term HRT should be reserved for the prevention and treatment of osteoporosis. Prevention of CHD was an indication for long-term HRT in the past, but this indication has been challenged by recent clinical trial data suggesting a possible harmful effect of estrogen, at least in the setting of secondary CHD prevention.

Unopposed estrogen is indicated for women who have undergone hysterectomy, since there is currently no known role for adding a progestin other than to prevent the increased risk of estrogen-induced endometrial cancer. If unopposed estrogen is used in women with an intact uterus, routine endometrial sampling is essential. Bleeding patterns in women on unopposed estrogen are unpredictable, since these women may experience regular withdrawal bleeding,

Table 48-1
Indications for Hormone Replacement Therapy

Indications	Rationale	Treatment	Onset	Duration	Other
Menopausal symptoms	Symptom relief	Oral or transdermal estrogen (.625 mg conjugated estrogens or equivalent) with cyclic or continuous progestin; titrate estrogen dose to symptoms relief	When symptoms become bothersome to patient during perimenopause or after menopause	6 months to several years	Taper estrogen over 6 to 12 months when discontinuing use; slower taper if symptoms recur
Genitourinary atrophy	Symptom relief or prevention of recurrent postmenopausal urinary tract infections	Oral or transdermal estrogen (as above) or vaginal estrogen	When symptoms become bothersome to patient	Indefinitely	Progestins warranted with long-term vaginal use if serum estradiol level >30 pg/ml
Prevention of osteoporosis	Risk reduction	Oral or transdermal estrogen (.625 mg conjugated estrogen or equivalent) with appropriate progestin cycling; .3 mg with calcium may be effective	Ideally within 6 to 12 months of menopause; preferably within 5 years of menopause	Uncertain; at least 8 years to produce significant reduction in osteoporosis risk	
Treatment of osteoporosis	Prevention of future fractures	Oral or transdermal estrogen (.625 mg conjugated estrogens or equivalent) with appropriate progestin cycling	At diagnosis of osteoporosis	Indefinite	Ensure adequate calcium, vitamin D intake, and exercise
Treatment of premature menopause	Relief of any symptoms; prevention of premature osteoporosis and coronary artery disease	Oral or transdermal estrogen (.625 mg conjugated estrogens or equivalent) with appropriate progestin cycling	At diagnosis	At least until age 50; generally 5 to 8 years beyond expected menopause	

irregular bleeding, or amenorrhea. The pattern of bleeding does not predict endometrial histologic characteristics in this group.

A variety of estrogen preparations are available (Table 48-2). The standard unopposed estrogen regimen is conjugated equine estrogens (Premarin) 0.625 mg daily or on days 1 to 25 of the calendar month. There is evidence that the risk of endometrial cancer associated with uninterrupted use of estrogens is no different from that with regimens incorporating a 1-week interruption.

Cyclic use of combined estrogen and progestin is recommended for most postmenopausal women with an intact uterus. The most popular regimen in the United States has been conjugated estrogen, 0.625 mg given daily, (or days 1 to 25 of the calendar month) with 5 mg of medroxyprogesterone acetate for 12 consecutive days each month. However, the recent trend has been to decrease the dose of progestin, to minimize metabolic effects while maximizing endometrial protection. Several alternative forms of progestins are now available (Table 48-2).

One of the major drawbacks of the cyclic regimens is that 85% to 90% of women have monthly withdrawal bleeding. In an effort to avoid menses there has been recent emphasis on the use of **continuous combined estrogen and progestin regimens.** In the United States, continuous conjugated estrogen 0.625 mg is given with daily medroxyprogesterone acetate 2.5 mg (Table 48-2). Although many studies now suggest that these regimens are protective of the endometrium, a beneficial effect on lipid profiles has not been firmly established. Of women using continuous combined regimens, 30% to 50% experience irregular bleeding that can last up to the sixth month of therapy. However, most women eventually have amenorrhea. The irregular bleeding seems to be more of a problem in perimenopausal women, and less of a problem in older postmenopausal women, who presumably have an atrophic endometrium before starting therapy.

Table 48-2
Types of Commonly Used Hormone Replacement Preparations

	Standard Dose	Frequency
Oral Estrogens		
Conjugated estrogens (Premarin; Cenestin)	0.625 mg	daily
Estradiol (Estrace)	1 mg	daily
Esterified estrogens (Estratab, Menest)	0.625 mg	daily
Estropipate (Ogen, Ortho-Est)	0.625 mg	daily
Transdermal Estradiol		
Alora, Esclim, Estraderm, Vivelle	0.05 mg/d	twice weekly
Climara	0.05 mg/d	once weekly
Vaginal Estrogen		
Conjugated estrogens (Premarin) cream	1 g	twice weekly
Estradiol vaginal (Estrace) cream	1 g	twice weekly
Estradiol vaginal tablets (Vagifem)	25 μg	twice weekly
Estring	7.5 μg/d	every 3 months
Progestins		
Medroxyprogesterone (Provera, Cycrin)	5 mg	daily for 12-14 days
or	2.5 mg	daily
Micronized progesterone (Prometrium)	200 mg	daily for 12-14 days
or	200 mg	daily
Crinone vaginal gel 4%	1 applicator	every other day for 12 days
Combination Preparations		
Oral		
Premphase		
conjugated equine estrogens	.625 mg	daily
with medroxyprogesterone	5 mg day 14-28	
Prempro 2.5, 5		
conjugated equine estrogens	.625 mg	daily
with medroxyprogesterone	2.5 or 5 mg	
Ethinyl estradiol 5 ug with norethindrone 1 mg (FemHRT)		daily
Estradiol 1 mg with norethindrone .5 mg (Activella)		daily
Estradiol 1 mg qd for 3 days, followed by estradiol 1 mg with		
norgestimate .09 mg for 3 days (Ortho Prefest)		daily
Esterified estrogens .625 mg with methyltestosterone 1.25 mg		daily
(Estratest HS)		
Transdermal		
Transdermal estradiol .5 mg		
with norethindrone, .14 or .25 mg (Combipatch)		twice weekly

BOX 48-3
BOX 48-3
Contraindications to Hormone Replacement Therapy

Absolute Contraindications
Known or suspected breast or uterine cancer
Active liver disease
Active thrombophlebitis or thromboembolic disorders

Relative Contraindications
Chronic hepatic dysfunction
Family history of breast cancer

BOX 48-4
Monitoring Hormone Replacement Therapy

Regimen	Indication for Endometrial Biopsy
Cyclic estrogen and progestin	Irregular bleeding (before day 6 of progestin)
Continuous estrogen and progestin	Heavy or prolonged bleeding Persistent bleeding after 6 months of therapy

Contraindications to postmenopausal estrogen use (Box 48-3) include a history of estrogen-dependent neoplasia (breast and endometrial cancer) or active liver disease. A history of thromboembolic event is considered to be a relative contraindication to estrogen use. If estrogen is used in this setting, transdermal estrogens should be considered, because of the lack of first-pass hepatic metabolism.

Use of **vaginal estrogen** is an alternative regimen in women with symptomatic genitourinary atrophy who are not candidates for systemic estrogens. A commonly used regimen is conjugated equine estrogen (Premarin) cream, one half to one applicator daily for 3 weeks, followed by one half applicator once or twice weekly. Progestins are not generally used with this dosing regimen; however, a serum estradiol level greater than 30 pg/ml during vaginal estrogen therapy warrants endometrial monitoring as for unopposed oral estrogens. Other available forms of vaginal estrogen therapy include a vaginal estradiol tablet and an estrogen-impregnated silicone ring (Estring) (Table 48-2). The latter has no detectable effect on serum estradiol levels within 48 hours of insertion and may be appropriate for women with contraindications to systemic estrogen who require treatment for vaginal atrophy.

Monitoring Therapy

When assessing response to treatment in a symptomatic patient, there is no reliable parameter to follow aside from symptom relief. It takes up to 3 to 4 weeks for patients to have complete relief of hot flushes. Therefore there is no role for increasing the dose before that time. Measuring serum FSH levels in general is not a useful way to monitor estrogen replacement, as extremely high doses of estrogen are necessary to suppress the FSH level into the premenopausal range. Estradiol level measurements are also not helpful in most instances, although persistent hot flushes with a serum estradiol level less than 20 pg/ml may suggest noncompliance. However, persistent flushes with an estradiol level greater than 150 pg/ml suggest another cause of the flushes.

Pelvic and breast examinations, as well as mammography, should be performed at baseline and at yearly intervals during HRT. Endometrial biopsies should be performed before treatment and annually while on treatment for women on unopposed estrogen because of the known increased risk of endometrial hyperplasia and carcinoma. It is now agreed that pretreatment biopsy is not necessary for women on combined hormone regimens, as these regimens have not

been associated with an increased risk of endometrial cancer. The American College of Obstetricians and Gynecologists (ACOG) has recommended that for the cyclic regimens biopsy should be performed if bleeding begins before the sixth day of progestin. For those on continuous regimens, biopsy recommendations are somewhat vague. However, most would agree that biopsy should be performed for heavy or prolonged bleeding, or bleeding that persists beyond the sixth month of therapy (Box 48-4).

Alternatives to Hormone Replacement Therapy for Menopausal Symptoms

Some women with menopausal symptoms are unable to have estrogen replacement because of other conditions, most commonly, breast cancer. Others prefer to use nonhormonal means of coping with symptoms such as hot flashes that may be bothersome but are self-limited.

A variety of **nonpharmacologic methods** of minimizing hot flashes are in common use, but have been little studied. Some of these methods involve avoidance of factors thought to precipitate hot flashes, including stress, hot weather or warm rooms, hot drinks, alcohol, caffeine, and spicy foods. Paced deep breathing, biofeedback, and other relaxation techniques have shown some evidence of effectiveness in controlled studies.

Alternative drug therapies for hot flashes when estrogen is not suitable include venlafaxine 75 mg, paroxetine 20 mg, clonidine (0.1 mg twice daily), and medroxyprogesterone acetate (Provera) 10 to 20 mg daily. Vaginal lubricants (such as Replens) are helpful for some women with symptomatic genitourinary atrophy.

BIBLIOGRAPHY

Barrett Connor E, Kritz-Silverstein D: Estrogen replacement therapy and cognitive function in older women, *JAMA* 269:2637, 1993.

Col NF et al: Patient-specific decisions about hormone replacement therapy in postmenopausal women, *JAMA* 277:1140, 1997.

Col NF et al: Individualizing therapy to prevent long-term consequences of estrogen deficiency in postmenopausal women, *Arch Intern Med* 159: 1458, 1999.

Collaborative Group on Hormonal Factors in Breast Cancer: Breast cancer and hormone replacement therapy: collaborative reanalysis of data from 51 epidemiologic studies of 52,705 women with breast cancer and 108,411 women without breast cancer, *Lancet* 350:1047, 1997.

Cushman M et al: Effect of postmenopausal hormones on inflammation-sensitive proteins: the Postmenopausal Estrogen/Progestin Interventions (PEPI) Study, *Circulation* 100:717, 1999.

Daly E et al: Risk of venous thromboembolism in users of hormone replacement therapy, *Lancet* 348: 977, 1996.

Ettinger B et al: Cyclic hormone replacement therapy using quarterly progestin, *Obstet Gynecol* 83:693, 1994.

Gapstur SM, Morrow M, Sellers TA: Hormone replacement therapy and risk of breast cancer with a favorable histology: results of the Iowa Women's Health Study, *JAMA* 281:2091, 1999.

Genant HK et al: Low-dose esterified estrogen therapy: effects on bone, plasma, estradiol concentrations, endometrium, and lipid levels, *Arch Intern Med* 157:2609, 1997.

Grady D et al. Postmenopausal hormone therapy increases risk for venous thromboembolic disease. The Heart and Estrogen/progestin Replacement Study, *Ann Intern Med* 132:689, 2000.

Grodstein F et al: Prospective study of exogenous hormones and risk of pulmonary embolism in women, *Lancet* 348: 983, 1996.

Grodstein F et al: Postmenopausal estrogen and progestin use and the risk of cardiovascular disease, *N Engl J Med* 335:453, 1996.

Grodstein F et al: Postmenopausal hormone use and risk for colorectal cancer and adenoma, *Ann Intern Med* 128:705, 1998.

Grodstein F, Newcomb PA, Stampfer MJ: Postmenopausal hormone therapy and the risk of colorectal cancer: a review and meta-analysis, *Am J Med* 106:574, 1999.

Gutthann, SP et al: Hormone replacement therapy and risk of venous thromboembolism: population based case-control study, *BMJ* 314:796, 1997.

Harlow BL, Signorello LB: Factors associated with early menopause, *Maturitas* 35:3, 2000.

Hirvonen E et al: Can progestin be limited to every third month only in postmenopausal women taking estrogen? *Maturitas* 21:39, 1995.

Hulley S et al for the Heart and Estrogen/progestin Replacement Study (HERS) Research Group: Randomized trial of estrogen plus progestin for secondary prevention of coronary heart disease in postmenopausal women, *JAMA* 280:605, 1998.

Jick H et al: Risk of hospital admission for idiopathic venous thromboembolism among users of postmenopausal oestrogens, *Lancet* 348:981, 1996.

Loprinzi CL et al: Pilot evaluation of venlafaxine hydrochloride for the therapy of hot flashes in cancer survivors, *J Clin Oncol* 16:2377,1998.

Lowe, G et al: Thrombotic variables and risk of idiopathic venous thromboembolism in women aged 45–64 years. Relationships to hormone replacement therapy, *Thromb Haemost* 84:530, 2000.

Mendelsohn ME, Karas RH: The protective effects of estrogen on the cardiovascular system, *N Engl J Med* 340:1801, 1999.

Mulnard RA et al: Estrogen replacement therapy for treatment of mild to moderate Alzheimer disease: a randomized controlled trial. Alzheimer's Disease Cooperative Study, *JAMA* 283:1007, 2000.

Pike MC et al: Estrogen-progestin replacement therapy and endometrial cancer, *J Natl Cancer Inst* 89:1110, 1997.

Recker RR, Davies M, Dowd RM, Heaney RP: The effect of low-dose continuous estrogen and progesterone therapy with calcium and vitamin D on bone in elderly women. A randomized, controlled trial, *Ann Intern Med* 130:897, 1999.

Ross RK, Paganini-Hill A, Wan PC, Pike MC: Effect of hormone replacement therapy on breast cancer risk: estrogen versus estrogen plus progestin, *J Natl Cancer Inst* 92:328, 2000.

Santen RJ, Petroni GR: Relative versus attributable risk of breast cancer from estrogen replacement therapy, *J Clin Endocrinol Metab* 84:1875, 1999.

Schairer C et al: Menopausal estrogen and estrogen-progestin replacement therapy and breast cancer risk, *JAMA* 283:485, 2000.

Shlipak MG et al: Estrogen and progestin, lipoprotein(a), and the risk of recurrent coronary heart disease events after menopause, *JAMA* 283:1845, 2000.

Weiderpass E et al: Risk of endometrial cancer following estrogen replacement with and without progestins, *J Natl Cancer Inst* 91:1131, 1999.

Whiteman MK et al: Low fibrinogen level: a predisposing factor for venous thromboembolic events with hormone replacement therapy, *Am J Hematol* 61:271, 1999.

The Writing Group for the PEPI Trial: Effects of estrogen or estrogen/progestin regimens on heart disease risk factors in postmenopausal women, *JAMA* 273:199, 1995.

Yaffe K et al: Estrogen therapy in postmenopausal women. Effects on cognitive function and dementia, *JAMA* 279:688, 1998.

CHAPTER 49

Pelvic Masses

Karen J. Carlson
Isaac Schiff

Evaluation of a pelvic mass by the primary care physician is required when an asymptomatic mass is detected during a routine pelvic examination or when a woman bothered by pelvic pain or other symptoms is found to have a mass on examination or imaging study. In either case the initial diagnostic priorities are to identify disorders that require urgent intervention (e.g., ectopic pregnancy) and to determine whether a malignant condition is present. The diagnostic approach is based on clinical data and noninvasive imaging studies, particularly the use of ultrasonography.

This chapter outlines the approach to evaluation of a pelvic mass by the primary care clinician. Evaluation of pelvic pain, sometimes accompanied by a pelvic mass, is discussed in detail in Chapter 55.

▦ EPIDEMIOLOGY

Pelvic masses may arise from the uterus, ovaries, fallopian tubes, bowel, peritoneum, or urinary tract (Box 49-1). The prevalence of benign and malignant masses varies according to age and menopausal status.

In women of **reproductive age,** one of the most common causes of an adnexal mass is a **functional ovarian cyst.** Such cysts may arise from the follicle or corpus luteum and sometimes are associated with pelvic pain. A dominant follicle often measures close to 2 cm in diameter before ovulation. Follicular cysts appear purely cystic on ultrasound; corpus luteum cysts may have a complex component. Functional ovarian cysts generally regress during the course of one or more menstrual cycles. Aside from use of the oral contraceptive pill, which is clearly protective, other factors affecting risk of cyst formation have not been defined.

An **ectopic pregnancy** is a less common but important diagnosis to consider in a reproductive-age woman with a pelvic mass presenting in the primary care setting. Bleeding and abdominal pain may not necessarily be present. A **tubo-ovarian abscess** is another critical diagnosis that sometimes presents as a pelvic mass, generally accompanied by pelvic pain, fever, and other signs of inflammation.

An **endometrioma** may sometimes manifest as a pelvic mass in the premenopausal woman, often accompanied by a history of dysmenorrhea and pelvic pain. An endometrioma

typically appears as a complex mass on ultrasound. Uterine **leiomyomas** may also present as a pelvic mass, most commonly with an enlarged irregular uterus but occasionally as an adnexal mass that is complex on ultrasound.

Ovarian cystadenomas are benign epithelial tumors that have been reported to undergo malignant transformation. Women with a family history of ovarian cancer have been found to have a higher prevalence of serous cystadenomas than do women without such a history. The probability of malignant transformation is unknown.

In **postmenopausal women, ovarian cancer** is a more common cause of a pelvic mass (Table 49-1). In published case series of postmenopausal women with adnexal masses who have undergone laparotomy, the prevalence of ovarian cancer has ranged from 30% to 60%. The annual incidence of ovarian cancer increases with age from approximately 20 per 100,000 in women younger than 50 years of age to 40 per 100,000 in women older than 50 years of age. The mean age at clinical presentation of ovarian cancer is 59 years. The strongest risk factor for ovarian cancer aside from age is a family history of the disease, but most cases of ovarian cancer occur in women without such a history.

The **postmenopausal enlarged ovary** is encountered with increasing frequency as use of diagnostic ultrasonography has expanded. The traditional teaching has been that a palpable ovary in a postmenopausal woman indicates a pathologic condition and requires further evaluation. However, it is now appreciated that the postmenopausal ovary is not totally quiescent and that benign ovarian cysts do occur in postmenopausal women.

◪ EVALUATION

History

The history focuses on assessment of reproductive factors, symptoms, and (particularly when the mass is adnexal) risk factors for ovarian cancer (Box 49-2). The first priority is to identify an acute process that requires urgent intervention, including ectopic pregnancy, pelvic inflammatory disease, ovarian torsion, or appendicitis.

A careful menstrual history is essential, including the date of the last and previous menstrual periods, sexual history, and use of contraception. Risk factors for pelvic inflammatory

BOX 49-1
Differential Diagnosis of Pelvic Masses

Benign
Ovarian
Simple cyst (follicle or corpus luteum)
Hemorrhagic cyst
Cystadenoma
Endometrioma
Teratoma
Other benign tumors: papilloma, fibroma
Nonovarian
Leiomyoma
Paraovarian cyst
Hydrosalpinx
Tubo-ovarian abscess
Ectopic pregnancy
Intrauterine pregnancy
Diverticulitis
Appendiceal abscess
Peritoneal inclusion cyst

Malignant
Ovarian
Epithelial ovarian carcinoma
Germ cell tumors of the ovary
Borderline tumors
Nonovarian
Leiomyosarcoma
Endometrial cancer
Carcinoma of fallopian tube
Colorectal carcinoma

Table 49-1
Risk Factors for Ovarian Cancer

Factor	Relative Risk
Age 50 yr	2
Familial ovarian cancer syndrome	Unknown; 20% to 60% lifetime risk
One first- or second-degree relative with ovarian cancer	3
Two or three relatives with ovarian cancer	5
Oral contraceptive pill use	0.65
Pregnancy	0.5

Modified from Carlson KJ, Skates SJ, Singer DE: *Ann Intern Med* 121:124, 1994.

BOX 49-2
Evaluation of Pelvic Mass

History
Reproductive factors
Menopausal status
Menstrual history
Sexual history: risk for pregnancy, pelvic inflammatory disease (PID)
Contraceptive use
Symptoms
Pelvic pain or discomfort
Bleeding
Gastrointestinal or urinary symptoms
Systemic symptoms: fever, weight loss, anorexia

Physical Examination
Vital Signs
Pelvic mass: size, shape, consistency, mobility, tenderness
Cervical, uterine tenderness; cervical discharge; bleeding
Abdominal and rectal examination

Diagnostic Tests
Complete blood count, differential
Serum beta-human chorionic gonadotropin (*b*-hCG)
Erythrocyte sedimentation rate (ESR)
Serum CA125 radioimmunoassay
Pelvic ultrasound

disease, such as previous sexually transmitted disease, also should be determined. The diagnosis of ectopic pregnancy and pelvic infection is discussed in more detail in Chapter 55.

Symptoms of pelvic pain or discomfort, abnormal vaginal bleeding, and gastrointestinal problems should be sought. The relationship of the symptoms to the menstrual cycle and other precipitating factors may provide useful clues. Women with ovarian torsion may report sudden onset of pain, sometimes with nausea and vomiting. Women with ovarian cancer may experience abdominal swelling or bloat-ing, nonspecific gastrointestinal complaints, and loss of appetite or weight loss.

Physical Examination

Differentiation of uterine enlargement and adnexal masses is the first step in the physical examination. Uterine enlargement is caused most commonly by uterine leiomyomas, adenomyosis, or intrauterine pregnancy. The characteristics of the pelvic mass should be noted, as well as the presence of other abnormalities (such as cervical or uterine tenderness, cervical discharge, or bleeding).

Diagnostic Tests

Pelvic ultrasonography is the single most important test in the evaluation of a pelvic mass. Ultrasound can differentiate a uterine from an adnexal mass, determine ovarian size and morphology, localize an ectopic pregnancy, identify extra-ovarian disease, and provide a preliminary assessment of the likelihood of malignancy in an ovarian mass. Transabdominal ultrasonography is helpful for identifying other abdominal process; transvaginal sonography provides better visualization of pelvic structures.

Several scoring systems having been developed to predict malignancy according to the characteristics of ovarian masses. Although there is no universally accepted system for classification according to the likelihood of malignancy, existing systems generally incorporate some combination of ovarian size, inner wall structure, wall thickness, presence of septation, and echogenicity (Table 49-2). In a premenopausal woman, a follicular cyst or other benign ovarian process can cause ovarian enlargement up to 10 cm. In a postmenopausal women, an ovarian diameter above 3 cm is considered abnormal.

Other imaging studies are sometimes appropriate. **Color-flow Doppler** techniques to detect tumor neovascularization improve the specificity of ultrasound. A recent meta-analytic review of imaging techniques for ovarian masses found that the combination of transvaginal gray scale ultrasound with color-flow Doppler imaging performed best for diagnosis of malignancy. **Computed tomography** and **magnetic resonance imaging** are used to define the anatomic features of pelvic masses and assess for lymphadenopathy before surgery.

The use of other diagnostic tests in the initial evaluation should be guided by the results of the history and physical examination. In any woman of reproductive age, a serum human chorionic gonadotropin level (beta-hCG) should be obtained, even if the possibility of pregnancy seems remote. A complete blood count with differential and an erythrocyte sedimentation rate are useful in assessing the possibility

of hemorrhage (as from a ruptured ectopic pregnancy) or infection.

The **CA125 radioimmunoassay** (CA125) is an important aid in the diagnosis of adnexal masses. CA125 is an antigenic determinant that is expressed by tissues derived from coelomic epithelium. It is shed in the blood by malignant cells arising from coelomic epithelium, and it is elevated in approximately 80% of ovarian cancers and advanced endometrial cancers, as well as in some pancreatic cancers and other solid tumors. CA125 is also elevated in women with certain benign gynecologic conditions, including endometriosis, uterine leiomyoma, pelvic inflammatory disease, early pregnancy, and benign ovarian cysts. Serum levels have been shown to fluctuate during the menstrual cycle. The normal level generally is set at less than 35 U/ml.

In premenopausal women, CA125 measurement has not been found to improve the diagnostic accuracy of ultrasound. A reasonable approach is to obtain a serum CA125 level if the ultrasonographic appearance of an adnexal mass is equivocal or if a benign-appearing cyst (particularly if larger than 4 cm) does not resolve during the course of one or two menstrual cycles, bearing in mind that endometriomas and uterine leiomyoma, as well as ovarian malignancies, can be associated with elevated CA125 levels.

In postmenopausal women, in whom the probability of ovarian cancer is considerably greater, a serum CA125 level should be obtained at the outset of the evaluation. On the basis of the published operating characteristics of serum CA125 (sensitivity 80%, specificity greater than 95%) in postmenopausal women with adnexal masses, obtaining an abnormal serum CA125 result shifts the estimated probability of malignancy from approximately 40% to more than 80%.

Table 49-2
Ultrasonographic Features of an Ovarian Mass* and Probability of Malignancy

| Feature | PROBABILITY OF MALIGNANCY | |
	Low	High
Inner wall	Smooth	Papillary
Wall thickness	Thin (<3 mm)	Thick (>3 mm)
Septation	None	Multiple
Echogenicity	Cystic (lucent)	Solid (echogenic)

*Normal ovarian volume: 7.5 cm³; enlarged ovary: 10 cm³.

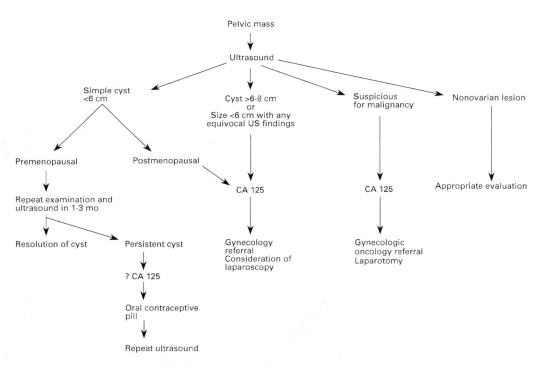

FIG. 49-1 Approach to the patient with a pelvic mass.

APPROACH TO THE PATIENT WITH A PELVIC MASS

The approach to the woman with a pelvic mass is guided by the patient's age and reproductive status, presenting complaints, and the results of history and physical examination. If the clinical findings are not suggestive of a process that requires urgent intervention (such as ectopic pregnancy, ovarian torsion, or abscess), the first step generally is to obtain an ultrasonogram of the pelvis (Fig. 49-1).

For a **premenopausal** woman with an ultrasound finding that indicates a simple cyst (less than 6 cm in diameter), it is appropriate for the primary care physician to repeat the physical and ultrasound examination in 1 to 3 months to assess resolution. Seventy percent of simple cysts will resolve in this interval. When the cyst persists (but has not grown), a trial of the oral contraceptive pill may promote resolution and prevent recurrence. A complex or solid mass on ultrasound, a simple cyst greater than 6 cm, or a simple cyst that does not resolve within 3 cycles should prompt referral to a gynecologist.

In a **postmenopausal woman** with a simple cyst less than 3 cm that has entirely benign ultrasonographic characteristics, a serum CA125 level should be obtained and gynecologic consultation arranged. Such women are often followed with serial ultrasound and CA125 measurement. Based on published observational studies, conservative management may also be appropriate when a simple cyst is 4 to 6 cm and CA125 level is normal. A simple cyst greater than 6 cm or a nonsimple cyst warrants consideration of laparoscopy. Finally, if a complex mass is present or the serum CA125 is elevated in a postmenopausal woman, referral directly to a gynecologic oncologist is appropriate.

BIBLIOGRAPHY

Aubert JM, Rombaut C, Argacha P: Simple adnexal cysts in postmenopausal women: conservative management, *Maturitas* 30:51, 1998.

Bailey CL et al: The malignant potential of small cystic ovarian tumors in women over 50 years of age, *Gynecol Oncol* 69:3, 1998.

Carlson KJ, Skates SJ, Singer DE: Screening for ovarian cancer, *Ann Intern Med* 121:124, 1994.

Finkler NJ et al: Comparison of serum CA125, clinical impression, and ultrasound in the preoperative evaluation of ovarian masses, *Obstet Gynecol* 72:659, 1988.

Grimes DA et al: Ovulation and follicular development associated with three low-dose oral contraceptives, *Obstet Gynecol* 83:29, 1994.

Kinkel K et al: Ultrasound characterization of ovarian masses: a meta-analysis, *Radiology* 217:803, 2000.

Luxman D et al: The postmenopausal adnexal mass: correlation between ultrasonic and pathologic findings, *Obstet Gynecol* 77:726, 1991.

Malkasian GD Jr et al: Preoperative evaluation of serum CA 125 levels in premenopausal and postmenopausal patients with pelvic masses: discrimination of benign from malignant disease, *Am J Obstet Gynecol* 159:341, 1988.

Parker WH, Berek JS: Management of the adnexal mass by operative laparoscopy, *Clin Obstet Gynecol* 36:413, 1993.

Roman LD et al: Pelvic examination, tumor marker level, and gray-scale and Doppler sonography in the prediction of pelvic cancer, *Obstet Gynecol* 89:493, 1997.

Russell DJ: The female pelvic mass. Diagnosis and management. *Med Clin North Am* 79:1481, 1995.

CHAPTER 50

Uterine Fibroids

Andrew J. Friedman
Karen J. Carlson

Uterine fibroids, otherwise known as myomas, fibromyomas, or leiomyomas, are the most common pelvic tumors in women. In the primary care setting, the clinician must be familiar with methods for the diagnosis of fibroids and for management of commonly associated symptoms, as well as with counseling the patient about the long-term clinical significance of newly diagnosed fibroids and about treatment choices for fibroids if symptoms become severe.

EPIDEMIOLOGY AND RISK FACTORS

It is estimated that 20% to 25% of women in the reproductive years will have fibroids that are clinically recognizable, although 40% of women will have myomas noted at autopsy. In one study where gross hysterectomy specimens were serially sectioned at 2-mm intervals, leiomyomas were detected in 77% of uteruses.

Uterine myomas most commonly are diagnosed in women between the ages of 30 and 50 years, with a peak incidence in the early 40s. These neoplasms are extremely rare before age 20. Uterine myomas are more common in African-American women than in Caucasians; annual incidence in one large prospective study was about 1% per year in white, Hispanic, and Asian women, and 3% per year in black women. Other factors associated with an increased risk of fibroids are obesity, including a significant weight gain after age 18; nulliparity; and family history. Oral contraceptive pill use and smoking have no apparent effect on risk of uterine myomas.

PATHOPHYSIOLOGY

Uterine myomas are benign neoplasms composed of smooth muscle cells and extracellular matrix (ECM). ECM consists primarily of collagen, proteoglycan, and fibronectin. The relative amounts of smooth muscle and ECM vary among fibroids, but most tumors are composed primarily of noncellular elements.

Fibroids generally are classified by their location within the uterus (Fig. 50-1). Subserosal myomas are found near the external or serosal surface of the uterus and produce a noticeable distortion of the external uterine contour. These tumors usually are easily palpated on bimanual examination, espe-cially when they are large. Intramural leiomyomas are located within the myometrium. Submucosal myomas are located near the endometrium and project into the uterine cavity. Most tumors span more than a single anatomic location. For example, a subserosal fibroid may have a significant intramural component. Only small intramural fibroids and those that are pedunculated in subserosal and submucosal locations may be classified as purely one fibroid subtype.

Uterine leiomyomas are believed to be monoclonal tumors resulting from somatic mutations in myocytes. Cytogenetic studies and analyses of X-linked glucose-6-phosphate dehydrogenase isoforms support the concept of leiomyomas as monoclonal tumors. The factor(s) responsible for the neoplastic transformation of myometrial cells are not known.

There is a growing body of evidence to suggest that an estrogenic milieu is necessary for the expression of this mutation and for the subsequent growth of these tumors, and some evidence that uterine myomas are more sensitive to estrogen than normal myometrium. Uterine fibroids are not seen in prepubertal girls, and myoma regression is noted in women after menopause. In addition, a number of in vitro experiments suggest that the intramyoma environment is relatively hyperestrogenic compared with adjacent myometrium. Treatment of women with gonadotropin-releasing hormone agonist (GnRH-a) will result in profound hypoestrogenemia, which, in turn, will lead to significant reductions in uterine and myoma size. It is not clear whether estrogen exerts its effects on these tumors directly or through growth factors such as epidermal growth factor, insulin-like growth factor-I, or platelet-derived growth factor. Finally, the role of other hormones such as progesterone, prolactin, and growth hormone in the pathogenesis of myomas is unclear.

Malignant leiomyosarcomas are present in 0.1% to 0.3% of cases of suspected uterine fibroids. Differences in karyotypic abnormalities between fibroids and leiomyosarcomas suggest that the latter arise from a distinct tumor precursor cell, rather than from degeneration of a benign fibroid. Leiomyosarcomas are not steroid sensitive and are characterized by a high mitotic index and cellular pleomorphism. These malignancies are rarely seen before age 40. The incidence of leiomyosarcomas increases with advancing age.

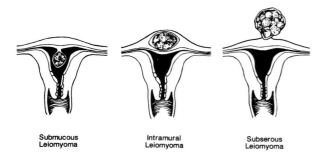

Submucous
Leiomyoma

Intramural
Leiomyoma

Subserous
Leiomyoma

FIG. 50-1 Leiomyomas classified according to their location in the uterus. (From Muto M, Friedman AJ: The uterine corpus. In Ryan KJ, Berkowitz RS, Barbieri RL, editors: *Kistner's gynecology: principles and practice,* ed 6, St Louis, 1995, Mosby.)

APPROACH TO THE PATIENT WITH SUSPECTED FIBROIDS

History and Symptoms

It is estimated that 20% to 50% of women with clinically recognizable fibroids have symptoms caused by these tumors. The presence of symptoms is dependent on the number, size, and location of these tumors. Approximately 30% of women with leiomyomas have **excessive uterine bleeding** (i.e., menorrhagia, hypermenorrhea), which is most common in women with intramural or submucous tumors. Intermenstrual bleeding is not typical of fibroids. Another 30% of women with leiomyomas have noncyclic **pelvic pain** produced by direct pressure on adjacent pelvic structures or acute myoma degeneration. Pelvic pressure, urinary frequency, and, rarely, constipation may result when subserosal or intramural tumors enlarge and press on adjacent pelvic organs. Rarely, acute pain may occur after degeneration or torsion of a pedunculated fibroid.

Reproductive dysfunction (e.g., infertility; spontaneous pregnancy loss; problems during pregnancy, labor, and delivery) is rarely caused by fibroids. Although myomas are present in 5% to 10% of infertile women, only 2% to 3% of infertile women have no other identifiable cause of infertility. Spontaneous pregnancy loss, abruption, and premature labor may be more common when the placenta implants on or near a submucous or intramural myoma.

It commonly is assumed that fibroids enlarge during pregnancy under the influence of increased circulating levels of estrogens. However, when serial sonographic measurements of fibroids are performed throughout pregnancy, some tumors are noted to grow, some remain unchanged, and some actually decrease in size. In general, if fibroids increase in size during pregnancy, most of the growth occurs in the first trimester. Occasionally rapid growth of fibroids during pregnancy may lead to acute degeneration of the tumor(s). When this occurs the woman often experiences severe pain and tenderness on palpation of the fibroid, and she may require narcotics for analgesia. Occasionally fibroid degeneration may precipitate premature labor.

Physical Examination and Differential Diagnosis

Uterine fibroids are usually first suspected at the bimanual examination that reveals an enlarged, often irregular uterus.

BOX 50-1

Differential Diagnosis of an Enlarged Pelvic Mass and Excessive Menstrual Flow

Enlarged Pelvic Mass
Benign
Pregnancy
Uterine myoma
Adenomyosis
Ovarian cyst/benign neoplasm/endometrioma
Hydrosalpinx
Diverticulitis
Pelvic abscess
Malignant
Uterine sarcoma
Ovarian carcinoma
Tubal carcinoma
Gastrointestinal carcinoma

Excessive Menstrual Flow
Uterine myoma
Adenomyosis
Coagulopathy (i.e., von Willebrand's disease, leukemia)
Aplastic anemia
Uterine malignancy
Cervical carcinoma
Dysfunctional uterine bleeding

Other gynecologic and nongynecologic disorders may give rise to an enlarged pelvic mass and to symptoms often attributed to myomas (Box 50-1).

Diagnostic Tests

Pelvic ultrasonography will confirm that the enlarged pelvic mass is of uterine origin and may allow discrete tumors to be visualized within the uterus, thus further supporting the presumed diagnosis of uterine myomas. **Magnetic resonance imaging** (MRI) will provide better resolution of the tumors as well as an improved ability to assess the ovaries, but it is rarely necessary, as ultrasonography usually provides adequate images and is far less expensive. MRI is more sensitive for differentiating fibroids and adenomyosis. If the clinical presentation suggests the possibility of a uterine malignancy (e.g., rapidly enlarging uterus and abnormal uterine bleeding in a postmenopausal woman), the physician should attempt to obtain a tissue specimen for further diagnosis. An outpatient endometrial biopsy may suffice to diagnose the cause of abnormal uterine bleeding; occasionally hysteroscopy with a directed biopsy is useful. A total abdominal hysterectomy plus bilateral salpingo-oophorectomy is appropriate treatment for a rapidly enlarging uterine mass in a postmenopausal woman; the incidence of sarcoma in such cases is 1% to 2%.

MANAGEMENT

Treatment options for women with uterine myomas have expanded over the last 20 years. In the past it was recommended that most women with symptomatic myomas or uterine size of 12 gestational weeks regardless of symptoms have hysterectomies; myomectomy, or removal of the tumor(s) with uterine reconstruction, was recommended only in women below age 40 who were interested in future childbearing. Clearly the acute relief of myoma-related symptoms, correction of anemia, and ruling out of uterine malignancy are the main goals of surgical or medical treatment. But first the physician must decide whether medical or surgical treatment is necessary.

The presence of an enlarged fibroid uterus that is not growing rapidly and is causing minor or no symptoms generally does not warrant treatment. When the patient's quality of life is not impaired and the likelihood that the pelvic mass is malignant is remote, close observation rather than intervention is preferable.

When a woman has bleeding symptoms and evidence of fibroids on examination, the possibility that bleeding may be caused by a coexisting condition, such as endometrial hyperplasia or cancer or an endometrial polyp, should be borne in mind. In women over 40 and in younger women with risk factors for endometrial cancer (such as obesity or chronic anovulation), an endometrial biopsy, as well as transvaginal ultrasound, should be performed before initiation of therapy for bleeding symptoms presumed due to fibroids.

In cases where intervention is necessary to treat moderate to severe myoma-related symptoms, the patient's goals of treatment should be explored in detail before embarking on a particular therapy, considering **symptom severity, childbearing plans,** and **proximity to menopause.** For some women preservation of the uterus for future childbearing or for nonreproductive reasons may be so important that they are willing to risk tumor recurrence or continued myoma-related symptoms. Others may wish to eradicate symptoms permanently and are less concerned about organ preservation. To decide the best way to proceed, the treatment goals of the physician and patient must be fully understood and discussed.

Choice of Therapy

Observation

The patient with an enlarged uterus that is not growing or slowly growing and is causing minor or no symptoms may be treated by close observation in many cases. A repeat outpatient visit is advisable 3 to 6 months after the original discovery of uterine myomas to assess whether the uterus and tumors have enlarged and symptoms have worsened. If there is no rapid increase of uterine size or symptoms, office visits may be made annually. Routine monitoring with pelvic ultrasonography is not recommended, but may sometimes be helpful for measurement of the uterus and myomas and assessment of ovarian size and architecture. If the severity of myoma-related symptoms worsens or the physician's suspicion of malignancy increases, imaging studies should be obtained.

The incidence of uterine sarcomas increases with each decade of life; these tumors may grow rapidly or slowly and may range in size at diagnosis from less than 6 gestational weeks to more than 20 weeks. Abnormal uterine bleeding may occur in women with leiomyosarcomas. However, endometrial biopsy or uterine curettage, which reliably leads to the diagnosis of endometrial adenocarcinoma, rarely yields the diagnosis of leiomyosarcoma. For these reasons the correct preoperative diagnosis of leiomyosarcoma is uncommon. The presence of an enlarging uterus with or without abnormal uterine bleeding in a postmenopausal woman should be viewed with great concern, and a tissue diagnosis should be obtained as rapidly as possible.

Medical Management

The general strategy behind the medical management of myomas consists of hormonal treatment directed at temporarily decreasing myoma and uterine size and menstrual blood flow. **Gonadotropic-releasing hormone (GnRH) agonists** are approved by the U.S. Food and Drug Administration for treatment of anemia in women with uterine fibroids before myomectomy or hysterectomy; they are sometimes used more broadly in clinical practice for short-term amelioration of menorrhagia caused by fibroids. By dramatically decreasing bioactive gonadotropin secretion by the pituitary, GnRH agonist therapy results in a hypogonadal state clinically resembling menopause. GnRH agonists are effective for symptom relief, but their use is limited by side effects of estrogen deficiency, and symptoms rapidly recur after discontinuation of therapy. These factors limit their utility in younger women with fibroids, but short-term use of GnRH agonists may play a role in alleviating symptoms in women nearing menopause, allowing them to avoid surgery. GnRH agonists are also used for 3 to 6 months as preoperative therapy to restore hemoglobin concentrations to normal; to decrease myoma and uterine size, which may facilitate vaginal rather than abdominal hysterectomy; and to create an atrophic endometrium, which will facilitate hysteroscopic surgery. Commonly used doses of GnRH agonists are shown in Table 50-1.

Myomas decrease in volume by 40% to 60% during treatment with a GnRH agonist for 3 to 6 months. Treatment with a GnRH agonist also results in amenorrhea in two thirds of women; the majority of the remaining women experience light irregular spotting. The decrease in menstrual bleeding results in dramatic improvements in hemoglobin concentrations in women with menorrhagia-associated anemia. Once GnRH agonist treatment is discontinued, however, uterine and myoma regrowth with return of pretreatment symptoms are usually noted within 3 to 6 months.

Vasomotor flushes occur in approximately 90% of women receiving GnRH agonists; 25% to 40% experience insomnia and symptoms of vaginal atrophy. GnRH agonist therapy for 6 months will also induce an average decrease in lumbar trabecular bone density of 6%, which is only partially reversible by discontinuation of treatment. **Add-back**

Table 50-1
Commonly Used GnRH-a in Clinical Practice*

Name	Dose
Leuprolide acetate (Lupron depot)	3.75 mg IM q4wk
Nafarelin acetate (Synarel)	1-2 whiffs (200-400 mg) intranasally twice each day
Goserelin acetate (Zoladex)	3.6 mg SC q4wk

*First dose usually administered cycle days 1-3 or in the middle to late luteal phase if the patient is known not to be pregnant.

therapy combined with a GnRH agonist is designed to restore sufficient estrogen to preserve bone and prevent other hypoestrogenic side effects, while preventing fibroid growth. There is growing evidence that use of low-dose estrogen replacement therapy (0.625 mg of conjugated equine estrogens or the equivalent) with a progestin prevents vasomotor symptoms and bone loss associated with GnRH agonists, as well as preventing excessive bleeding and fibroid growth.

Other hormonal treatments such as **danazol** or **low-dose oral contraceptives** may control excessive menstrual blood loss but will not reliably decrease uterine or myoma size. **Mifepristone (RU486),** an anti-progestin, shows promise as a hormonal therapy for fibroids. It appears to reduce uterine volume and bleeding while maintaining follicular phase levels of estrogen, which may minimize the adverse impact on bone density.

Nonsteroidal antiinflammatory drugs (NSAIDs) may reduce pelvic pain associated with fibroids, but do not reduce excessive bleeding caused by fibroids. Use of oral **iron supplements** (e.g., ferrous gluconate or ferrous sulfate 325 mg one to three times daily) may help to increase hemoglobin concentrations in women with menorrhagia-associated anemia.

Surgical Management

Myomectomy. Uterine myomectomy—surgical removal of myomas with subsequent uterine reconstruction—may be performed if the woman wishes to preserve her uterus for any reason. Myomectomies are most commonly performed through laparotomy; blood loss, complication rates, and hospital stays are similar to those occurring after abdominal hysterectomy.

Hysteroscopic myomectomy is an alternative procedure for women with submucous myomas that cause excessive uterine bleeding or reproductive dysfunction. The advantages of hysteroscopic myomectomy are considerable, since it is a same-day surgical procedure and requires 2 to 3 weeks for recovery, compared with 6 weeks for open myomectomy. Endometrial ablation can be performed concurrently in women who do not wish to preserve fertility and may further reduce menorrhagia.

Laparoscopic myomectomy is sometimes an alternative when there are a limited number of subserosal or intramural fibroids in a uterus 16 weeks size or smaller. Indications for laparoscopic myomectomy are evolving, with controversy about the potential for uterine rupture during a subsequent pregnancy.

Myomectomies are usually successful in alleviating preoperative symptoms. In a large retrospective series, 81% of women with menorrhagia had a significant decrease in menstrual flow after myomectomy; these findings have been confirmed by prospective studies. In addition, most women who have symptoms attributable to an enlarged pelvic mass experience resolution of these complaints after myomectomy.

The risk of recurrence of myomas is the major limitation of myomectomy. Clinically manifest myomas develop in 15% to 30% of women 5 years after myomectomy, and more than half will have ultrasonographic evidence of fibroids. The risk of recurrence is correlated positively with the numbers of myomas resected, not with myoma size.

Pregnancy and Myomectomy. A critical question for women with fibroids who are contemplating pregnancy is whether to undergo myomectomy before attempting conception. Myomectomy is often performed to preserve reproductive potential, yet only about 40% of women conceive after this operation. Postoperative adhesion formation involving the fallopian tubes or ovaries, or both, may render a woman infertile. A woman must be counseled about these risks before selecting a surgical treatment plan. Cesarean section is often recommended in women who conceive after myomectomy in which the uterine cavity was entered or extensive myometrial dissection was performed. Although the risk of uterine rupture during spontaneous labor in women who have previously undergone myomectomy is 1%, this recommendation is still made because of the potential catastrophic consequences to the mother and her baby, especially if rupture occurs outside a hospital setting.

There are also risks of not removing myomas in women who wish to conceive. It is estimated that 10% to 15% of women with infertility have myomas and that myomas are the primary cause of infertility in 2% to 3% of all infertile women. Women with myomas who conceive are at higher risk of having a spontaneous pregnancy loss than those without myomas. The incidence of spontaneous pregnancy losses in a large series of women undergoing myomectomy decreased from 41% preoperatively to 19% after this procedure. Uterine fibroids are also associated with higher rates of adverse pregnancy outcomes, including abruption, dysfunctional labor, and postpartum hemorrhage. In the absence of data from clinical trials, generalized treatment recommendations cannot be made about when preconception myomectomy is prudent.

During pregnancy it is generally recommended to avoid surgical treatment of symptomatic or asymptomatic uterine fibroids. Uterine blood flow is greatly increased during pregnancy; and myomectomy may result in significant blood loss, uterine irritability, premature labor, or infection and may jeopardize the fetus. In rare cases pedunculated subserosal fibroids with thin pedicles may undergo torsion leading to severe, unrelenting abdominal pain. In these cases myomectomy may be performed safely during pregnancy.

Hysterectomy. Hysterectomy is the only treatment of uterine myomas that guarantees a cure of the condition. Uterine myomas constitute the single largest diagnostic category of all hysterectomies performed in the United States, accounting for 27%, or 175,000, procedures annually.

Prospective observational studies have shown that hysterectomy is effective for relief of multiple symptoms related to fibroids, resulting in significant improvement in quality of life in women with moderate to severe symptoms before surgery. Hysterectomy permanently abolishes bleeding, and observational studies indicate that a variety of other symptoms (pelvic pain, dyspareunia, urinary symptoms, fatigue, and premenstrual symptoms) also improve after hysterectomy.

Abdominal hysterectomy must be viewed as a major surgical procedure requiring 4 to 8 weeks for full recovery; recovery from vaginal hysterectomy is shorter, typically 2 to 3 weeks. The most common postoperative complication is febrile morbidity, present in up to 32% of women. Transfusion with homologous blood is necessary in approximately

5% to 10% of cases; however, with a greater emphasis on preoperative blood donation and a greater willingness of physicians not to use transfusion for women with low hematocrits who are asymptomatic, this rate is declining. Serious postoperative complications, such as unplanned surgical procedures and pulmonary emboli, occur in 1% of women. The mortality rate of hysterectomy for all causes is 0.1% but is clearly much lower when malignant diagnoses are excluded.

Studies of long-term adverse effects of hysterectomy are limited, but do not suggest any negative effect of hysterectomy on mood, except possibly in women with a prior history of depression. Older studies of sexual function after hysterectomy have indicated improvement in the majority of women, with worsening in 15% to 25%. More recent studies of the effects of hysterectomy on sexual function have found that sexual functioning improves overall, with decreased dyspareunia, low libido, and anorgasmia; fewer than 5% of women develop these problems after hysterectomy. Vaginal dryness also decreases after hysterectomy overall, although about 10% of women develop this problem posthysterectomy.

Removal of the ovaries at hysterectomy is recommended only for perimenopausal or postmenopausal women and for those with ovarian abnormalities. If the ovaries are removed, estrogen replacement therapy should be considered unless contraindicated.

Innovative Treatments

Uterine Artery Embolization. Uterine artery embolization, a procedure used since the 1970s to treat postpartum hemorrhage, has recently been examined as a less invasive alternative to myomectomy for alleviating bleeding and other symptoms. Via a catheter inserted in the femoral artery, the interventional radiologist injects polyvinyl particles to occlude the blood supply to the myomas. Tumor volume shrinks by 50% or more. Case series report the procedure is moderately to completely effective in relieving menorrhagia in 85% to 90% of cases and is 70% to 90% effective in relieving pain and pressure symptoms. Complications such as infection and hematoma occur in 5%; ovarian failure has been reported in 1% to 5% of premenopausal women undergoing embolization. This investigational procedure generally requires an overnight hospital stay for pain management.

BIBLIOGRAPHY

Barbieri RL: Ambulatory management of uterine leiomyomata, *Clin Obstet Gynecol* 42:196, 1999.

Carlson KJ, Miller BA, Fowler FJ: The Maine Women's Health Study: I. Outcomes of hysterectomy, *Obstet Gynecol* 83:556, 1994.

Coronado GD, Marshall LM, Schwartz SM: Complications in pregnancy, labor, and delivery with uterine leiomyomas: a population-based study, *Obstet Gynecol* 95:764, 2000.

Cramer SF, Patel D: The frequency of uterine leiomyomas, *Am J Clin Pathol* 94:435, 1990.

Elder-Geva T et al: Effect of intramural, subserosal, and submucosal uterine fibroids on the outcome of assisted reproductive technology treatment, *Fertil Steril* 70:687, 1998.

Friedman AJ et al: Treatment of leiomyomata uteri with leuprolide acetate depot: a double-blind, placebo-controlled, multicenter study, *Obstet Gynecol* 77:720, 1991.

Friedman AJ et al: Recurrence of myomas after myomectomy in women pretreated with leuprolide acetate depot or placebo, *Fertil Steril* 58:205, 1992.

Friedman AJ, Haas ST: Should uterine size be an indication for surgical intervention in women with myomas? *Am J Obstet Gynecol* 168:751, 1993.

Hillis SD, Marchbanks PA, Peterson HB: Uterine size and risk of complications among women undergoing abdominal hysterectomy for leiomyomas, *Obstet Gynecol* 87:539,1996.

Kjerulff KH et al: Effectiveness of hysterectomy, *Obstet Gynecol* 95:319, 2000.

Leibsohn S et al: Leiomyosarcoma in a series of hysterectomies performed for presumed uterine leiomyomas, *Am J Obstet Gynecol* 162:968, 1990.

Marshall LM et al: Risk of uterine leiomyomata among premenopausal women in relation to body size and cigarette smoking, *Epidemiology* 9:511,1998.

Murphy AA et al: Regression of uterine leiomyomata in response to the antiprogesterone RU 486, *J Clin Endocrinol Metab* 76:513, 1993.

Parker WH, Fu YS, Berek JS: Uterine sarcoma in patients operated on for presumed leiomyoma and rapidly growing leiomyoma, *Obstet Gynecol* 83:414, 1994.

Reiter RC, Wagner PL, Gambone JC: Routine hysterectomy for large asymptomatic uterine leiomyomata: a reappraisal, *Obstet Gynecol* 79:481, 1992.

Rhodes JC et al: Hysterectomy and sexual functioning, *JAMA* 282:1934, 1999.

Thomas EJ: Add-back therapy for long-term use in dysfunctional uterine bleeding and uterine fibroids, *Br J Obstet Gynaecol* 103 (Suppl 14):18, 1996.

Vercellini P et al: Hysterescopic myomectomy: long-term effects on menstrual pattern and fertility, *Obstet Gynecol* 94:341,1999.

Worthington-Kirsch RL, Popky GL, Hutchins FL: Uterine arterial embolization for the management of leiomyomas:quality of life assessment and clinical response, *Radiology* 208:625, 1998.

CHAPTER 51

Vaginitis

May M. Wakamatsu

Complaints of vaginitis constitute a significant proportion of office visits to adult primary care health care providers. Recent advances in understanding disease mechanisms have refined diagnostic criteria of specific vaginal disorders. Nonetheless diagnosis and management of vaginitis, particularly recurrent or chronic vaginitis, can be frustrating and time consuming for the patient and the clinician.

Diagnosis may be difficult because the three most common vaginal disorders, bacterial vaginosis, candida vaginitis, and trichomonas vaginitis, have overlapping symptoms. Although there are "classic" symptoms and signs for each, the vaginitis may be atypical or asymptomatic.

Moreover, since vaginitis is generally not considered a serious medical problem, the diagnosis may be inaccurate because it is based on the patient's symptoms and gross examination of the vaginal discharge. Other times the initial vaginitis is diagnosed correctly, but subsequent complaints are treated as recurrences of that disorder. When treatment fails, patients are labeled as having "chronic yeast infections" or "recurrent bacterial vaginosis" without a sound basis. Ultimately both the patient and the health care provider's practice suffer.

The diagnosis of vaginitis may also be hampered by incomplete understanding of normal vaginal physiologic characteristics. Some patients believe that any discharge is abnormal; Godley demonstrated that 4 to 6 cm^2 of daily discharge is normal. Similarly, patients may notice a relative increase in vaginal discharge during and after ovulation or after discontinuation of oral contraceptives and interpret it as vaginitis. Fluctuating hormone levels during the menstrual cycle and higher endogenous estrogen levels than those associated with oral contraceptives may produce relative increases in vaginal discharge.

Educating patients about the characteristics and differences of normal and abnormal vaginal discharge can offer significant relief to the patient and prevent unnecessary phone calls and visits to the health care provider. Diagnosis may require repeated evaluations to develop a picture of the clinical problem. It is best not to presume a diagnosis but to insist that the patient seek proper evaluation, particularly in cases of treatment failure. As our understanding of the causes and pathogenesis of vaginitis and vaginosis increases, it is important to use that information methodically to diagnose and treat vaginal disorders.

This chapter will consider and contrast normal vaginal physiologic characteristics and flora with the characteristics of the vaginal disorders most diagnosed. The diagnosis and treatment of bacterial vaginosis, *Candida* vaginitis, *Trichomonas* vaginitis, atrophic vaginitis, and cytolytic vaginosis will be highlighted.

THE NORMAL VAGINA

It is important to understand that the vaginal milieu is a delicate ecosystem that is easily unbalanced by insult. The normal pH of 3.8 to 4.2 is thought to be the first line of defense against pathogenic bacteria, fungi, and protozoa and helps to maintain cornification of the vaginal epithelium. The acidic pH is predominantly maintained by the metabolism of glycogen to lactic acid in the vagina. This is accomplished primarily by the lactobacilli present in a normal vagina, but other bacteria probably contribute as well.

Besides lactobacilli, the normal vagina contains a variety of aerobic and anaerobic bacteria (Table 51-1). The types and numbers of the different bacteria are not static and have been demonstrated to fluctuate throughout a menstrual cycle. Although most of these bacteria in a normal vaginal environment are nonpathogenic, if vaginal defenses are weakened these same endogenous bacteria can participate in pelvic inflammatory disease, amnionitis during pregnancy, or vaginitis. Alteration of the normal flora may also result in the proliferation of opportunistic fungi.

Normal vaginal discharge may appear clear or white, or even flocculent, but is odorless and does not cause pruritus or irritation. Asymptomatic women average 1.6 g of discharge every 8 hours.

The tools to distinguish normal vaginal discharge from abnormal and to make the diagnosis of a vaginal disorder are not expensive or complex. Most diagnoses can be made by examining the patient, testing the pH, and examining a wet preparation of the vaginal secretions; occasionally culturing the discharge is necessary (Table 51-2). It is important to keep in mind that malignancies of the fallopian tube, uterus, cervix, and vagina can also cause abnormal discharge. Unusual causes such as sigmoid-utero fistulas secondary to diverticular disease or appendiceal-fallopian tube fistulas secondary to appendicitis have been reported.

Table 51-1
Bacterial Vaginal Flora among Asymptomatic Women Without Vaginitis

Organism	Range of Recovery (%)
Facultative Organisms	
Gram-positive rods	
Lactobacilli	50-75
Diphtheroids	40
Gram-positive cocci	
Staphylococcus epidermidis	40-55
Staphylococcus aureus	0-5
b-Hemolytic streptococci	20
Group D streptococci	35-55
Gram-negative organisms	
Escherichia coli	10-30
Klebsiella spp.	10
Other organisms	2-10
Anaerobic Organisms	
Peptococcus spp.	5-65
Peptostreptococcus spp.	25-35
Bacteroides spp.	20-40
Bacteroides fragilis	5-15
Fusobacterium spp.	5-25
Clostridium spp.	5-20
Eubacterium spp.	5-35
Veillonella spp.	10-30

From Eschenbach DA: *Clin Obstet Gynecol* 26:187, 1983.

BACTERIAL VAGINOSIS

Bacterial vaginosis is currently the most common cause of vaginitis in the United States. The incidence ranges from 15% in private practice settings to 65% in sexually transmitted disease clinics.

Previously, bacterial vaginosis was known as "nonspecific vaginitis," since it was essentially a diagnosis of exclusion. It was believed that the condition was associated with a specific bacterium whose name changed taxonomically over time: *Haemophilus vaginitis, Corynebacterium vaginitis,* and *Gardnerella vaginitis.* However, now it is understood that bacterial vaginosis is not caused by a single bacterium, but by multiple types of bacteria, thus giving rise to the new name, bacterial vaginosis.

Pathophysiology

It is now accepted that bacterial vaginosis is caused by the overgrowth of many different types of anaerobic bacteria, including *Peptostreptococcus, Bacteroides,* and *Mobiluncus* species. These anaerobes produce aminopeptidase, which breaks down peptides to amino acids and decarboxylases and then to amines. These amines, putrescine, cadaverine, and trimethylamine, produce the characteristic "fishy" odor of bacterial vaginosis, particularly on alkalinization of vaginal secretions. The numerous bacteria cling to the epithelial cell surfaces, producing the "clue cell" on a normal saline solution wet mount preparation. Concomitant with the overgrowth of anaerobic bacteria is a decrease of the normal, "protective" lactobacilli.

Risk factors for development of bacterial vaginosis are undetermined. Thomason reviewed the literature and identified two probable risk factors: the presence of an intrauterine device and the number of different sexual partners during the month before diagnosis. Possible risk factors for bacterial vaginosis, such as age, lifetime number of sexual partners, abnormal Papanicolaou smears, and diaphragm use, were not consistently associated with bacterial vaginosis. Evidence for sexual transmission includes decreased incidence of bacterial vaginosis in monogamous couples, coital transmission of bacteria associated with bacterial vaginosis, and acquisition of new bacterial strains in women in whom bacterial vaginosis develops. Evidence against sexual transmission includes the demonstration that bacterial vaginosis does occur in virgins and that treatment of the partners of sexually active women in general is not beneficial.

History and Physical Examination

Patients will most often complain of an increased, malodorous vaginal discharge. Less frequently vulvovaginal irritation is also present. However, up to 50% of patients can be asymptomatic even though the findings of bacterial vaginosis can be demonstrated. Classically the discharge is gray.

Diagnostic Tests

Diagnosis can be made when three of the following four findings are present: increased vaginal discharge; pH >4.5; "clue cells" (epithelial cells heavily stippled with bacteria that obscure the cell border) (Fig. 51-1); or release of an amine odor with potassium hydroxide (KOH) 10% solution. The most sensitive and specific sign is the clue cell, but this finding is dependent on the skill of the examiner. Clue cell presence is usually determined by examining a normal saline solution wet mount preparation.

Cultures generally are not helpful in diagnosis as the associated bacteria can be found in women who do not have bacterial vaginosis.

Gram stain can be used to aid in the diagnosis of bacterial vaginosis, since clue cells can be recognized and the dominance or nondominance of lactobacilli can be determined.

✤ MANAGEMENT

The standard treatment for bacterial vaginosis is metronidazole 500 mg orally twice daily or 250 mg three times daily for 7 days. This therapy yields an 80% to 90% cure rate. Previously the literature has not supported shorter duration treatment regimens. However, a meta-analysis of oral metronidazole therapies supports the use of a 2-g, single-dose regimen. But higher rates of recurrence have been reported.

As oral metronidazole is not tolerated by all patients and is relatively contraindicated in the first trimester of pregnancy, other therapies have been investigated. Clindamycin, 300 mg orally twice a day for 7 days, or topical vaginal therapy with 2% clindamycin cream (5 g once daily for 7 days) or 0.75% metronidazole gel (5 g for 5 days) have been shown to be as effective as metronidazole orally. A three day course of topical clindamycin suppositories achieves similar early cure rates.

Ampicillin has been used to treat bacterial vaginosis; however, it yields a 50% to 60% cure rate. Given the efficacy of clindamycin and its safety in the pregnant patient, ampicillin is rarely used (Table 51-3).

Table 51-2
Differential Diagnosis of Vaginitis

	Symptoms	Volume of Discharge	Appearance of Discharge	Wet Mount	pH	Culture
Normal vagina	None	4-6 cm³/day	Clear, white	Squamous epithelial cells	<4.5	Normal vaginal flora
Bacterial Vaginosis	Asymptomatic, irritation	Increased	Homogenous, gray	NS: clue cells KOH: amine odor	>4.5	Nondiagnostic
Candida Vaginitis	Pruritus, burning	Usually increased	Cottage cheese-like, white	KOH: pseudohyphae	4-5	90% sensitive
Trichomonas Vaginitis	Pruritus	Increased	Frothy, green or gray	NS: trichomonads, increased polys	>4.5	95% sensitive
Atrophic Vaginitis	Irritation, pruritus, dyspareunia	None or increased	Watery, yellow or green	Increased polys	>4.5	Normal vaginal flora
Cytolytic Vaginosis	Burning, irritation, dyspareunia	Increased	Clumpy, white	Cytolysis of squamous epithelial cells	>4.5	Nondiagnostic

NS, Normal saline solution; *KOH,* potassium hydroxide 10% solution; *polys,* polymorphonuclear leukocytes.

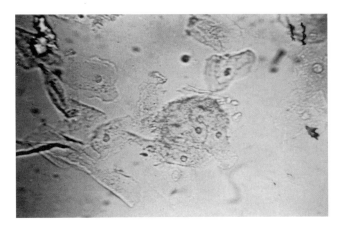

FIG. 51-1   Clue cells characteristic of bacterial vaginosis, squamous epithelial cells whose borders are obscured by bacteria.

CANDIDA VAGINITIS

Candida vaginitis is the second most common vaginitis in the United States with an estimated 1.3 million cases annually. The incidence of candida vaginitis doubled from 1980 to 1990. Many health care providers are familiar with patients with recurrent or chronic candida vaginitis necessitating frequent visits for evaluation and treatment. These patients often have dyspareunia, which may significantly disrupt their personal lives, and their constant symptoms are a reminder that they are not "normal." Although candida vaginitis is not life-threatening, recurrent candida is frustrating for the patient and clinician and can consume health care resources.

Pathophysiology

Candida vaginitis is caused by the growth of the fungus *Candida* in the vagina. Most commonly *Candida albicans* is the causative fungal species, but over the last 20 years the in-cidence of non-*Candida albicans* species vaginitis has been increasing. Currently 20% of candida vaginitis may be non-*Candida albicans.* The clinical significance is that the symptoms may not be classic and some species may be slightly more resistant to the standard anticandidal treatments.

The familiar signs and symptoms, erythema, edema, burning, and pruritus, are probably a result of the alcohol that is produced by the fungal metabolism of sugar. Any condition that raises the sugar substrate availability may be a risk factor, such as diabetes and pregnancy. Other risk factors include conditions in which depressed cellular immunity is present, such as regimens of steroids or immunosuppressive agents. Any alteration of the normal vaginal flora, such as occurs with antibiotic treatment, often results in especially difficult to treat vaginal candidiasis. It is unclear whether oral contraceptives are really a risk factor since the literature both supports their role and shows no association. Occlusive clothing has traditionally been suspected of creating a more favorable climate for candida growth, and one study has shown a significant association between pantyhose use and candida vaginitis. Sexual transmissibility of candida vaginitis has been difficult to determine as well. Bisschop and Merkus showed no effect of treating the male partner of female patients with candida vaginitis. However, these patients did not have a history of recurrent candidiasis, the male partners were not cultured for *Candida* spp., and follow-up observation was only 4 weeks. Conversely, Horowitz and colleagues studied 33 couples in which the female patient had a history of recurrent candida vaginitis and were able to demonstrate a decrease in recurrence rate after the partner was treated. *Candida* spp. were cultured more frequently from the oral cavities and ejaculates of male partners of the female study group. There was no difference in the rectal cultures of male partners in the study versus those of the control group. After treatment 31 of 33 patients followed for 1 year had no recurrent candida vaginitis.

Table 51-3
Treatment of Vaginitis

Type	Treatment
Bacterial vaginosis	Metronidazole 500 mg PO qd for 7 days
	Metronidazole 0.75% gel intravaginally bid for 5 days
	Clindamycin 300 mg PO bid for 7 days
	Clindamycin 2% cream intravaginally qd for 7 days
Candida vaginitis	Miconazole 2% cream intravaginally qd for 3-7 days
	Miconazole 200-mg vaginal suppositories qd for 3 days
	Clotrimazole 1% cream intravaginally qd for 3-7 days
	Butoconazole 2% cream intravaginally qd for 3-6 days
	Tioconazole 6.5% cream intravaginally as a single dose
	Terconazole 0.8% cream intravaginally qd for 3 days
	Terconazole 80-mg vaginal suppositories qd for 3 days
	Terconazole 0.4% cream intravaginally qd for 7 days
	Fluconazole 150 mg PO once
Chronic suppression	Ketoconazole 400 mg qd for 5 days monthly or 100 mg qd
	Fluconazole 150 qd once a month
	Clotrimazole 500-mg suppositories once weekly
Trichomonas vaginitis	Metronidazole 2 g PO as single dose, or 250 mg tid for 7 days
Atrophic vaginitis	Estradiol cream 0.25 mg (1/4 applicator) intravaginally twice weekly (or equivalent)
	Oral conjugated estrogens 0.3-0.625 mg qd (with progestin cycling when appropriate) or equivalent
Cytolytic vaginosis	Sodium bicarbonate douche (30-60 g/L warm water) 2-3 times weekly, then 1-2 times weekly as needed

Chronic or Recurrent Candida Vaginitis

The pathophysiologic characteristics of chronic or recurrent candida vaginitis in women without obvious risk factors such as diabetes or immunosuppression are highly debated. Traditional theories include the hypothesis that the intestinal tract acts as a reservoir from which the vagina can be reseeded; the "vaginal relapse theory," in which yeast colonies are so low after treatment that the patients are culture-negative, but candida is still present and can then multiply and become symptomatic later; and the theory of sexual transmission of candida. More recently it has been suspected that some women may have a localized vaginal allergic response to candida that results in decreased cellular immunity, which then predisposes them to recurrent symptoms and infections.

History and Physical Examination

Classically candida vaginitis manifests a cottage cheese-like white discharge and pruritus. However, it can also exhibit no apparent increase of vaginal discharge, and patients may complain of "burning" instead of pruritus. These latter symptoms may be more characteristic of non-*Candida albicans* candidal infections.

On examination the vulva and vagina may be erythematous, edematous, and covered with a characteristic discharge. Fissuring of the vulva may occur if the infection has been present for a long time.

Diagnostic Tests

Diagnosis can be made by the presence of pseudohyphae or spores on examination of a KOH 10% solution wet mount preparation; however, the sensitivity of wet mounts is only 50%. Cultures are 90% sensitive and thus are a more reliable method to make the diagnosis. Cultures also offer the opportunity to determine the species in cases of recurrent or chronic candida vaginitis.

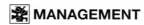 MANAGEMENT

Currently many therapeutic choices are available. Choice of therapy should be determined by the patient's preference, history, severity of disease, and presence of risk factors.

For mild, nonrecurrent candida vaginitis in a patient without additional risk factors such as immunosuppression, the over-the-counter clotrimazole and miconazole creams are easily available and effective with a greater than 85% cure rate. In addition, creams are probably preferable to suppositories when candida vulvitis is also present.

If a patient has simple candida vaginitis with symptoms of short duration, single-dose therapies that may result in better compliance can be offered. However, the cure rate, 70%, may be slightly lower than that of longer duration therapies. If the patient has been treated with antibiotics, has a long duration of symptoms, or complains of severe symptoms, one should consider the 3- or 7-day therapies. Cure rates do not significantly differ among the intravaginal imidazoles: clotrimazole, miconazole, butoconazole, and tioconazole. Most cure rates are above 85%.

Terconazole offers the theoretic advantages of being more specific for the fungal cytochrome P-450, having less tendency to induce its own metabolism, and having increased contact with the fungal membrane. However, studies have shown either little or no increase in cure rate for terconazole when compared to that of the imidazoles. Terconazole may offer an advantage in treating non-*Candida albicans* species, such as *C. glabrata* and *C. torulopsis.* With its greater specificity for the fungal cytochrome P-450, one would expect adverse reactions to occur less often; however, clinically terconazole does not seem to be significantly different.

Oral therapy has been used for chronic or recurrent candida vaginitis, theoretically decreasing reseeding rates from the "intestinal reservoir." Previously ketoconazole has been used as the oral agent of choice, but a review of studies comparing the newer oral triazole, fluconazole, 150 or 200 mg once, to standard intravaginal therapies and to ketoconzole shows that fluconazole is as effective as ketoconazole and has fewer adverse effects. Fluconazole is well absorbed given orally, has a lower risk of hepatotoxicity, and has a long half-life of approximately 25 hours. However, the risk of adverse effects from fluconazole therapy is still higher than that of local intravaginal therapy, so it should probably be reserved for chronic or recurrent cases.

Itraconazole has variable oral absorption and a higher risk of hepatotoxicity and therefore does not appear to offer an advantage over fluconazole.

Recurrent or chronic candida vaginitis can be successfully suppressed with intermittent intravaginal or oral antifungals. For chronic suppression oral therapy is usually preferred by the patient because of convenience. Ketoconazole, 400 mg daily for 5 days monthly or 100 mg daily, can reduce recurrence rates. Fluconazole may become the oral drug of choice for suppression. Fluconazole, 150 mg orally once a month, reduces recurrence rates by 50%.

Local therapy in the form of clotrimazole, 500-mg suppositories, has been used monthly and weekly for suppression. Monthly regimens have not shown to be effective, but weekly treatment may reduce recurrence rates similar to regimens using daily ketoconazole. When choosing therapy, the convenience of oral therapy, which may result in better patient compliance, must be weighed against the higher risks of oral therapy when compared to local therapy. Patients should participate in determining their suppressive therapy.

It is unclear from the literature whether treating the partner of patients with recurrent candida vaginitis will reduce recurrence rates. However, if other risk factors are ruled out and other treatment regimens have failed to reduce recurrence rates, it is worth a trial. As Horowitz and colleagues showed, it is important to identify the reservoirs of candida in the partner and direct treatment accordingly. When this was done, recurrence rates were reduced.

Finally, hyposensitization may be considered when treating difficult, recurrent candida. A small trial of 10 women with a history of recurrent candida vaginitis were hyposensitized to candida; the result was a decrease in the recurrence rate from every 5 months to every 15 months, and when an infection occurred the symptoms were reported as less severe and more amenable to treatment. However, as there is little literature on hyposensitization as a form of treatment, it should be reserved for the difficult, recurrent cases in which other treatment modalities have been tried.

TRICHOMONAS VAGINITIS

Trichomonas vaginitis is the third most common vaginitis with an estimated five million cases each year in the United States. Its incidence is actually decreasing, probably largely as a result of the effectiveness of metronidazole.

Pathophysiology

Trichomonas vaginitis is caused by the infection of the flagellated protozoan *Trichomonas vaginalis.* It is a sexually transmitted disease. There have been scattered reports documenting the viability of trichomonads on potential infective surfaces, such as toilet seats. However, whether actual transmission can occur via these surfaces remains conjectural.

History and Physical Examination

Most patients complain of vaginal and vulvar pruritus and an increased vaginal discharge. The discharge may be green, copious, and frothy. Edema and erythema of the vulva and particularly of the vagina may be present. The "strawberry" cervix is a classic finding resulting from punctate mucosal hemorrhages of the cervix.

Diagnostic Tests

Diagnosis can be made by several methods. The normal saline solution wet mount preparation is most commonly used. This method is inexpensive, is convenient, and gives immediate results. However, a normal saline solution wet mount preparation has a wide range of sensitivity, 45% to 95%, because it is dependent on the experience of the microscopist. If the motile, flagellated trichomonads are identified, wet mount diagnosis is 100% specific.

Diagnosis by culture of trichomonas is more sensitive than that of the wet mount, 92% to 95%. Additionally, susceptibility testing can be performed if necessary. However, cultures are more costly, and results are not available for several days, delaying treatment. Culture should be considered if the wet mount preparation finding is negative and trichomonas vaginitis is suspected.

Trichomonads can be found incidentally on Papanicolaou's smear in asymptomatic patients undergoing routine examination. It is debated whether asymptomatic trichomonads should be treated, although most clinicians favor treatment, as its risks are not great.

Several new diagnostic tests are not yet available for clinical use but probably will be in the near future. A direct immunofluorescence assay has been developed, but it is still only available in research settings. It is more sensitive than the wet mount, but less sensitive than a culture, 80% to 90%. The specificity is lower than that of both the wet mount and culture, 99%. A monoclonal-based enzyme-linked immunosorbent assay may become available, with the advantages of an in-office test with greater sensitivity than that of the wet mount. A latex agglutination test may also offer higher sensitivity than the wet mount, but the reliability has not yet been established.

✴ MANAGEMENT

Because trichomoniasis is a multifocal infection of the vaginal epithelium, Skene's glands, Bartholin's gland, and urethra, systemic treatment is necessary for cure. The standard therapy is metronidazole, 2 g orally, in a single dose. An alternative therapy for patients who have experienced significant nausea with the single-dose regimen is metronidazole,

250 mg orally three times a day for 7 days. Both regimens usually yield cure rates of more than 90%.

The incidence of trichomonas infection in the male partner has not been well defined. In an unpublished study in which only the male urethra was examined, 8% of the male contacts of infected women had positive results. The yield may have been higher if prostatic and seminal secretions had been examined. Up to 24% of women will be reinfected if their partners are not treated, so treatment of the male partner is recommended even when he is asymptomatic.

Resistant and Recurrent Trichomonas Vaginitis

Resistance to metronidazole is uncommon, although reports in the literature of cases have been increasing since 1982. Most metronidazole-resistant cases can be cured with larger doses of metronidazole, since resistance is relative. If failure of initial therapy occurs the course should be repeated (with concomitant treatment of the partner). If the infection is persistent, 2 to 4 g daily for 5 to 14 days can be given; however, with higher doses of longer duration the incidence and severity of adverse effects increase. These include nausea and vomiting, a metallic taste, glossitis, stomatitis, urticaria, vertigo, and, rarely, convulsive seizures and peripheral neuropathy that is reversible but may last months. Severely resistant cases should be managed in conjunction with susceptibility testing and in consultation with a specialist experienced in treating resistant cases.

VAGINITIS IN PREGNANCY

As many as 16% of pregnant women have bacterial vaginosis. Metronidazole is relatively contraindicated in pregnancy particularly in the first trimester because of its potential teratogenic effects. Clotrimazole given intravaginally can be used during pregnancy for symptomatic relief if the vaginitis is secondary to candida. Cure rates are generally less than 60%. Saline solution 20% douches have been reported anecdotally to relieve symptoms as well. Povidone-iodine douches should not be used in pregnancy because absorption of the iodine may result in neonatal hypothyroidism. Acidification of the vagina through either vaginal jelly (Aci-Jel) or acetic acid washes would probably be safe, but efficacy and safety have not been documented.

Recent studies have shown that spontaneous abortion, preterm labor, premature birth, preterm rupture of the membranes, amniotic fluid infection, postpartum endometritis, and postcesarean wound infections are increased because of infection with bacterial vaginosis during pregnancy (replacement of the normal hydrogen peroxide producing *Lactobacillus* sp. in the vagina with high concentrations of characteristic sets of aerobic and anaerobic bacteria). Clinical trials have demonstrated reduction in all these events with appropriate screening and intervention with antibiotics safe during pregnancy. Therefore early screening of all pregnant women, appropriate treatment, and follow-up for cure are now recommended by the American College of Obstetricians and Gynecologists.

ATROPHIC VAGINITIS

Atrophic vaginitis primarily affects postmenopausal women but may occur in any woman who is in a low estrogenic state (i.e., women who are breastfeeding or using oral contraceptives). As women now live one third of their lives after menopause and expect to continue to have fulfilling sexual lives, vaginal atrophy has become a significant disorder that can affect quality of living.

Pathophysiology

Atrophic vaginitis is the result of estrogen deprivation of the estrogen-dependent tissues of the genital tract. The most common cause is the postmenopausal state. Because the atrophic changes occur very gradually, women often do not notice any symptoms until 5 to 10 years after menopause. Without estrogen the vulvar and vaginal epithelium become very thin, sensitive, and nonlubricated. Other hypoestrogenic states that may cause atrophic vaginitis include breastfeeding, oral contraceptive use, and gonadotropin-releasing hormone (GnRH) agonists for endometriosis.

History and Physical Examination

Women with atrophic vaginitis often complain of dyspareunia, which may be mild or severe relative to the amount of atrophy present. They may complain of "feeling dry" and uncomfortable even if not sexually active. Pruritis is another common symptom. Less often "postmenopausal bleeding" may send the patient to the physician's office. The site of bleeding may not be obvious, necessitating an endometrial biopsy to rule out endometrial cancer. Occasionally patients complain of a watery discharge along with some of the symptoms mentioned.

Diagnosis can usually be made by examination. The vulvar and vaginal epithelium appear less pink, thinner, and dryer, and vaginal rugae are absent.

Diagnostic Tests

In patients who have complaints consistent with atrophy but have more subtle changes that are difficult to see, a vaginal Papanicolaou's test for a maturation index can be done. The *maturation index* is the percentage of basal, intermediate, and superficial cells present in the smear. In atrophy there is an increasing dominance of basal and intermediate cells. This test may be useful in women with vaginitis complaints who are using oral contraceptives or are breastfeeding when the diagnosis is uncertain.

It is important to rule out other causes that may have similar manifestations. The vulvar dystrophies, lichen sclerosus and squamous cell hyperplasia, may have a similar clinical picture. Diagnosis can be made by biopsy of the affected epithelium (see Chapter 44).

MANAGEMENT

Estrogen replacement is the treatment of choice for atrophic vaginitis. Estrogen administered either orally or locally results in maturation of the vaginal epithelium. If systemic hormone replacement therapy is not indicated, excellent response can be achieved by using estradiol cream 0.25 mg (or the equivalent dose in any of the other estrogen vaginal cream preparations) intravaginally twice a week. This dose has been shown to have a minimal systemic effect. Some women can achieve a satisfactory response on a once-a-week regimen. Vaginal estrogen can also be administered via estradiol vaginal tablets and an estradiol-impregnated silicone ring (Estring). The latter, which is inserted and removed by the patient, causes no detectable effect on serum estradiol levels.

In patients for whom estrogen is contraindicated, for example women with a history of breast cancer, treatment alternatives are often ineffective. Vaginal lubricating agents can relieve vaginal dryness and dyspareunia secondary to vaginal dryness. Acidifying agents may help decrease the risk of infection by maintaining the vaginal pH in the normal acidic range (4.5) and may help to cornify the epithelium, thus possibly lessening epithelial sensitivity. Many over-the-counter products that combine lubricating and acidifying properties are available. For patients who have mild symptoms, for example those who are recently postmenopausal, using oral contraceptives, or breastfeeding, a lubricating agent may be satisfactory. Generally, however, patients with moderate to severe atrophy are not satisfied with these agents as their effect on maturation of the epithelium, the underlying problem, is negligible.

CYTOLYTIC VAGINOSIS

Another vaginosis from which other types of vaginitis should be differentiated is cytolytic vaginosis. This vaginosis was previously known as Doderlein's cytolysis but more recently has been further characterized by Cibley and Cibley. It is a condition that is often misdiagnosed as other vaginal infections, particularly recurrent candida. The typical patient is a woman referred for "recurrent candida" that has not been alleviated by multiple therapies.

Pathophysiology

The pathogenesis of cytolytic vaginosis is unclear. It is hypothesized that overgrowth of vaginal *Lactobacillus* spp. results in an environment that is too acidic and produces the symptoms. However, further studies are needed to elucidate the cause.

History and Physical Examination

Symptoms may be very similar to those of candida vaginitis, including pruritus, vulvar dysuria, dyspareunia, and a clumpy white discharge. The "typical" patient may have "a shopping bag full of partially used medications" that have failed. Some women may note that their symptoms occur or worsen during the luteal phase of the menstrual cycle.

Diagnostic Tests

The current diagnostic criteria are absence of trichomonas vaginitis, candida vaginitis, or bacterial vaginosis; increased vaginal discharge, which is usually white, frothy, or cheesy; a pH between 3.5 and 4.5 and an increased number of lactobacilli on a normal saline solution wet mount preparation; evidence of cytolosis; and few polymorphonuclear cells. Culture would not be helpful since it would only reveal "normal vaginal flora."

MANAGEMENT

The recommended treatment of cytolytic vaginosis is douching with a sodium bicarbonate solution, 30 to 60 g of sodium bicarbonate in 1 L of warm water two to three times per week and then once or twice a week as needed. In patients who experience cyclic symptoms, prophylactic sodium bicarbonate douches 1 to 2 days before anticipated symptoms are recommended.

OTHER VAGINAL DISORDERS

There are other less common causes of vaginitis, some of which are controversial and others that are rarely seen in the United States.

Normal vaginal flora contains a fluctuating variety of aerobic and anaerobic bacteria. Bacteria that are potential pathogens in other parts of the body may be harmless in the vagina. However, it may be possible that overgrowth of certain types of bacteria such as *Streptococcus pyogenes* or *Escherichia coli* may result in vaginitis. It is important to rule out any other possible causes before treatment, since this hypothesized cause is controversial and remains unconfirmed.

Amoebic vaginal infections are extremely rare in the United States, but if the patient has recently returned from a country where amoebiasis is prevalent and complains of a malodorous, serosanguinous, or bloody discharge with necrotic tissue fragments and vaginal ulcers, amoebiasis should be ruled out.

Retained foreign bodies, such as forgotten tampons, diaphragms, or contraceptive sponges, or the use of pessaries usually cause a malodorous, profuse, watery discharge. The discharge may be bloody because of vaginal erosions or fissures caused by pressure necrosis from the foreign body. Removal of the foreign body usually results in prompt resolution of symptoms. Management of discharge secondary to pessary use involves using intravaginal estrogen cream and acidifying agents and ruling out other causes of vaginitis.

Psychosomatic vaginitis is rarely encountered in a routine practice and is uncommon even at referral centers. Patients may have a chronic history of symptoms and multiple treatments without resolution and complain of dyspareunia resulting in abstinence. When they are examined repeatedly no pathologic findings can be demonstrated. There may be a background of psychologic problems that may not always be apparent at the beginning of the investigation. These patients must be differentiated from those with vulvar vestibulitis, as some of the symptoms are similar. Patients with psychosomatic vaginitis will respond to psychotherapy and not to any nerve blocks or topical anesthetics, to which vestibulitis patients usually respond temporarily.

BIBLIOGRAPHY

American College of Obstetricians and Gynecologists: ACOG committee opinion: bacterial vaginosis screening for prevention of preterm delivery. Number 198, February 1998. Committee on Obstetric Practice. American College of Obstetricians and Gynecologists, *Int J Gynaecol Obstet* 61:311, 1998.

Andres FJ et al: Clindamycin vaginal cream versus oral metronidazole in the treatment of bacterial vaginosis: a prospective double-blind clinical trial, *South Med J* 85:1077, 1992.

Bisschop MPJM, Merkus JMWM: Co-treatment of the male partner in vaginal candidosis: a double-blind randomized control study, *Br J Obstet Gynaecol* 93:79, 1986.

Cates W et al: Estimates of the incidence and prevalence of sexually transmitted diseases in the United States, *Sex Tran Dis* 261(suppl):52, 1999.

Carey JC et al: Metronidazole to prevent preterm delivery in pregnant women with asymptomatic bacterial vaginosis. National Institute of Child Health and Human Development Network of Maternal-Fetal Medicine Units, *N Engl J Med* 342:534, 2000.

CDC: 1998 guidelines for treatment of sexually transmitted diseases, *MMWR* 47:1, 1998.

Carr PL et al: Evaluation and management of vaginitis, *J Gen Intern Med* 13:335, 1998.

Cibley LJ, Cibley LJ: Cytolytic vaginosis, *Am J Obstet Gynecol* 165:1245, 1991.

Ernest JM: Topical antifungal agents, *Obstet Gynecol Clin North Am* 19:587, 1992.

Eschenbach DA: Vaginal infections, *Clin Obstet Gynecol* 26:187, 1983.

Eschenbach DA et al: Diagnosis and clinical manifestations of bacterial vaginosis, *Am J Obstet Gynecol* 158:819, 1988.

Godley MJ: Quantitation of vaginal discharge in healthy volunteers, *Br J Obstet Gynaecol* 92:739, 1985.

Greaves WL et al: Clindamycin versus metronidazole in the treatment of bacterial vaginosis, *Obstet Gynecol* 72:799, 1988.

Hauth JC et al: Reduced incidence of preterm delivery with metronidazole and erythromycin in women with bacterial vaginosis, *N Engl J Med* 333:1732, 1995.

Heidrich FE, Berg AP, Bergman JJ: Clothing factors and vaginitis, *J Fam Pract* 19:491, 1984.

Hillier S et al: Efficacy of intravaginal 0.75% metronidazole gel for the treatment of bacterial vaginosis, *Obstet Gynecol* 81:963, 1993.

Horowitz BJ, Edelstein SW, Lippman L: Sexual transmission of candida, *Obstet Gynecol* 69:883, 1987.

Kaufman RH, Faro S, editors: *Benign diseases of the vulva and vagina*, ed 4, St Louis, 1994, Mosby.

Livengood CH, Thomason JL, Hill GB: Bacterial vaginosis: treatment with topical intravaginal clindamycin phosphate, *Obstet Gynecol* 76:118, 1990.

Lossick JG, Kent HL: Trichomoniasis: trends in diagnosis and management, *Am J Obstet Gynecol* 165:1217, 1991.

Lugo-Miro VI, Green M, Mazur L: Comparison of different metronidazole therapeutic regimens for bacterial vaginosis, *JAMA* 268:92, 1992.

McGregor JA, French JI: Bacterial vaginosis in pregnancy, *Obstet Gynecol Surv* 55: S1, 2000.

Mettler L, Olsen PG: Long-term treatment of atrophic vaginitis with low-dose oestradiol vaginal tablets, *Maturitas* 14:23, 1991.

Patel HS, Peters MD, Smith CL: Is there a role for fluconazole in the treatment of vulvovaginal candidiasis? *Ann Pharmacother* 26:350, 1992.

Rosedale N, Browne K: Hyposensitization in the management of recurring vaginal candidiasis, *Ann Allergy* 43:250, 1979.

Slavin MB et al: Single dose oral fluconazole vs. intravaginal terconazole in treatment of candida vaginitis: comparison of pilot study, *J Fla Med Assoc* 79:693, 1992.

Sobel JD et al: Treatment of complicated candida vaginitis: comparison of single and sequential doses of Fluconazole, *Am J Obstet Gynecol* 185:363, 2001.

Sobel JD: Pathogenesis and treatment of recurrent vulvovaginal candidiasis, *Clin Infect Dis* 14(suppl l):448, 1992.

Thomason JL: Clinical evaluation of terconazole: United States experience, *J Reprod Med* 34:597, 1989.

Thomason JL, Gelbart SM, Scaglione NJ: Current review with indications for asymptomatic therapy, *Am J Obstet Gynecol* 1665:1210, 1991.

CHAPTER **52**

Abnormal Vaginal Bleeding

Soheyla Dana Gharib
Stephanie A. Eisenstat

In the course of caring for women, every primary care physician is confronted with questions from patients about alterations in patterns of menstruation. Whether it is irregular and unpredictable bleeding in an adolescent, midcycle bleeding in a mature woman, or spotting in a postmenopausal woman, unexpected changes in vaginal bleeding can be alarming for patients and can pose a diagnostic challenge for their physicians.

In approaching the woman with abnormal bleeding, the physician should pose the following screening questions:

- Is the patient pregnant?
- At what stage of the reproductive life cycle is the patient (adolescence, mature cycle, perimenopausal, or postmenopausal)?
- Is the bleeding occurring in the setting of an ovulatory cycle?
- What is the pattern of abnormal bleeding?

The answers to these questions will direct the evaluation and determine whether the patient will need referral to a gynecologist.

NORMAL MENSTRUAL CYCLE

Menstruation is a bloody, vaginal discharge that occurs as the result of endometrial shedding after ovulation when fertilization has not occurred. Changes in the interval between menses, the duration of menses, or the amount of menstrual flow can cause women to visit their physicians. In the normal menstrual cycle there is a regularity to the interval of menstrual bleeding, usually between 24 and 35 days (only one sixth of cycles are exactly the lunar cycle of 28 days). The duration of normal, ovulatory menses is 3 to 7 days, with the average blood loss being 33 ml. More than 80 ml of blood loss is considered excessive. Inquiries about the number of pads or tampons used usually are made to assess the amount of blood loss—use of a pad or tampon per hour suggests unusually vigorous bleeding. Patients' estimates of blood loss, however, correlate poorly with measured blood loss.

The physiology of the menstrual cycle is reviewed in Chapter 43.

EVALUATION
Clinical Presentation
History

The history, physical, and pelvic examinations take place in a focused fashion to determine the site of bleeding and its cause (Box 52-1). The pace of the evaluation is determined by the patient's complaints. The physician should seek to understand whether the bleeding is an annoyance, if it is interfering with the patient's lifestyle, or if it is a dramatic change in the patient's baseline that is alarming to her.

The *age* of the patient can point the clinician in the proper direction to reach the appropriate diagnosis. In adolescent patients, acute menorrhagia is attributed usually to anovulation. In patients in their reproductive years, the cause of bleeding often is related to pregnancy. In perimenopausal patients the cause of excessive bleeding most likely is anovulation secondary to ovarian failure. Finally, in postmenopausal women, the concern is that abnormal bleeding is secondary to hyperplasia or a neoplastic process.

The *timing, duration,* and *amount* of the vaginal bleeding should first be determined. As already noted, the particular pattern of bleeding abnormality may furnish clues about the underlying diagnosis. The interval of bleeding may be abnormal: increased (polymenorrhea), decreased (oligomenorrhea), or irregular (metrorrhagia); the duration may be increased (hypermenorrhea) or decreased (hypomenorrhea); or the amount may be altered—increased (menorrhagia) or decreased (hypomenorrhea) (Table 52-1).

It is important to establish whether the abnormal bleeding is occurring in a patient who usually has menstrual bleeding at regular intervals. If the patient has bleeding at regular intervals (24 to 35 days) with molimina (menstrual cramps, back pain, mood changes), it is likely that she has ovulatory cycles (Box 52-2). If the patient usually has ovulatory cycles and has had an isolated episode of abnormal bleeding, the most important diagnosis to consider is pregnancy. The patient should be asked the date of her last menstrual period, whether she has had unprotected intercourse, and if the symptoms of pregnancy are present (amenorrhea, breast tenderness, anorexia, or nausea).

The patient's menstrual and gynecologic history, from the time of menarche to the present, should be taken carefully. If the patient has had irregular menses without molimina, a diagnosis of polycystic ovary syndrome is likely. A history of hirsutism makes this diagnosis even more likely.

Table 52-1
Definitions for the Changes in Menstrual Flow

Parameter	Definition
Interval of Bleeding	
Polymenorrhea	Increase in interval of bleeding
Oligomenorrhea	Decrease in interval
Metrorrhagia	Irregularity of interval
Duration of Bleeding	
Hypermenorrhea	Increase in the duration of flow
Hypomenorrhea	Decrease in the duration of flow
Amount of Bleeding	
Menorrhagia	Increased amount of bleeding
Hypomenorrhea	Decreased amount of bleeding

BOX 52-1

Evaluation: Key Factors in the History

Age
Timing, duration, and amount of menses
Pattern of abnormal menses
Last menstrual period
Pain associated with the bleeding
Evidence of ovulatory cycling
Past gynecologic surgical procedures
Contraceptive history
Other medical symptoms:
  Symptoms of hypothyroidism
  Symptoms for blood dyscrasias
Medication history:
  Oral contraceptives, Norplant, medroxyprogesterone (Depo-Provera)
  Coumadin, aspirin, nonsteroidal antiinflammatory drugs
  Postmenopausal hormonal therapy

BOX 52-2

Evidence of Ovulatory Cycling

Regular menstrual intervals (24-35 days)
Moliminal symptoms
  Breast tenderness
  Fluid retention
  Menstrual cramps
  Back pain
  Mood changes
Midcycle cervical mucus
Increase in basal body temperature: 0.2°-0.6°
Luteal phase progesterone 0.3 ng/ml
Secretory changes on endometrial biopsy

If the patient has always had heavy, prolonged menses, a coagulopathy may be present. Past gynecologic procedures may suggest a preexisting anatomic lesion (cervical carcinoma, fibroids, polyps) that may be causing the present episode of bleeding. Contraception use also can be associated with abnormal bleeding. Oral contraceptives can cause midcycle bleeding, and the most common complaint of patients who use intrauterine devices is prolonged menstrual bleeding.

The presence of *pain* during a bleeding episode can suggest a number of diagnoses. The most important diagnosis to consider is ectopic pregnancy. The classic presentation is vaginal bleeding with unilateral pelvic pain after an episode of amenorrhea, but the diagnosis can elude even the most experienced clinician because of the many variations of presentation (a detailed discussion on ectopic pregnancy appears in Chapter 65). Intermenstrual cramps with or without bleeding can occur in patients with endometrial polyps. Degenerating fibroids, endometritis, persistent corpus luteum, and adenomyosis (endometrial tissue in the myometrium, or endometriosis interna) also can be associated with varying degrees of pain (see Chapter 55).

The *past medical history* of the patient is important. A history of liver or renal disease may explain abnormal patterns of bleeding. In patients with chronic renal failure who are undergoing hemodialysis, menorrhagia may be observed (see Chapter 25). Hypothyroidism commonly is associated with prolonged, heavy menses. A careful drug history should be obtained because the use of certain medications (oral contraceptive pills, anticoagulants, aspirin,) commonly cause abnormal bleeding patterns.

Physical Examination

A complete physical examination of any patient with abnormal bleeding is essential (Box 52-3). The patient's *body habitus* should be noted. Patients who are under the 10th percentile in body weight, whether because of anorexia nervosa/bulimia or chronic disease, may have oligomenorrhea because of hypothalamic dysfunction. Obese patients often have irregular, anovulatory bleeding because of increased circulating levels of estrogen as a result of conversion of androgens to estrogen in adipose tissue. The *pattern of hair distribution* should be checked because hirsutism can be associated with polycystic ovary syndrome, a cause of oligomenorrhea. The *skin* should be checked for petechiae

---

BOX 52-3

Evaluation of Abnormal Vaginal Bleeding:
Key Factors in the Physical Examination

Body habitus
Hair distribution
Presence or absence of petechiae
Thyroid examination
Presence or absence of galactorrhea
Breast examination
Pelvic examination with speculum and bimanually
Rectovaginal examination

and other findings that might suggest an abnormal clotting mechanism. *Breast examination* should include inspection and palpation for milky discharge. A thorough general physical examination should detect any signs of thyroid and liver disease.

A careful examination of the vagina and cervix may identify the source of the bleeding. Vaginal atrophy and cervical lesions (cervicitis, polyps, or carcinoma) can explain postcoital bleeding. Blood coming from the os confirms a higher source of the bleeding (uterus or fallopian tubes). Products of conception may be found in the vaginal vault or in the cervical os. Bimanual examination may identify uterine myomata, ovarian masses, or ectopic pregnancy. A rectal examination may reveal hemorrhoids that have been mistaken by the patient as vaginal bleeding. Rectovaginal examination also can detect nodules suggestive of endometriosis.

Differential Diagnosis

One of the important goals in the evaluation of abnormal vaginal bleeding is to determine whether the bleeding is originating from the gynecologic tract. On rare occasions patients may mistake slight bleeding from the rectum or urethra for vaginal bleeding.

The findings of a careful history and physical examination should provide the clinician with adequate data on which to form a differential diagnosis and then proceed with an appropriate diagnostic evaluation.

There is a vast list of diagnoses that can cause abnormal vaginal bleeding, but a list is not always helpful in organizing an evaluation. A far more productive way to think about the differential diagnoses is to subdivide this cumbersome list into diagnoses that are likely to affect women at specific points in their reproductive life cycle (pregnancy versus the nonpregnant state), and if not pregnant, ovulatory cycling and specific pattern of vaginal bleeding (Box 52-4). A list of differential diagnoses in terms of these parameters appears in Table 52-2. It is important to remember that certain diagnoses, notably trauma and neoplasia, may be the underlying cause of vaginal bleeding in any female patient, whether or not she is pregnant, or whether she is premenopausal or postmenopausal.

Pregnancy

In a pregnant patient the two most common times of bleeding are in the first and third trimesters (Box 52-5). Usually only patients in the first trimester will seek the care of a primary care physician. The causes of first-trimester bleeding include spontaneous abortion ("missed," incomplete, or complete), ectopic pregnancy, and "implantation bleeding."

The most *important* of these diagnoses for the clinician is **ectopic pregnancy,** which is treatable but life-threatening if missed. The classic presentation of ectopic pregnancy is a history of amenorrhea followed by abnormal vaginal bleeding and unilateral pelvic pain. (For a detailed discussion regarding the diagnosis and management of ectopic pregnancy see Chapter 65.)

The most common cause of bleeding in the first trimester of pregnancy is spontaneous abortion. An abortion is called missed when products of conception are retained after a fetal death has occurred. The patient's pregnancy test is positive and weeks of amenorrhea are followed by vaginal bleeding. Ultrasound examination may reveal an empty ges-

tational sac or the presence of a fetus without a heartbeat. An incomplete abortion is defined as the expulsion of fetus or the placenta, or both. When the placenta, in whole or in part, is retained in the uterus, bleeding ensues to produce the profuse bleeding of incomplete abortion. A complete abortion is the complete expulsion of the products of gestation.

Implantation bleeding is a general phrase that applies to any bleeding that occurs in the first weeks of pregnancy. Implantation occurs approximately 6 days after conception

---

BOX 52-4
Factors Affecting Abnormal Vaginal Bleeding

Pregnancy status
Stage of reproductive life cycle
Presence of ovulatory cycling
Pattern of vaginal bleeding

Table 52-2
Differential Diagnosis: Abnormal Vaginal Bleeding

Factors	Diagnosis
General	Trauma
	Neoplasia
Specific to reproductive cycle	
Pregnancy	
First trimester	Spontaneous abortion
	Ectopic implantation
Third trimester	Placenta previa
	Placental abruption
	Premature labor
Ovulatory cycles present	Shortened follicular luteal phase
	Anatomic lesion
	Endometrial polyps
	Cervical polyps
	Adenomyosis
	Fibroids
	Systemic disease
	Coagulopathies
	Intrauterine device
	Cervical cancer
	Sarcomas
	Pelvic inflammatory disease
Anovulatory cycles	Immature hypothalamic regulation
	Polycystic ovary syndrome
	Perimenopausal changes
	Endometrial hyperplasia
	Endometrial carcinoma
	Postmenopausal hormone replacement
	Dysfunctional uterine bleeding (no pelvic organ disease or systemic disorder)
	Endometriosis

BOX 52-5

Differential Diagnosis of Abnormal Vaginal Bleeding in Pregnant Women

First Trimester	**Third Trimester**
Implantation bleeding	Placenta previa
Abortion	Placenta abruption
Threatened	Premature labor
Complete	Choriocarcinoma
Incomplete	
Missed	
Ectopic pregnancy	
Neoplasia	
Hydatidiform mole	
Cervix	

Table 52-3
Abnormal Vaginal Bleeding: Pattern of Bleeding for Nonpregnant Women

Bleeding Pattern	Differential Diagnosis
Ovulatory	
Polymenorrhea	Shortening follicular luteal phase
	Pelvic inflammatory disease
	Endometriosus
	Dysfunctional uterine bleeding
Menorrhagia	Endometrial polyps
	Adenomyosis
	Fibroids
	Intrauterine device
	Sarcoma
	Blood dyscrasias
	Systemic lupus erythematosus
	Hypothyroidism
	Persistent corpus luteum
	Dysfunctional uterine bleeding
Hypomenorrhea	Oral contraceptive pills
	Hyperthyroidism
	Renal failure
Metrorrhagia	Endometritis
	Polyps
	Physiologic
	Oral contraceptive pills
Anovulatory	
Oligomenorrhea	Hypothalamic dysfunction
	Chronic illness
	Stress
	Anorexia
	Polycystic ovary
Delayed menses	Any anovulatory state with polymenorrhagia

(day 20 of the woman's menstrual cycle) and sometimes is associated with spotting, which may be mistaken for an early menstrual period. However, bleeding also can occur in the subsequent weeks of a viable, early pregnancy, and the cause of this bleeding is not known. It may be secondary to continued invasion of the trophoblast into the decidua. Abnormal bleeding in early pregnancy is discussed in detail in Chapter 65.

Pregnant patients in the third trimester are less likely to see a primary care physician unless they are unaware that they are pregnant. Causes of third-trimester bleeding include placenta previa, placental abruption, and premature labor. Of course, pregnant patients also can have causes of bleeding that are unrelated to the pregnancy, such as neoplasia or trauma.

Ovulatory Cycles

If clinical data suggest that a nonpregnant patient ovulates (Box 52-2), abnormal bleeding should be considered evidence for an anatomic lesion or a systemic illness (liver or renal disease, a thyroid disorder, or a coagulopathy). Anatomic lesions may arise from the vagina (laceration, carcinoma, atrophy), cervix (polyps, carcinoma, or cervicitis), uterus (tumor, endometritis, ovulatory bleeding, myomata, or endometriosis), fallopian tubes (tumor), or the ovary (tumor or persistent corpus luteum). Patients who have ovulatory cycles also may have hormonal derangements that can lead to polymenorrhea (shortened follicular or luteal phases) (Table 52-2).

Pattern of Abnormal Bleeding. The pattern of abnormal bleeding can give important clues to the diagnosis, especially in the woman with ovulatory cycles. The history usually reveals that the bleeding has changed in terms of its frequency, duration, or amount, or any combination of these characteristics (Table 52-3).

Polymenorrhea (cycle lengths of 16 to 22 days) can result from the shortening of the follicular or luteal phase. Luteal phase defects can occur in the setting of hypothyroidism or hyperprolactinemia. Decreased menstrual frequency, or **oligomenorrhea,** usually is the result of hypothalamic dysfunction. Stress, anxiety, starvation, chronic illness (such as renal failure), and anorexia nervosa can turn off the gonadotropin-releasing hormone (GnRH) pulse generator, so that the characteristic gonadotropin-pulsatile secretion is disrupted, and menses may occur infrequently or cease altogether. Hypothalamic dysfunction also can occur idiopathically. In addition, there are peripheral causes of oligomenorrhea, including polycystic ovary and other hyperandrogenic disorders. Oligomenorrhea can be the result of oligoovulation or infrequent anovulatory bleeding (Table 52-2).

Alterations in the duration of menses or in the amount of its flow suggest other diagnoses. Increased duration or flow, **menorrhagia,** is seen in blood dyscrasias, hypothyroidism, systemic lupus erythematosus, uterine fibroids, irregular menstrual shedding, and persistence of the corpus luteum. The blood dyscrasias that cause abnormal menstrual bleeding are usually platelet abnormalities and often are detected at menarche. Claessens and Cowell reported 59 cases of abnormal bleeding in adolescents and noted that 44 (77%) patients were anovulatory and 11 had bleeding disorders. Irregular menstrual shedding is characterized by prolonged menses that result from an unusually long desquamation phase. This diagnosis can be made only by endometrial

BOX 52-6

Signs and Symptoms of Anovulatory Cycles

Prolonged bleeding at irregular intervals after several months of amenorrhea

No increase in basal body temperature after time of ovulation

Luteal phase progesterone 3 ng/ml

Proliferative changes on endometrial biopsy

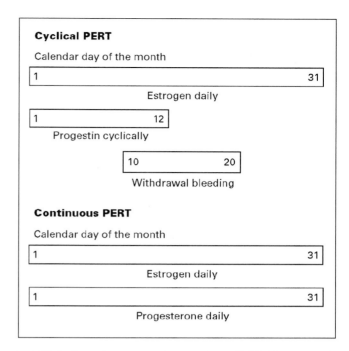

FIG. 52-1 Progestin-estrogen replacement therapy (PERT). (From Matzen R, Lang R: *Clinical preventive medicine,* St Louis, 1993, Mosby.)

biopsy or curettage on the fifth or sixth day of bleeding, which can reveal the simultaneous presence of secretory and proliferative endometrium. Persistent corpus luteum is a rare syndrome that can be mistaken for ectopic pregnancy. In both there is unilateral pain, adnexal mass, and abnormal bleeding. In persistent corpus luteum, however, the human chorionic gonadotropin-beta subunit (*b*-hCG) is negative. The problem is self-limited and may last only a week, but the bleeding is profuse.

Decreased duration or flow of menses (**hypomenorrhea**) occurs most commonly in patients who take oral contraceptive pills. The reduced estrogen content of most preparations causes the endometrium to be thinner than in ovulatory women, and thus there is less to shed. Hypomenorrhea also can be seen in patients with hyperthyroidism, renal failure, or tuberculous endometritis.

Irregular menstrual bleeding, or **metrorrhagia,** is a characteristic of endometritis. It also may be seen in patients with retained products of gestation or with endometrial cancer. Patients who report intermenstrual bleeding, especially postcoital bleeding, should be evaluated for cervical polyps and cervical carcinoma. Midcycle bleeding can be physiologic (bleeding at ovulation) or the result of oral contraceptive use. Usually, midcycle bleeding that occurs in patients who take oral contraceptive pills occurs only in the first three cycles.

Anovulatory Cycles

If the patient has a history of anovulation (Box 52-6), her age will be an important factor in determining the likely diagnosis (Table 52-2).

Adolescent girls and young women often have irregular, anovulatory bleeding as a result of hypothalamic immaturity. As already noted, even 5 years after menarche a substantial number of women (20%) still experience anovulatory menstrual cycles.

Anovulatory cycles also can be seen in more mature women, often a result of polycystic ovary syndrome. These patients often are amenorrheic or oligomenorrheic, obese, and hirsute and have enlarged ovaries, with elevated levels of ovarian (testosterone, androstanedione) or adrenal androgen (dehydroepiandrosterone). Polycystic ovary syndrome has been associated with a number of disorders, including hyperprolactinemia, hypothalamic dysfunction, increased androgen production by the adrenal glands, and increased risk of type II diabetes over one's lifetime (see Chapter 46).

In perimenopausal women, cycles become anovulatory as the number and quality of remaining follicles diminish and estrogen production declines in spite of rising levels of

follicle-stimulating hormone (FSH). The low levels of estrogen, in the absence of progesterone, produce a persistently secretory endometrium that will periodically shed when estradiol levels decline. Menses may be irregular for a period of months to years. When no viable ovarian follicles remain, menses stop and the woman enters the menopause.

In the postmenopausal woman, all bleeding should be considered secondary to neoplasia until proved otherwise. More benign causes of bleeding in this group of patients include obesity, trauma, and iatrogenic factors. Obese women may have enough circulating estrogen from the aromatization of adrenal androgens by fat cells to cause irregular bleeding from endometrial hyperplasia, which may be a precursor to endometrial carcinoma. The other important cause of vaginal bleeding in this age-group is atrophic vaginitis, which usually results from coital trauma.

Patients who are receiving hormone replacement therapy may experience irregular bleeding during the initiation of exogenous hormonal therapy. There are two commonly used methods of administering estrogen replacement therapy. In the first, oral conjugated estrogens, or oral or transdermal estradiol, are taken daily, and a progestational agent is taken for 10 to 12 days of the month (Fig. 52-1). Approximately 3 days after the progestational agent is stopped, withdrawal bleeding ensues. In the second method, estrogen is taken daily with a low daily dose of a progestational agent. With this method of hormonal replacement, there is very irregular, unpredictable bleeding for 3 to 6 months, after which most women become amenorrheic. If irregular bleeding persists after 6 months, a full evaluation to explore anatomic causes of bleeding should be pursued (see Chapter 48).

It is important to remember that patients with anovulatory cycles may still have anatomic causes of abnormal bleeding. Neoplasia and trauma should be considered in every patient with abnormal vaginal bleeding.

Diagnostic Tests

After the differential diagnosis is considered, the following ancillary tests may be necessary to confirm a suspected diagnosis or to make a diagnosis in cases that remain a mystery after the clinical evaluation (Box 52-7).

Determination of Pregnancy

The first test that should be performed in all premenopausal patients is a pregnancy test. The urine pregnancy test, which can be completed easily in the office, has the advantage of providing immediate results. The sensitive enzyme-linked immunoassays for urine hCG are 99% accurate in diagnosing intrauterine pregnancy by the time of the first missed period. This test is not quantitative; the result is positive if the serum b-hCG level is greater than 25 mIU/ml. The serum b-hCG assay is more sensitive, detecting levels of b-hCG subunit as low as 5 mIU/ml. Levels below the limit of assay detection are never consistent with pregnancy. The serum assays are extremely sensitive and are capable of detecting "chemical" pregnancies, in which b-hCG is present in the serum but there is no evidence of a pregnancy on ultrasound examination. False-positive results can occur because of the cross-reactivity with luteinizing hormone. The specificity varies among assays and depends on the antibodies used.

BOX 52-7
Key Diagnostic Tests for Evaluation of Abnormal Vaginal Bleeding

---

To Determine Pregnancy
Pregnancy test
Urine b-hCG
Serum b-hCG
Ultrasound (if clinically indicated)

To Determine Ovulation
Basal body temperature charts
Serum progesterone (obtained after ovulation during the luteal phase in cycle)
Endometrial biopsy (to evaluate for cancer or to establish anovulation)

Other Tests
Pap smear
Cervical cultures for chlamydia/gonorrhea
Hematocrit value, red blood cell indexes, platelet count, PT/PTT

When Clinically Indicated
TSH, LFT
FSH (to confirm PCO, ovarian failure, or menopause)
Testosterone, DHEAS, follicular phase 17-hydroxyprogesterone (for suspected hirsuitism)
Prolactin (if galactorrhea)
DST (for suspected Cushing's syndrome)

PT, Prothrombin time; *PTT,* partial thromboplastin time; *TSH,* thyroid-stimulating hormone; *LFT,* liver function test; *FSH,* follicle-stimulating hormone; *PCO,* polycystic ovary; *DHEAS,* dehydroepiandrosterone sulfate; *DST,* dexamethasone suppression test.

Determination of Ovulatory Status

There are several methods of determining whether the patient is ovulating. First, and least expensive, the physician may ask the patient to fill out **basal body temperature charts.** The patient should record her temperature each morning before getting out of bed. Ovulation thermometers are available at most pharmacies, but digital thermometers also are accurate and are easier for patients to use. The patient makes note of days that bleeding occurred. When graphed against time in days, ovulatory cycles exhibit a biphasic curve, with higher temperatures present in the latter half of the cycle, or after ovulation. If the patient detects a rise in temperature, she can ascertain that ovulation did in fact occur by using a nonprescription **ovulation kit.** These kits use antibodies to luteinizing hormone (LH) to detect secreted LH during the LH surge.

Serum progesterone levels greater than 3 ng/ml also can be used to confirm that ovulation has occurred. In a normal cycle, peak progesterone secretion occurs on day 20, or about a week after ovulation. The blood test for progesterone should be timed so that it takes place after ovulation is thought to have occurred, using information either from the patient's symptoms or from the basal body temperature chart.

The definitive test to prove whether a patient has ovulated is the **endometrial biopsy.** The presence of a secretory endometrium at the start of menses definitively proves that ovulation has occurred. The pathologist dates the secretory endometrium based on the changes seen in a typical 28-day cycle. An endometrium that is reported to be more than 2 days out of phase with the actual cycle day of the biopsy is considered diagnostic of a luteal-phase defect.

Other Diagnostic Tests

Other laboratory tests that may be of value include the hematocrit value, red blood cell indexes, platelet count, prothrombin time (PT) and partial thromboplastin time (PTT), cervical cultures for chlamydia and gonorrhea, and a Pap smear. When indicated by the history or physical examination, liver function tests, thyroid function tests, and levels of LH, FSH, estradiol, progesterone, and prolactin may be helpful. If the LH value is more than twofold greater than that of FSH, the patient may have polycystic ovary syndrome. An FSH concentration that is greater than that of LH can be the earliest sign of ovarian failure.

If the patient is pregnant and is experiencing abnormal bleeding, an ultrasound examination should be performed, which can confirm an intrauterine pregnancy but cannot rule out ectopic pregnancy. Ultrasound findings also can provide information about whether a spontaneous abortion is occurring. If the pregnancy is greater than 6 weeks' gestation, a fetal heartbeat should be detectable if the pregnancy is viable. If there is no heartbeat and the bleeding is occurring at about 6 weeks of gestation, the ultrasound should be repeated in a week to determine if there has been a missed abortion (see Chapter 66).

APPROACH TO THE PATIENT WITH ABNORMAL VAGINAL BLEEDING

The two goals in the management of abnormal uterine bleeding are to control the acute bleeding episode and to prevent recurrent episodes. For the woman with massive vaginal hemorrhaging and hypotension, the first step is to stabilize the patient's condition (Box 52-8). This includes a focused physical and pelvic examination in addition to establishing an intravenous access, obtaining blood for type and cross match, and completing initial hematologic studies (hematocrit, platelet estimate) and serum pregnancy test. After the cause is established, often suction curettage by a gynecologist will stop the bleeding unless the causative factor is a blood dyscrasia or a carcinoma.

If the bleeding is not severe, the first step is to determine if the patient with abnormal vaginal bleeding is pregnant. This can be accomplished by performing a simple urine test. Sometimes if the vaginal bleeding occurs within 2 to 10 days after a reported missed period, the urine test is negative for pregnancy. In this event, if the physician still suspects pregnancy (especially an ectopic pregnancy), a serum b-hCG level should be obtained. In fact, 1% to 2% of patients with ectopic pregnancies have serum b-hCG levels below 25 mIU/ml, and thus the urine pregnancy test would miss the diagnosis. Therefore, if results of the urine test are negative and the patient is complaining of unilateral abdominal pain with bleeding, which would heighten the suspicion of ectopic pregnancy, a pelvic ultrasound examination should be performed. In addition, ultrasound examination is appropriate if there is no time to wait for results of the serum pregnancy tests. If the serum b-hCG level is greater than 2000 mIU/ml, ultrasound examination should show a gestational sac in an intrauterine pregnancy (see Chapter 65).

The ultrasound findings are unlikely to be helpful if the serum b-hCG level is less than 2000 mIU/ml because a gestational sac will not be present even if the pregnancy is intrauterine. In these early cases of pregnancy with bleeding, the stability of the patient's condition will dictate management. The patient whose condition is unstable (severe pain, hypotension, massive bleeding) should undergo laparoscopy on an emergent basis. If the serum b-hCG level is less than 2000 mIU/ml and the patient is clinically stable, she should be observed and the hCG level should be obtained again in 48 hours. If the hCG level fails to double and the patient continues to have bleeding and pain, laparoscopy should be performed.

As mentioned before, other causes of abnormal bleeding in patients with positive pregnancy test results include complete and incomplete abortion and molar pregnancy. In both molar pregnancy and abortion, serum b-hCG levels are higher than expected for a given gestational age. Because bleeding after complete abortion is usually minimal, continued bleeding usually indicates that gestational products have been retained. If bleeding does not resolve within 1 week, these patients should be evaluated by a gynecologist for possible dilation and curettage.

If the patient is not pregnant but is ovulating, she may have a systemic illness, a hormonal disruption of normal physiology, or an organic lesion. As mentioned before, the most common cause of abnormal bleeding in ovulatory patients, after pregnancy, is blood dyscrasia, the most common of which is von Willebrand's disease. Acute bleeding episodes in these patients are managed by administering factor VIII. Abnormal vaginal bleeding that occurs as the result of other systemic illnesses, such as chronic renal failure, systemic lupus erythematosus, liver disease, and thyroid disease, can be expected to improve by treating the underlying disease. When a systemic illness or blood dyscrasia cannot be detected in ovulatory patients, a thorough search for an anatomic lesion should be performed.

Finally, patients can have alterations in the frequency of menses but still have ovulatory cycles. Polymenorrhea that results from shortened follicular phase can occur in adolescence and usually will correct with time. Shortened luteal phases, or inadequate luteal phase, can be treated with progesterone beginning the day after ovulation. When an anatomic lesion is suspected, the patient should be referred to a gynecologist.

Anovulatory bleeding results from chronic unopposed estrogen stimulation of the endometrium. Management and treatment of dysfunctional uterine bleeding are discussed in Chapter 53. Management and treatment of abnormal bleeding associated with polycystic ovary syndrome is discussed in Chapter 46.

BIBLIOGRAPHY

American College of Obstetricians and Gynecologists: Management of anovulatory bleeding. *ACOG Practice Bulletin 14*, Washington, DC, 2000, ACOG.

Barbieri RL, Smith S, Ryan KJ: The role of hyperinsulinemia in the pathogenesis of ovarian hyperandrogenism, *Fertil Steril* 50:197, 1988.

Bayer SR, DeCherney AH: Clinical manifestations and treatment of dysfunctional uterine bleeding, *JAMA* 269:1823, 1993.

Chan WY, Hill JC: Menstrual prostaglandin levels in nondysmenorrheic and dysmenorrheic subjects, *Prostaglandins* 15:365, 1978.

Claessens EA, Cowell CA: Acute adolescent menorrhagia, *Am J Obstet Gynecol* 139:277, 1981.

Cowan BD, Morrison JC: Management of abnormal genital bleeding in girls and women, *N Engl J Med* 324:1710, 1991.

Emans SJ, Grace E, Goldstein DP: Oligomenorrhea in adolescent girls *J Pediatr* 97:815, 1980.

Falone T et al: Dysfunctional uterine bleeding in adolescents, *J Reprod Med* 39:761, 1994.

Fraser IS, McCarron G, Markham R: A preliminary study of factors influencing perception of menstrual blood loss volume, *Am J Obstet Gynecol* 149:788, 1984.

Fraser IS et al: Measured menstrual blood loss in women with menorrhagia associated with pelvic disease of coagulation disorder, *Obstet Gynecol* 68:630, 1986.

Givens JR et al: Dynamics of suppression and recovery of plasma FSH, LH, androstenedione, and testosterone in polycystic ovarian disease using an oral contraceptive, *J Clin Endocrinol Metab* 37:407, 1973.

BOX 52-8
Management of Acute Vaginal Hemorrhage

Hemodynamic Instability
IV access and fluid resuscitation and determine pregnancy
Blood type and cross matching
Initial hematologic screen
Suction curettage

Hemodynamic Stability and No Pregnancy
Conjugated equine estrogen 25 mg IV q4h (maximum of 6 doses)
Estradiol/norgestrel oral contraceptive (2 pills of Ovral) 50 mg/0.5 mg
    pills bid for 3-5 days until bleeding stops; then remaining pills 1/day

Hallberg L et al: Menstrual blood loss: a population study, *Acta Obstet Gynecol Scand* 45:320, 1966.

Hamilton JV, Knab DR: Suction curettage: therapeutic effectiveness in dysfunctional uterine bleeding, *Obstet Gynecol* 45:47, 1975.

Keye WR: Dysfunctional uterine bleeding. In Glass R, editor: *Office gynecology,* Baltimore, 1988, Williams & Wilkins.

Long CA, Gast MJ: Menorrhagia, *Obstet Gynecol Clin North Am* 17:343, 1990.

Matzen R, Lang R: *Clinical preventive medicine,* St Louis, 1993, Mosby.

Mishell DR et al: Oral contraception for women in their 40s, *J Reprod Med* 35(suppl):447, 1990.

Sherman BM, Korenman SG: Hormonal characteristics of the human menstrual cycle throughout reproductive life, *J Clin Invest* 55:699, 1975.

Wentz AC: Abnormal uterine bleeding. In Jones HW, Wentz AC, Burnett LS, editors: *Novak's testbook of gynecology,* Baltimore, 1988, Williams & Wilkins.

Wilansky DL, Greisman B: Early hypothyroidism in patients with menorrhagia, *Am J Obstet Gynecol* 160:673, 1989.

Winter JSD, Fairman C: The development of cyclic pituitary-gonadal function in adolescent females, *J Clin Endocrinol Metab* 37:714, 1973.

CHAPTER 53

Dysfunctional Uterine Bleeding

Karen J. Carlson
Raja A. Sayegh
Johnny T. Awwad

Dysfunctional uterine bleeding (DUB) is a diagnosis of exclusion that indicates excessive uterine bleeding in the absence of an organic uterine pathologic condition, abnormalities of other reproductive organs, or systemic condition. The term *DUB* sometimes is used to denote noncyclic, anovulatory bleeding; in this chapter, menorrhagia (heavy menstrual bleeding) and idiopathic intermenstrual bleeding are considered as forms of DUB. The management of idiopathic postmenopausal bleeding also is addressed.

The pathophysiology of DUB is poorly understood, but most cases are believed to result from dyssynchronized sex steroid action on the endometrium. Although chronic anovulation at any age may be associated with DUB, most commonly it is observed at the extremes of reproductive age, perimenarche, and perimenopause. Less frequently, DUB can occur in ovulatory cycles and manifest as menorrhagia, midcycle bleeding, or irregular menses.

The parameters of normal menstrual function are shown in Box 53-1. The repetitiveness and constancy of any given set of parameters define normal menstrual function for each woman. Any perceived deviation from the usual interval, duration, or flow pattern often prompts a woman to seek medical attention.

GOALS OF MANAGEMENT

It is essential to rule out endocrinopathies, abnormal pregnancy, and an organic pathologic condition of the uterus and ovaries before making a diagnosis of DUB. Chapter 52 describes the evaluation of abnormal uterine bleeding.

Once a diagnosis of DUB is made, management is guided by consideration of the woman's age and the presence of ovulatory or anovulatory cycles (Table 53-1). The primary management goals are to alleviate excessive bleeding, to correct anemia if it exists, and to monitor response to treatment in order to detect the rare case of occult disease missed on the initial diagnostic evaluation.

ADOLESCENCE

The interval between menarche and the establishment of regular ovulatory cycles is variable and depends on the rate of maturation of the hypothalamic-pituitary-ovarian axis. During this period, acyclic ovarian activity prevails, and unopposed estrogen action on the endometrium may extend over several months. The proliferating endometrium reaches a critical height beyond which it cannot maintain its structural integrity. Fragmented endometrial shedding occurs, causing DUB that at times may be heavy and prolonged.

Choice of Therapy

The choice of therapy for DUB in the adolescent is dictated by the severity and frequency of bleeding and the need for contraception. A large proportion of patients have a self-limited course with a few episodes of light to moderate bleeding that can be reliably managed until regular ovarian cycles are established. Others may have frequent, heavy, and painful episodes of bleeding, and iron-deficiency anemia may develop. In this case a regimen of hormonal therapy that prevents prolonged unopposed estrogen action and ensures regular menstrual shedding is used.

The **combination oral contraceptive pill** that contains a progestin along with 30 to 35 mg of ethinyl estradiol generally is the first choice of therapy. This provides predictable 28-day cycles, as well as reliable contraception. There is no evidence that maturation of the hypothalamic-pituitary-ovarian axis is delayed or adversely affected by oral contraceptives.

Another option is to simulate a luteal phase with **oral progestins.** A typical regimen is medroxyprogesterone acetate 10 mg daily, or its equivalent (Box 53-2), for 10 to 13 days. Patients completing the first course of treatment must be cautioned to expect a heavy episode of bleeding as a result of the shedding of a thick endometrial build-up. Nonsteroidal antiinflammatory drugs (NSAIDs) are helpful to control the discomfort that often coexists with such heavy flow. The course of progestins may be repeated in 6 weeks unless spontaneous menses occurs, signaling a remission of anovulation. The clinician should recognize that concerns about future fertility are common in adolescent women with irregular bleeding. These concerns should be addressed directly, and the transient nature of this condition should be emphasized.

BOX 53-1

Parameters of Normal Menstrual Function

Cycle interval (days)	21-35
Duration of flow (days)	2-8
Blood loss/cycle (ml)	30-80

BOX 53-2

Equivalent Daily Doses of Oral Progestins for the Treatment of Dysfunctional Uterine Bleeding

Medroxyprogesterone acetate (Provera, Cycrin)	10 mg
Micronized progesterone (Prometrium)	400 mg
Norgestrel (Ovrette)	150 μg
Norethindrone acetate (Micronor, Nor-QD)	0.7-1.0 mg

Table 53-1
Management of Dysfunctional Uterine Bleeding

Bleeding Pattern	Cause	Treatment
Ovulatory DUB		
Heavy menstrual bleeding	Imbalance in endometrial prostacyclins and prostaglandins	Nonsteroidal antiinflammatory drugs Combination oral contraceptive pill Progestin intrauterine device Endometrial ablation
Midcycle spotting	Periovulatory estrogen decline	None
Delayed menses	Persistent corpus luteum	None (rule out pregnancy)
Anovulatory DUB		
Irregular menses	Unopposed estrogen stimulation of endometrium	Combination oral contraceptive pill Cyclic progestins Endometrial ablation
Postmenopausal bleeding	Endometrial atrophy	Hormone replacement therapy Endometrial ablation

DUB, Dysfunctional uterine bleeding.

REPRODUCTIVE YEARS
Ovulatory Dysfunctional Uterine Bleeding

It is estimated that 15% of women with DUB are ovulatory. The presence of molimina (breast tenderness, pelvic cramping, bloating, edema) and cycle regularity generally indicate the presence of ovulatory cycles. Basal body temperature charting over a 1- to 2-month period may be used to document ovulation. The postovulatory rise in progesterone causes a sustained elevation in basal body temperature of at least 0.5° C throughout the luteal phase. In equivocal situations, ovulation can be confirmed by measuring serum progesterone between cycle day 18 and 24; a level greater than 3 ng/ml is indicative of ovulation. Results of an endometrial biopsy that demonstrate secretory changes also indicate ovulation and progesterone production.

Menorrhagia

Menorrhagia in the absence of any anatomic abnormality or systemic illness is considered to be a form of DUB caused by an imbalance between endometrial prostacyclin and prostaglandin production. Although menstrual blood loss in excess of 80 ml is considered abnormal, there are no practical objective means to assess the severity of menstrual bleeding other than the presence of iron-deficiency anemia. Women's subjective reports of heavy bleeding and patterns of sanitary protection use correlate poorly with measured menstrual blood loss. The passing of blood clots is one clinical indicator of excessive menstrual bleeding. Another useful clinical criterion for gauging bleeding severity is whether bleeding repeatedly interferes with a woman's important daily activities. Menorrhagia should be treated when it produces iron-deficiency anemia or when it is bothersome to the woman's comfort.

Options for initial treatment of menorrhagia include prostaglandin synthetase inhibitors or the oral contraceptive pill. **Prostaglandin synthetase inhibitors** such as mefenamic acid, naproxen sodium, or ibuprofen have been shown in randomized trials to reduce blood loss up to 50%. They have the additional benefit of relieving dysmenorrhea. The usual dose is 1 to 1.5 g daily of any of the aforementioned agents divided in two to three oral doses, started 1 day before the onset of menses. The main side effect of prostaglandin synthetase inhibitors is gastric irritation, which is less likely if medication is taken with food.

Estrogen-progestin combination oral contraceptives generally produce a reduction in menstrual flow and are particularly appropriate for initial treatment when contraception is needed. Another treatment option is a **levonorgestrel-impregnated intrauterine device** (IUD) that delivers the progestin locally and renders the endometrium atrophic, thus effectively reducing menstrual blood loss. The progestin-medicated IUD is an option for women desiring contraception who are not candidates for the oral contraceptive pill and have no contraindications to the IUD (see Chapter 58).

Iron replacement with ferrous sulfate or gluconate, 300 mg two to three times a day, should be given when iron-deficiency anemia is present.

Women whose menorrhagia is not controlled by medical therapy should be referred to a gynecologist for further management. Alternatives include **endometrial ablation, gonadotropin-releasing hormone (GnRH) agonists,** or **hysterectomy** (described in the next section).

Persistent Corpus Luteum

Another cause of DUB in ovulatory cycles is a persistent corpus luteum, or Halban's syndrome. In this instance the life span of the corpus luteum is longer than the usual 10 to 16 days, and menstrual withdrawal bleeding is delayed and unpredictable. The etiology of this condition is unknown, and the important differential diagnosis is pregnancy, which can be ruled out with a serum chorionic gonadotropin (b-hCG) level. The condition often is self-limited, and no treatment is necessary.

Midcycle Spotting

Midcycle spotting that occurs in the periovulatory period is attributed to a transient physiologic decline in serum estradiol level after ovulation. Such bleeding may be associated with *mittelschmerz,* or acute midcycle abdominal pain. Midcycle spotting usually is self-limited and requires no intervention.

Anovulatory Dysfunctional Uterine Bleeding

The pathophysiology of anovulatory DUB in the reproductive years is similar to that in the adolescent, namely prolonged, unopposed estrogen action on the endometrium and breakthrough bleeding. Anovulation in the reproductive years (approximately ages 16 to 44 years) may be idiopathic and self-limited, in which case it often is ascribed to central nervous system or hypothalamic dysfunction associated with stress, heavy exercise, or rapid weight changes. Up to 90% of women in the fifth decade of life experience increased variability in their menstrual cycles before the onset of menopause. A dwindling ovarian reserve, abnormal folliculogenesis, and altered hypothalamic feedback result in frequent anovulatory cycles and unopposed estrogen action on the endometrium. The menopausal transition may extend over several years and may be punctuated by episodes of DUB.

Idiopathic Anovulation

Women with DUB caused by idiopathic anovulation may be treated with cyclic progestins or the combination oral contraceptive pill. The purpose of treatment is to provide predictable flow, to avoid heavy episodes of bleeding, and to prevent the increased risk of endometrial hyperplasia and cancer associated with prolonged unopposed estrogen action. Because spontaneous ovulation and conception can occur during cyclic progestin therapy, oral contraceptives may be preferred when contraception is needed.

In women of reproductive age, the **combination oral contraceptive** (30 to 35 mg of ethinyl estradiol or the equivalent) is appropriate for healthy nonsmoking women without contraindications to oral contraceptive pill use. (Use of the oral contraceptive pill is discussed in detail in Chapter 58.)

In perimenopausal women, **low-dose oral contraceptives** (containing 20 mg of ethinyl estradiol) have several advantages over cyclic progestins, including predictable cycle control, decrease in perimenopausal symptoms (such as mood swings, irritability, decreased libido, and hot flashes), reliable contraception, and, possibly, the prevention of accelerated bone mineral loss that is believed to start in the perimenopausal years. Most women complete the menopausal transition by age 50 to 52 years, at which time it is reasonable to switch to conventional postmenopausal hormone replacement therapy.

Cyclic progestin therapy is an alternative when the low-dose oral contraceptive pill is contraindicated, not tolerated, or not desired. A widely used regimen is oral medroxyprogesterone acetate, 10 mg daily for 10 to 13 days every 6 weeks to 3 months. One general rule is to start with a course of progestins every 8 weeks and to ask the patient to keep a record of the amount of withdrawal bleeding. Heavy bleeding indicates the need to shorten the interval; scant bleeding suggests that the interval may be increased. No bleeding, in the absence of pregnancy, indicates that the perimenopausal transition may have been completed and treatment can be stopped or replacement estrogen added.

Premature Ovarian Failure and Polycystic Ovary Syndrome

Oral contraceptives are the preferred treatment of DUB in premature ovarian failure, in which estrogen deficiency is likely. The oral contraceptive pill (30 to 35 mg ethinyl estradiol or equivalent) is also the optimal choice for treatment in polycystic ovary syndrome because it suppresses ovarian androgen production and helps control the androgenic manifestations of the disorder.

Women with anovulatory DUB who do not respond to hormonal therapy should be further examined for an occult, focal, intrauterine pathologic condition (small submucous myomas, endometrial polyps, or focal endometrial hyperplasia or carcinoma) that could not be identified on initial investigation. Women older than 40 years old who have already undergone endometrial biopsy before treatment should be referred for hysteroscopic examination or dilation and curettage. Small-caliber fiberoptic hysteroscopes can be introduced transcervically without anesthesia, making this a relatively easy office procedure. The procedure is preferably performed during nonbleeding intervals because visibility may be impaired otherwise. Focal lesions often require the use of operative hysteroscopy for resection and histologic evaluation. Women younger than 40 years old whose bleeding is not controlled by hormonal therapy should undergo endometrial evaluation by endometrial biopsy, hysteroscopy, or dilation and curettage.

Endometrial ablation is a conservative surgical alternative for the treatment of DUB in women who have completed childbearing. This procedure uses laser or electrocautery under hysteroscopic guidance to destroy the endometrium. Endometrial ablation offers significant advantages over hysterectomy: a shorter duration of surgery and hospital stay, and return to work within 2 to 3 weeks; the main disadvantage is the potential for recurrence of bleeding. The effectiveness of endometrial ablation by any method for reducing or abolishing excessive bleeding is 80% to 90%; 30 to 40% of women become amenorrheic. Pelvic pain is decreased in 50%. An alternative method for ablation, the thermal balloon, has been approved for use in the United States. Its overall effectiveness is similar to other ablation techniques, although the number of women rendered amenorrheic is lower.

Bleeding recurs, however, in up to 40% of women over 5 years; 10% to 20% require additional procedures. Perioperative complications of ablation occur in 10% to 15% of cases. The long-term risks of these procedures are not known. There has been theoretical concern about the potential for endometrial tissue remnants to undergo estrogenic stimulation and hyperplasia, yet escape detection through the usual symptom of vaginal bleeding. For this reason, any woman treated with ablation who subsequently receives estrogen replacement therapy should also receive a progestin. Pregnancy is unlikely, but not impossible, after endometrial ablation.

GnRH agonists may provide an alternative treatment for women who do not respond to the aforementioned therapies. GnRH agonists, delivered by the intramuscular, subcutaneous, or intranasal routes, produce a profound hypoestrogenic state within a few weeks of initiation. Endometrial atrophy and amenorrhea or oligomenorrhea occur. Use of GnRH agonists for DUB currently is limited by systemic complications of hypoestrogenemia (particularly decreased bone density), which occur after as little as 6 months of use. At present GnRH agonists are used primarily in women whose medical conditions preclude hormonal therapy (e.g., after liver transplantation). Long-term use may become feasible with "add-back" hormone replacement therapy, which in some studies has appeared to maintain bone density while preventing recurrence of DUB. GnRH agonists are not approved by the United States Food and Drug Administration for the treatment of dysfunctional uterine bleeding.

Hysterectomy may be necessary for treatment of severe, functionally limiting menorrhagia that is refractory to conservative treatment in women who do not wish to preserve fertility. Randomized trials in the United Kingdom comparing hysterectomy with endometrial ablation have shown significantly higher levels of satisfaction with hysterectomy at 1 and 2 years, with equivalent levels of satisfaction at 3 and 4 years. Outcomes of hysterectomy are discussed further in Chapter 50.

Management of Acute Bleeding

Management of DUB that is severe and prolonged requires rapid control of bleeding and hemodynamic resuscitation as needed to restore effective circulation. Women with evidence of severe hypovolemia (orthostatic hypotension or tachycardia) or anemia (hematocrit less than 25%) require hospitalization. Outpatient management is appropriate if the woman has no signs of significant hypovolemia, can take medications orally, and is able to maintain close follow-up monitoring.

Initial treatment to control bleeding is either high-dose medroxyprogesterone acetate (30 mg/day in three divided dosages) or intramuscular injection of 150 mg depot medroxyprogesterone acetate. The latter preparation maintains endometrial atrophy for 2 to 3 months, providing adequate contraception and significant relief from anovulatory DUB, but it also can cause DUB through endometrial atrophy.

In some instances, patients who have been bleeding heavily for weeks do not respond to progesterone, possibly because of a denuded endometrial lining. High-dose estrogens can be added if bleeding has not diminished within 24 hours of initiating progestin therapy. A convenient form of adding estrogens is use of an oral contraceptive that contains 35 mg ethinyl estradiol; the dosage is one tablet every 4 to 6 hours given over 2 to 3 days. Although the mechanism of action of bolus estrogen is not very well understood, its effect is thought to be mediated via accelerated proliferation of the endometrial basal layer, which seals the bleeding vessels.

Once the acute bleeding is brought under control, long-term management should aim at restoring depleted iron stores with oral iron replacement and preventing recurrences by use of cyclic progestins or conventional doses of oral contraceptives. Failure to achieve tight cycle control in the ensuing months necessitates further evaluation, for example, endometrial biopsy, office hysteroscopy, or dilatation and curettage.

If the acute episode is not controlled within 24 hours of hormonal therapy, hospital admission and surgical dilatation and curettage are advisable, both for diagnostic value and immediate therapeutic effects. However, occult pathologic conditions such as polyps and submucous myomas may be missed with blind curettage. Dilatation and curettage has no role in the long-term treatment of DUB, as menstrual loss rapidly returns to previous levels.

The use of continuous flow hysteroscopy provides a panoramic view of the uterine cavity and is an invaluable diagnostic and therapeutic adjunct to curettage when such focal endometrial abnormality is suspected. Hysteroscopically directed resections of endometrial lesions can be safely performed, with low morbidity and good outcome. In certain instances a lesser curettage may be performed on an ambulatory basis with a Karman suction apparatus and the patient under light sedation and with local cervical anesthesia. In extremely rare circumstances, when all conservative medical and surgical efforts have failed and life-saving measures are needed, a hysterectomy may be necessary.

POSTMENOPAUSAL YEARS

Menopause is associated with amenorrhea as a result of cessation of ovarian estrogen production and an inactive, atrophic endometrium. In some postmenopausal women, however, sufficient estrogen is produced from peripheral conversion of ovarian and adrenal androgens to stimulate the endometrial lining and cause resumption of bleeding. An endometrial biopsy that shows evidence of endometrial activity (proliferative endometrium, hyperplasia, or cancer) in postmenopausal women necessitates a thorough search for estrogen- or androgen-producing tumors of the ovary and adrenal gland. In the absence of such a pathologic condition, endometrial activity in postmenopausal women usually is caused by excessive peripheral production of estrogens, commonly observed in obese women who are at increased risk of developing endometrial hyperplasia and cancer. These women can be treated with cyclic progestins as already described.

Postmenopausal uterine bleeding in the absence of any endometrial activity is due mostly to endometrial atrophy, but focal uterine disease may coexist with atrophy and is best ruled out with hysteroscopic examination in the office. Treatment of atrophic DUB is not necessary unless bleeding is bothersome, recurrent, or severe. Treatment options include hormone replacement therapy, hysteroscopic endometrial ablation, or hysterectomy. Bleeding from an atrophic endometrium rarely is severe enough to warrant surgical intervention. However, postmenopausal women with certain chronic medical illnesses (e.g., renal failure and liver disease) may have coexistent coagulopathies that may predispose them to heavy bleeding from an atrophic endometrium. These women are appropriate candidates for endometrial ablation rather than hormonal therapy or hysterectomy.

BIBLIOGRAPHY

Alexander DA et al: Randomised trial comparing hysterectomy with endometrial ablation for dysfunctional uterine bleeding: psychiatric and psychosocial aspects, *BMJ* 312:280,1996.

American College of Obstetricians and Gynecologists: Management of anovulatory bleeding. ACOG Practice Bulletin 14. ACOG 2000; Washington, DC.

Baird DT, Glasier AF: Drug therapy: hormonal contraception, *N Engl J Med* 328:1543, 1993.

Casper RF et al: The effect of 20 μg ethinyl estradiol/1 mg norethindrone acetate(minestrin), a low dose oral contraceptive, on vaginal bleeding patterns, hot flushes and quality of life in symptomatic perimenopausal women, *Menopause* 4:139, 1997.

Cooper KG et al: Two-year follow-up of women randomized to medical management or transcervical resection of the endometrium for heavy menstrual loss: clinical and quality of life outcomes, *Br J Obstet Gynaecol* 106:258, 1999.

Crosignani PG et al: Levonorgestrel-releasing intrauterine device versus hysteroscopic endometrial resection in the treatment of dysfunctional uterine bleeding, *Obstet Gynecol* 90:257, 1997.

Iyer V, Farquhar C, Jepson R: The effectiveness of oral contraceptive pills versus placebo or any other medical treatment for menorrhagia. In *The Cochrane Library*, Issue 2, 2000, Oxford: Update Software.

Kleerekoper M et al: Henry Ford Hospital Osteoporosis Research Group: oral contraceptive use may protect against low bone mass, *Arch Intern Med* 151:1971, 1991.

Lethaby A, Augood C, Duckitt K: Nonsteroidal anti-inflammatory drugs vs either placebo or any other medical treatment for heavy menstrual bleeding (menorrhagia). In *The Cochrane Library*, Issue 2, 2000. Oxford: Update Software.

Lethaby AE, Cooke I, Rees M: Progesterone/progestogen releasing intra-uterine systems versus either placebo or any other medication for heavy menstrual bleeding. In *The Cochrane Library*, Issue 2, 2000. Oxford: Update Software.

Lethaby AE et al: Endometrial resection and ablation versus hysterectomy for heavy menstrual bleeding. In *The Cochrane Library*, Issue 2, 2000. Oxford: Update Software.

Lindsay R, Tohme J, Kanders B: The effect of oral contraceptives use on vertebral bone mass in pre- and postmenopausal women, *Contraception* 34:333, 1986.

Metcalf MG: Incidence of ovulatory cycles in women approaching the menopause, *J Biosci Sci* 11:39, 1979.

Meyer WR et al: Thermal balloon and rollerball ablation to treat menorrhagia: a multicenter comparison, *Obstet Gynecol* 92:98, 1998.

Serden SP, Brooks PG: Preoperative therapy in preparation for endometrial ablation, *J Reprod Med* 37:679, 1992.

Thomas EJ, Okuda KJ, Thomas NM: The combination of a depot gonadotropin releasing hormone agonist and cyclical hormone replacement therapy for dysfunctional uterine bleeding, *Br J Obstet Gynaecol* 98:1155, 1991.

CHAPTER 54

Incontinence and Pelvic Organ Prolapse

May M. Wakamatsu

Urinary incontinence, although not a life-threatening disorder, can significantly decrease the quality of a woman's life. A woman may stop exercising, traveling, or even visiting friends because of the fear of urinary incontinence. Approximately 60% to 70% of urinary incontinence can be treated primarily without surgery.

This chapter reviews the pathophysiology, primary diagnosis, and treatment of urinary incontinence, with a focus on the two most common types, stress and urge incontinence. Genital prolapse is discussed in terms of symptoms, complications of prolapse, and primary treatment.

▦ EPIDEMIOLOGY

A total of 15 to 19 million individuals are affected by urinary incontinence in the United States. In all, 30% of the ambulatory elderly and 50% of nursing home patients experience incontinence.

Types of Incontinence

The two most common forms of incontinence are stress incontinence and detrusor instability, also called "urge" incontinence (Table 54-1).

Stress incontinence results from damage to the "continence mechanism system," which includes the nerves, muscles, and connective tissues of the pelvic floor. Normally, a hammock of muscle and connective tissue supports the urethrovesical junction and urethra. When pressure from a cough or sneeze compresses the bladder, it also applies pressure to the urethra. If the hammock is intact, it allows the urethrovesical junction and urethra to be compressed closed so that urine does not escape. If the hammock is weakened by muscle or connective tissue stretching or breaking, or if there is sufficient nerve damage to weaken muscle integrity, compression does not occur, and stress incontinence results.

Childbirth is the most common risk factor for stress incontinence. The first vaginal delivery usually causes the most damage to the pelvic floor; subsequent deliveries may or may not add to pelvic floor dysfunction. Other risk factors are advanced age, atrophy, cigarette smoking, and work that requires heavy lifting.

The patient will usually present complaining of incontinence that occurs with coughing, sneezing, lifting, or exercise. She may complain of needing larger and larger pads, having to change them more often, or even overflowing the pads.

Detrusor instability (urge incontinence) occurs when the detrusor muscle is not inhibited at the appropriate moment by conscious will; the detrusor muscle contracts even when the woman does not want to void. There are many different triggers for detrusor overactivity, including hearing running water or feeling water; changing position; cold ambient temperature; being near a toilet; or anticipating voiding. In addition, caffeine, excessive fluid intake, and diuretics may make frequency and urge incontinence more likely.

The most common cause for detrusor instability incontinence is idiopathic; there is no overt neurologic disorder. However, it is seen more commonly in the elderly, so presumably the aging cortex plays a role in poor bladder control. Detrusor instability can occur with diabetes, multiple sclerosis, Parkinson's disease, and any type of central nervous system injury. The pathophysiology for detrusor instability is poorly understood.

Patients with urge incontinence complain of urinary frequency, often voiding every hour or more; nocturia (voiding more than twice during the night); and "not making it to the toilet on time." When women experience urge incontinence, they usually respond by voiding more frequently. This behavior, however, worsens the frequency and urge incontinence and "trains" the bladder to hold smaller and smaller volumes of urine. The problem worsens until the bladder controls the patient, rather than the patient choosing when to void. Patients often state, "I know where every bathroom is in my town" or they are afraid to leave the house or travel.

Approximately, one third of women have pure stress incontinence, one third have pure urge incontinence, and one third have both forms, so-called "mixed" incontinence. These patients complain of leaking both with a cough or a sneeze, and "on the way to the toilet."

Functional incontinence may be the third frequent form of incontinence seen in primary care practice. The patient

Table 54-1
Differential Diagnosis of Stress Incontinence vs. Detrusor Instability

	Stress Incontinence	Detrusor Instability
Typical symptoms	Urine loss at instant of physical stress, cough, sneeze	Urgency, frequency, urge incontinence, incontinence without sensation
Volume of urine lost	Variable but limited spurt or gush	Large volume of urine over several seconds
Effect of bladder volume	Occurs even soon after voiding	More likely when moderately full
History of bladder disorders	In general, no history of functional disorders of bladder control, except related to pregnancy	May have "lifelong" history of voiding and voiding difficulties, including childhood enuresis

with two hip replacements or severe arthritis whose bathroom is on a different floor experiences incontinence because she cannot ambulate quickly enough to the toilet. It can be difficult to determine whether the incontinence is due to a functional problem, detrusor instability, or both.

Overflow incontinence is not commonly seen in the general population. Usually there is a history of a significant neurologic deficit such as stroke or spinal cord injury. The detrusor muscle no longer contracts strongly enough to empty the bladder adequately; as more urine enters the already full bladder, overflow occurs, resulting in incontinence. Sensory impairment may be present as well, so that the patient does not feel the urge to void at normal bladder capacity. Symptoms of overflow incontinence can be similar to urge incontinence—frequency and leaking on the way to the toilet. In addition, the patient may complain of leaking when she gets up from a chair or walks. She may also complain of feeling like she has a "full bladder all the time."

Detrusor hyperactivity with impaired contractility is a paradoxical bladder dysfunction that generally occurs in the elderly. The detrusor muscle contracts when the patient is not prepared to void, so she experiences urge incontinence, but when she wants to void, the detrusor muscle is unable to mount a strong enough contraction to empty the bladder adequately. Clinically, the patient complains of paradoxical symptoms that can be diagnostically challenging; "I leak on the way to the toilet, but when I get there, I can't go." This type of urinary incontinence can be treated by anticholinergic medications (such as oxybutinin or tolterodine) and by teaching the patient to self-catheterize two to three times each day.

EVALUATION

History

The history should assess the duration and severity of the symptoms and whether the incontinence is progressive or stable. Good indicators of the **severity** of the problem are whether the patient wears protective pads, and the size and type of pad.

There are two different types of pads, pads for menstruation and pads for urine loss. The pad for urine loss is significantly different from the menstrual pad; it has a gel that helps wick urine away from the skin and holds more fluid. In fact, the gel can be so effective that sometimes patients cannot tell when they are leaking. To differentiate the type of incontinence, it may be necessary to ask the patient to go without a pad so that she can tell when she is leaking.

Specific questions regarding **when the incontinence occurs** can help differentiate between stress and urge incontinence. Does the patient leak when she coughs, sneezes, lifts, runs, or exercises? Or does she run to the toilet frequently (more often than every 2 hours) and leak on the way to the toilet? Does she get up more than twice at night to void?

The clinician should inquire about factors that worsen or alleviate the incontinence, specifically daily **caffeine** and **total fluid intake.** Many women consume 6 to 8 glasses of water daily as well as several cups of coffee, tea, or caffeinated soda. With these patients, simply adjusting their fluid intake to a normal amount, 48 to 64 oz/day, and decreasing or discontinuing the caffeine can sometimes resolve the problem. Excessive alcohol intake may also aggravate incontinence because of its diuretic effect.

Most patients, however, are really not sure of their actual fluid intake so a **voiding and fluid intake diary** can be useful. The patient is given a form and a measuring "hat" and asked to keep a record of fluid intake and of every voiding and leakage episode for 1 to 3 days (not necessarily consecutive) (Fig. 54-1). The diary will accurately show the patient's urinary frequency and incontinence episodes, as well as the activity associated with the incontinence, which can help the provider differentiate between stress and urge incontinence.

If a reversible cause of incontinence is found, it should be treated and the incontinence then reevaluated (Box 54-1). **Medication use** is a common reversible cause of incontinence; examples include diuretics and terazosin, an alpha-antagonist that can relax the urethra, resulting in stress or urge incontinence symptoms.

A medical history to rule out **neurologic causes** of incontinence is important. If a neurologic condition exists, referral directly for urodynamic testing is appropriate.

An inquiry should be made about **fecal** or **flatus incontinence.** Up to 30% of patients with urinary incontinence experience regular or intermittent fecal incontinence. Pelvic floor (Kegel) exercises and bulking agents, such as psyllium (Metamucil) or methylcellulose (Citrucel), can reduce fecal incontinence. If these measures are not adequate, the patient should be referred to a colorectal surgeon (ideally one with a special interest in fecal incontinence) or to a urogynecologist for biofeedback or possible anal sphincter repair.

Examination

Assessment of the **general mental status and cognitive ability** of the patient is important. It is extremely difficult

Date	Time	Voided Amount	Fluid Intake	Leak Amount	Activity with leak	Urge Present? Yes or No

FIG. 54-1 Voiding and fluid intake diary.

BOX 54-1
Reversible Causes of Urinary Incontinence, "DIAPPERS"

Delirium (confusional state)
Infection, urinary
Atrophic urethritis or vaginitis
Pharmaceuticals (sedatives, diuretics, alpha receptor antagonists)
Psychologic disorder, especially depression (rare)
Excess urine output (especially elderly at night, congestive heart failure)
Restricted mobility
Stool impaction

Adapted from Resnick NM: *Urol Clin North Am* 23:55, 1996.

---

for patients with impaired memory or cognition to do bladder training or even Kegel exercises. A general assessment of the patient's **mobility** is also important to assess whether a functional component is contributing to incontinence.

On gynecologic examination, any **genital atrophy** should be noted. It is useful to examine the patient before she empties her bladder. Before the speculum is placed, the patient is asked to bear down to check for **prolapse.** Next, the patient is instructed to cough in an effort to **observe the timing of leakage.** If incontinence is seen at the exact moment of cough, the diagnosis of stress incontinence can be made. If incontinence occurs after coughing, the patient may have detrusor instability, as the cough may trigger a detrusor contraction.

The patient is instructed to empty her bladder; then a bimanual pelvic examination is performed to rule out a **pelvic mass.** However, pelvic masses such as fibroids are rarely the true cause of bladder control dysfunction. The anterior vaginal wall should be examined carefully looking for masses that might indicate a urethral diverticulum, an infrequent cause of incontinence.

The patient is then instructed to perform the Kegel exercise and the **strength of the pelvic floor muscles** is assessed. Many patients perform pelvic floor exercises incorrectly, by tightening up the buttock or thigh muscles or by performing the Valsalva maneuver, which only worsens the problem. The **anal wink reflex,** an indicator of S3-S4 function, is checked to rule out neurologic causes of incontinence.

If urinary retention is a concern, after the pelvic examination a **postvoid residual** can be checked by straight catheterization or bladder ultrasound. If a catheter sample is obtained, it is sent for urinalysis and culture. If a catheter sample is not obtained, a clean-catch midstream sample should be sent.

MANAGEMENT

Many bladder control problems seen in primary care practice will resolve by educating the patient about bladder physiology, lifestyle habits, and Kegel exercises. The following general management strategies are useful for patients with any type of incontinence.

If maceration and irritation of the perineal epithelium are noted on examination, the patient may be using a menstrual pad; she should be instructed to use **incontinence pads** instead. A **protective ointment,** such as Balmex or Desitin, can help prevent skin irritation and breakdown. The patient should be instructed to gently clean the area, pat dry, use a blow dryer on the cool setting, and then apply the ointment.

By improving the integrity of vulvar and vaginal tissues in postmenopausal women, **topical estrogen therapy** can significantly alleviate symptoms of atrophy that are often aggravated by urinary incontinence. In some cases, bladder control may also improve markedly. The dose of conjugated estrogen cream is 1 g at bedtime twice weekly; no progesterone is needed, as endometrial hyperplasia does not occur at this dose.

If the history reveals excessive fluid or caffeine intake, the patient should be instructed to **decrease fluid intake** to 48 to

---

BOX 54-2
Grading Strength of Pelvic Floor Muscle Contraction

0 = Cannot feel any contraction of muscle
1 = Can barely feel a contraction
2 = Can easily feel a contraction
3 = There is resistance to palpation of the muscle
4 = There is very strong resistance to palpation
5 = There is complete resistance to very strong palpation

BOX 54-3
Medications for Detrusor Instability

- Tolterodine 1 or 2 mg QD or BID
- Oxybutynin, extended release 5, 10 or 15 mg QD
- Oxybutynin 5 mg 1/2 to 1 tablet BID-TID
- Hyoscyamine extended release 0.375 mg 1 capsule QD or BID
- Imipramine 10 to 20 mg QHS
- Propantheline 15 mg 1/2 to 1 tablet BID-TID

---

64 ounces daily and **limit caffeine intake** to 1 cup/day or less. In many instances, normalizing fluid intake and minimizing caffeine intake will resolve the bladder control problem.

TREATING STRESS INCONTINENCE
Kegel Exercises

In addition to the preceding management strategies, strengthening the pelvic floor muscles and teaching patients *how* to use the pelvic floor muscles are key to successfully treating stress incontinence.

Many women try to do Kegel exercises, but perform them incorrectly. A correct Kegel exercise will feel like the anus is being pulled up or inward; the patient will not feel much movement in the bladder area. Useful prompts are "it should feel like you are pulling in the anal area," "like stopping gas from escaping," or "tighten around my fingers" (during the pelvic examination). If the patient does the Kegel exercise properly, the posterior vaginal wall will become firmer and elevate. A grade can be assigned so that pelvic floor strength can be monitored (Box 54-2).

After the patient has been taught to do pelvic floor exercises correctly, she is taught when to use them. She is instructed to do the Kegel maneuver at the time of a cough or sneeze, or with lifting or laughing. This activates the hammock effect at the time it is needed: at the moment the pressure hits the bladder. Follow-up is very important. The patient should return in 4 to 6 weeks to check the quality of the Kegel maneuver. Improvement of bladder control due to Kegel exercises may require 3 months.

Insertion of a **tampon** before attempting activities that provoke stress incontinence has been shown to reduce incontinence episodes. Tampon use is appropriate when symptoms are infrequent, but predictable, for example, when stress incontinence occurs primarily during exercise.

TREATMENT OF URGE INCONTINENCE
Bladder Training

If normalizing fluid and caffeine intake has not resolved urinary frequency and urge incontinence, bladder training should be instituted.

The first step of bladder training is to have the patient complete a voiding/intake diary. The diary is assessed for voiding intervals, fluid intake, and leaking episodes. The rough average of the shortest voiding interval is determined. This interval is the starting point for the patient's bladder training. She is instructed to void at this interval "by the clock," not when she feels the urge. When she is able to void at that interval comfortably without experiencing urge incontinence, she lengthens the interval by 15 to 30 minutes. She continues to lengthen the intervals until she can wait a minimum of 3 hours. Normal voiding intervals are 3 to 8 hours during the daytime. During the sleep hours, the patient can get up and void whenever she feels the need. Eventually bladder training during the day lengthens the voiding intervals at night.

Kegel exercises can also help the patient control urge incontinence. The more often the patient controls her bladder, the easier the control becomes.

Medical Therapy

Many patients can carry out bladder training without medication, but some patients may become frustrated with slow progress or even experience increased incontinence during treatment. Even in motivated patients, medication can expedite progress, so it may be desirable to start medication at the initiation of bladder training. Newer, improved anticholinergic medications for urge incontinence (such as tolterodine and extended-release oxybutynin) have greatly improved patient acceptance and compliance. Box 54-3 lists commonly used medications and doses.

All of these medications can cause side effects of dry mouth and eyes, dyspepsia, headache, and constipation; side effects tend to be less frequent with tolterodine and extended-release oxybutinin. Anticholinergic medications should be used with caution in the elderly, as they can cause drowsiness, cognitive impairment, blurred vision, and impaired memory. Tolterodine does not pass the blood-brain barrier readily and may be the drug of choice in the elderly.

Indications for Referral

Specialist referral is appropriate if the patient's symptoms do not respond to the measures described here. **Urodynamic testing** is generally performed first to determine the type of incontinence, assess urethral function, and guide further treatment. Testing is performed in the office in 10 to 20 minutes and is not usually painful for the patient.

Other indications for referral and urodynamic testing are severe incontinence, pelvic organ prolapse, a prior history of surgery for incontinence, and significant neurologic disease.

ADDITIONAL TREATMENT FOR URINARY INCONTINENCE
Physical Therapy

Various forms of physical therapy can be effective for further strengthening pelvic floor muscles in the patient with weak muscle tone despite her best efforts.

Biofeedback uses balloon pressure or electromyogram (EMG) probes placed in the vagina to measure the strength of pelvic floor contractions. This measurement is displayed on a computer screen viewed by the patient as she performs the Kegel exercise. Office and home systems are available. In addition to biofeedback, the EMG probe can provide **electrical stimulation** to produce contractions and strengthen muscles of the pelvic floor. This approach is useful for the patient initially unable to perform the Kegel exercise.

Another form of biofeedback is **vaginal cones,** which consist of sets of four or five progressively heavier cones. The patient places the cone into the vagina and must contract the pelvic floor muscles strongly enough to keep the cone in while walking. Once she is able to retain the first cone in the vagina for 15 minutes twice each day, she advances to the next, slightly heavier, cone. This form of biofeedback is relatively inexpensive and more convenient for some patients than office-based physical therapy.

Another form of physical therapy is **extracorporeal magnetic stimulation.** A focused magnetic field is generated in the seat of a chair. When the patient sits on the chair, the nerves in the pelvic floor are stimulated and muscle contractions occur. Preliminary trials suggest that effectiveness is approximately 60% for stress and urge incontinence.

A **peripheral nerve stimulator,** the Sensory Afferent Nerve Stimulator (SANS), is also available. A needle is placed into the posterior tibial nerve and stimulated electrically on a weekly basis. This treatment can be effective for patients with frequency and urge incontinence.

A major barrier to use of these advanced forms of physical therapy is limited insurance coverage in some cases.

Pessaries and Other Devices

The **pessary** has long been used to treat incontinence in patients with pelvic organ prolapse. Standard pessaries often do not provide enough support to the bladder neck; modified pessaries have been developed specifically for incontinence. Their effectiveness depends on the type and severity of incontinence and the patient's anatomy. Patients are usually able to place and remove these pessaries themselves.

An external device in the shape of a **cap** (Capsure) made of soft silicone can be used for mild to moderate stress incontinence. It is placed over the external urethral meatus and removed for voiding. There is a small risk of urethral mucosal prolapse, and patient acceptance tends to be low.

A **urethral insert** (Femsoft), a device that is inserted by the patient into the urethra, is also available for stress incontinence. There is a significant risk of urinary tract infection with use of this device.

Injection Therapy

Collagen can be injected around the bladder neck via cystoscopy to increase coaptation of the urethral mucosa for patients with poor urethral function. These patients often have a history of pelvic radiation or multiple surgeries or are quite elderly. The procedure can be performed with the patient under local anesthesia. The disadvantage of collagen therapy is that it is not permanent; the effect wears off in 1 to 7 years and the injection must be repeated.

A newer product, **Duraspheres,** consists of graphite beads suspended in a gelatin matrix that is injected around the bladder neck. Its effect should be permanent, but long-term effectiveness is unknown.

Surgical Therapy

A variety of surgical procedures are performed to stabilize the urethrovesical junction or provide a hammock for it. A recent advance is the **laparoscopic urethropexy procedure,** which allows faster recovery and causes less postoperative pain. Another minimally invasive procedure is a modification of the urethrovesical sling procedure, the **tension free vaginal tape.** This procedure can be performed with the patient under local or spinal anesthesia and is very effective.

TREATMENT FOR REFRACTORY FREQUENCY AND URGE INCONTINENCE

For patients with severe detrusor instability who do not respond to medication, bladder training, and physical therapy, **bladder augmentation** or **urinary diversion** can be offered. However, after bladder augmentation the patient must self-catheterize on a long-term basis. Urinary diversion has obvious drawbacks for patients, who must learn to cope with a drainage bag.

A newer form of therapy for refractory detrusor instability is **chronic stimulation of S3,** InterStim. The patient undergoes a trial of this therapy by having an electrode placed percutaneously (in the office while under local anesthesia) into the S3 foramina. This electrode is attached to a small stimulator box that the patient wears for 1 to 2 weeks. If her symptoms respond, she is a candidate for implantation of a neurostimulator, performed while she is under general anesthesia. The implant is similar to a cardiac pacemaker and must have its battery changed every 6 to 10 years. InterStim therapy is also effective for patients with idiopathic urinary retention.

PELVIC ORGAN PROLAPSE

Mild to moderate pelvic organ prolapse has been documented in 50% of women seeking routine gynecologic care; approximately 3% have severe prolapse. Although lesser degrees of prolapse may be quite tolerable, significant prolapse can seriously impair a woman's quality of life.

Symptoms

The most common presentation is **uterine prolapse** together with the bladder **(cystocele)** and rectum **(rectocele).** The clinician may detect prolapse on examination before the patient has noticed any symptoms. The patient may complain of "something bulging" from the vaginal canal. She may also experience lower abdominal or back pain or pressure, or even pelvic cramping. Symptoms may worsen during the course of the day. Occasionally, bleeding from erosions on the prolapsed vaginal wall or cervix prompts a patient to seek care.

Other symptoms that may accompany a cystocele are urinary incontinence, frequency, or urinary hesitancy. Patients with a rectocele may complain of constipation, although on detailed history they actually have difficulty evacuating their rectum when they have the urge to move their bowels. Some women discover that by manually supporting the posterior

> **BOX 54-4**
> **Pelvic Floor Muscle Exercises**

- Check patient's contraction for quality and strength; correct if patient is performing the contraction incorrectly
- Patient should perform 30 to 40 contractions daily spread out over the day, holding each contraction for 5 to 10 seconds
- Stress incontinence: patient should do Kegel exercise when she coughs, sneezes, or lifts
- Urge incontinence: With the urge to void, patient should stand still, perform Kegel exercise to prevent leakage, wait until the strong urge subsides, then walk to toilet under control

vaginal wall or perineum (splinting) they are able to evacuate the rectum more easily.

Treatment

If prolapse is not advanced (that is, the prolapsed part is protruding only intermittently), Kegel exercises may help (Box 54-4). The patient should be instructed to perform the Kegel maneuver whenever lifting. If there is no improvement with Kegel exercises, a pessary or surgery should be considered.

Pessaries come in a variety of shapes and sizes and are made of silicone. Finding the appropriate pessary may take several office visits. Sometimes patients can be taught to remove and replace the pessary. This is especially necessary if the patient is sexually active.

Pessary users should ideally use estrogen cream twice weekly to prevent vaginal wall erosions, discharge, and odor. Occasionally, odor is a persistent problem. The patient can be instructed to use Trimosan jelly, an over-the-counter vaginal jelly that is mildly antibacterial.

Many patients are able to use the pessary indefinitely. Others may experience recurrent erosions or stress incontinence. These patients should strongly consider surgery. Before surgery, the patient's continence system should be evaluated to determine if anti-incontinence surgery is needed at the time of prolapse repair.

BIBLIOGRAPHY

DeLancey JOL: Structural support of the urethra as it relates to stress urinary incontinence: the hammock hypothesis, *Am J Obstet Gynecol* 170:1713, 1994.

Elia G, Bergman A: Estrogen effects on the urethra: Beneficial effects in women with genuine stress incontinence, *Obstet Gynecol Surv* 48:509, 1993.

Fantl JA et al: Efficacy of bladder training in older women with urinary incontinence, *JAMA* 265:609, 1991.

Jackson SL: Fecal incontinence in women with urinary incontinence and pelvic organ prolapse, *Obstet Gynecol* 89:423, 1997.

Onuora CO et al: Vaginal estrogen therapy in the treatment of urinary tract symptoms in postmenopausal women, *Int Urogynecol J* 2:3, 1991.

Resnick NM: Geriatric incontinence, *Urol Clin North Am* 23:55, 1996.

Resnick NM: Initial evaluation of the incontinent patient, *J Am Geriatr Soc* 38:311, 1990.

Sultan AH et al: Anal-sphincter disruption during vaginal delivery, *N Engl J Med* 329:1905, 1993.

Ulmsten U et al: A three-year follow up of tension free vaginal tape for surgical treatment of female stress urinary incontinence, *Br J Obstet Gynaecol* 106:345, 1999.

CHAPTER 55

Pelvic Pain

Karen J. Carlson
Kathleen F. Thurmond

Pelvic pain is a common problem in the primary care of women. In recent years there has been an explosion of scientific knowledge and technology allowing early diagnosis of acute pelvic pain. However, there is a relative dearth of clinical research on the causes of and treatments for chronic pelvic pain, particularly in view of the prevalence of this disorder according to recent population-based surveys.

The problem of pelvic pain presents challenges in both diagnosis and treatment. The challenge in diagnosing pelvic pain is to identify causes that, inadequately treated, may lead to serious short-term sequelae (internal hemorrhage and fulminant infection) or long-term complications (chiefly infertility). The management of chronic pelvic pain, in view of the uncertainty about the cause of this complex problem and sparse scientific evidence to guide treatment, presents an equally challenging clinical task.

The evaluation of pelvic pain begins with differentiating acute and chronic pelvic pain. This chapter addresses the evaluation of acute and chronic pelvic pain and the management of chronic (idiopathic) pelvic pain and dysmenorrhea.

ACUTE PELVIC PAIN

Acute pelvic pain is pain below the level of the umbilicus that has been present for hours or days; in some cases pain may develop over the course of a few weeks. Causes of acute pelvic pain are listed in Box 55-1.

Differential Diagnosis

Ectopic Pregnancy

An ectopic pregnancy is a pregnancy that implants in a location other than the endometrial cavity of the uterus. Almost all ectopic pregnancies are located in the fallopian tube. An ectopic pregnancy and an intrauterine pregnancy can coexist, although heterotopic pregnancy is very rare.

The incidence of ectopic pregnancy has been increasing over the past three decades, likely related to the increasing number of women who have had pelvic inflammatory disease (PID). The primary care clinician must maintain a high index of suspicion for this diagnosis in any woman of reproductive age presenting with pelvic pain. The strongest risk factors for ectopic pregnancy are previous ectopic pregnancy

(which is associated with a 15% likelihood of subsequent ectopic pregnancy), tubal surgery or known tubal pathology, diethylstilbestrol (DES) exposure, previous PID, and infertility. Less potent risk factors are multiple sexual partners, smoking, douching, and use of an intrauterine device (IUD).

Spontaneous Abortion

An early abortion is loss of a pregnancy before the completion of 22 gestational weeks. About 10% of all pregnancies over 6 menstrual weeks spontaneously abort; earlier pregnancy losses are even more common.

Adnexal Cyst or Mass

Adnexal cysts or masses may cause acute pelvic pain if their location results in stretching of tissue or pressure on adjacent organs, if rapid growth occurs, or if rupture or torsion occurs.

Pelvic Inflammatory Disease

PID, the commonly used term for active infection or chronic inflammation of the endometrium, tubes, or ovaries (with or without a pelvic abscess), is a frequent cause of acute pelvic pain. The pathogens most frequently implicated in PID are *Neisseria gonorrhoeae, Chlamydia trachomatis,* anaerobic and facultative anaerobic bacteria (particularly *Bacteroides* spp., *Escherichia coli,* and groups B and D *Streptococcus* spp.). The most important risk factors for PID are multiple sexual partners, a new or symptomatic sexual partner, age under 35 (peak frequency of PID is between ages 15 and 25), and use of nonbarrier contraception.

Appendicitis

Appendicitis must always be considered as a potential cause of pelvic pain. Appendicitis reaches its maximum incidence in the second and third decades of life. The female to male ratio is about 2:3 until after age 25, when the incidence begins to equalize between the sexes.

Urinary Tract Disorders

Lower urinary tract infection and urethritis can cause acute suprapubic pressure, pain, or a pulling sensation that intensifies with urination. Other common symptoms are

BOX 55-1
Causes of Acute Pelvic Pain

More Common
Ectopic pregnancy
Spontaneous, incomplete, or threatened abortion
Adnexal mass or cyst
Pelvic inflammatory disease
Appendicitis
Urinary tract infection

Less Common
Degenerating fibroid
Ureteral obstruction
Intestinal obstruction
Diverticulitis

dysuria, frequency, urgency, and hesitancy. Evaluation and management of acute dysuria are discussed in Chapter 23.

⚖ EVALUATION

The first task in evaluating a woman with acute pelvic pain is to assess whether a potentially life-threatening condition, such as internal hemorrhage caused by a ruptured ectopic pregnancy or septic shock related to a ruptured ovarian abscess, is present. Signs of significant hypovolemia, hypotension, or peritonitis should prompt immediate referral for emergency laparotomy or laparoscopy.

When there is no immediate evidence of a life-threatening condition, the evaluation of acute pelvic pain focuses on rapid assessment for potentially serious conditions. These include ectopic pregnancy, PID, appendicitis, and rupture or torsion of an ovarian cyst (Table 55-1).

Table 55-1
Evaluation of Acute Pelvic Pain

Cause	History	Physical Examination	Diagnostic Tests
Ectopic pregnancy	Nonspecific pelvic pain with or without abnormal vaginal bleeding	Normal or low blood pressure; orthostatic hypotension Normal pulse or tachycardia; orthostatic tachycardia Blood in vagina Adnexal tenderness Peritoneal signs	Hct and Hb normal or low Serum β-hCG > 10 mIU/ml Ultrasound showing empty uterus and possibly adnexal mass or cyst
Spontaneous abortion	Cramping pelvic pain, abnormal vaginal bleeding	Enlarged uterus Cervical os open or closed Blood or tissue in cervix or vagina	Ultrasound showing intrauterine pregnancy or tissue
Adnexal mass or cyst	Unilateral pelvic pain	Unilateral mass or fullness Adnexal tenderness	Ultrasound showing mass
Pelvic inflammatory disease	Diffuse pelvic pain; may be lateralized if tubo-ovarian abscess present Vaginal discharge	Normal or elevated temperature Vaginal or cervical discharge Diffuse pelvic and/or cervical motion tenderness Adnexal mass (tubo-ovarian abscess)	Normal or increased WBC Normal or increased ESR Increased POLYS in cervical secretions Ultrasound may show tubo-ovarian abscess
Appendicitis	Epigastric or periumbilical pain localizing to right lower quadrant Diffuse abdominal pain Anorexia, nausea, vomiting	Normal or elevated temperature Right lower quadrant tenderness and/or mass	Normal or increased WBC Left shift in differential cell count

Hct, Hematocrit; *Hb*, hemoglobin; β-*hCG*, beta-human chorionic gonadotropin; *WBC*, white blood cell count; *ESR*, erythrocyte sedimentation rate; *POLYS*, polymorphonuclear leukocytes.

History

An **ectopic pregnancy** must be ruled out in any woman of reproductive age who has pelvic pain or abnormal vaginal bleeding. Pain and abnormal bleeding are sometimes, but not always, present. Pain is caused by localized bleeding, which occurs when the trophoblast invades blood vessels and the serosa is stretched. Pelvic pain may be dull or sharp, localized or diffuse.

Many patients with ectopic pregnancy have some abnormal bleeding; however, the absence of bleeding does not rule out ectopic pregnancy. When taking a menstrual history, it is important to determine the last menstrual period (LMP) and to confirm that it was normal in flow, length, and onset. The same information should be obtained about the previous menstrual period (PMP). Otherwise, aberrant bleeding that occurred any time up to 4 weeks before the evaluation may be erroneously considered a normal LMP.

Spontaneous abortion may produce pelvic pain (typically uterine cramping) and abnormal vaginal bleeding as the products of conception are expelled. A threatened abortion is characterized by light bleeding and mild cramping without evidence of passed tissue; the cervical os remains closed.

Pain from an **adnexal mass** or cyst is usually lateralized, unless the involved adnexa is in the midline, in which case mid-lower abdominal pain may be present.

PID typically causes diffuse lower abdominal pain, which may be more severe on one side if there is a unilateral tubo-ovarian abscess. Increased vaginal discharge, fever, chills, nausea, and vomiting may be present.

In **appendicitis** the typical sequence of symptoms is pain in the epigastrium or around the umbilicus, followed by anorexia, nausea, and sometimes vomiting. Although the pain typically localizes to the right lower quadrant, it may remain diffuse. Approximately 45% of patients experience atypical pain.

Physical Examination

Physical findings in **ectopic pregnancy** span the spectrum from an entirely normal examination to hypotension with obvious peritoneal signs. On pelvic examination there may be blood in the vagina with or without cervical motion tenderness. Adnexal tenderness may be present, with or without a mass, on the side of the ectopic pregnancy or on the side of the corpus luteum, which may be contralateral to the pregnancy.

Depending on gestational age and stage of abortion the physical examination in **spontaneous abortion** can reveal an enlarged uterus, an adnexal mass associated with a corpus luteum cyst, and evidence of uterine bleeding with an open or closed cervical os.

In **PID** the abdominal examination typically reveals diffuse lower abdominal tenderness. Peritonitis, if present, can result in rebound and guarding. Right upper quadrant pain or tenderness suggests that perihepatic inflammation is present (Fitz-Hugh–Curtis syndrome). Pelvic examination often indicates increased vaginal discharge, cervical motion tenderness, and bilateral adnexal tenderness. A palpable mass should alert the clinician to a possible tubo-ovarian abscess.

Appendicitis may manifest without fever, even when rupture has occurred. There is either diffuse or right lower quadrant tenderness, sometimes with guarding or rebound.

Rectal examination may elicit right lower quadrant tenderness, and occasionally a right lower quadrant mass is palpable. Some manifestations of appendicitis may be difficult to distinguish from PID, especially when the woman has diffuse abdominal pain and pelvic examination reveals cervical motion tenderness and diffuse pelvic tenderness.

Diagnostic Tests (Box 55-2)

The basic laboratory evaluation of pelvic pain includes a complete blood count with differential, sedimentation rate, serum beta human chorionic gonadotropin (β-hCG), and urinalysis. Tests for chlamydia and gonorrhea and a specimen of vaginal fluid for microscopic examination should be obtained during the pelvic examination to evaluate for PID. Pelvic ultrasonography is one of the most useful diagnostic tests in the evaluation of acute pelvic pain.

When an **ectopic pregnancy** exists, the serum β-hCG is always greater than 10 IU/ml; β-HCG is also elevated in **spontaneous abortion.** If the initial β-hCG level is less than 1500 IU/L, β-hCG levels should be measured every 2 days, preferably in the same laboratory; the level doubles about every 2 days in a normal pregnancy. In an ectopic pregnancy the level of serum β-hCG is often less than what would be expected for a normal pregnancy at the same gestational age. The hematocrit and hemoglobin may be normal, or low if significant bleeding has occurred.

A pelvic ultrasound should be performed if ectopic pregnancy is suspected as soon as the β-hCG reaches a level of 1500 to 2000 IU/L (depending on the operating characteristics of the ultrasonographer). An intrauterine pregnancy (IUP) will be detectable by ultrasound at this point; if no intrauterine gestational sac is evident, ectopic pregnancy is highly probable. Ultrasonography should also be performed for suspected spontaneous abortion; it may show an intrauterine pregnancy or some pregnancy tissue in the uterus or vagina.

Leukocytosis and an elevated erythrocyte sedimentation rate (ESR) are present in more severe cases of **PID** but may be lacking in mild cases. A saline wet mount of vaginal secretions has a sensitivity 80% for detection of PID (an abnormal result is defined as ≥3 wbc/hpf). Although no single

---

BOX 55-2
Diagnostic Tests in Acute Pelvic Pain

Laboratory
CBC with differential
ESR
Serum β-hCG
Urinalysis

Pelvic Examination
Testing for chlamydia and gonorrhea infection
Saline preparation of vaginal secretions for microscopy

Radiology
Transvaginal ultrasound

CBC, Complete blood count; *ESR*, erythrocyte sedimentation rate; β-*hCG*, human chorionic gonadotropin.

diagnostic test has adequate sensitivity for detecting PID, the combination of a normal ESR, normal white blood count, and negative microscopic examination of vaginal secretions has a very high negative predictive value. Pelvic ultrasonography should be performed if there is any suggestion of pelvic mass on examination; it may reveal a tubo-ovarian abscess.

Although the white blood count is most often elevated in **appendicitis,** it is estimated that 30% of patients have a normal white blood count. However, there is usually a left shift in the differential, even when the total white blood count is not elevated. Ultrasonography may be abnormal in appendicitis if there is a markedly enlarged appendix or appendiceal abscess; an abdominal computed tomography (CT) scan has greater sensitivity.

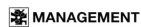 MANAGEMENT

Ectopic Pregnancy

If a woman has a positive pregnancy test result, an ultrasound without evidence of an intrauterine pregnancy, and pelvic pain, immediate referral to a gynecologist is necessary. Early diagnosis and intervention increase the likelihood that medical management will be possible, allowing preservation of the tube. Medical and surgical management of ectopic pregnancy is discussed in Chapter 65. Because a woman's risk of ectopic pregnancy is increased by its initial occurrence, it is important to instruct her to seek medical attention early in any future pregnancy for serial serum β-hCG titers and appropriately timed ultrasonography.

Spontaneous Abortion

Management of threatened, incomplete, and complete abortion is discussed in Chapter 66.

Adnexal Mass

Further evaluation and management of an adnexal mass are discussed in Chapter 49.

Pelvic Inflammatory Disease

The diagnosis of PID is a clinical one, based on the presence of risk factors, a suggestive examination, and negative pregnancy test. In accordance with current recommendations of the Centers for Disease Control and Prevention, a low threshold for empiric treatment of suspected PID is appropriate, even while other diagnostic possibilities continue to be considered. Outpatient treatment for PID is indicated when the woman can take oral medication, is available for follow-up evaluation, and has no signs of severe infection. The patient should be reassessed after 48 to 72 hours of outpatient antibiotic therapy, and sexual partners should be examined and treated for sexually transmitted diseases. Admission for intravenous antibiotics is needed when there is evidence of a tubo-ovarian abscess, when nausea or vomiting precludes use of oral antibiotics, in pregnancy, or when there are signs of a severe infection. Detailed treatment recommendations for PID are given in Chapter 22.

Appendicitis

A woman with suspected appendicitis should be referred for laparoscopy or laparotomy, depending on the certainty of the diagnosis.

CHRONIC PELVIC PAIN

The term *chronic pelvic pain* has been used to denote the symptom of recurrent pelvic discomfort and also as a specific diagnosis (characterized by pelvic pain present for at least 6 months with no evidence of an organic cause after thorough evaluation, including laparoscopy). The prevalence of chronic pelvic pain in population-based studies in the United States and the United Kingdom ranges from 4% to 15%. Conditions causing pelvic pain that is persistent or recurrent over months to years are listed in Box 55-3.

Causes

Dysmenorrhea

Primary dysmenorrhea is cyclic uterine pain that occurs before or during menses in the absence of any significant pelvic abnormality. It is thought to be caused by prostaglandins produced by the endometrium. Secondary dysmenorrhea may be caused by endometriosis, adenomyosis, and fibroids (if clots large enough to produce cramps are passed). Hematometrium, a collection of menstrual blood distending the endometrial cavity in the presence of cervical stenosis, is a rare cause of secondary dysmenorrhea.

Endometriosis

Endometriosis is a condition in which endometrial tissue implants in extrauterine locations, such as the pelvic peritoneum, uterine ligaments, ovaries, tubes, cervix, bowel, bladder, and rarely more distant sites. Endometriosis is discussed in detail in Chapter 45.

Adenomyosis

Adenomyosis is the presence of endometrial tissue ectopically located within the myometrium. Adenomyosis is common, occurring in more than 50% of uteruses in some series, but often asymptomatic. Uterine leiomyomas often

---

BOX 55-3
Causes of Chronic Pelvic Pain

Gynecologic Disorders
Primary dysmenorrhea
Endometriosis
Adenomyosis
Adhesions
Fibroids
Retained ovary syndrome posthysterectomy
Previous tubal ligation
Chronic pelvic infection

Musculoskeletal Disorders
Myofascial pain syndrome

Gastrointestinal Disorders
Irritable bowel syndrome
Inflammatory bowel disease

Urinary Tract Disorders
Interstitial cystitis
Nonbacterial urethritis

coexist with adenomyosis. Adenomyosis is more common in women who have borne children than in nulliparous women.

Adhesions

Adhesions, or scar tissue, are thought to cause pelvic pain by producing abnormal adherence between adjacent organs. Adhesions are more common when there has been prior pelvic infection or surgery. The mechanism for pain related to adhesions is unclear, and there is some controversy about whether adhesions are an unequivocal cause of pelvic pain. The prevalence of adhesions (15% to 20%) is similar in women with no history of pelvic pain undergoing laparoscopy for infertility and those undergoing laparoscopy for pelvic pain. Laparoscopic lysis of adhesions has been reported to reduce symptoms in 40% to 75% of cases.

Fibroids

Fibroids (leiomyomas), benign fibromuscular growths within the uterus, are thought to cause chronic pelvic pain by pressure on adjacent organs or, in the case of degenerating fibroids, by outgrowing their blood supply. Fibroids are discussed in detail in Chapter 50.

Pelvic Pain after Gynecologic Surgery

Retained ovary syndrome is a syndrome of recurrent adnexal pain after hysterectomy. Pelvic adhesions, follicular cysts, and hemorrhagic corpus luteum cysts within the retained ovaries are among the suggested explanations. The only known treatment is oophorectomy.

Studies of late sequelae of tubal ligation have found chronic pelvic pain in a small number of women after tubal ligation. The mechanism is unclear; torsion of the ovary and ischemia have been proposed as possible causes.

Pelvic Pain with a History of Abuse

A subgroup of women with chronic pelvic pain has associated psychosocial conditions, particularly a history of sexual or physical abuse. The prevalence of childhood sexual abuse in women with chronic pelvic pain has been reported at 20% to 60%, and of childhood physical abuse at 40%. High levels of dissociation, somatization, and substance abuse have been reported in women with chronic pelvic pain who have a history of sexual or physical abuse. The mechanism for this association is not well understood but may involve abnormal autonomic reactivity and heightened sensitivity to pain stimuli, based on recent studies documenting dysfunction of pituitary-adrenal and autonomic responses to stress in women after sexual and physical abuse in childhood.

Other Causes

A report of the multidisciplinary evaluation of chronic pelvic pain in women with negative laparoscopy findings by Reiter and Gambone indicates that other frequent causes are **myofascial pain syndrome** or **fibromyalgia, irritable bowel syndrome,** chronic **pelvic infection,** and **urinary tract disorders.**

▣ EVALUATION

A woman with chronic pelvic pain can also have an acute cause of pelvic pain. Once the causes of acute pain (de-

scribed previously) have been ruled out, the evaluation of chronic pelvic pain can proceed in a stepwise fashion (Table 55-2).

History

In addition to characterizing the symptom of pain, gynecologic history (pelvic infections, tubal ligation, pelvic or abdominal surgery), and any other gynecologic symptoms (such as irregular or excessive vaginal bleeding), the history should also address other organ systems that may be responsible for pelvic pain. Associated gastrointestinal symptoms such as diarrhea, constipation, and more generalized abdominal discomfort should be sought. Urinary symptoms such as dysuria, urgency, and frequency (with a negative urine culture result) may suggest interstitial cystitis or nonbacterial urethritis. Low back pain, unilateral or bilateral leg pain, or coccygeal pain may suggest a musculoskeletal process.

The woman's general health, nutritional status, and exercise habits should be assessed. The clinician should inquire about unrelated somatic symptoms and the extent of any past evaluation. A careful exploration of psychosocial factors is essential. The clinician must become comfortable in inquiring in a sensitive way about a history of abuse and should be alert to the presence of depression (see Chapters 81 and 87) or a somatization disorder (see Chapter 82). Indications for referral are shown in Box 55-4.

Endometriosis may cause cyclic pelvic pain, which may not be relieved by nonsteroidal antiinflammatory drugs (NSAIDs) or oral contraceptives. If adhesions or an endometrioma has developed, pelvic pain can occur throughout the menstrual cycle. The pain may be unilateral or diffuse. Dyspareunia may be present if there are significant uterosacral ligament implants, adhesions, or an endometrioma.

Adenomyosis classically presents as menorrhagia and dysmenorrhea in women between 40 and 50 years old. Pain attributed to **adhesions** can occur without provocation, or with activities that put tension on the adhesions, such as intercourse, exercise, defecation, ovulation, or filling or emptying of the bladder. The nature of the pain is nonspecific.

Physical Examination

The pelvic examination in endometriosis may be normal or may reveal diffuse or localized tenderness. Physical findings characteristic of endometriosis are uterosacral ligament abnormalities (nodularity, thickening, or tenderness), lateral displacement of the cervix, and cervical stenosis. The classic finding of nodularity on rectovaginal examination may be absent. A pelvic mass suggests the presence of an endometrioma. In adenomyosis the uterus is typically diffusely enlarged (though not generally above 12 weeks' gestational size) and soft. Adhesions may produce no abnormality on examination. Fibroids are typically palpable as a bulky enlarged uterus, or a midline or adnexal mass, but may not be detectable on examination.

Diagnostic Testing

Initial laboratory testing includes a complete blood count with differential, urinalysis, testing for chlamydia and gonorrhea, and a serum β-hCG. Microscopic examination of vaginal secretions for leukocytes may be helpful in suspected PID.

Table 55-2
Evaluation of Chronic Pelvic Pain

Cause	History	Physical Examination	Diagnostic Tests
Primary dysmenorrhea	Cyclic uterine cramping	Normal pelvic examination finding	None
Endometriosis	Cyclic or constant pelvic pain, unilateral or diffuse Dyspareunia Premenstrual spotting	Pelvic examination result may be normal Adnexal tenderness or mass Tender nodules on rectovaginal examination Uterus with limited mobility	Ultrasound may show endometrioma; findings often normal Laparoscopy required for definitive diagnosis
Adenomyosis	Progressively worsening cyclic cramping Heavy menstrual bleeding	Mildly enlarged, soft uterus	Sometimes detectable by MRI
Adhesions	Previous pelvic or abdominal surgery Nonspecific pain, sometimes related to specific activities	Often normal Diffuse or localized tenderness	Requires laparoscopy for definitive diagnosis
Chronic pelvic infection	Risk factors for PID Localized or diffuse noncyclic pain	Normal or elevated temperature Diffuse pelvic tenderness Adnexal tenderness or mass Cervical motion tenderness	Normal or increased WBC, ESR Culture or antigen detection test for *Chlamydia* and gonorrhea
Fibroids	Heavy menstrual bleeding Cyclic or constant pelvic pressure or pain	Uterine enlargement Adnexal or midline mass Pelvic examination result may be normal	Hct/Hb result normal or decreased Ultrasound showing single or multiple myomas
Idiopathic	Unilateral or diffuse cyclic or noncyclic pain	Diffuse or localized pelvic tenderness, no masses	Diagnosed by exclusion of other causes

MRI, Magnetic resonance imaging; *PID*, pelvic inflammatory disease; *WBC*, white blood cell count; *ESR*, erythrocyte sedimentation rate; *Hct*, hematocrit; *Hb*, hemoglobin.

Pelvic **ultrasonography** should be performed to detect fibroids and to rule out a pelvic mass as the cause of pain. **Magnetic resonance imaging** (MRI) is more sensitive than ultrasound for the diagnosis of adenomyosis. Use of unselected radiographic studies such as barium enema and intravenous pyelography has been shown to have limited value. Barium enema or colonoscopy should be reserved for evaluation of gastrointestinal symptoms when the diagnosis of irritable bowel syndrome is uncertain.

The standard approach to evaluation of chronic pelvic pain that is undiagnosed after the initial evaluation is **laparoscopy.** Laparoscopy has been shown to identify pelvic abnormality in 60% to 80% of women with chronic pelvic pain, compared to 30% of those undergoing tubal ligation. An alternative approach limits use of laparoscopy in the context of a multidisciplinary evaluation that includes psy-

chologic, nutritional, and physical therapy assessments. In this setting laparoscopy was found to have an unimportant role in diagnosis and treatment in one randomized trial.

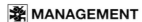 **MANAGEMENT**

Dysmenorrhea

Initial treatment for dysmenorrhea is **NSAIDs.** The effectiveness of NSAIDs for relieving primary dysmenorrhea is approximately 70%. There are no data on the relative efficacy of different NSAIDs for this condition. Commonly used regimens include naproxen sodium, 375 to 750 mg twice a day; ibuprofen, 200 to 800 mg four times a day; and mefenamic acid, 250 to 500 mg twice a day. Effectiveness is greater when medications are started 1 day in advance of expected onset of pain. The **oral contraceptive pill** is also ef-

BOX 55-4
Indications for Referral

Acute Pelvic Pain
Signs of intraabdominal hemorrhage or peritonitis
Known or suspected ectopic pregnancy
Spontaneous, incomplete, or threatened abortion
Pelvic inflammatory disease with tubo-ovarian abscess
Suspected appendicitis

Chronic Pelvic Pain
Dysmenorrhea refractory to NSAIDs and/or oral contraceptive pill or with suspected endometriosis
Consideration of laparoscopy when diagnosis uncertain after initial evaluation
Symptomatic uterine fibroids
Idiopathic chronic pelvic pain, for multidisciplinary management

NSAIDs, Nonsteroidal antiinflammatory drugs.

fective for dysmenorrhea. It acts to reduce endometrial prostaglandin production by decreasing the amount of endometrium that is built up in each cycle.

Pain that is not relieved by trials of multiple NSAIDs or the oral contraceptive pill warrants consideration of laparoscopy to rule out endometriosis.

Adenomyosis

The only definitive treatment for adenomyosis at present is hysterectomy. Data on the effectiveness of limited surgical procedures, such as endometrial ablation and laparoscopic myometrial electrocoagulation, are very limited but suggest these procedures may be effective in some patients.

Adhesions

Laparoscopic lysis of adhesions has variable effectiveness for improving pelvic pain symptoms, ranging from 40% to 75% in published case series; the likelihood of recurrence has been estimated at 25%.

Idiopathic Chronic Pelvic Pain

The clinician should approach treatment of idiopathic chronic pelvic pain by appreciating that the causes of pain are complex, and that scientific data to guide therapy are limited. Principles for treatment of any chronic pain syndrome are applicable here. These include (1) the establishment of an ongoing relationship and contacts between clinician and patient, independent of the presence of pain symptoms; (2) an empathic attitude in the clinician and validation of the woman's experience of pain; (3) a focus on learning to adapt to pain symptoms, including use of relaxation techniques and exercise; and (4) an expressed willingness of the clinician to reopen a diagnostic evaluation when new evidence warrants.

A **multidisciplinary approach** to chronic pelvic pain is most effective. A randomized trial of multidisciplinary treatment showed that attention to somatic, psychologic, nutritional, environmental, and physical conditioning factors (with selective use of laparoscopy) was more effective at

1 year than standard care that emphasized medications and laparoscopy. Provision of specialized care in a multidisciplinary setting may reduce the stigma associated with psychologic evaluation and treatment and enhance a woman's ability to address the nonsomatic aspects of her condition. Although multidisciplinary units are not widely available, these findings suggest that treatment of chronic pelvic pain by individual clinicians should include psychologic evaluation (and therapy when indicated), referral for physical therapy (if therapists are experienced in treatment of chronic pelvic pain), and nutritional assessment.

Medical therapy of chronic pelvic pain is reasonable as one component of management. Treatment typically is initiated with NSAIDs or (particularly when cyclic pain is present) the oral contraceptive pill. Use of narcotic analgesics should be avoided because of the high risk of dependency.

A few studies have reported the results of other empiric therapies for chronic pelvic pain. A randomized trial of depot leuprolide (Lupron) in women with chronic pelvic pain and clinically suspected endometriosis (after workup as outlined previously, not including laparoscopy) demonstrated a significant improvement in pain symptoms after 3 months; since 80% of the patients in this sample ultimately proved to have endometriosis, this finding is consistent with other studies of GnRH agonists (see Chapter 45). A 6-week controlled trial of sertraline found no benefit for chronic pelvic pain. Other medical therapies for chronic pain, as outlined in Chapter 29, may be tried.

Surgical therapy for chronic pelvic pain has included nerve ablation procedures and hysterectomy (with or without bilateral salpingo-oophorectomy). Studies of neurectomy procedures, including laparoscopic uterine nerve ablation and presacral neurectomy, have been performed largely in women with endometriosis; they are have not been studied sufficiently in controlled trials in women with idiopathic pelvic pain.

After hysterectomy for chronic pelvic pain, 5% to 20% of women report persistent pain more than a year after surgery. Age less than 30 years and a history of chronic PID are factors associated with a higher failure rate. Consideration of hysterectomy should take place only after more conservative medical therapy has failed, and after thorough psychologic evaluation has ruled out a somatization disorder, a posttraumatic disorder, and depression.

BIBLIOGRAPHY

Ankum WM et al: Risk factors for ectopic pregnancy: a meta-analysis, *Fertil Steril* 65:1093, 1996.

Badura AS et al: Dissociation, somatization, substance abuse, and coping in women with chronic pelvic pain, *Obstet Gynecol* 90:405, 1997.

Barbieri RL, Propst AM: Physical examination findings in women with endometriosis: uterosacral ligament abnormalities, lateral cervical displacement and cervical stenosis, *J Gynecol Technol* 5:157, 1999.

Carson SA, Buster JE: Ectopic pregnancy, *N Engl J Med* 329:1174, 1993.

Check JH, Weiss RM, Lurie D: Analysis of serum human chorionic gonadotropin levels in normal singleton, multiple and abnormal pregnancies, *Hum Reprod* 7:2176, 1992.

Engel CC et al: A randomized, double-blind crossover trial of sertraline in women with chronic pelvic pain, *J Psychosom Res* 44:203, 1998.

Heim C et al: Pituitary-adrenal and autonomic responses to stress in women after sexual and physical abuse in childhood, *JAMA* 284:592, 2000.

Hillis SD, Marchbanks PA, Peterson HB: The effectiveness of hysterectomy for chronic pelvic pain, *Obstet Gynecol* 86:941, 1995.

Hurd WW: Criteria that indicate endometriosis is the cause of chronic pelvic pain, *Obstet Gynecol* 92:1029, 1998.

Ling FW: Randomized controlled trial of depot leuprolide in patients with chronic pelvic pain and clinically suspected endometriosis, *Obstet Gynecol* 93:51, 1999.

Peipert JF et al: Laboratory evaluation of acute upper genital tract infection, *Obstet Gynecol* 87:730, 1996.

Peters A et al: A randomized clinical trial to compare two different approaches in women with chronic pelvic pain, *Obstet Gynecol* 77:740, 1991.

Reiter RC, Gambone JC: Nongynecologic somatic pathology in women with chronic pelvic pain and negative laparoscopy, *J Reprod Med* 36:253, 1991.

Saferins S et al: Long-term sequelae of acute pelvic inflammatory disease, *Am J Obstet Gynecol* 166:1300, 1992.

Scialli AR: Evaluation chronic pelvic pain: a consensus recommendation, *J Reprod Med* 44:945, 1999.

Steege JF, Stout AL: Resolution of chronic pelvic pain after laparoscopic lysis of adhesions, *Am J Obtet Gynecol* 165:278, 1991.

Walker EA et al: Psychiatric diagnoses and sexual victimization in women with chronic pelvic pain, *Psychosomatics* 36:531, 1995.

Wood C: Surgical and medical treatment of adenomyosis, *Hum Reprod Update* 4:323, 1998.

Zondervan KT et al: Prevalence and incidence of chronic pelvic pain in primary care: evidence from a national general practice database, *Br J Obstet Gynaecol* 106:1149, 1999.

CHAPTER 56

Premenstrual Syndrome

Kathleen Hubbs Ulman
Karen J. Carlson

DEFINITION

In recent years the term *premenstrual syndrome* (PMS) has come to be used in everyday parlance to refer to a variety of unpleasant symptoms associated with the menstrual cycle. The diagnostic criteria and nomenclature for premenstrual syndrome are often unclear to both physicians and patients.

Premenstrual dysphoric disorder (PMDD) is a severe cyclical mood disorder causing functional impairment, with prospective documentation of symptoms limited to the luteal phase of most menstrual cycles and without evidence for another disorder. The *Diagnostic and Statistical Manual of Mental Disorders (DSM-IV)* includes "premenstrual dysphoric disorder" in the category of research criteria needing further study (Box 56-1). "Premenstrual dysphoric disorder" is not yet a clinical psychiatric diagnosis. *DSM-IV* suggests that "depressive disorder not otherwise specified" be used when symptoms severely interfere with a woman's everyday functioning and that the term *premenstrual syndrome* be used to describe less severe symptoms.

Premenstrual syndrome is used to describe a chronic mood disorder of mild to moderate severity, sometimes with physical symptoms and behavioral changes, occurring during the luteal phase and remitting after onset of menses. Premenstrual syndrome is listed as a diagnosis in the ICD-10 (International Classification of Disease, 10th edition).

Consideration of an individual woman's sociocultural context is important in determining the significance of reported cyclic emotional and physical events on a continuum ranging from normal fluctuations to functionally disruptive symptoms. Studies of cultures as diverse as Nigeria, China, and India suggest the universal existence of distressing premenstrual symptoms, but the significance of these for an individual woman will vary according to her social context.

▦ EPIDEMIOLOGY

Large population-based studies indicate that approximately 1% to 5% of women experience serious premenstrual symptoms. Increased severity of symptoms has been associated with younger age. There have been no consistent associations of PMS with parity, use of the oral contraceptive pill, socioeconomic factors, or personality attributes. Twin studies suggest a substantial familial linkage. Some studies have reported an increased lifetime prevalence of major depression in women with PMDD; however, careful follow-up studies do not substantiate this association. There does appear to be an increased lifetime prevalence of postpartum depression in women with PMDD.

Although the association of PMS personality problems is unfounded, certain underlying psychiatric illness can be exacerbated in the premenstrual phase of the cycle. Symptoms of major depression may be worse premenstrually. Women with PMS show an increased susceptibility to panic symptoms in challenge studies. An increased frequency of premenstrual binge eating may occur in women with bulimia. Existing studies do not indicate an increased premenstrual use of drugs or alcohol in women with a history of substance abuse.

CAUSES

A growing body of research indicates that central neurotransmitter dysregulation plays a central role in PMS. The work of Rubinow, Schmidt, and colleagues indicates that cylic changes in estrogen and progesterone may trigger premenstrual symptoms, but only in susceptible women; that is, women with PMS are differentially sensitive to normal levels of ovarian hormones. There are no differences in luteal phase hormone levels in women with PMS versus unaffected women. Suppression of normal ovarian function with GnRh agonists, followed by adding back estrogen or progesterone, reproduces symptoms in women with PMS but not in normal women. Other research documents disturbances in circadian rhythms and seasonal patterns of symptoms in women with PMS.

There is some evidence that PMS is not simply a variant form of depression. Irritability, anxiety, and tension are often prominent, rather than depressed mood. Unlike major depression, PMS is a chronic disorder that does not remit spontaneously. Finally, response to specific antidepressants varies markedly in PMS compared to depression.

BOX 56-1
Diagnostic Criteria for Premenstrual Dysphoric Disorder

Symptoms occur cyclically and occurred in most cycles during the past year

At least five of the following are present (including at least one of the first four):

- Markedly depressed mood, feelings of hopelessness, or self-deprecating thoughts
- Marked anxiety, tension
- Marked affective lability
- Persistent and marked anger or irritability or increased interpersonal conflicts
- Decreased interest in usual activities
- Subjective sense of difficulty concentrating
- Lethargy, easy fatigability, or marked lack of energy
- Marked change in appetite, overeating, or food cravings
- Hypersomnia or insomnia
- Physical symptoms, such as breast pain, bloating, headaches

Symptoms are serious enough to interfere with activities and relationships

Symptoms are not an exacerbation of an underlying disorder

Symptoms are confirmed by prospective daily ratings during two cycles

Modified from *Diagnostic and statistical manual of mental disorders,* ed 4, Washington DC, 1994, American Psychiatric Association.

BOX 56-2
Evaluation of Premenstrual Symptoms

History
Nature, timing, and severity of symptoms
Symptom course over time; precipitating events
Effect of symptoms on daily functioning
Psychiatric history
Family history of psychiatric illness
Personal history of psychiatric illness
Alcohol and drug use
Social history
Diet and exercise habits

Physical Examination
General examination
Pelvic examination

Diagnostic Tests
Daily symptom recording for two cycles
Selective laboratory tests: TSH, CBC

TSH, Thyroid-stimulating hormone; *CBC,* complete blood count.

EVALUATION

The goals of the initial evaluation are to clarify the nature and timing of the premenstrual symptoms, to determine whether an underlying medical or psychiatric illness is present, and to enlist the woman's active participation in evaluation and treatment to enhance her sense of control.

History and Physical Examination

The history should collect information about the nature, timing, and severity of symptoms and the woman's perception of their relationship to the menstrual cycle (Box 56-2). Variability in the intensity of symptoms over time and changes in symptom patterns during the course of reproductive life are commonly seen. A detailed psychiatric history is important to determine whether an underlying or exacerbating condition is present. Understanding the context of the woman's current life, as well as the significance of menstrual events in the woman's family and culture, is essential to formulating an effective approach to treatment.

The physical examination focuses on identifying any underlying systemic disorders that may mimic PMS (e.g., anemia) or any anatomic causes of symptoms (such as endometriosis, fibroids, or other gynecologic disorders that may contribute to pelvic pain). Medical conditions whose symptoms may overlap those of PMS include thyroid and adrenal disorders, hyperprolactinemia, chronic fatigue syndrome, fibromyalgia, and irritable bowl syndrome. A number of medical disorders may be exacerbated during the premenstrual phase, including migraine headaches, seizure disorders, asthma, allergy, and urticaria.

Diagnostic Tests

Prospective daily symptom recording is essential for diagnosis. Some women incorrectly attribute symptom changes to the menstrual cycle, and others are unaware of a relationship between specific symptoms and the menstrual cycle. Women with severe PMS are less likely to report their symptoms incorrectly than women with mild to moderate symptoms. Because of underlying biologic variability in the menstrual cycle, it is necessary to record symptoms for a minimum of two cycles to discern the symptom pattern.

Laboratory tests are of little value in the diagnosis of PMS, except to rule out other disorders such as hypothyroidism or anemia.

MANAGEMENT

When the diagnosis of PMS has been established through careful assessment of prospective symptom records and exclusion of other medical or psychiatric disorders, a spectrum of treatment approaches should be considered. These include changes in lifestyle, psychoeducational groups and other techniques for coping with stress, diet, vitamin and mineral supplements, and medical therapy directed at specific symptoms or constellations of symptoms.

Diet and Exercise

The first level of intervention for women with PMS involves modification of diet and exercise habits and development of effective techniques for coping with stress. The rationale underlying these interventions derives from epidemiologic studies of factors associated with PMS, rather than from randomized trials; however, they have little risk or cost, and clinical experience supports their beneficial effects for some women.

Women with PMS consume significantly more caffeine and concentrated sweets than control subjects. Improvement in PMS symptoms has been observed after consumption of evening meals high in carbohydrates during the luteal phase; the mechanism may be alterations in serotonin level. Evidence from a randomized trial indicates that a strict low-fat diet) reduces cyclic breast pain. Finally, moliminal symptoms have been observed to diminish after sedentary women begin a regular exercise program. The recommended interventions based on these observations are outlined in Box 56-3.

Psychosocial Interventions

An important adjunct to modifications in diet and exercise is the development of techniques for actively coping with premenstrual symptoms and with stress in general. This can be accomplished most effectively through meeting with an individual counselor or participating in a time-limited psychoeducational group.

These psychosocial interventions should focus on (1) the development of an awareness of the relationships among external stress, internal responses, and behavior; (2) the development of an active problem-solving attitude toward the symptoms; and (3) the implementation of behavior changes and coping strategies that diminish the symptoms. Individual or group interventions such as these will provide a supportive setting in which to diagnose, as well as to treat, PMS. Through the use of prospective symptom recording and discussion, a woman has the opportunity to determine the relationships among her menstrual cycle, external events, internal psychologic states, her behavior, and premenstrual symptoms. In addition the individual therapist or group leader can provide education about lifestyle changes and support to help each woman implement these changes.

When available, time-limited psychoeducational groups are preferable to individual counseling sessions. In addition to the benefits of education and discussion previously listed, group meetings provide the unique opportunity for women with PMS to meet and work with other women who share similar experiences. This shared experience promotes group cohesiveness and reduces the sense of shame and isolation many women experience. Over time many group members derive a sense of hope and energy from the group process that helps them to take an active role in developing new behavior and techniques to diminish their premenstrual symptoms and to decrease the overall stress in their lives.

If a psychoeducational group is offered, the group leader should be experienced in group psychotherapy. Each member should have at least one pregroup interview to review her complaints and determine suitability for the group. All women who complain of PMS and who are not psychotic or paranoid can be included. Each member should be willing to make a commitment to attend all 12 sessions. At the time of the interview the patient can be asked to start charting her symptoms daily so that she will go to the first meeting of the group with some data about the relationship between her symptoms and her menstrual cycle.

A group meeting for 12 weeks' duration works well. It allows time for each woman to go through several menstrual cycles while in the group and time for the members to establish some comfort with each other. To include time for both diagnosis and treatment, each meeting can be divided roughly into thirds. At the start of each meeting, members can be given time to relate the status of their symptoms for the past week, discuss the ways they reacted to their symptoms, and outline and readjust goals for the upcoming week. The group leader can then spend some time (about one-half hour) presenting some educational material. Areas that are useful to cover are the physiologic characteristics of the menstrual cycle, questionnaires that assess areas of stress, methods of relaxation and stress management, nutrition, and behavioral management of stress at home and work. In addition the leader should save time each week (about one-half hour) to allow for unstructured discussion of feelings regarding PMS. Many women who have felt out of control premenstrually may never have discussed the extent of their symptoms with anyone. This time allows the group to develop a sense of commonality that will reduce shame and isolation and increase the likelihood that the members will implement behavioral changes.

Randomized trials have documented the effectiveness of formal relaxation training as well as time-limited cognitive behavioral therapy in reducing symptoms of PMS. Another nonpharmacologic therapy that shows evidence of effectiveness from randomized trials is light therapy, using 30 minutes of 10,000 lux evening light during the luteal phase.

Vitamin and Mineral Supplements

Several vitamin and mineral supplements have been evaluated as treatments for PMS in randomized controlled trials (Box 56-3). The results of studies of vitamin B_6, a cofactor in serotonin metabolism, are conflicting, but overall suggest a modest benefit. A large randomized trial has confirmed earlier reports of the effectiveness of calcium supplements in alleviating both physical and psychologic symptoms of PMS. The mechanism of calcium's beneficial effect is unknown. There is some evidence that abnormalities of calcium and vitamin D regulation across the menstrual cycle may affect the manifestations of PMS. Since most American women ingest less than the recommended amounts of calcium, calcium supplements should be one of the first interventions suggested to women presenting for treatment of PMS.

Choice of Therapy

In critically evaluating the evidence for effectiveness of medical therapy for PMS, it is important to bear in mind the

---

BOX 56-3
Initial Interventions for Women with Premenstrual Syndrome

Lifestyle Modifications
Frequent small meals
Adequate protein and complex carbohydrates
Elimination of concentrated sweets, caffeine, and alcohol
Regular aerobic exercise for 20 to 45 minutes, at least three times weekly
Stress management

Vitamin and Mineral Supplements
Calcium (elemental) 1200 mg/day
Vitamin B_6 50-100 mg/day
Magnesium 200 mg/day

factors that complicate interpretation of research on this subject. Consensus on the definition of PMS for research purposes has evolved only in recent years, and many studies differ in their definitions of PMS and their methods for measuring symptoms. The duration of therapy is rarely more than two or three cycles. The large placebo effect observed in many studies of PMS virtually requires that clinical decisions about the effectiveness of treatment be based on randomized trials, particularly when those treatments are associated with potential adverse effects or significant costs.

Studies of treatments for PMS include symptom-specific therapy, hormonal therapy generally involving ovarian suppression, and psychotropic medications. The evidence for the effectiveness of each of these forms of treatment, derived from published randomized controlled trials, is summarized in the following sections, and clinical recommendations for their use are presented in Table 56-1.

Symptom-Specific Therapy

For symptoms of bloating and edema, **spironolactone** taken during the luteal phase is effective. Metolazone shows similar effectiveness, but chlorthalidone does not.

Cyclic breast pain is reduced by **bromocriptine,** which may be used in low doses during the luteal phase. Evidence

to support a benefit from vitamin E is lacking, although it is widely used clinically and has little apparent toxicity.

The effectiveness of **nonsteroidal antiinflammatory drugs** for cyclic pelvic pain is well known. Some evidence for a beneficial effect of these agents on fatigue, mood swings, and headache also exists.

Hormonal Therapy

The results of studies of **progesterone** for premenstrual syndrome do not support its use to treat PMS. Other hormone interventions based on ovulation suppression have shown more consistent evidence for effectiveness, but their use is limited by short- and long-term side effects. **Gonadotropin-releasing hormone (GnRH) analogs** have generally reduced both physical and psychologic symptoms; however, use for more than 6 months is precluded by their negative effects on bone density. Studies of "add-back" therapy with replacement-level doses of estrogen and progestin, designed to minimize long-term risks of GnRH analogs, appear promising. The high cost of GnRH analogs further limits their use.

Danazol, which also results in ovulation suppression and eventual amenorrhea, alleviates a range of premenstrual symptoms but is often associated with bothersome side effects, including hirsutism, acne, and hot flashes. **The oral**

Table 56-1
Interventions for PMS with Evidence of Benefit from Controlled Trials

Nonpharmacologic

Relaxation training
Cognitive therapy
Moderate aerobic exercise
Light therapy: 30 minutes of 10,000 lux evening light during luteal phase

Pharmacologic

Treatment of Specific Symptoms

Fluid retention	Spironolactone	50-100 mg/day, luteal phase
Breast pain	Bromocriptine	2.5-5 mg/day, luteal phase
Pelvic pain	Any NSAID	

Treatment of Multiple Symptoms
Antidepressants and other psychotropic agents

	Fluoxetine	10-60 mg/day
	Sertraline	50-150 mg/day
		50-150 mg/day in luteal phase
		50-100 mg/day in week before menses
	Paroxetine	20 mg/day
	Citalopram	10-30 mg/day
		5 mg/day follicular phase, 10-30 mg/day luteal phase
	Clomipramine	25 mg/day-50 mg bid
	Alprazolam	0.25-1 mg tid, luteal phase

Hormonal therapy

Danazol 200-400 mg/day or in luteal phase
  (not effective for contraception)
GnRH analogs acetate 3.75-7.5 mg IM monthly
  Nafarelin acetate
  Leuprolide nasal spray 200 mg bid-tid
  Begin first dose at start of menses; limit use to 6 months
With estrogen/progestin "add-back":
  Conjugated estrogens 0.625 mg/day
  Medroxyprogesterone 5 mg day 1-12

contraceptive pill affects only a limited number of premenstrual symptoms; a trial may be appropriate in women who also need contraception, although the published literature shows no good evidence for benefit in PMS.

Psychotropic Agents

Studies demonstrating a consistent benefit from **selective serotonin reuptake inhibitors (SSRIs)** support the hypothesis that some premenstrual symptoms may be mediated through alterations in the neurotransmitter serotonin. **D-fenfluramine,** which also acts by affecting serotonin levels, has been shown to alleviate depression and reduce premenstrual calorie, fat, and carbohydrate consumption in women with PMS, but is not currently available in the United States.

Studies of **alprazolam** indicate that both anxiety and depression, as well as somatic symptoms, are reduced with use of the agent during the luteal phase or throughout the cycle. The potential for dependency is minimized by confining use to the luteal phase. Limited evidence supports the use of **atenolol** for irritability, particularly in women also bothered by premenstrual migraine.

Parry has investigated innovative approaches to reducing premenstrual symptoms through alterations in circadian rhythms. Controlled trials have demonstrated improvements in depression with **bright light treatments** throughout the cycle or **late sleep deprivation** (awakening at 2 AM) at symptom onset. These approaches need further study but may be offered to women with prominent affective symptoms who wish to avoid pharmacologic therapy.

Treatment options for women with clear evidence of PMS who do not respond to more conservative measures are listed in Table 56-1. If the patient and physician believe that further treatment is indicated, the patient should understand that the current state of medical knowledge about PMS is limited and that predicting response to treatment is difficult.

Hysterectomy with bilateral oophorectomy is a drastic measure for which there is some limited evidence of effectiveness for relief of premenstrual symptoms. Surgery should be considered only if the diagnosis has been prospectively established and confirmed, underlying psychiatric disorders have been ruled out through formal psychiatric evaluation, symptoms have not responded to multiple trials of medical and behavioral therapy, and symptoms substantially affect quality of life.

BIBLIOGRAPHY

Brown CS et al: Efficacy of depot leuprolide in premenstrual syndrome: effect of symptom severity and type in a controlled trial, *Obstet Gynecol* 84:779, 1994.

Campbell EM et al: Premenstrual symptoms in general practice patients: prevalence and treatment, *J Reprod Med* 42:637, 1997.

Freeman EW et al: Differential response to antidepressants in women with premenstrual syndrome/premenstrual dysphoric disorder. A randomized controlled trial, *Arch Gen Psychiatry* 56:932, 1999.

O'Brien PM, Abukhalil IE: Randomized controlled trial of the management of premenstrual syndrome and premenstrual mastalgia using luteal phase-only danazol. *Am J Obstet Gynecol* 180:18, 1999.

Parry BL et al: Light therapy of late luteal phase dysphoric disorder: an extended study, *Am J Psychiatry* 150:1417, 1993.

Ramcharan S et al: The epidemiology of premenstrual syndrome in a population-based sample of 2650 urban women: attributable risk and risk factors, *J Clin Epidemiol* 45:377, 1992.

Roca CA, Schmidt PJ, Rubinow DR: A follow-up study of premenstrual syndrome, *J Clin Psychiatry* 60:762, 1999.

Schmidt PJ et al: Differential behavioral effects of gonadal steroids in women with and in those without premenstrual syndrome, *N Engl J Med* 338:209, 1998.

Thys-Jacobs S et al: Calcium carbonate and the premenstrual syndrome: effects on premenstrual and menstrual symptoms, *Am J Obstet Gynecol* 179:444, 1998.

Wang M et al: Treatment of premenstrual syndrome by spironolactone: a double-blind, placebo-controlled study, *Acta Obstet Gynecol Scand* 10:803, 1995.

Wood SH et al: Treatment of premenstrual syndrome with fluoxetine: a double-blind, placebo-controlled crossover study, *Obstet Gynecol* 80: 339, 1992.

Wyatt KM et al: Efficacy of vitamin B-6 in the treatment of premenstrual syndrome: systematic review, *BMJ* 318:1375, 1999.

Yonkers KA: Anxiety symptoms and anxiety disorders: how are they related to premenstrual disorders? *J Clin Psychiatry* 58S:62, 1997.

Yonkers KA et al: Symptomatic improvement of premenstrual dysphoric disorder with sertraline treatment, *JAMA* 278:983, 1997.

CHAPTER 57

Sexual Dysfunction

Linda Shafer

In our society not only is sexual fulfillment important to people, it is closely linked to emotional and physical well-being. Although the exact incidence of sexual dysfunction in the general population is unknown, a recent study reported that sexual dysfunction is widespread, and is influenced by both psychosocial and organic factors. Surprisingly, sexual problems were found to be more prevalent in females, affecting 43% of women and 31% of men. Yet, despite its high prevalence, most psychophysiologic research has been done on males, and knowledge of female sexuality is primarily based on the male. With the Food and Drug Administration (FDA) approval of sildenafil (Viagra) in 1998 to treat erectile dysfunction, there has been an upsurge of interest in female sexual dysfunction, especially its pharmacologic treatment.

The first part of this chapter discusses the causes of sexual dysfunction, evaluation, and approach to treatment from the perspective of heterosexual relationships. The second section addresses what is known of sexual dysfunction in lesbian relationships.

FEMALE SEXUAL DISORDERS
Hypoactive Sexual Desire Disorder (Low Libido)

The condition of *hypoactive sexual desire disorder* has been defined as persistently deficient or absent sexual fantasies and desire for sexual activity. This disorder is the most common sexual disorder in women. According to one recent study, 33% of all women, twice as many as men, reported a lack of interest in sex. It is caused by either psychologic or organic factors. Hormone deficiencies caused by natural menopause, surgical or medically induced menopause, or other endocrine disorders, should be ruled out in every case.

The role of testosterone in libido in women is a subject of growing recent interest. Research suggests that female sex drive is governed by multiple cyclic hormones, including testosterone, estrogen, and progesterone. Diurnal and monthly variations in these hormones and their interactions make study of their effects difficult. In addition, measurement issues complicate the interpretation of much of the existing research, which was done using total rather than biologically active free testosterone levels. The available studies suggest that testosterone, together with other andro-gens such as DHEA, promotes sexual drive in women, as well as affecting mood and overall sense of well being. Progesterone appears to blunt this effect.

Sexual Aversion Disorder

Sexual aversion disorder has been defined as a persistent or recurrent extreme aversion to and avoidance of all or almost all genital sexual contact with a sexual partner. The exact incidence of this disorder is unknown, but it is one of the more common sexual disorders presenting for treatment. Primary sexual aversion seems more prevalent in men, and secondary is more common in women. The disorder is generally psychologically based, resulting from such causes as childhood trauma, such as physical or sexual abuse. The syndrome is associated with phobic avoidance of sexual activity or even the thought of sexual activity. Of patients with sexual phobias and aversions, 25% meet the criteria for panic disorder. Most people with this disorder respond fairly naturally to sex, if they can get past the high anxiety associated with the initial dread. Typically the frequency of intercourse is only once or twice a year.

Sexual Arousal Disorder (Arousal Phase Disorder)

Female sexual arousal disorder is defined as a persistent or recurrent partial or complete failure to attain or maintain the lubrication swelling response of sexual excitement until the completion of the sexual activity. Although the exact incidence of this problem is unknown, a recent study reported the disorder in 19% of women and increasing to 27% of women over age 50. The condition includes lack of or diminished vaginal lubrication, decreased clitoral and labial sensation, or lack of vaginal smooth muscle relaxation. Although the condition may be caused by psychologic factors, there is often an underlying organic basis, such as prior pelvic trauma, pelvic surgery, and/or side effects of medication. The disorder is often linked to problems with sexual desire and dyspareunia.

Orgasmic Dysfunction (Orgasm Phase Disorder)

Orgasmic dysfunction is defined as a persistent or recurrent delay in or absence of orgasm despite a normal desire and arousal phase. Some women find it difficult to reach orgasm during intercourse but can do so with direct clitoral contact. This is usually a normal variant of response and does not justify the diagnosis of orgasmic dysfunction. Claims that stimulation of an area in the anterior wall of the vagina, called the G spot (Grafenberg spot), will trigger female orgasm and ejaculation have never been substantiated.

Anorgasmia in all of its forms occurs in about 25% of females. The incidence runs from about 5% to 8% of women who are totally unable to achieve orgasm to 30% to 40% of women who are unable to achieve orgasm without clitoral stimulation or during intercourse alone. The capacity for orgasm increases with experience. It is important to evaluate the partner, who may have premature ejaculation, which contributes to the female's anorgasmia.

Vaginismus (Sexual Pain Disorder)

Vaginismus is defined as recurrent or persistent involuntary spasm of the musculature of the outer third of the vagina (pubococcygeus muscles) that makes sexual intercourse impossible, difficult, or painful. Although the exact frequency of vaginismus is not known, it probably accounts for less than 10% of female sexual disorders. Vaginismus often develops as a conditioned response to painful penetration or secondary to psychologic factors. Because there is a high incidence of pelvic abnormality associated with this condition, a careful gynecologic examination is warranted and is the only definitive way to make the diagnosis. Secondary impotence in the male partner may develop. Vaginismus is the sexual disorder most often found in long-term unconsummated marriages.

Dyspareunia (Sexual Pain Disorder)

Dyspareunia is defined as a recurrent or persistent genital pain before, during, or after sexual intercourse. The overall prevalence of dyspareunia in the general population is about 15%. A recent study reported that young single women had the most pain during sex, probably resulting from instability of sexual relationships, along with general inexperience. Women over age 50 were found to be one third less likely to have pain during sex. This disorder can develop secondary to organic conditions such as vestibulitis or vaginal atrophy or vaginal infection, and/or can be the result of psychologic factors.

CAUSES OF SEXUAL DYSFUNCTION

The vast majority of sexual problems are caused by a multitude of factors, often a combination of biologic and psychogenic. Thus it is important to evaluate each individual carefully for organic and psychogenic contributions, so that proper treatment can be prescribed.

Table 57-1 lists some of the more common medical and surgical conditions that can cause sexual difficulties.

Table 57-2 provides a list of some drugs that are either known to affect the female sexual response or believed to cause female sexual dysfunction, on the basis of studies done on males.

There are many psychogenic issues leading to sexual problems, ranging from superficial causes such as anxiety over performance or fears of "letting go" to more deep-seated issues in which sex is unconsciously equated with danger. There are no rigid correlations between certain

Table 57-1
Medical and Surgical Conditions Causing Female Sexual Problems

Disorder	Sexual Impairment
Endocrine Diabetes; thyroid, adrenal, pituitary glands	Reduced vaginal lubrication, vaginal infection (diabetes)
Vascular Sickle-cell anemia Cardiac: MI, angina	Decreased arousal and orgasm Fear of death, decreased frequency
Neurologic Spinal cord damage Multiple sclerosis	Decreased arousal, orgasm, and genital lubrication
Gynecologic Vaginitis, PID, uterine prolapse, fibroids	Vaginismus, dyspareunia endometriosis, Decreased arousal and desire
Renal Renal failure (on dialysis)	Decreased arousal and desire Electrolyte and hormone imbalance
Musculoskeletal Arthritis Sjögren's syndrome	Chronic pain, limited motion Decreased lubrication
Surgery Gynecologic oophorectomy, episiotomy	Decreased estrogen levels and lubrication Tightness of vaginal opening
Other Mastectomy, colostomy	Self-esteem issues, fears of discomfort

MI, Myocardial infarction; *PID,* pelvic inflammatory disease.

background factors and dysfunctional syndromes. However, most sexual disorders can be related to prior experiences that place an individual at risk of having a sexual disorder. These may include negative family attitudes about sex, inadequate information or education about sex, and past traumatic sexual experiences such as rape or incest. There is usually an acute precipitant that will actually trigger the problem, causing the patient to seek help. Examples of such precipitating causes are childbirth, marital infidelity, a depression or other psychiatric problem, or a sexual problem in the partner. Moreover, there may be maintaining factors that prevent the problem from being solved such as ongoing communication issues, lack of cooperation, financial problems, and lack of foreplay. Sometimes latent homosexuality may be the basis for the complaint.

▨ EVALUATION

It has been estimated that approximately 15% to 25% of medical outpatients consult primary care physicians for sexual complaints. However, it has been clearly demon-

Table 57-2
Medications that Affect Female Sexuality

Drug	Side Effect
Antihypertensives	
Methyldopa, reserpine, clonidine propranolol, spironolactone	Decreased libido, anorgasmia
Anticholinergics	
Propantheline, methantheline	Decreased lubrication
Hormones	
Estrogen, progesterone, steroids, androgen	Decreased libido (variable) Increased libido
Psychotropics	
Sedatives—alcohol, barbiturates	Higher dose—sexual problems
Anxiolytics—diazepam, alprazolam	Anorgasmia
Antipsychotics—thioridazine	Anorgasmia
Antidepressants	
MAO inhibitors— phenelzine	Anorgasmia
Tricyclics—imipramine, clomipramine	Anorgasmia
SSRIs—fluoxetine, sertraline	Low libido, anorgasmia
Atypical—trazodone	Anorgasmia
Lithium	Decreased libido
Opiates	
Morphine, codeine, methadone	Anorgasmia, decreased libido
Miscellaneous	
Phenytoin, indomethacin, clofibrate, cimetidine, carbamazepine	Decreased libido

MAO, Monoamine oxidase; *SSRI,* selective serotonin reuptake inhibitor.

strated that the incidence of sexual problems treated in any medical office is directly associated with those clinicians who routinely take a sexual history. Since discussions of sexuality still cause shame and embarrassment for many people, the presentation of sexual problems may take on many covert forms. These include somatic symptoms that have no medical cause, including headaches, low back pain, generalized pelvic pain, and vulvar pruritis.

A brief **sexual history** should be a required part of every medical evaluation, both for its positive clinical value and for its moral and legal implications during this current acquired immunodeficiency syndrome (AIDS) crisis. It can be done most easily in conjunction with the gynecologic and menstrual review in women, but the physician should remember to display an open nonjudgmental attitude. Helpful screening questions include: "Have there been any changes in your sex life?" "Would you like to change anything about your sexual functioning?" "Have you been sexually active (or involved) with a partner?" "Do you practice safer sex?"

Careful history taking sometimes helps distinguish an organic cause from a psychogenic one. Moreover, a sexual history helps delineate which further diagnostic tests are indicated and helps determine the treatment approaches that

will be needed. Failure to take a sexual history and educate the patient about risk factors for human immunodeficiency virus (HIV) infection and safer sex practices may leave the physician open to charges of negligence.

Few **diagnostic tests** are indicated in female sexual disorders beyond the physical examination, which should include a thorough gynecologic examination. In cases of vaginal dryness, a serum follicle-stimulating hormone level and a vaginal maturation index may be done, especially in perimenopausal women, to determine whether ovarian failure has begun. (See Chapter 48 for more information on assessment of menopausal status.) For dyspareunia, a complete blood count, sedimentation rate, and cervical culture should be done to rule out pelvic inflammatory disease, especially if the pain is greatest on deep penetration. A Papanicolaou's smear should be done to rule out malignancy. Pelvic ultrasonography may help define a suspected pelvic mass, and referral for laparoscopy may help make the diagnosis of endometriosis, adhesions, or an adnexal mass.

For complaints of low sexual desire, a serum testosterone level may be obtained. Normal total testosterone levels in premenopausal women are between 20 and 80 ng/dl; levels vary according to cycle phase. In premenopausal women, circadian rhythms have a much greater effect on testosterone level than changes during the cycle, with levels 80% higher in the morning than in the evening. Normal total testosterone levels in postmenopausal women range from 10 to 40 ng/dl. Existing research shows inconsistent relationships of endogenous testosterone levels to sexual drive and behavior.

The development of more sophisticated diagnostic testing, primarily for male sexual disorders, has led to the overall conclusion that sexual problems once thought to be psychogenic in origin have been found to have an organic basis. Psychophysiologic research into women's sexual problems is now underway to measure female genital blood flow, vaginal pH, vaginal compliance, and genital vibratory thresholds. Early data indicate that the sympathetic nervous system may be more important for female than for male sexual arousal.

MANAGEMENT

Often the primary care physician is the first person to be consulted about a sexual complaint. Aside from estrogen replacement and androgen replacement therapy in postmenopausal women, pharmacologic treatment is still in experimental phases in women, with mixed results. A recent report of a large clinical trial of sildenafil in women yielded the disappointing results that the drug was not effective in treating female sexual arousal disorder, although more studies are pending.

Table 57-3 lists drugs and medical devices currently being studied as treatments for female sexual dysfunction (in pilot or preclinical studies).

Sex therapy, a psychobehavioral short-term treatment of sexual symptoms, has proved useful in treating female sexual dysfunction. Because many levels of intervention may be helpful to patients, even physicians without formal training in sex therapy may enable patients to deal effectively with sexual problems. Physicians can help patients by giving permission and reassurance, providing information, and correcting misinformation. If this is insufficient, specific suggestions can be given to the patient and the partner. These

Table 57-3
Medications and Medical Devices for the Treatment of Female Sexual Dysfunction

Drug	Potential Benefits
Estrogen Replacement Therapy Oral, topical, estradiol ring (Estring)	In menopausal women, improves clitoral sensitivity, increases libido, decreases pain during intercourse.
Methyl Testosterone Oral, topical, patch; combined with estrogen (Estratest)	In menopausal women, improves clitoral sensitivity increases libido, decreases pain during intercourse.
Sildenafil (Viagra) Oral, nasal spray, topical	Increases blood flow to vagina to treat FSAD; useful in SSRI-induced anorgasmia.
Phentolamine (Vasomax) Oral, vaginal suppository (Vasofem)	Increases blood flow to vagina to treat FSAD.
Apomorphine (Uprima) Sublingual	Stimulates brain centers to facilitate arousal and desire.
Alprostadil (Prostaglandin E$_1$) Vaginal suppository, cream (Femprox)	Increases blood flow to vagina to treat FSAD.
L-Arginine Oral	Precursor to formation of NO; increases vascular smooth muscle relaxation to treat FSAD.
EROS-CTD Clitoral therapy device (FDA approved)	Gentle suction directly to clitoris to increase blood flow to genitalia; improves sensation, lubrication, orgasm, satisfaction.

FSAD, Female sexual arousal disorder; *NO,* nitric oxide.

encompass the behavioral techniques used in sex therapy. Although there are specific techniques used to treat particular kinds of dysfunctions, some general principles of behavior therapy include increasing communication between partners, decreasing performance anxiety or "spectatoring" by changing the goal of the sexual activity away from emphasis on orgasm and more toward giving pleasure and feeling good, relieving the pressure to perform at any sexual encounter, and encouraging sexual experimentation. A trial of this kind of therapy is certainly reasonable where there is no evidence of more serious underlying psychopathologic condition or organic disease and/or until vasoactive agents are demonstrated to be effective and safe in women.

INDICATIONS FOR REFERRAL

Behavior therapy often leads to improvement in sexual functioning without the need for referral. If the condition does not improve, this may be a sign that the patient needs more intensive therapy. A consultation with a mental health expert trained in sex and marital therapy may be indicated. Often a direct referral to a specialist may be indicated for patients known to have chronic psychologic issues, who experience gender confusion, or who have never had a period of satisfactory functioning.

SPECIFIC PSYCHOBEHAVIORAL TREATMENT TECHNIQUES

Hypoactive Sexual Disorder

Positive sexual experiences help increase sexual desire, although most cases require some insight into background influences and are difficult to treat.

1. Sensate focus exercises (nondemand pleasuring techniques) to enhance enjoyment without pressure.
2. Use of erotic material.
3. Masturbation training with fantasy to help individuals become aware of conditions necessary for a positive sexual experience.

Sexual Aversion Disorder

1. Same as for hypoactive sexual desire (i.e., systematic desensitization with sensate focus exercises).
2. Where phobic/panic-type symptoms are displayed, the addition of antipanic medication (tricyclic antidepressants such as imipramine, or benzodiazepines such as alprazolam) may be helpful when used for 3 or 4 months and offers an excellent prognosis.

Female Arousal Disorder

Because female arousal disorder usually results from a more severe psychopathologic condition, it usually requires referral for treatment.

1. Supplemental use of lubrication, such as water-soluble lubricant jelly or saliva, can be suggested for vaginal dryness.
2. Postmenopausal women with atrophic vaginal mucosa may benefit from topical estrogen therapy.

Orgasmic Dysfunction

Totally Anorgastic

1. Education and encouragement of self-exploration, including masturbation and use of fantasy material, offer excellent prognosis.
2. Kegel vaginal exercises to increase frequency of orgasm (contraction of pubococcygeus muscles).

Anorgastic with Partner

1. Sensate focus exercises (from nongenital stimulation to genital stimulation).
2. Intercourse and orgasm prohibited at this time to take away performance pressure.
3. Use of back protected position (male in seated position with female between his legs with back against his chest) to allow the female to control the stimulation and eliminate self-consciousness).

4. Pelvic thrusting explored in nondemanding way, beginning with female superior position, followed by lateral position that allows for mutual freedom of movement.
5. Use of the above yields a success rate of 70% to 80%.

Anorgastic During Intercourse
1. Use of "bridge technique," in which clitoris is stimulated manually or with a vibrator after insertion of the penis into the vagina, is successful in 30% to 50% of couples.

Vaginismus
1. Demonstrate to woman (and her partner) that the condition is involuntary and not willfully contrived, typically shown by inserting a gloved finger into the vagina, which has involuntary spasm.
2. Encourage the woman to insert larger and larger objects into the vagina in a gradual step-by-step fashion. Use of one finger, then several, to approximate the penis.
3. Use of Hegar graduated vaginal dilators to control dilation without pain. Syringe containers of different sizes make good alternative dilators.
4. In female superior position woman uses erect penis as her dilator to insert gradually into vagina, in conjunction with extravaginal lubricant (K-Y jelly).
5. Kegel vaginal exercises to develop sense of control.
6. Behavior modification yields an excellent success rate of about 95%.

Dyspareunia
1. Treat underlying gynecologic problem first.
2. If accompanying vaginismus, use previously mentioned techniques.
3. Treat insufficient lubrication as described.
4. Variable prognosis depends on organic factors involved and ability to treat them.

SEXUAL DYSFUNCTION IN LESBIANS

On the basis of available studies, the percentage of gay men and lesbians in the general population is somewhere between 2% and 10%. The clinician should expect to encounter some lesbian patients and be prepared to deal with their sexual complaints. A patient may spontaneously reveal her sexual orientation, or during the review of systems, the clinician may ask the patient directly with sexual screening questions.

As a group, lesbian couples have not been well researched. However, studies show that, like heterosexual women, lesbians value relationships highly. Single lesbians have less sex and fewer partners than do gay men. Lesbians are more sexually responsive and more satisfied with sex than are heterosexual women.

Lesbians have not been reported to have significant rates of orgasmic dysfunction, dyspareunia, or vaginismus, probably because of sexual technique. There is less emphasis on genital organs and orgasm and more on sensuality. However, lesbians do have low rates of sex within long-term committed relationships and often consult the clinician with a complaint of low sexual desire. Often they prefer nongenital physical contact (e.g., hugging) to genital sex. In one study, half the couples with a low frequency of genital sex were dissatisfied, leading to one partner's having an affair and the resulting dissolution of the relationship. Lesbian women tend to equate sexual attraction with love, moving from one relationship to another. They are not comfortable with sex outside the context of a relationship. Such relationships, which are not given much time to develop and lack the opportunity for the couple to explore their compatibility, have a high failure rate.

SAFER SEX FOR AIDS PREVENTION

Lack of knowledge of safer sex practices can contribute to the spread of AIDS. Increasing numbers of women have become infected with HIV through heterosexual intercourse. There should be an active attempt to eroticize safe sex behavior including holding, hugging, massage, mutual masturbation, use of vibrators, and dry kissing. The physician should be prepared to discuss the advantages of long-term relationships, the use of condoms, and spermicides containing nonoxynol-9 in minimizing the AIDS risk. Patients in high-risk groups such as intravenous drug users and those at above-average risk with multiple partners should be encouraged to modify their behavior. The risk of sexual transmission of HIV among lesbians is low. See Chapter 22 for more information on counseling about safer sex practices.

BIBLIOGRAPHY
Basson R et al: Efficacy and safety of sildenafil in estrogenized women with sexual dysfunction associated with female sexual arousal disorder, *Obstet Gynecol* 95(4 Suppl 1):S54, 2000.

Basson R: Report of the International Consensus Conference on Female Sexual Dysfunction: definitions and classifications, *J Urol* 163:888, 2000.

Bell R: ABC of sexual health: homosexual men and women, *BMJ* 318:452, 1999.

Berman JR, Berman LA, Goldstein I: Female sexual dysfunction: incidence pathophysiology, evaluation and treatment option, *Urology* 54:385, 1999.

Berman JR: Sildenafil in postmenopausal women with sexual dysfunction, *Urology* 54:578, 1999.

Crenshaw TL, Goldberg JP: *Sexual Pharmacology,* New York, 1996, W Norton.

Davis S: The clinical use of androgens in female sexual disorders, *J Sex Marital Ther* 23:153, 1998.

Kaplan HS: *The sexual desire disorders: dysfunctional regulation of sexual motivation,* New York, 1995, Brunner/Mazel.

Kaplan SA et al: Safety and efficacy of sildenafil in postmenopausal women with sexual dysfunction, *Urology* 53:481, 1999.

Laumann EO, Paik A, Rosen RC: Sexual dysfunction in the United States: prevalence and predictors, *JAMA* 281:537, 1999.

Leiblum SR, Rosen RC: *Principles and practice of sex therapy, update for the 1990s,* ed 2, New York, 1989, Guilford Press.

Maurice W: *Sexual medicine in primary care,* New York, 1999, Mosby.

Meston CM, Heiman JR: Ephedrine-activated physiological sexual arousal in women, *Arch Gen Psychiatry,* 55:652, 1998.

Nichols M: Lesbian relationships: implications for the study of sexuality and gender. In McWhirter DP et al, editors, *Homosexuality/heterosexuality,* New York, 1990, Oxford University Press.

Read S, King M, Watson J: Sexual dysfunction in primary medical care: prevalence, characteristics and detection by the general practitioner, *J Public Health Med* 19:387, 1997.

Rosen RC et al: Prevalence of sexual dysfunction in women results of a survey study of 329 women in an outpatient gynecological clinic, *J Sex Marital Ther* 19:171, 1993.

Segraves RT: Psychiatric drugs and inhibited female orgasm, *J Sex Marital Ther* 14:202, 1988.

Shafer LC: Approach to the patient with sexual dysfunction. In Goroll AH, May LA, Mulley, AG Jr., editors: *Primary care medicine,* ed 3, Philadelphia, 1995, JB Lippincott.

Shafer LC: Approach to the patient with sexual dysfunction, In Stern TA, Herman JB, Slavin PL, editors: *The MGH guide to psychiatry in primary care,* New York, 1998, McGraw-Hill.

Shafer LC: The denial of the risk of AIDS in heterosexuals coming for treatment of sexual disorders. In Rutan JS, editor: *Psychotherapy for the 1990s,* New York, 1992, Guilford Press.

Shen WW, Urosevich Z, Clayton DO: Sildenafil in the treatment of female sexual dysfunction induced by selective serotonin reuptake inhibitors, *J Reprod Med* 44:535, 1999.

Spector IP, Carey MP: Incidence and prevalence of the sexual dysfunctions: a critical review of the empirical literature, *Arch Sex Behav* 19:389, 1990.

Wincze JP, Carey MP: *Sexual dysfunction,* New York, 1991, Guilford Press.

RESOURCES

Patients have many questions and concerns about sexuality and may benefit from and find reassurance from the following suggested self-help books:

Barbach LG: *For yourself: the fulfillment of female sexuality,* New York, 1975, Doubleday.

Berzon B: *The intimacy dance: a guide to long-term success in gay and lesbian relationships,* New York, 1997, Plume.

Heiman J, LoPiccolo J: *Becoming orgasmic: a sexual growth program for women,* New York, 1988, Prentice-Hall.

Kaplan HS: *The real truth about women and AIDS: how to eliminate the risks without giving up love and sex,* New York, 1987, Simon & Schuster.

Rako S: *The hormone of desire: the truth about testosterone, sexuality, and menopause,* New York, 1999, Three Rivers Press.

Reichman J: *I'm not in the mood,* New York, 1998, William Morrow.

Winks C, Semans A: *The new good vibrations guide to sex,* ed 2, San Francisco, 1997, Cleis Press.

CHAPTER **58**

Contraception

Karen J. Carlson
Rapin Osathanondh
Michael R. Stelluto

Preventing unwanted pregnancy is a multifactorial process. The willingness and ability to use contraception are influenced not only by the efficacy of the methods, but also by cost, availability, personality, life circumstances, and culture. Although the range of prescription and nonprescription contraceptive options is large, including hormonal methods, barrier methods, intrauterine devices, and sterilization, no method is ideal. It is a challenging and complex task to assist women in making choices that are appropriate for a particular stage of life and medical and social circumstances.

This chapter describes a framework for approaching the female patient who desires contraception and outlines the physiology, effectiveness, benefits, and risks of available contraceptive methods.

EPIDEMIOLOGY

A woman's life expectancy is inversely proportional to the number of pregnancies she experiences. All contraceptive methods available in the United States are safer than carrying a pregnancy to term. Theoretically, the safest contraceptive practice for a monogamous woman is the diaphragm or condom, followed by early, legal abortion should one of those methods fail.

Effectiveness in prevention of pregnancy (Table 58-1) is a critical attribute of any contraceptive method, although it is only one of several factors that must be weighed in the selection of the optimal birth control method for an individual woman. Theoretic effectiveness rates reflect the ideal that can be achieved under ideal conditions. The actual or use effectiveness depends on many individual factors that introduce error.

APPROACH TO THE WOMAN WHO DESIRES CONTRACEPTION

Effective contraceptive management requires time for education and counseling. Because conflicting primary data about the sequelae of various methods have confused many women, education about risks and benefits is crucial to clarify what is known and what remains controversial. Counseling explores values and life circumstances, including marital status, partner(s), work or educational opportunity, home re-sponsibilities, future childbearing plans, sexuality and body image, and the need for security versus the willingness to risk pregnancy or side effects.

Informed consent, in nontechnical terminology and in the woman's native language, should be obtained for any prescription method of contraception and before any invasive procedures. Informed consent recognizes that contraceptive interventions that involve hormones, devices, or surgery expose healthy people to known and unknown risks. Beyond delineating medicolegal and ethical responsibilities, informed consent provides useful information for assisting women in selecting a contraceptive method and in gaining the confidence to use it.

The screening history is directed toward the gynecologic and obstetric history, review of systems to establish potential contraindications and risk factors for complications, and personal history to elicit lifestyle preferences. Similarly, the screening physical examination and laboratory studies uncover potential contraindications or risks for complications of chosen contraceptive methods.

HORMONAL METHODS
Oral Contraceptive Pill

There are two types of oral contraceptive pills (OCPs). Combination or combined pills contain a synthetic estrogen, ethinyl estradiol (or its methyl ester, mestranol) and a progestin. Combination pills are packaged in 21- or 28-day cycles; the last seven tablets in 28-day packs are hormonally inert and may contain iron. Monophasic pills contain the same amount of estrogen and progestin in the 21 hormonally active tablets. Efforts to lower the total exposure to steroids while mimicking the patterns of the physiologic menstrual cycle led to the marketing of multiphasic (biphasic and triphasic) pills. They contain 35 mg or less of estrogen in each active tablet, and varying amounts of progestin. There is also a multiphasic preparation with a gradually increasing amount of estrogen and a fixed amount of progestin. The clinical advantages of these varying formulations have not been established in controlled studies.

The progestins have differing levels of androgenic and estrogenic activity. The newer progestins desogestrel and norgestimate have decreased androgenic activity and fewer

Table 58-1
Effectiveness Rates of Contraceptive Methods

Method	Theoretical Effectiveness (%)	Use Effectiveness (%)
Oral Contraceptive Pill		
Combination	99.9	97
Progestin only	99.5	97
Injectable Hormonal Regimens		
Depo Provera	99.7	99.7
Norplant	99.96	99.96
Barrier Methods		
Condoms	98	88
Diaphragm	94	82
Cervical cap	94	82
Spermicides	97	79
Intrauterine Device		
Copper T380	99.2	97
Progestasert	98	97
Sterilization		
Male	99.9	99.9
Female	99.8	99.6

Data adapted from Trussel J et al: *Obstet Gynecol* 76:558, 1990.

effects on blood pressure and carbohydrate and lipid metabolism than older progestins. Table 58-2 shows the relative androgenic and estrogenic activity of combination pills containing 35 mg or less of estrogen.

Progestin-only pills, also called the "mini pill," contain a small dose of progestin and no estrogen.

Mechanism of Action

Estrogens and progestins in low daily dosage synergistically prevent ovulation by inhibiting the midcycle surge of the gonadotropins—luteinizing hormone (LH) and follicle-stimulating hormone (FSH). This suppresses endogenous ovarian estrogen and progesterone production, which then inhibits endometrial proliferation. Bleeding occurs in response to progestin withdrawal, which mimics monthly menstrual periodicity.

Progestins decrease tubal function, diminish endometrial receptiveness to implantation, and render the cervix less permeable to penetration by sperm. Progestins alone can provide adequate contraceptive effects but do not totally suppress LH surges or ovarian estrogens, which accounts for their higher failure rate compared to combined pills. In addition, the irregular bleeding that is sometimes a side effect of progestin-only pills contributes to noncompliance.

Benefits

A principal benefit of the OCP is its very high effectiveness rate (97% to 99%). Daily pill-taking is dissociated from the sexual act, which may make compliance easier for some women. The combination pill protects the user from ectopic pregnancy, reduces primary dysmenorrhea, and reduces the incidence of fibrocystic breast disease and functional ovarian cysts. Increased cycle regularity is another potential benefit of the combination pill, particularly for women approaching

Table 58-2
Progestational and Androgenic Activity of Combination Oral Contraceptive Pills Containing 35 mg or Less of Ethinyl Estradiol

	PILLS WITH LOW ESTROGEN ACTIVITY	
Level of Activity	**Progestational**	**Androgenic**
Low	TriLevlen/Triphasil/ Trivora **Alesse/Levlite**	**Demulen 1/35/Zovia 1/35** Mircette*
Intermediate	Lo-Ovral/Low-Ogestrel Levlen/Nordette/ Levora	TriLevlen/Triphasil/ Trivora Lo-Ovral/Low-Ogestrel Levlen/Nordette/ Levora **Alesse/Levlite Lo-Estrin 1/20; Estrostep**
High	**Lo-Estrin 1/20; Estrostep Demulen 1/35/Zovia 1/35 Lo-Estrin 1.5/30** Mircette*	Lo-Estrin 1.5/30

	PILLS WITH INTERMEDIATE ESTROGEN ACTIVITY	
Level of Activity	**Progestational**	**Androgenic**
Low	Ortho-Tricyclen*; Ortho-Cyclen* Ovcon 35 Brevicon/Modicon/ Nelova 0.5/35/ Necon 0.5/35	Ortho-Tricyclen*; Ovcon 35 Desogen*/Orthocept*/ Apri*; Brevicon/Modicon/ Nelova 0.5/35/ Necon 0.5/35 Ortho-Cyclen
Intermediate	Tri-Norinyl OrthoNovum 777 Jenest OrthoNovum 10/11 Genora/Nelova/ Norethin/Norinyl/ OrthoNovum 1/35/ Necon 1/35	Tri-Norinyl OrthoNovum 777; OrthoNovum 10/11 Jenest Genora/Nelova/ Norethin/Norinyl/ OrthoNovum 1/35/ Necon 1/35
High	Desogen*/Orthocept*/ Apri*	

Pills in bold contain the equivalent of 20 μg ethinyl estradiol or less.
*Contains a third-generation progestin (desogestrel or norgestimate).

menopause. Use of the OCP is associated with a decreased risk of ovarian cancer and endometrial cancer, and there is some evidence of increased bone mineral density after several years of use.

Risks

Confusion about pill-associated morbidity and mortality stems from two major factors. First, studies conducted in the 1960s and 1970s were based on the use of pills with 50 mg or greater estrogen content. Lowering the amount of estrogen in the so-called "second generation" OCPs to 35 mg ethinyl estradiol diminished many unwanted effects. Second, long-term sequelae of oral contraceptive use, particularly neoplasia, may take 20 to 30 years to manifest; the original cohort of users is just entering that period.

Cardiovascular disease incidence was increased in early studies of the OCP, which showed higher rates of myocardial infarction, stroke, and thromboembolic disease in current users of the pill. The mechanism of **ischemic heart disease** was thought to be thrombosis, not atherosclerosis, mediated through the estrogen component of the pill. In these early studies, which mostly involved pills containing greater than 50 mg of ethinyl estradiol, risk was limited to current users; no studies have shown increased risk after cessation of the pill. Recent studies of current users of lower-dose pills (35 mg of ethinyl estradiol) have shown no increase in risk of cardiovascular disease in women under 30 or in nonsmokers without other risk factors. The risk of cardiovascular disease increases with age, and is heightened by smoking, particularly heavy smoking (15 or more cigarettes per day). Current practice, supported by recommendations of the American College of Obstetricians and Gynecologists, is to limit pill use beyond age 35 to nonsmokers. A recent consensus panel, while emphasizing the importance of smoking cessation interventions, has suggested that in some circumstances combination OCPs with the lowest estrogen doses (20 mg ethinyl estradiol) may be used in women over 35 who smoke fewer than 15 cigarettes per day.

Studies of **stroke** in users of second-generation OCPs have generally shown low or no excess stroke risk compared with earlier studies of OCPs with higher estrogen doses. A recent meta-analysis estimated that stroke risk for a healthy normotensive woman using the low-dose OCP increased from 4 to 8 per 100,000 per year.

Hypertension developed in about 5% of normotensive women after 3 months of older OCPs containing 50 mg ethinyl estradiol. More recent studies of low-dose OCPs indicate a lower risk of developing hypertension, approximately 4 cases per 1000 current users per year.

The risk of **venous thromboembolic disease** is mediated primarily through the estrogen component of the pill. Pooled data from numerous published studies indicate this risk is threefold or less for second-generation OCPs. Some studies of third-generation OCPs containing desogestrel or norgestimate have found a higher risk of thromboembolic disease (approximately fourfold to fivefold). Methodologic controversy has surrounded these findings; however, there is some evidence that the increase in risk with desogestrel and norgestimate may be clinically important, particularly in women with an inherited or acquired hypercoagulable state. Balancing these concerns are some studies that suggest the risk of ischemic heart disease may be reduced by third-generation OCPs and that any increased risk of thromboembolic disease would be offset by a lower likelihood of heart disease.

The pill is sometimes the cause of **lipid abnormalities.** Estrogens tend to increase high density lipoprotein (HDL) levels and decrease low density lipoprotein (LDL) levels; progestins generally have the opposite effect. The net effect is little or no change in total cholesterol, HDL, or LDL levels; triglycerides may increase, sometimes substantially.

Glucose intolerance is a consequence of the progestin component of the pill and occurs least with progestins having lower androgenic activity. There is evidence that combination OC use does not precipitate development of diabetes.

Recent data on the effect of OCP use on **breast cancer** risk indicate that there may be a slight increase in breast cancer risk with current use that abates after cessation. A reanalysis of 54 studies found that current use of the pill was associated with a 24% increase in risk (RR 1.24); 10 years after discontinuing OCP use, breast cancer risk was identical to that of women who never used OCPs. Risk was not affected by a family history of breast cancer, a personal history of benign breast disease, onset of OCP use in adolescence, dose of hormone, or duration of use.

Cervical dysplasia is increased twofold in pill users, even after controlling for factors such as frequency and age at onset of intercourse. Cervical epithelial abnormalities associated with OCP use predispose to infection with human papillomavirus, human immunodeficiency virus (HIV), and chlamydia.

The risk of **gallbladder disease** is increased approximately twofold in OCP users. **Hepatic adenomas** are rare benign vascular tumors associated with the oral contraceptive pill.

Management Issues

Most clinicians benefit from familiarity with a few of the many formulations of the oral contraceptive pill. When initiating OCP use, it is advisable to begin with a low-dose (30 to 35 mg ethinyl estradiol) pill. Because of concern about greater thromboembolic risk, we generally avoid pills containing third-generation progestins when initiating OCPs. The choice of pill may be modified by a history of estrogen-sensitive symptoms (premenstrual breast tenderness, bloating, weight gain), for which a progestin with low estrogenic activity is best, or of hirsutism or acne, for which a progestin with low androgenic activity is preferred (Table 58-2).

Women over 40 who do not smoke are good candidates for the lowest dose estrogen pills (those with 20 mg of ethinyl estradiol). Good cycle control and relief of vasomotor symptoms are potential benefits in this age group, although sometimes breakthrough bleeding occurs. A baseline mammogram and lipid profile should be obtained.

Postpartum women who desire oral contraceptives should be given the lowest estrogen preparations. Controversy exists regarding the appropriate commencement time. Manufacturers recommend delaying the start of OCP use until 4 to 6 weeks postpartum. However, many authorities feel that the benefits of an early start outweigh the risks (principally venous thromboembolism) because ovulation can occur as early as 2 weeks postpartum. Combination OCPs reduce the amount of breast milk. Breastfeeding women should consider a barrier method of contraception. Alternatively, progestin-only pills have long been used in lactating women.

Women with diabetes should be discouraged from using the pill if they have elevated blood pressure, nephropathy, or retinopathy. **Hypertensive women** generally are not candidates for combination oral contraceptives, although the pill can be considered with close monitoring when blood pressure is well controlled. The progestin-only pill may also be used, with careful monitoring of lipid levels.

Women with migraine headaches often experience an increase in the frequency or severity of headaches, particularly women with menstrual migraines. To avoid this problem, as well as the possible slight increase in risk for stroke, a progestin-only pill is a reasonable alternative.

Box 58-1 lists absolute and relative contraindications to OCP use.

Basic guidelines for pill use should be reviewed. The woman should begin the pill on the first day of her next menstrual period, which provides greater immediate effectiveness than the traditional Sunday start date. A backup method for the first cycle is generally recommended because common minor problems with side effects or forgetfulness may occur. If a woman forgets one pill, she should be advised to take her previous day's pill with her current one. If she forgets two consecutive pills, she should take two pills for 2 days and resume one pill daily for the remainder of the cycle; a barrier method should also be used. If the woman forgets three or more consecutive pills, she must be considered unprotected; the pill may not be an appropriate method for her.

A woman beginning the OCP should be evaluated after three cycles to review pill use, measure blood pressure, and assess the presence of any side effects (Box 58-2). Thereafter she should be seen annually to monitor for side effects.

Breakthrough bleeding is a common problem, occurring in approximately 15% of women beginning OCP use. If it has not resolved after the third cycle, the pill should be changed according to the timing of the bleeding. Late cycle bleeding responds to an increase in progestin, while early cycle bleeding is often a consequence of inadequate estrogen effect. Bleeding that develops after prolonged pill use may be related to inadequate estrogen, but should always be evaluated to rule out infection, neoplasia, and pregnancy (see Chapter 52).

Amenorrhea occurs after long-term pill use in 1% to 3% of women. When pregnancy has been ruled out, the woman can be reassured that it is safe to continue the OCP. If the absence of a menstrual period is bothersome to the woman, a change to a higher estrogen preparation is reasonable. Post-pill amenorrhea is said to be present if the menstrual cycle does not resume 6 months after cessation of pill use. A full evaluation (see Chapter 43) is necessary.

Nausea is thought to be related to the estrogenic component of the pill. Taking the pill with the evening meal or at bedtime may help. If not, a change to a lower estrogen formula is appropriate.

Drug interactions with the oral contraceptive pill are listed in Appendix VI. The effect of the OCP on laboratory measures is outlined in Appendix VII.

Emergency Contraception

Emergency contraception should be discussed at routine office visits since many women are unaware of this option. Several postcoital contraceptive methods have been approved by the U.S. Food and Drug Administration and are now widely available, in some states without requiring an office visit. These methods are effective when used within 72 hours of unprotected intercourse, preventing pregnancy in 94% to 99.5% of women, with earlier use within this interval associated with greater effectiveness.

Postcoital contraceptive methods using high-dose estrogens act by preventing implantation. In addition to high-dose estrogens, progestins alone, danazol, and mifepristone (RU 486, a progestin antagonist) have been used for postcoital prevention of pregnancy. Emergency contraception methods available in the United States are listed in Table 58-3. Mifepristone is not approved for postcoital use but has

---

BOX 58-1
Contraindications to Oral Contraceptive Pill Use

History of cardiovascular disease or stroke
History of thromboembolic disease
Known coagulation disorder: protein C or S deficiency, antithrombin III deficiency
Severe liver disease
Known or suspected malignancy of breast or endometrium
Undiagnosed genital bleeding
Known or suspected pregnancy

Relative Contraindications

Smoking in women over 30	Migraine headaches
Hypertension	Seizure disorder
Diabetes	Sickle cell anemia
Hypertriglyceridemia	

BOX 58-2
Side Effects of Oral Contraceptive Pill Use

Estrogen-related	Progestin-related
Nausea	Increased appetite
Breast tenderness	Depression
Fluid retention	Fatigue
Weight gain	Decreased libido
Headaches	Acne
	Headaches

Table 58-3
Postcoital Contraception

Preparation	Content Per Tablet	Dosage
Preven	100 mg ethinyl estradiol and 0.5 mg levonorgestrel	2 tablets every 12 hours for 2 doses
Ovral	100 mg ethinyl estradiol and 0.5 mg levonorgestrel	2 tablets every 12 hours for 2 doses
Plan B	0.75 mg levonorgestrel	1 tablet every 12 hours for 2 doses
Ovrette	1 tablet = 0.075 mg levonorgestrel	10 tablets every 12 hours for 2 doses
Danazol	1 capsule = 200 mg	2 capsules every 12 hours for 3 doses

been shown to be 100% effective in a dose of 600 mg administered within 72 hours of intercourse and has a fewer side effects than other regimens. Use of mifepristone for medical abortion is discussed in Chapter 59.

A careful menstrual history (and testing, when indicated) to exclude an existing pregnancy is important; however, there is no evidence that the fetus is harmed if a pregnancy is present. Nausea and vomiting are common side effects and may be minimized by concurrent administration of an antiemetic. Bleeding usually occurs within a few days after administration; a pregnancy test should be performed if bleeding has not occurred within 4 weeks.

Injectable Hormonal Contraception

Progestins can be injected intramuscularly or subdermally to provide prolonged contraception for 1 month to up to 5 years. Two long-acting injectables are intramuscular medroxyprogesterone acetate (Depo-Provera) and subdermal levonorgestrel (Norplant). Both are highly effective, with failure rates of less than 1% per year (Table 58-1). A third long-acting regimen combines medroxyprogesterone acetate and estradiol cypionate (Lunelle) in a monthly intramuscular injection.

Mechanism of Action

Injectable progestins act by inhibiting ovulation and impairing sperm transport and implantation. After one injection of 150 mg, Depo-Provera remains measurable in the circulatory system for 8 to 9 months. Estradiol levels during Depo-Provera treatment are suppressed to the level in the early follicular phase of the normal cycle. Norplant provides a blood level of levonorgestrel similar to that in a progestin-only pill or one-fourth to one-half of combination oral contraceptives.

Benefits

The principal benefits of the injectable hormonal regimens are ease of compliance and high effectiveness. Progestin-only regimens allow avoidance of estrogen-related side effects and are particularly valuable for use in women with heart disease, a history of thromboembolic disorders, diabetes, sickle cell disease, seizure disorders, or systemic lupus erythematosus (SLE) and in women over 35 who smoke.

Risks

Depo-Provera completely disrupts the menstrual cycle, causing amenorrhea in about 70% of women after 2 years and irregular bleeding in 30% of women, particularly during the first 3 months of use. Increased appetite, weight gain, acne, and depression can also occur. Another problem is that resumption of fertility may not occur for a year or longer in some cases. Prolonged use over years may result in mildly decreased bone density, a concern primarily in adolescents.

Breakthrough bleeding is a common side effect of Norplant; an average of 100 days of irregular bleeding occurs during the first year of use. Other side effects include weight gain, headaches, and occasionally androgenic effects. In several studies, discontinuation of Norplant was requested by 10% to 20% of its users because of side effects. Many women have regular menstrual cycles while taking Norplant; a missed period in such women should prompt a preg-

nancy test. Resumption of menses occurs within a month after cessation.

Lunelle is associated with less irregular bleeding than Depo-Provera and fewer side effects such as weight gain and headache. Fertility returns within 3 to 4 months of discontinuation.

Management Issues

Depo-Provera is administered by intramuscular injection of 150 mg every 3 months. The initial dose should be given during the first 5 days of menses and pregnancy should be excluded. A pregnancy test should also be performed if more than 14 weeks elapse between injections.

Lunelle is administered by intramuscular injection every 28 to 30 days after the previous injection. A pregnancy test should be performed if the patient presents for a follow-up injection after day 33.

The insertion technique for the Norplant system involves placement of six polymeric silicone rods in a fan-shaped arrangement under the skin. It is a fairly simple technique but does require special training.

BARRIER METHODS
Condoms

The male condom is the most popular contraceptive method. The recent introduction of a female condom provides women with another option for protection from pregnancy and sexually transmitted diseases. Effectiveness rates are 85% to 95%; male condoms prelubricated with spermicide have an estimated effectiveness rate of, 96%.

Mechanism of Action

Male condoms cover the penis during coitus and serve as a reservoir to prevent the deposit of semen in the vagina. Female condoms consist of a polyurethane pouch held in place by an outer and an inner ring.

Benefits

Condoms are inexpensive, available without prescription, and free of systemic side effects. Condoms made of polyurethane or latex may be effective in preventing viral transmission.

Risks

Allergic reactions to latex may occur. Use of the female condom or male condoms made of polyurethane avoids such reactions.

Intravaginal Devices

The **diaphragm** is a dome of latex rubber or polyurethane inserted in the vagina to cover the cervix. A spermicide containing nonoxynol-9 is applied at the time of insertion and before repeated intercourse. The diaphragm is sized according to the diameter of the circular rim; the three sizes in the middle range (65, 70, and 75 mm) will fit most women. The **cervical cap** is a rubber dome that fits tightly over the cervix and is also used with spermicide at the time of insertion. It is much smaller than the diaphragm, with a diameter of 22 to 35 mm. The theoretic effectiveness rates of intravaginal devices range from 91% to 94% (Table 58-1).

Mechanism of Action

All intravaginal devices provide a mechanical barrier to sperm transport, which is augmented by spermicide.

Benefits

Intravaginal devices allow avoidance of systemic side effects while achieving fairly high effectiveness rates in motivated users. Nonoxynol-9 has microbicidal properties that reduce the risk of sexually transmitted diseases, including HIV, gonorrhea, and chlamydial infection.

Compared to the diaphragm, the cervical cap has the advantage of providing effective contraception while being left in place for 1 to 2 days without insertion of additional spermicide.

Risks

The diaphragm can increase the risk of urinary tract infections because of urethral compression; this problem can sometimes be avoided by use of the wide-seal diaphragm. Odor, discharge, and partner discomfort are occasional problems.

Spermicides

Most vaginal spermicides contain nonoxynol-9, a detergent that immobilizes sperm. It is available as cream, jelly, aerosol foam, a foaming tablet, and film that dissolves into a gel. Because spermicides alone result in failure rates of over 20%, they are not generally recommended as the sole contraceptive method.

THE INTRAUTERINE DEVICE

The intrauterine device (IUD) represents a highly effective means of birth control for a select group of women. In the United States two kinds are available: the Copper T380 (Paragard) and the progestin-releasing IUDs, which release progesterone (Progestasert) and levonorgestrel (Mirena). The Copper T380 is effective for 10 years; Progestasert is replaced annually, and the levonorgestrel IUD, every 5 years.

Mechanism of Action

The IUD prevents fertilization and implantation by several mechanisms, all of which are promptly reversible on removal of the device.

Benefits

The IUD has high effectiveness rates and long-term ease of use, without unwanted metabolic effects. The progestin-releasing IUDs have the additional benefit of reducing menorrhagia and dysmenorrhea.

Risks

The chief complication of IUD use is pelvic infection, which may lead to tubal infertility. The risk appears to limited to the first few months after insertion and is low in women without other risk factors for pelvic infection. Women at high risk for developing pelvic inflammatory disease (PID), including those with a prior history of PID or sexually transmitted disease, multiple sexual partners, and nulliparous women under age 25, should be discouraged from using the IUD. The IUD is most appropriate for parous women in a stable and mutually monogamous relationship.

A high incidence of ectopic pregnancy has been observed among women who conceive while using an IUD, particularly the progestin-containing IUD. Other problems, primarily with the copper IUD, include an increase in dysmenorrhea and menstrual bleeding.

Management Issues

Dysmenorrhea and increased menstrual flow may improve with short-term intermittent use of a nonsteroidal anti-inflammatory drug such as ibuprofen. If these problems persist or worsen, an alternative method should be used.

Actinomyces-positive Pap smears are occasionally found in women with IUDs. If the woman is asymptomatic, no treatment is required.

Women using an IUD should be instructed to immediately report any lower abdominal pain, unusual vaginal bleeding, dyspareunia, or vaginal discharge.

NATURAL METHODS

A variety of methods to prevent unwanted pregnancy are in common use, all of which have high failure rates. The **rhythm method** (periodic abstinence) involves avoidance of coitus during the woman's fertile period; the fertile period is estimated from the calendar, basal body temperature, or cervical mucus. Factors that limit this method's effectiveness are individual variations in cycle length, length of survival of sperm, and compliance. **Prolonged breastfeeding** is also unreliable because the resumption of ovulation may occur before the first menstrual period. **Withdrawal** of the penis before ejaculation fails because conception can occur from preejaculatory release of seminal fluid.

STERILIZATION

Sterilization permanently blocks or removes the male or female genital tracts so that fertilization will not occur. From a couple's standpoint, the safest and most effective method of permanently preventing pregnancy is male sterilization (vasectomy).

Permanency should be the main consideration for any individual who contemplates a surgical method of contraception. Reversal of sterilization requires major surgery and is successful in only two thirds of women and half of men.

Vasectomy is an ambulatory surgical procedure to occlude a portion of the vas deferens. It requires local anesthesia and usually takes 15 minutes. Semen analysis is required 3 months later to confirm success. Complications include hematomas and sperm leakage leading to granulomas. Initial concerns about increased rates of testicular or prostate cancer have not been substantiated in subsequent studies.

Tubal sterilization in the female can be performed by two routes: the vaginal approach through colpotomy or culdoscopy, and the abdominal approach through laparoscopy or minilaparotomy. Laparoscopy is the most commonly used method in the United States. It is usually performed under general endotracheal anesthesia as an ambulatory surgical procedure. The operative risk in a healthy woman is approximately 1 in 10,000. The failure rate is 2% to 5% of procedures over 10 years.

BIBLIOGRAPHY

Baird DT, Glasier AF: Hormonal contraception, *N Engl J Med* 328:1543, 1993.

Chasan-Taber L, Stampfer MJ: Epidemiology of oral contraceptives and cardiovascular disease, *Ann Intern Med* 128:467, 1998.

Collaborative Group on Hormonal Factors in Breast Cancer: Breast cancer and hormonal contraceptives: collaborative re-analysis of individual data on 53,297 women with breast cancer and 100,239 women without breast cancer from 54 epidemiological studies, *Lancet* 347:1713, 1996.

Douketis JD et al: A reevaluation of the risk for venous thromboembolism with the use of oral contraceptives and hormone replacement therapy, *Arch Intern Med* 158:1522, 1997.

Gillum LA, Mamidipudi SK, Johnston SC: Ischemic stroke risk with oral contraceptives: a meta-analysis, *JAMA* 284:72, 2000.

Jick H et al: Risk of idiopathic cardiovascular death and non-fatal venous thromboembolism in women using oral contraceptives with differing progestagen components, *Lancet* 346:1589, 1995.

Kjos SL et al: Contraceptive and the risk of type 2 diabetes mellitus in Latina women with prior gestational diabetes mellitus, *JAMA* 28:533, 1998.

LeBlanc ES, Laws A: Benefits and risks of third-generation oral contraceptives, *J Gen Intern Med* 14:625, 1999.

Peterson HB et al: The risk of menstrual abnormalities after tubal sterilization, *N Engl J Med* 343:1681, 2000.

Peterson HB et al: The risk of pregnancy after tubal sterilization: findings from the U.S. Collaborative Review of Sterilization, *Am J Obstet Gynecol* 174:1161, 1996.

Pettiti DB et al: Stroke in users of low-dose oral contraceptives, *N Engl J Med* 335:8, 1996.

Rosing J et al: Low-dose oral contraceptives and acquired resistance to activitated protein C: a randomized cross-over study, *Lancet* 354:2036, 1999.

Schiff I et al: Oral contraceptives and smoking, current considerations: recommendations of a consensus panel, *Am J Obstet Gynecol* 180:S383, 1999.

Sidney S et al: Myocardial infarction and use of low-dose oral contraceptives: a pooled analysis of 2 US studies, *Circulation* 98:1058, 1998.

Trussel J et al: A guide to interpreting contraceptive efficacy studies, *Obstet Gynecol* 76:558, 1990.

WHO Collaborative Study of Cardiovascular Disease and Steroid Hormone Contraception: Acute myocardial infarction and combined oral contraceptives: results of an international multicentre case-control study, *Lancet* 349:1202, 1997.

CHAPTER 59

Abortion

Martha Ellen Katz
Rapin Osathanondh

More than 1 million therapeutic abortions have been reported annually in the United States for two decades. Each year, nearly half of the 6.3 million pregnancies in the United States were reported as "unintended" and half of those were terminated (a rate of one abortion in four pregnancies). In addition, office procedures to remove products of conception around the time of the menses (menstrual extraction) are performed but are not reported.

This chapter outlines the care of women who undergo one of the most common types of procedures, first-trimester abortion by dilation and suction evacuation. The chapter also describes pharmacotherapeutic agents that soften the cervix and expel the products of conception, which are used as adjuncts and alternatives to surgical abortion. Pregnancy loss (spontaneous abortion), also called miscarriage, is reviewed in Chapter 66.

Although this chapter focuses on the clinical aspects of induced abortion, ongoing political controversies constrain the ability to obtain this service. Legislation curtailing abortion rights, restrictions by public and private insurers for induced abortion, harassment and violence against providers and patients at abortion facilities, as well as the dearth of abortion providers, limit access to abortion services. In the United States 86% of counties have no known abortion provider. In 36 states, laws, regulations, or constitutional amendments limit public financial coverage for elective induced abortion, providing coverage for the procedure for health reasons only. Many of these states include coverage for cases of rape and incest; some states only include cases of life endangerment.

TYPES OF ABORTION PROCEDURES

Abortion procedures differ by the trimester in which the procedure is performed. The gestational age is based on the onset of the last menstrual period (LMP) and thus 2 weeks earlier than the actual time of fertilization and age of the embryo. First-trimester abortions represent approximately 95% of the total and are performed from weeks 5 or 6 to week 13; second-trimester procedures, fewer than 5% of the total, are performed between weeks 13 through 24. Approximately 1% of therapeutic abortions are performed after week 20, and rarely after week 24, usually for severe fetal anomalies or lethal maternal diseases.

There are two major types of therapeutic abortions: suction evacuation and labor induction. Minor methods involve the use of pharmacotherapeutic agents and ultrasound-assisted procedures.

Ninety-nine percent of surgical abortions, all first-trimester and most second-trimester, employ the suction evacuation technique. From week 6 or 7 of gestation through week 22, dilation is necessary to open the internal cervical os before suction. Consequently, this procedure is called *dilation and evacuation (D&E)*. Between weeks 5 and 7, suction evacuation may be accomplished without cervical dilation; some call this *menstrual extraction, menstrual regulation, vacuum aspiration, miniabortion or minisuction*. Only 1% of all abortion procedures and 7% of second-trimester pregnancy terminations are performed by inducing labor. Although some use the term D&C (dilation and curettage) and D&E interchangeably, D&C specifically refers to dilating and removing the uterine contents without the use of vacuum aspiration. D&E was the procedure used for elective pregnancy terminations until the advent of vacuum suction and continues to be used for gynecologic diagnosis and treatment.

EPIDEMIOLOGY

Although it might be inferred that some women use abortion in place of contraception, the relationship between contraception and abortion is a dynamic one. When populations are learning to control their fertility, such as in the United States between 1880 and 1900—and now among the young or unmarried—the use of contraception and the use of abortion rise concomitantly. With the subsequent falling birth rate, however, abortion levels tend to peak. Thereafter, when contraceptives are available and abortion laws are liberalized, the rate of contraceptive use continues to rise and abortion rates fall. Easy access to both contraception and abortion lowers the abortion rate but, because of unavoidable contraceptive failures, the need for abortion never is eliminated.

An accurate report of the illegal abortion rate is almost impossible to obtain. Most societies have a range of drugs, herbs, and procedures used by women on themselves and by unlicensed persons to end an unwanted pregnancy or to bring on a delayed menses. With the repeal of restrictive abortion laws in the United States and Europe the 1970s, it has been postulated in New York, England, and Wales that the total number of abortions did not change greatly. Rather, previously illegal operations were transferred into the legal sector.

Induced abortion today is a safe procedure. The number of maternal deaths declined more than 20-fold since abortion was legalized. Abortion is safe when compared with pregnancy. In 1996, only 8 deaths occurred (1/167,000 legal abortions) whereas maternal mortality was approximately 10/167,000, and the rate of death from ectopic pregnancy was 1/2000 cases. The mortality risk of childbearing approaches the risk of an abortion at 20 weeks' gestation.

SPECIFIC PROCEDURES
Suction Evacuation
Dilation and Evacuation

In D&E, tapered metal rods of increasing diameter are inserted through and just beyond the internal cervical os to dilate it. Some practitioners open the cervical canal with osmotic dilators (see next section) for 2 to 4 hours before first trimester procedures and most practitioners use osmotic dilators overnight for early second trimester procedures. After the dilation, a transparent plastic suction cannula large enough for the size of the gestation is inserted into the uterine cavity. It is then attached to an electric or hydrostatic pump that produces adequate vacuum pressure for aspirating the pregnancy tissue into a container such as a gauze bag or a syringe. This vacuum aspiration causes the uterus to contract when it is empty, which feels like strong menstrual cramps. The surgeon then grossly inspects the aspirated products of conception (POC) to ensure completion of the procedure and help determine the age of the pregnancy. Microscopic examination of the specimen may be useful clinically and is required in many states. The POC consist of chorionic villi, gestational sac and yolk, and decidua (hypertrophic gestational endometrium). The fetus of nine weeks' gestation is less than 1 cm and amorphic, that of 10 weeks' gestation approximately 1.5 cm and has recognizable parts. An incomplete procedure removed only the decidua and/or a fragment of the total chorionic villi.

Surgical abortion during the first trimester is a 5- to 15-minute procedure and can be performed in one visit. The woman recuperates for about 1 hour and may then be discharged home to rest. At home she may participate in activities depending on medications used for anesthesia and analgesia. Women usually return to their routines within 1 to 2 days.

Menstrual Extraction

Menstrual extraction terminates pregnancy at or before the time of the expected menses up to 7 weeks from the patient's LMP. Usually an office procedure, menstrual extraction may be performed without cervical dilation or electric or hydrostatic pump. A soft and flexible 3- or 4-mm diameter plastic suction cannula may be inserted into a gravid uterus without stretching the cervical canal; a self-locking or bulb syringe provides adequate suction. When these procedures fail, it is often because it is difficult to visualize the

complete POC. The failure rate may be reduced if an ultrasound is done after the procedure.

Many authorities recommend a pregnancy test on the day of the procedure and at the postoperative visit several weeks afterward to evaluate for an extrauterine gestation or unrecognized continuation of an intrauterine pregnancy.

Labor Induction

Labor induction may be preferred for pregnancy termination beyond 18 weeks of gestation when fetal biparietal diameter measure 50 to 55 mm, although experienced operators may terminate pregnancies safely by D&E until the maximum legal gestational age. On the day after the gradual dilation of the cervix by inserting osmotic dilators such as laminaria tents (see next section), uterine contractions are induced by a variety of oral, intravaginal, intraamniotic, or intravenous pharmacotherapeutic protocols. One method instills carboprost tromethamine, a synthetic prostaglandin, into the amniotic fluid, followed immediately by saline. The intraamniotic injection, similar to diagnostic amniocentesis, produces fewer side effects than the extraamniotic route. Another method uses misoprostol, a methyl analog of prostaglandin E_1, orally after the overnight laminaria. Myometrial contractions begin within an hour. If the cervical effacement reaches 90% and the last dose of prostaglandin was administered at least 2 hours previously, a high-dose intravenous oxytocin infusion is started. Induction to delivery time averages 8 hours, but the patient is allowed to labor until her cervix and lower uterine segment are favorable for instrumental extraction of the fetus. After delivery of the placenta, uterine exploration and sharp curettage are routinely performed to remove the remaining decidual tissue. Most patients undergoing prostaglandin-induced abortion are discharged the same day.

Agents for Softening the Cervix

Osmotic, gas-sterilized, mechanical cervical dilators (Fig. 59-1) gently swell and stretch the cervix open to dilate it before the abortion procedure. They are inserted in the cervical canal 2 to 4 hours before first-trimester D&E and overnight for second-trimester procedures. As they slowly open the cervix, they may produce moderate, crampy pain. At the time of the procedure, the enlarged and softened dilators are removed. This pretreatment decreases the incidence of cer-

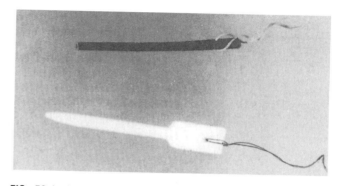

FIG. 59-1 Laminaria tent *(dark)* shown in comparison to synthetic dilator (Lamicel) *(white)*. (From Ryan KJ, Berkowitz R, Barbieri R, Dunaif, A, editors: *Kistner's gynecology and women's health,* ed 7, St Louis, 1999, Mosby.)

vical laceration, cervicovaginal fistula, uterine perforation, and excessive hemorrhage if cervical dilation is accomplished by inserting metal dilators at the time of D&E procedures. In addition to their mechanical action, the use of laminaria is associated with increasing blood levels of prostaglandin metabolites and thus may shorten the induction-to-delivery time in prostaglandin labor-induction procedures. The primary risk of dilation by laminaria is infection caused by leaving them in place more than 48 hours.

Several varieties of osmotic dilators are available. Laminaria tents are 6-cm dried stems of seaweed in diameter sizes of 2 to 6 mm. They swell to three or four times their original width. Several brands of synthetic dilators are also available. In addition to osmotic devices, intracervical or vaginal prostaglandin E$_2$ and other prostaglandin derivatives have been used successfully to soften the closed cervix.

Pharmacotherapeutic Methods

Various agents are available that disrupt chorionic villi or promote cervical softening and uterine contractions. These agents are used in conjunction with oral or vaginal prostaglandins or surgical methods to terminate pregnancy. *Mifepristone,* also known as *RU486,* is the only pharmacotherapeutic agent currently approved by the U.S. Food and Drug Administration (FDA) to terminate a normal pregnancy, although drugs approved for other indications have been used for this purpose.

Agents That Disrupt Chorionic Villi

Three different types of agents disrupt chorionic villi: progesterone receptor blockers, of which mifepristone is the prototype; inhibitors of progesterone biosynthesis, such as aminoglutethimide, epostane, and trilostane; and inhibitors of folate reductase, such as the antimetabolite methotrexate. Mifepristone represents the greatest advance as well as perpetual controversy.

Mifepristone. Mifepristone, an antiprogesterone derivative of norethindrone (a 19-nor steroid), was synthesized by the Roussel Uclaf pharmaceutical company in 1981. It has been approved for use in China, England, France, and Scandinavian countries as an abortifacient in the first 7 weeks of pregnancy and in the induction of labor after fetal death. It also has been used in the treatment of Cushing's syndrome. Under the aegis of the Population Council, a private agency with the patent rights to the drug in the United States, mifepristone underwent satisfactory clinical trials as an oral abortifacient in conjunction with misoprostol, a prostaglandin analog, for pregnancy termination up to 7 weeks' gestation.

MECHANISM OF ACTION. Mifepristone disrupts pregnancy primarily, but not exclusively, by blocking the effects of progesterone. It displaces progesterone from its receptors on the secretory endometrium, causing the chorionic villi to detach and, consequently, blood levels of progesterone and human chorionic gonadotropin to fall. Mifepristone stimulates endogenous prostaglandins and sensitizes uterine myometrium to them, inducing a fivefold increase in myometrial sensitivity to exogenous prostaglandins between 30 and 60 hours after oral administration. The cervix softens and opens, and

24 to 36 hours after a 600-mg dose, uterine contractions begin.

EFFICACY AND SAFETY. In earlier trials, after a single oral 600-mg dose of mifepristone, 80% of patients completely expelled the gestational products. The remaining cases required further treatment for retained POC. Now, more successful protocols add a single dose of the oral prostaglandin, misoprostol, 2 days after the mifepristone, which acts synergistically to induce uterine cramping and bleeding and potentiates the expulsion of pregnancy products. Women are asked to collect expelled tissue at home. The recovery rate of POC varies among different clinical trials. Overall, the success rate with the two-drug regimen approaches 96%, with greater success at earlier gestational ages. Up to 5% of patients require uterine evacuation, and fewer than 1% may lose enough blood to require transfusion. The adjunctive drug misoprostol may cause nausea, vomiting, or diarrhea, and may cause birth defects (cranial and limb reduction) if the medical protocol were unsuccessful and the pregnancy were to continue. The effect of mifepristone on the developing fetus is unknown. No cases of fetal abnormalities have yet been documented among the few cases of continuing pregnancy, although significant concentrations of the drug have been shown to cross the placenta. Because progesterone opposes the effects of endogenous estrogens, it is possible, but not known whether repeated blockade of progesterone receptors would eventually lead to any estrogen-related or other disorders. Clinically mifepristone is being evaluated for treatment of endometriosis, uterine leiomyoma, meningioma, and certain cancers.

Medical abortion with mifepristone followed by misoprostol is most suited to women in locals where surgical abortion is unavailable and for women who prefer the privacy of a medical visit or who are reluctant to undergo surgical procedures. Acceptability studies have shown variations with different regions and cultures. Concurrent with a controversy about the availability, restrictions, and marketing of mifepristone, enthusiasm for the drug is tempered by several concerns. The method may not allow for routine examination of POC, bleeding may be prolonged, and the cost may be high for multiple visits, medications, and sonography (see Internet site: www.earlyoptionpill.com).

Inhibitors of Progesterone Biosynthesis

Aminoglutethimide, epostane, and trilostane inhibit progesterone biosynthesis by blocking steroidogenic enzymes. High doses (epostane 800 mg/day for a week, for instance) are usually required for pregnancy termination up to 7 weeks of gestation. Inhibitors of progesterone biosynthesis are only moderately effective abortifacients and do not appear as promising as the progesterone receptor blockers. Furthermore, these drugs may also have unacceptable secondary effects: in addition to adrenocortical suppression, they may depress the central nervous system and activate hepatic microsomal enzymes.

Inhibitors of Folate Reductase

Methotrexate. Inhibitors of folate reductase, such as the antimetabolite methotrexate, have been used in a single oral dose to terminate a normal intrauterine pregnancy, although to date they appear more valuable in the pharmacotherapy of small ectopic pregnancies, destroying abnormal or ectopic trophoblastic cells. Methotrexate, however, as an adjunct in terminating early intrauterine pregnancies appears to potentiate the uterotonic effect of misoprostol. Induced first-trimester abortion by methotrexate may be followed by oral or vaginal administration of misoprostol 5 to 7 days afterwards to expel the POC. This method has been found to be approximately 80% to 90% effective. Practical limitations of the methotrexate/misoprostol regimen are the long "window period" between methotrexate and misoprostol administration as well as prolonged vaginal bleeding. Furthermore, the use of methotrexate as an abortifacient is controversial because of the potential long-term risk. Its effects on hepatic and bone marrow stem cells is unknown, although if hepatic enzymes do rise, they usually return to normal after the drug is withdrawn. A fatal, idiosyncratic reaction may occur in certain patients when methotrexate is administered with nonsteroidal anti-inflammatory drugs.

Uterotonic Agents. Prostaglandins, oxytocin, and intraamniotic hypertonic solutions cause contraction of the gravid uterus. They are used singly or in combination for inducing labor and delivery in therapeutic abortions. Prostaglandins and oxytocin are naturally occurring compounds that have been synthesized for use in pharmacologic doses.

Prostaglandins. Prostaglandins that induce contractions of the gravid uterus include the prostaglandin E_1 methyl analog, misoprostol; prostaglandin E_2, dinoprostone, and its synthetic derivatives such as meteneprost potassium and 15-methyl-prostaglandin F_2a, carboprost tromethamine. Side effects vary among the different compounds, but each carries risks. Cardiovascular complications of certain prostaglandins can be life threatening.

Misoprostol, approved in the United States for the treatment of peptic ulcer disease, causes contractions of the gravid uterus at doses of 200 mg or higher by the oral or intravaginal route. It has been widely used for illegal pregnancy termination in Africa and in South America because it is less expensive than other prostaglandins. Tolerable gastrointestinal side effects may occur, but if administered in unmonitored circumstances, hemorrhage and infection may follow. Furthermore, if the abortion were incomplete the uninterrupted pregnancy may result in congenital malformations of the brain and cranium, skin, and bones including limb reduction defects.

Recent reports in the United States of a combination of oral methotrexate and intravaginal misoprostol to terminate pregnancies at less than 10 weeks' gestation resulted in complete abortion in 90% of cases. Further studies of safety and efficacy will determine its ultimate value and use.

Dinoprostone, a vaginal suppository in wax or gel form, has been approved by the FDA for labor induction for a fetal demise up to 28 weeks' gestation. The recommended dosage of 5 to 20 mg is readily absorbed through the vaginal mucosa into the systemic circulation and stimulates the smooth muscle of the gravid uterus and, in some cases, those in the intestine and milk ducts. However, because it also may stimulate the smooth muscle of the gastrointestinal tract as well as disturb the body's thermoregulatory center, it may cause nausea, vomiting, diarrhea, and fever. Unlike carboprost

tromethamine, dinoprostone dilates bronchial and vascular smooth muscle when large doses are used. Thus for patients with active asthma or compromised cardiopulmonary status, dinoprostone is preferred.

Carboprost tromethamine, approved by the FDA for treatment of postpartum hemorrhage by intramuscular injection, is used for intraamniotic abortion in combination with hypertonic saline. The injection-to-abortion time for second-trimester pregnancies averages 8 hours if used after laminaria preparation of the cervix. When 1.5 mg of carboprost tromethamine and 64 to 100 ml of 23% saline are administered via the intraamniotic route, there are minimal or no systemic effects when compared with the use of dinoprostone vaginal suppositories. Untoward effects, some caused by accidental leakage of a large amount of carboprost tromethamine into the systemic circulation, may include cardiac arrhythmias, bronchoconstriction, pulmonary hypertension, increased intrapulmonary shunting, and arterial oxygen desaturation.

Oxytocin. Endogenous oxytocin, a neurohypophysial octapeptide hormone, is released by suckling and, it is believed from animal data, by cervical dilation. It has been synthesized for the induction of labor near term. Oxytocin and prostaglandins work synergistically: the uterine muscle becomes more sensitive to prostaglandins with advancing gestational weeks, and prostaglandins themselves may induce an increase in the number of oxytocin receptors. However, clinically, when these two drugs are administered concomitantly to induce labor, the combination may be too potent. Uterine rupture has been reported.

Hypertonic Solutions. When hypertonic solutions such as 23.4% saline, 30% or 40% hyperosmolar urea, or antiseptic acridine orange are injected into the amniotic sac, they induce a cascade of events leading to prostaglandin release in local tissues. Effective uterine contractions occur within several hours. However, if too large or too concentrated a volume of saline solution is accidentally injected into the uterine circulation, complications such as life-threatening disseminated intravascular coagulation, intravascular hemolysis, or hypernatremia may occur.

ANESTHESIA AND ANALGESIA

Parenteral and local drugs given before surgical abortion allow the woman to be comfortable and minimize movement inasmuch as changing position increases the risk of trauma and uterine perforation by sharp instruments. Local (paracervical) anesthesia with or without intravenous (IV) conscious sedation is preferable to general anesthesia because blood loss and uterine perforation are reduced. Recently, most complications from legal abortion in the United States are drug-related. Toxic reactions and overdose occur with efforts to medicate the patient with vasopressors to reduce uterine bleeding and with barbiturates to relieve anxiety. A specially trained nurse, counselor, family member, or friend who accompanies the woman before and during the procedure can help relax the patient with emotional support, relaxation, focused breathing, and verbal distraction.

Women generally are instructed to take nothing by mouth for 6 hours before the procedure to prevent aspiration of gastric contents in the event that a complication should require general anesthesia. Although no special indications support the use of general anesthesia for the procedure, some women may request it despite the small increased risk.

Paracervical Local Anesthesia

Most D&Es up to 12 weeks can be performed with paracervical local anesthesia only. Chloroprocaine, an ester anesthetic, or lidocaine, an amide anesthetic, may be used. Chloroprocaine is more expensive but has a wider safety margin and longer duration of action than does lidocaine. Acute drug reactions occur if a toxic dose is erroneously administered, if the anesthetic is too rapidly absorbed into the highly vascular gravid tissue, or if the operator inadvertently injects the anesthetic into the maternal circulation. The nervous system may become excited or depressed; similarly the cardiorespiratory system may react with myocardial depression, arrhythmias, hypotension, or even cardiac or respiratory arrest.

Intravenous Sedation

IV sedation with short-acting benzodiazepines and opioids reduces anxiety, produces retrograde amnesia, and blunts discomfort. At our institution we use midazolam, not exceeding 2 mg, plus fentanyl, not exceeding 100 μg. Midazolam may prevent a rare syndrome of chest wall stiffness caused by intravenous (IV) injection of an opioid such as fentanyl. Excessive fentanyl or opioids may lead to dose-related respiratory depression. Excitement, dizziness, tachycardia, and hypotension, as well as nausea and vomiting, have also been known to occur as a result of these agents. Some of these reactions may be potentiated by the increase in vagal tone that can accompany manipulation of the cervix. Occasionally 25 mg of diphenhydramine may be required for its mild anticholinergic effects. Pulse oximetry during and after the procedure allows monitoring for potential complications of intravenous sedation. Antidotes to sedatives should be readily available: flumazenil for midazolam and naloxone for opioids.

PROPHYLAXIS
Antimicrobial

A therapeutic abortion is a clean procedure; only the portion of instruments entering the uterine cavity are kept sterile. Opening the cervical os exposes the endometrium to vaginal flora and subsequent range of infection from mild febrile morbidity to sepsis. Infections are polymicrobial: pathogens responsible for postoperative endomyometritis include aerobic and anaerobic gram-negative bacilli, aerobic streptococci, anaerobic gram-positive cocci, and mycoplasmas. Controversy surrounds the value of screening for genital infection before the procedure or treating all or at-risk patients with prophylactic antibiotics before, or afterward, or both because most clinical trials are uncontrolled or lack inadequate statistical power. Those who recommend screening point out that it is more cost-effective than universal prophylaxis. Without treatment, as many as 63% of women whose preoperative screening for chlamydia were positive later become infected. Advocates of perioperative prophylactic treatment reason that compliance is best with IV doses. Those who recommend routinely treating patients intraoper-

atively or postoperatively note that in high-prevalence populations (>10%), treatment is cost-effective. Despite concerns about the overuse of broad-spectrum antibiotics in the absence of a specific infecting organism, a survey of members of the National Abortion Federation showed that over 90% used prophylactic antibiotics routinely for first-trimester procedures.

Although universal prophylactic antibiotic use is controversial, most agree that antimicrobial prophylaxis is appropriate for women at high risk. According to the literature review, a large at-risk population includes those with fetal death, placenta previa, tattoo, Asherman's syndrome, an intrauterine device, an orthopedic or a cardiac prosthesis, or cervical cytologic findings of trichomonads or koilocytosis. We also treat women with a history of multiple abortions, pelvic inflammatory disease, sexually transmitted disease, tubal pregnancy, intravenous drug use, or multiple male partners, as well as adolescents, diabetics with vascular complications, women who are human immunodeficiency virus (HIV) positive, women with sickle cell trait or disease or chronic hepatitis, and women in correctional institutions. In addition, we also prescribe antibiotics after excessive blood loss during the procedure if myometrial injury is suspected, or if a procedure takes longer than 20 minutes (Box 59-1).

Preoperative prophylaxis against bacterial endocarditis is recommended not only for patients with valvular heart disease or septal defects but also for IV drug users.

RH Sensitization

To prevent Rh isoimmunization, anti–D immune globulin such as RhoGAM or MICRhoGAM should be administered within 72 hours to all Rh-negative, Du-negative women who are undergoing induced abortion. Approximately 4% of these women would otherwise become sensitized after therapeutic abortion beyond 7 weeks' gestation. The incidence of RH isoimmunization increases with advancing gestational age. The standard dose for first-trimester abortions is

---

BOX 59-1

Suggested Antibiotic Prophylaxis Regiments for Therapeutic Surgical Abortions

Doxycycline 100 mg bid × 7 days.

Doxycycline 100 mg bid + metronidazole* 500 mg bid × 5 days

Ampicillin 2 g + gentamicin 100 mg + clindamycin 900 mg or metronidazole 500 mg*†

Doxycycline 100 mg 1 hour before the procedure and 200 mg one-half hour afterward‡

Metronidazole 400 mg 1 hour before and 4 and 8 hours afterward§

Aqueous penicillin G 2 million units IV, or doxycycline 100 mg PO one hour before the procedure, and 200 mg one-half hour afterward; second trimester, cefazolin 1 g IV¶

---

*Use metronidazole if a malodorous vaginal discharge suggests nonspecific vaginosis or if trichamonads are present.

† Centers for Disease Control: Morbidity and Mortality Weekly Reports, vol 42, 1993.

‡ Levallois P, Rioux JE: *Am J Obstet Gynecol* 158:100, 1988.

§ Heisterberg L, Petersen K: *Obstet Gynecol* 65:371, 1985.

¶ *Met Lett Drugs Ther* 41:1060, 1999.

50-mg anti–D immune globulin and 300 mg for procedures after week 13.

During medical abortion with mifepristone and prostaglandin or during menstrual extraction abortion, fetomaternal hemorrhage occurs, although less frequently than with dilated surgical procedures. It is safe and inexpensive to administer anti-D immune globulin to all women with Rh or Du negativity at or before the time of menstrual extraction or at the time of the oral prostaglandin dose after mifepristone.

COMPLICATIONS
Abortion Facilities

Almost all D&E procedures may be safely accomplished at an outpatient facility. Mortality has been found to be equivalent in hospital and licensed outpatient settings. Patients with medical or technical risks should be referred to a hospital center with ancillary and emergency services and a surgeon with particular expertise. Candidates for specialty referral include women with uterine anomalies or leiomyoma restricting easy access to the uterus, severe cardiac or pulmonary disease, coagulopathies, or mental diseases that prevent cooperation. Previous cesarean section or other pelvic surgery may not be a contraindication to outpatient first-trimester abortion. Intraoperative ultrasound guidance has been advocated by several authors to minimize complications, particularly in cases of anatomic abnormalities.

Second-trimester pregnancies also may be safely terminated in an outpatient setting by a specifically trained physician with preoperative dilation with osmotic dilators and blood products available on site. Although the potential for major complications is small, licensed outpatient facilities are required to have pulse oximetry, resuscitative and ultrasound equipment, and appropriate drugs available, as well as a way to expeditiously transport patients to a hospital if needed.

Risk

The most important determinants of mortality and morbidity as a result of abortion are the gestational age of the conceptus and the operator's experience. It has been shown repeatedly that the safest induced abortions are performed between 7 and 12 weeks' gestation; morbidity and mortality rates of these procedures are approximately one-tenth those of later abortions. Increased risk of uterine trauma and hemorrhage occur in procedures performed by inexperienced physicians. The type of operation and method of cervical dilation, age of the patient, type of anesthesia, obstetric history, and body habitus also contribute to complications (Box 59-2).

Common and Rare Complications

Complications occur in 0.11% of all abortions. The most common complications are retained tissue and mild infection (Table 59-1). Inaccurate assessment of uterine size and prolonged procedures by inexperienced operators often contribute to these complications.

Catastrophic and rare complications that occur in the perioperative period include laceration of uterine vessels, with subsequent expanding hematoma and hypovolemia, and uterine perforation and bowel injury leading to generalized peritonitis. These complications may be fatal and require prompt surgical exploration and treatment.

Other rare complications primarily associated with second-trimester D&E and labor-induction procedures include hematometra, also called postabortal, or redo, syndrome, which is characterized by dark, clotted blood in the uterus. Also, often in the setting of fetal demise, an unusual respiratory embarrassment associated with forceful uterine contractions may occur, causing transient coughing and bronchospasm. Amniotic fluid embolism may occur after the disruption of the placental bed with surgical instruments and resultant leakage of a large volume of amniotic fluid into the uterine circulation usually is associated with cardiopulmonary collapse and disseminated intravascular coagulopathy. Finally, Asherman's syndrome, a rare condition characterized by destruction and scarification of the endometrium with adhesions and synechiae, may be related to a genetic propensity coupled with an as yet unrecognized endometrial infection or hematometra.

Table 59-1 Complications of First-Trimester Abortion	
Complication	**Ratio**
Serious	
Incomplete	1:3,617
Sepsis	1:4,722
Uterine perforation	1:10,625
Vaginal bleeding	1:14,166
Inability to complete	1:28,333
Ectopic pregnancy	1:42,500
TOTAL	1:1,405
Minor	
Mild infection	1:216
Repeat procedure, same day	1:553
Repeat procedure, subsequently	1:596
Cervical stenosis	1:6,071
Cervical tear	1:9,444
Underestimation of gestational age	1:15,454
Seizure	1:25,086
TOTAL	1:118

Modified from Hakim-Elahi E, Tovell HM, Burnhill MS: *Obstet Gynecol* 76:929, 1990.

BOX 59-2

Factors that Decrease Risk of Uterine Perforation in Dilation and Evacuation Abortion

7 to 12 weeks' gestation
Use of laminaria
Patient older than 17 years of age (all gestational ages)
Use of local anesthesia
History of a prior abortion
Nulliparous patient
Patient not obese
Performed by attending physician
No cesarean scars

APPROACH TO THE WOMAN CONSIDERING AN ABORTION

When a woman presents requesting a pregnancy termination, the goal of the visit is to confirm the diagnosis of intrauterine pregnancy, estimate the age of the conceptus, support the decision for abortion, review and select the appropriate type of termination, and schedule the abortion. When a woman seeks care for a suspected pregnancy, confirmation of the pregnancy and decision making about the potential outcome may proceed simultaneously. After the abortion, medical follow-up and evaluation include assessment that the procedure was complete, bleeding has not been excessive, infection has not occurred, and that the woman is emotionally secure and has selected a reliable form of contraception.

Counseling

Pregnancy option counseling plays a critical role in the development of quality abortion services. Factors that may be explored in the decision to terminate or to continue a pregnancy include number of children, nature of the relationship with the father, and, in the case of adolescents, nature of the relationship with parents, emotional or financial ability to care for a child, medical risks, toxin or environmental exposures, and career or educational plans. During pregnancy option counseling, it is particularly important for the practitioner to refrain from inadvertently or subtly conveying his or her own values because this impedes a woman's decision-making process. Medical risks associated with carrying a pregnancy to term and with abortion are reviewed. Family or professional support is assessed. Screening for psychiatric illness, substance use, and abusive relationships will help determine if additional support is needed. Carrying the pregnancy to term or adoption is presented as options.

Once the decision to terminate a pregnancy is made, guidance about the anticipated medical and emotional experience prepares the woman for the procedure. Sometimes an unplanned pregnancy precipitates a life crisis with relationships or career plans. If the woman feels ambivalent, her anxieties may be relieved if the provider describes the decision as complex but not wrong and offers empathic, nonjudgmental listening. Preabortion counseling differentiates ambivalence from confusion. Although some ambivalence is common, confusion requires further counseling or education to resolve.

A woman also may choose to terminate a second-trimester pregnancy for fetal structural defects or for chromosomal or metabolic abnormalities detected by amniocentesis. These pregnancies are likely to be at 15 weeks' gestation or more and are usually under the care of an obstetrician.

History and Physical Examination

A directed history and a physical examination confirm the diagnosis of intrauterine pregnancy and estimates the gestational age. Findings also determine reproductive problems, elicit underlying disease, and uncover conditions that create risks for the abortion procedure or analgesia (Box 59-3). Estimation of gestational age may be made by a combination of the date of the LMP, the timing of intercourse, symptoms of pregnancy, and results of the abdominal and pelvic examination. The history and physical findings may be corroborated with ultrasound examination and, if necessary, quantitative serum human chorionic gonadotropin (hCG) levels. Error in the bimanual examination increases with parity, obesity, fibroids, and prior pelvic surgery.

Error in establishing the LMP is highest in women who become pregnant postpartum or while using or after discontinuing oral contraceptives, because the intervals for ovulation are variable. Other causes for error in the LMP occur when vaginal bleeding or spotting follows implantation of the blastocyst, which may be misinterpreted as a menstrual period, especially when menses are irregular. Furthermore, according to World Health Organization (WHO) studies, one in five adolescents is uncertain of her LMP. Accuracy in the estimation of fetal age is crucial inasmuch as pregnancies before and after week 7, week 13, or week 18 may be handled differently. Ultrasound examination only improves accuracy in dating first trimester pregnancy ±1 week. However ultrasound imaging does successfully identify 100% of cases past the first trimester even if the LMP and a bimanual examination indicate otherwise.

Diagnostic Tests

A positive result of a urine or serum test for hCG confirms the pregnancy. Nonprescription and commonly used laboratory qualitative urine tests show positively at 4 to 5 weeks from the LMP. Current commercial tests are highly sensitive.

Serum quantitative pregnancy tests measure the level of total hCG using an antibody to its beta-subunit. hCG is detectable in the maternal circulation about 6 to 9 days after ovulation, or approximately 3 weeks from LMP. A single quantitative serum test result may give a crude estimate of gestational age. hCG levels are higher in patients carrying multiple or molar pregnancies and are lower in those with missed abortion, complete abortion, or ectopic pregnancy than those in women carrying a single intrauterine pregnancy.

If a discrepancy is found between the LMP and uterine size by bimanual examination, the use of ultrasound is indicated to determine the gestational age. A full bladder improves ultrasound resolution.

An extrauterine (ectopic) pregnancy is suspect if the uterus feels small for the LMP, there is pain, an adnexal mass is palpated, or a quantative serum hCG level does not correspond to the clinical findings. In this case, a transvaginal ultrasound scan is indicated. If copious vaginal bleeding or clots have been expelled and abdominal pain is present, particularly if the cervical os is found to be open, a spontaneous or incomplete miscarriage can be ruled out by use of an ultrasound, as well. If the suspicion of ectopic pregnancy or incomplete miscarriage is low, quantative hCG levels should be obtained serially at appropriate intervals (Table 59-2). During the first month of gestation, serum levels of hCG double approximately every 2 days. The doubling time varies greatly with the age of gestation as well as with the individual. Because standards differ, the same laboratory should be used for serial tests.

Preoperative diagnostic and screening tests are listed in the Box 59-4.

Patients may have personal requests, such as having a companion in the procedure room, which is permitted in

BOX 59-3

History and Physical Examination Before Abortion

History
Age
Obstetric history
Gravidity and parity:
    Prior spontaneous or elective abortions (gestational age, complications)
    Prior ectopic pregnancies
Obstetric outcomes:
    Method of delivery/cesarean section
    Complications
Gynecologic history
Menarche, interval, last normal menstrual period and duration
Pelvic inflammatory disease
Sexually transmitted disease
Abnormal Pap smear
Fibroids
Congenital anomalies
Diethylstilbestrol exposure (DES)
Pelvic surgery
Reproductive history
    Contraceptive history
    Number and sexual history of partners
    Frequency of intercourse
Future childbearing plans
Medical history
    Diabetes
    Hepatitis
    Heart disease/rheumatic heart disease/heart murmur
    Hypertension
    Neurologic problems/seizures
    Phlebitis/thromboembolic disease
    Hematologic disorders
    Thyroid disorders/endocrine problems
    Asthma
    Urinary disorders/kidney problems

Human immunodeficiency virus (HIV) status
Allergies
Medication(s)
Surgery
Anesthesia
Blood transfusions
Habits
    Alcohol/drug use
    Smoking—packs per day
Family history
Psychosocial history
Psychiatric or social problems, including family violence/abuse
Father of pregnancy (involved, supportive)
Marital status
Schooling/Job/Occupation
Social supports
Current symptoms and duration
    Breast tenderness
    Nausea
    Bleeding/spotting
    Pain
Physical examination
    Blood pressure/pulse
    Height/weight
    Head/eyes/ear/nose/throat
    Skin
    Thyroid
    Breasts and axilla
    Heart
    Lungs
    Abdomen
    Genitalia/pelvic

Table 59-2

Pregnancy Dating by Ultrasound and Quantative Serum Human Chorionic Gonadotropin

Measure by Gestational Sac (Age/LMP Diameter)	Serum hCG (Second System of Units) 2nd International Reference (2nd IRP)	Transabdominal Sonographic Scanning	Transvaginal Sonographic Scanning
	0-180 mIU/ml	No sac	No sac
	500-1000 mIU/ml		Gestational sac usually seen
	≥1000 mIU/ml		Gestational sac consistently seen
5½ wks	≥3600 mIU/ml		Yolk sac
	≥5400 mIU/ml		Embryo
4-6 wks	1800-10,000 mIU/ml	Gestational sac only	
5-6 wks	≥10,000 mIU/ml	Embryo	
5-7 wks		Cardiac activity	Cardiac activity
5-10 wks		Yolk sac	
5-16 wks		Amnion separate from chorion	Amnion separate from chorion
Up to 15 wks		Corpus luteum cyst	Corpus luteum cyst

Courtesy Peter M. Doubilet, MD, PhD, Boston, Mass.

many facilities. Some women are curious about the size and form of the POC. Those who wish to see them at the time of the procedure may be encouraged to ask the surgeon. Future contraception should be discussed at the time of preoperative counseling.

Informed Consent

Many states require written informed consent before performing the abortion. Review of the information that describes the procedure and potential adverse outcomes provides an opportunity to answer questions and to prepare the patient regarding what to expect. In all but 13 states, adolescents need parental consent or notification for abortion procedures. In certain circumstances, a judicial waiver can bypass the parental notification requirements. Specific consent is required if the POC will be used for medical research.

Referral

Nearly all women who want to terminate their pregnancy in the first trimester are good candidates for an outpatient surgical procedure under local anesthesia. The patient may elect IV sedation to augment local paracervical block.

Second-trimester abortion procedures up to 22 weeks may be performed by specially trained operators at certain outpatient sites. Women who require late second-trimester procedures should undergo ultrasound imaging to accurately size the pregnancy. If the biparietal diameter is greater than 50 to 55 mm, the woman generally is referred to a facility that performs labor-induction procedures.

Referral by the primary care physician to the clinician who performs the abortion includes the results of the physical examination and pregnancy test(s), the ultrasound scan if obtained, and the estimated period of amenorrhea (LMP). The referral indicates any need for antibiotic, cardiac, or Rh prophylaxis, results of screening tests for infection, prior reactions to anesthetic agents, underlying diseases, allergies, and medications.

Patients with Medical Problems and Those on Long-Term Drug Therapy

Women on chronic medications should take the recommended dosages, described in the following, on the morning of the procedure with a small amount of water. Patients with stable, well-controlled diabetes (no ketoacidosis or recent

---

BOX 59-4
Diagnostic Tests

Human chorionic gonadotropin (hCG)
Hematocrit and platelets
Blood type (ABO and Rh) and antibodies
Gonorrhea and chlamydia*
Hepatitis B*
Rapid plasma reagin (RPR)*
Human immunodeficiency virus (HIV)*
Pap smear*
Rubella

---

*For screening or if clinically indicated.

insulin adjustments) can undergo an abortion in an outpatient setting. If the woman is fasting all morning, it is recommended that she take half her normal insulin or oral hypoglycemic dose on the day of the procedure. Perioperative monitoring of glucose determines therapy afterward. Diabetic women should have an intravenous line in place and be well hydrated. Women with brittle diabetes and those with renal or vascular complications should have a hospital-based procedure and receive antibiotic prophylaxis.

Patients with mild or moderate hypertension may undergo an abortion in an outpatient setting. If medicated, the woman should take her usual dose the morning of the procedure. Oxytocin is the drug of choice for a hypertensive woman if bleeding occurs after the procedure as a result of uterine atony rather than Ergotalkaloids (e.g., methylergonovine maleate or Ergotrate maleate). Preoperative potassium levels are useful in the event of surgical complications that require general anesthesia. For the woman with uncontrolled hypertension, an elective abortion should be deferred until elevated blood pressures are successfully treated.

Patients with symptomatic cardiac disease and those with artificial heart valves, previous myocardial infarction, coronary heart disease, or a history of bacterial endocarditis should undergo abortion procedures in a hospital setting. Intraoperative and postoperative cardiac monitoring may be required. Women with valvular heart disease or septal defects require antibiotic prophylaxis against bacterial endocarditis and may undergo an outpatient abortion if they are free of symptoms.

Women with severe or active asthma are most safely cared for in a hospital facility. Preoperative glucocorticoids and/or diphenylhydramine may be used for prophylaxis. Sympathomimetic agents are contraindicated because they can confound the accurate assessment of cardiopulmonary status.

Women with hemorrhagic disorders or conditions that alter blood clotting, such as uremia or lupus erythematosus, should undergo abortion procedures in a hospital facility.

Women with well-controlled seizure disorders may undergo an outpatient abortion. If a woman is on a daily medication regimen, she should take her usual morning dose with a small amount of water. If the woman has a history of poorly controlled seizures, she should be referred for abortion at a facility where endotracheal intubation is available.

Disease secondary to HIV does not contraindicate an outpatient abortion. Platelet function and coagulation studies should be assessed before the procedure. Women receiving nucleoside or oncolytic therapy may continue their use if hematologic parameters are stable. Antibiotic prophylaxis is recommended for HIV-positive women.

For mentally incompetent or psychiatric patients, complete control with neuropsychiatric medications is vital before they enter the abortion facility. This can be accomplished once the decision to terminate the pregnancy is certain, and thus the effects of the medication on the fetus are inconsequential. A consent form signed by the legal guardian or authority is required. These women should be accompanied by their guardian on all visits.

Vaginitis with trichomonads or bacterial vaginosis should be treated before and after the abortion with metronidazole. Candidiasis may be treated before the procedure or after the follow-up visit.

Women taking aspirin or aspirin-containing drugs should discontinue their use for 7 days before surgery. Women taking long-term nonsteroidal anti-inflammatory medications should temporarily discontinue the drug 3 days before the surgical procedure.

Women taking warfarin should discontinue it 2 days before the procedure or convert to heparin anticoagulation on the two preceding nights, depending on the clinical situation. Generally, for patients with a mechanical valve, heparin is preferred.

AFTER THE PROCEDURE

After the procedure, the woman is discharged from the center with instructions to participate in activities as tolerated and refrain from intercourse, swimming, bathing, and vaginal insertions (i.e., tampons) for 2 weeks. After a procedure under intravenous sedation or general anesthesia, the woman must be escorted home.

Iron may have been prescribed if bleeding during the procedure were excessive or if the patient had a low preoperative hematocrit. At some procedure sites, iron supplementation is routine for a hematocrit less than 32%. Unfortunately, this may complicate the diagnosis of a non-iron-deficiency anemia. If bleeding during the procedure were excessive, a short course of an oral ergot alkaloid may have been prescribed. Oral antibiotics for prophylaxis against pelvic infections and nonsteroid anti-inflammatory medications for pain and cramping may have also been prescribed. Oral contraceptives may be started on the Sunday after the procedure. Pills low in estrogen should be selected for women in whom a relatively hypercoagulable state is suspected after pregnancy termination (Box 59-5). Medroxyprogesterone acetate injection or insertion of a long-acting levonorgestrel implant may be done just after the procedure.

The Postabortion Visit

The routine postabortion visit may be scheduled 2 to 3 weeks after the procedure to detect complications, give emotional support, and answer questions about birth control and return to sexual activity (Box 59-6).

Bleeding and pain should have ceased by the postoperative visit. The physical examination will determine if there is fever, if the uterus has involuted, and if a pelvic mass or tenderness is present, signs that might indicate infection, retained POC, ectopic pregnancy, or endoparametritis. The serum hCG should be undetectable at 4 weeks after a first-trimester abortion and 2 weeks after a second-trimester abortion, although it is not routinely checked (Fig. 59-2).

For menstrual extraction procedures, some authorities recommend obtaining a routine postoperative hCG level to rule out retained POC. Most retained POC will be expelled spontaneously, but 1% to 2% of menstrual extraction procedures fail, resulting in the continuation of an intrauterine pregnancy.

Most women experience relief in the weeks after an abortion, although many initially feel emotionally labile. Even if the woman were certain about her decision to terminate the pregnancy, she may subsequently feel doubt or recrimination about the loss. Most grief reactions resolve; few are prolonged. Women who are uncertain about relationships or life goals or who do not have dependable social supports are at greater risk for depression. Adolescents are particularly vulnerable to psychologic problems. Postpartum depression,

---

> **BOX 59-5**
> **Risk Factors for Coagulation Abnormalities**
>
> **Activated Clotting**
> Malignant disease or occult malignancy
> Obesity
> Oral contraceptive use
> Intravenous drug use
> Repetitive pregnancy loss (antiphospholipid antibodies)
> Chronic abruptio placentae
> Early fetal demise
>
> **Depressed Clotting**
> Mild/occult von Willebrand's disease
> Aspirin or nonsteroidal anti-inflammatory drug use
> Red wine three or more times a day
> Human immunodeficiency virus
> Uremia
> Acute abruptio placentae
> Late fetal demise

> **BOX 59-6**
> **The Postabortion Visit**
>
> **Information from the Abortion Provider**
> Estimated gestational age after the procedure
> Results of laboratory testing (usually includes hematocrit, blood type)
> Type of anesthesia or sedation used
> Complications
> If Rh and anti–D immuneglobulins administered
> Discharge medications (antibiotics, ergot alkaloids, analgesics)
> Type of contraceptive anticipated or prescribed
> Pathology report
>
> **Information from the Patient**
> Symptoms of ongoing pregnancy
> Pain, bleeding, fever
> Medications taken after procedure
> Emotional status and support
> Resumed intercourse
>
> **Physical Examination**
> Temperature/blood pressure/pulse
> Abdomen
> Genitalia/pelvic
>
> **Laboratory**
> Quantitative hCG (routine for menstrual extractions only)
>
> **Counseling/Education/Prescription**
> Contraceptive method
> Emotional support

especially after a second-trimester abortion, may have hormonal components, but this is unproven. Nevertheless, if distress is prolonged or severe, the woman should be referred for professional counseling or psychiatric evaluation. Women who are uneasy about their decision to have terminated the pregnancy in relation to their religious beliefs may be referred to Clergy for Choice.

The postabortion visit includes establishing a realistic, usable form of contraception. An unplanned pregnancy helps some women to become more consistent and assertive with partners in the use of contraception (see Chapter 58).

Evaluation of Complications

Patients with a persistent fever of 38° C (100.4° F), bleeding that soaks one pad every 1 to 2 hours or that increases over 2 days, or severe persistent pain, require evaluation for infection, perforation, retained POC, or ectopic pregnancy. Furthermore, if the microscopic examination of the suctioned uterine contents reports no villi or implantation site, the patient must be evaluated for complete miscarriage or ectopic pregnancy.

The most common cause of heavy postabortal bleeding is retained POC. This occurs in 0.2% to 0.6% of cases and may be diagnosed by ultrasound scan. Most excessive bleeding occurs within 1 week, although it occasionally occurs several weeks after the procedure. Severe pain, pelvic tenderness, or bleeding may suggest infection or inflammation. One-half of one percent of abortion complications present with uterine tenderness. In the absence of retained POC, bleeding from infection and inflammation owing to a subinvoluted uterus usually is modest. If fever accompanies uterine tenderness, with or without an open cervical os,

postabortal endometritis is suspect and may require uterine respiration.

Endometritis requires antibiotic treatment and if reevacuation is indicated, only experienced surgeons should perform the procedure, as the risk of perforating a necrotic or inflamed uterine wall is greater than in the initial procedure. Patients with fevers above 38° C (100.4° F) and signs of peritoneal irritation require hospitalization to be observed for potential progression of intra-abdominal infection and receive intravenous antibiotics against anaerobes, gonorrhea, and chlamydia. Outpatient treatment with doxycycline, 100 mg twice daily for 7 to 14 days, should be reserved for patients whose signs and symptoms are confined to the empty uterus.

Dysfunctional uterine bleeding after abortion without signs or symptoms of retained POC or infection may be treated with three cycles of oral contraceptives. Curettage rarely is necessary unless bleeding is heavy, prolonged, or causes symptoms and signs of acute blood loss. A slowly expanding broad-ligament hematoma requires immediate attention from an experienced gynecologic surgeon.

Thromboembolic complications usually occur within 1 or 2 weeks after the abortion.

Ectopic pregnancy occurs in 0.5% to 1% of all pregnancies. From 1972 to 1985, the rate of ectopic pregnancy concurrent with induced abortion was 1.36/1000 abortions. An ectopic pregnancy is suspect if no trophoblastic tissue is evacuated during the procedure.

Early clinical presentation may include pain, bleeding, and an adnexal mass; late presentation is hypotension and shock. Transvaginal, rather than transabdominal, ultrasound is the procedure of choice to rule out an early ectopic pregnancy because of the proximity of the probe to the adnexae. A transvaginal ultrasound compared to transabdominal can visualize a smaller yolk sac and embryo one-half week earlier and at lower levels of hCG. If the transvaginal scan demonstrates a lower uterine-segment fibroid or suggests a higher pelvic mass, then an abdominal ultrasound is indicated. Transabdominal scan may also be done routinely after the transvaginal one. The diagnosis of ectopic pregnancy is certain if the ultrasound scan shows an embryo outside the uterine cavity. If ultrasound results show an intrauterine pregnancy, the likelihood of ectopic is less than 1:8000. Likewise, this probability is low if there is a clearly demonstrated simple ovarian cyst. The probability is high in the absence of intrauterine pregnancy and the presence of a complex adnexal mass and/or free fluid.

Hematometra may occur 1 or 2 days after D&E. The tense, tender, and globular uterus contains dark liquid and clotted blood. The patient looks distressed and is tachycardic and sweating, but vaginal bleeding is not excessive. Repeat suction evacuation of the uterine cavity is the recommended treatment. Although the cause of this problem is unknown at this time, an ergot alkaloid and antibiotic is usually prescribed for prophylaxis. Other rare complications primarily associated with second trimester abortions were discussed earlier.

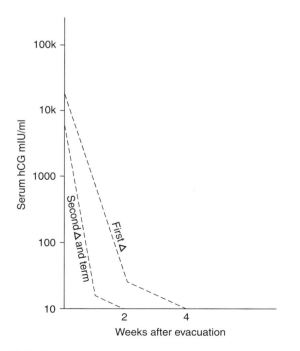

FIG. 59-2 Disappearance of human chorionic gonadotropin after termination of normal pregnancy. (Modified from Osathanondh R: *Current problems in obstetrics and gynecology,* Chicago, 1980, Year Book Medical Publishers.)

Late Complications

Delayed complications of induced abortion include degrees of postabortal infection: endoparametritis to pelvic septic thrombophlebitis to septicemia/shock, and thromboembolic events. Infection usually is associated with retained POC or a continuing pregnancy. Common symptoms are crampy pain with prolonged vaginal bleeding and a low-grade fever. The uterus is tender, slightly enlarged, and boggy.

Ultrasound may confirm or exclude the diagnosis of retained POC. Treatment of late infections include intravenous antibiotics and an ergot. Repeat uterine evacuation may be required. Patients with a continuing pregnancy or retained POC do require a D&E under ultrasound guidance. Of note, these women may have a previously unrecognized uterine anomaly. Postabortal, painless amenorrhea may be related to Asherman's syndrome. Hysteroscopic surgery is required to confirm the diagnosis and initiate treatment.

Long-Term Sequelae

Repeat first-trimester abortions by vacuum aspiration are not associated with fertility problems or subsequent abnormal pregnancies including ectopics. Evidence from the 1970s suggested that two or more induced abortions increase the risk of subsequent first- and second-trimester spontaneous abortion, prematurity, and low–birth-weight infants. With current surgical techniques these findings have been disputed. In 1994 a case-control study was reported which demonstrated an increased risk of developing breast cancer in women who had an induced abortion. This has been shown to be insignificant.

REPEATED REQUESTS FOR ABORTION

It is widely believed that women who repeatedly request abortions are noncompliant with birth control or substitute abortion for contraception. During the 1980s, approximately 1.2 million live births per year occurred because of mistimed or unwanted pregnancies, many despite the use of contraception. Among one sample of abortion patients, 51% were using a method of contraception during the month in which they conceived. Studies examining the rate of abortion relative to the use of contraception indicate that contraceptive failure constitutes the major cause of repeat abortion.

Two general populations of women who request abortions have been identified. The first group has access to contraception. These women tend to use abortion as an adjunct to other family planning methods to postpone first births or to prevent late or higher parity order offspring, usually after the second child. Another group does not have easy access to contraception. These women use abortion to prevent late pregnancies or to increase birth spacing, usually after four or more children. The first group of women tends to rely on abortion for contraceptive failures, whereas the second group, composed of women still struggling to control their fertility, uses contraceptives intermittently and therefore depends on abortion instead of contraception to terminate unwanted or mistimed births.

BIBLIOGRAPHY

Atrash HK, Cheek TG, Hogue CJR: Legal abortion mortality and general anesthesia, *Am J Obstet Gynecol* 158:420, 1988.

Atrash HK, Lawson HW, Smith JC: Legal abortion in the US: trends and mortality, *Contemp Obstet Gynecol* 35:58, 1990.

Birgerson L et al: Termination of early human pregnancy with epostane, *Contraception* 35:111, 1987.

Buehler JW et al: The risk of serious complications from induced abortion: do personal characteristics make a difference? *Am J Obstet Gynecol* 153:14, 1985.

Creinin MD, Vittinghoff E: Methatrexate and misoprostol vs. misoprostol alone for early abortion, *JAMA* 272:15, 1994.

Daling JR et al: Ectopic pregnancy in relation to previous induced abortion, *JAMA* 253:1005, 1985.

Daling JR et al: Risk of breast cancer among young women: relationship to induced abortion, *J Natl Canc Inst* 86:1585, 1994.

Darj E, Stralin EB, Nilsson S: The prophylactic effect of doxycycline on postoperative infection rate after first trimester abortion, *Obstet Gynecol* 70:755, 1987.

Darney PD, Sweet RL: Routine intraoperative ultrasonography for second trimester abortion reduces incidence of uterine perforation, *J Ultrasound Med* 8:71, 1989.

Forrest JD, Henshaw SK: Providing controversial health care: abortion services since 1973, *Women's Health Institute* 152, 1993.

Freedman MA et al: Comparison of complication rates in first trimester abortions performed by physician assistants and physicians, *Am J Public Health* 76:550, 1986.

Freeman EW: Abortion: subjective attitudes and feelings, *Fam Plann Perspect* 10:150, 1978.

Grimes DA, Cates W Jr, Selik RM: Abortion facilities and the risk of death, *Fam Plann Perspect* 13:30, 1981.

Grimes DA, Schulz KF, Cates W Jr, Tyler CW Jr: Local versus general anesthesia: which is safer for performing suction curretage abotions? *Am J Obstet Gynecol* 135:1030, 1979.

Hakim-Elahi E, Tovell HMM, Burnhill MS: Complications of first-trimester abortion: a report of 170,000 cases, *Obstet Gynecol* 76:129, 1990.

Henshaw SK, Silverman J: The characteristics and prior contraceptive use of U.S. abortion patients, *Fam Plann Perspect* 20:158, 1988.

Henshaw SK, Van Vort J, editors: *The abortion fact book,* New York, 1992, Alan Guttmacher Institute.

Henshaw, SK: Abortion incidence and services in the United States, 1995-1996, *Fam Plann Perspect* 30:6, 1998.

Henshaw SK: Unintended pregnancy in the United States, *Fam Plann Perspect* 30:24, 46, 1998.

Hogue CJR, Cates W Jr, Tietze C: The effects of induced abortion on subsequent reproduction, *Epidemiol Rev* 4:66, 1982.

Hogue CJR: Impact of abortion on subsequent fecundity, *Clin Obstet Gynecol* 13:95, 1986.

Hornstein M et al: Ultrasound guidance for selected dilatation and evacuation procedures, *J Reprod Med* 31:947, 1986.

Houang ET: Antibiotic prophylaxis in hysterectomy and induced abortion, *Drugs* 41:19, 1991.

Kleinman RL, editor: *Family planning handbook for doctors,* London, 1988, International Planned Parenthood Federation.

Koonin LM, Smith JC, Ramick M: Abortion surveillance—United States, 1990, *MMWR* 42:SS-6, 1993.

Landy U: Abortion counselling—a new component of medical care, *Clin Obstet Gynecol* 13:33, 1986.

Landy U, Lewit S: Administrative, counselling and medical practices in National Abortion Federation facilities, *Fam Plann Perspect* 14:257, 1982.

Lawson H, Atrash HK, Safflas A: Ectopic pregnancy surveillance—United States, 1970-1989, *MMWR* 42:SS6, 1989.

Lichtenberg ES, Paul M, Saporta V: *Provider clinical survey: first trimester surgical abortion practice,* Washington DC, 1997, National Abortion Federation.

Mackay HT, Schulz KF, Grimes DA: Safety of local versus general anesthesia for second-trimester dilatation and evacuation abortion, *Obstet Gynecol* 66:661, 1985.

National Abortion and Reproductive Rights/NARAL: *Who decides? Public funding for abortion.* Washington, DC, 1999, NARAL.

National Abortion Federation: *Summary of annual complication statistics, 1992,* Washington, DC, 1993.

Osathanondh R: *Conception control.* In Ryan KJ, Berkowitz R, Barbieri R, Dunaif A, editors: *Kistner's gynecology and women's health,* ed 7, St Louis, 1999, Mosby.

Osathanondh R: Endocrine tests in obstetrics and gynecology, Part I. *Current problems in obstetrics and gynecology,* Chicago, 1980, Year Book Medical Publishers.

Peterson WF et al: Second-trimester abortion by dilatation and evacuation: an analysis of 11,747 cases, *Obstet Gynecol* 62:185, 1983.

Potts M, Diggory P, Peel J: *Abortion,* Cambridge, 1977, Cambridge University Press.

Rosenberg L: Induced abortion and breast cancer: more scientific data are needed, *J Natl Canc Inst* 86:1569, 1994.

Sawaya GF et al: Antibiotics at the time of induced abortion: the case for universal prophylaxis based on meta-analysis, *Obstet Gynecol* 87:884, 1996.

Smith N et al: Screening for chlamydia infection, *Lancet* 342:687, 1993 (letter).

Spitz IM, Bardin CW, Benton L, Robbins A: Early pregnancy termination with mifepristone and misoprostol in the United States, *N Engl J Med* 338:1241, 1998.

Steinhoff PG et al: Women who obtain repeat abortions: a study based on record linkage, *Fam Plann Perspect* 11:30, 1979.

Stevenson MM, Radcliffe KW: Preventing pelvic infections after abortion, *Int J STD AIDS* 6:305, 1995.

Stockley IH: Methotrexate-NSAID interactions, *Drug Intell Clin Pharm* 21:546, 1987.

Stotland NL: The myth of the abortion trauma syndrome, *JAMA* 268:2078, 1992.

Stubblefield PG, Grimes DA: Septic abortion, *N Engl J Med* 331:310, 1994.

Stubblefield PG et al: Fertility after induced abortion: a prospective follow-up study, *Obstet Gynecol* 62:186, 1984.

Whitfield CR: Future challenges in the management of rhesus disease. In Studd, J, editor: *Progress in obstetrics and gynecology,* ed 3, Edinburgh, 1982, Churchill Livingstone.

Williams L, Pratt WF: *Wanted and unwanted childbearing in the United States 1973-88,* Hyattsville, Md, 1990, National Center for Health Statistics.

RESOURCES

Abortion Clinics On-Line
www.gynpages.com

Alan Guttmacher Institute (AGI)
New York
120 Wall Street
21st Floor
New York, NY 10005
Tel: (212) 248-1111
Fax: (212) 248-1951
Washington, DC
1120 Connecticut Avenue, NW
Suite 460
Washington, DC 20036
Tel: (202) 296-4012
Fax: (202) 223-5756
www.agi-usa.org

Catholics for a Free Choice
1436 U Street NW, Suite 301
Washington, DC 20009
Tel: (202) 968-6093
Fax: (202) 332-7995
E-mail: cffa@catholicsforchoice.org
www.catholicsforchoice.org

Center for Disease Control and Prevention (CDC)
www.cdc.gov

Center for Reproductive Law and Policy
New York
120 Wall Street
New York, NY 10005
Tel: (917) 637-3600
Fax: (917) 637-3666
info@crlp.org
Washington DC
1146 19th Street NW
Washington, DC 20036
Tel: (202) 530-2975
Fax: (202) 530-2976
dcinfo@crlp.org
www.crlp.org

Mifeprex
Tel: 1-877-432-7596
www.earlyoptions.com

The National Abortion Federation (NAF)
1755 Massachusetts Avenue, NW Suite 600
Washington, DC 20036
Tel: (202) 667-5881
www.prochoice.org

Planned Parenthood Federation of America
810 Seventh Avenue
New York, NY 10019
Tel: (212) 541-7800
Fax: (212) 245-1845
communications@ppfa.org
www.plannedparenthood.org

CHAPTER **60**

Benign Breast Disease

Barbara L. Smith

Benign breast disease and its symptoms bring many women to their physician's office. Many additional breast abnormalities are discovered during the course of routine physical examination and mammography. Management of these benign problems can be challenging, and it may be difficult to distinguish benign from malignant breast lesions.

Breast problems seen commonly in clinical practice include abnormalities detected on clinical or self-examination including discrete palpable masses, vague thickening or nodularity, breast pain, nipple discharge, infections, and abnormalities detected by screening mammography.

Failure to diagnose breast cancer is one of the most common causes of litigation in medical practice. From a medicolegal and risk management perspective, as well as for good medical practice, it is important to document any recommendations for mammography, ultrasound, biopsy, referral, or follow-up visits in each patient's chart. It is also essential to discuss these recommendations in detail with the patient herself.

OFFICE EVALUATION OF BREAST PROBLEMS

Evaluation of a breast problem requires a detailed history of the presenting complaint, a review of prior breast problems, a review of risk factors for breast carcinoma, a thorough physical examination of the breasts, appropriate imaging studies, and evaluation of the patient's general medical condition.

Physical Examination

Physical examination of the breasts includes inspection of the skin, palpation of the breasts, examination of the nipples for discharge, and palpation of the axillary and supraclavicular lymph node areas. The breasts should be inspected with the patient sitting with her hands behind her head and her elbows back to look for asymmetry, dimpling of the skin, and any areas of erythema or edema. The breasts should then be palpated in a systematic fashion with the patient supine and sitting, examining tissue from the clavicle to below the inframammary fold, and from the sternum to the posterior axillary line, taking care to include the subareolar area. If an abnormal area is identified, a careful description of its size, contour,

texture, tenderness, and position should be recorded. A diagram of the location of any abnormality noted is extremely useful for future reference.

The nipples and areolae are best examined with the patient in the supine position, first inspecting for any areas of skin breakdown, and then squeezing gently to check for discharge.

The axillary nodes lie beneath the hair-bearing skin of the axilla and are examined pressing the examiner's fingers inward and upward to check for enlarged nodes. Supraclavicular nodes may be examined in the supine or sitting position. Should any enlarged nodes be discovered, their size, mobility, and number should be recorded. Tenderness of enlarged nodes, which may be more suggestive of a reactive process, should be noted.

Breast Imaging Studies

Evaluation of many but not all breast problems may require the use of imaging studies. Mammography, ultrasound and, increasingly, breast magnetic resonance imaging (MRI) are useful in characterizing breast lesions.

Mammography is the primary diagnostic imaging modality in evaluation of breast problems. It has been suggested that mammography is appropriate in the workup of a breast problem in women over the age of 35, and may be used at an earlier age for breast problems in younger, high-risk women.

Despite its overall value in the evaluation of breast problems, it must be remembered that 10% to 15% of palpable breast cancers will not be visualized by mammography. In such cases the cancer is not producing calcifications or a density radiographically different from surrounding normal breast tissue. For this reason, a negative mammogram does not eliminate the need for biopsy of a palpable breast abnormality. Inappropriate reliance on a negative mammogram can result in delays in diagnosis of a breast malignancy.

Ultrasound

Ultrasound is useful in determining whether a lesion identified by physical examination or mammography is cystic or solid, and to better define its size, contour, and internal texture. However, ultrasound fails to detect calcifications, may fail to detect some breast masses, and may misinterpret irregularities in normal breast texture as masses. As is the case for mammography, a negative ultrasound does not eliminate the need to biopsy a palpable mass.

Magnetic Resonance Imaging and Other Imaging Modalities

MRI is a promising addition to breast imaging options. With gadolinium contrast, many malignant lesions enhance relative to normal breast parenchyma. Although some benign lesions such as fibroadenomas also enhance with gadolinium, malignant lesions appear to enhance more rapidly and often to a greater extent.

The sensitivity and specificity of MRI in distinguishing benign from malignant lesions are still being defined. Its main approved use is in identifying leaks in silicone breast implants, where it can identify the ruptured silicone membrane within the silicone gel. MRI is also proving useful in assessing the extent of vaguely defined tumors, in identifying unsuspected multifocal disease, and in helping to identify those patients not eligible for breast-conserving surgery. It also appears that MRI can distinguish locally recurrent tumor from surgical scarring and radiation change after lumpectomy and radiation, although it does not provide reliable readings until 18 months or more after completion of surgery or radiation therapy. The utility of MRI in screening young, high-risk women with mammographically dense breast tissue is being explored.

Nuclear medicine studies such as sestimibi scintimammography and positron emission tomography remain primarily investigational tools. There is currently no role for thermography or xerography in the evaluation of breast problems.

⚕ MANAGEMENT OF COMMON BREAST PROBLEMS

Palpable Abnormalities

Palpable breast lesions include discrete palpable masses, vague thickenings, and generalized nodularity.

Discrete Palpable Masses

Cysts

Clinical examination is not accurate in distinguishing a cyst from a solid mass. Rosner and Baird found that physical examination correctly identified only 58% of 66 palpable cysts. A palpable mass suspected to be a cyst should be confirmed as such by aspiration or ultrasound (Fig. 60-1). Aspiration may also be appropriate to confirm that the palpable mass corresponds to the lesion seen on ultrasound. Removal of the mass by aspiration also permits a more thorough examination of the surrounding breast tissue.

Bloody cyst fluid, or a mass that persists after aspiration, is worrisome for malignancy and the aspirated fluid should be sent for cytologic analysis. Biopsy is generally indicated in this setting even if the cytologic analysis is negative for malignancy. If cyst fluid is not bloody, and no mass remains after aspiration, there is little chance of malignancy, and the fluid need not be sent for cytology. Ciatto et al found no malignancies among 6747 nonbloody cyst aspirations.

If a cyst is aspirated without prior ultrasound documentation that it was a simple cyst, the patient should be re-examined in 4 to 8 weeks. Fewer than 20% of simple cysts will recur after a single aspiration, and fewer than 9% will recur after two or three aspirations. When the same cyst recurs rapidly after aspiration, it should be reaspirated and the cyst contents sent for cytologic analysis. A biopsy should be performed if the cytology is suspicious or if the cyst recurs. Appearance of a new cyst in a different area of breast tissue, however, does not require this additional workup, and should be evaluated and aspirated as a new problem. Additional cysts may be expected in more than half of patients.

Solid Masses

Discrete masses within the breast that are solid, either by ultrasound criteria or by failing to yield fluid on aspiration attempts, require a tissue diagnosis to exclude malignancy. Physical examination alone correctly identifies a mass as malignant in only 60% to 85% of cases, and experienced examiners will often disagree on the need for biopsy of a particular lesion. Boyd et al found that four surgeons uniformly agreed on the need for biopsy of only 73% of 15 palpable masses later shown on biopsy to be malignant.

Before biopsy, it is appropriate to order a mammogram in a woman over 35 to look for synchronous lesions. It must be emphasized that a normal mammogram and/or ultrasound does not eliminate the need for a biopsy of a discrete palpable mass since as many as 10% to 15% of palpable cancers will not be visualized by mammography. Options for biopsy of palpable lesions include fine needle aspiration (FNA) biopsy, core needle biopsy, and open surgical biopsy.

Vague Thickening or Nodularity

Normal breast texture is often heterogeneous, particularly in premenopausal women. These variations in texture may create areas that feel firmer to palpation than surrounding tissue, and may or may not be tender. Such areas are of particular concern, as it may be difficult to rule out a malignancy such as lobular carcinoma, which produces only a vague mass.

In evaluating an area of concern, it should first be compared with the corresponding area of the opposite breast for symmetry. Symmetric areas of thickening are rarely pathologic. Asymmetric areas, particularly those that are tender, often represent fibrocystic disease and will often resolve spontaneously. To avoid unnecessary biopsies, such vague areas occurring in premenopausal women should be re-examined after one or two menstrual cycles. For postmenopausal women on hormone replacement, the hormone replacement may be discontinued for a month, and the patient reexamined. If the asymmetry resolves, the finding was most likely due to a benign process, and the patient may return to a routine follow-up schedule. Areas of asymmetry that persist, however, must be viewed with some suspicion. Such patients should be referred to a surgeon for evaluation and potential biopsy. In addition, postmenopausal women who are not taking hormone replacement are unlikely to have a physiologic reason for asymmetric thickening, and should be promptly referred to a surgeon for evaluation.

It is appropriate to order a mammogram to rule out synchronous lesions in a woman over 35 who has not had a mammogram within the past 6 months. Once again, a negative mammogram does not eliminate the need for biopsy of any persistent asymmetry. FNA biopsy is generally not

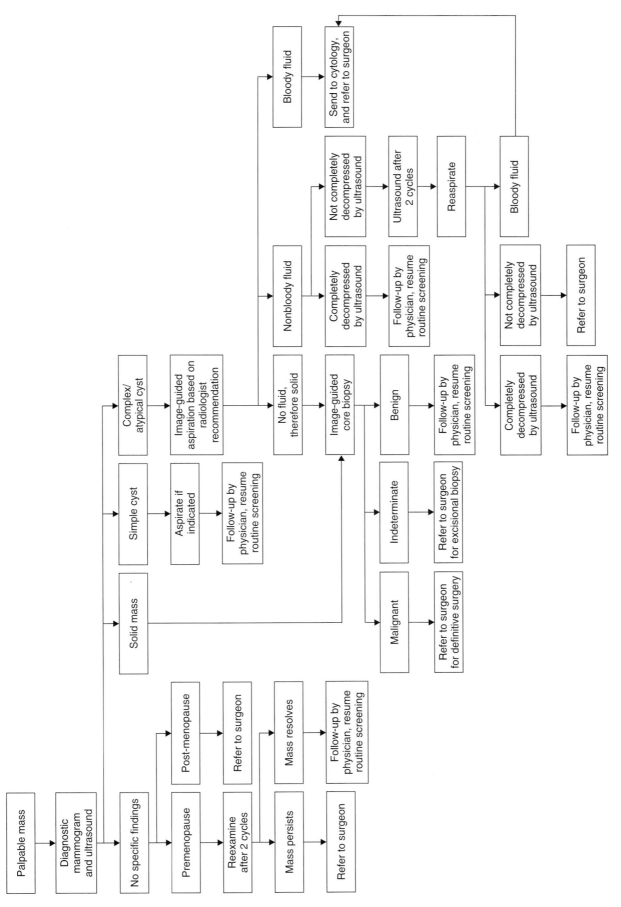

FIG. 60-1 Palpable mass algorithm. (From Risk Management Foundation of the Harvard Medical Institutions.)

appropriate in this setting, as tumors that produce only vague masses often have intermingled normal tissue and sampling error can be high. Open surgical biopsy is generally required for adequate sampling to rule out malignancy.

Breast Pain

Breast pain is one of the most common breast symptoms experienced by women and brings many women to their physicians (Fig. 60-2). Most often, it is concern that the pain is indicative of a more serious condition such as breast cancer that motivates the visit. Physiologic breast tenderness varies with the menstrual cycle, with greatest tenderness immediately before the menstrual period, or for some women, mid-

cycle. Noncyclic pain may also be observed. The pain may be intermittent or continuous and is often described by the patient as "burning." The pain may be diffuse or primarily in a localized area and may be asymmetric.

Although breast pain is poorly understood, its cyclic nature and its resolution at menopause suggest a hormonal cause. Several studies have measured estrogen levels in women with breast pain and have shown no difference in circulating estrogen levels compared with pain-free control subjects. It has been postulated that progesterone levels may be decreased in women with breast pain, and that the relative balance of estrogen and progesterone influences breast pain. It has also been suggested that thyroid hormones may

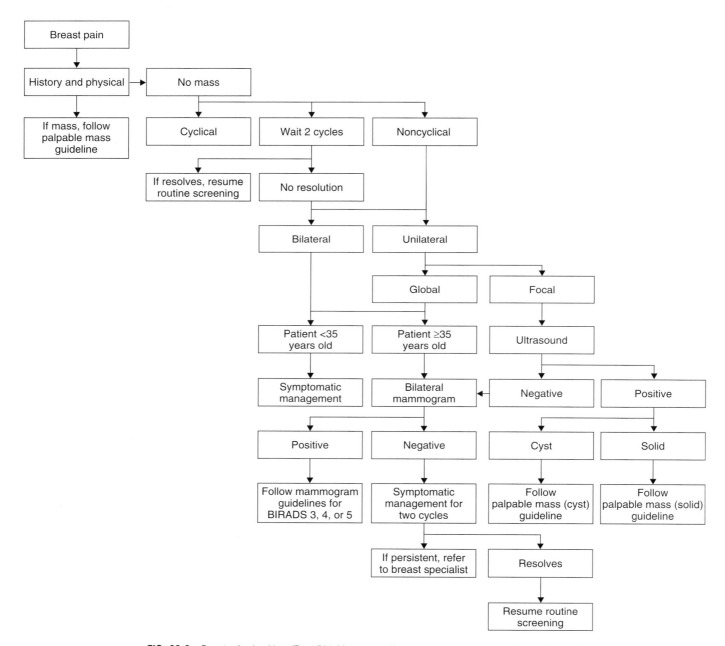

FIG. 60-2 Breast pain algorithm. (From Risk Management Foundation of the Harvard Medical Institutions.)

impact on breast pain, as it was observed that the administration of thyrotrophin-releasing factor resulted in a marked increase in prolactin release in a large group of women with breast pain compared to asymptomatic control subjects.

Although breast pain is rarely indicative of a breast cancer, evaluation of the patient with breast pain first requires that malignancy be ruled out. A careful physical examination should be performed and any palpable masses present evaluated as described previously. A mammogram should be performed in any woman over the age of 35 with persistent, noncyclic breast pain, particularly if the pain is asymmetric. It is also important to rule out causes of pain that do not arise from the breast itself, including muscle strain, costochondritis, and pain of pleural or mediastinal origin. Once these less common causes of pain are excluded, efforts should be directed at symptom management.

For the majority of women presenting with breast pain, reassurance that the workup has shown no evidence of breast cancer or other serious abnormality is the only treatment necessary. The patient may also be reassured that breast pain is usually self-limited, most often resolving within a few months. During the periods of more severe breast tenderness, symptomatic relief may usually be obtained with the use of non-narcotic analgesics, in particular, nonsteroidal antiinflammatory agents. Maneuvers such as elimination of caffeine, chocolate, or salt from the diet, while harmless, are of no proven benefit.

Other remedies may be helpful in women with significant breast pain. Evening primrose oil, one or two capsules orally twice a day, has been reported to produce significant or complete pain relief in half of women with cyclic mastalgia. The oil is obtained from the evening primrose flower, is high in polyunsaturated oils, and may have some prostaglandin-inhibiting effects. Vitamin E at 400 to 800 IU daily and vitamin B_6 at 50 IU daily will also reduce breast pain in some women.

It is advisable to reexamine the patient with new symptoms of breast pain after one or two menstrual cycles to be sure that no palpable abnormality is evolving, and to assess her response to conservative treatment. For the rare patient whose breast pain is severe and unresponsive to conservative measures, pharmacologic therapy may be instituted. Agents that have been used to treat breast pain include danazol, bromocryptine, and tamoxifen. It should be emphasized that such pharmacologic interventions are only rarely required. For pain of this severity it would be appropriate to consult a breast specialist.

Nipple Discharge and Other Nipple and Areola Pathology

Discharge may be expressed from the nipples of as many as 60% to 70% of healthy women. Physiologic nipple discharge is usually bilateral, appears from multiple ducts, is yellow to green in color, and is observed only with attempts to express it rather than spontaneously. This is to be distinguished from galactorrhea, which is bilateral, often spontaneous, milky discharge. Galactorrhea, which is almost never caused by a breast malignancy, may be distinguished from physiologic discharge under the microscope by the presence of fat in the secretions. As many as one-third of women with galactorrhea will have pituitary tumors, particularly if there is associated amenorrhea. Other causes of galactorrhea include hypothyroidism, chest wall trauma, and certain pharmacologic agents. The evaluation of galactorrhea includes measurement of serum prolactin levels and thyroid function tests. If the prolactin level is elevated, an MRI scan of the head should be performed to rule out a pituitary adenoma.

Pathologic nipple discharge is most often unilateral and spontaneous and may be bloody (Fig. 60-3). Although the most common cause of pathologic nipple discharge is a papilloma or other benign process, such discharge may also indicate malignancy and should be evaluated further. A mammogram should be performed in the evaluation of pathologic nipple discharge for any woman over 35 years old.

Careful physical examination should be performed to identify any palpable masses present. The position of the duct from which discharge is obtained should be documented. Of most concern is spontaneous, single duct discharge, or any discharge that is bloody.

Cytology analysis of nipple discharge is rarely useful, as surgical evaluation is required whether the cytology is positive or negative. Ductograms are rarely useful for the same reason, as they rarely provide data that changes the need for surgery, or the surgical procedure performed. Excision of the duct from which the discharge is arising is performed to rule out malignancy.

Erosion or chronic crusting of the nipple raises the suspicion of Paget's disease of the nipple, a variant of infiltrating or intraductal carcinoma that arises in the terminal ducts to involve the surface of the nipple itself. A biopsy is required to distinguish Paget's disease from benign lesions, such as nipple adenomas, or dermatologic conditions, such as eczema, that may also involve the nipple and areola.

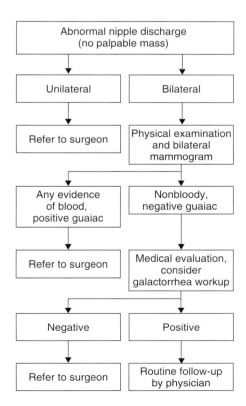

FIG. 60-3 Abnormal nipple discharge algorithm. (From Risk Management Foundation of the Harvard Medical Institutions.)

Breast Infections

Infections of the breast fall into two general categories, lactational infections (which are discussed in Chapter 79) and chronic subareolar infections associated with duct ectasia.

In women who are not lactating, the subareolar ducts of the breast may develop a chronic relapsing form of infection variously known as periductal mastitis or duct ectasia. This condition appears to be associated with smoking and diabetes. The infections that result are most often mixed infections that include both aerobic and anaerobic skin flora. A series of infections with resulting inflammatory changes and scarring may lead to retraction or inversion of the nipple, masses in the subareolar area, and, occasionally, in a chronic fistula from the subareolar ducts to the periareolar skin. Palpable masses and mammographic changes that mimic carcinoma may result.

Such infections may initially present with subareolar pain and mild erythema. If treated at this stage, warm soaks and oral antibiotics may be effective. Antibiotic treatment should cover both aerobic and anaerobic skin flora. Antibiotic treatment is often unsuccessful unless anaerobic coverage is included. If an abscess has developed, treatment in the acute phase is incision and drainage with antibiotics that cover both aerobic and anaerobic skin flora. Repeated infections are treated by excision of the entire subareolar duct complex after the acute infection has completely resolved, with intravenous antibiotic coverage during the perioperative period. A few patients will have recurrent infections requiring excision of the nipple and areola.

Abnormalities on Screening Mammography

The use of screening mammography has led to an increase in the number of nonpalpable breast lesions identified. The majority of abnormal mammographic findings, however, will be benign. In the past, open surgical biopsy with preoperative wire localization was required if biopsy of a nonpalpable mammographic- or ultrasound-detected lesion was recommended. For many women, stereotactic 11- or 14-gauge core needle biopsy or ultrasound-guided core needle biopsy is now a less invasive and less costly alternative to open surgical biopsy. The location and nature of the lesion to be biopsied, for example, its size, and whether it is a mass or just faint calcifications determine the feasibility and advisability of core needle biopsy.

It is important for the ordering clinician to recognize the limitations of core biopsy to be able to correctly interpret its results. Even in skilled hands, there is a false-negative rate of core biopsy in identifying a malignancy. If the core biopsy pathology is discordant with the mammographic findings—for example, only benign breast tissue is identified after core biopsy of a suspicious, spiculated mass—the biopsy should be repeated or the patient referred for open surgical biopsy.

In addition, it must be recognized that pathologic interpretation of certain lesions may difficult on core biopsy. The small tissue fragment size and potential distortion resulting from core biopsy make the differentiation of atypia versus carcinoma in situ extremely difficult. The finding of atypia on core biopsy requires open surgical biopsy to rule out malignancy, with up to half of such subsequent open biopsies showing carcinoma in situ.

For patients who choose or require open surgical biopsy of a nonpalpable lesion, preoperative wire localization of the lesion using mammographic or ultrasound guidance is required to direct the surgeon to the appropriate area. The surgeon then removes a piece of tissue around the wire so as to include the lesion with a rim of surrounding normal breast tissue, usually under local anesthesia. A specimen radiograph of the excised tissue is obtained before the patient leaves the operating room to be sure that the lesion is contained within the specimen.

BREAST IMPLANTS

It is estimated that more than 1 million women in the United States have silicone or saline breast implants in place, most of which were placed for cosmetic purposes. A smaller number of women have had implants placed as part of breast reconstruction after mastectomy.

Physical Examination

For cosmetic breast augmentation, implants are now usually placed beneath the greater pectoral muscle. In this situation, all native breast tissue is pushed forward and remains accessible to physical examination. Implants also have been placed in the retromammary position, behind native breast tissue but superficial to the greater pectoral muscle. Because more prominent capsule formation and contraction often occur with an implant in this position, this technique is now used infrequently. In addition, since the implant is within, rather than behind, the breast, some areas of breast tissue may be less accessible to physical examination.

On physical examination, the implant capsule may result in a firm-to-hard breast texture but does not create masses or nodularity. All palpable masses in women with implants must be viewed as suspicious masses and should be biopsied.

Mammography

With either subpectoral or retromammary implant positioning, native breast tissue may be significantly compressed, decreasing mammographic sensitivity. In addition, silicone-filled implants are radiopaque. Even with special techniques using multiple tangential views, it is estimated that a significant proportion of breast tissue is not well seen. Although saline implants are less radiodense, they still significantly obscure adjacent breast tissue on mammographic examination. Despite these limitations, it is still advisable for a woman with implants to undergo screening mammography and physical examination as appropriate for her age.

Complications of Breast Implants
Capsule Formation
All implants will have dense fibrous capsules form around them in a standard foreign-body reaction. Over time, there is a variable degree of contraction of this capsule, which tends to force the implant into a more hemispheric shape and may result in migration of the implant upward or laterally on the chest wall. In some cases discomfort may be associated with capsule formation and contracture. Severe contracture occurs in only a small fraction of implants placed.

Silicone Implant Leaks

It is not known with certainty how frequently silicone breast implants leak. Rupture of the implant's outer membrane with free leakage of silicone into the body's fibrous capsule may be detected by physical examination as a change in the shape of the augmented breast. MRI is the most accurate way to confirm implant rupture. Such gross rupture generally requires replacement of the implant.

Concern about potential medical problems created by degradation of polyurethane implant coverings, silicone gel bleed, and gross silicone leakage resulted in a number of lawsuits against implant manufacturers and led the Food and Drug Administration (FDA) to place a moratorium on the placement of silicone implants in 1992. This moratorium was subsequently modified to allow silicone implant use for breast reconstruction or for cosmetic purposes in the setting of a scientifically conducted study. Nearly all breast implants placed since 1992 have been saline-filled.

Despite initial concerns, scientific review failed to confirm a link between silicone implants and any autoimmune disorder. A meta-analysis by Janowsky found no evidence of an association between breast implants and collagen, vascular, rheumatic, or autoimmune diseases. One large study found a slight increase in self-reported connective-tissue disease in women with silicone implants. There continues to be a consensus that silicone implants currently in place need not be removed unless specific medical problems or complications develop.

Infections

Infection of breast implants is estimated to occur in only a small percentage of women. Infections require removal of the implant and antibiotic therapy.

Implants and Breast Cancer

There is no evidence that either silicone or saline breast implants are carcinogenic or teratogenic. In a study of 3111 women with breast implants in place, no increase in the frequency of breast carcinomas was observed. A small increased risk of sarcomas was observed.

In the past, if breast carcinoma developed in a woman with implants in place, mastectomy, with or without reconstruction was usually recommended. There is, however, increasing experience with lumpectomy and radiation in women with implants. The risk of infection with breast surgery in the presence of implants is only minimally increased and skin necrosis is rarely a problem after surgery and radiation.

The main complication of radiation therapy in women with breast implants is increased capsule formation and contracture. This may result in increased firmness of the breast and potential migration of the implant. Follow-up monitoring for local recurrence after lumpectomy and radiation is made more difficult by the limitations of physical examination and mammography already discussed. Each woman and her physician must weigh these factors in making their decisions about breast cancer management.

BIBLIOGRAPHY

Baker H, Snedecor P: Clinical trial of danazol for benign breast disease, *Am Surg* 45:727, 1979.

Ballo MS, Sneige N: Can core needle biopsy replace fine-needle aspiration cytology in the diagnosis of palpable breast carcinoma: a comparative study of 124 women, *Cancer* 78:773, 1996.

Berkell H, Birdsell DC, Jenkins H: Breast augmentation: a risk factor for breast cancer? *N Engl J Med* 326:1649, 1992.

Boyd NF et al: Prospective evaluation of physical examination of the breast, *Am J Surg* 142:331, 1981.

Brody GS et al: Consensus statement on the relationship of breast implants to connective-tissue disorders, *Plast Reconstr Surg* 90:1102, 1992.

Brook I: Microbiology of nonpuerperal breast abscesses, *J Infect Dis* 157:377, 1988.

Cady B et al: Evaluation of common breast problems: guidance for primary care providers, *Cancer* 48:49, 1998.

Ciatto S, Cariaggi P, Bulgaresi P: The value of routine cytologic examination of breast cyst fluids, *Acta Cytol* 31:301, 1987.

Deapen DM, Brody GS: Augmentation mammoplasty and breast cancer: a 5-year update of the Los Angeles study, *Plast Reconstr Surg* 89:660, 1992.

Devitt JE: Management of nipple discharge by clinical findings, *Am J Surg* 149:789, 1985.

Fentiman et al: Double-blind controlled trial of tamoxifen therapy for mastalgia, *Lancet* 1:287, 1986.

Food and Drug Administration General and Plastic Surgery Devices Panel Meeting, February 18-20, 1992, Freedom of Information Services Inc documents 100714, 107031, and 107032.

Hamed H et al: Follow-up of patients with aspirated breast cysts is necessary, *Arch Surg* 124:253, 1989.

Hennekens CH et al: Self-reported breast implants and connective-tissue diseases in female health professionals. A retrospective cohort study, *JAMA* 275:616, 1996.

Hughes LE, Bundred NJ: Breast macrocysts, *World J Surg* 13:711, 1989.

Janowsky EC, Kupper LL, Hulka BS: Meta-analysis of the relation between silicone breast implants and the risk of connective-tissue diseases, *N Engl J Med* 342:781, 2000.

Leis HP Jr: Gross breast cysts: significance and management, *Contemp Surg* 39:13, 1991.

Mansel R, Preece P, Hughes L: A double-blind trial of the prolactin inhibitor bromocriptine in painful benign breast disease, *Br J Surg* 65:724, 1978.

Meyer JE et al: Evaluation of nonpalpable solid breast masses with stereotaxic large-needle core biopsy using a dedicated unit, *Am J Roentgenol* 167:179, 1996.

Parker SH et al: Stereotactic breast biopsy with a biopsy gun, *Radiology* 176:741, 1990.

Pashby NL et al: A clinical trial of evening primrose oil in mastalgia, *Br J Surg* 68:801, 1981.

Passaro ME et al: Lactiferous fistula, *J Am Coll Surg* 178:29, 1994.

Petrakis NL: Physiologic, biochemical, and cytologic aspects of nipple aspirate fluid, *Breast Cancer Res Treat* 8:7, 1986.

Rosner D, Baird D: What ultrasonography can tell in breast masses that mammography and physical examination cannot, *J Surg Oncol* 28:308, 1985.

Smith BL: Duct ectasia, periductal mastitis, and breast infections. In Harris JR et al, editors: *Breast diseases,* Philadelphia, 1991, JB Lippincott.

Walker AP et al: A prospective study of the microflora of nonpuerperal breast abscess, *Arch Surg* 123:908, 1988.

Watt-Boolsen S, Eskildsen P, Blaehr H: Release of prolactin, thyrotropin, and growth hormone in women with cyclical mastalgia and fibrocystic disease of the breast, *Cancer* 56:500, 1985.

Wisbey J, Mansel R, Pye J: Natural history of breast pain, *Lancet* 2:672, 1983.

CHAPTER **61**

Use of Medications in Pregnancy and Lactation

Stephanie A. Eisenstat

Prescribing medications for a pregnant or lactating woman can be complicated by the risk of adverse effects on the fetus or in the infant if the mother is breastfeeding. The timing of medication use during pregnancy influences the potential risk. Often primary care clinicians avoid all medications during pregnancy because of fear of harm to the fetus and thus may undertreat certain medical conditions in the pregnant woman.

Difficult decisions—weighing the benefit to the pregnant or lactating woman against the potential risk to the fetus or infant—often must be made in the absence of adequate research data. Toxic effects of medications are most important during the first trimester, when the fetus is developing, and at the time of delivery, when medications may have an adverse effect on the course of labor or result in neonatal depression. Certain medications that are clearly detrimental during pregnancy are safe during the breastfeeding period (e.g., warfarin).

The purpose of this chapter is to summarize the major clinical issues in prescribing classes of medications not discussed elsewhere in this book. For a more detailed discussion of specific medications, the reader is referred to standard references listed at the end of this chapter.

CLASSIFICATION OF MEDICATIONS

There are many problems in evaluating the effects of drugs in pregnancy and in implementing prospective studies. For many medications, research data are available only in animals. Many drugs have been released by the Food and Drug Administration (FDA) for which safety during pregnancy has not yet been established. To assist in the classification of medications, the FDA developed a classification system based on known risk factors for the fetus (Box 61-1).

Category A drugs have been shown to be safe in the first trimester of pregnancy in controlled studies, and the potential harm to the fetus is remote. The actual number of medications that fall into this category is small. **Category B** drugs are commonly used by physicians. For these medications, animal studies have revealed no detrimental effects in the fetus but no controlled studies in pregnant females exist, or detrimental effects found in animal studies have not been

shown in controlled studies in pregnant women. **Category C** drugs are classified as such because animal studies demonstrate clear detrimental effects, but there are no controlled studies in pregnant women. Because of the particular risk to the fetus, these drugs should be given only if potential benefit justifies the risk. **Category D** drugs have been shown to have adverse effects for the fetus but in certain life-saving situations would be considered acceptable for use despite the risk to the fetus. **Category X** drugs are contraindicated in pregnancy because studies in animals and human beings have demonstrated severe fetal risk (Box 61-2). The FDA is proposing revamping the present system of classification to enhance its relevance for clinical practice.

Generally, one should recommend the use of a medication during pregnancy with clear clinical indications and withhold all unnecessary medications. Dosing of drugs may need to be changed for the pregnant female because of the increased volume of distribution and renal and hepatic drug clearance of medications during pregnancy.

TYPES OF MEDICATION
Analgesics

The appropriate medication for pain relief during pregnancy is a common clinical question for the primary care clinician. The pregnant woman may have a mild headache, backache, or other minor discomfort and may request advice on analgesic use. Generally, *acetaminophen (Tylenol)* has been shown to be safe during pregnancy and lactation. Even though it crosses the placenta and is present in breast milk, controlled studies have shown that the levels attained in prescription doses are safe to the fetus. There is potential harm in high doses such as those seen in overdose cases. When given close to the time of delivery, *salicylate (aspirin)* has the potential for increased bleeding abnormalities during labor and in the fetus because of the effect on platelets and the prolongation of the bleeding time (even with small doses). A few studies have suggested the occurrence of fetal malformations from first-trimester exposure, but this conclusion is controversial. The American Academy of Pediatrics recommends caution in prescribing aspirin. In some instances the use of aspirin may outweigh the potential risk, such as in the possible

---

BOX 61-1

Drug Classification System of the Food and Drug Administration

A Controlled studies in women fail to demonstrate risk to fetus in first trimester and fetal harm remote

B Animal reproduction studies have not demonstrated risk to fetus, but no controlled studies in pregnant females; or animal studies have shown effect but no controlled studies in pregnant females

C Animal studies have revealed adverse effects in fetus; no controlled studies in women; *should be given only if potential benefit justifies risk*

D Evidence for fetal risk, but benefits may be acceptable in pregnant females despite risk (e.g., life-saving situation)

X Studies in animals and humans demonstrate fetal risk; contraindicated in pregnancy

Modified from Food and Drug Administration: *Federal Register* 44:37434, 1980.

---

prevention of preeclampsia and the treatment of rheumatoid arthritis during pregnancy. *Ibuprofen* products (Motrin, Naprosyn) have been shown to be safe, but there is potential risk when used during the third trimester because of risk of bleeding (through prolongation of the bleeding time). Prolonged *narcotic* use can be a problem for the fetus because of the risk for respiratory depression or addiction, but in terms of risk for development of fetal malformations, all but codeine are considered safe. *Codeine* has been associated with fetal malformations, including circulatory and cardiac abnormalities, pyloric stenosis, inguinal hernia, and cleft lip and palate, and should be used with caution during pregnancy. *Demerol* is relatively safe and, except for the risk of neonatal depression in higher doses at the time of labor, is acceptable for use during pregnancy. All narcotic medications have abuse potential. Whether the potential for abuse is higher because of the effect of pregnancy on drug metabolism is unknown. Current recommendations for analgesic use are summarized in Table 61-1.

Asthma Medications

For many medications commonly used in the treatment of asthma, the adverse effects on the fetus are unknown. There is no indication that the fetus suffers from serious effects except when exposed to corticosteroids. The potential detrimental effects from corticosteroids during the first trimester are not clearly delineated and may be greater for the oral preparations than for aerosolized forms. In addition, the risk of hypoxia to the fetus from an untreated episode of asthma is probably far greater than the risk from use of the medication during pregnancy. Beta-adrenergic agonists and theophylline are safe for use during pregnancy. A summary of the commonly used medications and recommendations for use appears in Table 61-2. For a more detailed discussion on treatment of asthma in pregnancy see Chapter 70.

Antimicrobial Agents

Most of the commonly used antimicrobial agents such as penicillin, dicloxacillin, and erythromycin (except for erythromycin estolate) are safe during pregnancy. Erythromycin estolate has been associated with cholestatic hepatitis in the

---

BOX 61-2

Drugs Contraindicated in Pregnancy Because of Toxicity and Fetal Risk (Category X)

Alcohol
Fetal alcohol syndrome

Angiotensin-Converting Enzyme Inhibitors
Renal failure in neonates, decreased skull ossification, renal tubular dysgenesis

Cyclophosphamide
Central nervous system (CNS) malformations, secondary cancer

Danazol
Masculinization of female fetuses

Diethylstilbestrol (DES)
Female offspring: anatomic anomalies of genital tract, adenosis, and clear cell carcinoma; increased risk of breast cancer
Male offspring: anatomic abnormalities, reproductive dysfunction, infertility, increased risk of testicular cancer

Disulfiram
Anomalies: vertebral defects, imperforate anus, tracheoesophageal fistula, and radial and renal dysplasia (VATER)

Folic Acid Agonists
Malformations

Isotretinoin
Severe malformations

Lithium
Ebstein's anomaly

Quinine
CNS and limb defects

Trimethadione
Mental retardation, developmental delay, cleft palate/lip, intrauterine growth retardation; cardiac, urogenital, and skeletal abnormalities

Valproic Acid
Neural tube defects, congenital heart disease, facial changes, developmental delay

Warfarin
Skeletal and CNS defects, Dandy-Walker syndrome

Others

Measles, Mumps, Rubella Vaccine (MMR)
Viral transmission to fetus

Radioactive Iodine
Congenital hypothyroidism (cretinism)

Modified from Briggs G, Freeman RK, Yaffe SJ: *Drugs in pregnancy and lactation*, ed 5, Boston, 1999, Lippincott, Williams & Wilkins.

---

pregnant woman and should be avoided. Ciprofloxacin has been shown to be embryotoxic, resulting in arthropathy in animals, and is contraindicated for use during pregnancy and lactation. Many clinicians avoid the use of ciprofloxacin in women of reproductive age because 50% of all pregnancies are unplanned and the detrimental effects of the drug are significant. Other contraindicated antibiotics are tetracycline

Table 61-1
Commonly Used Medications and Their Safety in Pregnancy and Lactation

Drug	Category	Pregnancy/Fetal Risk	RECOMMENDATION FOR USE Pregnancy	RECOMMENDATION FOR USE Breastfeeding
Acetominophen	B	None in prescribed doses	Safe	Safe
Aspirin (during third trimester)	C	Possible fetal malformations	Caution	Caution
	D	Increased risk of neonatal hemorrhage		
Ibuprofen	B	None known	Safe	Safe
During third trimester	D			
Oxycodone	B	None	Safe	Caution
With prolonged use	D	Neonatal depression		
Codeine	C	Cardiac, circulatory malformations, pyloric stenosis inguinal hernia, cleft lip/palate	Caution	Caution
High dose at term	D	Neonatal depression	Safe	Safe
Demerol	B	Neonatal depression		

Modified from Berkowitz R, Mochizuki T: *Handbook for prescribing medications during pregnancy*, ed 3, Boston, 1998, Lippincott Williams & Wilkins Publishers; and Briggs GC, Freeman RK, Yaffe SJ: *Drugs in pregnancy and lactation*, ed 5, Boston, 1999, Lippincott Williams & Wilkins Publishers.

Table 61-2
Commonly Used Antiasthmatic Medications and Their Safety in Pregnancy and Lactation

Drug	Category	Pregnancy/Fetal Risk	RECOMMENDATION FOR USE Pregnancy	RECOMMENDATION FOR USE Breastfeeding
Beta adrenergic agonists	C	None	Safe	Safe
Steroid inhalers	C	Unknown	Use if medically indicated	Unknown
Oral steroids	C	Unknown	Use if medically indicated	Unknown
Cromolyn	B	None	Safe	Safe
Ipratropium (Atrovent)	B	None	Safe	Safe
Theophylline	C	None	Safe	Safe

Modified from Berkowitz R, Mochizuki T: *Handbook for prescribing medications during pregnancy*, ed 3, Boston, 1998, Lippincott Williams & Wilkins Publishers; and Briggs GC, Freeman RK, Yaffe SJ: *Drugs in pregnancy and lactation*, ed 5, Boston, 1999, Lippincott Williams & Wilkins Publishers.

(which causes dental dysplasia and inhibition of bone growth in the fetus) and trimethoprim-sulfamethoxazole (which is teratogenic in rats and increases the risk of kernicterus and hemolysis in the newborn). Antituberculous medications are all embryocidal in animals, but the benefit of treating active tuberculosis in the pregnant woman clearly outweighs the risk to the fetus. Zidovudine (AZT) used to prevent vertical transmission of human immunodeficiency virus from mother to fetus is safe in pregnancy. Recommendations for antibiotic use during pregnancy appear in Table 61-3.

Anticoagulation Therapy

Heparin does not cross the placenta and is therefore safe for use during pregnancy with respect to the fetus. *Warfarin (Coumadin)*, however, is not safe and is associated with the fetal warfarin embryopathy syndrome. Treatment of thromboembolic disorders of pregnancy is reviewed in Chapter 77. Unlike its use in pregnancy, Coumadin is the drug of choice during the breastfeeding period and does not pose undue threat to the fetus.

Anticonvulsant Therapy

Treatment of seizure disorders is complicated in the pregnant woman because there are no safe anticonvulsant thera-

pies. Physicians experienced in the management of these disorders should oversee anticonvulsant therapy during pregnancy. It is important to treat seizure disorders during pregnancy because of the risk of hypoxia to the fetus during a seizure. *Carbamazepine (Tegretol)* is considered the safest of the anticonvulsant therapies but is associated with multiple abnormalities, including craniofacial abnormalities, intrauterine growth retardation, microcephaly, and fingernail hypoplasia. *Phenytoin (Dilantin)* is associated with major birth defects as is *valproic acid (Depakene)*. The use of these medications in pregnancy is summarized in Table 61-4.

Antidepressant Therapy

Approximately 8% to 20 % of women suffer form depression. Older antidepressants such as amitryptiline (Elavil) have been associated with limb malformations. However, if treatment is clinically indicated, the newer selective serotonin reuptake inhibitors (SSRIs) appear to be safe for use in pregnancy. In a study by Chambers, the rate of spontaneous pregnancy loss did not differ significantly between women treated with fluoxetine and control women; a study by Goldstein supported the safety of this medication. More recent reports from seven teratogen centers in North America found no increased rate of malformations in women who

Table 61-3
Commonly Used Antimicrobial Agents and Their Safety in Pregnancy and Lactation

| Drug | Category | Pregnancy/Fetal Risk | RECOMMENDATION FOR USE | |
			Pregnancy	Breastfeeding
Antibacterial Agents				
Penicillins	B	None	Safe	Safe
Dicloxacillin	B	None	Safe	Safe
Erythromycin				
Estolate	B	Cholestatic hepatitis in mother	Contraindicated	Safe
Others	B	None	Safe	Safe
Cephalosporins	B	None	Safe	Safe
Trimethoprim-sulfamethoxazole	C	Folate antagonism; teratogenic in rats; hemolysis in newborn; increased risk of kenicterus; teratogenic in animals	Use other options	Safe
Quinolones	C	Arthropathy in animals	Contraindicated	Contraindicated
Aminoglycosides	C	Eighth nerve toxicity	Use other options	Contraindicated
Tetracycline	D	Tooth discoloration and dysplasia; inhibition of bone growth in fetus	Contraindicated	Contraindicated
Vancomycin	C	Unknown—possible auditory and renal	Use other options	Contraindicated
Metronidazole	B	Unknown	Contraindicated in first trimester; safe in second and third trimesters	Safe
Antituberculous Medications				
Isoniazid	C	Embryocidal	Caution	Caution
Rifampin	C	Teratogenic in animals	Caution	Caution
Ethambutol	B	None known—teratogenic in animals	Caution	Caution
Antiviral Agents				
Zidovudine	C	Unknown, but no apparent effects		

Modified from Berkowitz R, Mochizuki T: *Handbook for prescribing medications during pregnancy,* ed 3, Boston, 1998, Lippincott Williams & Wilkins Publishers; and Briggs GC, Freeman RK, Yaffe SJ: *Drugs in pregnancy and lactation,* ed 5, Boston, 1999, Lippincott Williams & Wilkins Publishers.

Table 61-4
Commonly Used Anticonvulsant Medications and Their Safety in Pregnancy and Lactation

| Drug | Category | Pregnancy/Fetal Risk | RECOMMENDATION FOR USE | |
			Pregnancy	Breastfeeding
Dilantin	D	Major birth defects, fetal hydantoin syndrome	Contraindicated	Caution
Phenobarbital	D	Risk of cleft palate and congenital heart disease; hemorrhagic disease in newborn	Contraindicated	Caution
Tegretol	C	Craniofacial abnormalities, IUGR, microcephaly, fingernail hypoplasia	Contraindicated	Caution
Valproic acid	X	Multiple malformations	Contraindicated	Safe

Modified from Berkowitz R, Mochizuki T: *Handbook for prescribing medications during pregnancy,* ed 3, Boston, 1998, Lippincott Williams & Wilkins Publishers. Briggs GC, Freeman RK, Yaffe SJ: *Drugs in pregnancy and lactation,* ed 5, Boston, 1999, Lippincott Williams & Wilkins Publishers.
IUGR, Intrauterine growth retardation.

took other SSRIs during pregnancy including clomipramine, paroxetine, and sertraline.

Nonprescription Medications

Frequently pregnant women ask the primary care clinician about the safety of nonprescription medications. Most over-the-counter preparations are safe during pregnancy with the exception of certain antihistamines, aspirin, nonsteroidal antiinflammatory drugs (as previously described), certain antiacids, and cathartics. The safety of commonly used nonprescription medications is summarized in Table 61-5.

Treating Dyspepsia and Nausea

The common medications used to treat dyspepsia, antiacids, cimetidine (*Tagamet*), ranitidine (*Zantac*), and famotidine (*Pepcid*) are all FDA category B and considered safe

Table 61-5
Commonly Used Nonprescription Medications and Their Safety During Pregnancy

Drug	TOXICITY DURING PREGNANCY	
	First Trimester	**Second and Third Trimesters**
Analgesics		
Acetaminophen (Tylenol)	Safe in recommended dose	Safe
Salicylates (aspirin)	Rare reports of malformations	Increased risk of neonatal hemorrhage
Ibuprofen (Motrin)	Safe	Risk of premature labor
Antihistamines*		
Dimenhydrinate (Dramamine)	Possibly teratogenic	Liver toxicity in fetus, premature labor
Diphenhydramine (Benadryl)	Oral clefts	
Clorpheniramine (Chlor-Trimeton)	Probably safe	Same as Dramamine
Pseudoephedrine (Sudafed)	Inguinal hernia, club foot	Safe
Bulk-forming Agents		
Agar, bran, methycellulose, psyllium	Safe	Safe
Belladonna Alkaloids	Safe	Safe
Cathartics		
Contact		
Antracene	—	All but aloe safe; aloe stimulates fetal
Aloe, cascara, senna		intestines, resulting increased meconium
Castor oil, bisacodyl	Safe	Safe
Saline		
Magnesium salts, Milk of magnesia epsom salts	Safe	Safe
Mineral Oil	Contraindicated	Contraindicated
Simethicone	Safe	Safe
Antacids		
Aluminum hydroxide	Risk of malformations	Safe
Calcium carbonate	Safe	Risk of fetal hypomagnesemia
Magnesium compounds	Unknown	Risk of fetal hypomagnesemia
Sodium bicarbonate	Contraindicated	Contraindicated because of increase in edema
Sympathomimetics		
Ephedrine, phenylephrine	Safe	Safe
Antitussive Agent		
Dextromethorphan	Safe	Safe

Modified from Berkowitz R, Mochizuki T: *Handbook for prescribing medications during pregnancy*, ed 3, Boston, 1998, Lippincott Williams & Wilkins Publishers.
*Inhibit lactation.

during pregnancy. Metoclopramide (*Reglan*) is a safe option for treating the nausea and gastroparesis associated with pregnancy.

BIBLIOGRAPHY

ACOG, ACAAI: The use of newer asthma and allergy medications during pregnancy. The American College of Obstetricians and gynecologists and the American College of Allergy, Asthma and Immunology, *Ann Allergy Asthma Immunol* 84:475, 2000.

ACOG educational bulletin. Antimicrobial therapy for obstetric patients. Number 245, March 1998, *Int J Gynaecol Obstet* 61:299, 1998.

Berkowitz R, Mochizuki T: *Handbook for prescribing medications during pregnancy*, ed 3, Boston, 1998, Lippincott, Williams & Wilkins.

Briggs GC, Freeman RK, Yaffe SJ: *Drugs in pregnancy and lactation*, ed 5, Boston, 1999, Lippincott, Williams & Wilkins.

Cefalo R, Moos M: *Preconceptional health care: a practical guide*, St Louis, 1995, Mosby.

Chambers CD et al: Birth outcomes in pregnant women taking fluoxetine, *N Engl J Med* 335:1010, 1996.

Cunningham FG et al: *Williams obstetrics*, ed 20, New York, 1997, McGraw-Hill Professional Publishing.

Duff P: Antibiotic selection on obstetric patients, *Infect Dis Clin North Am* 11:1, 1997.

Goldstein DJ, Corbin LA, Sundell KL: Effects of first trimester exposure on the newborn, *Obstet Gynecol* 89:713, 1997.

Hollingworth DR, Resnik R: *Medical counseling before pregnancy*, New York, 1988, Churchill Livingstone.

Ito S: Drug therapy for breastfeeding women, *N Engl JMed* 343:118, 2000.

Koren G, Pastuszak A, Ito S.: Drugs in pregnancy, *N Engl J Med* 338:1128, 1998.

Kulin N et al: Pregnancy outcome following maternal use of the new selective serotonin reuptake inhibitors. A prospective controlled multicenter study, *JAMA* 279:609, 1998.

Lawrence RA: *Breastfeeding: a guide for the medical profession,* ed 5, St Louis, 1998, Mosby.

Pastuszak AL et al: Pregnancy outcome following first trimester exposure to fluoxetine (Prozac), *JAMA* 269:2246, 1993.

Rayburn WF, Zuspan FP: *Drug therapy in obstetrics and gynecology,* ed 3, St Louis, 1992, Mosby.

Sontheimer DL, Ables AZ: Safety of antidepressant medications during pregnancy, *JAMA* 283:1139, 2000.

Wisner KL et al: Pharmacologic treatment of depression during pregnancy, *JAMA* 282:1264, 1999.

CHAPTER 62

Pregnancy in the Older Woman

Linda J. Heffner

▦ EPIDEMIOLOGY

Deliveries by older women have risen dramatically in the United States over the last 25 years, with a 460% increase in first births to women over 30 years of age since 1975. By 1998, 23% of first births and 35% of all births occurred in women over age 30 and 7% of first births and 13% of all births occurred in women over age 35. These high rates are expected to continue through at least the year 2010 when the youngest of the baby boomers reach menopause. Although the absolute numbers of women aged 30 to 44 have increased by 60% since 1970, the decision to delay childbearing until after the age of 30 has largely been responsible for the increase in births to older mothers.

In 1950 the term *elderly primigravida* was first used to describe a woman whose first birth occurs after her 35th birthday. In a landmark paper Waters and colleagues first raised the notion that pregnancy is a perilous journey, fraught with maternal and fetal risk, for the older parturient. Unfortunately for many older women contemplating bearing their first child, the notion that delayed childbearing was blatantly risky, even for healthy women, was widespread. Careful review of the literature on pregnancy outcome among older gravidas indicates that it can be quite good when the true risks are understood and managed. In this chapter each purported risk will be examined critically. Recommendations for addressing the real risks will conclude the discussion.

INFERTILITY

Actual fertility rates, defined as number of live births per 1000 women of the same age, have been increasing since the 1970s for women aged 30 to 39 as a result of the demographic characteristics of delayed childbearing. More accurately it is *fecundity,* or the ability of a couple to establish a pregnancy within a year, that appears to decline with age. This age-related decline in fecundity combined with the clinical definition of infertility (the inability of a couple to conceive despite 1 year of effort) results in a threefold increase in infertility rates in women over age 35 compared with women aged 20 to 29.

Because fecundity can be influenced by deliberate fertility control, it is necessary to study populations seeking pregnancies to evaluate the impact of age on fecundity. These populations can also suffer from conditions limiting fertility that may or may not be independent of age. Nonetheless, most studies do demonstrate a decline in fecundity with advancing maternal age that appears largely to be the result of a decline in oocyte quality. A decline in endometrial responsiveness to steroid hormones leading to implantation problems was earlier thought to be a major factor in age-related reproductive failure, but has not been documented. No age-related decline in fertility rates was found in women in their 40s undergoing in vitro fertilization (IVF) with oocytes donated by younger women.

Indeed, it is the high success rates of donor egg IVF in older women that has led to a recent and dramatic rise in the number of women over the age of 45 years giving birth. In 1998, the second year for which national statistics are available for women over age 50, 158 births were reported in women aged 50-54 years and 3624 in women aged 45-49 years. Accompanying this rise in births has been a disproportionate rise in the rate of multiple gestations among older gravidas due to the use of fertility treatments coupled with the spontaneous increase in twinning that occurs as women age. From 1980 to 1982 and 1996 to 1998, the twin birth rate rose from 22 to 38 per 1,000 (77% increase) among women aged 40 to 44 years and from 11 to 130 per 1000 in women aged 45 to 49 years. The triplet and higher order multiple birth rate rose from 59 to 332 per 100,000 (461% increase) in women in their 30s while rising 15-fold among women in their 40s (28 to 412 per 100,000 births).

MISCARRIAGE

Miscarriage (spontaneous abortion in the first half of pregnancy) is a common event, occurring in at least 15% of recognized pregnancies. More than 60% of first-trimester miscarriages are chromosomally abnormal. It is not surprising, therefore, that the miscarriage rate increases as the risk of chromosomal abnormalities increases with maternal age. Numerous studies have confirmed this finding; however, an increase in first-trimester spontaneous abortions of chromosomally normal (euploid) conceptions appears to occur in women over 35 as well. Unfortunately, gravidity, pregnancy order, and number of prior miscarriages, which affect miscarriage rates, were not adjusted for in this study. In a study of 3500 female British physicians, miscarriage rates increased with gravidity at the younger ages and decreased with pregnancy order with increasing age. This would argue against an age effect on euploid miscarriage. The investigators noted that the interval leading up to a miscarriage tended to be longer than that leading up to a live birth, suggesting that women whose first pregnancy miscarries may be older because of a more difficult time conceiving. An alternative explanation is that pregnancies preceded by a long interval are more likely to miscarry because the women are older. A progressive increase in spontaneous losses also occurs with increasing numbers of previous miscarriages to the point where women with three or more previous miscarriages suffer a threefold increase in the age-adjusted incidence of miscarriage.

Thus older women do have a clearly increased risk of aneuploid miscarriage and may have an increased risk of euploid miscarriage that probably results either from a nonchromosomal decline in oocyte quality or from enrichment by a population of recurrent spontaneous abortors who age as they continue to miscarry.

CHROMOSOMAL ABNORMALITIES

Chromosomal abnormalities in the conceptuses of older women are probably the best documented and most widely recognized risk of delayed childbearing. Karyotypes supporting the increased risk of aneuploidy come from multiple sources: miscarriages, induced abortions, midtrimester amniocenteses, liveborn infants, and stillbirths. All indicate a steadily increasing risk of chromosomal abnormalities throughout a woman's lifetime such that by the time she is 45 years old, she carries a 1:21 risk of an aneuploid fetus at delivery. Table 62-1 is an example of a risk chart used for genetic counseling of older women; the age entered for an individual woman is her age on her due date. The biologic basis for the increase in chromosomal abnormalities with increasing age is thought to be related to the fact that oocytes reach metaphase of meiosis I at about 5 months post conception and remain aligned on the metaphase plate throughout a woman's reproductive life until the oocyte is stimulated to divide just before ovulation. Over time the risk of nondisjunction, or the failure of the chromosomes to divide equally, increases.

CONGENITAL MALFORMATIONS

Although earlier evidence suggested an increased risk of nonchromosomal congenital malformations among the offspring of older mothers, more recent investigations have not confirmed this finding. In the largest early study, facial clefts, cardiac malformations, anorectal defects, and hypospadias were reported in a larger proportion of firstborn infants of mothers over 40 years of age than in those of younger mothers. The major limitation of this study, conducted from 1961 to 1966, is that chromosomal evaluation of the abnormal children was not possible. Although the investigators did exclude those infants with clinically apparent Down syndrome,

Table 62-1
Age-Specific Risks for Chromosomal Abnormalities in Liveborn Infants

Maternal Age at Delivery	Risk of Down Syndrome	Risk of Any Chromosomal Abnormality*
20	1/1667	1/526
22	1/1429	1/500
24	1/1250	1/476
26	1/1176	1/476
27	1/1111	1/455
28	1/1053	1/435
29	1/1000	1/417
30	1/952	1/385
31	1/909	1/385
32	1/769	1/322
33	1/602	1/286
34	1/485	1/238
35	1/378	1/192
36	1/289	1/156
37	1/224	1/127
38	1/173	1/102
39	1/136	1/83
40	1/106	1/66
41	1/82	1/53
42	1/63	1/42
43	1/49	1/33
44	1/38	1/26
45	1/30	1/21
46	1/23	1/16
47	1/18	1/13
48	1/14	1/10
49	1/11	1/8

Data modified from the maternal age-specific rates derived by Hook EB, Cross PK, Schreinemachers DM: *JAMA* 249:2034, 1983; Hook EB: *Obstet Gynecol* 58:282, 1981.
*Excludes 46,XXX for ages 20-32 because data are not available.

which is associated with cardiac defects, this genetic disorder may not be clinically apparent at birth. Several trisomies, as well as other chromosomal abnormalities, also can be associated with cardiac defects and facial clefts.

Recently 26,859 live-born children in British Columbia were surveyed for birth defects not associated with chromosomal abnormalities, single gene defects, maternal diabetes, alcoholism, or teratogen exposure. No increase in any of 43 birth defect categories was found for older mothers.

LOW BIRTH WEIGHT

The incidence of low birth weight (<2500 g) has been repeatedly shown to be higher in older than in younger gravidas; however, low birth weight can result from either prematurity or decreased intrauterine growth. The causes and long-term consequences of these two sources of low birth weight are quite different. Many of the early studies addressing maternal age and birth weight failed to distinguish between the two types of small infants. More recent studies indicate that the risk of having a premature infant does not appear to increase substantially with advanced maternal age if the data are controlled for the effects of multiple gestation on the prematurity rate. Twins, triplets, and higher order multiple gestations are at significantly elevated risk for delivering prematurely (4% of singleton births, 42% of twins, and 89% of triplets and higher order multiples delivered prematurely in 1998).

Low birth weight resulting from inadequate intrauterine growth has been even less well studied than prematurity, but the rate would appear to be increased with maternal age. A group of 127 Canadian women delivering after the age of 40 were found to have an 11% incidence of small-for-dates infants compared with 2% in women under 25. In a larger study of pregnancy outcomes in 4463 Swedish women aged 35 to 39 years, rates of low birth weight term infants were increased in the primigravid patients. Among well-educated, mostly white women in New York City over age 35, a 5% incidence of small-for-dates infants did not differ from that of the younger control subjects. Hypertension, which is a risk factor for low birth weight, has an increased incidence in older mothers (see later discussion), suggesting that the proportion of hypertensive women in the study population may influence the incidence of small-for-gestational-age infants. Cigarette smoking, a type of environmental exposure that can diminish intrauterine growth, has a more profound effect in older mothers. In light of the high proportion of studies that have reported an increase in births of low birth weight infants and the minimal change in the prematurity rate, more attention to fetal growth as a pregnancy outcome in older gravidas is warranted.

PERINATAL MORTALITY

Perinatal mortality is the sum of two components, fetal deaths in the second half of pregnancy (stillbirths) and neonatal deaths. Almost all large, controlled studies have shown an increased perinatal mortality rate with advancing maternal age such that women in their late 30s have a twofold risk that increases to a fourfold risk by age 45. The increase is essentially limited to stillbirths.

There are several explanations for the increased stillbirth rates in older mothers. First, older women have an increased incidence of medical complications, especially hypertension and diabetes, which can cause abnormal fetal growth and predispose to antenatal asphyxia and intrauterine death (see Medical Complications). In older black women with hypertension, perinatal mortality rate was substantially higher than that attributable to either age or hypertension alone. Healthy older gravidas experienced minimal increases in perinatal loss. Second, older women are at increased risk for fetal chromosomal abnormalities and chromosomally abnormal fetuses are at increased risk for fetal death in utero. Most older studies of perinatal outcome among older women did not control for the increased prevalence of chromosomally abnormal fetuses in that population.

Recently Fretts et al. reviewed stillbirth rates as a function of maternal age in a large cohort of Canadian women between 1961 and 1993. Over the 33-year interval, the stillbirth rate declined by more than 70%, in spite of increases in the reported prevalence of medical conditions that are associated with increased risk of fetal death. In the face of the declining stillbirth rate, advancing maternal age remained associated with an increased risk of stillbirth even after controlling for lethal anomalies, multiple gestation, hypertension, diabetes mellitus, placenta previa, placental abruption, previous abortion, and previous fetal death. In the most recent interval studied (1990–1993), women aged 35 to 39 years had almost twice the risk of stillbirth compared with women under age 30, whereas women 40 years and older had 2.4 times the risk. The exact causes of the additional stillbirths could not be determined, and hence the potential role of antepartum fetal surveillance in their prevention could not be ascertained.

The safety of allowing older women to carry their pregnancies past the 42nd week of gestation (postdates) has been investigated in a small number of pregnancies. Although there was no indication of antepartum fetal compromise before arrival on the labor suite, significantly more low 1-minute Apgar scores, intrapartum decelerations, and cesarean deliveries occurred in women over age 35. Five-minute Apgar scores of neonatal intensive care admissions did not differ between the older and younger parturients. Interestingly, in a much larger Swedish study of older gravidas, significantly fewer women over age 35 delivered at or after the 40th week of gestation compared to the 20- to 24-year-old control population. Current data support the induction of women between the 41st and 42nd week of gestation regardless of maternal age.

MEDICAL COMPLICATIONS

Hypertension

In most studies of hypertension in pregnancy, chronic hypertension, pregnancy-induced hypertension, and preeclampsia are all grouped together. All hypertensive disorders appear to be increased in older gravidas. All but two small studies of pregnant women over age 35 have shown at least a twofold elevation in risk for hypertensive complications for the older women regardless of parity. In the two largest studies, of 36,482 and 41,798 women, preeclampsia rates in women over 40 were double those in women under 30. Very significant increases in the frequency of all hypertensive disorders from 3% between ages 20 and 30 to 10% over age 40 have been reported. Since preeclampsia is more common in first pregnancies, the overall increase in hypertension with age is sustained by multiparas with chronic hypertension. In the latter study the increase in hypertensive complications was associated with maternal obesity.

Diabetes

Like that of hypertension, the prevalence of diabetes mellitus increases with advancing age. The incidence of gestational diabetes rises from a low of 0.3% to 2% in younger women to 1% to 4% in nulliparous women over 35. Again obesity and parity are additive risk factors. Although insulin-dependent diabetes antedating pregnancy is associated with increased rates of perinatal morbidity and mortality, it is unclear whether gestational diabetes is associated with additional fetal risk in older mothers. Gestational diabetes is associated with increased risk of large infants, which may predispose to more difficult labors and the risk of birth injury. Infants with birth weight over 4000 g are found in higher proportions among older gravidas; parity, obesity, and diabetes appear to account for most, but not all, of the excess.

OBSTETRIC COMPLICATIONS
Abnormal Bleeding

Bleeding in the third trimester can result from either placenta previa or placental abruption; such bleeding appears to occur about twice as frequently in older primigravidas. Women of any age who are hypertensive during pregnancy are at increased risk for a placental abruption; no measure of the independent contribution of maternal age is available. Postpartum hemorrhage in older women appears to be largely restricted to the multiparous patient.

Delivery Difficulties

Every study since 1963 reporting the incidence of cesarean section in women 35 years or older compared to those in their 20s has shown an increase of at least 70% in the older gravidas. Some of the increase may result from a decreased ability of the fetuses of older mothers to tolerate labor; however, the strong positive association between cesarean section and maternal age persists after adjustment for induction of labor, epidural anesthesia, meconium staining of the amniotic fluid, and fetal distress. In one study, advanced maternal age was the stated reason that 31% of the older women had primary cesarean section. It is not certain whether these higher cesarean section rates result from physiologic changes or from physician beliefs that somehow the infants of older women are more "precious" than those of younger women.

Maternal Death

Maternal death rates increase with maternal age, largely as a result of obstetric complications of high parity and of indirect deaths resulting from underlying medical problems. Fortunately unlike fetal death, maternal death is a very rare complication of pregnancy, which had dropped to less than 8/100,000 live births by the mid-1980s compared to perinatal mortality, which has averaged 18/1000 total births between 1982 and 1992. Maternal death rates among women aged 35 and older are double those of 25-year-olds and quadruple by age 45. Nonwhite race is a more significant risk for maternal death than age, beginning at age 20. Healthy women over 35 who desire a baby should not be concerned about having a greater risk of dying than their younger counterparts because of the rarity of maternal death.

COUNSELING THE OLDER GRAVIDA

In older women with preexisting medical conditions, counseling should be individualized to the specific medical problems encountered. Hypertension is among the most commonly encountered medical problems. These women carry a disproportionate amount of the risk for an adverse pregnancy outcome. This is largely manifested as higher perinatal morbidity and mortality rates from low birth weight that result from either prematurity or poor intrauterine growth. Maternal health is infrequently directly affected.

For the healthy, motivated woman who delays childbearing until after age 35, the likelihood of a good outcome is high with careful attention to the areas of greatest risk. Increasing clinical experience shows that the prospect of a good outcome can be extended to include healthy women in their late 40s and early 50s with such attention. The following specific points are useful in counseling older gravidas about delayed childbearing.

First, a delay in successful establishment of a pregnancy may result from the modest decline in fecundity with advancing maternal age. The presence of the "biologic reproductive clock" may be felt acutely by these women. It is generally recommended that older couples who have been trying unsuccessfully for 6 months to establish a pregnancy seek the advice of a medical professional. Although many will delay the start of complete infertility testing until a full year has passed, several simple tests of sperm quality and ovulatory capacity can be performed early. Ovulation induction and assisted reproduction techniques such as IVF are associated with a high rate of multiple gestation. Multiple gestations in older women should be managed by an obstetrician with expertise in the area.

Second, the risk of chromosomal abnormalities clearly increases with advancing maternal age. Fetal karyotyping after amniocentesis or chorionic villus sampling should be offered to all women age 35 and over. It is important in counseling not to equate use of prenatal diagnosis with willingness to undergo pregnancy termination for positive results, as this is not the only option available to couples with chromosomally abnormal fetuses. Adoptive families are available for children born with chromosomal abnormalities if the biologic parents feel they would not be able to raise the child themselves but do not wish to terminate the pregnancy. Pregnancies conceived with donor eggs carry the risk of the donor, not the recipient.

Third, all women age 35 and older should be screened for gestational diabetes by using a 50-g oral glucose challenge. A plasma glucose value greater than 140 mg/dl should be followed by a diagnostic 3-hour glucose tolerance test. If the woman is obese a screen should be performed at the initial prenatal visit and again at 24 to 28 weeks of gestation even if the initial screen finding is negative. Normal-weight women should be screened at 24 to 28 weeks of gestation.

Liberal use of ultrasound and antepartum testing is appropriate if obstetric complications develop or abnormal fetal growth is suspected. Cigarette smoking should be discouraged; fetal growth should be carefully monitored in older women who continue to smoke. There is no information on the usefulness of routine antepartum surveillance in preventing stillbirth in healthy older women with normally grown fetuses. Intrapartum electronic fetal monitoring in labor is reasonable for all older women.

Finally the need for genetic counseling, glucose screening, and careful surveillance and treatment for obstetric complications in all older women is likely to mean more interaction with the health care system than some women anticipate. Anxiety and disappointment later in pregnancy can be minimized if women are counseled about the expected content of their prenatal care and are prepared for this in advance.

BIBLIOGRAPHY

Atrash HK et al: Maternal mortality in the United States, 1979-1986, *Obstet Gynecol* 76:1055, 1990.

Baird PA, Sadovnick AD, Yee IML: Maternal age and birth defects: a population study, *Lancet* 337:527, 1991.

Berkowitz GS et al: Delayed childbearing and the outcome of pregnancy, *N Engl J Med* 322:659, 1990.

Cnattinguis S et al: Smoking, maternal age, and fetal growth, *Obstet Gynecol* 66:449, 1985.

Federation CECOS, Schwartz D, Mayaux MJ: Female fecundity as a function of age, *N Engl J Med* 306:404, 1982.

Forman MR, Meirik O, Berendes HW: Delayed childbearing in Sweden, *JAMA* 252:3135, 1984.

Fretts RC et al: Increased maternal age and the risk of fetal death, *N Engl J Med* 333:953, 1995.

Grimes DA, Gross GK: Pregnancy outcomes in black women aged 35 and older, *Obstet Gynecol* 58:614, 1981.

Hansen JP: Older maternal age and pregnancy outcome: a review of the literature, *Obstet Gynecol Surv* 41:726, 1986.

Harlop S, Shiono PH, Ramcharan S: A life table of spontaneous abortions and the effect of age, parity, and other variables. In Porter IH, Hook EB, editors: *Embryonic and fetal death,* New York, 1980, Academic Press.

Hay S, Barbano H: Independent effects of maternal age and birth order on the incidence of selected congenital malformations, *Teratology* 6:271, 1972.

Hook EB, Cross PK, Schreinemachers DM: Chromosomal abnormality rates at amniocentesis and in live-born infants, *JAMA* 249:2034, 1983.

Hook EB: Rates of chromosomal abnormalities at different maternal ages, *Obstet Gynecol* 58:282, 1981.

Kajii T et al: Anatomic and chromosomal anomalies in 639 spontaneous abortuses, *Hum Genet* 55:87, 1980.

Kajonoia P, Widholm: Pregnancy and delivery in women aged 40 and over, *Obstet Gynecol* 51:47, 1978.

Kane SH: Advancing age and the primigravida, *Obstet Gynecol* 29:409, 1967.

Kirz DS, Dorchester W, Freeman RK: Advanced maternal age: the mature gravida, *Am J Obstet Gynecol* 152:7, 1985.

Lehman DK, Chism J: Pregnancy outcome in medically complicated and uncomplicated patients aged 40 years or older, *Am J Obstet Gynecol* 157:738, 1987.

Machin GA: Chromosome abnormality and perinatal death, *Lancet* 1:549, 1974.

Martel M et al: Maternal age and primary cesarean section rates: a multivariate analysis, *Am J Obstet Gynecol* 156:305, 1987.

Morrison I: The elderly primigravida, *Am J Obstet Gynecol* 121:465, 1975.

Navot D et al: Poor oocyte quality rather than implantation failure as a cause of age-related decline in female fertility, *Lancet* 337:1375, 1991.

Postponed childbearing—United States, 1970-1987, *JAMA* 263:360, 1990.

Roman E, Alberman E: Spontaneous abortion, gravidity, pregnancy order, age and pregnancy interval. In Porter IH, Hook EB, editors: *Embryonic and fetal death,* New York, 1980, Academic Press.

Sauer MV, Paulson RJ, Lobo RA: Reversing the natural decline in human fertility, *JAMA* 268:1275, 1992.

Shapiro H, Lyons E: Late maternal age and postdate pregnancy, *Am J Obstet Gynecol* 160:909, 1989.

Spellacy WN, Miller SJ, Winegar A: Pregnancy after 40 years of age, *Obstet Gynecol* 68:452, 1986.

Stein Z et al: Maternal age and spontaneous abortion. In Porter IH, Hook EB, editors: *Embryonic and fetal death,* New York, 1980, Academic Press.

Stovall DW et al: The effect of age on female fecundity, *Obstet Gynecol* 77:33, 1991.

Tuck SM, Yudkin PL, Turnbull AC: Pregnancy outcome in elderly primigravidae with and without a history of infertility, *Br J Obstet Gynecol* 95:230, 1988.

Tysoe FW: Effect of age on the outcome of pregnancy, *Trans Pacific Coast Obstet Gynecol Soc* 38:8, 1970.

Ventura SJ et al: Births: final data for 1998, *Natl Vital Stat Reports* 48:1, 2000.

Waters EG, Wager HP: Pregnancy and labor experiences of elderly primigravidas, *Am J Obstet Gynecol* 59:296, 1950.

CHAPTER 63

Preconception Counseling and Nutrition

Stephanie A. Eisenstat

Good prenatal care may reduce the risk for obstetric complications and result in improved pregnancy outcome. Although not all causes of low birth weight, infant mortality, and obstetric complications can be prevented, risk for certain birth defects can be markedly decreased if women of reproductive age receive preconception counseling as well as prenatal care. Supplementation of folate before conception can decrease the risk of fetal neural tube defects. Abstinence from alcohol can prevent fetal alcohol syndrome, and cessation of smoking can decrease the risk of intrauterine growth retardation. Cocaine use has been associated with congenital anomalies and birth complications. Prevention needs to start before the woman becomes pregnant.

It is important for the primary care clinician to discuss ways to improve pregnancy outcome with all women of reproductive age who may become pregnant. The effort at risk reduction before and during pregnancy involves collaboration between the obstetrician-gynecologist and primary care clinician and should be a continuous process that occurs at each visit for routine preventive care and, it is hoped, before and during pregnancy.

The essential components of preconception care in the primary care setting encompass risk assessment, health promotion, and intervention. Specific areas for preconception counseling are outlined in Box 63-1. This chapter summarizes aspects of preconception counseling in nutrition, substance abuse, alcoholism, and smoking. Other components of preconception care include the identification and treatment of women at risk for adverse psychologic outcomes (see Chapters 80 and 81), domestic violence (see Chapter 87), for preventable infectious diseases such as human immunodeficiency virus (HIV) (see Chapter 21), hepatitis, rubella, and toxoplasmosis (see Chapter 67), and for medical conditions such as hypertension and diabetes (see Chapters 3 and 11). The key recommendations for preconception counseling are summarized in Table 63-1.

NUTRITION AND VITAMIN SUPPLEMENTATION

The nutritional status of a woman has an impact on maternal and fetal health throughout pregnancy. Women who are underweight before conception have a higher risk of low-birth-weight infants. The first trimester is the time when critical development of the fetus occurs; normal development depends partially on adequate maternal nutrition. An accurate assessment of a woman's nutritional status is important in identifying women at risk.

Nutritional Assessment

History

The first goal is to assess whether the woman is adhering to a balanced diet. The basic food groups and components of a healthy diet are covered in Chapter 85 and listed in Table 63-2. Dietary practices that potentially carry additional risk to the fetus include pica (ingestion of nonnutritional substances, most commonly dirt or clay), bulimia and anorexia, specific dietary restrictions, vegetarianism, vitamin and mineral supplementation, and lactose intolerance. Each of these clinical situations affects the woman's ability to maintain an adequately balanced diet and is an indication for further nutritional counseling and more active monitoring during pregnancy.

Physical Examination

Expected weight for height can be estimated by use of standard charts as appear in the Appendix and guidelines for weight gain during pregnancy (Box 63-2). Although these estimates consist of averages, they serve as a baseline as the practitioner sets goals with the patient. If a woman falls above or below the range for ideal body weight, alteration in dietary patterns may be warranted. If the clinician has a concern about the patient, more intensive evaluation by a nutritional expert should be arranged.

Diagnostic Tests

Iron deficiency anemia is common among menstruating women. As the iron demands of pregnancy increase, it is also common to develop iron deficiency anemia during the pregnancy even if it has not previously existed. It is still unclear if anemia during pregnancy is correlated with poor birth outcome (e.g., preterm birth, low birth weight, and increased perinatal mortality), as some observational studies have suggested, or if supplementation with iron makes a difference in fetal outcome. Although routine screening for anemia in the nonpregnant female is not recommended by the U.S. Preventive Health Services Task Force, assessment for iron stores is recommended at the first prenatal visit and if clinically suspected should be assessed in the preconception period as well. The status of iron stores is also a good measure for overall nutritional status. Screening for iron deficiency anemia usually is measured by the hematocrit level. If the level is low (less than 36% to 38% for women), iron studies (iron and total iron-binding capacity [TIBC]) can be ordered to identify iron deficiency anemia. If the test results are equivocal, iron stores can be measured by use of ferritin. For more detailed discussion on iron deficiency anemia, detection, and treatment see Chapter 20.

General Nutritional Requirements During Pregnancy

The recommended daily allowance (RDA) for the pregnant woman, developed by various government research groups, provides the clinician with guidelines on basic nutritional requirements (Table 63-3). Protein is important in the development of fetal tissue, especially brain tissue. The RDA of protein in pregnancy is 60 g/day. Amino acids must be ingested in adequate but not excessive amounts. Large doses of aspartame (Nutrasweet or Equal), which contains com-

mercially produced L-aspartate and L-phenylalanine, have been found to cause hypothalamic neuronal destruction in rats but have not been shown to be teratogenic in human beings. It is generally recommended that pregnant women use the substance in moderation.

The effects of various vitamin and mineral deficiencies and excesses are summarized in Table 63-4.

FOLATE SUPPLEMENTATION TO DECREASE RISK OF NEURAL TUBE DEFECTS

EPIDEMIOLOGY

Recent evidence has shown that supplementation of the water-soluble vitamin folate is particularly important in preventing neural tube defects. Each year more than 4000 infants are born with a neural tube defect, most commonly spina bifida. The recurrence rate in the subsequent pregnancies is estimated at 2% to 10%.

The RDA for pregnant adult women is 0.4 mg (400 μg) folate. Most multivitamins contain 0.4 mg. Prenatal vitamins contain 0.8 mg folate. Most women consume an average 0.2 mg folate in the usual diet, which is less than both the RDA and the Food and Drug Administration (FDA)-RDA for the pregnant woman. Because almost 50% of all pregnancies are unplanned and most women do not obtain the minimum daily requirements of folate in their diet alone, the FDA began requiring folate supplementation in flour. How much folate should be contained in supplemented food sources remains controversial.

Retrospective studies and randomized controlled trials clearly support folate supplementation. In one randomized controlled trial, women who had a previous pregnancy resulting in a fetus with a neural tube defect were followed from before conception through 6 weeks of gestation. They received high-dose folate (4 mg/day) 1 month before conception through 6 weeks of gestation. This intervention was associated with a 60% reduction in risk for neural tube defects. These results were corroborated in a multicenter study by the Medical Research Council Vitamin Study Research Group using a similar intervention that documented a 70% reduction in risk for neural tube defect.

Two nonrandomized intervention studies also were completed in a similar population (women with a prior history of neural tube defect–affected pregnancy) using supplementation with 5 mg folate. These studies also showed that folate supplementation decreased the recurrence rate for subsequent pregnancies (85% reduction in risk).

Based on all of these results, in 1991, the Centers for Disease Control and Prevention (CDC) issued recommendations for women who had a *previous* pregnancy resulting in an infant with neural tube defect: to consume 4 mg folate at least 1 month before conception and to continue for the first 3 months of pregnancy.

A recent carefully controlled randomized double-blind study was conducted that involved healthy women contemplating pregnancy who did not have a history of neural tube defect–affected pregnancy. Supplementation with 0.8mg (800 μg) folate (a dose seen in most prenatal vitamins), along with supplemental vitamins and minerals and trace elements, was begun 1 month before conception through 6 weeks of gestation. The control group received only trace

Table 63-1
Summary of Recommendations for Preconception Counseling

Area for Prevention	Potential Adverse Events	Recommendation
Nutrition	LBW, IUGR	Balanced diet with increased protein and iron
Folate supplementation	Neural tube defects	For women with prior history of neural tube defect–affected pregnancy: 4 mg folate or higher based on recommendation of physician
		For women contemplating pregnancy: 0.4 mg folate 2 mo before conception through 6 weeks of gestation
		For all women of reproductive age: dietary guidelines
Ingestion of caffeinated products	SAB, IUGR, microcephaly	Less than 2-3 cups per day
Adverse health behaviors		
Alcohol	Fetal alcohol syndrome, SAB	There is no safe level; advise to limit drinking and attempt to quit
Smoking	Increased risk of abruption LBW, IUGR, SAB, cleft palate, cardiovascular and urogenital malformations	Smoking cessation including nicotine gum/patch if not pregnant
Illicit drugs	Increased risk of placental abnormalities Urogenital malformations IUGR, LBW, placental abnormalities Neurobehavioral abnormalities	Drug rehabilitation and detoxification
Domestic violence	Fetal fractures, premature labor Infectious disease	Resources and social service assessment and psychologic risk
Rubella	Congenital rubella	Screening and immunization if necessary (before pregnancy)
Hepatitis	Fulminant hepatitis	Screening for hepatitis B (HBsAg), with vaccination for seronegative patients at high risk
Sexually transmitted diseases	Transmission to infant	Screening and intervention based on symptoms and risk profile
HIV	Transmission to infant	Education on HIV transmission; testing after informed consent
		Education on safe sex practices
Medical conditions		
Diabetes	Macrosomia, preeclampsia	For diabetic women, optimal control of glucose and normalization of hemoglobin A_{1c}
	Congenital malformations	For women without prior history of diabetes, screening based on symptoms before pregnancy; oral GTT after 24-28 weeks' gestation

LBW, Low birth weight; *IUGR*, intrauterine growth retardation; *SAB*, spontaneous abortion; *HBsAg*, hepatitis B surface antigen; *GTT*, glucose tolerance test.

elements. The group that received the folate supplementation experienced close to one half the rate of neural tube defects.

The CDC extrapolated from these data and issued updated guidelines in 1992 with the following recommendations.

All women of childbearing age in the United States who are capable of becoming pregnant should consume 0.4 mg (400 mg) of folic acid per day for the purpose of reducing their risk of having a pregnancy affected with spina bifida or other neural tube defects. Because the effects of high intakes are not well known but include complicating the diagnosis of vitamin B_{12} deficiency, care should be taken to keep total folate consumption at less than 1 mg/day, except under the supervision of a physician. Women who have had a prior neural tube defect–affected pregnancy are a high risk of having a subsequent affected pregnancy. When these women are planning to become pregnant, they should consult their physician, may recommend the high dose (4 mg) used in most of the studies.

The effect of folate deficiency is particularly pronounced in women with twin pregnancies, in those taking anticonvulsants, and in those with hemoglobinopathies inasmuch as the need for folate is increased in these situations.

In support of this effort, a controlled study of mothers in North America whose infants had neural tube defects as compared with mothers of children with other malformations has demonstrated that ingestion of 0.4 mg folate reduced the risk by almost 60% in the cohort of women from 1988 to 1991 and that 0.4 mg should be the recommended amount to protect all women contemplating pregnancy.

Counseling

Although the proportion of US women who are aware of the present recommendations has increased since 1995, a recent study from 1998 indicates that only a small percentage

Table 63-2
Recommended Daily Food Guide

Food Group	Source	RECOMMENDED MINIMUM SERVINGS PER DAY	
		Nonpregnant	Pregnant or Breastfeeding
Protein (also source of vitamin B_6, iron, zinc; animal protein also has B_{12} and vegetable protein has folic acid, magnesium and fiber)	*Animal Protein:* meat, fish poultry, seafood	4	6
	Vegetable Protein: cooked dry beans, tofu, peanuts, peanut butter	1	1
Milk Products (also source of protein and calcium, vit A, B_{12}, riboflavin, and zinc. Fortified milk contains vitamin D)	Milk, yogurt, cream soups, cheese	2	4
Breads, Cereals, Grains (all provide carbohydrates, some protein, and thiamine, riboflavin, niacin, and iron. Whole grains provide B_6, folic acid, vitamin E, magnesium, zinc and fiber)	Bread, bagels, cereal, noodles, rice, pancake, waffle, muffins, crackers	6	7
Vitamin C-rich Fruits and Vegetables (also provide fiber, vitamin A, B_6 and folic acid)	Oranges, tomatoes, vegetable juice, strawberries, broccoli, cabbage, canteloupe	1	5
Vitamin A-rich Fruits and Vegetables (also sources of beta-carotene, fiber and dark green vegetables provide vitamin B_6, folic acid and magnesium)	Apricots, canteloupe, carrots, greens, spinach, tomatoes	1	5
Other Fruits and Vegetables (also, carbohydrates or fiber)	Fruit juice, apple, banana, berries, cherries, peach, grapes, watermelon, dried fruit, asparagus, beans, celery, peas, lettuce	3	3
Folic Acid Rich Foods	Beans, lentils, liver, peanuts, yeast		4
Non-dairy Calcium	Almonds, baked beans, broccoli,		
Rich Foods	Turnips, greens, salmon		

BOX 63-2
Guidelines for Weight Gain in Pregnancy

Prepregnancy BMI (kg/m²)	Total Weight Gain (lb)
19.8-26 (normal)	25-35
<19.8 (underweight)	28-40
>26.1-29 (overweight)	15-25
>29 (obese)	15
Twin gestation	35-45
Triplet gestation	60

BMI, Body mass index = weight (kg) divided by height (m) squared.
Modified from Nutrition during pregnancy. ACOG Technical Bulletin 179, April, 1993, *Intl J Gyneacol Obstet,* 1993.

of women were aware of the potential benefits of periconceptional intake of folic acid. During a focus group carried out by the CDC of 58 health care providers who spent at least 50% of their time caring for women of reproductive age, many reported lack of knowledge regarding the benefit of folic acid, limited time with patients to review potential benefits, and lack of educational materials to support their counseling of women. Remarkably, in a nonrandomly controlled study conducted by the March of Dimes of attendees to grand rounds at selected academic teaching centers with residencies in obstetrics and gynecology, 30% of the attendees reported a lack of knowledge regarding the recommended daily requirements of folate for women and less than 70% reported recommending folic acid to their female patients.

Table 63-3
Recommended Daily Dietary Allowances*

Nutrient (unit)	ADULT WOMAN[†]		Post-partum Breastfeeding
	Nonpregnant	Pregnant	
Protein (g)	46-50	60	65
Carbohydrates (g)	100	250	
Vitamins			
A (μg)	800	800	1300
D (μg)	5-7.5[‡]	10	10
E (mg)	8	10	12
K (μg)	65	65	65
Folic acid (μg)	180[§]	400	280
Thiamine (B$_1$) (mg/day)	1.1	1.5	1.6
Riboflavin (B$_2$) (mg/day)	1.3	1.6	1.8
Niacin (mg niacin equivalent)	15	17	20
Pyridoxine (B$_6$) (mg/day)	1.6	2.2	2.1
Cyanocobalamin (B$_{12}$) (mg/day)	2.0	2.2	2.1
Pantothenic acid (mg)	10	4-7	
Ascorbic acid (vitamin C) (mg/day)	60	70	95
Minerals			
Calcium (mg/day)	1000[¶]	1200	1200
Phosphorus (mg/day)	800	1200	1200
Magnesium (mg/day)	280	320	355
Iron (mg/day)	15	30-60	15
Zinc (mg/day)	12	15	19
Iodine (mg/day)	150	175	200
Selenium (mg/day)	55	65	75
Copper (mg/day)	2	1.5-3.0	

Modified from National Research Council: *Recommended dietary allowances*, ed 10, Washington, DC, 1989, National Academy Press.
* Since 1997, referred to as Dietary Reference Intakes (DRIs). These values are goals for individuals and is based on the estimated average requirement (EAR). It is the daily dietary intake level that is sufficient to meet the nutrient requirement of 97% to 98% of all healthy individuals in a group.
[†] U.S. RDA (National Nutrition Consortium): *Nutrition labeling: how it can work for you*, Bethesda, Md, 1975, The Consortium.
[‡] 7.5 μg = 300 International Units (IU). A recent report *New England Journal of Medicine* March 1998 indicates all adults should be receiving 20-25 μg of vitamin D per day.
[§] Women contemplating pregnancy should increase folate to 400 μg/day.
[¶] After menopause, women who do not take hormonal replacement therapy should increase their intake of calcium to 1200 mg/day.

The data clearly support the recommendation that women with a history of neural tube defect–affected pregnancy should take supplemental folate and high doses (0.8 mg and higher if indicated by the individual physician). For those contemplating pregnancy (and possibly even all women of reproductive age), the lowest dose of 0.4 mg 2 months before conception to 6 weeks of gestation is adequate and can be obtained in most over-the-counter multivitamins or prenatal vitamins (these contain 0.8 mg of folate). Because many pregnancies are unplanned, a daily multivitamin is recommended if the woman does not have adequate intake from the diet alone.

The only potential risk of folate supplementation is masking B$_{12}$ deficiency with doses higher than 1.0 mg/day.

Caffeine

Data on the risks to the fetus from caffeine ingestion during pregnancy remain inconclusive, although minimal intake of 1 to 2 cups a day does not appear to be associated with spontaneous miscarriage or birth defects.

Caffeine consumption increases circulating catecholamines, which is thought to be a possible mechanism for causing birth defects. Its metabolites readily cross the blood-brain barrier in adults and fetuses and act by blocking adenosine A1 and A2a receptors, which leads to secondary effects on many classes of neurotransmitters. Animal studies have shown an increased incidence of skeletal defects in offspring of rats fed extremely high amounts of caffeine (equivalent to more than 50 cups of coffee per day), decreased brain weight, and alterations in brain development, learning, and memory. With lower intake of caffeine (4, 8, and 28 cups per day), no birth defects occurred in the pregnant rats' offspring.

Results from human studies have been inconsistent. In a prospective study of more than 400 pregnant women, moderate caffeine intake (less than 3 cups per day) was not associated with an increased risk for spontaneous abortion, intrauterine growth retardation, or microcephaly. More than 3 cups per day did appear to increase the risk for intrauterine growth retardation, although the outcome events were small. However, in a case-controlled study of caffeine consumption among 331 women who suffered fetal loss, there was a significantly increased risk for spontaneous abortion with consumption of only 1 to 2 cups per day; high consumption

Table 63-4
Effect of Nutrient, Vitamin, and Mineral Excess and Deficiency During Pregnancy

Nutrient	Excess	Deficiency
Protein	For aspartame, data inconclusive in humans	Poor fetal growth and development in humans
Vitamins		
Fat-soluble		
A	Malformation of urinary tract, first trimester CNS/liver damage Skin changes	—
D	Hypercalcemia Supravalvular aortic stenosis Cranial/facial abnormalities in first trimester (elfin facies), growth retardation	—
E	—	High rate of CNS and skeletal defects and spontaneous abortion in rats
K	Skeletal abnormalities in rats	—
Water-soluble		
Folic acid	Masks B_{12} deficiency	Increased risk of neural tube defects and spontaneous abortion
Thiamine (B_1)	—	Severe fetal abnormalities and infant beriberi
Riboflavin	—	—
Niacin	—	—
Pyridoxine (B_6)	Neuropathy in mother	Hypoplasia of thymus and spleen; diminished neonatal immunocompetence in animals; mental retardation in humans
Cyanocobalamin	—	Megaloblastic anemia, coma, hyperpigmentation
Pantothenic acid	—	—
Ascorbic acid	—	Congenital scurvy, spontaneous abortion and premature births
Minerals		
Iron	—	Anemia Increased risk of premature delivery in some observational studies
Calcium	—	Neonatal hypocalcemia Abnormal fetal bone development and mineralization ? Increased preeclampsia
Zinc	In rats, fetal loss and growth retardation	Congenital lesions Low levels associated with pregnancy-induced hypertension
Chromium		Low levels associated with glucose intolerance
Iodine	Congenital goiter Hypothyroidism Mental retardation	Cretinism
Copper	—	In rats, increased congenital malformations

Modified from Hollingsworth DR, Resnik R: *Medical counseling before pregnancy,* New York, 1988, Churchill Livingstone.

(more than 3 cups) further increased the risk. Klebanoff and associates used a biologic marker of caffeine intake, the levels of the caffeine metabolite paraxanthine in serum, to estimate exposure and found an association between spontaneous abortion, primarily in the second trimester, and unusually high levels of caffeine consumption of more than the equivalent of 6 cups of coffee a day.

There are no standard recommendations at this time regarding caffeine intake, but prudent intake (less than 2 cups a day of coffee, tea, or cola drinks or chocolate, which also contains caffeine) probably should be advised.

SUBSTANCE ABUSE
Alcohol

▦ EPIDEMIOLOGY

Alcohol intake during pregnancy occurs commonly. According to the National Household Survey on Drug Abuse, 73% of women between 12 and 34 years old expose their fetuses to alcohol at some time during pregnancy. The prevalence of fetal alcohol syndrome is 2 per 1000 live births.

BOX 63-3

Alcohol-Related Physical Problems Associated with Prenatal Alcohol Exposure

Dysmorphic features
Characteristic facial features, low-set ears, palmar creases

Intraoral Deformities
Cleft palate, malocclusions, poor dental alignment

Hearing
Chronic otitis media, permanent hearing loss

Vision
Eyeground malformations, optic nerve hypoplasia, strabismus, ptosis, nystagmus, myopia

Cardiac
Heart murmurs, patent ductus arteriosus

Skeletal Malformations
Congenital hip dislocation, scoliosis, bilateral halluces

Genitourinary
Hydronephrosis, labial hypoplasia

Growth Retardation
Microcephaly, weight/height (less than 10% normal), failure to thrive

Immune System Deficits
T cell loss, allergies

Modified from Coles C: *Clin Obstet Gynecol* 36:255, 1993.

BOX 63-4

Fetal Alcohol Syndrome

Prenatal or Postnatal Growth Retardation

Facial Features (at least 2 or 3 abnormalities)
Absent philtrum
Thinned upper vermilion
Hypoplastic midface
Low nasal bridge
Epicanthal fold
Shortened palpebral fissure
Low-set ears
Microcephaly

Central Nervous System Dysfunction
Neurologic abnormalities
Mental deficiency
Developmental delays

Modified from Jones KL, Smith DW: *Lancet* 2:999, 1973.

Effects of Alcohol on Conception and Pregnancy

Alcohol has profoundly negative effects on the fetus. Alcohol abuse during pregnancy is the third leading cause of mental retardation. Alcohol-related effects (Box 63-3) include physical effects, as well as risk of intrauterine death, prenatal and postnatal growth retardation, low birth weight, central nervous system abnormalities, and behavior deficits. A relationship between alcohol consumption and the development of the fetal alcohol syndrome has clearly been established. Fetal alcohol syndrome is defined as prenatal or postnatal growth retardation (less than 10th percentile in body weight, length, and head circumference), two or three characteristic facial abnormalities (microcephaly, microphthalmia, underdeveloped philtrum, thin upper lip, maxillary hypoplasia, and central nervous system dysfunctions such as neurologic abnormalities, mental deficiency, and developmental delays) (Box 63-4). An increased incidence of fetal alcohol syndrome has been found in women who have consumed more than four drinks per day. It is not clear whether less than that amount also is associated with increased risk.

Mental retardation, hyperactivity, and developmental delays have all been reported in children of mothers who consume large amounts of alcohol. However, controlled studies on the long-term consequences of maternal alcohol ingestion during pregnancy are few. One study suggested that moderate drinking (one drink per day during pregnancy) was associated with attention deficit disorder in the children of moderate drinkers compared with occasional drinkers and nondrinkers. Alcohol consumption is associated with an increased risk of spontaneous abortion in the first trimester and an increased risk of abruptio placentae.

Although there is agreement that heavy drinking is detrimental, there is no agreement about the effects of lower levels of alcohol consumption. Evidence exists that the risk is markedly decreased if a woman stops drinking alcohol during pregnancy. It appears that the timing of alcohol consumption is important, with the greatest negative impact being at the time of conception through the first month of pregnancy.

Counseling

It is important that the clinician who counsels a woman before conception obtains a clear history of alcohol consumption. Methods for obtaining an accurate history of alcohol intake are described in Chapter 90. It is clear that heavy ingestion is detrimental to the developing fetus and that cessation of alcohol intake, especially early in the pregnancy, can decrease the risk of fetal anomalies.

No level of alcohol consumption has been proved to be safe. For this reason many clinicians recommend complete abstinence. Explaining what is known of the effects of alcohol use on pregnancy outcome is important. In women with identified alcohol abuse, referral for treatment before conception and maintaining close follow-up throughout pregnancy can prevent the development of major birth anomalies and obstetric complications.

Smoking

▦ EPIDEMIOLOGY

In the United States, 26% of women are smokers, most of whom are of reproductive age. Maternal smoking is a major preventable cause of low birth weight and perinatal mortality. Studies have shown that as many as 40% of infants born with low birth weight can be attributed to maternal smoking. Smoking also is associated with infertility, menstrual disorders, spontaneous abortions, ectopic pregnancies,

---

BOX 63-5
Effects of Smoking on Conception and Pregnancy

Fertility
Delay in conception
Risk of tubal pregnancy

Birth Defects
Cleft palate
Cardiovascular and urogenital abnormalities

Obstetric Complications
Intrauterine growth retardation
Low birth weight
Spontaneous abortion
Placenta previa
Abruptio placentae
Vaginal bleeding

Long-Term Consequences
Increased respiratory infections
Sudden infant death syndrome

---

placental irregularities, and increased childhood morbidity (Box 63-5).

According to data from the National Health Interview Survey, completed by the U.S. Department of Health and Human Services, 32% of women were found to be smokers before pregnancy and 21% quit during the pregnancy. In other studies almost 70% of women who stopped smoking during their pregnancies resumed after completing the pregnancy, and 25% of all women continue to smoke during pregnancy.

Pathophysiology

The pathophysiology of the negative effects include exposure to nicotine and various by-products and additives in the cigarettes, such as polycyclic aromatic hydrocarbons and carbon monoxide. Nicotine causes vasoconstriction and vasospasm, hydrocarbons interfere with maternal fetal transport, and the carbon monoxide displaces the oxygen. Not only are there direct effects on the fetus, but the adequacy of the placenta is affected by abnormal microcirculation.

Effects of Smoking on Conception and Pregnancy

Review of the data on the effect of smoking on fertility has clearly shown that fertility is adversely affected by smoking, and the effect is worse in women who smoke more than 16 cigarettes per day. A delay in conception for women who smoke is three times more likely than for nonsmokers, and it can take smokers more than 1 year to conceive. There is also a reported increased risk in ectopic pregnancy. After cessation of smoking, the risk for infertility is the same as for nonsmokers.

Although the data are inconsistent, some studies have found an increased incidence of birth defects, including cleft palate and cardiovascular and urogenital abnormalities in infants of mothers who smoke during pregnancy.

Many studies have shown that intrauterine growth retardation and low birth weight are causally related to smoking and are dose-dependent, with heavy smokers being at increased risk for low-birth-weight infants as compared with occasional smokers. There is also an increase in risk for spontaneous abortion, and the risk increases with heavier smoking patterns. Preterm birth (less than 37 weeks of gestation) has been shown to be more common in smokers, especially in those who consume more than one pack per day, and placental complications, including placenta previa, abruptio placentae, and vaginal bleeding, also are more prevalent. Long-term consequences of increased respiratory infections in the infant and a link between smoking and sudden infant death syndrome exist as well.

Counseling

Counseling women on cessation of smoking is important especially if the woman is contemplating pregnancy. Even if women acknowledge the perinatal risks of cigarettes and want to quit, many continue smoking throughout the pregnancy. Chapter 89 discusses in detail methods for approaching smoking cessation. If the woman is pregnant, behavioral methods usually are most appropriate inasmuch as nicotine gum is contraindicated in pregnancy. The safety of the nicotine patch, which provides a lower, continuous release of nicotine, has not been established for pregnant women, but recent pilot studies suggest that the patch can be safely used if the level of nicotine is kept less than would be the case with smoking.

Cocaine Use

▦ EPIDEMIOLOGY

Prevalence of cocaine use among pregnant women is difficult to estimate. Approximately 5% of women of reproductive age reported cocaine ingestion in the 1990 National Household Survey on Drug Abuse. It is estimated that anywhere from 3% to 17% of pregnant women use cocaine.

Pathophysiology

Cocaine has potent effects on both the peripheral and central nervous systems. The mechanism of the deleterious effects of maternal cocaine ingestion on the fetus has been outlined by Volpe. In the mother, increased peripheral catecholamine production results in vasoconstriction, uterine contraction, and decreased placental flow. Fetal effects also are mediated by placental transfer of catecholamines, decreased nutrients, and decreased oxygen transfer, leading to focal cerebral ischemia and decreased cerebral blood flow. These factors result in severe interruption in the development of the fetal nervous system and increased risk of obstetric complications.

Effects of Cocaine on Conception and Pregnancy
(Box 63-6)

Conflicting data exist on the effects of cocaine use during early pregnancy. Effects of cocaine use reported in some studies include an increased rate of spontaneous abortion, retardation in fetal growth, and congenital anomalies, particularly in the genitourinary tract. In addition, intrauterine exposure to cocaine significantly affects human brain development (Table 63-5).

Later in pregnancy, there appear to be higher rates of placental abruption, abnormal labor, and premature rupture of membranes. Other effects on the fetus include an increase in

Table 63-5
Disturbances in Human Brain Development Reported after Intrauterine Exposure to Cocaine

Event	PEAK GESTATIONAL Period	Abnormality
Neural tube formation	3-4 wk	Myelomeningocele Encephalocele
Prosencephalic development	2-3 mo	Agenesis of corpus callosum; agenesis of septum pellucidum; septooptic dysplasia
Neuronal proliferation	3-4 mo	Microcephaly
Neuronal migration	3-5 mo	Schizencephaly, neuronal heterotopias
Neuronal	5 mo-postnatal	Abnormal cortical differentiation neuronal cytodifferentiation (preliminary)
Myelination	After birth	None

Modified from Volpe J: *N Engl J Med* 327:399, 1992.

BOX 63-6
Effects of Cocaine on Conception and Pregnancy

Birth Defects
Congenital urogenital malformations

Obstetric Complications
Intrauterine growth retardation
Low birth weight
Spontaneous abortion
Placental abruption
Abnormal labor
Premature rupture of membranes

Other Effects on Fetus
Behavioral abnormalities
Sudden infant death syndrome
Necrotizing enterocolitis
Cerebrovascular accidents
Long-term neurodevelopmental problems

Comorbidities
Malnutrition
Sexually transmitted diseases
Hepatitis B
HIV
Other addictions

---

sudden infant death syndrome, necrotizing enterocolitis, and cerebrovascular accidents. Severe long-term effects also have been demonstrated, including behavioral problems as children are followed into their school years.

The direct effects of cocaine for any user regardless of pregnancy include myocardial ischemia, cerebrovascular accidents, subarachnoid hemorrhage, hypertension, seizures,

---

BOX 63-7
Effects of Diabetes on Conception and Pregnancy

Birth Defects
Ventricular septal defects
Neural tube defects
Caudal regression syndrome

Other Fetal Effects
Macrosomia

Obstetric Complications
Preeclampsia
Urinary tract infections
Premature labor

---

intestinal ischemia, pulmonary edema, and sudden death. Associated comorbidities that result in a riskier pregnancy include malnutrition; increased rate of sexually transmitted diseases, hepatitis B, and HIV; and other drug addictions.

Counseling

Chapter 91 reviews methods for identifying cases of substance abuse. Referral and treatment before pregnancy are important but often are unavailable because of limited resources and programs. When a woman becomes pregnant, intervention becomes even more difficult because many programs do not accept pregnant women. A list of available resources appears in Appendix XIV.

DOMESTIC ABUSE

Domestic abuse increases during pregnancy and is associated with complications late in pregnancy such as abruptio placentae and premature rupture of membranes. It is important to elicit a history of domestic abuse during all routine visits and provide appropriate preventive intervention. This topic is covered in detail in Chapter 87.

DIABETES AND HYPERTENSION

Preconception counseling has clearly been shown to improve a pregnancy outcome in a woman with hypertension and diabetes (Box 63-7). The incidence of congenital malformations in infants of diabetic women is 6% to 10%. Common malformations include ventricular septal defects, neural tube defects, and caudal regression syndrome. Macrosomia increases the risk for birth trauma and the need for cesarean section. In addition, the risk is increased for preeclampsia, susceptibility to urinary tract infections and pyelonephritis, and progression of preexisting diabetic nephropathy and retinopathy. Multiple studies have demonstrated that monitoring and control of glucose before conception and during early pregnancy result in a decrease in the likelihood of more serious malformations and early pregnancy complications. The incidence of major congenital fetal defects is clearly correlated with hemoglobin A_{1c} measurements during early pregnancy. Control of the glucose throughout pregnancy is correlated with improved pregnancy outcomes, including a decrease in risk of fetal macrosomia, premature labor, and stillbirth. Oral hypoglycemic agents should be discontinued before pregnancy because of the association with increased risk of congenital malformations, and it is difficult to obtain optimal glucose control. Those requiring insulin may need to increase their usual dose to maintain glycemic control and, if insulin resistant, changes may approach up to 90% of the prepregnancy dose. Chapters 11 and 3, respectively, cover in detail diabetes and hypertension during pregnancy.

BIBLIOGRAPHY

General

Burrow G, Duffy T: *Medical complications during pregnancy,* ed 5, Philadelphia, 1999, WB Saunders.

Cefalo R, Moos M: *Preconception health care: a practical guide,* ed 2, St Louis, 1995, Mosby.

Hollingsworth DR, Resnik R: *Medical counseling before pregnancy,* New York, 1988, Churchill Livingstone.

Jack B, Culpepper L: Preconception care risk reduction and health promotion in preparation for pregnancy, *JAMA* 264:1147, 1990.

Nutrition

ACOG committee opinion: Vitamin A supplementation during pregnancy. Number 196, January 1998. Committee on Obstetric Practice. American College of Obstetricians and Gynecologists, *Int J Gynaecol Obstet* 61: 205, 1998.

ACOG educational bulletin: Nutrition and women. Number 229, October 1996. Committee on Educational Bulletins of the American College of Obstetricians and Gynecologists, *Int J Gynaecol Obstet* 56:71, 1997.

Council Report: Aspartame: review of safety issues, *JAMA* 254:400, 1985.

DiGuiseppi C, Atkins D, Woolf S: *Guide to clinical preventive services. Report of the US preventive services task force,* ed 2. Alexandria, Vn, 1997, International Medical Publishing, Inc.

Institute of Medicine: *Dietary reference intake: folate, other B vitamins and choline,* Washington DC, 1998, National Academy Press.

Kim I et al: Pregnancy nutrition surveillance system—United States 1979-1980, *MMWR* 41:25, 1992.

National Research Council: *Recommended dietary allowances,* ed 10, Washington, DC, 1989, National Academy Press.

Nelson J et al: *Mayo Clinic diet manual: a handbook of nutrition practices,* St Louis, 1994, Mosby.

Nutrition during Pregnancy: ACOG Technical Bulletin, Number 179, April 1993. *Int J Gyneacol Obstet* 43:67, 1993.

US Preventive Health Services Task Force (policy statement): Routine iron supplementation during pregnancy, *JAMA* 270:2846, 1993.

Folate Supplementation

American Academy of Pediatrics: Folic acid for the prevention of neural tube defects, *Pediatrics* 104:325, 1999.

Bower C, Stanley FJ: Dietary folate as a risk factor for neural tube defects: evidence from a case-control study in Western Australia, *Med J Aust* 150:613, 1989.

Centers for Disease Control: Use of folic acid for prevention of spina bifida and other neural tube defects 1983–1991, *MMWR* 40:513, 1991.

Centers for Disease Control: Recommendations for the use of folic acid to reduce the number of cases of spina bifida and other neural tube defects, *MMWR* 41(RR-14):1, 1992.

Czeizel A, Dudas I: Prevention of the first occurrence of neural tube defects by periconceptual vitamin supplementation, *N Engl J Med* 327:1832, 1992.

Daly S et al: Minimum effective dose of folic acid for food fortification to prevent neural tube defects, *Lancet* 350:1666, 1997.

Dietary reference intakes for thiamin, riboflavin, niacin, vitamin B₆, folate, vitamin B₁₂, pantothenic acid, biotin, and choline: a report of the Standing Committee on the Scientific Evaluation of Dietary Reference Intakes and its Panel on Folate, Other B Vitamins, and Coline and Subcommittee on Upper Reference Levels of Nutrients. Washington DC, 1998, National Academy Press.

Laurence KM et al: Double blind randomized controlled trial of folate treatment before conception to prevent recurrence of neural tube defects, *Br Med J* 282:1509, 1981.

Medical Research Council Vitamin Study Research Group: Prevention of neural tube defects: results of the Medical Research Council vitamin study, *Lancet* 338:131, 1991.

Mills JL et al: The absence of a relation between the periconceptional use of vitamins and neural tube defects, *N Engl J Med* 321:430, 1989.

Mills JL: Fortification of foods with folic acid—how much is enough? *N Engl J Med* 342:1442, 2000.

Milunsky A et al: Multivitamin folic acid supplementation in early pregnancy reduces the prevalence of neural tube defects, *JAMA* 262:2847, 1989.

MMWR: Use of folic acid-containing supplements among women of childbearing age—United States, 1997, *JAMA* 279: 1998.

MMWR: Knowledge and use of folic acid by women of childbearing age—United States, 1995 and 1998, *JAMA* 281: 1999.

Mulinare J et al: Periconceptional use of multivitamins and the occurrence of neural tube defects, *JAMA* 260:3141, 1988.

Oakley G: Folic acid–preventable spina bifida and anencephaly, *JAMA* 269:1292, 1993.

Oakley G: Prevention of neural tube defects, *N Engl J Med* 341:1546, 1999.

Lawrence JM et al: Trends in serum folate after food fortification, *Lancet* 354:915, 1999.

Smithells RW et al: Further experiences of vitamin supplementation for the prevention of neural tube defect recurrences, *Lancet* 1:1027, 1983.

Subcommittee on Dietary Intake and Nutrient Supplements During Pregnancy: *Nutrition during pregnancy,* Washington, DC, 1990, National Academy Press.

Vergel RG et al: Primary prevention of neural tube defects with folic acid supplementation: Cuban experience, *Prenat Diagn* 10:149, 1990.

Werler M, Shapiro S, Mitchell A: Periconceptional folic acid exposure and risk of occurrent neural tube defects, *JAMA* 269:1257, 1993.

Caffeine

Cnattingius S et al: Caffeine intake and the risk of first-trimester spontaneous abortion, *N Engl J Med* 343:1839, 2000.

Eskenazi B: Caffeine during pregnancy: grounds for concern? *JAMA* 270: 2973, 1993.

Eskenazi B: Caffeine—filtering the facts, *N Engl J Med* 341:1688, 1999.

Grimm VE, Freider B: Prenatal caffeine causes long-lasting behavioral and neurochemical changes, *Int J Neurosci* 41:15, 1988.

Hatch EE, Bracken MB: Caffeine use during pregnancy: what is safe? *JAMA* 270:47, 1993.

Infante-Rivard C et al: Fetal loss associated with caffeine intake before and during pregnancy, *JAMA* 270:2940, 1993.

Klebanoff MA et al: Maternal serum paraxanthine, a caffeine metabolite and the risk of spontaneous Abortion, *N Engl J Med* 341:1639, 1999.

Mills JL et al: Moderate caffeine use and the risk of spontaneous abortion and intrauterine growth retardation, *JAMA* 269:593, 1993.

Spiller J, editor: The methylxanthine beverages and foods: chemistry, consumption and health effects. In *Progress in clinical and biological research,* vol. 158, New York, 1984, Alan Liss.

Substance Abuse

Alcohol

Abel EL: *Fetal alcohol syndrome,* New York, 1986, Praeger Publication Text.

Alcohol and the fetus—is zero the only option? *Lancet* 1:682, 1983.

Coles C: Impact of prenatal alcohol exposure on the newborn and the child, *Clin Obstet Gynecol* 36:255, 1993.

Council on Scientific Affairs: Fetal effects of maternal alcohol use, *JAMA* 249:2517, 1983.

Day N, Cottreau C, Richardson G: The epidemiology of alcohol, marijuana and cocaine use among women of childbearing age and pregnant women, *Clin Obstet Gynecol* 36:232, 1993.

Ernhart C et al: Alcohol-related birth defects: syndromal anomalies, intrauterine growth retardation, and neonatal behavioral assessment, *Alcoholism: Clin Exp Res* 9:447, 1985.

Ernhart C et al: Alcohol teratogenicity in the human: a detailed assessment of specificity, critical period and threshold, *Am J Obstet Gynecol* 156:33, 1987.

Hanson JW, Jones K, Smith D: Fetal alcohol syndrome, *JAMA* 235:1458, 1976.

Hanson JW, Streissguth AP, Smith DW: The effects of moderate alcohol consumption during pregnancy on fetal growth and morphogenesis, *Pediatrics* 92:457, 1978.

Harlap S, Shiono PH: Alcohol, smoking and the incidence of spontaneous abortions in the first and second trimester, *Lancet* 2:173, 1980.

Jones KL, Smith DW: Recognition of the fetal alcohol syndrome in early infancy, *Lancet* 2:999, 1973.

Jones KL et al: Pattern of malformation in offspring of chronic alcoholic mothers, *Lancet* 1:1267, 1973.

Kaufman MH: Ethanol induced chromosomal abnormalities at conception, *Nature* 302:258, 1983.

Kline J et al: Drinking during pregnancy and spontaneous abortion, *Lancet* 2:176, 1980.

Landesman-Dwyer S, Ragozin AS, Little RE: Behavioral correlates of prenatal alcohol exposure: a four year follow-up study, *Neurobehav Toxicol Teratol* 3:187, 1981.

Marbury MC et al: The association of alcohol consumption with outcome of pregnancy, *Am J Public Health* 73:1165, 1983.

National Institute on Drug Abuse: *National household survey on drug abuse: 1990 population estimates,* US Public Health Service Pub No ADM 91-1732, Washington, DC, 1991, US Government Printing Office.

Ouellette E et al: Adverse effects on offspring of maternal alcohol abuse during pregnancy, *N Engl J Med* 297:528, 1977.

Rosett HL: A clinical perspective of the fetal alcohol syndrome, *Alcoholism: Clin Exp Res* 4:119, 1980.

Rosett HL, Weiner L: *Alcohol and the fetus: a clinical perspective,* New York, 1984, Oxford University Press.

Rosett HL et al: Patterns of alcohol consumption and fetal development, *Obstet Gynecol* 61:539, 1983.

Streissguth AP, Clarren SK, Jones KL: Natural history of the fetal alcohol syndrome: a 10 year follow-up of eleven patients, *Lancet* 2:85, 1985.

Streissguth AP et al: Teratogenic effects of alcohol in humans and laboratory animals, *Science* 209:353, 1980.

Streissguth AP et al: Fetal alcohol syndrome in adolescents and adults, *JAMA* 265:1961, 1991.

Smoking

American College of Obstetricians and Gynecologists. *Technical Bulletin: Smoking and women's health,* No. 240. Washington DC, 1997, American College of Obstetricians and Gynecologists.

Baird DD, Wilcox AJ: Cigarette smoking associated with delayed conception, *JAMA* 253:2979, 1985.

Benowitz NL: Nicotine replacement therapy during pregnancy, *JAMA* 266:3174, 1991.

Fedrick J, Alberman ED, Goldstein H: Possible teratogenic effect of cigarette smoking, *Nature* 231:529, 1971.

Fingerhut LA, Kleinman JC, Kendrick JS: Smoking before, during and after pregnancy, *Am J Public Health* 80:541, 1990.

Floyd RL et al: Smoking during pregnancy: prevalence, effects, and intervention strategies, *Birth* 18:48, 1991.

Hackman R, Kapur B, Koren G: Use of the nicotine patch by pregnant women, *N Engl J Med* 341:1700, 1999.

Himmelberger DU, Brown BW, Cohen EN: Cigarette smoking during pregnancy and the occurrence of spontaneous abortion and congenital abnormalities, *Am J Epidemiol* 108:470, 1978.

Lambers DS, Clark KE: The maternal and fetal physiologic effects of nicotine, *Semin Perinatol* 20:115, 1996.

Meyer MB, Jonas BS, Tonascia JA: Perinatal events associated with maternal smoking during pregnancy, *Am J Epidemiol* 103:464, 1976.

MMWR: Trends in pregnancy-related smoking rates in the United States 1987-1996, *JAMA* 283:2000.

Mullen PD, Quinn VP, Ershoff DH: Maintenance of nonsmoking postpartum by women who stopped smoking during pregnancy, *Public Health Briefs* 80:992, 1990.

Nieberg et al: The fetal tobacco syndrome, *JAMA* 253:2998, 1985.

Rosenberg MJ: *Smoking and reproductive health,* St Louis, 1987, Mosby.

Shiono P, Klebanoff M, Rhoads G: Smoking and drinking during pregnancy, *JAMA* 255:82, 1986.

Stillman R, Rosenberg M, Sachs B: Smoking and reproduction, *Fertil Steril* 46:545, 1986.

US Department of Health and Human Services: *The health consequences of smoking for women: a report of the surgeon general,* DHHS Pub No CDC89-8411, Washington, DC, 1989, US Government Printing Office.

Cocaine

Allen P, Sandler M: Critical components of obstetric management of chemically dependent women, *Clin Obstet Gynecol* 36:347, 1993.

Baciewicz G: The process of addiction, *Clin Obstet Gynecol* 36:223, 1993.

Chasnoff I: Drugs, *Alcohol, pregnancy and parenting,* Boston, 1988, Kluwer Academic Publishers.

Chasnoff I et al: Cocaine use in pregnancy, *N Engl J Med* 313:666, 1985.

Chasnoff I et al: Temporal patterns of cocaine use in pregnancy, *JAMA* 261:174, 1989.

Chavez G, Mulinare J, Coredero J: Maternal cocaine use during early pregnancy as a risk factor for congenital abnormalities, *JAMA* 262:795, 1989.

Cregler L, Mark H: Medical complications of cocaine, *N Engl J Med* 315:1495, 1986.

Dicke J, Verges D, Polakoski K: Cocaine inhibits alanine uptake by human placental microvillous membrane vesicles, *Am J Obstet Gynecol* 169:515, 1993.

Gillogley K et al: The perinatal impact of cocaine, amphetamine, and opiate use detected by universal intrapartum screening, *Am J Obstet Gynecol* 163:1535, 1990.

Glantz JC, Woods J: Cocaine, heroin and phencyclidine: obstetric perspectives, *Clin Obstet Gynecol* 36:279, 1993.

Little B et al: Cocaine abuse during pregnancy: maternal and fetal implications, *Obstet Gynecol* 73:157, 1989.

MacGregor S et al: Cocaine use during pregnancy: adverse perinatal outcome, *Am J Obstet Gynecol* 157:686, 1987.

MacGregor S et al: Cocaine abuse during pregnancy: correlation between prenatal care and perinatal outcome, *Obstet Gynecol* 74:882, 1989.

Mayes L et al: The problem of prenatal cocaine exposure: a rush to judgment, *JAMA* 267:406, 1992.

Ness RB et al: Cocaine and tobacco use and the risk of spontaneous abortion, *N Engl J Med* 340:333, 1999.

Ryan L, Ehrlich S, Finnegan L: Cocaine abuse in pregnancy: effects on the fetus and newborn, *Neurotoxicol Teratol* 9:295, 1987.

Slutsker L: Risks associated with cocaine use during pregnancy, *Obstet Gynecol* 79:778, 1992.

Smith C, Asch R: Drug abuse and reproduction, *Fertil Steril* 48:355, 1987.

Vega W et al: A prevalence and magnitude of perinatal substance exposures in California, *N Engl J Med* 329:850, 1993.

Volpe J: Effect of cocaine use on the fetus, *N Engl J Med* 327:399, 1992.

Warner E: Cocaine abuse, *Ann Intern Med* 119:226, 1993.

Zuckerman B et al: Effects of maternal marijuana and cocaine use on fetal growth, *N Engl J Med* 320:762, 1989.

Diabetes

Coustan D: Pregnancy in diabetic women, *N Engl J Med* 319:1663, 1988.

Gold A, Reilly R: The effect of glycemic control in the pre-conception period and early pregnancy on birth weight in women with IDDM, *Diabetes Care* 21:535, 1998.

Frankel N, Dooley S, Metzger B: Care of the pregnant woman with insulin dependent diabetes mellitus, *N Engl J Med* 313:96, 1985.

Hollingsworth D: *Pregnancy, diabetes and birth: management guide,* Baltimore, 1984, Williams & Wilkins.

Hollingsworth D, Resnik R: *Medical counseling before pregnancy,* New York, 1988, Churchill Livingstone.

Kitzmiller J et al: Preconception care of diabetes: glycemic control prevents congenital abnormalities, *JAMA* 265:731, 1991.

Miller E et al: Elevated maternal HbA_{1c} in early pregnancy and major congenital anomalies in infants of diabetic mothers, *N Engl J Med* 304:1331, 1981.

Mills JL, Baker L, Goldman AS: Malformations in infants of diabetic mothers occur before the seventh gestational week, *Diabetes* 28:292, 1979.

Mills JL et al: Incidence of spontaneous abortion among normal women and insulin dependent diabetic women whose pregnancies were identified within 21 days of conception, *N Engl J Med* 319:1617, 1988.

HIV Prevention and Pregnancy

ACOG educational bulletin: Human immunodeficiency virus infections in pregnancy. American College of Obstetricians and Gynecologists, *Int J Gynaecol Obstet* 57:73, 1997.

American Academy of Pediatrics, Committee on Pediatric AIDS: Technical report: perinatal human immunodeficiency virus testing and prevention of transmission, *Pediatrics* 106:E88, 2000.

Garcia PM et al: Maternal levels of plasma human immunodeficiency virus type 1 RNA and the risk of perinatal transmission, *N Engl J Med* 341: 394, 1999.

Lallemant M et al: A trial of shortened zidovudine regimens to prevent mother-to-child transmission of human immunodeficiency virus type 1, *N Engl J Med* 343:982, 2000.

Mofenson LM et al: Risk factors for perinatal transmission of human immunodeficiency virus type 1 in women treated with zidovudine, *N Engl J Med* 341:385, 1999.

Rogers MF, Shaffer N: Reducing the risk of maternal-infant transmission of HIV by attacking the virus, *N Engl J Med* 341:441, 1999.

The International Perinatal HIV Group: The mode of delivery and the risk of vertical transmission of human immunodeficiency virus type 1—a meta analysis of 15 prospective cohort studies, *N Engl J Med* 340:977, 1999.

Wade NA, Birkhead GS, Warren BL: Abbreviated regimens of zidovudine prophylaxis and perinatal transmission of the human immunodeficiency virus, *N Engl J Med* 339:1409, 1998.

CHAPTER **64**

Hyperemesis

Stephanie A. Eisenstat
Joseph A. Hill

The most common problems in early pregnancy, hyperemesis, vaginal bleeding (Chapter 65), and spontaneous abortion (Chapter 66), can have a significant impact on the early pregnancy experience and in some cases may be life-threatening. Understanding the pathophysiologic mechanisms involved in these disorders will enable women's health care providers to diagnose and manage these conditions effectively. This chapter covers the key features of hyperemesis gravidarum.

HYPEREMESIS GRAVIDARUM

Hyperemesis gravidarum is a pathologic state of persistent nausea and vomiting during pregnancy with resultant dehydration, ketosis, electrolyte imbalance, inadequate caloric intake, and poor weight gain or even weight loss.

▦ EPIDEMIOLOGY AND RISK FACTORS

Between 30% and 90% of pregnant women experience symptoms of nausea and vomiting during their pregnancy; 0.5% to 2% have symptoms severe enough to be considered hyperemetic. The incidence of hyperemesis is reported to be higher in developed countries. Even though there may be selection bias in the reporting, it is becoming increasingly clear that different lifestyles and stress factors play an important role in the development of this condition.

Several risk factors for hyperemesis gravidarum have been proposed, although the cause of the disorder remains poorly understood. Younger age, first pregnancy, high body weight, other eating disorders, previous history of hyperemesis gravidarum, single marital status, and *Helicobacter pylori* infection are all associated with an increased risk of hyperemesis. Racial and socioeconomic factors may also play a role, as hyperemesis is more common in Caucasians of high socioeconomic status. The psychologic profile of many patients with hyperemesis is that of a young, unmarried, immature, and dependent pregnant woman. These individuals are often ambivalent about their pregnancy. Identified hormonal risk factors include increased serum estradiol and the beta (*b*) subunit of human chorionic gonadotropin (*b*-hCG) levels. This may explain the association between hyperemesis gravidarum and pregnancies with multiple gestations or hydatidiform mole. More thorough analysis comparing hyperemetics with age- and gestation-matched control subjects has determined that serum estradiol levels and not *b*-hCG levels are related to hyperemesis gravidarum. Although most pregnant women can tolerate pregnancy levels of serum estradiol with only occasional episodes of nausea and vomiting, some women have lower tolerance secondary to psychologic and perhaps physiologic differences that may lead to a cycle of uncontrolled nausea and vomiting. In most cases, the symptoms either abate or markedly improve after 12 to 14 weeks of pregnancy, but up to 20% will continue to have significant symptoms throughout gestation.

Pathophysiology

Attempts to identify the pathophysiology of this disorder have been limited. Current knowledge is primarily based on retrospective studies that have examined the psychologic profile of affected women. A review of the literature suggests that hormone (estradiol and perhaps others) levels accentuated by pregnancy act on the emetic centers of the brain to produce nausea and vomiting. Women of a particular emotional state during their pregnancy have a lower threshold for symptoms, suggesting a psychologic component. However, it remains a matter of speculation whether the mind set of these individuals directly contributes to the condition or whether it is the lack or the excess of some factor that either prevents or predisposes to disease development. It is also unclear why some women have hyperemesis, whereas others of similar emotional and hormonal profile do not. More studies are needed before definitive statements can be made.

Differential Diagnosis

Many women experience nausea and vomiting after 6 to 10 weeks of a missed period. A pregnancy test should be obtained regardless of the frequency of symptoms. Once pregnancy is determined, the clinician should make an attempt to determine whether the patient is having normal pregnancy-related symptoms of nausea and vomiting or hyperemesis. This is often determined by frequency and severity of symptoms. If the patient requires hospitalization or intensive outpatient management to prevent dehydration and electrolyte imbalances in the absence of other medical

---

BOX 64-1
Diagnostic Evaluation of the Expected Hyperemetic Patient

History: Young primigravida, single parent, ambivalent about pregnancy, Caucasian, high socioeconomic class, dependent personality
Physical: Postural vital signs, dry mucous membranes, poor skin turgor, in severe cases hepatocellular jaundice, generally clear lungs, nontender abdomen and no costovertebral angle tenderness, normal uterine size for gestational age but may be enlarged secondary to multiple gestation or molar pregnancy
Laboratory: Serum-positive pregnancy test (*b*-hCG), hypokalemia, hyponatremia, hypochloremia, metabolic alkalosis, elevated blood urea nitrogen (BUN) and creatinine, urine ketosis and elevated specific gravity of urine
Other differential diagnoses:
  Medical conditions: gallbladder disease, hepatitis, pancreatitis, gastroenteritis, appendicitis, pyelonephritis
  Pregnancy conditions: molar pregnancy, twin gestation

---

conditions that may cause her symptoms, she has hyperemesis gravidarum. It is sometimes difficult to quantify vomiting since any amount is distressing. The clinician must therefore rely on history and physical examination along with appropriate laboratory testing to determine the need for medical intervention and possible hospitalization. Associated medical or pregnancy-related conditions must also be excluded to determine treatment options. Box 64-1 lists the findings in the history, physical examination, and laboratory assessment that suggest the diagnosis of hyperemesis. Other associated medical and pregnancy-related conditions are also listed.

✴ MANAGEMENT
Outpatient Therapy

Outpatient therapy should be reserved for patients with mild dehydration and with only minor electrolyte abnormalities. Furthermore, these patients should be able to tolerate clear fluids and small quantities of bland food. The goal of therapy is to correct mild dehydration and to initiate antiemetic therapy that will raise the threshold for nausea and vomiting. The patient may be started on any of the standard antiemetics, such as prochlorperazine (Compazine, 5 to 10 mg orally four times a day, or 25 mg rectally every 12 hours), trimethobenzamide (Tigan, 250 mg orally four times a day, or 200 mg rectally every 6 to 8 hours), promethazine (Phenergan, 25 to 50 mg orally/rectally every 4 to 6 hours), or metoclopramide (Reglan, 10 mg orally 1 hour before a meal and before bedtime). Both oral and rectal suppository forms of one of these medications should be given. If one medication does not successfully relieve symptoms, often another medication will. Other than metoclopramide (Reglan), the safety of these antiemetics as demonstrated by controlled trials in humans is lacking. Thus caution should be used and antiemetic medication use limited to cases of unrelenting symptoms. With all the antiemetics, retrospective reviews have failed to show teratogenicity directly linked to these medications in humans. As with any medication used during pregnancy, caution dictates that use be limited to individuals who do not respond to more conservative dietary measures. These drugs do cross the placenta at least at term, but most studies have shown the drugs to be safe. In addition to antiemetics, patients should be instructed to eat small frequent meals of bland foods rich in carbohydrates. It is helpful to consult a social worker or psychologist for evaluation of underlying emotional factors that may be contributing to disease severity. Psychotherapeutic techniques such as stimulus control, imagery conditioning, and hypnosis have been tried with reported success, as have acupressure and acupuncture; but studies of these therapies have been of insufficient sample size, poorly controlled, and confounded by questionable diagnosis and other treatments. Patients should be instructed to keep a chart of symptoms and daily weight with frequent follow-up visits.

Inpatient Therapy

Patients admitted to the hospital for hyperemesis gravidarum often are dehydrated and have electrolyte imbalance. Furthermore, they may be unable to tolerate any food or even liquids. Therapy should be directed toward restoring fluid and electrolyte balance. Intravenous therapy with dextrose and half normal saline solution with supplemental potassium chloride, as indicated by serum electrolyte levels, is standard. Antiemetic agents are given intravenously or as rectal suppositories. Oral food intake may begin once fluid and electrolyte balances have been restored and symptoms of nausea have ceased. Oral intake should begin slowly, starting with liquids and then advancing to solid bland food taken as small frequent meals. Initially, patient isolation from visitors and avoidance of other hospital stimulation such as television may be required on an individualized basis. Patient evaluation by social services or psychiatry may disclose underlying stress factors that may be managed by support aimed at relieving environmental stress. Tranquilizers may be necessary to treat anxiety states. Individuals admitted for hyperemesis gravidarum should be evaluated by a dietitian to determine their nutritional status and assist in recommending enteral or total parenteral nutrition needs, especially in those patients who do not respond to more conservative management and exhibit continued weight loss. Even patients who respond quickly to medical therapy often have frequent relapses and need a dietary management plan to optimize their nutritional status during pregnancy.

Daily weight measurement is the best guide for following therapeutic efficacy. Serum electrolyte levels and vital signs are also important treatment outcome variables.

Pregnancy Outcome

The effect of hyperemesis on pregnancy outcome is dependent on the amount of weight loss. Early reports stressed favorable pregnancy outcomes in hyperemetic women because of the reduced risk of early pregnancy loss. This association, however, may be secondary to selection bias in which pregnancies with sustained levels of estrogen and perhaps *b*-hCG may be more prone to hyperemesis. More recent studies have shown an increased risk of low birth weight and growth retardation in pregnant patients whose weight loss during pregnancy is 5% or whose symptoms are severe.

BIBLIOGRAPHY

Boyce RA: Enteral nutrition in hyperemesis gravidarum: a new development, *J Am Diet Assoc* 92:733, 1993.

Carlsson CP et al: Manual acupuncture reduces hyperemesis gravidarum: a placebo-controlled, randomized single blind crossover study, *J Pain Symptom Manage* 20:273, 2000.

Chin RKH, Lao TT: Low birth weight and hyperemesis gravidarum, *Eur J Obstet Gynecol Reprod Biol* 28:179, 1988.

Depue RH et al: Hyperemesis gravidarum in relation to estradiol levels, pregnancy outcome, and other maternal factors: a seroepidemiologic study, *Am J Obstet Gynecol* 156:1137, 1987.

Eliakim R, Abulafia O, Sherer DM: Hyperemesis gravidarum: a current review, *Am J Perinatol* 17:207, 2000.

Franko DL, Spurrell EB. Detection and management of eating disorders during pregnancy, *Obstet Gynecol* 95:942, 2000.

Gross S, Librach C, Cecutti A: Maternal weight loss associated with hyperemesis gravidarum: a predictor of fetal outcome, *Am J Obstet Gynecol* 160:906, 1989.

Jacoby EB, Porter KB: *Helicobacter pylori* infection and persistent hyperemesis gravidarum, *Am J Perinatol* 16:85, 1999.

Long MD, Simone SS, Tucker JJ: Outpatient treatment of hyperemesis gravidarum with stimulus control and imagery procedures, *J Behav Ther Exp Psychiatry* 17:105, 1986.

Meltzer D: Selections from current literature. Complementary therapies for nausea and vomiting in early pregnancy, *Fam Pract* 17:570, 2000.

Milkovich L, Vanden Berg CJ: An evaluation of the teratogenicity of certain antinauseant drugs, *Am J Obstet Gynecol* 125:244, 1976.

Moya F, Thorndike V: Passage of drugs across the placenta, *Am J Obstet Gynecol* 84:1778, 1962.

Russo-Stieglitz KE et al: Pregnancy outcome in patients requiring parenteral nutrition, *J Matern Fetal Med* 8:164, 1999.

Weigel RM, Weigel MM: Nausea and vomiting of early pregnancy and pregnancy outcome: a meta-analytical review, *Br J Obstet Gynaecol* 96:1312, 1989.

Wu CY et al: Correlation between *Helicobacter pylori* infection and gastrointestinal symptoms in pregnancy, *Adv Ther* 17:152, 2000.

CHAPTER 65

Vaginal Bleeding in Pregnancy and Ectopic Gestation

Mylene W. M. Yao

Joseph A. Hill

Vaginal bleeding in the first trimester is common and occurs in up to 20% of all pregnancies. The differential diagnoses of vaginal bleeding in the presence of a positive pregnancy test include intrauterine pregnancy, ectopic pregnancy, coincidental structural lesions such as cervical polyp, and molar pregnancy. The diagnosis of ectopic pregnancy should not be missed, as this is potentially fatal and is the leading cause of maternal mortality in the first trimester. History and physical examination are often inconclusive and a diagnostic protocol consisting of serum quantitative human chorionic gonadotropin (hCG), ultrasound, and sometimes pathology from endometrial sampling is required to determine the diagnosis and management plan.

Significant progress has been made in the past few decades to transform the typical treatment of ectopic pregnancy from emergency laparotomy with blood transfusion, to laparoscopic surgery with tubal preservation and medical treatment with methotrexate (MTX) for eligible patients. We first discuss the diagnostic protocol for first trimester vaginal bleeding and ectopic pregnancy, then focus on the current surgical and medical management of ectopic pregnancy.

DIAGNOSTIC PROTOCOL OF FIRST TRIMESTER VAGINAL BLEEDING

On presentation of vaginal bleeding in early pregnancy, the patient should first be assessed to ensure **hemodynamic stability.** A complete history will provide information on gestational age, risk factors for ectopic pregnancy or spontaneous abortion, and severity of symptoms. Although patients with ectopic pregnancy can present with bleeding, abdominal pain, shoulder pain, presyncope, or syncope, they may be asymptomatic. Further, bleeding and abdominal pain are also common presenting symptoms of spontaneous abortion. On physical examination, localized abdominal tenderness is suspicious for ectopic pregnancy; in addition, peritoneal signs indicate that a hemoperitoneum may be present and that care in an emergency setting is required. Estimation of gestational age based on the uterine size on pelvic examination can be misleading, as conditions such as fibroids, molar pregnancy, and twin gestation can lead to an overestimation of gestational age. However, one can determine whether bleeding is via the cervical os or due to structural lesions such as a cervical polyp on speculum examination. The finding of a dilated cervical os is highly reliable in indicating that the gestation has arrested and spontaneous or incomplete abortion is in evolution. However, if no tissues of conception have been passed and the patient is stable, it is advisable to document fetal demise on ultrasound to ease the patient's psychological acceptance of the diagnosis.

A **transvaginal ultrasound** (TVUS) is the first step in the diagnostic protocol. An intrauterine sac with a yolk sac or a fetal pole is evidence of an intrauterine pregnancy; fetal cardiac activity further confirms viability of an intrauterine pregnancy. In contrast, a yolk sac or fetal cardiac activity seen outside of the uterus signifies an ectopic pregnancy and treatment should be initiated. Even in the absence of fetal cardiac activity or a sac, the combined observation of a complex adnexal mass noncontiguous with the ovary, an empty uterus, and a positive hCG is 99% specific for an ectopic pregnancy (with positive and negative predictive values 96% and 95%, respectively) so that further diagnostic workup is not necessary. All other findings make the TVUS indeterminate and mandate further evaluation with serial serum quantitative hCG levels.

Current **serum and urine tests** involve immunoassays to detect the beta-subunit of hCG and can detect concentrations of hCG as low as 5 and 20 to 50 IU/L, respectively. In the past, hCG levels were reported as First and Second International Standard Units, but now are reported as the First International Reference Preparation (1st IRP) or the Third International Standard (3rd IS). The reference of the assay must be known to interpret the values correctly. Serum hCG is first detected before the expected menses at 7 to 9 days after the luteinizing hormone surge or 6 to 8 days after ovulation. Urine hCG is detected by the day of the expected menses, when serum hCG reaches 100 IU/L. Thereafter, it approximately doubles every 48 hours. The doubling time increases significantly after 20 days postovulation, and then increases even further after 30 days postovulation. As hCG rises, its rate of rise decreases, so that it reaches its peak levels of 50,000 to 100,000 IU/L at 8 to 0 weeks of gestation, after which it remains at 10,000 to 20,000 IU/L for the remainder of pregnancy. While an abnormal rise in hCG of

<66% over 48 hours increases the likelihood of an abnormal pregnancy, 15% of viable intrauterine pregnancies have an abnormal rise, and 15% of ectopic pregnancies can have a normal rise of >66% in 48 hours. Thus, an abnormal hCG rise cannot be used to differentiate between an arrested intrauterine pregnancy and an ectopic pregnancy.

In a patient with mild or no symptoms, stable hematocrit, and no significant amount of free fluid on TVUS to indicate hemoperitoneum, serial quantitative hCG levels are followed until they plateau (doubling time of 7 days) or reach 1500 to 2000 IU/L. An intrauterine sac corresponding to 5 to 5.5 weeks of gestation should be seen on TVUS at a discriminatory serum hCG level of 1500 IU/L. An indeterminate TVUS at the discriminatory hCG level or plateauing hCG level reflects a nonviable gestation and necessitates exclusion of an ectopic pregnancy. Tissues obtained by uterine curettage (dilatation and curettage, D&C) should be subjected to pathologic examination for the presence of chorionic villi, which would confirm an intrauterine arrested gestation. Once an arrested intrauterine gestation is diagnosed, no further treatment is required except to monitor the hCG level until it becomes negative. If chorionic villi are absent, the diagnosis of presumed ectopic pregnancy is made. Surgical diagnosis is not mandatory and surgery is performed only as indicated by clinical condition, contraindication to medical treatment, or patient's request. If the hCG levels remain low (<200 IU/L) or drop rapidly (>50% in 48 hours), then expectant management is reasonable for a spontaneously resolving presumed ectopic pregnancy.

The evidence for the use of this diagnostic protocol is based on the finding of Barnhart and colleagues finding that a serum hCG of 1500 IU/L in the absence of an intrauterine pregnancy on TVUS was 100% sensitive and 99.9% specific in diagnosing an ectopic pregnancy. Further, below the hCG discriminatory cut-off of 1500 IU/L, the diagnostic accuracy of TVUS was only 29%. Each institution should set its own discriminatory hCG level according to the hCG immunoassays and the experience of the ultrasonographers.

Uterine findings on TVUS such as endometrial thickness is not discriminative between intrauterine and ectopic pregnancies. Similarly, although an endometrial cavity containing fluid, echogenic material, or saclike structures on TVUS is more likely found with an arrested intrauterine gestation, ectopic pregnancy cannot be excluded on that basis. Of 26 patients who had indeterminate TVUS scans showing endometrial contents, 19% had no chorionic villi found on D&C, and the diagnosis of presumed ectopic pregnancy was made. Conversely, if there is no adnexal mass, one should not diagnose patients with an empty uterus on TVUS routinely as having presumed ectopic pregnancy, as almost half of such patients would have chorionic villi on D&C. Indeed, presumed ectopic pregnancy is a new clinical entity that is well treated with MTX, but it is difficult to estimate what proportion of these cases are truly ectopic and not missed abortion, as most of them are successfully treated with MTX. Therefore, vigilance is required to avoid overdiagnosis, which results in unnecessary treatment with a chemotherapeutic agent.

The search is still on for the ideal, single biochemical test to diagnose ectopic pregnancy. Candidates have included creatine kinase, CA125, and vascular endothelial growth factor. Unfortunately, no discriminatory cut-off has been identified for these tests. A single serum progesterone level >25 pg/ml is 98% predictive of a viable intrauterine pregnancy, and <5 pg/ml was proposed to be 100% diagnostic for either an arrested gestation or an ectopic pregnancy. Unfortunately, most patients have a serum progesterone level between 5 and 25 pg/ml, which is nondiagnostic. Therefore, we do not use the single serum progesterone test, as it has limited availability as a rapid test, and does not contribute further to the diagnostic protocol described previously.

ECTOPIC PREGNANCY
Incidence and Risk Factors
Ectopic pregnancy is a common condition in women of reproductive age that is associated with both short- and long-term morbidity. In 1992, the incidence of ectopic pregnancy was 2% of all reported pregnancies; moreover, it was the cause of 9% of all pregnancy-related deaths. Tubal disease secondary to infection or chronic inflammation is the primary risk factor. Although tubal mucosal damage is most commonly attributed to *Chlamydia trachomatis,* severe endometriosis, history of ruptured appendix, postsurgical adhesions, and luteal phase defects have all been implicated as risk factors. Recently, smoking as a risk factor has been substantiated by the finding of decreased tubal motility in response to cigarette smoke/nicotine. Most ectopic pregnancies are located in the ampullary, or distal third of the fallopian tube, but they can be found in the more proximal portion as well; rarely, they can be located in the interstitium or even outside the tube.

Surgical Treatment
Laparoscopic surgery has been demonstrated by prospective, randomized trials to be superior to laparotomy and has become the "gold standard" in treatment of ectopic pregnancy in hemodynamically stable patients. More than 85% to 90% of ectopic pregnancies are amenable to laparoscopic surgery. The surgical blood loss is minimal (<100 ml) and the duration of hospital stay is typically less than 48 hours. However, the surgical complication rate of laparoscopic surgery for ectopic pregnancy is 12% to 14%, which may reflect the individual surgeon's learning curve, as this procedure becomes more widely practiced and more patients with ruptured ectopic pregnancy are included.

If the patient does not wish to preserve fertility, the tube is badly damaged or hemostasis is not controlled, then the tube may be removed (salpingectomy) at laparoscopy. If the tubal condition and hemostasis are favorable, then the tube is usually preserved (salpingostomy) for patients who wish to maintain the option of natural conception. The risks of preserving the tube include persistent ectopic pregnancy and recurrence.

Persistent Ectopic Pregnancy
Persistent, ectopic gestational tissues occur in approximately 8% to 10% of salpingostomies; therefore, weekly follow-up evaluation of serum quantitative hCG levels are mandatory postoperatively. If the hCG levels are plateaued, then persistent ectopic pregnancy is diagnosed, irrespective of the presence of symptoms or TVUS findings. The treatment of persistent ectopic pregnancy in stable patients is single-dose, intramuscular (IM) MTX (Box 65-1). Medical

---

BOX 65-1

Intramuscular Methotrexate Protocol for the Treatment of Ectopic Pregnancy

---

Indication:

Diagnosis of proven, presumed, or persistent ectopic pregnancy.

Contraindications:

1. Clinical or sonographic evidence of hemoperitoneum, impending tubal rupture, or hemodynamic instability.
2. Serum hCG > 15,000 mIU/ml.
3. Patient does not give informed consent or will not comply with follow-up.
4. Breastfeeding.
5. Abnormal liver, renal, or hematologic profiles; any chronic liver disease or alcoholism; history of blood dyscrasias (i.e., bone marrow hypoplasia, leukopenia, thrombocytopenia, or significant anemia); clinical or laboratory evidence of immunodeficiency.
6. Known sensitivity to MTX.
7. Active pulmonary disease.
8. Peptic ulcer disease.
9. Coexisting viable intrauterine pregnancy.

Relative Contraindications:

1. Extrauterine fetal cardiac activity on ultrasound.
2. Declining serum hCG levels.
3. Patient is symptomatic or moderate tenderness is elicited on abdominal palpation.

Pretreatment or Baseline Tests:

1. CBC
2. SGOT/SGPT
3. BUN/Creatinine
4. Blood type
5. Serum quantitative hCG level
6. Transvaginal ultrasound
7. Endometrial sampling if indicated

Protocol:

1. Obtain results from pretreatment tests, height and weight.
2. Day 1: methotrexate 50 mg/m^2 intramuscular
3. Give RhoGAM if Rh negative
4. Days 4 and 7: serum hCG levels
5. If there is >10% decline in serum hCG between days 4 and 7, then follow serum hCG weekly until it is < assay.
6. If there is <10% decline in serum hCG between days 4 and 7, and patient is clinically stable, give a second dose of methotrexate 50 mg/m^2 IM on day 7. Repeat serum hCG levels on days 11 and 14. If the decline in serum hCG between days 11 and 14 is less than 5%, a third dose of methotrexate 50 mg/m^2 IM or surgical treatment should be considered. Serum hCG is followed weekly until it is < assay.
7. Pelvic examinations should not be done.
8. Follow-up monitoring should be arranged.
9. If the patient develops abdominal pain, then repeat clinical assessment, TVUS, and repeat CBC should be performed. If indicated, the patient should be admitted for observation until hemodynamic stability is assured.

Instructions to Patients:

1. Do not drink alcohol for 2 weeks after receiving methotrexate.
2. Do not take aspirin or aspirin-like medications such as ibuprofin (Advil or Motrin) for 2-3 weeks after receiving methotrexate.
3. Avoid exposure to sun or sunlamps for 4 weeks after methotrexate therapy.
4. Avoid pelvic examinations and intercourse until complete resolution of the ectopic pregnancy as indicated by a negative pregnancy blood test.
5. Use birth control for the next 2 months.

Avoid vitamin preparations containing folic acid until the ectopic pregnancy is resolved.

---

hCG, Human chorionic gonadotropin; *MTX,* methotrexate; *CBC,* complete blood count; *SGOT,* serum glutamic-oxaloacetic transaminase; *SGPT,* serum glutamatepyruvate transaminase; *BUN,* blood urea nitrogen.

treatment of persistent disease is successful in 97% of cases obviating further medical or surgical treatment. Routine treatment with single-dose IM MTX postoperatively has been proposed to reduce persistent disease from 15% to 2% after laparoscopic surgery. Although MTX prophylaxis for noncompliance is understandable, its routine postoperative use is unclear given the high success rate of treatment of persistent disease by MTX.

RECURRENT ECTOPIC PREGNANCY AND LONG-TERM REPRODUCTIVE OUTCOMES

Overall, the most important prognostic factors for a subsequent intrauterine pregnancy (IUP) are history of infertility, contralateral tubal status at time of surgery, and age. The subsequent rates of IUP and ectopic pregnancy were 60% and 15%, respectively, based on a review of 12 studies involving 1514 patients who attempted to conceive after laparoscopic

Finally, although it is encouraging that conservative surgical and medical treatments for extratubal ectopic pregnancies are reported with higher efficacy, there is a possibility of reporting bias, so that unsuccessful cases are less likely to be reported. Therefore, the morbidity of these unusual ectopic pregnancies should still be considered very high, and prudent care must be exercised when managing these cases, especially when medical options are chosen.

BIBLIOGRAPHY

Atri M et al: Ectopic pregnancy: evolution after treatment with transvaginal methotrexate, *Radiology* 185:749, 1992.

Barnhart KT et al: Diagnostic accuracy of ultrasound above and below the beta-hCG discriminatory zone, *Obstet Gynecol* 94:583, 1999.

Barnhardt K et al: Prompt diagnosis of ectopic pregnancy in an emergency department setting, *Obstet Gynecol* 84:1010, 1994.

Benifla JL: Alternative to surgery of treatment of unruptured interstitial pregnancy:15 cases of medical treatment, *Eur J Obstet Gynecol Reprod Biol* 70:151, 1996.

Brown DL, Doubilet PM: Transvaginal sonography for diagnosing ectopic pregnancy: positivity criteria and performance characteristics, *J Ultrasound Med* 12:259, 1994.

Brown DL et al: Serial endovaginal sonography of ectopic pregnancies treated with methotrexate, *Obstet Gynecol* 77:406, 1991.

Castles A et al: Effects of smoking during pregnancy. Five meta-analyses, *Am J Prev Med* 16:208, 1999.

Centers for Disease Control: Current trends: ectopic pregnancy–United States, 1990-1992, *CDC MMWR Weekly* 44:46, 1995.

Check JH et al: Analysis of serum human chorionic gonadotropin levels in normal singleton, multiple and abnormal pregnancies, *Hum Reprod* 7:1176, 1992.

Clasen K et al: Ectopic pregnancy: let's cut! Strict laparoscopic approach to 194 consecutive cases and review of literature on alternatives, *Hum Reprod* 12:596, 1997.

Daniel Y et al: Levels of vascular endothelial growth factor are elevated in patients with ectopic pregnancy: is this a novel marker? *Fertil Steril* 72:1013, 1999.

Dart R et al: The utility of a dilatation and evacuation procedure in patients with symptoms suggestive of ectopic pregnancy and indeterminate transvaginal ultrasonography, *Acad Emerg Med* 6:1024, 1999.

Dela Cruz A et al: Factors determining fertility after conservative or radical surgical treatment for ectopic pregnancy, *Fertil Steril* 68:871, 1997.

DiCarlantonio G, Talbot P: Inhalation of mainstream and sidestream cigarette smoke retards embryo transport and slows muscle contraction in oviducts of hamsters (Mesocricetus auratus), *Biol Reprod* 61:651, 1999.

Everett C: Incidence and outcome of bleeding before the 20th week of pregnancy: prospective study, *BMJ* 315:32, 1997.

Fernandez H et al: The hidden side of ectopic pregnancy: the hormonal factor, *Hum Reprod* 11:243, 1996.

Fernandez H et al: Methotrexate treatment of ectopic pregnancy: 100 cases treated by primary transvaginal injection under sonographic control, *Fertil Steril* 59:773, 1992.

Frates MC, Laing FC: Sonographic evaluation of ectopic pregnancy: an update, *AJR* 165:251, 1995.

Glock JL et al: Efficacy and safety of single-dose systemic methotrexate in the treatment of ectopic pregnancy, *Fertil Steril* 62:716, 1994.

Graczykowski JW et al: Methotrexate prophylaxis for persistent ectopic pregnancy after conservative treatment by salpingostomy, *Obstet Gynecol* 89:118, 1997.

Gross Z et al: Ectopic pregnancy: non-surgical, outpatient evaluation and single-dose methotrexate treatment, *J Reprod Med* 40:371, 1995.

Hajenius PJ et al: Randomised trial of systemic methotrexate versus laparoscopic salpingostomy in tubal pregnancy, *Lancet* 350:774, 1997.

Hajenius PJ et al: Serum human chorionic gonadotropin clearance curves in patients with interstitial pregnancy treated with systemic methotrexate, *Fertil Steril* 66:723, 1996.

Hillis SD et al: Recurrent chlamydial infections increase the risks of hospitalization for ectopic pregnancy and pelvic inflammatory disease, *Am J Obstet Gynecol* 176:103, 1997.

Hoppe DE et al: Single-dose systemic methotrexate for the treatment of persistent ectopic pregnancy after conservative surgery, *Obstet Gynecol* 83:51, 1994.

Horrigan TJ et al: Methotrexate pneumonitis after systemic treatment for ectopic pregnancy, *Am J Obstet Gynecol* 176:714, 1997.

Kadar N et al: A method for screening for ectopic pregnancy, *Obstet Gynecol* 58:162, 1981.

Kadar N et al: Discriminatory hCG zone: its use in the sonographic evaluation for ectopic pregnancy, *Obstet Gynecol* 58:156, 1981.

Kjer JJ, Iversen T: Malignant trophoblastic tumours in Norway. Fertility rate after chemotherapy, *Br J Obstet Gynecol* 97:623, 1990.

Korhonen J et al: Serum human chorionic gonadotropin dynamics during spontaneous resolution of ectopic pregnancy, *Fertil Steril* 61:632, 1994.

Kung FT et al: Subsequent reproduction and obstetric outcome after methotrexate treatment of cervical pregnancy: a review of original literature and international collaborative follow-up, *Hum Reprod* 12:591, 1997.

Landstrom G et al: Treatment, failures and complications ectopic pregnancy: changes over a 20 year period, *Hum Reprod* 13:203, 1998.

Lau S, Tulandi T: Conservative medical and surgical management of interstitial ectopic pregnancy, *Fertil Steril* 72:207, 1999.

Lipscomb GH et al: Management of separation pain after single-dose methotrexate therapy for ectopic pregnancy, *Obstet Gynecol* 93:590, 1999.

Lipscomb GH et al: Predictors of success of methotrexate treatment in women with tubal ectopic pregnancies, *N Engl J Med* 341:1974, 1999.

Lundorff P et al: Laparoscopic surgery in ectopic pregnancy: a randomized trial versus laparotomy, *Acta Obstet Gynecol Scand* 70:343, 1991.

Marcus SF et al: Heterotopic pregnancies after in-vitro fertilization and embryo transfer, *Hum Reprod* 10:1232, 1995.

Mol BW et al: Are gestational age and endometrial thickness alternatives for serum human chorionic gonadotropin as criteria for the diagnosis of ectopic pregnancy, *Fertil Steril* 72:643, 1999.

Murphy AA et al: Operative laparoscopy versus laparotomy for the management of ectopic pregnancy: a prospective trial, *Fertil Steril* 57:1180, 1992.

Predanic M: Differentiating tubal abortion from viable ectopic pregnancy with serum CA-125 and beta-human chorionic gonadotropin determinations, *Fertil Steril* 73:522, 2000.

Seifer DB et al: Persistent ectopic pregnancy: an argument for heightened vigilance and patient compliance, *Fertil Steril* 68:402, 1997.

Seinera P et al: Ovarian pregnancy and operative laparoscopy: report of eight cases, *Hum Reprod* 12:608, 1997.

Shalev E et al: Spontaneous resolution of ectopic tubal pregnancy: natural history, *Fertil Steril* 63:15, 1995.

Sotrel G et al: Heterotopic pregnancy following Clomid treatment, *J Reprod Med* 15:78, 1976.

Stovall TG et al: Single-dose methotrexate: an expanded clinical trial, *Am J Obstet Gynecol* 168:1759, 1993.

Stovall TG et al: Improved sensitivity and specificity of a single measurement of serum progesterone over serial quantitative beta-human chorionic gonadotropin in screening for ectopic pregnancy, *Hum Reprod* 7:723, 1992.

Tal J et al: Heterotopic pregnancy after ovulation induction and assisted reproductive technologies: a literature review from 1971 to 1993, *Fertil Steril* 66:1, 1996.

Tulandi T et al: Rupture of ectopic pregnancy in women with low and declining serum β-hCG levels, *Fertil Steril* 56:786, 1991.

Urbach DR, Cohen MM: Is perforation of the appendix a risk factor for tubal infertility and ectopic pregnancy? An appraisal of the evidence, *Can J Surg* 42:101, 1999.

Ushakov FB et al: Cervical pregnancy: past and future, *Obstet Gynecol Surv* 52:45, 1996.

Vandermolen DT: Serum creatine kinase does not predict ectopic pregnancy, *Fertil Steril* 65:916, 1996.

Vermesh M et al: Management of unruptured ectopic gestation by linear salpingostomy: a prospective, randomized clinical trial of laparoscopy versus laparotomy, *Obstet Gynecol* 73:400, 1989.

Walden PAM, Bagshawe KD: Reproductive performance of women successfully treated for gestational trophoblastic tumors, *Am J Obstet Gynecol* 125:1108, 1976.

Wu MY et al: Heterotopic pregnancies after controlled ovarian hyperstimulation and assisted reproductive techniques, *J Formos Med Assoc* 94:600, 1995.

Yao M, Tulandi T: Surgical and medical management of tubal and nontubal ectopic pregnancies, *Curr Opin Obstet Gynecol* 10:371, 1998.

Yao M and Tulandi T: Current status of surgical and nonsurgical management of ectopic pregnancy, *Fertil Steril* 67:421, 1997.

CHAPTER **66**

Miscarriage and Recurrent Spontaneous Pregnancy Loss

Mylene W.M. Yao
Joseph A. Hill

⊞ EPIDEMIOLOGY AND DEFINITION OF ABORTION

In approximately 70% of human conceptions fetal viability is not achieved, and an estimated 50% are lost before the first missed menses. The actual rate of pregnancy loss after implantation may be as high as 31%. Spontaneous abortion, defined as the loss of a clinically recognized (blood test or ultrasound) pregnancy before 20 weeks' gestation, occurs in 10% to 15% of all clinically established pregnancies. Approximately 60% of pregnancy losses before 8 weeks' gestation are chromosomally abnormal; trisomies are the most common abnormality. However, the most common single abnormality is monosomy X.

Spontaneous abortions are subdivided into threatened abortion, inevitable abortion, incomplete abortion, complete abortion, missed abortion, and recurrent abortion. Threatened abortion is a viable clinical pregnancy accompanied by vaginal bleeding. Inevitable abortion occurs during pregnancy in the presence of a dilated internal cervical os or in cases of ruptured membranes. In an incomplete abortion some but not all fetal-placental tissue has passed through the internal cervical os; in a complete abortion all fetal-placental tissue has been spontaneously passed through the internal cervical os. A missed abortion is a pregnancy in which the fetus is no longer viable in the absence of vaginal bleeding. Symptoms of pregnancy (nausea, breast tenderness) may or may not be present at the time of pregnancy loss. Pelvic examination and ultrasound assessment will usually lead to the proper diagnosis.

DEFINITION OF RECURRENT PREGNANCY LOSS

Recurrent pregnancy loss (RPL), classically defined as three or more consecutive pregnancy losses before 20 weeks of gestation, affects 1% to 3% of couples annually in the United States. This definition of RPL has been challenged, since most clinicians currently recommend diagnostic evaluation following two consecutive spontaneous abortions. Given the high incidence of sporadic miscarriages in the general population (occurring in 12% of pregnant women below age 20, and in 26% of those over age 40), it is important to consider that the incidence of RPL is higher than that expected based on the spontaneous abortion rate. This suggests that specific causes of repeated pregnancy failure exist. It is clear that RPL is not a specific disease, but rather a symptom that can be observed in association with several potential abortifacient conditions.

The calculated risks for recurrent pregnancy loss are based on epidemiologic surveys. These surveys indicate that after one spontaneous abortion the recurrence risk is 24%; after two, 30%; after three, 35%; and after four consecutive clinical losses, approximately 40%.

CAUSES
Chromosomal Abnormalities

Parental chromosomal abnormalities remain the only uncontested cause of recurrent pregnancy loss and occur in approximately 5% of couples seeking evaluation. Other associations with recurrent pregnancy loss have been made, including müllerian or anatomic anomalies (10%), endocrinologic abnormalities (17%), infections (5%), and autoimmunity (3%). The potential cause in the majority of cases however, remains unexplained (60%) after a thorough conventional evaluation (Box 66-1).

The most common inborn parental chromosomal abnormality contributing to recurrent abortion is balanced translocation. Pericentric chromosomal inversion and sex chromosome mosaicism have also been associated with recurrent abortion. Other genetic causes of abortion include multifactorial inheritance of autosomal recessive genes and X-linked disorders.

Congenital and Acquired Anatomic Causes (Box 66-2)

Anatomic causes can be divided into both congenital and acquired lesions. Congenital anomalies include incomplete müllerian fusion or septum resorption defects, diethylstilbestrol (DES) exposure, and uterine artery anomalies. Women with a septate uterus may have a 62% risk for spontaneous abortion. Second trimester losses are most commonly seen; however, first trimester abortions may be caused if the embryo implants on the intrauterine septum since the endometrium overlying a septum is poorly developed and blood supply to this area is often limited. Therefore abnormal placentation may occur, potentially culminating in an abortion. DES exposure in utero can lead to uterine developmental anomalies, most commonly hypoplasia, later causing both first and second trimester abortions. DES exposed women also have a predisposition to development of incompetent cervix and premature labor. Isolated cases of uterine artery anomalies have been reportedly associated with recurrent abortion, most likely caused by compromised blood flow to the implanting blastocyst and developing placenta. Acquired anatomic lesions potentially predisposing to recurrent abortion include uterine synechiae (adhesions), and leiomyomata (fibroids). These associations with abortion are tenuous, but theoretic mechanisms that may be involved include interference with blood supply.

Endocrinologic Abnormalities

Endocrinologic abnormalities associated with recurrent abortion include luteal phase insufficiency, thyroid disorders, and diabetes mellitus. The early maintenance of pregnancy is dependent on progesterone production by the corpus luteum until the placenta takes over progesterone production between 7 and 9 weeks' gestation. Spontaneous abortion could ensue if (1) the corpus luteum fails to produce significant quantities of progesterone, (2) progesterone delivery to the uterus is compromised, or (3) progesterone use within endometrial/decidual tissue is disordered. Thyroid disorders, most commonly hypothyroidism, have also been associated with recurrent abortion, most likely because of ovulation disorders that lead to corpus luteum insufficiency. The mechanism of abortion in women with diabetes mellitus is unclear but may be caused by compromised blood flow to the developing conceptus, especially in cases of advanced disease. Elevated hemoglobin A1c levels in peripheral blood before conception have also been associated with pregnancy failure.

Maternal Infections

Maternal infections have been tenuously associated with recurrent abortion. The most commonly reported association between infection and pregnancy loss has been cervical colonization with mycoplasma, Ureaplasma, chlamydia and Group B streptococcus. Casual mechanisms are poorly described but one theoretic possibility may involve immunologic activation.

Environmental Factors

Other poorly established associations include environmental factors such as exposure to heavy metal toxicity, carbon tetrachloride, and trichloroethylene benzene; drugs such as caffeine, folic acid antagonists, nicotine, ethanol, and inhalation anesthetic agents; ionizing radiation; and chronic medical illnesses such as cardiac and renal diseases or any other disorder that compromises uterine blood supply. It is important to reassure patients that exposure to video display terminals and microwave ovens does not cause abortion.

Thrombophilic Factors

Pregnancy is an acquired hypercoagulable state and inherited thrombophilias have recently been associated with recurrent pregnancy loss. The precise prevalence of these disorders in women with recurrent pregnancy loss remains incompletely understood, although an increased incidence of pregnancy loss in women with antithrombin III, protein C, and protein S deficiencies and in women with factor V Leiden mutation has been reported. Individuals with the C677TY mutation in the MTHFR gene causing elevated homocysteine levels predisposing to early development of arteriosclerosis have also been reported to have a higher prevalence of pregnancy loss than individuals without this mutation. The mechanism of loss in these individuals involves thrombosis; however, not all placental bed biopsies obtained from spontaneous abortions in these women demonstrate placental pathology. Anticoagulant therapy, especially in cases where placental pathology has been previously confirmed in prior losses should be considered; however, the clinical utility of these assays and therapy remains to be definitely established.

Immunologic Phenomena

Immunologic phenomena involving allogenic immunity and autoimmunity have also been associated with reproductive failure. The immune system is a complex integrated system that has evolved to protect the individual from nonself tissue. The immune system can be simplistically divided into the humoral immune system, which is mediated by antibody secreting plasma cells derived from B-lymphocytes, and the cellular immune system, which is mediated by cytokines secreted by activated macrophages, T-lymphocytes, and natural killer cells.

Autoimmune Mechanisms of Pregnancy Loss

Of all the immunological theories proposed for recurrent pregnancy loss, only the theory involving antiphospholipid antibody to cardiolipin has fulfilled most of the criteria for causality. The association of anticardiolipin antibody with one or more of the clinical features listed in Box 66-3 has been termed the antiphospholipid syndrome. It is thought that placental coagulopathy mediates fetal loss occurring generally after week 10 of gestation in women with the antiphospholipid syndrome. The median time of pregnancy loss in these women is week 20.5 of gestation. The incidence of the antiphospholipid syndrome is controversial as it depends on which antiphospholipid antibodies are measured and the methods used to define a positive value. From well-defined clinical and laboratory criteria, a conservative estimate of the incidence of the antiphospholipid syndrome is <5% in women with recurrent pregnancy loss. The anticardiolipin antibody test, which uses defined cardiolipin standards to calculate positive values, is the only well-standardized assay applicable for testing antiphospholipid antibodies.

Lupus anticoagulant tests (activated PTT, Russell viper venom time) have also been used to diagnose the antiphospholipid syndrome. These tests must differentiate whether prolonged clotting in vitro is due to clotting factor deficiency (false positive) or an inhibitor (true positive) after addition of normal control serum. The pathophysiological mechanisms involved potentially in anticardiolipin-related pregnancy loss include increased platelet aggregation, decreased endogenous anticoagulant activity, increased thrombosis, and vasoconstriction resulting from immunoglobulin, specifically IgG binding to endothelial membrane cardiolipin within placental tissues.

Autoimmunity to other phospholipids and cellular components has also been proposed as a mechanism for recurrent pregnancy loss, although in most cases cause versus effect have not been adequately differentiated, with the possible exception of antibodies against the phospholipid phosphatidylserine. Antibodies, specifically IgM, against this phospholipid inhibit intercellular fusion of trophoblast cell lines in vitro and impair both trophoblast hormone production and invasion in vitro.

Women with low or unsustained moderate concentrations of anticardiolipin antibodies are no more likely to develop phospholipid related disorders, including pregnancy loss, than are women without these antibodies. Similarly, autoantibody testing of subfertile women, including those undergoing repeated implantation failure after IVF-ET, is not justified clinically since women with high titers of anticardiolipin antibody, such as women with the antiphospholipid syndrome or women with systemic lupus erythematosus, do not have difficulty in establishing pregnancy.

Alloimmune Mechanisms of Pregnancy Loss

One alloimmune hypothesis proposed for some cases of reproductive difficulty in women concerns immunodystrophism involving Th1 cytokines such as gamma-interferon (IFN-γ) and tumor necrosis factor (TNF), which may have embryotoxic effects. The fundamental hypothesis underlying this novel alloimmune disorder is that immune and inflammatory cells residing in the uterus may become activated in response to either microbial antigens or to reproductive antigens such as invading cytotrophoblast. A byproduct of activation is the secretion of a wide variety of immunological growth factor/cytokines by these cells. It is hypothesized that, in successful pregnancies, homeostasis among these growth-modulating proteins is achieved. In cases in which Th1 cytokines predominate, limited trophoblast invasion may occur, culminating in intrauterine growth restriction or preeclampsia, or in severe cases, pregnancy loss. In cases in which the amount of Th1 cytokines produced is too small, unrestricted trophoblast invasion may occur culminating theoretically in placenta accreta, percreata mand increnta, or perhaps to invasive and persistent trophoblast disease. These hypotheses remain to be substantiated.

The actions of these growth-regulating proteins are mediated by cell surface receptor binding and human cytotrophoblast expresses receptors for all of these cytokines providing an anatomical basis for this theory. Additional evidence in support of this theory comes from the finding that IL-12 mRNA is observed more commonly in the decidua of spontaneously aborted pregnancies compared with elective pregnancy terminations of the same gestational age. This may be an important observation, since IL-12 is known to initiate Th1 immunity. Whether this observation provides evidence that IL-12 is involved in pregnancy loss or is merely an effect of fetal demise requires further studies correlating with fetal karyotype assessments.

Evaluation of Women With History of Recurrent Abortion

The diagnostic evaluation of couples experiencing recurrent abortion should begin with a general history: medical, surgical, genetic, and psychologic. A description and sequence of all prior pregnancies is important as is whether histologic and karyotypic assessment of prior abortions was performed. The practitioner should also ask about chronic illnesses, uterine instrumentation, infection, DES exposure, and exposure to drugs, radiation, and possible environmental pollutants.

A general physical examination of the woman should look for signs of metabolic illness. On pelvic examination the examiner should look for signs of infection, DES, exposure, or previous cervical lacerations. A bimanual examination should be performed to determine the size, shape, and contour of the uterus.

Potentially useful laboratory measurements include (1) peripheral blood karyotype of both partners; (2) a uterine structural study, such as hysterosalpingogram or sonohysterogram followed by hysteroscopy and laparoscopy, if indicated; (3) luteal phase endometrial biopsy, ideally 10 days after the luteinizing hormone (LH) surge or after cycle day 24 of an idealized 28-day cycle. If the biopsy is out of phase by more than 2 days according to established criteria then repeat assessment in a subsequent cycle should be considered to definitively make the diagnosis of luteal phase insufficiency. In cases of an abnormal biopsy result, a serum prolactin and androgen profile should also be determined; (4) antibody and antiphosphatidylserine antibody; (5) lupus anticoagulant (a partial thromboplastin time [PPT] or Russell viper venom time); and, perhaps as a last resort, (6) a cervical culture for mycoplasma, Ureaplasma, chlamydia, and Group B β streptococcus. Investigative measures that are of no benefit in the evaluation of recurrent pregnancy loss include (1) antinuclear antibodies, (2) antipaternal cytotoxic antibodies, (3) parental HLA profiles, and (4) CD56 immunophenotype profiles. Further work is needed before suppressor cell/factor determinations, cytokine, oncogene, and growth factor measurements or Th1 embryotoxic factor assessment can be clinically justified and available.

✳ MANAGEMENT

Therapy should include appropriate measures for the individual known groups. Antibiotic therapy is indicated only if findings on the cervical culture warrant treatment. Normalization of ovulation, and synchronization of ovulation and sperm deposition should be advised. Early diagnosis and close monitoring during the first trimester may also be therapeutic. Serial human chorionic gonadotropin determinations for the β subunit of hCG (β-hCG) should be performed after the first period is missed. Ultrasound assessment should be performed to confirm an intrauterine pregnancy once the β-hCG attains 1000 to 5000 mIU/ml or 5 to 6 weeks' gestation, because women with recurrent spontaneous abortion have a 2% to 4% risk of ectopic gestation. A repeat pelvic ultrasound to confirm fetal viability should be performed every 2 weeks through the first trimester or past the point in gestation whether the individual's abortions have previously occurred. This may help alleviate the couple's anxiety and to allow intervention for karyotype assessment should fetal demise occur.

Immunotherapy

Both immunostimulating and immunosuppressive therapies have been proposed for recurrent spontaneous abortion depending on whether the maternal immune system was thought to be hyporesponsive or hyperresponsive to paternal-fetal antigen stimulation. Immunostimulation using a variety of agents, including leukocytes, trophoblast membrane vesicle extracts, and seminal plasma, has been performed historically based on the theory of blocking antibody deficiency. However, the rationale behind this theory has been disputed. Among the clinical risks of such therapy are sensitization to HLA, other leukocyte, platelet, or blood group antigens and other transfusion related risks including bacterial, viral and prion disease transmission. Based on meta-analyses of available published, double-blind, placebo-controlled trials, such therapy does not appear to be effective. The most recent double-blinded, placebo-controlled trial indicated that the outcome of women immunized with paternal leukocytes had significantly worse pregnancy outcomes than women receiving the placebo.

Thus alternative immunomodulating therapies have been proposed for unexplained recurrent spontaneous abortion. Most prominent among these has been intravenous immunoglobulin (IVIG). IVIG has many potential immunomodulating effects. However, the clinical trials published to date have lacked sufficient power to allow a definitive conclusion resulting from their limited sample size. These studies were neither prestratified by age nor number of prior losses. Few of these studies were randomized properly, placebo-controlled or corrected for concomitant therapy. Many included women with only two prior losses and did not have strict inclusion and exclusion criteria possibly resulting in a heterogeneous group of subject. Meta-analysis of these data have not suggested efficacy. In addition to lack of efficacy, other compelling reasons not to use IVIG include the potential for adverse long-term side effects such as Creutzfeldt-Jakob, Mad Cow disease and other prion-related diseases. Although these may only be remote possibilities, it is important to realize that blood from approximately 150 donors is needed to produce one vial of IVIG. The financial cost of this unsubstantiated and potentially dangerous therapy is $7,000 to $14,000 over the course, which further diminishes enthusiasm for its use. Evidence does indicate that aspirin (81 mg/day) and heparin (10,000 units bid) are efficacious in preventing abortion and other malobstetric outcomes except in cases of the antiphospholipid antibody syndrome. Aspirin (81 mg/day) may also be worthwhile in women who have had pregnancy loss after 13 weeks' gestation but is not of benefit in women with recurrent pregnancy loss occurring during the first trimester of pregnancy.

For women with recurrent spontaneous abortion believed to be caused by autoimmune or cellular maternal immune responses to the developing conceptus, immunosuppressive therapy has also been advocated. Corticosteroids have been recommended by some for pregnancy loss resulting from antiphospholipid antibodies, although they are not always effective. The potential adverse side effects of corticosteroids also temper their use in treating presumed immunologic reproductive failure. Low dose aspirin (81 mg/day)

Table 66-1
Prognosis for Live Birth

Cause	% Success
Genetic (chromosomal)	30-60
Anatomic	60-70
Endocrinologic	90
Unknown (other)	30-90

and heparin (5,000 units twice a day) are currently recommended for the treatment of autoimmune reproductive failure in women with antiphospholipid antibodies.

Safe and effective treatment modalities are needed for couples who are experiencing recurrent abortion. The rationale for therapy, however, must be scientifically well founded and more innocuous than the disease. Practicing physicians should refrain from using or recommending immunotherapy for their patients with recurrent abortion until the rationale for such therapy has been proved and the safety and efficacy of potential regimens have been scientifically tested in double-blind, randomized, appropriately controlled trials.

PROGNOSIS FOR LIVE BIRTH

The prognosis for a subsequent live birth in couples with a history of recurrent abortion is not necessarily dismal (Table 66-1). Most chromosomally abnormal pregnancies abort before achieving fetal cardiac activity. Once fetal cardiac activity has been ultrasonically detected between 5 and 6 weeks' gestation, the risk of subsequent loss is approximately 23%. Although this is significantly higher than the 4% incidence in the general population, knowledge that a 77% chance of fetal viability exists once fetal cardiac activity has been detected can be tremendously reassuring to the couple who has experienced multiple miscarriages and helps establish a more realistic prognosis for pregnancy success.

BIBLIOGRAPHY

Alberman E: The epidemiology of repeated abortion. In Sharp F, editor: *Early Pregnancy Loss: Mechanisms and Treatment,* New York, 1988, Springer-Verlag.

Antiphospholipid syndrome. ACOG Technical Bulletin 2000.

Boue J, Boue A, Lasar P: Retrospective and prospective epidemiologic studies of 1,500 karyotyped spontaneous abortions, *Teratol* 11:11, 1975.

Ecker JL, Laufer MR, Hill JA: Measurement of embryotoxic factors is predictive of pregnancy outcome in women with a history of recurrent abortion, *Obstet Gynecol* 81:84, 1993.

Hill JA, Anderson DJ, Polgar K: T helper 1-type cellular immunity to trophoblast in women with recurrent spontaneous abortion. *JAMA* 273: 1933, 1995.

Hill JA: Sporadic and recurrent spontaneous abortion. In Creasey RK, Resnik R, editors: *Maternal-Fetal Medicine,* Philadelphia, 1999, WB Saunders.

Hill JA et al: Evidence of embryo and trophoblast toxic cellular immune response(s) in women with recurrent spontaneous abortion, *Am J Obstet Gynecol* 166:1044, 1992.

Laufer MR, Ecker JL, Hill JA: Pregnancy outcome following ultrasound documented fetal cardiac activity in women with a history of multiple spontaneous abortions, *J Soc Gynecol Invest* 1994.

Triplett DA: Obstetrical implications of anti phospholipid antibodies, *Bailliere Clin Obstet Gynecol* 6:507, 1992.

Warburton D, Fraser FC: Spontaneous abortion rate in man: data from reproductive histories collected in a medical genetics unit, *Am J Hum Genet* 16:1, 1963.

Wilcox AJ et al: Incidence of early loss of pregnancy, *N Engl J Med* 319: 189, 1988.

CHAPTER 67

Infectious Exposure and Immunization

Stephanie A. Eisenstat

A number of infectious diseases in the pregnant woman can have devastating consequences for the fetus. To evaluate and counsel pregnant women who have been exposed to or have contracted specific infections the primary care clinician needs to be familiar with the effects of these diseases. Although there are vast observational data, controversy remains regarding screening for most of these infectious diseases; thus standard protocols have been difficult to implement. This chapter reviews the major issues in identification and prevention of the more common infectious diseases during pregnancy that have serious consequences for the fetus. The subject of human immunodeficiency virus (HIV) infection and pregnancy is discussed in Chapter 21 and sexually transmitted diseases in Chapter 22.

PATHOPHYSIOLOGY
Fetal Immunity

The fetal immune system is immature until after 20 weeks of gestation. Because of the lack of maturity across all cell lines, there is a decrease in function in the T-cell-mediated processes (delayed hypersensitivity, T-cell help for B-cell differentiation, and cytokine production) and in B-cell line function (resulting in poorly functioning neutrophils and an inability to produce antibodies to bacterial polysaccharides). Most of the immunoglobulin present is immune globulin G (IgG) synthesized by the mother and subsequently transferred across the placenta. The fetus is able to produce IgM, but relies on the mother's immunocompetence. Other cells such as natural killer (NK) cells are present but immature and not completely functional.

SCREENING DURING PREGNANCY

Screening for certain infectious diseases during pregnancy is an important part of routine prenatal care. The most common infections that have adverse fetal outcome are toxoplasmosis, rubella, cytomegalovirus, and herpes simplex viruses (TORCH). In some diseases, such as hepatitis B, early identification in the mother followed by immunoprophylaxis of the newborn can prevent severe neonatal morbidity. Routine serologic screening to detect a variety of infections has been advocated by some during both the preconception and the early prenatal periods. Serologic diagnosis is based on the demonstration of a significant rise in antibody titer against the specific causative infectious agent. Many clinicians obtain prepregnancy antibody measurements to improve the ability to detect an antibody rise should primary infection occur during pregnancy.

However, the sensitivity of the serologic tests and the cost effectiveness of routine screening have been controversial. The U.S. Preventive Health Services Task Force, after reviewing the data regarding the efficacy of certain screening interventions in pregnancy, concluded that serologic testing for rubella antibodies should be performed in *all* pregnant and nonpregnant women of reproductive age who are unclear about their immune status. Blood tests for hepatitis B surface antigen also should be performed at the time of the first prenatal visit and repeated during the third trimester for women at high risk for contracting hepatitis B. Prenatal screening for hepatitis C remains controversial. Routine screening for toxoplasmosis and cytomegalovirus was not reviewed by the U.S. Preventive Health Services Task Force. A proposal for systematic screening was developed by Wilson and Remington and McCabe and Remington but has remained difficult and controversial to implement because of lack of quality control, difficulty in diagnosing the affected fetus, and lack of therapy of proved efficacy. Other infections for which routine screening during pregnancy has been advocated include syphilis, chlamydia, and gonorrhea in high-risk populations (see Chapter 22).

HERPES SIMPLEX VIRUS

Some sexually transmitted diseases can have significant effects on the fetus. It is well known that infection with herpes simplex virus (HSV) (usually type 2, occasionally type 1) contracted from passage through an infected birth canal can result in severe disseminated herpes infection in the neonate, including central nervous system infection leading to mental retardation or death. It is estimated that one in five pregnant women has had HSV-2 infection, and the incidence of neonatal infection from herpes virus may be as high as 1 in 20,000 live births. The spectrum of genital herpes infection includes primary infection, recurrent infection (with or without symptoms), and asymptomatic viral shedding without clinical disease. Studies have shown that the risk of contracting herpes by the fetus is higher (more than 50%) if the mother has an active primary herpes infection than if she has recurrent infection (less than 5%). Transmission rates are lowest for women with asymptomatic viral shedding. Most cases of neonatal herpes result from contact with mothers who have asymptomatic viral shedding at the time of delivery.

The risk for the development of the more severe consequences of herpes in the newborn relates directly to the extent of viral shedding at the time of delivery. Thus the standard recommendation is cesarean delivery when examination at the time of rupture of membranes and labor reveals herpes lesions (primary or secondary). Although screening for herpes can be helpful in the mother with recurrent infection, routine screening cultures have shown poor predictive value for identifying the patient who will be shedding at delivery. For this reason, and because the transmission rates are low for women without a history of recurrent disease, routine viral cultures are not currently recommended.

For primary herpes infection during pregnancy, treatment with acyclovir is recommended to prevent severe disease in the mother. Because these infections are associated with high rates of viral shedding and reactivation, some groups advocate weekly cervical cultures. If viral shedding continues at the time of labor (assumed by the presence of genital lesions or persistent seropositive surveillance cultures in the pregnant woman with primary herpes infection), delivery by cesarean section may be indicated in this subgroup. Treatment for herpes infection is the same for pregnant women as for nonpregnant women and is reviewed in Chapter 22. Prevention of herpes infection is important during pregnancy. Sexual contact with infected partners should be avoided, and patients should be counseled about safe sex practices.

SYPHILIS

Congenital syphilis, caused by the organism *Treponema pallidum,* is on the rise in the United States with an incidence of 1 in 10,000 live births. Congenital infection includes hepatosplenomegaly, jaundice, hemolysis, and lymphadenopathy. If untreated, there is also an increased risk of miscarriage, stillbirth, and premature delivery.

Regardless of sexual history, all pregnant women should be routinely screened for syphilis with a nontreponemal antibody test: Venereal Disease Research Laboratories (VDRL) or rapid plasma reagin (RPR). Screening should be performed as early as possible, preferably at the first prenatal visit. On the basis of the risk profile, screening may need to be repeated during the second and third trimesters of pregnancy and near the time of delivery.

In the case of a pregnant woman who shows evidence of clinical disease or has been exposed to an infected partner but whose VDRL or RPR test results are negative, the recommendation is to treat for primary syphilis and repeat the VDRL or RPR in 3 to 6 weeks because of the high likelihood of fetal infection. The standard treatment protocols for the nonpregnant woman (see Chapter 22) should be used for the pregnant woman with the exception of the alternative treatment for the penicillin-allergic patient. In the nonpregnant woman, erythromycin is the drug of choice for the patient with penicillin allergy but, because of the high failure rates, the current recommendation is to conduct skin testing to the major and minor penicillin determinants; in cases of positivity the pregnant patient should undergo desensitiza-

tion to penicillin. This usually is performed in a controlled setting in consultation with an allergist. Close follow-up monitoring is mandatory with monthly syphilis serologic screening throughout pregnancy. Because eradication of the infection is paramount, retreatment should be implemented if there is not a fourfold decrease in the nontreponemal titer over 3 months in a patient whose initial test results were positive. It is important for partners to be treated.

CHLAMYDIA AND GONORRHEA

Infection with *Chlamydia trachomatis* and *Neisseria gonorrhoeae* is associated with a number of sequelae for the fetus as well as the pregnant woman: increased risk for cervicitis, endometritis, peritonitis, perihepatitis, and disseminated infection and an associated risk for prematurity, premature rupture of membranes, intrauterine growth retardation, and chorioamnionitis. Neonatal infection with gonorrhea can result in eye (ophthalmia neonatorum), scalp, and disseminated infection. Multiple studies have estimated the prevalence of asymptomatic infection during pregnancy at 2% to 5%. Many clinicians recommend screening for both chlamydia and gonorrhea during early pregnancy and repeated screening in patients at high risk of contracting the infections. Treatment for gonorrhea is the same as in the nonpregnant woman. Alternatives to the tetracycline medications that are used for treatment of chlamydia but are contraindicated during pregnancy include erythromycin and amoxicillin, but high relapse rates exist. For a detailed discussion of the treatment of gonorrhea and chlamydial infection see Chapter 22.

CYTOMEGALOVIRUS

Cytomegalovirus (CMV) is a herpes virus infection that in adults generally causes no symptoms or manifests a syndrome similar to mononucleosis. Because CMV is endemic, many women have preexisting immunity, although the actual percentage of pregnant women who are immune is difficult to determine. Approximately 2% of susceptible women develop asymptomatic primary CMV infection during pregnancy; 40% of the infants of these mothers develop infection. The consequences for these infants can be devastating, including stillbirth, deafness, neurologic complications, developmental learning disabilities, and multiple physical defects, with an incidence of 1% in all newborns whose test results are positive, 10% of whom are seriously affected. In a study by Stagno et al., the rate of transmission of CMV from mother to fetus was almost 50% in the pregnant woman with primary CMV infection; 20% of those infants showed obvious clinical disease at birth. Most of the infants who developed complications later in childhood had visible disease at the time of delivery. Infants of mothers with primary infection are at greater risk for congenital CMV infection, although infants of mothers who are immune can still contact CMV infection, with a 0.5% to 1% incidence of congenital infection caused by recurrent CMV in the mother and a less than 1% chance of clinically apparent disease at birth. A later prospective study of 3700 women by Stagno et al. showed that immunity in woman who had CMV infection before pregnancy partially protected her baby and that congenital CMV occurred less frequently with less severe consequences than in offspring of women with primary CMV infection during pregnancy.

Because there is no effective drug intervention and the actual risk of infection to the fetus is low, routine screening has been controversial. Unfortunately the methods for confirming primary infection in the fetus of the infected mother at present are inaccurate. Therefore there are no recommendations for universal screening for infants. Recommendations for prevention for high-risk women (i.e., daycare center workers) include good hand-washing and hygienic measures. There has been much discussion in the medical community concerning the development of a CMV vaccination as the ideal method for prevention. Counseling the woman who is currently infected is difficult. Demonstration of fetal infection often can be made by amniocentesis or umbilical blood sampling. How to use that information is more problematic because many fetal infections do not lead to long-term sequelae.

HEPATITIS

Hepatitis B virus (HBV) is a growing public concern. Data from the Centers for Disease Control and Prevention (CDC) estimate that 22,000 infants are born annually to women with chronic HBV. Acute HBV occurs in 1 to 2 per 1000 pregnancies. The incidence of acute HBV in the newborn population is rising. Women at highest risk for contracting HBV include those with a history of intravenous drug use, history of multiple sexual partners, employment in health care, or household contact with HBV. If the mother contracts the disease early in the pregnancy, the rate of vertical transmission to the infant is 10% but rises to 50% to 60% if contracted during the third trimester. Multiple studies have shown that women who are chronic carriers, with positive hepatitis B surface antigen (HBsAg) only or positive HBsAg and hepatitis Be antigen (HBeAg) have a 12% to 25% and 70% to 90% neonatal infection rate, respectively. Infants with neonatal hepatitis are at highest risk for becoming chronic carriers of hepatitis.

At present the American College of Obstetricians and Gynecologists (ACOG) and other groups recommend screening all pregnant women for HBsAg during the first prenatal visit to identify those infants who will need intervention for the prevention of perinatal HBV infection. If the woman is in a high-risk group, the test should be repeated during the third trimester and at the time of delivery. Testing for HBeAg can be helpful in assessing the degree of infectivity and risk, but the intervention with immunoprophylaxis is the same regardless of the presence of the e antigen. All infants of mothers who have active or chronic hepatitis should receive 0.5 ml of hepatitis B immune globulin during the first 12 hours of life. They should then be immunized with hepatitis B vaccine (Heptavax-B) during the first week of life, 1 month later, and a final dose at 6 months of age, which is now standard practice for all newborn infants.

Hepatitis C (HCV) is the current name for one of the parenterally transmitted non-A non-B hepatitides. The actual incidence of HCV infection during pregnancy and fetal transmission rate is unknown. Women at highest risk for contracting HCV are those with a history of multiple blood transfusions, personal use of intravenous illicit drugs, or intimate contact with a partner with a history of risk factors for HCV. The ability to identify HCV has improved recently with new methods for identification of the virus in the blood. Recent studies by Ohto et al. have shown that HCV is vertically transmitted and that the risk of transmission is correlated with high titers of HCV RNA in the mothers. Vertical transmission is estimated at 5% and is higher for those mothers co-infected with virus. There are no drugs available to treat established HCV infections in mothers and infants to prevent vertical transmission. Further research is necessary before standard recommendations regarding screening for HCV can be made.

Hepatitis A is an uncommon complication of pregnancy and is not associated with perinatal transmission. Hepatitis E is rare in the United States and is similar to hepatitis A. In contrast, there have been reported cases of perinatal transmission of hepatitis E.

PARVOVIRUS B19

Parvovirus B19, which causes mild systemic symptoms and distinct facial rash in children and susceptible adults (erythema infectiosum or fifth disease), can result in nonimmune fetal hydrops and death in infected infants. The greatest risk to the fetus occurs during the first 20 weeks of pregnancy, which coincides with the major development of erythroid precursors. A prospective study from the Public Health Laboratory of Great Britain monitored 190 pregnant women who were identified as having recent parvovirus infection (IgM antibody positivity). Approximately 82% delivered healthy infants, and 30 (15%) fetal deaths were reported in this study. There have been no reported cases of congenital anomalies in live births after in utero exposure to parvovirus. The fetal risk during pregnancy from maternal exposure is low, and most women have been exposed before pregnancy.

Routine screening for parvovirus B19 is not recommended, but if infection is suspected, IgM and IgG antibodies for parvovirus can be obtained. Newer methods using B19 DNA-specific polymerase chain reaction tests are being developed for future use. The recommendation at this time is follow-up of pregnant women with serial ultrasound examinations to reveal any signs of fetal anemia or impending hydrops and if the initial IgM antibody test results are positive, to repeat determinations of alpha-fetoprotein.

RUBELLA

Most pregnant women are protected against contracting rubella because of their own childhood vaccination. According to reports from CDC, during the years 1988 to 1990, there was an increase in the number of reported cases of congenital rubella caused by lack of immunization of younger women. Consequences consist of an increase in congenital rubella syndrome, which includes intrauterine growth retardation (IUGR), prematurity, and increased risk for spontaneous abortion and stillbirth, as well as severe neurologic, ophthalmologic, and cardiac complications. Not all sequelae manifest at birth. Hearing loss and other central nervous system problems have been identified years after in utero exposure. The greatest risk to the infant is exposure during the first trimester. The risk of *congenital rubella infection* in fetuses born to mothers with rubella is 90% before 11 weeks of gestation, 25% if infected during weeks 23 to 26, and 67% after 31 weeks of gestation. Before 11 weeks of gestation, the incidence of *birth defects* in infected infants approaches 100%.

It is recommended that all women of reproductive age be screened for rubella antibodies and, if seronegative, receive immunization. If rubella infection is suspected in the pregnant woman, the clinician should obtain acute and convalescent antibody titers 10 to 14 days apart that reveal a greater than or equal to fourfold rise between the two titers. The presence of rubella-specific IgM antibody also is diagnostic of acute infection but needs to be obtained within 7 days after the onset of the rubella rash. If an acute infection is documented—especially if earlier than 13 weeks of gestation—the patient needs to discuss options with the obstetrician or primary care clinician. There is a role for high-dose immune globulin for those women who are unable to terminate their pregnancy, but the efficacy and protective effect for the fetus are unpredictable. Inasmuch as rubella is a live attenuated virus, it should not be administered during pregnancy or within 3 months of a planned pregnancy. Because as many as 50% of women will have unplanned pregnancy and there exists a theoretic risk of the fetus contracting congenital rubella from a vaccine (the CDC has no reported cases of the fetus developing congenital rubella syndrome after maternal vaccination during pregnancy), it is important to administer the vaccine at the time of menstruation if the woman is not taking an oral contraceptive pill. (For a detailed discussion on management of acute rubella disease during pregnancy see Remington and Klein.)

VARICELLA-ZOSTER VIRUS

Most women have been infected with chickenpox as children because of its high communicability and thus are immune to the development of infection with primary varicella infection during pregnancy. The incidence of chickenpox during pregnancy is estimated at 1.3 to 7 cases per 10,000 pregnancies. There is a small chance of reactivation of the virus resulting in clinical varicella-zoster virus (VZV) in the pregnant woman. If primary varicella infection (chickenpox) develops, some studies have shown a greater risk for the development of severe maternal complications such as varicella pneumonia.

The effect on the fetus depends on the timing of the infection during pregnancy. Although infection before 20 weeks of gestation can result in severe congenital varicella syndrome (skin lesions, limb paresis, chorioretinitis, and limb hypoplasia), the actual incidence was rare (<1% to 2%) in a recent prospective study of more than 3000 infected pregnant women. The greatest risk posed to the fetus is the mother's infection with primary varicella during the later part of the pregnancy, especially around the time of delivery. Consequences in the fetus of maternal infection at this time include neonatal VZV and disseminated varicella. The risk for disseminated varicella infection is 30% when the mother develops the chickenpox rash between 5 days before and 2 days after delivery. Although disseminated varicella is associated with severe neonatal morbidity and mortality, it may be prevented by use of the VZV immune globulin. If the maternal infection occurs after delivery, the infant is at risk for developing chickenpox. Although this disease is usually mild, there is a small increase in risk for a severe case of chickenpox in the newborn.

Diagnosis of chickenpox is usually straightforward because of the classic presentation of the rash, but if the diagnosis is in question, varicella-specific IgM antibodies can be helpful in diagnosing recent infection and varicella-specific IgG for assessing long-term immunity. The IgM test will not show positivity for at least several days after the onset of the rash. If a pregnant woman has been exposed to varicella but is seronegative, she should receive varicella-zoster immune globulin (VZIG) intramuscularly in a dose of 0.125 ml/kg. After that period the mother will have mounted her immune response and passed her antibodies to the fetus. Infants born to mothers who have contracted chickenpox between 5 days before and 2 days after delivery should receive VZIG to decrease the risk of disseminated varicella.

GROUP B STREPTOCOCCAL INFECTION

Group B streptococcus (GBS) is present in the vaginal and rectal areas of 15% to 40% of pregnant women. Although clinical disease in women is uncommon, the newborn can suffer consequences from contact with an infected maternal birth canal, including meningitis, neurologic complications, and death. Of the neonates born to women who are carriers of GBS, colonization occurs in 40% to 73%, but clinical disease develops in only 1 in 50 infants born to women in whom colonization has occurred. Neonatal sepsis from GSB develops in approximately 1 in 1000 infants, with a 50% mortality rate. The risk of neonatal disease is increased for those fetuses born to mothers who have preterm delivery, multiple gestations, prolonged rupture of membranes, heavy colonization of GBS, and low maternal levels of circulating antibodies to GBS.

In 1992, the ACOG recommended that routine cultures of the urine, the outer third of the vagina, and the rectum be obtained in the pregnant women with a history of a *previous child* with GBS infection or in a pregnant woman with risk factors such as preterm labor, preterm premature rupture of membranes, prolonged rupture of membrane, or fever during delivery. Studies of treatment of this subgroup of women with positive cultures have demonstrated a significant reduction in vertical transmission of GBS and neonatal mortality from group B streptococcal sepsis. Even though carriage of GBS is common in women (especially in those with the aforementioned risk factors), the carrier status often changes spontaneously during pregnancy. Thus screening cultures are not always reliable, even in women at high risk. Cultures negative for GBS are not uncommon for many women who may in fact show GBS colonization. ACOG, in recent considerations of the prevention of neonatal GBS infection, proposed that empiric treatment be initiated without culturing in pregnant women with any of the aforementioned risk factors. The American Academy of Pediatrics' (AAP) committees on infectious diseases in the fetus and newborn have recommended that screening with vaginal and anorectal cultures occur for *all* pregnant women between 26 and 28 weeks of gestation. If surveillance cultures are positive for GBS near the time of delivery and if the woman has risk factors at the time of labor (preterm labor, preterm premature rupture of membranes, prolonged rupture of membranes, or maternal fever during labor), intravenous penicillin (or erythromycin if the patient is allergic to penicillin) should be administered.

By 1996, a uniform set of recommendations was issued by the CDC, the ACOG, and the AAP. Recommendations included the use of either prenatal screening with cultures of vaginal and rectal specimens or a risk-based strategy to identify candidates for intrapartum antibiotic prophylaxis. Since implementation of these recommendations, hospitals in compliance have experienced a significant decrease in early onset disease.

TOXOPLASMOSIS

Toxoplasma gondii is a protozoan infection to which most adults have been exposed as children and have antibody protection. The cat is the predominant host for *T. gondii.* When adults contract toxoplasma infection, it usually is asymptomatic or associated with mild constitutional symptoms and lymphadenopathy except in the immunocompromised host. The actual prevalence of seropositive pregnant women varies depending on the geographic area and mode of exposure to the sources of *T. gondii:* cats or raw meat. Primary infection during pregnancy can be detrimental to the fetus, resulting in seizures, hydrocephaly, microcephaly, and jaundice. Approximately 4100 of 4.1 million infants born each year in the United States have congenital toxoplasma infection. The more severe cases of toxoplasmosis usually are seen in fetuses exposed earlier in pregnancy, and there can be a 60% reduction in the rate of sequelae of infection if treated. Long-term consequences of exposure are unpredictable. The incidence of contracting infection among seronegative women is 5%.

Although many groups have advocated routine prenatal screening and identification of seronegative women, universal screening has not been established because it has not been shown to be cost effective, and laboratory measurements of antibody levels have been difficult to standardize and interpret. The advent of fetal blood sampling has improved the ability for diagnosing potentially affected fetuses.

At present, primary infection can be identified by any one of a number of antibody tests. To determine that the infection is primary, it is necessary to show a conversion of a titer from negative to positive or a rise in titer from low to high. The timing of the serologic test is important inasmuch as the peak of the titer may be missed if blood is drawn late after the clinical presentation. Because of the lack of sensitivity of many commonly used measurements of IgM, it also is important to use methods that are adequate in differentiating IgM toxoplasmosis from natural IgM, rheumatoid factor, and antinuclear antibody. Capture IgM, enzyme-linked immunosorbent assay (ELISA), and IgM-ISAGA are more sensitive measures. Remington and Klein indicated that any patient with a Sabin-Feldman dye test or an indirect fluorescent antibody (IFA) test titer of greater than 300 IU/ml or 1:1000 and an IgM IFA test titer of 1:80 or higher or a capture IgM ELISA of 2 or greater is presumed to have recently acquired infection. When primary infection is

identified after 14 weeks of gestation, treatment should be instituted with pyrimethamine and sulfadiazine plus leucovorin. Safety of treatment with these drugs before 14 weeks has not been established. Prevention should be the goal, and advising pregnant women to avoid undercooked meat or contact with materials contaminated with cat feces is important.

Table 67-1 summarizes the current recommendations regarding evaluation and management of those infections already discussed that occur during pregnancy.

LYME DISEASE

The prevalence of Lyme disease has been increasing. The disease is caused by the spirochete *Borrelia burgdorferi* and results from the bite from an infected tick of the genus *Ixodes.* Congenital Lyme borreliosis syndromes include miscarriage (40% risk if mother left untreated), severe early congenital disease (20% risk if mother left untreated), and late congenital disease (2% to 3% risk if mother left untreated), so it is important to aggressively treat the pregnant woman suspected on having Lyme disease.

Any pregnant woman who develops an illness consistent with Lyme borreliosis should have serologic confirmation if possible. Identification of the disease is done by obtaining an ELISA test, either polyvalent or IgM or IgG, and, if positive, confirmed with Western blot assay. If positive, treatment options for the pregnant female include amoxicillin, 500 mg taken orally three times a day for 14 to 21 days, or cefuroxime axetil, 500 mg taken orally twice a day for 20 days.

TUBERCULOSIS

Tuberculosis (TB) has experienced a recent resurgence due to the rise in HIV infection in women and immigration from countries where TB is endemic. The disease is contracted through inhalation of *Mycobacterium tuberculosis,* which results in a granulomatous reaction in lung tissue. Although congenital TB is rare, it can be fatal.

Screening all pregnant women for TB remains controversial. Experts agree that skin testing should be performed for those in high-risk groups (Box 67-1).

The preferred antigen is purified protein derivative (PPD) in the intermediate strength of 5 tuberculin units and placed subcutaneously. The threshold for a positive test depends on the patient's risk for tuberculosis (Box 67-2).

Once a positive test is identified, the patient should receive a chest radiograph during pregnancy (with abdomen shielded). If the radiograph is negative, then no prophylactic treatment is necessary until after delivery.

Because of the increased risk of isoniazid (INH) associated hepatitis during pregnancy, unless the patient is at high risk for reactivation (recent converters have 3% incidence of active infection in the first year and in study of HIV positive drug abusers with seroconversion the incidence was 4% over 21 months), INH prophylaxis should wait until after delivery and then be started using the standard recommended dose (300 mg daily with vitamin B_6 for 1 year). Nursing is not a contraindication to preventive therapy with INH.

Active disease is always treated with at least two tuberculostatic drugs. Several first-line drugs appear to be safe in pregnancy and are reviewed in Chapter 61.

Table 67-1
Evaluation and Management of Common Infectious Diseases During Pregnancy

Infectious Disease	Clinical Symptoms in Pregnant Woman	Clinical Manifestations in Fetus	Fetal Infection Rate	General Guidelines for Management
Cytomegalovirus	None	CMV infection, progressive deafness, learning disabilities, cerebral palsy, hydrocephalus, eye problems, increased risk of prematurity, LBW, IUGR	40%-50% in fetuses exposed to mother with primary infection	Hand washing/hygienic measures for high-risk groups (e.g., women working in day-care centers) No routine screening because no specific preventive treatment
Genital herpes simplex (HSV-2, HSV-1)	Painful vesicular lesions but can be asymptomatic carriers	First trimester: spontaneous abortion, severe congenital malformations Second and third trimesters: increase perinatal mortality	Possibly 8% in fetuses exposed to recurrent HSV	Inspection of female genital tract before delivery; if lesions present, delivery by cesaran section
Chlamydia and gonorrhea	Acute disease (see text) or asymptomatic carrier	? prematurity, PROM, IUGR, chorioamnionitis, disseminated infection		Screening with cervical cultures CDC advocates early in pregnancy; repeat during third trimester for high-risk women
Syphilis	Primary syphilis, secondary syphilis or asymptomatic	Congenital syphilis Increased risk for miscarriage and stillbirth		Screen all pregnant women with VRDL at first prenatal visit; repeat screening during second and third trimesters if high risk. Treat using standard protocols, and follow nontreponemal titers once a month for 3 mo. If there is not fourfold decrease, repeat treatment
Rubella (German measles)	Asymptomatic, slight fever, swollen lymph glands	Congenital rubella syndrome: cardiac defects, sensorineural and hearing loss, cataracts Risk for LBW, IUGR	Up to 50% during first 8 wk of pregnancy	Screening and immunization of all seronegative women of reproductive age; immunization contraindicated if pregnant or 3 mo. before conception because rubella vaccine is live attenuated virus
Varicella (chickenpox and zoster)	If contracted during pregnancy, high rate of varicella pneumonia and mortality	First trimester: ? association with limb hypoplasia, cutaneous scars, chorioretinitis, cataracts, cortical atrophy, microcephaly Within 5 days of onset of rash at delivery: neonatal varicella with associated high death rate	30% develop neonatal varicella if within 5 days of exposure at time of delivery	If exposed within 5 days of delivery, administer VZIG at delivery or within 24 hrs of delivery Screening for IgG antibody titers only if mother has negative history for chickenpox and has been exposed to infection. If seronegative, administer VZIG after exposure
Parvovirus B19	Asymptomatic or constitutional symptoms and rash	Increased risk of nonimmune fetal hydrops before 20-wk gestation	Approximately 15% fetal death rate (United Kingdom study)	Offer IgM and IgG antibody testing. Counsel woman on risks to fetus. Monitor pregnancy with serial ultrasound and alpha-feto protein measurements

Data from Remington JS, Klein JO, editors: *Infectious diseases of the fetus and newborn infant*, ed 4, Philadelphia, 1995, WB Saunders.
LBW, Low birth weight; *IUGR*, intrauterine growth retardation; *PROM*, premature rupture of membranes.

Table 67-1
Evaluation and Management of Common Infectious Diseases During Pregnancy—cont'd

Infectious Disease	Clinical Symptoms in Pregnant Woman	Clinical Manifestations in Fetus	Fetal Infection Rate	General Guidelines for Management
Toxoplasmosis	Asymptomatic	Seizures, hydrocephaly, microcephaly jaundice, chorioretinitis Increased risk of prematurity, LBW, IUGR		Treatment with pyrimethamine and sulfadiazine after 14 wk gestation. Routine prenatal screening impractical at this time. See text
Hepatitis B	Active disease; chronic carrier state	Acute fulminant hepatitis	10% during first trimester; 50%-60% during third trimester	Obtain serology in all pregnant women for HBsAg during first trimester; repeat if at high risk during third trimester and at delivery If positive, administer 0.5 ml of hepatitis immune globulin during first 12 hr of life; then proceed with immunization with Heptavax during wk 1, 1 mo later, and at 6 mo.
Group B streptococcal infection	Asymptomatic carriers	Meningitis, neurologic complications, death	1 in 1000 live births develop neonatal sepsis	Pregnant women at high risk should be screened with vaginal and anorectal cultures and treated during labor with penicillin if positive, for GBS Screening all pregnant women during gestational wk 26-28 has been advocated by some but still remains controversial

---

BOX 67-1
High-Risk Groups Recommended for Tuberculosis Screening During Pregnancy

HIV
Close contact with known case or person who has been exposed
Medical risk factors increasing risk of disease
Immigrants from countries with high prevalence of TB
Medically underserved
Low-income patients
Alcoholics
Those with substance abuse
Residents of long-term care facilities, correctional institutions, mental institutions, nursing home facilities, and residential facilities

Modified from Centers for Disease Control and Prevention, 1990, Screening for Tuberculosis and tuberculosis infection in high risk populations. Recommendations of the Advisory Committee on the Elimination of Tuberculosis, *MMWR* 39:1, 1990.

BOX 67-2
Positive PPD

Risk Category	Degree of Induration (mm)
Very-high risk patients	5 mm = positive
■ HIV positive	
■ Abnormal chest radiograph	
■ Recent contact with an active case	
High-risk patients	10 mm = positive
■ Foreign born	
■ Intravenous drug users who are HIV negative	
■ Low-income populations	
■ Medical conditions that increase risk if contract TB	
None of the above risk factors	15 mm = positive

American Thoracic Society and Centers for Disease Control and Prevention, 1990.

IMMUNIZATION

Immunization is important for all women of reproductive age; the objective should be to immunize women before pregnancy. In 1991 the ACOG issued recommendations regarding immunization during pregnancy. The updated recommendations concluded that immunization during pregnancy should be reserved for the specific situations summarized in Table 67-2 and that if a pregnant woman requires an immunization, she should not receive vaccines containing live virus such as measles, mumps, or rubella. If a woman is in an endemic area and she is at high risk for exposure, then poliomyelitis and yellow fever vaccines may be administered.

Text continued on p. 497

Table 67-2
Immunization During Pregnancy

Immuno-biologic Agent	Risk from Disease to Pregnant Woman	Risk from Disease to Fetus or Neonate	Type of Immunizing Agent	Risk from Immunizing Agent to Fetus	Indications for Immunization During Pregnancy	Dose Schedule	Comments
Live Virus Vaccines							
Measles	Significant morbidity, low mortality; not altered by pregnancy	Significant increase in abortion rate; may cause malformations	Live attenuated virus vaccine	None confirmed	Contraindicated (see immune globulins)	Single dose SC, preferably as measles-mumps-rubella*	Vaccination of susceptible women should be part of post-partum care
Mumps	Low morbidity and mortality; not altered by pregnancy	Probable increased rate of abortion in first trimester	Live attenuated virus vaccine	None confirmed	Contraindicated	Single dose SC, preferably as measles-mumps-rubella	Vaccination of susceptible women should be part of post-partum care
Poliomyelitis	No increased incidence in pregnancy, but may be more severe if it does occur	Anoxic fetal damage reported; 50% mortality in neonatal disease	Live attenuated virus (oral polio vaccine [OPV]) and enhanced-potency inactivated virus (e-IPV) vaccine†	None confirmed	Not routinely recommended for women in U.S., except persons at increased risk of exposure	Primary: 2 doses of e-IPV SC at 4-8 wk intervals and a 3rd dose 6-12 mos after the 2nd dose. Immediate protection: 1 dose OPV orally (in outbreak setting)	Vaccine indicated for susceptible pregnant women traveling in endemic areas or in other high risk situations
Rubella	Low morbidity and mortality; not altered by pregnancy	High rate of abortion and congenital rubella syndrome	Live attenuated virus vaccine	None confirmed	Contraindicated	Single dose SC, preferably as measles-mumps-rubella	Teratogenicity of vaccine is theoretic, not confirmed to date; vaccination of susceptible women should be part of postpartum care
Yellow fever	Significant morbidity and mortality; not altered by pregnancy	Unknown	Live attenuated virus vaccine	Unknown	Contraindicated except if exposure is unavoidable	Single dose SC	Postponement of travel preferable to vaccination, if possible

Continued

From ACOG technical bulletin, no. 160, Oct 1991.
SC, subcutaneously; *PO,* orally; *IM,* intramuscularly; *ID,* intradermally.
*Two doses necessary for adequate vaccination of students entering institutions of higher education, newly hired medical personnel, and international travelers.
†Inactivated polio vaccine recommended for nonimmunized adults at increased risk.

Table 67-2
Immunization During Pregnancy—cont'd

Immuno-biologic Agent	Risk from Disease to Pregnant Woman	Risk from Disease to Fetus or Neonate	Type of Immunizing Agent	Risk from Immunizing Agent to Fetus	Indications for Immunization During Pregnancy	Dose Schedule	Comments
Inactivated Virus Vaccines							
Influenza	Possible increase in morbidity and mortality during epidemic of new antigenic strain	Possible increased abortion rate; no malformations confirmed	Inactivated virus vaccine	None confirmed	Women with serious underlying diseases; public health authorities to be consulted for current recommendation	One dose IM every yr	
Rabies	Near 100% fatality; not altered by pregnancy	Determined by maternal disease	Killed virus vaccine	Unknown	Indications for prophylaxis not altered by pregnancy; each case considered individually	Public health authorities to be consulted for indications, dosage, and route of administration	
Hepatitis B	Possible increased severity during third trimester	Possible increase in abortion rate and prematurity; neonatal hepatitis can occur; high risk of newborn carrier state	Recombinant vaccine	None reported	Pre- and post-exposure for women at risk of infection	Three- or four-dose series IM	Used with hepatitis B immune globulin for some exposures; exposed new-born needs vaccination as soon as possible
Inactivated Bacterial Vaccines							
Cholera	Significant morbidity and mortality; more severe during third trimester	Increased risk of fetal death during third-trimester maternal illness	Killed bacterial vaccine	None confirmed	Indications not altered by pregnancy; vaccination recommended only in unusual outbreak situations	Single dose SC or IM, depending on manufacturer's recommendations when indicated	
Plague	Significant morbidity and mortality; not altered by pregnancy	Determined by maternal disease	Killed bacterial vaccine	None reported	Selective vaccination of exposed persons	Public health authorities to be consulted for indications, dosage, and route of administration	
Pneumo-coccus	No increased risk during pregnancy; no increase in severity of disease	Unknown	Polyvalent poly-saccharide vaccine	No data available on use during pregnancy	Indications not altered by pregnancy; vaccine used only for high-risk individuals	In adults, 1 SC or IM dose only; consider repeat dose in 6 yrs for high-risk individuals	

Typhoid	Significant morbidity and mortality; not altered by pregnancy	unknown	Killed or live attenuated oral bacterial vaccine	None confirmed	Not recommended routinely except for close, continued exposure or travel to endemic areas	Killed: Primary: 2 injections SC at least 4 wks apart Booster: Single dose SC or ID (depending on type of product used) every 3 yrs Oral: Primary: 4 doses on alternate days Booster: Schedule not yet determined	
Toxoids							
Tetanus diphtheria	Severe morbidity; tetanus mortality 30%, diphtheria mortality 10%; unaltered by pregnancy	Neonatal tetanus mortality 60%	Combined tetanus-diphtheria toxoids preferred: adult tetanus-diphtheria formulation	None confirmed	Lack of primary series, or no booster within past 10 yrs	Primary: 2 doses IM at 1-2-mo interval with a 3rd dose 6-12 mos after the 2nd Booster: Single dose IM every 10 yrs, after completion of primary series	Updating of immune status should be part of antepartum care
Specific Immune Globulins							
Hepatitis B	Possible increased severity during third trimester	Possible increase in abortion rate and prematurity; neonatal hepatitis can occur; high risk of carriage in newborn	Hepatitis B immune globulin	None reported	Postexposure prophylaxis	Depends on exposure; consult Immunization Practices Advisory Committee recommendations (IM)	Usually given with HBV vaccine; exposed newborn needs immediate post-exposure prophylaxis

Continued

From ACOG technical bulletin, no. 160, Oct 1991.

SC, subcutaneously; *PO*, orally; *IM*, intramuscularly; *ID*, intradermally.

*Two doses necessary for adequate vaccination of students entering institutions of higher education, newly hired medical personnel, and international travelers.

†Inactivated polio vaccine recommended for nonimmunized adults at increased risk.

Table 67-2
Immunization During Pregnancy—cont'd

Immunobiologic Agent	Risk from Disease to Pregnant Woman	Risk from Disease to Fetus or Neonate	Type of Immunizing Agent	Risk from Immunizing Agent to Fetus	Indications for Immunization During Pregnancy	Dose Schedule	Comments
Specific Immune Globulins—cont'd							
Rabies	Near 100% fatality; not altered by pregnancy	Determined by maternal disease	Rabies immune globulin	None reported	Postexposure prophylaxis	Half dose at injury site, half dose in deltoid	Used in conjunction with rabies killed virus vaccine
Tetanus	Severe morbidity; mortality 21%	Neonatal tetanus mortality 60%	Tetanus immune globulin	None reported	Postexposure prophylaxis	One dose IM	Used in conjunction with tetanus toxoid
Varicella	Possible increase in severe varicella pneumonia	Can cause congenital varicella with increased mortality in neonatal period; very rarely causes congenital defects	Varicella-zoster immune globulin (obtained from the American Red Cross)	None reported	Can be considered for healthy pregnant women exposed to varicella to protect against maternal, not congenital, infection	One dose IM within 96 hrs of exposure	Indicated also for newborns of mothers who developed varicella within 4 days prior to delivery or 2 days following delivery; approx. 90-95% of adults are immune to varicella; not indicated for prevention of congenital varicella
Standard Immune Globulins							
Hepatitis A	Possible increased severity during third trimester	Probable increase in abortion rate and prematurity; possible transmission to neonate at delivery if mother is incubating the virus or is acutely ill at that time	Standard immune globulin	None reported	Postexposure prophylaxis	0.02 ml/kg IM in one dose of immune globulin	Immune globulin should be given as soon as possible and within 2 wks of exposure; infants born to mothers who are incubating the virus or are acutely ill at delivery should receive one dose of 0.5 ml as soon as possible after birth
Measles	Significant morbidity, low mortality; not altered by pregnancy	Significant increase in abortion rate; may cause malformations	Standard immune globulin	None reported	Postexposure prophylaxis	0.25 ml/kg IM in one dose of immune globulin, up to 15 ml	Unclear if it prevents abortion; must be given within 6 days of exposure

From ACOG technical bulletin, no. 160, Oct 1991.

Routine vaccination with tetanus and diphtheria toxoids and influenza is safe during pregnancy. Because prolonged viral shedding after immunization can occur up to 3 months, women of reproductive age who receive live vaccines should be advised to use contraception to avoid pregnancy, although fetuses with sequelae of infection from live virus vaccination have never been reported.

BIBLIOGRAPHY

General

Cefalo R, Moos M: *Preconceptional health care: a practical guide,* ed 2, St Louis, 1995, Mosby.

Charles D: *Obstetrical and perinatal infections,* St Louis, 1993, Mosby.

Remington JS, Klein JO, editors: *Infectious diseases of the fetus and newborn infant,* ed 4, Philadelphia, 1995, WB Saunders.

U.S. Preventive Health Task Force: *Guide to clinical preventive services,* ed 2, Alexandria, 1996, International Medical Publishing, Inc.

Cytomegalovirus

Daffos F et al: Prenatal management of 746 pregnancies at risk for congenital toxoplasmosis, *N Engl J Med* 318:271, 1988.

Fowler KB et al: The outcome of congenital cytomegalovirus infection in relation to maternal antibody status, *N Engl J Med* 326:663, 1992.

Hunter K et al: Prenatal screening of pregnant women for infections due to cytomegalovirus, Epstein Barr, herpes, rubella and *Toxoplasma gondii,* *Am J Obstet Gyncol* 145:269, 1983.

Medearis D: CMV immunity: imperfect but protective, *N Engl J Med* 306:985, 1982.

Nankervis G et al: A prospective study of maternal cytomegalovirus infection and its effect on the fetus, *Am J Obstet Gynecol* 149:435, 1984.

Stagno S: Characteristics of CMV infection in pregnancy, *N Engl J Med* 313:1270, 1985.

Stagno S et al: Congenital cytomegalovirus infection: occurrence in an immune population, *N Engl J Med* 296:1254, 1977.

Stagno S et al: Congenital cytomegalovirus infection: the relative importance of primary and recurrent maternal infection, *N Engl J Med* 306:945, 1982.

Yow M, Demmler G: Congenital cytomegalovirus disease—20 years is long enough, *N Engl J Med* 326:702, 1992.

Group B Streptococcal Infection

American Academy of Pediatrics, Committee on Infectious Diseases and Committee on Fetus and Newborn: Guidelines for prevention of group B streptococcal (GBS) infection by chemoprophylaxis, *Pediatrics* 90:775, 1992.

American Academy of Pediatrics, Committee on Infectious Diseases and Committee on Fetus and Newborn: Revised guidelines for prevention of early-onset group B streptococcal (GBS) infection, *Pediatrics* 99:489, 1997.

Boyer KM, Gotoff SP: Prevention of early onset neonatal group B streptococcal disease with selective intrapartum chemoprophylaxis, *N Engl J Med* 314:1665, 1986.

Centers for Disease Control: Prevention of perinatal group B streptococcal disease: a public health perspective, *MMWR* 45:1, 1996.

Centers for Disease Control: Early onset Group B streptococcal disease-United States, 1998-1999, *JAMA* 284:1508, 2000.

McKenzie H et al: Risk of preterm delivery in pregnant women with group B streptococcal urinary infections or urinary antibodies to group B streptococcal and *E. coli* antigens, *Br J Obstet Gynaecol* 101:107, 1994.

Schuchat A: Neonatal group B streptococcal disease—screening and prevention, *N Engl J Med* 343:209, 2000.

Strickland D, Yeomans E, Hankins G: Cost effectiveness of intrapartum screening and treatment for maternal group B streptococci colonization, *Am J Obstet Gynecol* 163:4, 1990.

Turow J, Spitzer A: Group B streptococcal infection early onset disease controversies in prevention guidelines, and management strategies for the neonate, *Clin Pediatr* 39:317, 2000.

Yancey M et al: Peripartum infection associated with vaginal group B streptococcal colonization, *Obstet Gynecol* 84:816, 1994.

Hepatitis

ACOG educational bulletin. Viral hepatitis in pregnancy. Number 248, July 1998.

ACOG committee opinion. Breastfeeding and the risk of hepatitis C virus transmission. Number 220, August 1999. Committee on Obstetric Practice. American College of Obstetricians and Gynecologists. *Int J Gynaecol Obstet* 66:307, 1999.

American College of Obstetricians and Gynecologist, *Int J Gynaecol Obstet* 63:195, 1998.

Burns DN, Minkoff H: Hepatitis C: screening in pregnancy, *Obstet Gynecol* 94:1044, 1999.

Centers for Disease Control and Prevention: Maternal hepatitis B screening practices—California, Connecticut, Kansas, and United States, 1992-1993, *JAMA* 271:1819, 1994.

Conte D et al: Prevalence and clinical course of chronic hepatitis C virus (HC infection) and rate of HCV vertical transmission in a cohort of 15,250 pregnant women, *Hepatology* 31:751, 2000.

Leikin E et al: Epidemiologic predictors of hepatitis C virus infection in pregnant women, *Obstet Gynecol* 84:529, 1994.

Ohto H and the Vertical Transmission of Hepatitis C Virus Collaborative Study Group: Transmission of hepatitis C from mothers to infants, *N Engl J Med* 330:744, 1994.

Silverman N et al: Hepatitis C virus in pregnancy: seroprevalence and risk factors in infection, *Am J Obstet Gynecol* 169:583, 1993.

Snydman D: Hepatitis in pregnancy, *N Engl J Med* 313:1398, 1985.

Zanetti AR, Tanzi E, Newell ML: Mother-to-infant transmission of hepatitis C virus, *J Hepatol* 31:96, 1999.

Herpes Virus Infections

ACOG practice bulletin. Management of herpes in pregnancy. Number 8, October 1999. Clinical management guidelines for obstetricians-gynecologists, *Int J Gynaecol Obstet* 68:165, 2000.

Baker DA: Herpes and pregnancy: new management, *Clin Obstet Gynecol* 33:253, 1990.

Brown ZA et al: Genital herpes in pregnancy: risk factors associated with recurrences and asymptomatic viral shedding, *Am J Obstet Gynecol* 153:24, 1985.

Brown ZA et al: Effects on infants of a first episode of genital herpes during pregnancy, *N Engl J Med* 317:1246, 1987.

Brown ZA et al: Neonatal herpes simplex virus infection in relation to asymptomatic maternal infection at the time of labor, *N Engl J Med* 324:1247, 1991.

Cone RW et al: Frequent detection of genital herpes simplex virus DNA by polymerase chain reaction among pregnant women, *JAMA* 272:792, 1994.

Harger JA et al: Characteristics and management of pregnancy in women with genital herpes simplex virus infection, *Am J Obstet Gynecol* 145:784, 1983.

Kulhanjian JA et al: Identification of women at unsuspected risk of primary infection with herpes simplex virus type 2 during pregnancy, *N Engl J Med* 326:916, 1992.

Prober CG: Herpetic vaginitis in 1993, *Clin Obstet Gynecol* 36:177, 1993.

Prober CG et al: Use of routine viral cultures at delivery to identify neonates exposed to herpes simplex virus, *N Engl J Med* 318:887, 1988.

Randolph AG, Washington AE, Prober CG: Cesarean delivery for women presenting with genital herpes lesions: efficacy, risks and costs, *JAMA* 270:77, 1993.

Stagno S, Whitley R: Herpesvirus infections of pregnancy. I. Cytomegalovirus and Epstein-Barr virus infections, *N Engl J Med* 313:1270, 1985.

Stagno S, Whitley R: Herpesvirus infections of pregnancy. II. Herpes simplex virus and varicella zoster virus infection, *N Engl J Med* 313:1327, 1985.

Lyme Disease

American College of Obstetricians and Gynecologists: Lyme disease during pregnancy. ACOG Committee opinion: Committee on Obstetrics: Maternal and Fetal Medicine. Number 99-November 1991, *Int J Gynaecol Obstet* 39:59, 1992.

Smith LG, Pearlman M: Lyme disease: a review with emphasis on the pregnant woman, *Obstet Gynecol Surv* 46:125, 1991.

Steere AC: Lyme disease, *N Engl J Med* 321:586, 1989.

Parvovirus B19

Hall CJ: Parvovirus B19 infection in pregnancy, *Arch Dis Child* 71:F4, 1994.

Kirchner J: Erythema infectiosum and other parvovirus B19 infections, *Am Family Phys* 50:335, 1994.

Public Health Laboratory Service Working Party on Fifth Disease: Prospective study of human parvovirus (B19) infection in pregnancy, 300:1166, 1990.

Torok T: Human parvovirus B19 infection in pregnancy, *Pediatr Infect Dis J* 9:772, 1990.

Rubella

American College of Obstetricians and Gynecologists: *Rubella and pregnancy* (Tech Bull No 171), Washington, DC, 1992, The College.

Centers for Disease Control, Immunization Practices Advisory Committee: Increase in rubella and congenital rubella syndrome, United States 1988-1990, *MMWR* 40:93, 1991.

Miller E, Cradock-Watson JE, Pollack TM: Consequences of confirmed maternal rubella at successive stages of pregnancy, *Lancet* 2:781, 1982.

Syphilis

Centers for Disease Control: Guideline for the prevention and control of congenital syphilis, *MMWR* 37:51, 1988.

Centers for Disease Control: Sexually transmitted disease treatment guidelines, *MMWR* 38:5, 1989.

Dorfman DH, Glaser JH: Congenital syphilis presenting in infants after the newborn period, *N Engl J Med* 323:1299, 1990.

McFarlin B et al: Epidemic syphilis: maternal factors associated with congenital infection, *Am J Obstet Gynecol* 170:535, 1994.

Wendel GD Jr, et al: Penicillin allergy and desensitization in serious infections during pregnancy, *N Engl J Med* 312:1229, 1985.

Toxoplasmosis

American College of Obstetricians and Gynecologists: *Perinatal viral and perinatal infections* (Tech Bull No 177), Washington, DC, 1992, The College.

Guerina N et al: Neonatal serologic screening and early treatment for congenital *Toxoplasma gondii* infection, *N Engl J Med* 330:1858, 1994.

McCabe R, Remington JS: Toxoplasmosis: the time has come, *N Engl J Med* 318:313, 1988 (editorial).

Wilson CB, Remington JS: What can be done to prevent congenital toxoplasmosis? *Am J Obstet Gynecol* 138:357, 1980.

Tuberculosis

American Thoracic Society/Centers for Disease Control: Diagnostic standards and classification of tuberculosis, *Am Rev Respir Dis* 142:725, 1990.

American Thoracic Society/Centers for Disease Control: Targeted tuberculin testing and treatment of latent tuberculosis infection, *Am J Respir Crit Care Med* 161:221, 2000.

Boggess KA, Myers S: Antepartum or postpartum isoniazid treatment of latent tuberculosis infection, *Obstet Gynecol* 96:757, 2000.

Centers for Disease Control: Screening for tuberculosis and tuberculosis infection in high risk populations. Recommendations of the Advisory Committee for Elimination of Tuberculosis, *MMWR* 39:1, 1990.

Riley L: Pneumonia, tuberculosis and urinary tract infections in pregnancy, *Curr Clin Top Infect Dis* 19:181, 1999.

Selwyn PA et al: A prospective study of the risk of tuberculosis among intravenous drug users with human immunodeficiency virus infection, *N Engl J Med* 320:544, 1989.

Snider DE et al: Treatment of tuberculosis during pregnancy, *Am Rev Respir Dis* 122:65, 1980.

Varicella

Enders G et al: Consequences of varicella and herpes zoster in pregnancy: prospective study of 1739 cases, *Lancet* 343:1548, 1994.

Paryani SG, Arvin AM: Intrauterine infection with varicella-zoster virus after maternal varicella, *N Engl J Med* 314:1542, 1986.

Sauerbrei A, Wutzler P: The congenital varicella syndrome, *J Perinatol* 20:548, 2000.

Immunization in Pregnancy

American College of Obstetricians and Gynecologists: *Immunization during pregnancy* (Tech Bull No 160), Washington, DC, 1991, The College.

American College of Physicians: Adult immunizations 1994, *Ann Intern Med* 121:540, 1994.

Fedson D: Adult vaccination: summary of the National Vaccine Advisory Committee Report, *JAMA* 272:1133, 1994.

CHAPTER 68

Amniocentesis and Prenatal Genetics

Louise Wilkins-Haug

During the last 20 years, prenatal genetics has evolved from a field of specialized testing into an integral component of routine obstetric care. Greater use of antepartum genetic testing has resulted from two major advances: (1) improved screening to identify those women with increased risk and (2) advancements in the techniques for diagnosing genetic disorders.

SCREENING
Chromosome Abnormalities

A positive correlation between the frequency of chromosomally abnormal fetuses and maternal age is well recognized. Although women at all ages are at risk for an infant with Down syndrome (trisomy 21), at age 25 the risk is 1/890 pregnancies, increasing to a risk of 1/250 at 35 years and 1/90 at 40 years of age. This risk is higher in early pregnancy, as many fetuses with chromosomal abnormalities are lost as early or late miscarriage (Table 68-1). In 1966 amniocyte culture provided a means for examining fetal chromosomes. Amniocentesis, the removal of a small quantity of amniotic fluid containing fetal cells, can provide a karyotype of the fetus during the second trimester but is associated with approximately a 1/200 risk of miscarriage. Thus only women with a risk of having an affected fetus equal to or greater than the risk of complication from the procedure (1/300) have been offered amniocentesis. Traditionally, a maternal age of 35 years or greater at delivery (risk of trisomy 21 = 1/250) has been the screening parameter used to identify women at sufficient risk to justify offering an invasive diagnostic test such as amniocentesis.

Maternal age as a screening parameter, however, has limitations. On average 5% to 7% of pregnant women are 35 years or older at delivery and thus have a "positive" maternal age screen for trisomy 21. However, only 20% of infants with Down syndrome are born to women over 35 years old. Furthermore, although acceptance of amniocentesis may vary on the basis of cultural and religious beliefs, by some reports acceptance of amniocentesis in women 35 or older may be as low as 50%, in part as a result of the risk associated with the procedure.

Maternal Serum Alpha-Fetoprotein

Additional screening programs have been developed to identify women, other than those older than 35 at delivery, who are at an increased risk for a chromosomally abnormal fetus. Quantification of maternal serum alpha-fetoprotein (MSAFP) level, which is produced by the fetal liver, was first shown to be at lower levels in fetuses with chromosomal abnormalities. As MSAFP quantification is now routinely offered for neural tube defect screening (see later discussion), the concomitant use of low MSAFP for trisomy 21 screening is also recommended. However, prospective studies of MSAFP screening for trisomy 21 in women less than age 35 at delivery have shown that a positive screen detects only 20% of affected fetuses.

Human Chorionic Gonadotropin and Unconjugated Estriol

In many centers screening for trisomy 21 risk has been expanded with the addition of other pregnancy hormones including human chorionic gonadotropin (hCG) and unconjugated estriol (UE3) determinations. The American College of Obstetricians and Gynecologists (ACOG) now recommends trisomy 21 screening be performed with two or more maternal serum markers. In addition, ACOG recommends that ultrasound be used preferentially for gestational age determination, ideally by biparietal diameter measurement. Repeat of the abnormal value is not encouraged. For women over 35 years old, serum screening is not equivalent to diagnostic testing by amniocentesis but is a reasonable screening test.

In pregnancies with a trisomy 21, fetal hCG levels are higher than expected and estriol levels are lower. For an individual maternal blood sample, the likelihood that the fetus has trisomy 21 can be calculated on the basis of the results of a triple panel (AFP, hCG, and estriol). This likelihood ratio in combination with the maternal age yields a new risk for trisomy 21 in any individual women. A triple panel risk for a trisomy 21 fetus of greater than 1/250 is considered a positive result. Approximately 7% of women below the age of 35 have a positive serum panel result. Women with a positive serum panel finding then have ultrasound confirmation

Table 68-1
Risk of Aneuploidy by Maternal and Gestational Age

Age (yrs)	9-14 Weeks Gestation			15-20 Weeks Gestation			Livebirths		
	Trisomy 21	Trisomy 18	Trisomy 13	Trisomy 21	Trisomy 18	Trisomy 13	Trisomy 21	Trisomy 18	Trisomy 13
20	1/696	1/2193	1/6125	1/1025	1/4576	1/15656	1/1529	1/15507	1/36148
25	1/616	1/1939	1/5414	1/906	1/4045	1/13839	1/1352	1/13708	1/31954
30	1/415	1/1306	1/3646	1/610	1/2724	1/9320	1/910	1/9232	1/12520
35	1/175	1/552	1/1542	1/258	1/1152	1/3942	1/385	1/3905	1/9102
40	1/51	1/162	1/452	1/76	1/338	1/1156	1/113	1/1145	1/2668
45	1/13	1/41	1/114	1/19	1/85	1/292	1/29	1/289	1/675

of gestational age, as the results of the three assays vary greatly with gestational week. In general only 3% of the originally screened population will continue to have positive serum triple panel findings after correction by ultrasound for inaccurate gestational age. From prospective studies in women less than 35 years at delivery, a positive triple assay serum screen detects 57% of the trisomy 21 fetuses at a 5% initial serum screen positive rate. For women older than 35 years, approximately 25% will have an initial screen positive for a detection rate of 75% to 89% of trisomy 21.

Given an initial screen positive rate of anywhere from 5% to 25% depending on maternal age and use of ultrasound, the patient's understanding of the screening process becomes critical. Unfortunately, many patients confuse screening with diagnostic studies and despite use of ancillary materials, the finding of a positive initial serum screen generates considerable anxiety. Recent surveys of women who have had both positive and negative initial serum screens are illustrative of this confusion. In one large study as many as 50% of women informed of a positive serum screen felt the chance their fetus had trisomy 21 was 50%, and 7% of women felt the chance their infant had trisomy 21 was 100%. In these same studies, women who had negative screens were overly optimistic as to the strength of a negative screen, as between 50% and 67% felt there was 100% reassurance their infant did not have trisomy 21 despite prior discussions of the sensitivity of the serum screen in the range of 75% to 80%.

Recently, additions to the second trimester serum screen have been introduced to try to decrease the initial screen positive rate as well as increase sensitivity. Most important among these has been the addition of inhibin. Comparative study of the standard triple panel (MSAFP/hCG/estriol) with a quad panel (the addition of inhibin) indicates an increase from a 69% to a 85% sensitivity. Further study is needed to validate whether this increased sensitivity is replicated in other prospective trials and if the cost and difficulty of inhibin assays can be overcome.

Attempts to move maternal serum screening into the first trimester have also been recently introduced. The Royal College of Obstetricians and Gynecologists in 1997 felt there existed sufficient evidence to consider moving serum screening to the first trimester. Such screening has primarily involved the use of "pregnancy associated plasma protein A" (PAPP-A) and free beta-hCG. The latter appears to have a greater advantage at the earlier gestational ages. Modeling of the use of two markers in the first trimester in conjunction with maternal age indicates at a 5% screen positive rate such screening would detect from 62% to 69% of trisomy 21 fetuses. However, some have questioned whether this first trimester screening preferentially selects for those trisomy 21 fetuses that were destined to miscarry, as 55% of trisomy 21 fetuses identified at 10 weeks of gestation will miscarry before the end of the second trimester. One constraint of first-trimester screening, however, is the extreme sensitivity to accurate gestational age. Although sensitivity for detection of trisomy 21 is 71.6% at 9 weeks, this decreases to 46% at 13 weeks. Recent prospective studies of first-trimester screening have indicated the additional of nuchal lucency measurements can produce a screening program with a 3.3% screen positive rate for detection of 85% of trisomy 21. These encouraging results need to be replicated in multiple centers where availability and skill at nuchal lucency measurement as well as varied gestational ages may well play an important role. Finally, integrated screening, incorporating first-trimester nuchal lucency, first-trimester serum screening, and second-trimester serum screening is currently undergoing large multicenter trials. This approach obtains information throughout the first and second trimester for a resultant lower screen positive rate (0.9%) in the second trimester with a 85% detection of Down syndrome at 16 weeks of gestation.

Screening for Neural Tube Defects

Determination of maternal serum alpha-fetoprotein level at 16 to 18 weeks of gestation was established in the late 1970s for neural tube defect (NTD) screening. Elevated MSAFP levels (>2.5 MoM [multiple of the median]) lead to the detection of approximately 80% of infants with NTDs and 90% of those with anencephaly. In an average obstetric population, approximately 3% of patients have an elevated MSAFP level. Generally half of these positive screen results can be explained by ultrasound findings such as twins, demise, or erroneous gestational age. Among the remainder, however, 1 in 15 will have an infant with a NTD. In many centers improved ultrasound resolution is now being considered in the counseling of patients with an elevated MSAFP level. Women with significantly elevated MSAFP (generally cited as >3.5 MoM) warrant amniocentesis to evaluate other possible causes such as congenital Finnish nephrosis, which can not be accurately diagnosed by ultrasound.

POPULATION-SPECIFIC DISEASE SCREENING

Couples who have a common heritage, such as both individuals of northern European, Ashkenazi Jewish, Mediterranean, or African-American ancestry are more likely than individuals from two different heritages to share common recessive genes. For a child to be affected with a recessive disease, both alleles of the gene pair must be abnormal. Thus the parents of someone with a recessive condition are known as carriers; they have one normal allele and one abnormal allele for the gene in question. A carrier will not have any signs of the disorder. However, if both parents carry the same altered gene, the chance their child will inherit both abnormal genes is 1 in 4 (25% for each pregnancy). Carrier testing involves checking whether a person carries one of the two abnormal genes that can produce a specific recessive disorder. This is usually done by a blood test or cells collected from the inside of the cheek. Testing is possible for many but not all genetic conditions. Also, the implications of being a carrier for a genetic condition can vary.

There are thousands of genetic disorders although for most conditions the genes remain unknown. It is, therefore, impossible to test for every possible disorder with current technology. Instead it is necessary to choose those disorders for which tests can be performed and for which a person has a reasonable chance of being a carrier. Also considered is the severity of the disease produced.

Carrier screening and interpretation is influenced by many factors. Among them are the following:

- Detection rate of carrier testing: For a few genetic conditions, testing can detect nearly all mutations. However, for others, only some of the gene changes can be identified. In practical terms this means that if a person is identified as a carrier, or has a "positive" result, the results are highly accurate. However, if the result is "negative," there is a chance the genetic change is present but not be detected by current testing. Depending on the specific genetic condition, carrier tests can lower an individual's carrier risk but never make this risk zero.

- Ethnicity: Carrier tests identify the changes in the gene found most commonly in a specific ethnic group. For example, cystic fibrosis carrier testing can identify 90% of the gene changes causing disease in persons of northern European ancestry, but only 30% of changes in persons of Asian-American ancestry. Ethnicity is important to consider when deciding on carrier testing.

- Severity of specific disorders: Information can be provided for the more common disorders for which carrier screening is currently available. This list will likely expand in coming years. An overall understanding of the disease, treatment, and outcome is important when considering carrier screening.

Tay-Sachs Disease

Tay-Sachs disease is a degenerative neurologic condition caused by a deficiency of hexosaminidase A. The disorder first appears in infancy with signs of progressive neurologic damage, including blindness, deafness, seizures, and spasticity, with eventual demise in childhood. Tay-Sachs disease is inherited as an autosomal recessive trait with the gene most prevalent in the Ashkenazic Jewish population. Approximately 1 in 22 Ashkenazic Jewish individuals carry the

gene for Tay-Sachs disease. Ninety percent of the Jewish population in the United States is estimated to have Ashkenazic background. Descendants of French Canadians also have an increased prevalence of the Tay-Sachs gene, 1/14 in some areas of Canada. Carrier detection can be accurately accomplished by detection of decreased serum hexosaminidase A levels. In nonpregnant individuals (not on oral contraceptives) serum levels are accurate, in pregnancy white blood cell enzyme levels should be studied. Enzyme levels will detect essentially all carriers regardless of their heritage. Although testing primarily for DNA mutations is effective in the majority of Ashkenazi Jewish individuals (98%), in non-Ashkenazi persons, DNA mutations are known in less than 50% of carriers. The American College of Obstetrics and Gynecology as of 11/1995 maintains "serum screening before pregnancy if both partners are Ashkenazi Jewish, French Canadian, or of Cajun descent; in women who are pregnant or on oral contraceptives, leukocyte testing must be used."

Table 68-2 indicates other disorders that have an increased frequency in the Ashkenazi population. Screening for Canavan disease is also currently recommended by the ACOG.

Sickle-Cell Disease

Sickle hemoglobin results from a point mutation in the gene producing the beta chain of hemoglobin A (a tetramer of two alpha and two beta chains). Persons with two copies of the sickle-cell gene (SS) have a chronic hemolytic anemia that can be symptomatic with painful crises, a lowered resistance to infection, jaundice, and leg ulcers. Approximately 1 in 10 persons of African black ancestry carries one copy of the sickle-cell gene. Hispanic individuals as well as persons from the Middle East, Mediterranean, and parts of India also have a higher frequency of the sickle-cell gene than other populations. Couples in which both partners are carriers of the sickle-cell gene have a 25% chance of an affected child. Prenatal diagnosis from chorionic villus sampling (CVS) or amniocentesis can be offered to couples at risk.

Another variant, hemoglobin C, is also prevalent worldwide. Like the mutation producing sickle-cell hemoglobin, the genetic defect producing hemoglobin C is located in the beta chain. However, unlike sickle-cell disease, hemoglobin C in the homozygous state results in a mild anemia without associated painful crises. More common than homozygotic CC disease, however, is hemoglobin SC. Occurring in approximately 1/1250 black Americans, SC disease can result in a chronic anemia. Couples in which one partner is a carrier of hemoglobin C and the other of hemoglobin S are at risk for a child with SC hemoglobin.

Thalassemia

The major hemoglobin component of adult blood, hemoglobin A (Hb A), is a tetramer of two alpha and two beta hemoglobin chains. The thalassemias are hemoglobin disorders characterized by decreased numbers of structurally normal alpha or beta chains. Beta-thalassemia with decreased or absent beta chain production can result from more than 30 molecular defects and is inherited as an autosomal recessive disorder. Persons homozygotic for the beta-thalassemia gene have Cooley's anemia, or beta-thalassemia major. Af-

Table 68-2
Autosomal Recessive Diseases with Increased Frequency among Ashkenazi Population

Disease	Typical Course	Carrier Rate	DNA mutations Ashkenazi Population	DNA Mutations-non-Ashkenazi Population	Alternative Carrier Testing in non-Ashkenazi Population
Tay-Sachs	Neurologic deterioration, death in early childhood, juvenile and late onset forms	1/30	3 mutations = 92-98%	Carrier rate- 1/300 50%	Hexosaminidase (serum/leukocyte) 100% sensitivity
Canavan ("spongy degeneration of CNS")	Neurologic deterioration, death during early childhood, some survivors into teens	1/40	2 mutations = 98%	Carrier rate- ?? 60%	Aspartoacylase activity (skin fibroblasts)
Cystic fibrosis	Chronic pulmonary disease, pancreatic insufficiency, variable survivorship	1/29	5 mutations = 97%	Caucasian = 1/29 92% with 72 mutations >400 mutations identified	None
Gaucher	Type I- variable severity, hepatospleno-megaly, bone crises, anemia; asymptomatic individuals with limited genotype/pheno type correlation	1/15	5 mutations = 97%	>30 mutations = 70%;	Enzymatic activity (urine/fibroblasts) normal and carriers overlap
Niemann-Pick	Type A- neurologic deterioration with death during early childhood Type B- hepatospleno-megaly, pulmonary, no neurologic involvement	1/90	3 mutations = 92% type A 1 mutation = 50% type B	Unique mutations	Enzyme levels problematic

fected individuals become symptomatic at about 3 months of age when the switch from fetal hemoglobin (Hb F) to adult hemoglobin (Hb A) normally occurs. Deficient beta chain production is reflected by a decrease in hemoglobin A (2 alpha/2 beta, an increased level of A2 (2 alpha/2 delta chains), and an increased hemoglobin F (2 alpha/2 gamma chains). A chronic anemia results and affected individuals are transfusion-dependent with problems secondary to transfusion-related iron overload (Table 68-3).

Prenatal diagnosis for beta-thalassemia is possible. Although the disease can be caused by a combination of more than 110 point mutations; among any one racial group usually the majority of mutations (90%) can be accounted for by less than 6 mutations. For prenatal testing, the abnormal hemoglobin in the parents should be verified by hemoglobin electrophoresis and parental DNA studies initiated to identify the specific mutations involved. This then permits fetal DNA studies from CVS or amniocentesis samples. If direct

Table 68-3
Frequency of Beta-Thalassemia Carriers

Population	Beta-Thalassemia Carrier Frequency
Mediterranean	1/10
Southeast Asian	1/20
Indian, Pakistanian	1/70
African, African ancestry	1/70

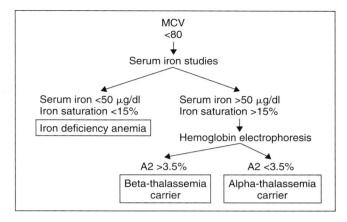

FIG. 68-1 Screening for thalassemias using MCV (mean corpuscular volume).

mutations are not known, then haplotype testing and linkage can be used, although an umbilical blood sample may be necessary for quantification of the abnormal hemoglobin.

The homozygotic state for alpha-thalassemia results in a four-gene deletion producing a fetus with Bart's hydrops fetalis. With alpha chains deficient, the fetus is unable to produce fetal hemoglobin (2 alpha/2 gamma) or any adult hemoglobin. Only Bart's hemoglobin (4 gamma), which has a higher oxygen affinity and thus a lower release of oxygen to fetal tissue resulting in hypoxia, is produced. The affected fetus has high output failure, hydrops, and stillbirth. If a three-gene deletion is present, non-transfusion-dependent anemia, thalassemia intermedia, occurs. Two gene deletions produce alpha-thalassemia minor with a mild anemia often confused with iron deficiency anemia because of its micro-cytic, hypochromic nature. Effective screening can be accomplished with a mean corpuscular volume (MCV) followed by a hemoglobin electrophoresis if needed (Fig. 68-1). Prenatal diagnosis for the thalassemia is now available through CVS or amniocentesis.

Prenatal diagnosis for alpha thalassemia is more complicated. Ethnicity is an important variable as only those individuals of Southeastern Asian ancestry are at risk for severe fetal hydrops (Barts). Among African American with alpha thalassemia, no cases of Barts have been reported due to the different configuration of the alpha gene deletions in this population, (Table 68-4).

Cystic Fibrosis

Cystic fibrosis (CF) is the most common autosomal recessive disorder among the white population. Approximately 1 in 29 Caucasians is a carrier of the CF gene, although persons of other ethnic distributions can also be carriers (Hispanics 1/45, African-Americans 1/60, Asians 1/90). Affected individuals have a median life expectancy of 28 years, although this is increasing as medical interventions are improving. Pancreatic insufficiency, respiratory infections, and inspissation of bronchial secretions characterize the disease. In persons with CF, an abnormal protein, the CF transmembrane regulator (CFTR) has been isolated and sequenced.

Carrier testing by DNA analysis from any source (cheek brushes, peripheral blood, and archival cells) is possible and more than 600 mutations are known. The frequencies of the various mutations are specific to the ethnicity of the individual (Table 68-5). Consensus as to who should be screened for cystic fibrosis should not be reached. An NIH consensus panel in 4/1996 felt the prenatal population and all couples planning pregnancy should be screened after written consent and education to include natural history, range of severity,

improvement in survival rates, quality of life for patients and families, range of therapeutic modalities, and range of reproductive options. The American Board Medical genetics (1/1998) conveys the sentiment that general population screening is premature, but education and screening models should be initiated now to assimilate this screening practice over the next 1 to 3 years. A definitive statement from the ACOG is currently pending.

At this time, Caucasians undergoing carrier screening should understand that approximately 15% of the mutations causing CF have not been identified. Practically, this implies that couples in which one partner is identified as a carrier and the other as a noncarrier (but with a 15% chance of an undetected mutation) have a risk of 1/666 for an affected offspring. Although it is a relatively small risk, in these cases prenatal diagnosis would not be able to differentiate carrier from affected fetuses. This is in contrast to the situation in which two individuals with identified CF mutations, most commonly delta 508, have a 1/4 (25%) risk of an affected fetus and for whom prenatal diagnosis, either CVS or amniocentesis, can accurately identify affected fetuses.

PRENATAL DIAGNOSIS OF GENETIC DISEASES

A diagnostic study of a fetus at risk for a genetic disorder is commonly undertaken because one of the screening tests described yields a positive result. The most frequent indication for both amniocentesis and chorionic villus sampling has traditionally been maternal age of 35 years at delivery. Recently, with the increased use of maternal serum panels for trisomy 21 risk assessment in women less than 35, a positive serum screen has become the second most frequent indication. Heterozygotic couples identified as a result of population-specific screening (Tay-Sachs disease, sickle-cell disease, thalassemia, CF) or a positive family history compose a small fraction of the invasive prenatal genetic studies of the fetus.

An increasingly common indication for diagnostic studies of the fetus has emerged with improvements in ultrasound resolution. A fetus with multiple malformations has a significant risk of being chromosomally abnormal. Specific collections of findings as well as some isolated malformations are associated with a higher rate of chromosomal

Table 68-4
Alpha-Thalassemia Carrier Frequencies

Clinical State	Manifestations	Genotype	Population Specificity	Carrier Rate
Silent carrier	Not clinically significance	-a/aa		
Trait carrier	Mild anemia, microcytosis	--/aa	Southeast Asian, China, Filipinos	1/5-1/20
		--/aa	Mediterranean	1/20
		-a/-a	African	1/50
Hemoglobin H	Chronic anemia of variable severity	--/-a		
Barts hydrops fetalis	Nonviable	--/--	Not seen with African ancestry	

Table 68-5
Detection of Cystic Fibrosis Mutations by Ethnicity

Delta 508		Detection Rate with 70 Mutation Panel
Caucasian	70%	90%
Ashkenazi Jewish	30%	97%
Hispanics	46%	57%
African American	48%	75%
Asian American	30%	30%

abnormality. In addition, with improved resolution more subtle alterations in fetal structure can be detected. In the first trimester, abnormal nuchal lucency measurements have been shown to be a risk factor not only for aneuploidy but also for structural malformations. At a 5% screen positive rate, a combination of nuchal lucency measurements and maternal age has a reported sensitivity of 73% for trisomy 21; however, efforts to duplicate these findings at other centers have not been promising.

Although minor alterations, such as choroid plexus cysts and mild hydronephrosis, may be normal variants and disappear in follow-up ultrasounds, such findings also may occur with increased frequency in chromosomally abnormal fetuses. Whether to offer amniocentesis for chromosome evaluation of every fetus with such minor alterations has been a continuing debate. In recent studies when choroid plexus cysts were identified in an otherwise structurally normal fetus, the chance of a chromosome abnormality may have been equal to or less than the risk of the diagnostic test. On the other hand, a collection of seemingly innocent ultrasound findings in the same fetus can denote an increased risk for chromosomal abnormality. Alterations of femur length, humeral length, renal pelvis size, and nuchal fold thickness have all been associated with an increased risk for trisomy 21. As an indication for diagnostic studies of the fetus, the role of ultrasound is currently expanding beyond the isolated identification of major malformations to an integrated picture of the fetus.

Diagnostic Technologies

Chorionic Villus Sampling

CVS was first attempted in 1973 in women scheduled for pregnancy termination. Ultrasound guidance of CVS did not occur until the early 1980s. The procedure involves obtaining a sample of placental tissue via a catheter placed trans-

cervically or transabdominally. The trophoblastic tissue obtained can be prepared for chromosome analysis or DNA studies. However, amniotic fluid components such as alpha-fetoprotein or acetylcholinesterase cannot be evaluated. Performed at 10 to 12 completed weeks of gestation, CVS provides the earliest detection of a genetically abnormal fetus. Additionally, in cases of third-trimester pregnancies with fetal anomalies in which amniotic fluid is not available (such as oligohydramnios) or in which a fetal blood sampling is not possible, CVS for karyotype analysis has been used with minimal risk to the fetus.

Karyotype analysis from a chorionic villus sample can be obtained from a direct preparation of the rapidly dividing cytotrophoblasts in 2 days. Most centers, however, now also elect to analyze the results of cultured trophoblasts; analysis may take an additional 10 to 14 days. In approximately 2% of CVS samples a *mosaic*—a combination of karyotypically normal and abnormal cells—is identified. As the CVS reflects the chromosomal makeup of the placenta, amniocentesis to provide further information concerning the karyotype of the fetus is warranted. Although only a third of CVS mosaicisms are confirmed in the fetus, karyotypically abnormal cell lines confined to the placenta (confined placental mosaicism [CPM]) have been associated with an increased rate of pregnancy loss and fetal growth retardation.

In two large collaborative studies of the safety of transcervical CVS, the rate of pregnancy loss was noted to be 0.6% and 0.8% higher after CVS than after amniocentesis; in neither study were these numbers significant. Likewise the safety of transabdominal CVS appears to be comparable to that of transcervical procedures. Complications include bleeding, rupture of membranes, and infection that may lead to pregnancy loss.

A possible association of limb reduction defects and oromandibular malformations with CVS sampling was first reported in 1991. Subsequent reports have both supported and refuted an increased incidence of such birth defects in association with CVS. Proposed mechanisms of action include possible vasoconstrictive events in the fetus as a result of the CVS procedure.

Amniocentesis

Amniocentesis involves the removal of amniotic fluid from around the developing fetus. Fetal cells in the fluid can be analyzed for either chromosomal complement or specific DNA studies. Traditionally amniocentesis has been performed at 16 to 20 weeks of gestation. At this gestational age the amount of fluid removed (20 ml) is only 1/10 of the total volume. In most centers, pregnancy loss after a second-trimester amniocentesis has been approximately 1 in 300.

Early amniocentesis, performed at 10 to 14 weeks, is now considered to have a complication and loss rate possibly equal to that of CVS. Technically the procedure is the same as standard amniocentesis, although incomplete fusion of the amnion and chorion at the earlier gestational ages can occasionally hamper needle insertion. With the earlier procedures, less fluid is removed, although the relative proportion to the total amniotic fluid volume is greater.

Karyotype analysis of amniotic fluid cell cultures typically requires 2 weeks to obtain sufficient cells for evaluation. The application of molecular cytogenetics to amniocentesis has provided a means of obtaining results in 24 to 48 hours. With traditional karyotype analysis, dividing cells are required in order for the chromosomes to be sufficiently condensed to facilitate recognition. However, fluorescent in situ hybridization (FISH) using tagged segments of DNA allows determination of the chromosomal makeup of a nondividing cell. With FISH probes, the number of copies of a specific chromosome can be visually detected in the undivided interphase cell. Specificity and sensitivity of FISH on interphase cells have varied.

Percutaneous Umbilical Blood Sampling

In the early 1980s ultrasound replaced fetoscopy as the method used in guiding percutaneous umbilical blood sampling (PUBS). Performed from approximately 18 weeks until term, PUBS provides access to the fetus for diagnostic studies of a peripheral blood sample (cytogenetic, hematologic, immunologic, DNA) as well as for treatment (transfusions). In some centers PUBS has been proposed for acid/base and lactate evaluations in growth-retarded fetuses. An anterior placenta facilitates obtaining the specimen from close to the insertion site of the cord into the placenta. Immobilization of the fetus with pancurarium is not needed for the short period required to obtain a fetal blood sample. The procedure has approximately a 1% to 2% risk of fetal loss. Other complications leading to preterm delivery can occur in another 5%. Fetal bradycardias, the majority of which resolve without incident, occur. Damage to the umbilical cord with laceration or hematoma formation has been reported but is a relatively rare complication.

Preimplantation Biopsy

Removing an individual cell early in gestation without subsequent harm to the developing fetus is possible at the four-cell stage in the mouse and at the eight-cell stage in the human. In women at risk for X-linked recessive disorders, identification of Y chromosome DNA in a single cell biopsy specimen from an embryo prepared for in vitro fertilization has allowed for the transfer of only XX-containing embryos. DNA study of the second polar body in humans has been another approach to preimplantation diagnosis. Produced during meiosis II, the second polar body contains basically the same genetic material as the ovum and is extruded into the zona pellucida. For a woman who is a carrier for a specific disorder, polymerase chain reaction (PCR) analysis of the polar body will discern whether the mutant allele is present in the polar body and thus also present in the oocyte. Only oocytes with a normal allele, by analysis of the polar body, would be used for the fertilization. Such a technique has been used in couples at risk for CF, alpha-$_1$-antitrypsin, and hemophilia.

A study has shown that preimplantation genetic diagnosis (PGD) screening for chromosomal abnormalities can increase the chances that a woman over the age of 40 who is undergoing in vitro fertilization will have a successful pregnancy. The biopsy procedure itself is not thought to be associated with an increased rate of congenital malformations most likely because, at the early stage of biopsy, the majority of cells are destined to be trophoblastic and contribute to placental development.

Fetal Cells in Maternal Blood

Whether by CVS, amniocentesis, PUBS, or preimplantation biopsy, accurate diagnosis of genetic diseases in the fetus has traditionally relied on invasive tests associated with risk to the pregnancy. The ability to obtain fetal DNA through noninvasive studies has been an area of continued research since the late 1970s. Although small numbers of fetal cells are known to be present in the maternal circulation in all pregnancies (approximately 20 fetal cells in a 20 ml maternal sample of blood), their use for diagnostic studies has previously been precluded by an inability to accurately identify and separate fetal from maternal cells as well as perform studies on extremely small quantities of DNA. During the 1980s, however, advances in molecular genetics rekindled interest in the detection of fetal cells in the maternal circulation. Use of PCR can now facilitate the identification of minute quantities of DNA. In addition improvements in the ability to sort fetal cells on the basis of cell surface markers of fetal red blood cells have now been described. Fetal cells sorted from a maternal blood sample can also be studied with the FISH technique and chromosomally abnormal fetuses detected. While still a technically difficult procedure, FISH analysis of fetal cells obtained from a maternal blood sample has identified at least one fetus with trisomy 18. Recently, the finding of fetal DNA fragments in maternal blood has received increased attention as another source of fetal evaluation without invasive testing.

BIBLIOGRAPHY

Benacerraf BR et al: Sonographic scoring index for prenatal detection of chromosomal abnormalities, *J Ultrasound Med* 11:449, 1992.

Bianchi DW et al: Isolation of fetal DNA from nucleated erythrocytes in maternal blood, *Proc Natl Acad Sci USA* 87:3279, 1990.

Cuckle H: Established markers in second trimester maternal serum, *Early Hum Dev* 47(Suppl):S27, 1996.

Cuckle HS: Effect of maternal age curve on the predicted detection rate in maternal serum screening for Down syndrome, *Prenat Diagn* 18:1127, 1998.

Cuckle HS, van Lith JM: Appropriate biochemical parameters in first-trimester screening for Down syndrome, *Prenat Diagn* 19:505, 1999.

Daffos F, Capella PM, Forestier F: Fetal blood sampling during pregnancy with use of a needle guided by ultrasound: a study of 606 consecutive cases, *Am J Obstet Gynecol* 153:655, 1985.

Djalali M et al: Introduction of early amniocentesis to routine prenatal diagnosis, *Prenat Diagn* 12:661, 1992.

Gekas J et al: Informed consent to serum screening for Down syndrome: are women given adequate information? *Prenat Diagn* 19:1, 1999.

Grewal GK et al: Factors affecting women's knowledge of antenatal serum screening, *Scott Med J* 42:111, 1997.

Firth HV et al: Limb abnormalities and chorion villus sampling, *Lancet* 338:51, 1991 (letter).

Firth HV et al: Severe limb abnormalities after chorion villus sampling at 56-66 days' gestation, *Lancet* 337(8744):762, 1991.

Haddow JE et al: Prenatal screening for Down's syndrome with use of maternal serum markers, *N Engl J Med* 327:588, 1992.

Haddow, JE et al: Screening of maternal serum for fetal Down's syndrome in the first trimester, *N Engl J Med* 338:955, 1998.

Handyside AH et al: Pregnancies from biopsied human preimplantation embryos sexed by Y-specific DNA amplification, *Nature* 344:768, 1990.

Henry GP, Miller WA: Early amniocentesis, *J Reprod Med* 37:396, 1992.

Holzgreve W, Miny P, Schloo R: 'Late CVS' international registry compilation of data from 24 centres, *Prenat Diagn* 10:159, 1990.

Hook EB, Cross PK, Regal RR: The frequency of 47, +21, 47, +18, and 47, +13 at the uppermost extremes of maternal ages: results on 56,094 fetuses studied prenatally and comparisons with data on livebirths, *Hum Genet* 68:211, 1984.

Geraedts J et al: ESHRE Preimplantation Genetic Diagnosis (PGD) Consortium: preliminary assessment of data from January 1997 to September 1998. ESHRE PGD Consortium Steering Committee, *Hum Reprod* 14: 3138, 1999.

Gianaroli L et al: Preimplantation diagnosis for aneuploidies in patients undergoing in vitro fertilization with a poor prognosis: identification of the categories for which it should be proposed, *Fertil Steril* 72:837, 1999.

Johnson JM et al: Technical factors in early amniocentesis predict adverse outcome. Results of the Canadian Early (EA) versus Mid-trimester (MA) Amniocentesis Trial, *Prenat Diagn* 19:732, 1999.

Kalousek DK et al: Confirmation of CVS mosaicism in term placentae and high frequency of intrauterine growth retardation association with confined placental mosaicism, *Prenat Diagn* 11:743, 1991.

Klinger K et al: Rapid detection of chromosome aneuploidies in uncultured amniocytes by using fluorescence in situ hybridization (FISH), *Am J Hum Genet* 51:55, 1992.

Lo YM et al: Increased fetal DNA concentrations in the plasma of pregnant women carrying fetuses with trisomy 21, *Clin Chem* 45:1747, 1999.

Macintosh MC et al: The selective miscarriage of Down syndrome from 10 weeks of pregnancy [published erratum appears in *Br J Obstet Gynaecol* 1996 Nov;103:1172-3], *Br J Obstet Gynaecol* 103:1172, 1996.

Medical Research Council European Trial of Chorion Villus Sampling: MRC working party on the evaluation of chorion villus sampling, *Lancet* 337:1491, 1991.

Merkatz IR et al: An association between low maternal serum alpha-fetoprotein and fetal chromosomal abnormalities, *Am J Obstet Gynecol* 148:886, 1984.

Multicentre randomised clinical trial of chorion villus sampling and amniocentesis: First report: Canadian Collaborative CVS-Amniocentesis Clinical Trial Group, *Lancet* 1:1, 1989.

Nadel AS et al: Isolated choroid plexus cysts in the second-trimester fetus: is amniocentesis really indicated? *Radiology* 185:545, 1992.

Ng IS et al: Methods for analysis of multiple cystic fibrosis mutations, *Hum Genet* 87:613, 1991.

Nicoladies KH et al: Down syndrome screening with nuchal translucency [letter; comment], *Lancet* 349:438, 1997.

Penso CA et al: Early amniocentesis: report of 407 cases with neonatal follow-up, *Obstet Gynecol* 76:1032, 1990.

Phillips OP et al: Maternal serum screening for fetal Down syndrome in women less than 35 years of age using alpha-fetoprotein, hCG, and unconjugated estriol: a prospective 2-year study, *Obstet Gynecol* 80:353, 1992.

Price JO et al: Prenatal diagnosis with fetal cells isolated from maternal blood by multiparameter flow cytometry, *Am J Obstet Gynecol* 165: 1731, 1991.

Riordan JR et al: Identification of the cystic fibrosis gene: cloning and characterization of complementary DNA, *Science* 245:1066, 1989.

Rommens JM et al: Identification of the cystic fibrosis gene: chromosome walking and jumping, *Science* 245:1059, 1989.

Tabor A et al: Randomised controlled trial of genetic amniocentesis in 4606 low-risk women, *Lancet* 1:1287, 1986.

Ttsukerman GL et al: Maternal serum screening for Down syndrome in the first trimester: experience from Belarus, *Prenat Diagn* 19:499, 1999.

Verlinsky Y et al: Analysis of the first polar body: preconception genetic diagnosis, *Hum Reprod* 5:826, 1990.

Wald NJ et al: Maternal serum screening for Down's syndrome in early pregnancy, *Br Med J* 297:883, 1988.

Wald NJ et al: Antenatal maternal serum screening for Down's syndrome: results of a demonstration project, *Br Med J* 305:391, 1992.

Wald NJ et al: Serum screening for Down syndrome between 8 and 14 weeks of pregnancy. International Prenatal Screening Research Group [see comments], *Br J Obstet Gynaecol* 103:407, 1996.

Wald NJ et al: Antenatal screening for Down syndrome, *Health Technol Assess* 2:1, 1998.

Wald NJ et al: Integrated screening for Down syndrome on the basis of tests performed during the first and second trimesters [see comments], *N Engl J Med* 341:461, 1999.

Wenstrom KD et al: Prospective evaluation of free beta-subunit of human chorionic gonadotropin and dimeric inhibin A for aneuploidy detection, *Am J Obstet Gynecol* 181:887, 1999.

Wilton LJ, Shaw JM, Trounson AO: Successful single-cell biopsy and cryopreservation of preimplantation mouse embryos, *Fertil Steril* 51:513, 1989.

Winsor EJ et al: Cytogenic aspects of the Canadian early and mid-trimester amniotic fluid trial (CEMAT), *Prenat Diagn* 19:620, 1999.

CHAPTER 69

Preeclampsia

Erin E. Tracy

Preeclampsia, traditionally identified by the classic triad of hypertension, proteinuria, and edema, is a common source of morbidity and mortality in obstetrical patients. Pulmonary embolism is the only condition resulting in more maternal deaths in the United States. Preeclampsia is also a leading cause of fetal growth restriction, intrauterine fetal demise, and indicated preterm birth. The definitive cause of preeclampsia remains elusive. Although there are many temporizing methods of treatment, the only cure is placental delivery. The inadequacy of effective therapeutic interventions largely stems from our limited understanding of the etiology and pathophysiology of this disease.

DEFINITIONS

Historically, many terms have been used to describe this disorder, including pregnancy-induced hypertension, pregnancy-aggravated hypertension, preeclampsia, toxemia, preeclamptic toxemia, gestational hypertension, and edema-proteinuric-hypertensive gestosis. The American College of Obstetricians and Gynecologists recognize two distinct categories of disease: chronic hypertension and pregnancy-induced hypertension (PIH). There is considerable overlap between the two categories, as patients with the former have an increased risk of developing manifestations of the latter. Specific subsets of PIH are preeclampsia (proteinuria secondary to renal involvement), eclampsia (seizures secondary to nervous system involvement), and HELLP syndrome (*H*emolysis, *E*levated *L*iver enzymes and *L*ow *P*latelets, secondary to hematologic and hepatic involvement).

▦ EPIDEMIOLOGY

Preeclampsia complicates 5% to 7% of pregnancies beyond 20 weeks of gestation. Preeclampsia is rare in the first half of pregnancy and is usually associated with a fetal abnormality (i.e., gestational trophoblastic disease or nonimmune hydrops). Eclampsia develops in 0.1% of all pregnancies. The disorder primarily affects primigravidas. Subsequent gestations of the same paternity are afforded some degree of adaptive protection from recurrence. If paternity changes, however, the risk of development of preeclampsia approaches that of the primigravida, suggesting a role for immunologic mechanisms. Other risk factors for the development of preeclampsia include extremes of maternal age, gestations with large placental mass (e.g., twins, molar gestation), associated medical disorders (e.g., chronic hypertension, renal disease, autoimmune diseases, and diabetes mellitus), African-American race, angiotensinogen gene T235 carriers, and a family history of preeclampsia (Box 69-1). Recent studies suggest a possible association between preeclampsia and hereditary thrombophilias, presumably owing to an increase in placental fibrin deposition and placental infarcts.

PATHOPHYSIOLOGY

Although historically a variety of theories have been proposed, current areas of investigation focus on those described in the following sections.

Abnormal Eicosanoid Metabolism

In vitro studies have demonstrated an increased thromboxane to prostacyclin ratio. Some studies demonstrate a change in the renal excretion of these substances, whereas others show a decrease in placental or endothelial prostacyclin production. The net effect of this imbalance leads to vasoconstriction and platelet aggregation, which could contribute to the hypertension and end-organ changes associated with preeclampsia.

Circulating Toxins

Reports have shown increased levels in circulating lipid peroxides and free radicals in preeclamptic patients. These substances may inhibit endogenous nitric oxide, a potent vasodilator, eventually leading to vasoconstriction and clinical hypertension.

Endothelial Factors

Vascular endothelial injury may also be contributory. One author showed that serum from preeclamptic patients was cytotoxic to endothelial cells in vitro. Several authors also reported a decrease in endothelium-derived relaxing factor (EDRF, nitric oxide), and others described an increase in endothelin, a potent vasoconstrictor.

BOX 69-1
Risk Factors for Preeclampsia

Primigravida
Extremes of maternal age
Gestations with large placental mass (e.g., twins, molar pregnancy)
Chronic hypertension
Diabetes
Renal disease
Autoimmune disease
Family history
Preeclampsia in prior pregnancy
African-American
Angiotensinogen gene T235
Nonimmune hydrops fetalis

BOX 69-2
Criteria for Severe Preeclampsia

Systolic blood pressure >160 to 180 mm Hg
Diastolic blood pressure 110 mm Hg
Proteinuria (5 g/24-hr)
Visual disturbances (scotomata, blindness, diplopia)
Headache
Epigastric pain
Pulmonary edema
Oliguria (<500 ml urine/24-hr)
Laboratory abnormalities: elevated liver transaminases, elevated serum creatinine, thrombocytopenia, hyperbilirubinemia
Microangiopathic hemolysis
Fetal growth restriction or oligohydramnios
Grand mal seizures (eclampsia)

Immunologic Factors

The clinical manifestations of preeclampsia could be attributed to an immune vasculitis caused by circulating immune complexes. A vasculitic cause unifies the preceding theories in the pathogenesis of preeclampsia. To date, however, the evidence supporting an immune complex vasculitis in preeclampsia is inconsistent.

DIAGNOSIS
Clinical Presentation
Mild Preeclampsia

Hypertension is defined as a systolic blood pressure of 140 or a diastolic pressure of 90 mm Hg on two separate occasions, at least 6 hours apart. Although an increase of systolic and diastolic blood pressure of 30 and 15, respectively, was historically considered diagnostic, new studies suggest that the majority of patients experience transient increases in this range, with no untoward effects. Although criteria used in the literature vary considerably, most authors consider the minimal proteinuric requirement to be 300 mg in a 24-hour collection. Many studies indicate the limited utility of urinary dipsticks for protein quantification. Patients often exhibit elevations in serum uric acid levels and hemoconcentration is common. The latter finding is often an early indicator of plasma volume contraction, one of the most consistent findings in this condition. Although traditional texts list nondependent edema as a clinical criterion for preeclampsia, its presence is so common (i.e., up to 80% of normotensive pregnancies) that it is not a clinically useful tool. Sudden increases in weight gain, however, should be investigated.

Preeclampsia has a wide clinical spectrum ranging from mild disease, with minimal hypertension and proteinuria, to severe multiorgan, systemic disease. The majority of patients with preeclampsia have mild disease, present in the late third trimester, and their condition resolves completely postpartum.

Severe Preeclampsia

Clinical indicators of severe preeclampsia include systolic blood pressure >160 to 180 mm Hg or a diastolic pres-

---

BOX 69-3
Laboratory Assessment of Preeclampsia

Serum creatinine
Uric acid
Liver transaminases
Complete blood count (including platelets)
Coagulation profile
24-hr urine collection for total protein and creatinine clearance
Blood type and screen

---

sure of 110 mm Hg, oliguria, pulmonary edema, symptoms indicating multiorgan involvement (e.g., visual disturbances, epigastric pain, headache), fetal indicators (e.g., intrauterine growth restriction, oligohydramnios), or eclamptic seizures (Box 69-2). Laboratory result abnormalities associated with severe preeclampsia include elevated liver transaminases, thrombocytopenia, hyperbilirubinemia, increased creatinine, 24-hour urine collection with at least 5 g of urinary protein, or an abnormal coagulation profile (secondary to microangiopathic hemolysis) (Box 69-3). HELLP syndrome can be associated with disseminated intravascular coagulation. Paradoxically, there is no consistent relationship between the severity of preeclampsia and the manifestations of HELLP syndrome.

Differential Diagnosis

Given the prevalence of preeclampsia, patients should have blood pressure measurements and close follow-up evaluation in the third trimester. Whenever patients report nonspecific findings, it should be considered, given the risk of atypical presentations of this disorder. Any patients who present with the presumptive diagnosis of liver or renal disease, cholecystitis, hemorrhage, immune thrombocytopenia purpura, or heart failure must have the diagnosis of severe preeclampsia ruled out before initiating conservative treatment measures. This is especially important, as delivery is the only cure for preeclampsia, and may not be indicated otherwise in these conditions. In evaluating a pregnant patient with any of these findings, the importance of considering preeclampsia as the primary diagnosis cannot be overemphasized (Box 69-4).

Complications

Complications of preeclampsia result in a maternal mortality rate of 3/100,000 live births in the United States. Maternal morbidity may include central nervous system complications (e.g., strokes, seizures, intracerebral hemorrhage, and blindness), disseminated intravascular coagulation, hepatic failure or rupture, and abruptio placentae, leading to maternal hemorrhage and acute renal failure. Placental abruption occurs in ~9% of cases, often resulting in significant deleterious fetal effects. Fetal morbidity may also include intrauterine growth retardation, acidemia, and complications of indicated preterm delivery (e.g., respiratory distress syndrome, intraventricular hemorrhage, and necrotizing enterocolitis).

✳ MANAGEMENT

The only definitive treatment for preeclampsia is delivery. Obstetric management is determined by the severity of the disease, gestational age, fetal pulmonary maturation (may be confirmed by amniocentesis), and assessment of the maternal cervix (as it relates to the predicted utility of labor induction). If there is evidence of intrauterine fetal distress, delivery is usually indicated, regardless of the gestational age or fetal pulmonary maturity. Some investigators advocate conservative management of severe preeclampsia when diagnosed at a very early gestational age, but there is general consensus that if delivery is not to be imminently planned, close observation is mandatory in an inpatient setting in a tertiary care center. Serious maternal sequelae including acute renal failure, disseminated intravascular coagulation, HELLP syndrome, abruption, eclampsia, and intrauterine fetal death have been reported with conservative therapy of severe preeclampsia. Patients with preterm gestations and mild preeclampsia, however, can successfully continue their pregnancies for weeks with close maternal and fetal observation.

Factors influencing early intervention in these patients include the subsequent development of severe preeclampsia, nonreassuring fetal status, and fetal pulmonary maturation.

Antepartum Conservative Management of Preeclampsia

Although some authors advocate outpatient management of mild preeclampsia, patients must be selected carefully for conservative management, with frequent outpatient visits. Many patients are hospitalized for bed rest and observation. Patients should be closely observed for evidence of worsening blood pressure, edema, laboratory parameters, or symptoms of severe preeclampsia. Intermittent 24-hour urine protein collections may be followed. Baseline liver and renal function tests, hematocrit, platelets, and coagulation studies are recommended. Repeat laboratory evaluation is based on clinical assessment of the patient's status. Weekly or semiweekly fetal surveillance, such as nonstress testing or fetal biophysical profile, is advised. Fetal ultrasound evaluation for interval growth and amniotic fluid volume is performed approximately every 2 to 3 weeks. Antepartum antihypertensive agents in preeclamptic patients being managed expectantly should be reserved for severe increases in blood pressure (i.e., diastolic pressure >110 mm Hg), and loop diuretics should be used only in the setting of cardiac decompensation, given the volume-contracted state. Hydralazine and labetolol are two of the agents most widely studied. Antepartum glucocorticoid therapy should be considered before 34 weeks of gestation.

If the decision if made to proceed with delivery, cervical ripening agents may be used (e.g., prostaglandins) if necessary before to pitocin therapy. Cesarean delivery should be planned only in cases remote from immediate delivery with suspected fetal distress, other obstetric indications (e.g., transverse lie or placenta previa), or rapidly deteriorating maternal status.

Intrapartum Management of Preeclampsia
Magnesium Sulfate

Magnesium sulfate has been used for seizure prophylaxis in this condition since 1925. Recent studies support its efficacy in comparison to phenytoin therapy. Magnesium is administered during labor induction, delivery, and for at least 24 hours postpartum. In the absence of renal disease, an intravenous loading dose of 4 g is infused, followed by a 2 to 3 g/hr continuous maintenance dose (Box 69-5). Urine output should be monitored hourly as oliguria can lead to toxic serum levels. Signs of magnesium overdose include loss of deep tendon reflexes, visual blurring or diplopia, respiratory depression or paralysis, and, at levels greater than 25 mEq/L, cardiac arrest (Box 69-6). Magnesium should be administered by a pump, to permit careful regulation of the infusion rate. In the event of acute magnesium toxicity, magnesium infusion should be discontinued immediately, airway and oxygenation maintained, and 1 g calcium gluconate administered slowly intravenously (over 3 minutes). Occasionally repeated doses of calcium gluconate may be required, as well as mechanical ventilation.

Fluid Balance

Careful monitoring of fluid balance is critical in these patients. Preeclampsia is associated with decreased intravascular volume, which can lead to oliguria. Unfortunately many

---

BOX 69-5

Magnesium Sulfate Infusion for Preeclampsia

Loading dose: Mix 4 g magnesium sulfate in 100 ml normal saline solution. Infuse over 20 min.

Maintenance dose: Mix 2 g magnesium sulfate per 100 ml normal saline solution. Infuse at a rate of 2-3 g/hr.

Monitoring: Check serum magnesium level 6 hr after the loading dose. Therapeutic levels considered to range from 4 to 7 mEq/L.

BOX 69-6

Acute Magnesium Toxicity: Signs and Symptoms

Clinical Findings	Serum Level (mEq/L)
Seizure prophylaxis	4-7
Loss of deep tendon reflexes	10
Respiratory depression	12
Respiratory paralysis	15
Cardiac arrest	25

BOX 69-7

Summary Table of Intrapartum Management of Preeclampsia Complication Recommended Intervention

Seizure prevention	Magnesium sulfate Loading dose: 6 g Maintenance dose: 1-2 g/hr Continuous IV infusion
Fluid balance	Placement of Foley catheter Careful fluid monitoring with total IV fluid rate 100 ml/hr
Hypertension	Hydralazine 5-10 mg IV push, then repeated every 20 minutes as needed to total of 40 mg Labetalol 20 mg IV then 40-80 mg IV every 10 minutes to total of 300 mg, follow with IV infusion 1-2 mg/min if necessary titrated to desired blood pressure Nifedipine 10-20 mg sublingual Nitroglycerin IV with starting dose 5 mg/min Consider arterial line
Labor and delivery	Anesthesia consultation Continuous intrapartum fetal heart rate monitoring

IV, Intravenous; *BP,* blood pressure.

---

patients also have capillary leak that predisposes them to pulmonary edema. A Foley catheter is helpful in monitoring urine output. Generally, total hourly intravenous fluid rate should be less than 100 ml/hr. If oliguria develops and is unresponsive to a 500-ml bolus of crystalloid, invasive hemodynamic monitoring with a Swan-Ganz catheter should be considered.

Treatment of Hypertension

Intrapartum severe hypertension (persistent diastolic blood pressure of 110 mm Hg or systolic blood pressure of 180 mm Hg) may be controlled with **hydralazine,** 5 to 10 mg IV push, then repeated every 20 to 30 minutes, as needed, to a total of 40 mg. It is important to recognize that the onset of action of hydralazine is not instantaneous; thus repeat doses should not be given more frequently than every 20 minutes to observe for hemodynamic effect. Intravenous **labetalol,** 20 mg initially then 40 to 80 mg every 10 minutes to a total of 300 mg, may be administered as an alternative to hydralazine. The maximal effect of a dose of labetalol occurs within 5 minutes. A continuous intravenous infusion of 1 to 2 mg/min may be titrated to the desired blood pressure. Labetalol has the advantage of faster onset of action, causing less reflex tachycardia, headaches, and hypotension than hydralazine. Care should be exercised not to reduce the blood pressure either too abruptly or too far, as decreased intravascular volume and poor uteroplacental perfusion may lead to acute fetal distress. Continuous hemodynamic monitoring with an arterial line is usually not necessary. Other agents useful in controlling acute hypertension include **nifedipine,** 10 to 20 mg sublingual, and intravenous **nitroglycerin** starting at 5 mg/min. In using sublingual nifedipine, however, one must be wary of the variable rate of absorption of sublingual agents and the potential for the magnesium potentiation of calcium channel blockers, resulting in a precipitous, significant decrease in blood pressure. Before delivery sodium nitroprusside is not recommended because of theoretic concerns regarding cyanide toxicity to the fetus.

Labor and Delivery

Anesthesia consultation in labor and delivery is strongly recommended. In general, epidural anesthesia may be used in preeclamptic patients, although caution should be exercised to prevent significant sympathetic blockade and acute hypotension, which can result in acute fetal distress. If the patient manifests disseminated intravascular coagulation or severe thrombocytopenia, epidural anesthesia is to be avoided. When platelet counts are starting to decline, an early epidural can be considered.

Continuous intrapartum fetal heart rate monitoring is advised, as fetal acidemia secondary to poor uteroplacental perfusion is common in these patients. Patterns suggestive of fetal compromise include persistent tachycardia, decreased short- and long-term variability, and recurrent late decelerations not responsive to standard resuscitative measures (Box 69-7).

Postpartum Management

Most postpartum eclamptic seizures occur within the first 24 hours after delivery. Magnesium sulfate seizure prophylaxis is thus continued during this period, regardless of the mode of delivery. Occasionally magnesium sulfate is continued for an additional 12 to 24 hours in patients considered at greatest risk for postpartum eclamptic seizures, such as those with signs of central nervous system irritability. Several reports have described seizure activity or abnormal electroencephalograms in women with therapeutic magnesium levels, demonstrating the limited utility of overreliance on serum levels. Intravenous fluid replacement ($\sim$100 ml/hr) should continue with close attention to intake and output data. Clinical and laboratory findings of preeclampsia may worsen immediately postpartum, but usually begin to resolve within 24 to 48 hours postpartum and normalize within 1 to 2 weeks. Maternal diuresis often ensues shortly after placental delivery. Patients with persistent hypertension (i.e., diastolic blood pressure of 110 mm Hg) may require short-term antihypertensive therapy. Blood pressure should be reassessed in 1 to 2 weeks after delivery, at which time the antihypertensive agent may be discontinued.

RECURRENCE OF PREECLAMPSIA IN SUBSEQUENT GESTATIONS

Patients diagnosed with preeclampsia in their first pregnancy are at increased risk for recurrent hypertensive disease in a subsequent pregnancy. Sibai et al reported that, in women diagnosed with either severe preeclampsia or eclampsia in their first pregnancy, this recurrence risk can be as high as 45%. This is particularly true when severe preeclampsia occurred remote from term. There is some evidence that suggests a predisposition to the development of chronic hypertension in later life.

PREVENTION OF PREECLAMPSIA

In light of the previously described eicosanoid theory of preeclampsia, a number of clinical trials have evaluated the prophylactic use of low-dose aspirin therapy. Several randomized controlled clinical trials studies failed to show an improvement in perinatal morbidity. One large study found a slightly increased incidence of placental abruption in patients on aspirin therapy. Although one author reported a decrease in preeclampsia in calcium supplementation in a select high-risk population, a subsequent randomized control trial of calcium failed to reveal a benefit using calcium prophylaxis. Without a clear understanding of the pathophysiology of this condition, it remains a challenge to develop an effective prophylactic measure for preeclampsia prevention.

IMPLICATIONS FOR DEVELOPMENT OF ADULT HYPERTENSION

The hypertensive effects of preeclampsia generally resolve within the first week postpartum. Occasionally patients require antihypertensive therapy up to 12 weeks postpartum. Controversy exists as to the correlation between the clinical diagnosis of preeclampsia and the subsequent development of chronic hypertension. It is recommended that women with a history of preeclampsia be advised of a slightly increased risk of chronic hypertension and be monitored accordingly.

BIBLIOGRAPHY

American College of Obstetricians and Gynecologists: Hypertension in Pregnancy, ACOG mechnical bulletin No. 219, Washington, DC, 1996.

Atrash HK et al: Maternal mortality in the United States: 1979-1986, *Obstet Gynecol* 76:1055, 1990.

Barton JR, Sibai BM: Acute life-threatening emergencies in preeclampsia-eclampsia, *Clin Obstet Gynecol* 35(2):402, 1992.

Belizan JM et al: Calcium supplementation to prevent hypertensive disorders of pregnancy, *N Engl J Med* 325:1399, 1991.

Collaborative Low-Dose Aspirin Study in Pregnancy Collaborative Group: CLASP: a randomized trial of low-dose aspirin for the prevention and treatment of preeclampsia among 9364 pregnant women, *Lancet* 343: 619, 1994.

Cunningham FG et al, editors: *Williams obstetrics,* ed 19, East Norwalk, Conn, 1993, Appleton & Lange.

Cunningham F, Lindheimer MD: Current concepts: hypertension in pregnancy, *N Engl J Med* 326:927, 1992.

Eclampsia Trial Collaborative Group: Which anticonvulsant for women with eclampsia: evidence from the Collaborative Eclampsia Trial, *Lancet* 345:1455, 1995.

Gabbe SG et al, editors: *Obstetrics: normal and problem pregnancies,* ed 3, Churchill Livingstone, 1996.

Goodlin RC: Severe pre-eclampsia: another great imitator, *Am J Obstet Gynecol* 125:747, 1976.

Hubel CA et al: Lipid peroxidation in pregnancy: new perspectives on preeclampsia, *Am J Obstet Gynecol* 161:1025, 1989.

Imperiale TF, Petrulis AS: A meta-analysis of low-dose aspirin for the prevention of pregnancy-induced hypertensive disease, *JAMA* 266:261, 1991.

Italian Study of Aspirin in Pregnancy: Low-dose aspirin in prevention and treatment of intrauterine growth retardation and pregnancy-induced hypertension, *Lancet* 341:396, 1993.

Kupferminis MF et al: Severe preeclampsia and high frequency of genetic thrombophilic mutations, *Obstet Gynecol* 96:45, 2000.

Lucas MF et al: A comparison of magnesium sulfate with phenytoin for the prevention of eclampsia, *N Engl J Med* 333:201, 1995.

Martin JN et al: Pregnancy complicated by preeclampsia-eclampsia with the syndrome of hemolysis, elevated liver enzymes, and low platelet count: how rapid is postpartum recovery? *Obstet Gynecol* 76:737, 1990.

Morris JF et al: A randomized controlled trial of aspirin in patients with abnormal uterine artery blood flow, *Obstet Gynecol* 87:74, 1996.

Niswander KR et al: Fetal morbidity following potential anoxigenic obstetric conditions, *Am J Obstet Gynecol* 98:871, 1967.

O'Brien WF: Predicting preeclampsia, *Obstet Gynecol* 75:3, 1990.

Roberts JM et al: Preeclampsia: an endothelial cell disorder, *Am J Obstet Gynecol* 161:1200, 1989.

Rochat RW et al: The maternal mortality collaborative. Maternal mortality in the United States: report from the Maternal Mortality Collaborative, *Obstet Gynecol* 72:91, 1988.

Rodgers GM et al: Preeclampsia is associated with a serum factor cytotoxic to human endothelial cells, *Am J Obstet Gynecol* 159:908, 1988.

Sadeh M: Action of magnesium sulfate in the treatment of preeclampsia-eclampsia, *Stroke* 20:1273, 1989.

Sanchez-Ramos L et al: Calcium supplementation in mild preeclampsia remote from term: a randomized double-blind clinical trial, *Obstet Gynecol* 85:915, 1995.

Schiff E et al: The use of aspirin to prevent pregnancy-induced hypertension and lower the ratio of thromboxane A2 to prostacyclin in relatively high risk pregnancies, *N Engl J Med* 321:351, 1989.

Sibai BM et al: Effect of magnesium sulfate on electroencephalographic findings in preeclampsia-eclampsia, *Obstet Gynecol* 64:261, 1984.

Sibai BM, El-Nazer A, Gonzalez-Ruiz A: Severe preeclampsia-eclampsia in young primigravid women: subsequent pregnancy outcome and remote prognosis, *Am J Obstet Gynecol* 155:1011, 1986.

Sibai BM et al: Maternal and perinatal outcome of conservative management of severe preeclampsia in midtrimester, *Am J Obstet Gynecol* 152: 32, 1985.

Sibai BM et al: A protocol for managing severe preeclampsia in the second trimester, *Am J Obstet Gynecol* 163:733,1990.

Sibai BM: Diagnosis and management of chronic hypertension in pregnancy, *Obstet Gynecol* 78:451, 1991.

Sibai BM et al: Aggressive versus expectant management of severe preeclampsia at 28 to 32 weeks' gestation: a randomized controlled trial, *Am J Obstet Gynecol* 171:318,1994.

Sibai BM et al: Prevention of preeclampsia with low-dose aspirin in healthy, nulliparous pregnant women, *N Engl J Med* 329:1213, 1993.

Villar MA, Sibai BM: Clinical significance of elevated mean arterial blood pressure in second trimester and threshold increase in systolic and diastolic blood pressure during third trimester, *Am J Obstet Gynecol* 160:419, 1989.

Walsh SW: Preeclampsia: an imbalance in placental prostacyclin and thromboxane production, *Am J Obstet Gynecol* 152:335, 1985.

Witlin AG, Sibai BM: Magnesium sulfate therapy in preeclampsia and eclampsia, *Obstet Gynecol* 92:883, 1998.

CHAPTER **70**

Asthma in Pregnancy

Phyllis Jen

▦ EPIDEMIOLOGY

Asthma is the most common respiratory disease in pregnancy and occurs in about 4% of all pregnancies. The course of asthma in pregnancy is unpredictable, with one third noting no change, one third noting improvement and one third noting a slight tendency for asthma to worsen in the second and third trimester. Asthma exacerbations during pregnancy can cause maternal hypoxia, hypocapnia, and alkalosis and resulting fetal hypoxia. Studies suggest that the severity of asthma during pregnancy (as indicated by steroid dependence) correlates with perinatal mortality, prematurity, and low birth weight. However, women who receive steroids and are able to avoid status asthmaticus have a better outcome than women who are undertreated and develop status asthmaticus. Of note is that congenital abnormalities do not occur in severe asthmatics at increased frequencies.

❋ MANAGEMENT
Goals

The goals of managing the pregnant woman with asthma are similar to those for the nonpregnant woman. The report of the Working Group on Asthma and Pregnancy emphasize four components of effective therapy:

- Monitoring of maternal lung function: Although spirometry measurement of baseline pulmonary function can be helpful, home monitoring of peak expiratory flow rates is recommended and can detect changes in lung function before the onset of symptoms
- Environmental controls, including avoidance of allergen and irritant exposure
- Patient education
- Pharmacologic therapy: The general principles of therapy of pregnant asthmatics are similar to those in nonpregnant asthmatics. Most drugs used in treatment of asthma are categorized in the Food and Drug Administration (FDA) Use-in-Pregnancy Rating Scale category B or C (Table 70-1).

CHOICE OF THERAPY
Chronic Asthma

Women with chronic asthma maintained on medications should continue those medications that are safe to use during pregnancy (Table 70-1). Inhaled agents are generally preferable to oral agents. Treatment approaches are summarized in Table 70-2.

Acute Asthma

When a pregnant woman has an asthma exacerbation, additional therapies are necessary. Rapid improvement of symptoms can often be achieved with inhaled beta-agonist therapy with minimal side effects. The addition of a spacer device can often improve delivery of the medication. Although beta-agonists such as terbutaline, albuterol and metaproterenol are probably safe, they may, even in the inhaled form, inhibit uterine contractions and they should be avoided, if possible, in late pregnancy or at term. If symptoms cannot be controlled with inhaled beta-agonists, methylxanthines (theophylline or aminophylline) are safe to use in pregnancy, although transient neonatal tachycardia and irritability have been noted. The use of epinephrine is somewhat more controversial because of studies showing a slight reduction in placental blood flow, and the Working Group on Pregnancy and Asthma has recommended that epinephrine be avoided during pregnancy.

If an acute asthma exacerbation does not respond to bronchodilator therapy, oral corticosteroids should be used to speed remission and prevent status asthmaticus. A short course of steroids (<2 weeks) is not associated with any adverse outcomes. Patients with severe asthma requiring chronic steroids, however, have an increased incidence of premature delivery (<37 weeks) and low-birth-weight infants (<2500 g). Steroid-dependent asthmatics who experience status asthmaticus during pregnancy have an increased incidence of low-birth-weight infants. Chronic inhaled steroid therapy, for patients with less severe disease, has been shown to reduce the frequency of acute exacerbations and to lower airway reactivity. There is no increased incidence of fetal mortality or congenital malformations when inhaled

Table 70-1
Food and Drug Administration Use-in-Pregnancy Rating Scale for Drugs to Treat Asthma

Drug Class	Specific Drug	FDA Category
Beta-adrenergic agonists	Albuterol	C
	Epinephrine	C
	Metaproterenol	C
	Pirbuterol	C
	Salmeterol	C
	Terbutaline	B
Methylxanthines	Theophylline	C
Corticosteroids	Prednisone (systemic)	Not classified
	Beclomethasone (inhaled)	C
	Budesonide	C
	Flunisolide (inhaled)	C
	Fluticasone (inhaled)	C
	Triamcinolone (inhaled)	C
Anticholinergic drugs	Ipratropium	B
Cromoglycates	Cromolyn sodium	B
	Nedocromil	B
Agents affecting leukotrienes	Zafirlukast	B
	Montelukast	B
	Zileuton	C
Antihistamines	Chlorpheniramine, etc.	Not classified
	Loratadine	B
	Fexofenadine	C
	Cetirizine	B
Decongestants	Pseudoephedrine, etc.	Not classified

Table 70-2
Management of Asthma in Pregnancy

Chronic

Mild intermittent (symptoms <2 days/wk)	Inhaled β_2-agonist as needed
Mild persistent (symptoms 3 to 6 days/wk)	Inhaled low-dose steroid or cromolyn
Moderate persistent (symptoms daily)	Inhaled medium-dose steroid Long acting inhaled β_2-agonist
Severe persistent (symptoms continual)	Inhaled high-dose steroid Long acting inhaled β_2-agonist Oral steroid at lowest effective dose
All patients	Inhaled short acting β_2-agonist

Acute Exacerbation

	Inhaled short acting β_2-agonist hourly Systemic steroid Oxygen

Management During Labor

	Continue same medication For steroid dependant patients, intravenous steroid If asthma symptoms increase during labor, treat as above for acute exacerbations

beclomethasone is used. Newer inhaled steroids have not been studied, but are likely to be safe. A relationship between steroid use and cleft palate demonstrated in rabbits has not been found in humans. Cromolyn therapy can also reduce airway reactivity, especially in the atopic patient with seasonal disease. Adverse fetal effects have not been noted. Agents that affect the leukotriene pathway have not been adequately studied in humans, but animal data have not shown teratogenicity. Iodide-containing expectorants may cause fetal goiter and should be avoided.

Use of Antibiotics and Immunizations

Antibiotics such as penicillins, cephalosporins, and erythromycin can be given to patients with infectious upper respiratory infections. Macrolides are probably safe and are in FDA category B or C. Sulfa-containing antibiotics when given near term can cause kernicterus. Tetracycline must be avoided because it causes staining of teeth and delayed fetal bone growth. Quinolones should be avoided because they have caused fetal arthropathy. Influenza immunization should be given, preferably in the second or third trimester.

MANAGEMENT DURING LABOR

Because minute ventilation during labor can increase two times, asthma symptoms should ideally be controlled before the onset of labor. Patients who are steroid dependent or who have recently been on a prolonged course of steroids should receive stress-dose hydrocortisone coverage when labor begins.

BIBLIOGRAPHY

Demissie K, Breckenridge MB: Infant and maternal outcomes in the pregnancies of asthmatic women, *Am J Respir Crit Care Med* 158:1091, 1998.

National Asthma Education Program. Report of the Working Group on Asthma and Pregnancy. *Management of asthma during pregnancy,* National Institute of Health (no. 93-3279A), Bethesda, MD, 1993.

Schatz M: Asthma and pregnancy, *Lancet* 353:1202, 1999.

Schatz M et al: Safety of asthma and allergy medications during pregnancy, *J Allergy Clin Immunol* 100:301, 1997.

CHAPTER 71

Diabetes in Pregnancy

Michael F. Greene
Stephanie A. Eisenstat

Diabetes mellitus has always been recognized as a serious complication in pregnancy. Dr. Elliott Joslin's first published series of diabetes in pregnancy in 1915 (7 years before the discovery of insulin) detailed 10 pregnancies among 7 women. There were only three surviving children, and four of the women died. The prognosis for diabetic women and their offspring has improved steadily and dramatically since the introduction of insulin. The incidence of maternal mortality has become so small that it is difficult to measure. Significant morbidity such as hypoglycemia, diabetic keto-acidosis, hypertension, and exacerbations of nephropathy and retinopathy still occur with greater frequency during pregnancy. Perinatal mortality is now less than one tenth of what it was shortly after insulin was introduced, but it is still twice that for the nondiabetic population. Although it is difficult to separate the elements of care for these patients to quantitate how each improvement has contributed to the improved prognosis for pregnancy, it is probably fair to say that no single intervention has been as important as improved metabolic control of the underlying disease.

PATHOPHYSIOLOGY
Metabolic Changes Associated with Pregnancy

Compared with the nonpregnant state, normal pregnancy is associated with a fall in fasting blood glucose levels but a rise in postprandial glucose levels. The net result of these changes is a modest rise in mean daily blood glucose levels throughout pregnancy. These changes occur in the presence of insulin levels, which are elevated above nonpregnant levels and rise throughout pregnancy. The occurrence of relative postprandial hyperglycemia despite relatively high insulin levels is, by definition, insulin resistance and has led to the characterization of pregnancy as a "diabetogenic" state. The hormones chiefly responsible for the insulin resistance are cortisol, growth hormone, and chorionic somatomammotropin. Blood amino acid levels are lower during pregnancy than in the nonpregnant state. A relatively brief fast (overnight) during the later half of pregnancy will result in higher levels of the ketones acetoacetate and β-hydroxy-butyrate than in the nonpregnant state. The rapid switch to fatty acids as an energy source after a brief fast, which is reflected by this ketone body formation, has been termed the accelerated starvation of pregnancy.

CLASSIFICATION OF DIABETES IN PREGNANCY

The classification of diabetes in adults has undergone reclassification over the years to decrease confusion, increase uniformity of definition, and reflect current knowledge about what we understand about the etiology of diabetes (see Chapter 11). The problem of diabetes complicating pregnancy can be broadly classified into overt diabetes, which antedates pregnancy (either type I or type II), and gestational diabetes. A modification of the classification system for diabetes in pregnancy originally proposed by White is presented in the Box 71-1.

Gestational Diabetes

Gestational diabetes mellitus (GDM) was redefined in 1984 as "carbohydrate intolerance of variable severity with onset or first recognition during the present pregnancy." The original definition of GDM by glucose tolerance testing in the 1960s was intended to identify women with relatively modest impairment of carbohydrate tolerance that developed later in pregnancy as a result of the physiologic changes of pregnancy. It was defined as glucose values 2 standard deviations above the mean for the population tested and validated by its association with an increased risk for the development of type 2 diabetes later in life. The new definition is so broad that it includes a wide variety of potentially very different patients. It includes patients with type 2 diabetes antedating pregnancy who possibly should have been receiving insulin or oral agents but who were not previously diagnosed. Harris found, for example, that at age 40 years, 8% of nonpregnant women had a degree of carbohydrate intolerance that would be classified as gestational diabetes. Occasionally type 1 diabetes develops coincidently during a young woman's pregnancy, and this too would be classified as gestational diabetes.

PRECONCEPTION CARE OF WOMEN WITH DIABETES

Clinical trials of preconception care to achieve optimal blood glucose control in the preconception period and during the

---

BOX 71-1

Classification of Diabetes in Pregnancy

GDM non-I

Non-insulin-requiring gestational diabetes	Abnormal carbohydrate tolerance in pregnancy; no insulin required

GDM I

Insulin-requiring gestational diabetes	Abnormal carbohydrate tolerance in pregnancy; insulin required

A Abnormal carbohydrate tolerance before pregnancy; no insulin required before or during pregnancy

B Insulin-requiring diabetes; onset after 20 years of age and duration <10 yr; no vascular complications

C Insulin-requiring diabetes; onset 10-19 yr of age and duration <20 yr or duration 10-20 yr with onset after age 20

D Insulin-requiring diabetes with either onset before 10 yr of age or duration >20 yr regardless of age at onset or associated with background retinopathy or associated with chronic hypertension

F Insulin-requiring diabetes with nephropathy (>500-mg proteinuria per day)

R Insulin-requiring diabetes with proliferative retinopathy

T Insulin-requiring diabetes with renal transplant

H Insulin-requiring diabetes with coronary artery disease

Modified from Hare JW, White P: *Diabetes Care* 3:394, 1980.

BOX 71-2

Criteria for the Diagnosis of Diabetes Mellitus in the Nonpregnant Female

Symptoms of diabetes (polyuria, polydipsia and weight loss) plus random plasma glucose level of >200 mg/dl *or*

Fasting plasma glucose >126 mg/dl (fasting = no caloric intake for at least 8 hours) *or*

2 hour plasma glucose >200 mg/dl during an OGTT (equivalent of 75 g oral glucose load)

---

first trimester of pregnancy have demonstrated clear dramatic reductions in rates of malformations compared with infants of diabetic women who did not participate in preconception care. Unfortunately more than two thirds of pregnancies of women with diabetes are unplanned. Therefore, health care providers who care for diabetic women of reproductive age should not only counsel women on the positive impact of tight glucose control on decreasing the development of the long-term medical complications associated with diabetes, but also the critical effect good metabolic control has on pregnancy outcome.

Preconception counseling involves education of the woman about the impact the hormonal changes of pregnancy on diabetic metabolic control, diabetic self-management skills, and more frequent laboratory monitoring of blood glucose and medical surveillance.

Criteria for the diagnosis of diabetes mellitus in the nonpregnant female appear in Box 71-2.

OVERT DIABETES
Maternal Complications
Hypoglycemia

Early pregnancy frequently is associated with some degree of anorexia, nausea, and vomiting, as well as lower fasting glucose levels as previously mentioned. In diabetic women taking a fixed daily dose of insulin, these changes often result in an increased frequency of insulin reactions in early pregnancy. Intensively treated diabetic patients often have a diminished awareness of and response to hypoglycemia. Diamond et al. recently showed this to be true for pregnant diabetic women, too. They compared the response to hypoglycemia in nine intensively treated diabetic women and seven nonpregnant nondiabetic age-matched women using a hypoglycemic insulin clamp technique. They found that the counterregulatory hormonal responses of glucagon, epinephrine, and growth hormone did not begin to rise until lower levels of blood glucose were reached; they rose more slowly; and they did not reach the same maximum levels of response in the diabetic pregnant women compared with the control subjects. Given the design of their study, it is impossible to determine the amount of difference caused as a result of pregnancy versus intensive insulin therapy.

The elevated progesterone levels of pregnancy are associated with delayed gastric emptying. In women with some degree of gastroparesis before pregnancy, this effect can be exacerbated. Delayed and unpredictable gastric emptying can make glycemic control, which depends on insulin injections timed to anticipate gastric emptying, difficult and result in wide swings in postprandial glucose values. At its worst in late pregnancy, it can lead to frequent vomiting, poor weight gain, and frequent hypoglycemia. Frequent vomiting of undigested meals 2 to 3 hours after eating is characteristic in these cases. Metoclopramide (Reglan) therapy has been quite helpful for these patients.

Severe hypoglycemia in the second half of pregnancy may be associated with a modest degree of fetal bradycardia—as low as 100 beats/min. This decrease reverses slowly as maternal blood glucose levels return to normal, with no obvious adverse consequences to the fetus. Recent data have suggested that overly zealous insulin therapy resulting in frequent symptomatic insulin reactions or chronic modest hypoglycemia may be associated with inadequate fetal growth.

Diabetic Ketoacidosis

It is often said that women with type 1 diabetes are at increased risk for the development of diabetic ketoacidosis (DKA) during pregnancy, but the relationship is not clear. It is clear that during pregnancy DKA may develop at much lower blood glucose levels than would normally be a problem in nonpregnant women. Vomiting frequently is associated with DKA during pregnancy and may confuse the diagnosis if the observed ketonuria is attributed to starvation because of protracted vomiting. Although DKA always has the potential to become a life-threatening emergency, it is particularly threatening to the fetus in the last half of pregnancy. Fetal death rates as high as 50% have been observed. Treatment of DKA should be aggressive and no different in principle than for nonpregnant persons. DKA often induces premature labor and is associated with nonreassuring fetal heart rate patterns. Both problems are best treated by vigorously addressing the metabolic disorder.

Retinopathy

Virtually all patients with diabetes of sufficient duration eventually develop some degree of retinopathy. Duration of diabetes, degree of glycemic control, and diastolic blood pressure have all been shown to correlate with the risk for development and progression of retinopathy. There has been considerable controversy over the years regarding the role of pregnancy as a risk factor for diabetic retinopathy. The best prospective and controlled study of this issue was reported by Klein et al. Pregnant diabetic women were matched with nonpregnant control subjects and monitored in a similar fashion over comparable periods. Serial fundus photographs were obtained, and the degree of retinopathy was graded by ophthalmologists without knowledge of the pregnancy status of the patients. Serial tests of visual acuity also were performed. The ophthalmologists concluded that on the basis of the fundus photographs, progression of retinopathy was more likely to occur in pregnant women than in nonpregnant subjects. Furthermore, women with more advanced disease in early pregnancy were more likely to have more dramatic progression. Pregnant women were significantly more likely to suffer a deterioration in visual acuity than the nonpregnant control group. This difference was minimal, however, at long-term postpartum follow-up examination.

Several studies have shown, and the Diabetes Control and Complications Trial (DCCT) has recently confirmed, that intensification of metabolic control is associated with an exacerbation of diabetic retinopathy over the short term. To what degree the progression of retinopathy during pregnancy can be attributed to improved efforts at metabolic control versus pregnancy is speculative.

Nephropathy and Hypertension

The microvascular diseases of diabetes have long been known to pose significant complications in pregnancy. As late as 1977, Pederson, in the second edition of his book, recommended that women with nephropathy be counseled to avoid pregnancy because they and their offspring would do poorly. Nephropathy clearly has a negative impact on pregnancy, but considerable controversy exists regarding the effect of intercurrent pregnancy on the course of nephropathy. It has been easier to define the effect of nephropathy on pregnancy because the pregnancy outcome variables are discrete and reached in relatively short follow-up periods. It is considerably more difficult to assess the influence of pregnancy on the course of nephropathy because the necessary follow-up periods are much longer and because the natural history is for progressive deterioration with time.

The incidence of nephropathy among pregnant diabetic women has been increasing. This trend can be traced in three published series from the Joslin Clinic. In 1957 Oppe et al. reported a series of 31 women among 767 (4%) whose pregnancies were complicated by nephropathy. Kitzmiller et al. found 26 cases of nephropathy among 258 (10%) between 1975 and 1978. In the most recently published series of pregnancies progressing beyond 20 weeks in 1983 through 1987, there were 55 cases of nephropathy (and 4 renal transplantations) among 420 pregnancies, for an incidence of 14%.

Pregnancies among women with diabetic nephropathy are complicated by increased incidences of dense proteinuria, hypertension, hypoalbuminemia, anemia, prematurity, and perinatal mortality. The 40% increase in plasma volume and parallel increase in cardiac output that accompany pregnancy place increased demands on the kidneys. Nondiabetic women with normal kidneys and renal function increase their creatinine clearances by approximately 30% and lose increasing quantities of protein in their urine in the third trimester. Diabetic women without overt nephropathy whose urine dipstick results are negative for urine protein in the first trimester lose considerably more protein in their urine in the third trimester than do their nondiabetic counterparts. The increase in creatinine clearance can be dramatic and exaggerated (to 200 ml/min and more) for patients who enter pregnancy in the hyperfiltration phase of developing nephropathy. Diabetic women who begin pregnancy with established nephropathy (proteinuria greater than 500 mg/day) tend not to experience the characteristic rise in creatinine clearance and have even more dramatic progressive urinary protein loss. As many as 70% of these women will have proteinuria in excess of 3 g/day before delivery. This generally returns to prepregnancy values by 6 to 8 weeks after delivery in most patients. Not surprisingly, proteinuria of this magnitude frequently leads to significant hypoalbuminemia and dependent edema. Occasionally this results in anasarca and pulmonary edema, which is refractory to therapy and necessitates delivery.

Among all diabetic women with pregnancies progressing beyond 20 weeks reported from the Joslin Clinic, the incidence of chronic hypertension antedating pregnancy was 6%, but among women with nephropathy one third were hypertensive. In most series of diabetic women, approximately one fourth have clinically significant hypertension during pregnancy. Among women with nephropathy, however, two thirds have significant hypertensive complications. Preeclampsia is defined as hypertension with proteinuria and edema developing after 24 weeks of pregnancy. All of these patients have proteinuria, and clinically significant edema is virtually universal in the last half of pregnancy. The diagnosis of preeclampsia among the third of patients with chronic hypertension is thus rather arbitrary. Even in the other third of patients in whom hypertension develops during pregnancy, many follow a rather prolonged and relatively benign course. Clearly, patients with evidence of other organ system involvement such as hemolysis, thrombocytopenia, or hepatocellular necrosis have preeclampsia. In the absence of these other systemic signs, the definition is imprecise and of little clinical utility.

Anemia Associated with Nephropathy. Anemia is common and may be quite profound with hematocrit values in the low 20s. In the series of Reece et al., 42% of patients had hemoglobin concentrations of less than 10 g/dl. Kitzmiller et al. found a mean third-trimester hematocrit of 29%, and 58% of the patients had values below 30%. The anemia usually is normocytic and normochromic, and the standard evaluation usually is unrewarding. Recently, erythropoietin levels have been found to be inappropriately low in some of these patients, and they have responded dramatically to therapy with recombinant human erythropoietin. Care must be taken not to raise the hematocrit too high too quickly or significant hypertension may result.

Premature Delivery

The incidence of delivery before 37 weeks in a general obstetric population is approximately 10%. Among diabetic women without nephropathy that risk is about 22%. In the series of Kitzmiller et al., 71% of the class F patients who did not spontaneously or electively abort delivered before 37 weeks. In the more recent Joslin Clinic series and that of Reece et al., that risk was 52% and 55%, respectively. In the Joslin series, almost half of these premature deliveries (14/31) were the direct result of the development of apparent preeclampsia.

The outlook for survival for the fetuses of these patients has improved steadily, although it still does not equal that for infants of nondiabetic women or even that for other diabetic women. In the 1981 series of Kitzmiller et al., the perinatal mortality was 110/1000. Reece et al. reported a 60/1000 perinatal mortality rate for their 1975-1984 series. The perinatal mortality rate for the Joslin Clinic series of 1983-1987 was 70/1000 for the patients with nephropathy compared with 27/1000 for the other patients in the series. These figures are comparable to a perinatal mortality rate in Massachusetts during this time of approximately 17/1000.

Treatment of Hypertension in Pregnancy

The antihypertensive agents traditionally used during pregnancy have been alpha-methyldopa and hydralazine. Although their use is safe during pregnancy, these agents are not particularly efficacious or well accepted by patients. Both must be given multiple times daily. In doses adequate to control significant hypertension, alpha-methyldopa often causes an unacceptable degree of somnolence. Hydralazine is ineffective as monotherapy in the outpatient setting but may be helpful when added to either alpha-methyldopa or a beta blocker. Neither drug is helpful in slowing the rate of progression of nephropathy or reducing proteinuria. Beta blockers have been used cautiously in diabetic patients because of concerns about damping the counterregulatory response to hypoglycemia. These agents, however, are quite effective in controlling hypertension; they are safe and efficacious during pregnancy, reduce proteinuria, seem to slow the progression of nephropathy, and are well accepted by patients. Metoprolol, atenolol, and most recently labetalol are becoming the antihypertensive agents of choice during pregnancy. Metoprolol and atenolol have been used as the primary antihypertensive agents in prenatal patients at the Joslin Clinic for the past decade with minimal problems with hypoglycemia.

Angiotensin converting enzyme (ACE) inhibitors are now the drugs of first choice for treating nephropathy and its associated hypertension in diabetic patients. Unfortunately these drugs should not be used in pregnancy because they cause a constellation of severe fetal and neonatal problems. Fairly extensive evidence has accumulated that ACE inhibitors cause deficient calcification of the bones of the fetal skull (hypocalvaria) and renal tubular dysgenesis that can lead to oligohydramnios in utero and renal insufficiency, failure, and death in the neonatal period. Thus these agents should be avoided during pregnancy. The toxicity seems confined to late-pregnancy exposure, and there do not appear to be any adverse consequences to early first-trimester exposure. Patients receiving long-term ACE inhibitor therapy should discontinue its use as soon as pregnancy is diagnosed early in the first trimester and should be reassured that this brief exposure is not known to be harmful. Diuretics are not ordinarily used during pregnancy, but occasionally they may be necessary in nephropathic patients with significant volume overload or severe edema. They frequently are helpful in the puerperium to resolve edema. The use of calcium channel blockers during pregnancy has not been studied adequately to make any recommendations.

No antihypertensive therapy has ever been shown to reduce the incidence of preeclampsia superimposed on chronic hypertension. Low-dose aspirin therapy (80 mg/day) appears to reduce the incidence of preeclampsia in patients at high risk for its occurrence or recurrence. No studies to date have specifically addressed diabetes or diabetic nephropathy in pregnant women, but a study is currently in progress at several centers funded by the National Institutes of Health.

Obstetric and Perinatal Complications

Spontaneous Abortion

The fertility of women with diabetes is unimpaired. There has been considerable debate, however, regarding the first-trimester spontaneous abortion rate among these women. It now seems clear that this rate is not increased for women in good metabolic control before and during very early pregnancy. The rate of first-trimester spontaneous abortions among clinically recognized pregnancies in the general population is 12% to 15%. The rate is the same for diabetic women with first-trimester glycosylated hemoglobin values up to 9 standard deviations above the nondiabetic mean. Several studies have now shown that first-trimester glycohemoglobin values greater than 9 standard deviations above the nondiabetic mean are associated with an increased incidence of spontaneous abortion. The poorest degrees of control are associated with a one-third risk of spontaneous abortion.

Major Malformations

Most large series of births to women with diabetes mellitus report a 6% to 9% incidence of major congenital malformations, which is significantly higher than the 2% to 3% incidence in the general population. These malformations are now the single greatest source of perinatal mortality for infants of diabetic mothers (IDM), accounting for 50% of all perinatal deaths. The anomalies found among IDM span the range of the anomalies found in the nondiabetic population. The most common are cardiac abnormalities, neural tube defects (anencephaly and spina bifida), and urinary tract anomalies. Some of these have been reported to occur at rates that are 10 or more times higher than in the general population. Careful examination of a timetable for normal human development reveals that all of these anomalies arise within the first 6 weeks from fertilization, or 8 weeks from last menstrual period.

The first large series to show a relationship between first-trimester metabolic control and risk for anomalies was that of Miller et al. from the Joslin Clinic. The researchers found that when patients were ranked according to first-trimester glycohemoglobin values, those in the lower half had a risk for major malformation of just over 3%, whereas those in the upper half had a risk of just over 20%. This was a highly statistically significant difference. Subsequently these findings have been confirmed in several other countries using a variety of glycosylated hemoglobin techniques, and these have been reviewed in detail elsewhere. Compilation of these data at the Joslin Clinic published in 1989 and ongoing studies, which include data from more than 700 diabetic gravidas, continue to support this relationship. The risk for major malformations does not rise with statistical significance from the 3% range until 12 standard deviations above the nondiabetic mean when the risk rises to 30% to 40%.

In summary, these data regarding the relationship between metabolic control and first-trimester events are both reassuring and worrisome for patients. They can be reassured that they do not need to be in perfect metabolic control to minimize their risks for spontaneous abortion and major malformations; good to fair control is adequate. Unfortunately, however, control is important. Women who conceive and spend the early first trimester in poor control face very high risks for spontaneous abortion and major malformation. In fact, at first-trimester glycosylated hemoglobin values of 12 or more standard deviations above the mean, a spontaneous abortion, a major congenital malformation, and a nonmalformed live birth are approximately equally likely probabilities. Thus the single most important element of care for diabetic women to optimize perinatal outcome is to spend the first 6 postovulatory weeks of pregnancy in good metabolic control. For women whose diabetes is not always in good control, it can take several weeks of effort on the part of patients, dietitians, teaching nurses, and physicians in adjusting diet, insulin therapy, and exercise to achieve good control. If those efforts are not initiated until after women recognize their pregnancies, this critical period of early embryologic development frequently passes before good control can be achieved. It is critically important therefore that diabetic women plan their pregnancies, using appropriate contraception when necessary, to be certain that they enter pregnancy in as good metabolic control as possible.

Several studies have now been published that report the results of demonstration projects to enroll diabetic women into programs of preconception care to optimize metabolic control and reduce the malformation rate. All apparently have been successful in that attenders consistently demonstrate malformation rates of 1% to 2%, whereas nonattenders have rates of 7% to 11%. These programs have been challenged on the basis that they may simply attract compliant women who would probably have entered pregnancy in good control regardless of the program, whereas noncompliant women do not voluntarily attend such programs. It has thus been argued that expensive health care resources are being thrown at women who need them least. It remains to be seen how successful these programs will be when applied to large populations.

Fetal Death

Fifty years ago 25% of the fetuses of diabetic women died in utero near term. Most of these fetuses were macrosomic with no malformations and no obvious cause for death. These deaths were blamed on asphyxia, and their number declined in frequency over the decades as the general level of metabolic control improved even without understanding the physiology of these losses. The unexplained stillbirth rate on large academic services for diabetic women is now approximately 1/300 to 1/400. Although this is now a relatively rare event on large services, the pathophysiology of uteroplacental insufficiency remains important and may claim fetuses.

Several factors may combine to render fetuses of diabetic women critically hypoxemic. Studies of placental perfusion using radiolabeled tracers have demonstrated a 35% to 45% decrease in uteroplacental blood flow index in diabetic women in general. This may be further exacerbated by microvascular disease. Glycosylated hemoglobin carries less oxygen molecule for molecule than does native hemoglobin. Furthermore, glycosylated hemoglobin binds that oxygen more tightly and releases it less well in the periphery at sites of lower oxygen tension, such as the placental bed. Hyperglycemic fetuses respond with hyperinsulinemia. Hyperinsulinemia in turn causes increased oxygen consumption in the fetus and results in an increased umbilical arteriovenous oxygen difference. These factors, which are associated with both acute and chronic hyperglycemia, may conspire to create a critical level of fetal hypoxemia.

Macrosomia

Excessive fetal growth (macrosomia) is characteristic of fetuses of diabetic women. In a general population, approximately 6% of delivered fetuses will weigh more than 4000 g, whereas in most series of IDM 20% to 25% of fetuses will be that large. As many as 60% of IDM will be greater than the tenth percentile for their gestational ages. The standard explanation for this excessive growth is the *Pedersen hypothesis.* Maternal hyperglycemia readily becomes fetal hyperglycemia as glucose passes through the placenta by facilitated diffusion. The fetus responds with hyperinsulinemia. Insulin is the most important growth hormone of the fetus, causing accretion of fat, muscle, and bone. This has been further expanded to include consideration of transplacental passage of amino acids that can act as insulin secretagogues. Improved metabolic control can help to reduce but not eliminate macrosomia. Although it has been known for some time that insulin will not cross the placenta, recently it has been demonstrated that insulin-anti-insulin antigen-antibody complexes can cross the placenta into the fetal circulation. Furthermore, the level of these antigen-antibody complexes correlates with the degree of fetal macrosomia. This observation helps to explain the fact that a few diabetic women in excellent control nonetheless have very large fetuses.

Macrosomia is important because larger fetuses are more likely to require either operative pelvic or cesarean delivery. Operative deliveries expose the mothers to greater risks for morbidity. These large fetuses also are at increased risk for birth trauma.

GESTATIONAL DIABETES MELLITUS

The definition of GDM, as already discussed, encompasses a wide range of physiologic factors. Most of these patients, however, have a relatively mild degree of carbohydrate intolerance, which develops later in pregnancy as the result of the physiologic changes (insulin resistance) of late pregnancy. The definition applies whether insulin or only diet modification is used for treatment, although those with GDM requiring insulin appear to be at higher risk for developing overt diabetes within 2 to 5 years postpartum.

The issue of GDM is surrounded by considerable controversy. Questions have been raised regarding both the amount of morbidity and mortality that it causes, as well as the quantity and quality of the data, suggesting that these can be modified by screening and treatment. Perinatal mortality is so low that it has been—and likely will remain—impossible to show that GDM significantly increases the risk for perinatal mortality. As the result of a major meta-analysis of available studies published in 1989, Hunter and Keirse concluded that "except for research purposes, all forms of glucose tolerance testing should be stopped." It is becoming increasingly clear, however, that GDM is associated with macrosomia and its complications—operative delivery, birth trauma, and pregnancy-induced hypertension. The occurrence of GDM is so closely associated with both age and obesity on a population basis that it is almost impossible to separate them. The argument has been made that the obstetric complications associated with GDM are caused primarily by obesity, which also causes GDM.

Epidemiology

GDM originally was defined as glucose tolerance testing results 2 standard deviations above the mean; therefore the incidence of the abnormality was 2.5% by definition. Those original data were collected from a mixed population in Boston. Subsequently, it has become obvious that the specified degree of carbohydrate intolerance may be found at very different incidences in different populations. Native Americans from the Southwest and Mexican Americans, for example, have much higher incidences of GDM. Approximately 7% of all pregnancies are complicated by GDM, resulting in more than 200,000 cases annually. Depending on the population studied and diagnostic tests used, the prevalence ranges from 1% to 14% of all pregnancies. In a prospective study by Solomon 1997, advanced maternal age, family history of diabetes mellitus, nonwhite ethnicity, higher body mass index, weight gain during early adulthood, and cigarette smoking were all found to be significant risk factors for GDM.

Screening (Table 71-1)

The major controversy surrounding GDM screening is identifying who should be screened biochemically with a glucose load. Before 1997, the American College of Obstetricians and Gynecologists recommended biochemical testing by means of a glucose load for patients with any of the following risk factors for GDM:

1. Maternal age 30 years or greater
2. Strong family history of diabetes
3. Previous history of GDM
4. Previous macrosomic infant
5. Previous stillbirth
6. Previous malformed infant
7. Marked obesity
8. Hypertension
9. Glycosuria

The American Diabetes Association and the Centers for Disease Control and Prevention had been advocating for universal screening of all pregnant women with a biochemical test regardless of risk factors, but in 1997 issued a more cost-effective modification of that position that has been generally instituted into routine practice. Women are categorized as high, average, or low risk for GDM. If a woman falls into one of the high-risk categories for GDM (Box 71-1), she should undergo glucose testing as soon as possible. If found not to have diabetes at the initial screening, she

Table 71-1
Screening and Diagnosis of Gestational Diabetes Mellitus

Plasma Glucose (mg/dl)	50 g Screening Test	100 g Diagnostic Test
Fasting	—	95-105
1-hour	140	180-190
2-hour	—	155-165
3-hour	—	140-145

Screening for GDM is not considered necessary in pregnant women who meet all of the following criteria: <25 years of age, normal body weight, no first-degree relative with diabetes, and not Hispanic, Native American, Asian or African American.

The 100 g diagnostic test is performed on patients who have a positive screening test. Two or more of the venous plasma concentrations must be met or exceeded for a positive diagnosis. The test should be done in the morning after an overnight fast between 8 and 14 hours and after at least 3 days of unrestricted diet (>150 g carbohydrate per day) and unlimited physical activity. The woman should remain seated and should not smoke throughout the test.

Modified from the American Diabetes Association: *Diabetes Care* 24:S78, 2001.

should still be retested between 24 and 28 weeks' gestation. Those at average risk should have testing done at 24 to 28 weeks' gestation and if low risk no testing at all. For a woman to be categorized as low risk, she must meet all the following criteria: age <25 years, weight normal before pregnancy, member of an ethnic group with a low prevalence of GDM, no known diabetes in first-degree relatives, no history of an abnormal glucose tolerance, and no history of poor obstetric outcome.

A two-stage biochemical screening procedure is recommended by the American Diabetes Association. Stage 1 of the Two-Step Approach is measuring a venous blood sample at 1 hour after a 50-g oral glucose load (glucose challenge test [GCT]). This glucose load can be administered in the fed or fasted state without prior dietary preparation. Values of 140 mg/dl or more should be followed by a full 3-hour 100-g oral glucose tolerance test (OGTT). This should be performed fasting after 3 days of dietary preparation with an unrestricted diet of at least 150 g of carbohydrate per day. The OGTT results are considered abnormal if two or more venous plasma glucose levels meet or exceed the following values: fasting 105 mg/dl, 1 hour 190 mg/dl, 2 hours 165 mg/dl, 3 hours 145 mg/dl. This two-step approach identifies approximately 80% of women with GDM. The yield is further increased to almost 90% if the criteria are more stringent with a cutoff of >130 mg/dl. Attempts to use determinations of glycosylated serum proteins or hemoglobin as screening tests have been too insensitive. Islet cell antibodies are found only in a small number of women with GDM (2% to 38% depending on the assay used) and therefore are not useful in screening for the condition (Box 71-3).

The insulin resistance of pregnancy increases with increasing gestational age; therefore the later in pregnancy that a population is tested, the greater the finding of abnormal carbohydrate tolerance. The later in pregnancy that a patient is diagnosed, however, the longer she may have had untreated carbohydrate intolerance and the less time there is left in pregnancy to attempt to improve outcome with proper therapy. Generally, patients should be screened once at 24 to 28 weeks of gestation, unless they meet the criteria for high or low risk.

BOX 71-3
Risk Categories and Clinical Screening for GDM

High Risk (one or more of the following)
Marked obesity
Diabetes in a first-degree relative
History of glucose intolerance
Previous infant with macrosomia
Current glycosuria
Screening recommendation: at initial antepartum visit or as soon as possible thereafter; repeat at 24 to 28 weeks if no diagnosis of gestational diabetes mellitus by that time

Average Risk
Neither high or low risk profile
Screening recommendation: between 24 and 28 weeks' gestation

Low Risk (all of the following)
Age <25 years
Belongs to low risk race or ethnic group (those other than Hispanic, black, Native American, South or East Asian, Pacific Islander or Indigenous Australian)
No diabetes in first-degree relatives
Normal prepregnancy weight and weight gain during pregnancy
No history of abnormal blood glucose concentrations
No prior poor obstetrical outcomes
Screening recommendation: not required

Modified from Kjos SL, Buchanan T: *N Engl J Med* 341:1749, 1999; Metzger BE, Coustan DM: *Diabetes Care* 21:S2, 1998.

The reproducibility of glucose tolerance testing is only fair. Only 40% of women with test results that are positive for GDM in one pregnancy will have this finding again in the next pregnancy. This fact has led many to criticize the validity of the testing procedure. As a practical matter, this means that women should be retested in subsequent pregnancies despite a prior pregnancy diagnosis of GDM. There are no data that address the question of whether testing should be performed with use of GLT followed by OGTT or directly by OGTT.

Management

Pregnancy

A diet should be prescribed according to ideal body weight with 30 kcal/kg in the first half of pregnancy and 35 kcal/kg in the second half. Approximately 50% of the calories should be provided as carbohydrate, and 1.3 g of protein per kilogram of body weight are allowed. The remainder of the daily calorie requirement is allocated to fat.

Any serious effort at achieving euglycemia must include home capillary blood glucose self-monitoring. Patients who cannot maintain fasting blood glucose values below 95 to 105 mg/dl, 1-hour postprandial below 140 mg/dl, and 2-hour postprandial values below 120 mg/dl should be treated with insulin. Stricter criteria for treatment have been advocated by some, but overtreatment may result in an increase in the rate of delivery of small-for-gestational-age infants. For treatment protocols appropriate for pregnancy, see Chapter 11. The number of patients who require insulin is determined in part by the diligence with which patients comply with their diets and the frequency with which their blood glucoses are checked. Between 30% and 50% of patients require insulin.

Postpartum

The purpose of the original study by O'Sullivan and Mahan was to define the relationship between abnormal carbohydrate tolerance in pregnancy and the later development of diabetes. In their Boston population they found a 22% cumulative prevalence of diabetes 8 years after a pregnancy with OGTT results greater than 2 standard deviations above the mean. This compared with a 4% prevalence for women with normal carbohydrate tolerance. Similar studies in various ethnic groups have been undertaken around the world confirming the relationship between GDM and later diabetes. Only the magnitude of the effect has varied. In Copenhagen, Damm et al. found a 17% prevalence of diabetes at follow-up evaluation (mean of 6 years) in women who had non–insulin-requiring GDM. In Los Angeles, Kjos et al. found a 40% prevalence at 36 months postpartum in an obese Mexican-American population. Among Zuni Indians in New Mexico, Benjamin et al. found a 30% prevalence at a mean follow-up period of 4.8 years.

Given the relatively high probability of developing diabetes usually within 2 to 5 years after a pregnancy complicated by GDM, patients should be educated about the risk, its relationship to obesity, and the symptoms of diabetes mellitus. It has been suggested that all patients in whom the diagnosis of GDM has been made should be evaluated with a 75-g OGTT 6 to 12 weeks postpartum. The results should be interpreted according to the standard criteria of either the National Diabetes Data Group or the World Health Organization. If the results are abnormal, then the patient should be treated accordingly. If they are normal, then the patient should be reevaluated periodically, although there are no solid data on which to recommend a specific follow-up interval. Attempts have been made to identify specific factors in GDM that would be more highly predictive for the development of later diabetes. Although such factors as a particularly high fasting glucose or 2-hour value on an OGTT or the area under the glucose curve on an OGTT identify women at higher risk, they are not sufficiently discriminatory to be useful.

Contraception and future pregnancies also should be discussed with GDM women postpartum. Despite some concerns raised by an early report, intrauterine devices are both safe and effective in women with diabetes and with former GDM. Although data are limited, modern low-dose combination oral contraceptives also appear to be safe, inducing minimal changes in cardiovascular risk factor lipoprotein markers. As noted already, future pregnancies are at increased risk for GDM. The degree to which weight reduction can reduce the risk for GDM in subsequent pregnancies is speculative but should be considered for obese patients.

BIBLIOGRAPHY

American Diabetes Association: Preconception care of women with diabetes, *Diabetes Care* 24:566, 2001.
American Diabetes Association: Gestational diabetes mellitus, *Diabetes Care* 24:S78, 2001.

American Diabetes Association: Report of the Expert Committee on the Diagnosis and Classification of Diabetes Mellitus. The Expert Committee on the Diagnosis and Classification of Diabetes Mellitus, *Diabetes Care* 20:1183, 1997.

Barr M Jr, Cohen M Jr: ACE inhibitor fetopathy and hypocalvaria: the kidney-skull connection, *Teratology* 44:485, 1991.

Benjamin E et al: Diabetes in pregnancy in Zuni Indian women: prevalence and subsequent development of clinical diabetes after gestational diabetes, *Diabetes Care* 16:1231, 1993.

Catalano PM, Tyzbir ED, Sims EAH: Incidence and significance of islet cell antibodies in women with previous gestational diabetes, *Diabetes Care* 13:478, 1990.

Damm P et al: Predictive factors for the development of diabetes in women with previous gestational diabetes mellitus, *Am J Obstet Gynecol* 167:607, 1992.

Diamond MP et al: Impairment of counterregulatory hormone responses to hypoglycemia in pregnant women with insulin-dependent diabetes mellitus, *Am J Obstet Gynecol* 166:70, 1992.

Danilenko-Dixon D, Van Winter J: Universal versus selective gestational diabetes screening: application of 1997 American Diabetes Association recommendations, *Am J Obstet Gynecol* 181:798, 1999.

Goldberg JD et al: Gestational diabetes: impact of home glucose monitoring on neonatal birth weight, *Am J Obstet Gynecol* 154:546, 1986.

Greene MF: Prevention and diagnosis of congenital anomalies in diabetic pregnancies. In Landon M, editor: *Clinics in perinatology,* Philadelphia, 1993, WB Saunders.

Greene MF et al: First-trimester hemoglobin A_1 and risk for major malformation and spontaneous abortion in diabetic pregnancy, *Teratology* 39:225, 1989.

Greene MF et al: Prematurity among insulin-requiring diabetic gravid women, *Am J Obstet Gynecol* 161:106, 1989.

Greene MF. Screening for gestational diabetes mellitus, *N Engl J Med* 337:1625, 1997.

Gregory R, Tattersall RB: Are diabetic pre-pregnancy clinics worthwhile? *Lancet* 340:656, 1992.

Hare JW, White P: Gestational diabetes and the white classification, *Diabetes Care* 3:394, 1980.

Harris MI: Gestational diabetes may represent discovery of preexisting glucose intolerance, *Diabetes Care* 11:402, 1988.

Hunter DJS, Keirse MJNC: Gestational diabetes. In Chalmers I, Enkin M, Keirse MJNC, editors: *Effective care in pregnancy and childbirth,* Oxford, 1989, Oxford University Press.

Imperiale TF, Petrulis AS: A meta-analysis of low-dose aspirin for the prevention of pregnancy-induced hypertension disease, *JAMA* 266:261, 1991.

Joslin EP: Pregnancy and diabetes mellitus, *Boston Med Surg J* 173:841, 1915.

Kitzmiller JL et al: Diabetic nephropathy and perinatal outcome, *Am J Obstet Gynecol* 141:741, 1981.

Kitzmiller JL et al: Preconception care of diabetes: glycemic control prevents congenital anomalies, *JAMA* 265:731, 1991.

Kjos SL et al: Serum lipids within 36 months of delivery in women with recent gestational diabetes, *Diabetes* 40:142, 1991.

Kjos SL, Buchanan T: Gestational diabetes mellitus, *N Engl J Med* 341:1749, 1999.

Klein BEK et al: Effect of pregnancy on progression of diabetic retinopathy, *Diabetes Care* 13:34, 1990.

Madsen H, Ditzel J: Changes in red blood cell oxygen transport in diabetic pregnancy, *Am J Obstet Gynecol* 143:421, 1982.

Magee MS et al: Influence of diagnostic criteria on the incidence of gestational diabetes and perinatal morbidity, *JAMA* 269:609, 1993.

Metzger BE, Coustan DM. Organizing Committee. Summary and recommendations of the fourth international workshop-conference on gestational diabetes mellitus, *Diabetes Care* 21:S2, 1998.

Miller E et al: Elevated maternal hemoglobin A_{1C} in early pregnancy and major congenital anomalies in infants of diabetic mothers, *N Engl J Med* 304:1331, 1981.

Milley JR et al: The effect of insulin on ovine fetal oxygen extraction, *Am J Obstet Gynecol* 149:673, 1984.

Molsted-Pedersen L, Skouby SO, Damm P: Preconception counseling and contraception after gestational diabetes, *Diabetes* 40:147, 1991.

Naylor CD, Sermer M, et al: Selective screening for gestational diabetes mellitus, *N Engl J Med* 337:1591, 1997.

Oppe TE, Hsia DY-Y, Gellis SS: Pregnancy in the diabetic mother with nephritis, *Lancet* 1:353, 1957.

O'Sullivan JB, Mahan CM: Criteria for the oral glucose tolerance test in pregnancy, *Diabetes* 13:278, 1964.

Pedersen J: Problems and management. In *The pregnant diabetic and her newborn,* ed 2, Baltimore, 1977, Williams & Wilkins.

Petersen KR et al: Effects of contraceptive steroids on cardiovascular risk factors in women with insulin-dependent diabetes mellitus, *Am J Obstet Gynecol* 171:400, 1994.

Reece EA et al: Diabetic nephropathy: pregnancy performance and fetomaternal outcome, *Am J Obstet Gynecol* 159:56, 1988.

Rubinstein P et al: HLA antigens and islet cell antibodies in gestational diabetes, *Hum Immunol* 3:271, 1981.

Solomon CG et al: A prospective study of pregravid determinants of gestational diabetes mellitus, *JAMA* 278:1078. 1997.

Steel JM, Irvine WJ, Clarke BF: The significance of pancreatic islet cell antibody and abnormal glucose tolerance during pregnancy, *J Clin Lab Immunol* 4:83, 1980.

Steinhart J, Sugarman J: Gestational diabetes is a herald of NIDDM in Navajo women, *Diabetes Care* 20:943, 1997.

Ylinen K et al: Risk of minor and major fetal malformations in diabetics with high haemoglobin A_{1C} values in early pregnancy, *Br Med J* 289:345, 1984.

CHAPTER 72

Hypertension in Pregnancy

Michael F. Greene
Stephanie A. Eisenstat

The hypertensive disorders of pregnancy are responsible for a disproportionate amount of maternal and perinatal morbidity and mortality. Although routine prenatal care, recognition of hypertension, and intervention have made maternal mortality rare in the United States, it is the most common cause of maternal mortality in many developing nations. Proper diagnostic categorization of the various disorders can be difficult and confusing, while their management can be challenging. The fundamental reason for difficulties in diagnosis and management is incomplete understanding of the basic etiologic pathophysiology of preeclampsia. Despite incomplete knowledge, interventions are necessary to prevent serious complications.

PHYSIOLOGY
Cardiovascular Changes with Pregnancy

During normal pregnancy there is a 40% increase in intravascular volume and a 20% increase in cardiac output, but a fall in peripheral vascular resistance. This results in a net fall in blood pressure in the second trimester. In the third trimester these changes result in a rise in blood pressure to first-trimester levels. The fall in peripheral vascular resistance is associated with reduced vascular responsiveness to pressors, including catecholamines and angiotensin II. Although the data regarding serum levels of catecholamines are somewhat ambiguous, it is clear that serum levels of angiotensin II and aldosterone are elevated. The vascular refractoriness to pressors is likely mediated by the prostaglandin system, and some investigators have found the urinary excretion of prostaglandin E_2 (PGE_2) and its metabolites to be increased substantially in pregnant women compared with nonpregnant control subjects.

Classification of Hypertensive Disorders in Pregnancy

Much of the confusion surrounding the treatment and prognosis for hypertension in pregnancy results from imprecision in its definition and diagnosis. Central to diagnosis is distinguishing hypertension that originates during pregnancy from hypertension that antedates pregnancy. If a patient is not seen for the first time until the midtrimester when blood pressure is normally somewhat lower, she may appear normotensive when she was really modestly hypertensive before pregnancy. The presence or absence of proteinuria is also a key diagnostic feature, and it cannot be assessed accurately without a 24-hour urine collection for quantitation. Semiquantitative urine protein diagnostic reagent dipsticks are not adequate.

During the 1980s the term *pregnancy-induced hypertension* (PIH) became popular, but it blurred some important distinctions and contributed more confusion than enlightenment. In 1990 the Working Group on High Blood Pressure in Pregnancy, convened by the National Heart, Lung and Blood Institute, reaffirmed the classification of hypertensive disorders in pregnancy proposed by the American College of Obstetricians and Gynecologists in 1972 which included four diagnostic categories of hypertensive disorders in pregnancy: chronic hypertension, preeclampsia-eclampsia, preeclampsia superimposed on chronic hypertension and transient hypertension. The most recent classification of hypertension in pregnancy is listed in Box 72-1.

SPECIFIC HYPERTENSIVE DISORDERS
Chronic Hypertension
Definition

Chronic hypertension is defined as hypertension (140/90 mm Hg or greater) that is observed before pregnancy or before 20 weeks' gestation. Retrospectively, patients whose hypertension persists beyond 42 days after delivery also are classified as having chronic hypertension. The vast majority of these patients have "essential" hypertension. A minority of these patients will have an assortment of relatively uncommon medical conditions complicated by hypertension, such as diabetic nephropathy, chronic glomerulonephritis, or systemic lupus erythematosus. A very small minority will have a variety of rare causes of hypertension, which are more or less surgically remediable, such as coarctation of the aorta, renal artery stenosis, Cushing's syndrome, or pheochromocytoma (see Chapter 3). The hallmark of chronic hypertension is that, although it may ameliorate postpartum, it persists beyond the puerperium.

Epidemiology

Estimates of the incidence of chronic hypertension among pregnant women are difficult to find. Most studies

---

BOX 72-1
Classification of Hypertension in Pregnancy*

Hypertension: Blood pressure >140 mm Hg systolic or 90 mm Hg diastolic occurring after 20 weeks in a woman who was normotensive before 20 weeks' gestation (Confirmed by two separate measurements)

Proteinuria: 300 mg/L protein in a random specimen or an excretion of 300 mg per 24 hours

Preeclampsia: Hypertension with proteinuria. *In the absence of proteinuria, highly suspected if:* increased blood pressure is accompanied by evidence of other systemic features of the condition

Chronic Hypertension: Blood pressure > or = 140/90 before the 20th week of pregnancy or if only diagnosed during pregnancy, persisting 6 weeks after delivery

Preeclampsia Superimposed on Chronic Hypertension: *Highly likely* in women with hypertension alone who develop new proteinuria, or in women with preexisting hypertension and proteinuria who have sudden increases in blood pressure or proteinuria, thrombocytopenia, or increases in hepatocellular enzymes

Gestational Hypertension: Hypertension without other signs of preeclampsia

---

From Report of the national high blood pressure education program working group on high blood pressure in pregnancy. *Am J Obstet Gynecol* 183, 2000.
* Removal of edema as a defining sign was an important change in this updated classification.

Table 72-1
Incidence of Intrauterine Growth Retardation (<10th Percentile) Among Hypertensive Patients

Reference	Type of Hypertension	*N*	%
Lin et al, 1982	Virtually all had PE	34/157	21.6
Sibai et al, 1983	Chronic HTN	10/190	5
	Chronic HTN and PE	7/21	32
Mabie et al, 1986	Chronic HTN	25/169	15
Ferrazzani et al, 1990	Chronic HTN	12/98	12
	Transient HTN	36/198	18
	PE	76/147	52
Rey and Courturier, 1994	Chronic HTN	52/337	15.5

HTN, Hypertension; *PE*, preeclampsia.

Table 72-2
Chronic Hypertension and Risk of Superimposed Preeclampsia

Reference	%
Landesman et al, 1957	34
Kincaid-Smith et al, 1966	38
Leather et al, 1968	33
Sandstrom, 1978	34
Curet and Olson, 1979	39
Welt et al, 1981	33
Sibai et al, 1983	10
Rubin et al, 1983	26
Mabie et al, 1986	34
Sibai et al, 1990	16
Rey and Couturier, 1994	21

---

are not population based but rather cohort studies of the natural history of the disease in pregnancy or clinical trials. Both types of studies have accumulated cases from large population bases of unknown size with unknown percentages of ascertainment. From the difficulties encountered in obtaining significant numbers of patients for study, it can be inferred that the incidence is rather low. Even among women with diabetes mellitus antedating pregnancy, the incidence of chronic hypertension is only 6% (Greene et al, 1989). The demographic characteristics of the population influence the incidence as a result of the well-known associations with race and age.

Maternal and Fetal Complications

The most important complication of chronic hypertension in pregnancy is the increased risk for perinatal mortality. Much of this risk in turn is due to or associated with other complications such as superimposed preeclampsia, prematurity, abruptio placentae, and intrauterine growth retardation (IUGR). The increased risk for perinatal mortality has been recognized for decades and has generally been approximately three to four times the risk in the general population from which the hypertensive patients were drawn. In a recent study from Quebec, for example, the perinatal mortality was 45/1000 among 337 pregnancies in 298 hypertensive women whereas it was 12/1000 during the same period in the general population (Rey and Couturier, 1994). Most of the increased risk for prematurity and cesarean section in these pregnancies is due to intervention to pre-

vent stillbirth in the setting of IUGR, preeclampsia, abruptio placentae, or other perceived threat to fetal well-being. The incidence of IUGR, defined as birth weight less than the 10th percentile for gestational age, has generally been reported to be 15% to 20% (Table 72-1). Estimates of the incidence of preeclampsia superimposed on chronic hypertension are often inaccurately high because patients recruited into studies relatively late in pregnancy are likely already to have some preeclampsia. Table 72-2 compiles the incidence of superimposed preeclampsia in patients with chronic hypertension in a number of studies. The incidence ranges from 10% to nearly 40%, with the best estimate being approximately 20%.

Patients with chronic hypertension frequently experience episodes of acutely elevated blood pressure, which some authors have termed "pregnancy aggravated" hypertensive episodes. It is difficult to show that these episodes are the proximate cause of any maternal or fetal morbidity, but they are anxiety provoking for the physician and frequently result in hospitalization of the patient and additional antihypertensive therapy.

Table 72-3
Summary of Major Randomized Controlled Trials of Antihypertensive Therapy in Pregnancy

Reference	Treatment (N)	Control (N)	Improved Gestational Age at Delivery	Effect on IUGR Incidence	Reduced PE
Leather et al, 1968	α-Methyldopa (52)	Routine care (48)	Yes	—	No
Redman et al, 1976	α-Methyldopa (117)	Routine care (125)	No	None	No
Sandstrom, 1978	Metoprolol (101)	Hydralazine (97)	No	None	No
Rubin et al, 1983	Atenolol (60)	Placebo (60)	No	None	Yes
Sibai et al, 1990	Labetalol (86)	No medication (90) α-Methyldopa (88)	No	None	No
Pickles et al, 1989	Labetalol (70)	Placebo (74)	No	None	No
Plouin et al, 1988	Labetalol (91) Hydralazine prn	α-Methyldopa (85) Hydralazine prn	No	None	No
Hogstedt et al, 1985	Metoprolol plus hydralazine (82)	Routine care (79)	No	None	No
Fidler et al, 1983	Oxprenolol (50)	α-Methyldopa (50)	No	None	No
Plouin et al, 1990	Oxprenolol plus hydralazine (78)	Placebo (76)	Yes	None	No
Gallery et al, 1985	Oxprenolol (96) Hydralazine prn	α-Methyldopa (87) Hydralazine prn	No	Reduced	No
Butters et al, 1990	Atenolol (15)	Placebo (14)	No	Increased	—

IUGR, Intrauterine growth retardation; *PE,* preeclampsia.

Management

Goals of Therapy

Patients with severely elevated blood pressures should be treated to prevent the potential maternal consequences of severe hypertension such as cerebrovascular accidents. Similarly, patients with preexisting renal disease should be treated to protect their kidneys from further damage. Controversy arises regarding the advisability of treating mild chronic hypertension in patients without renal disease. The goals of antihypertensive therapy should be to reduce the risks of the aforementioned perinatal complications. In the past 25 years a large number of trials have been published with rather consistently disappointing results (Table 72-3).

Antihypertensive Agents

Among the first agents used was *alpha-methyldopa (α-MD)* as epitomized in the studies of Leather et al and Redman et al. Although these investigators were able to achieve adequate blood pressure control with α-MD and other agents, there was no significant impact on the incidence of superimposed preeclampsia, the mean birth weight, or the mean gestational age at the time of delivery. It should be noted that the mean daily dose of α-MD necessary in the study of Redman, Beilin, and Bonnar was 1.9 g, with a maximum dose of 4 g/day. There were no adverse effects of the α-MD on either the mothers or their offspring followed through early childhood, thus firmly establishing its safety. Both studies found a reduced incidence of midtrimester loss associated with α-MD therapy. This was an unexpected finding with no obvious mechanism to explain it. Furthermore, no other studies have confirmed these initial studies.

The next group of drugs to be studied systematically comprised the *beta blockers.* Early reports suggested that they, particularly propranolol, were associated with a variety of fetal and neonatal complications, including IUGR and

hypoglycemia. With the exception of one very small study of 15 patients treated with atenolol, hundreds of patients have been treated with metoprolol, atenolol, and oxprenolol without evidence for an increased incidence of these complications (Table 72-3). Although the beta blockers were demonstrably efficacious in lowering blood pressure, they, like α-MD, produced no demonstrable improvement in perinatal outcome.

Most recently, labetalol, the combined alpha blocker and nonspecific beta blocker, has been studied in several large trials. The results of the trials indicate that labetalol is clearly both safe and effective for lowering blood pressure during pregnancy, but it does not improve perinatal outcome. It is clearly superior to α-MD in reducing pregnancy-aggravated hypertensive episodes and the frequency with which additional agents must be added to adequately control blood pressure.

The use of *calcium channel blockers* has been reported in some small series (Constantine et al, 1987). They appear to be safe and effective in reducing blood pressure, but there are not yet any trials to address their ability to change perinatal outcome. The use of *clonidine* has been reported in a small trial without convincing evidence that it improves perinatal outcome.

Diuretic therapy during pregnancy should be discouraged. There is considerable literature to suggest that successful pregnancy is associated with adequate expansion of intravascular volume, whereas severe hypertension, IUGR, and perinatal mortality are associated with inadequate volume expansion. It is not clear whether adequate volume expansion is causal for optimal pregnancy outcome or whether both result from some more proximate physiologic cause. In a small series Sibai et al have shown that patients who are maintained through pregnancy on their prepregnancy diuretic therapy fail to expand their blood volumes. The series was too small to recognize an adverse impact on perinatal outcome, nor was there evidence that if the diuretics had been discontinued, the blood volumes would have expanded. Nonetheless, diuretic therapy should be initiated during pregnancy only under unusual circumstances, such as pulmonary edema or anasarca associated with nephrotic syndrome, and not for blood pressure control. The issue of whether long-standing diuretic therapy, which is part of a balanced program of successful blood pressure control, should be discontinued with pregnancy is controversial. This author's practice is not to discontinue the therapy.

Angiotensin converting enzyme inhibitors deserve special mention because they are becoming very widely used in young diabetic women, and they should not be used during pregnancy. Although first-trimester exposure does not appear to be teratogenic, their use later in pregnancy can have devastating consequences, and the FDA has warned against their use in a *Medical Bulletin* issued in April 1992. Exposure in the second and third trimester has resulted in fetal renal tubular dysgenesis, oligohydramnios, severe IUGR, inadequate ossification of the calvarial plates, and transient or permanent neonatal renal insufficiency of severe or fatal degree.

The use of *nitroprusside* should also be avoided during pregnancy. Animal studies have shown that the cyanide, which results from the metabolism of nitroprusside, can accumulate in the fetal compartment to toxic levels.

In summary, severe hypertension and hypertension associated with renal disease should be treated to prevent maternal complications. Commonly used agents are summarized in Table 72-4. There is no convincing evidence, however, that treating hypertension during pregnancy reduces the incidence of IUGR, prematurity, superimposed preeclampsia, or perinatal mortality.

Prognosis

Women with chronic hypertension frequently experience exacerbation of their hypertension in late pregnancy. It usually requires several weeks after delivery for their blood pressure to return to prepregnancy levels. During that time they should be seen frequently because they may become hypotensive on the therapy that was increased in late pregnancy to control rising blood pressure.

A woman whose chronic hypertension complicates one pregnancy can expect subsequent pregnancies to be similarly affected. Complications of chronic hypertension, such as IUGR and superimposed preeclampsia, are more likely to recur in a patient (~20% for each) than to occur initially.

Preeclampsia-Eclampsia

Definition

Preeclampsia is unique to pregnancy, requiring the presence of trophoblastic tissue, and seems unique to human beings without any naturally occurring animal models. It is classically defined as the triad of hypertension, proteinuria, and edema in pregnancy. Edema is so common during pregnancy however, affecting 50% to 80% of pregnancies, that it is considered normal. The clinical diagnosis of edema is subjective and impossible to standardize or quantitate. Attempts to distinguish between "normal edema" and "pathologic edema" on the basis of either the rate or timing of development or anatomic distribution have not been successful. Furthermore, the clinical assessment of edema has not been useful prognostically with respect to the risk for perinatal mortality. Edema, therefore, is not a very useful diagnostic sign.

Hypertension is diagnosed on both relative and absolute criteria. Compared with the average values before 20 weeks'

Table 72-4
Antihypertensive Agents for Use in Pregnancy

Agent	Mechanism of Action	Daily Dose Range (mg)	Dosing Schedule	Comment
Methyldopa	Central sympatholytic	750-3000	tid-qid	Very safe. Slow onset of action. Often caused unacceptable degree of somnolence at therapeutic dose
Hydralazine	Direct relaxation of arterial smooth muscle	40-200	qid	Ineffective as chronic oral monotherapy. Useful when added to methyldopa oral beta blocker. Useful IV to acutely lower blood pressure (5 mg bolus at 15-min intervals or continuous infusion)
Metoprolol	Beta$_1$-blockade	100-400	bid	Effective, well tolerated, convenient dosing schedule
Atenolol	Beta$_1$-blockade	50-200	qd	Effective, well tolerated, convenient dosing schedule
Labetalol	Alpha blockade	300-1200	tid-qid	Effective, well tolerated. Useful IV to acutely lower blood pressure (20-80 mg bolus at 20- to 30-min intervals or continuous infusion)
Nifedipine	Calcium channel blocker	30-120	tid	Seems safe and effective although least available data. Useful administered sublingually to acutely lower blood pressure

gestation, a rise in systolic pressure of 30 mm Hg or more or a rise in diastolic pressure of 15 mm Hg or more is considered hypertension. If blood pressure early in pregnancy is not known, then a value of 140/90 or greater beyond 20 weeks' gestation is considered hypertension.

Significant proteinuria is defined as greater than or equal to 300 mg protein in a 24-hour urine collection. The 95% upper confidence limit for protein loss in apparently normal women in the third trimester is 200 mg in 24 hours. This gives a small margin of separation between the normal range for the excretion rate and that which must be diagnosed as pathologic.

Attempts to grade preeclampsia as mild versus moderate have been arbitrary and not useful. There are generally accepted criteria for severe preeclampsia, with all other cases classified as mild. The presence of any of the criteria listed in Box 72-2 would be considered diagnostic of severe preeclampsia.

Eclampsia is diagnosed when a patient with preeclampsia develops seizures that cannot be attributed to another cause.

It is well recognized that eclamptic seizures may occur in mildly hypertensive patients with proteinuria and in hypertensive patients who have not yet developed proteinuria. The aforementioned criteria, therefore, should not be applied too rigidly in daily practice. A high index of suspicion should be maintained, and overdiagnosis is preferable to underdiagnosis if progression to eclampsia is to be avoided. It should be obvious from this discussion that preeclampsia is a clinical diagnosis based on a constellation of findings, none of which is specific. It could be difficult to distinguish the first occurrence of lupus nephritis in pregnancy from preeclampsia. In women with diabetic nephropathy with hypertension, proteinuria, and edema antedating pregnancy, the diagnosis of preeclampsia is entirely arbitrary in the absence of some complication indicating severe preeclampsia. Although not specific, a serum uric acid level, which rises disproportionately to the degree of renal dysfunction, may also be helpful in making the diagnosis of preeclampsia.

Incidence

Preeclampsia occurs in 4% to 10% of all pregnancies progressing beyond the first trimester. The actual incidence depends on the criteria used for diagnosis and the demographics of the population being studied. It is severalfold more common among primigravidas than it is in subsequent pregnancies. It is more common in young women because young women are more likely to be primigravidas, but when parity is controlled, youth does not seem to be a risk. Obesity and carbohydrate intolerance are also risk factors. Advanced maternal age appears to be a risk factor, but this may be due to the association of chronic hypertension, obesity, and carbohydrate intolerance with advancing age and the risk for the superimposition of preeclampsia on chronic hypertension. Similarly, the higher incidence of preeclampsia among African-Americans may be due to their generally higher incidence of hypertension. The apparent relationship between low socioeconomic status and preeclampsia in the United States may be due to the relationship between race and socioeconomic status. In other countries, socioeconomic status does not appear to be a risk factor.

Eclampsia appears to be related to socioeconomic status. This probably is due to the fact that preeclampsia often can be prevented from developing into eclampsia by timely delivery in women receiving regular prenatal care. To the extent that women of lower socioeconomic status are more likely to receive less regular prenatal care, it is more likely that their preeclampsia will evolve into eclampsia.

A variety of medical and obstetric conditions cause a predisposition to preeclampsia. Women with insulin-requiring diabetes mellitus have a 20% to 40% risk of developing preeclampsia. Systemic lupus erythematosus and any preexisting renal disease increase the risk. Multiple gestations, hydatidiform moles, and hydropic fetuses of any cause also place women at high risk.

Maternal and Fetal Complications

Historically preeclampsia-eclampsia has been a major cause of maternal mortality. One of the most important benefits of routine prenatal care has been the early recognition of preeclampsia and intervention that now makes maternal mortality rare. Significant maternal morbidity, including intracranial hemorrhage, intrahepatic hemorrhage and rupture, abruptio placentae and hemorrhage, and renal cortical necrosis, can still result from severe preeclampsia.

A significant minority (10% to 15%) of patients with preeclampsia will develop a variant in which microangiopathic hemolysis, hepatocellular necrosis, or thrombocytopenia appear prior to or more prominently than hypertension and proteinuria. This variant, frequently referred to by the acronym HELLP (*H*emolysis, *E*levated *L*iver enzymes, and *L*ow *P*latelets syndrome), can be difficult to distinguish from a variety of other disease preocesses with which it overlaps. These include thrombotic thrombocytopenia purpura, hemolytic uremic syndrome, and systemic lupus erythematosis.

The cerebral circulation has the ability to autoregulate its own flow over a broad range of perfusion pressure. When the mean arterial pressure exceeds 140 mm Hg, however, that

---

> **BOX 72-2**
> **Criteria for the Diagnosis of Severe Preeclampsia**
>
> - Blood pressure consistently in excess of 160 mm Hg systolic or 110 mm Hg diastolic
> - Dense proteinuria—various criteria ranging from 2 to 5 g/day have been used
> - Oliguria or elevated serum creatinine levels ($\geq$1.2 mg/dl) in a patient previously known to have a normal serum creatinine
> - Thrombocytopenia (100,000 per ml) and/or evidence of hemolysis
> - Elevated hepatic enzymes (alanine aminotransferase (ALT) or aspartate aminotransferase (AST))
> - Epigastric pain and/or evidence of hepatocellular necrosis
> - Persistent headache and/or visual disturbance of apparently central origin
> - Retinal hemorrhages, exudates, or papilledema
> - Pulmonary edema
> - According to some authors, the presence of fetal growth retardation is a criterion

Modified from the National High Blood Pressure Education Program, Working Group Report on High Blood Pressure in Pregnancy, 2000.

range is exceeded and hypertensive encephalopathy may result. Associated with this is severe arteriolar vasospasm that limits perfusion, which can result in ischemia, infarction, and petechial or gross hemorrhage. Petechial hemorrhages are frequently seen in the cerebral cortex of women dying of severe preeclampsia. They are particularly prone to occur in the occipital (visual) cortex and may be responsible for the visual phenomenon of scintillations, which are frequently described. It is generally difficult to interpret the significance of headache because it is such a common complaint, both in general and during pregnancy. In the setting of preeclampsia, however, headaches may be ominous signs, occurring in 85% of eclamptic women before their seizures.

Swelling of the liver causes stretching of Glisson's capsule and epigastric pain. In the setting of preeclampsia, epigastric pain usually is due to hepatic swelling, which may be associated with intrahepatic hemorrhage. If this progresses to hepatic rupture, it is associated with a very high fatality rate.

The healthy left ventricle, faced with increased afterload, is capable of responding with a substantial increase in work to maintain cardiac output. This ability is not infinite, however, and faced with sufficiently high afterload for a sufficiently long period of time, the left ventricle will fail and pulmonary edema will result. Most of the hemodynamic data obtained from preeclamptic women who have undergone invasive monitoring indicate that their left ventricles are healthy and respond normally to increased afterload. Thus pulmonary edema in the preeclamptic patient, which occurs only rarely, is evidence of very severe disease. Much more commonly, pulmonary edema is seen in these patients as the result of overly zealous intravenous fluid therapy. Perinatal mortality is significantly increased in preeclamptic women. Because of the generally low incidence of perinatal mortality, large numbers of patients must be studied to obtain reliable estimates of risk. The Collaborative Perinatal Project followed more than 50,000 mother-infant pairs from enrollment during pregnancy between 1959 and 1965 through the seventh year of the children. Analysis of that data showed the important influences of both hypertension and proteinuria on perinatal mortality. Although those data are now 30 years old, and the overall rate of perinatal mortality has fallen sharply during that time, the risk of perinatal mortality for normal women relative to hypertensive and proteinuric women probably has not changed. Those data show quite clearly that the risk for perinatal mortality increased progressively with increases in both diastolic blood pressure and proteinuria. The risk of IUGR also was increased in preeclampsia, and the risk for perinatal mortality dramatically increased among those IUGR fetuses.

Management

Preeclampsia is a progressive disorder for which the only cure is delivery of the fetus. Although it can be stated with confidence that preeclampsia will not resolve until after delivery, the rate of progression is entirely unpredictable. The period of mild preeclampsia from first diagnosis until the appearance of complications that warrant the diagnosis of "severe" or seizures indicating eclampsia can be quite prolonged. In patients with mild preeclampsia remote from term, expectant management is appropriate for the benefit of both the mother and the fetus. The mother benefits because the likelihood that she will have a successful pelvic delivery increases with increasing gestational age. The fetus benefits from increased maturity, which reduces the likelihood of complications in the nursery. Expectant management is not without risks however. The risk of stillbirth is everpresent for the fetus, and the mother could suffer an intracranial hemorrhage with permanent sequelae. The development of virtually any of the complications already listed as criteria for "severe" preeclampsia, with the exceptions of dense proteinura and IUGR, is an indication for prompt delivery. All other patients should be managed expectantly when the neonatal risks of prematurity would be substantial. This risk-benefit analysis is dynamic and must be reevaluated frequently during the course of expectant management. Some of the most difficult decisions in obstetrics must be made in this setting.

A wide variety of therapies have been employed over the decades on the basis of an equally wide variety of theories regarding the pathophysiology of the disease to attempt to ameliorate the severity of preeclampsia and prevent eclampsia. These have included "lytic cocktails" of barbiturates and opiates, dietary therapy, antihypertensive therapy, volume expansion, dopamine, and others. Some have been harmful; none have been helpful. A detailed discussion of management is found in Chapter 69.

Preeclampsia Superimposed on Chronic Hypertension

Current understanding is that the pathophysiology, potential complications, and management of preeclampsia superimposed on chronic hypertension are no different than those for preeclampsia. The prognosis for recurrence in subsequent pregnancies may be much higher however. Sibai et al have documented that in women with severe preeclampsia very early in pregnancy the recurrence risk in subsequent pregnancies may be as high as 65%. The use of low-dose aspirin for successful prophylaxis against the development of preeclampsia in patients at high risk has been reported and is discussed in the next section.

Transient Hypertension

Definition

Transient hypertension is defined as hypertension of modest degree that first appears late in pregnancy or during the first 24 hours postpartum in a patient without evidence of preeclampsia or preexisting hypertension. There has been some difficulty in gaining recognition of this entity, which also has been termed *gestational hypertension* and *nonproteinuric pregnancy-induced hypertension*. The main argument against the utility of the diagnosis has been that a pregnancy can confidently be placed in this category only after it is over. Until then, the patient must be managed as though she were developing preeclampsia. Although there is certainly an element of truth to this argument, these patients often show characteristics that provide sufficient support for a prospective diagnosis. These patients tend to be older and more obese, with poorer carbohydrate tolerance and hyperinsulinemia. The problem tends to recur in subsequent pregnancies. These patients tend to have family histories of hypertension and are more likely to develop chronic hypertension themselves. It is not associated with IUGR or other complications.

Management

Antihypertensive therapy is not indicated for patients with transient hypertension. Large randomized trials have failed to demonstrate any benefit to bed rest for these patients. An organized program of expectant outpatient management can provide excellent outcomes while minimizing drug therapy, inpatient admissions, and inductions of labor. Generally these patients should be permitted to go to term and enter spontaneous labor with minimal intervention.

Aspirin Therapy

There has been considerable interest in recent years in the potential for low-dose aspirin therapy to provide prophylaxis against preeclampsia, IUGR, and fetal demise. The theory behind the therapy has been that platelet activation, with thromboxane production and endothelial cell damage, is central both to the development of preeclampsia and to many cases of IUGR and fetal death as a result of "uteroplacental insufficiency." By disabling platelets with chronic low-dose aspirin therapy, it is hoped that this chain can be broken. Studies to date can be divided into two broad categories: those enrolling high-risk patients and those enrolling low-risk primigravidas. Differences among the studies in subject selection criteria, gestational age at initiation of therapy, and drugs used (some added dipyridamole to the aspirin) make grouping the data and direct comparisons difficult. In summary it is fair to say, however, that multiple studies of high-risk patients have rather uniformly shown a benefit to therapy in reducing the incidences of both preeclampsia and IUGR in the aspirin-treated groups. In contrast, the studies in low-risk women have failed to demonstrate any benefit to aspirin therapy. One of the studies suggested that the aspirin may have caused an increased incidence of abruptio placentae, but the other two do not confirm that risk. Taken together, the studies are reassuring that the aspirin is at worst not helpful but not harmful to mother or fetus.

Patients most likely to benefit from prophylactic aspirin therapy are those with a history of a prior episode of severe preeclampsia, especially early in pregnancy, and those with a history of IUGR caused by uteroplacental insufficiency, with or without fetal demise. A dose of 80 mg per day is adequate. The aspirin must be started before the development of any signs of preeclampsia or IUGR. The Collaborative Low-Dose Aspirin Study in Pregnancy showed that aspirin is ineffective if started after the development of signs of preeclampsia.

Calcium

Calcium metabolism may be abnormal in women with preeclampsia sparking interest in the role of calcium supplementation in the prevention or treatment of preeclampsia. Recent metaanalysis of the studies on calcium supplementation did show some mild beneficial effect, but others argue that the studies reviewed were of inconsistent quality with many of the subjects having gestational hypertension, rather than preeclampsia. A larger NIH trial of calcium supplementation to prevent preeclampsia indicated no benefit in incidence or severity of preeclampsia or gestational hypertension, preterm birth or birthweight between those treated with calcium and the control group. Like aspirin, the results with calcium preventing preeclampsia have been discouraging.

Postpartum Counseling and Follow-up

Women who develop hypertension during pregnancy should have follow-up blood pressure check at the 6-week postpartum visit. If the woman had preeclampsia, her blood pressure and all lab abnormalities should return to normal by this time. If not, she should be reevaluated 6 weeks later and if the blood pressure is still abnormal, her hypertension should be considered chronic and she should be treated and counseled accordingly (see Chapter 3).

BIBLIOGRAPHY

Arias F, Zamora J: Antihypertensive treatment and pregnancy outcome in patients with mild chronic hypertension, *Obstet Gynecol* 53:489, 1979.

Barr M Jr, Cohen MM Jr: ACE inhibitor fetopathy and hypocalvaria: the kidney-skull connection, *Teratology* 44:485, 1991.

Beaufils M et al: Prevention of pre-eclampsia by early antiplatelet therapy, *Lancet* 1:840, 1985.

Benigni A et al: Effect of low-dose aspirin on fetal and maternal generation of thromboxane by platelets in women at risk for pregnancy-induced hypertension, *N Engl J Med* 321:357, 1989.

Bucher HC, Guyart GH, Cook RJ: Effect of calcium supplementation on pregnancy-induced hypertension and preeclampsia: a meta-analysis of randomized controlled trials, *JAMA* 275:1113, 1996.

Butters L, Kennedy S, Rubin PC: Atenolol in essential hypertension during pregnancy, *Br Med J* 301:587, 1990.

Caritis S et al: Low dose aspirin to prevent preeclampsia in women at high risk, *N Engl J Med* 338: 701, 1998.

Chua S, Redman CWG: Prognosis for pre-eclampsia complicated by 5 g or more of proteinuria in 24 hours, *Eur J Obstet Gynaecol Reprod Biol* 43:9, 1992.

Cockburn J et al: Final report of study on hypertension during pregnancy: the effects of specific treatment on the growth and development of the children, *Lancet* 1:647, 1982.

Collaborative Low-Dose Aspirin Study in Pregnancy Collaborative Group: CLASP: a randomised trial of low-dose aspirin for the prevention and treatment of pre-eclampsia among 9364 pregnant women, *Lancet* 343: 619, 1994.

Constantine G et al: Nifedipine as a second line antihypertensive drug in pregnancy, *Br J Obstet Gynaecol* 94:1136, 1987.

Crowther CA, Bouwmeester AM, Ashurst HM: Does admission to hospital for bed rest prevent disease progression or improve fetal outcome in pregnancy complicated by non-proteinuric hypertension? *Br J Obstet Gynaecol* 99:13, 1992.

Curet LB, Olson RW: Evaluation of a program of bed rest in the treatment of chronic hypertension in pregnancy, *Obstet Gynecol* 53:336, 1979.

Donaldson JO: *Neurology of pregnancy,* Philadelphia, 1978, WB Saunders.

Eskenazi B, Fenster L, Sidney S: A multivariate analysis of risk factors for preeclampsia, *JAMA* 266:237, 1991.

Ferrazzani S et al: Proteinuria and outcome of 444 pregnancies complicated by hypertension, *Am J Obstet Gynecol* 162:366, 1990.

Fidler J et al: Randomised controlled comparative study of methyldopa and oxprenolol in treatment of hypertension in pregnancy, *Br Med J* 286: 1927, 1983.

Friedman EA, Neff RK: *Pregnancy hypertension,* Littleton, Mass, 1977, PSG Publishing Co.

Gallery EDM, Ross MR, Gyory AZ: Antihypertensive treatment in pregnancy: analysis of different responses to oxprenolol and methyldopa, *Br Med J* 291:563, 1985.

Greene MF et al: Prematurity among insulin-requiring diabetic gravid women, *Am J Obstet Gynecol* 161:106, 1989.

Hauth JC et al: Low-dose aspirin therapy to prevent preeclampsia, *Am J Obstet Gynecol* 168:1083, 1993.

Hogstedt S et al: A prospective controlled trial of metoprolol-hydralazine treatment in hypertension during pregnancy, *Acta Obstet Gynecol Scand* 64:505, 1985.

Kincaid-Smith P, Bullen M, Mills J: Prolonged use of methyldopa in severe hypertension in pregnancy, *Br Med J* 1:274, 1966.

Kuo VS, Koumantakis G, Gallery EDM: Proteinuria and its assessment in normal and hypertensive pregnancy, *Am J Obstet Gynecol* 167:723, 1992.

Landesman R et al: Reserpine in toxemia of pregnancy, *Obstet Gynecol* 9:377, 1957.

Leather HM et al: A controlled trial of hypotensive agents in hypertension in pregnancy, *Lancet* 2:488, 1968.

Levine R et al: Trial of Calcium to prevent preeclampsia, *N Engl J Med* 337;69, 1997.

Lin C-C et al: Fetal outcome in hypertensive disorders in pregnancy, *Am J Obstet Gynecol* 142:255, 1982.

Mabie WC, Pernoll ML, Biswas MK: Chronic hypertension in pregnancy, *Obstet Gynecol* 67:197, 1986.

Magee LA, Ornstein MP, von Dadelszen P: Management of hypertension in pregnancy, *BMJ* 318:1332, 1999.

Mathews DD: A randomized controlled trial of bed rest and sedation or normal activity and nonsedation in the management of non-albuminuric hypertension in late pregnancy, *Br J Obstet Gynaecol* 84:108, 1977.

McParland P, Pearce JM, Chamberlain GVP: Doppler ultrasound and aspirin in recognition and prevention of pregnancy-induced hypertension, *Lancet* 335:1552, 1990.

National High Blood Pressure Education Program: Working group report on high blood pressure in pregnancy, *Am J Obstet Gynecol* 1831, 2000.

Phippard A et al: Early blood pressure control improves pregnancy outcome in primigravid women with mild hypertension, *Med J Aust* 154:378, 1991.

Pickles CJ, Broughton Pipkin F, Symonds EM: A randomised placebo controlled trial of labetalol in the treatment of mild to moderate pregnancy induced hypertension, *Br J Obstet Gynaecol* 99:964, 1992.

Pickles CJ, Symonds EM, Broughton Pipkin F: The fetal outcome in a randomized double-blind controlled trial of labetalol versus placebo in pregnancy-induced hypertension, *Br J Obstet Gynaecol* 96:38, 1989.

Plouin P-F et al: Comparison of antihypertensive efficacy and perinatal safety of labetalol and methyldopa in the treatment of hypertension in pregnancy: a randomized controlled trial, *Br J Obstet Gynaecol* 95:868, 1988.

Plouin P-F et al: A randomized comparison of early with conservative use of antihypertensive drugs in the management of pregnancy-induced hypertension, *Br J Obstet Gynaecol* 97:134, 1990.

Redman CWG, Beilin LJ, Bonnar J: Treatment of hypertension in pregnancy with methyldopa: blood pressure control and side effects, *Br J Obstet Gynaecol* 84:419, 1977.

Redman CWG et al: Fetal outcome in trial of antihypertensive treatment in pregnancy, *Lancet* 2:753, 1976.

Rey E, Couturier A: The prognosis of pregnancy in women with chronic hypertension, *Am J Obstet Gynecol* 171:410, 1994.

Roberts JM, D'Abarno: Effects of calcium supplementation on pregnancy induced hypertension, *JAMA* 276;1386, 1996.

Roberts JM: Prevention or early treatment of preeclampsia, *N Engl J Med* 337;124, 1997.

Roberts JM, Cooper DW: Pathogenesis and genetics of pre-eclampsia, *Lancet* 357:53, 2001.

Rubin PC et al: Placebo-controlled trial of atenolol in treatment of pregnancy-associated hypertension, *Lancet* 1:431, 1983.

Rubin PC et al: Obstetric aspects of the use in pregnancy-associated hypertension of the β-adrenoceptor antagonist atenolol, *Am J Obstet Gynecol* 150:389, 1984.

Sandstrom B: Antihypertensive treatment with the adrenergic beta-receptor blocker metoprolol during pregnancy, *Gynecol Obstet Invest* 9:195, 1978.

Schiff E et al: The use of aspirin to prevent pregnancy-induced hypertension and lower the ratio of thromboxane A_2 to prostacyclin in relatively high risk pregnancies, *N Engl J Med* 321:351, 1989.

Sibai BM, Abdella TN, Anderson GD: Pregnancy outcome in 211 patients with mild chronic hypertension, *Obstet Gynecol* 61:571, 1983.

Sibai BM, Grossman RA, Grossman HG: Effects of diuretics on plasma volume in pregnancies with long-term hypertension, *Am J Obstet Gynecol* 150:831, 1984.

Sibai BM, Mercer B, Sarinoglu C: Severe preeclampsia in the second trimester: recurrence risk and long-term prognosis, *Am J Obstet Gynecol* 165:1408, 1991.

Sibai BM et al: A comparison of no medication versus methyldopa or labetalol in chronic hypertension during pregnancy, *Am J Obstet Gynecol* 162:960, 1990.

Sibai BM et al: Prevention of preeclampsia with low-dose aspirin in healthy, nulliparous pregnant women, *N Engl J Med* 329:1213, 1993.

Solomon CG et al: Glucose intolerance as a predictor of hypertension in pregnancy, *Hypertension* 23:717, 1994.

Suhonen L, Teramo K: Hypertension and pre-eclampsia in women with gestational glucose intolerance, *Acta Obstet Gynecol Scand* 72:269, 1993.

Tuffnell DJ et al: Randomised controlled trial of day care for hypertension in pregnancy, *Lancet* 339:224, 1992.

Uzan S et al: Prevention of fetal growth retardation with low-dose aspirin: findings of the EPREDA trial, *Lancet* 337:1427, 1991.

Wallenburg HCS et al: Low-dose aspirin prevents pregnancy-induced hypertension and pre-eclampsia in angiotensin-sensitive primigravidae, *Lancet* 1:1, 1986.

Walsh SW: Preeclampsia: an imbalance in placental prostacyclin and thromboxane production, *Am J Obstet Gynecol* 152:335, 1985.

Welt SI et al: The effect of prophylactic management and therapeutics on hypertensive disease in pregnancy: preliminary studies, *Obstet Gynecol* 57:557, 1981.

CHAPTER **73**

Liver Disease in Pregnancy

Lori D. Olans
Jacqueline L. Wolf

Liver disease in pregnancy includes disorders present before pregnancy (which may be exacerbated during pregnancy) and disorders that may occur only during pregnancy. De novo liver function test abnormalities during pregnancy are uncommon, probably occurring in 5% or fewer of pregnant women in the United States. However, identification of their etiology is important because of the potential of high maternal and fetal mortality if conditions such as acute fatty liver, preeclampsia, and hepatic rupture remain unrecognized and untreated. The focus of this chapter is a discussion of liver disorders unique to pregnancy.

CLASSIFICATION OF HEPATIC DISORDERS OF PREGNANCY

Hepatic disorders during pregnancy may be categorized as those occurring in the pregnant or nonpregnant state and those occurring only in the pregnant state. Those disorders that may occur independent of pregnancy, such as viral hepatitis and cholelithiasis, present special therapeutic concerns for the mother and fetus when they occur during pregnancy. A discussion of these topics are found in Chapters 16, 18, and 67. Those disorders that occur only in the pregnant state include hyperemesis gravidarum (covered extensively in Chapter 64), intrahepatic cholestasis of pregnancy, fatty liver of pregnancy, preeclampsia/eclampsia (reviewed in Chapter 69), HELLP syndrome (Hemolytic anemia, Elevated Liver function tests and Low Platelets), and hepatic rupture.

■ LIVER FUNCTION TESTS DURING PREGNANCY

Many physiologic and systemic changes occur during pregnancy, and the liver is included among the organs affected. Even in uncomplicated pregnancies, liver function tests may differ from those found in the nonpregnant state. For example, alkaline phosphatase increases gradually during the first 7 months of pregnancy and then rises rapidly to peak at term. This elevation rarely exceeds two to four times the normal value and is principally of placental origin. In addition, serum albumin concentration may be decreased to values 10% to 60% below normal, largely owing to increased maternal blood volume during pregnancy. Transaminases and bilirubin, however, are generally not altered by pregnancy (Table 73-1).

■ EVALUATION OF THE PREGNANT WOMAN WITH ABNORMAL LIVER FUNCTION TESTS

History

The history obtained from a pregnant woman with abnormal liver function tests should include several symptoms that may have different implications or less importance in the nonpregnant patient. The time of symptom onset in relation to the weeks of gestation provides important clues to the etiology of the liver function test abnormalities. For example, severe nausea and vomiting are the key features of hyperemesis gravidarium during the first trimester. However, when these symptoms are accompanied by headache and peripheral edema in the third trimester, this may indicate preeclampsia; if these symptoms are accompanied by right upper quadrant abdominal pain with or without hypotension in late pregnancy, this may indicate hepatic rupture. Pruritis is the characteristic feature of intrahepatic cholestatsis of pregnancy. It typically involves the palms of the hands and soles of the feet initially and then involves the rest of the body. Jaundice, if present, follows the pruritis. Abdominal pain is a significant symptom. One should note the location of the pain, duration, character (colicky, sharp or dull, incidious or sudden), factors that induce or relieve the pain, and other associated symptoms. Right upper quadrant and mid abdominal pain have potential ominous implications, particularly if occurring in late pregnancy which may indicate acute fatty liver of pregnancy or hepatic rupture. Colicky pain with or without fever may indicate biliary colic and/or acute cholecystitis. Other symptoms important to elicit are headache, fever, peripheral edema, foamy urine, oliguria, insomnia, change in stools (i.e., acholic or diarrhea), malaise, weight loss or gain, dizziness, easy bruisability, or neurological symptoms.

A history of the present and past pregnancies may be helpful, for example, multiple versus single fetus, multiparous versus primiparous, similar symptoms in previous

Table 73-1
Liver Function Tests in Normal Pregnancy

Test	Effect	Trimester of Maximum Change
Albumin	↓20%	2nd
Gamma-globulin	nl to sl↓	3rd
Fibrinogen	↑50%	2nd
Transferrin	↑	3rd
Bilirubin	nl	3rd
Alkaline phosphastase	2- to 4-fold↑	3rd
SGOT/AST	nl	
SGOT/ALT	nl	
Cholesterol	2-fold↑	3rd

nl, Normal; *sl*, slight; *SGOT*, serum glutamic-pyruvic; *AST*, aspartate aminotransferase; ↑, increase; ↓, decrease; *ALT*, alanine aminotransferase.

pregnancies and time of onset of these symptoms, similar symptoms unassociated with pregnancies, and outcome of previous pregnancies (weight gain, maternal problems, weeks of gestation, health of newborn). The history should also include symptoms with ingestion of oral contraceptive pills, drug ingestion or injection, previous blood transfusions, alcohol use, a past history of hepatitis or liver function test abnormalities, diabetes mellitus, recent travel history, close contact with others with a similar illness, or pets at home. A family history of preeclampsia, oral contraceptive pill intolerance, pregnancy problems, or cholelithiasis is particularly pertinent.

Physical Examination

The physical examination by itself is rarely diagnostic. Some of the common stigmata of liver disease on physical examination are found in the normal pregnant female. Because of physiologic and hormonal changes such as spider angioma and palmar erythema can be seen in a normal healthy pregnant female and does not in and of itself indicate underlying liver pathology. Jaundice, enlargement of the liver, a tender liver, a hepatic friction rub or bruit, splenomegaly, a Murphy's sign, and excoriations are not normal in pregnancy. Other abnormal findings that might be associated with hepatic disorders of pregnancy are hypertension, orthostatic hypotension, peripheral edema, asterixes, hyperreflexia, or other neurologic findings, ecchymoses, and petechiae.

Diagnostic Tests

Laboratory Tests

The evaluation of abnormal liver function tests in pregnancy varies only slightly from that in nonpregnancy, with the exception of limiting radiation exposure.

Blood tests should include a complete blood count (CBC) with hemoglobin, hematocrit, white blood cell count, and specific chemistries including glucose, electrolytes, transaminases, lactic dehydrogenase, bilirubin, alkaline phosphatase, and uric acid. Also important is a protime, partial thromboplastin time, and fibrinogen. Uric acid elevation usually occurs in acute fatty liver of pregnancy and may occur in preeclampsia. Serum bile acid levels, which may be elevated before the onset of or in conjunction with intrahepatic cholestasis of pregnancy (IHCP) is helpful if the diagnosis of

IHCP is being considered. An amylase and lipase should be done if abdominal pain and/or jaundice are present. If a viral etiology is possible, one should obtain serologies for hepatitis including hepatitis A (immunoglobulin [Ig]M and IgG), hepatitis B (surface antigen, surface antibody, core antibody and if surface antigen is present "e" antigen and "e" antibody), and hepatitis C. In certain circumstances delta hepatitis antibody is indicated.

Other Diagnostic Tests

Abdominal ultrasound is safe in pregnancy and helpful in the evaluation of biliary tract disease, acute fatty liver of pregnancy, and hepatic rupture. However, if negative these diagnoses may not be ruled out. If there is a strong suspicion of biliary tract disease an endoscopic retrograde cannulation of the biliary ducts (ERCP) may be done safely with shielding by a skilled endoscopist. A computed tomography (CT) scan may be more sensitive than ultrasound in detection of acute fatty liver and hepatic rupture but, if necessary for diagnosis, must be limited to one or two views because of the potential risk of radiation exposure to the fetus. The utility and safety in pregnancy of an magnetic resonance imaging (MRI) has yet to be determined conclusively but is generally thought to be safe in pregnancy. An angiogram is occasionally needed for the diagnosis of hepatic rupture.

Differential Diagnosis

A complete discussion of the differential diagnosis is beyond the scope of this review. For a differential diagnosis by trimester of hepatic disorders most common in pregnancy and unique to pregnancy see Table 73-2.

HYPEREMESIS GRAVIDARUM (Table 73-3)

Hyperemesis gravidarum occurs principally during the first trimester and has been rarely associated with abnormal liver function, particularly in women with extreme illness. The clinical features of this disorder have been described in Chapter 64 and include severe nausea and vomiting, as well as dehydration, electrolyte disturbances, and ketosis. In affected women, slight elevations in bilirubin, transaminases, or alkaline phosphatase may occur. In autopsy series, liver histology is normal or shows fatty infiltration, whereas in liver biopsy series the histology is normal. Although the pathologic mechanism of liver injury is unknown, the combined systemic effects of hypovolemia, malnutrition, and lactic acidosis are believed to play a role. Treatment is mainly supportive.

INTRAHEPATIC CHOLESTASIS OF PREGNANCY
(Table 73-4)

IHCP is a cholestatic disorder specific to the second and third trimester of pregnancy. Pruritis, with or without jaundice, is a hallmark feature.

Epidemiology and Risk Factors

Worldwide, IHCP is a rare disorder occurring in 0.1% to 0.01% of deliveries. Wide geographic variation in frequency of IHCP has been observed. For example, IHCP is more common in Sweden and Chile, with incidence rates approximating 2% and 4%, respectively The incidence rate in Chile

Table 73-2
Differential Diagnosis for Transaminitis and/or Jaundice in Pregnancy

Trimester of Pregnancy	Differential Diagnosis
First	Normal pregnancy
	Infectious viral hepatitis
	Hyperemesis gravidarum
	Drug-induced hepatitis
	Gallstones
	Intrahepatic cholestasis of pregnancy (uncommon)
Second	Normal pregnancy
	Infectious viral hepatitis
	Gallstones
	Drug induced hepatitis
	Intrahepatic cholestasis of pregnancy
	Preeclampsia/eclampsia (uncommon)
	HELLP syndrome (uncommon)
Third	Normal pregnancy
	Intrahepatic cholestasis of pregnancy
	Infectious viral hepatitis
	Preeclampsia/eclampsia
	HELLP syndrome
	Acute fatty liver of pregnancy
	Gallstones
	Hepatic rupture
	Drug-induced hepatitis

HELLP, hemolytic anemia, elevated liver function tests, low platelets.

Table 73-3
Hyperemesis Gravidarum

Onset	Symptoms/Signs	Laboratory Tests
4-20 weeks	+Nausea	+Transaminases increase (1-2X)
	+Vomiting	+Alkaline phosphatase increase (1-2X)
Usually 1st trimester		+Bilirubin increase (<5 mg/dl)
		+Urine ketones

Table 73-4
Intrahepatic Cholestasis of Pregnancy

Onset	Symptoms/Signs	Laboratory Tests
25 weeks delivery	+Pruritis	+Transaminases increase (1-4X)
	+/−Jaundice	+Alkaline phosphatase increase (1-2X)
		+Bilirubin increase (<5 mg/dl)
Usually after 30 weeks		+Bile acids increase (30-100X)
		+/−Cholesterol increase
		+/−Triglycerides increase

administering estrogens, pruritis and jaundice may be precipitated. This suggests a potential etiologic role for estrogens. The precise mechanism by which estrogens lead to cholestasis remains unclear.

Familial and epidemiologic data have supported a role for genetic factors in contributing to the development of IHCP. For example, IHCP is more common in women with sisters or a mother with a history of IHCP. In addition, groups such as Araucanian Indians in Chile have a prevalence rate of 24%, a rate significantly higher than that of the general Chilean population. The etiology of IHCP is likely multifactorial, and estrogens and genetics play a major role.

Clinical Presentation

History and Physical Examination

The spectrum of clinical illness varies from pruritis gravidarum, defined as diffuse itching, to severe cholestasis with accompanying jaundice. The onset of IHCP is most common in the third trimester but can rarely occur before 25 weeks of gestation.

In almost all affected women, the presenting symptom is **pruritis,** which can involve any part of the body including the palms and soles. Often it is more severe at night resulting in significant emotional distress, insomnia, anorexia, and malaise. The pruritis generally resolves within 2 days of delivery. Because of the intense itching, excoriations are a common physical finding.

The frequency of **jaundice** associated with IHCP is approximately 20%. The jaundice generally follows the onset of pruritis by approximately 2 to 4 weeks and usually resolves by 1 to 2 weeks postpartum. Nausea, vomiting, and abdominal discomfort may rarely be associated with IHCP. Diarrhea resulting from fat malabsorption may result from cholestasis.

Diagnostic Tests

Laboratory tests reveal a variety of abnormalities. Serum bilirubin, mostly direct, may be elevated but rarely exceeds 5 mg/dl. Alkaline phosphatase may increase by twofold, consistent with the normal rise in pregnancy. Transaminases can increase by fourfold or rarely higher. Serum bile acids may increase 30- to 100-fold and postprandial cholic acid 10- to 70-fold. Serum bile acids may represent the first or only sign of IHCP in women with pruritis but without other

has decreased from 14% in 1975 to 4% in 1995 for unknown reasons. IHCP demonstrates seasonal variation, being more common in winter months. IHCP has been more frequently observed in women with a family or past history of IHCP or of cholestatic sensitivity to estrogens. Recurrence in subsequent pregnancies is 40% to 60%.

Pathogenesis and Etiology

The etiology of intrahepatic cholestasis of pregnancy has not been clearly delineated. A variety of theories and contributing factors have been postulated. Hormonal and genetic factors are suspected.

Women with intrahepatic cholestasis attributable to oral contraceptive use are more likely to develop IHCP. Furthermore, on rechallenging women with a history of IHCP by conventional liver function test abnormalities. Serum cholesterol and triglycerides may be higher than expected for normal pregnancy. Liver biopsy reveals cholestasis. Bile may be deposited within hepatocytes in a central-lobular pattern or may plug canaliculi. Minimal or no hepatocellular necrosis is present. It is not usually necessary to perform a liver biopsy because diagnosis can be made by history and physical examination.

Maternal and Fetal Outcomes

Maternal outcome is benign when compared with that of infants. Pruritis, at times severe, resolves quickly after delivery. The onset of ICHP has been associated with urinary tract infections. Steatorrhea-induced vitamin K deficiency was been postulated as a contributing factor to postpartum bleeding. Long-term follow-up in Sweden has demonstrated an increased incidence of gallstones and gallbladder disease. There is no permanent liver damage to the mother postpartum.

Maternal intrahepatic cholestasis has been associated with an increased incidence of prematurity, perinatal deaths, fetal distress, and meconium staining of amniotic fluid. The reason for the potentially poor fetal outcome is still unknown. Elevated levels of bile acids, which are measurable in maternal blood, amniotic fluid, and umbilical cord blood, may be a contributing factor. Careful monitoring, particularly during the third trimester, for maternal and fetal well-being is recommended. Physicians should have a low threshold for early delivery if signs of fetal or maternal distress develop.

✴ MANAGEMENT

Pruritis improves immediately after delivery. However, since IHCP does not significantly endanger maternal well-being, delivery before term is rarely first-line therapy. Instead, management strategies have focused on symptomatic relief for the mother, as well as careful monitoring for signs of fetal distress. General recommendations for alleviation of pruritis have included sleeping in a cool room and applying topical alcohol.

Antihistamines and phenobarbital have been ineffective in relieving pruritis. **Cholestyramine,** administered in maximum doses of 8 to 12 g/day, has met with variable success. Cholestyramine acts by binding bile acids in the intestinal lumen and thus decreasing systemic bile acid concentrations. It can produce relief within 1 to 2 weeks and usually works best in cases with moderately increased bile acid levels. Cholestyramine therapy, however may aggravate malabsorption of fat-soluble nutrients.

Ursodeoxycholic acid (UDCA) has been used successfully to treat cholestatic liver disease and has shown promise in the treatment of IHCP. Its proposed mechanisms of action include modification of the bile acid pool by replacement of more hydrophobic and cytotoxic bile salts within hepatocyte membranes, inhibition of intestinal absorption of more hydrophobic bile acids, and modification of immune-mediated liver injury. In several small case series as well as two small randomized, double-blind, placebo-controlled studies, UDCA was found to be effective in reducing pruritis and improving laboratory parameters without adverse maternal or fetal outcomes. The larger controlled study involved 24 patients with IHCP diagnosed before 33 weeks of gestation. Patients were randomized to receive 1 g/day orally of UDCA or placebo until delivery. Only 15 of 24 patients completed the study (8 patients had deliveries before completing 2 weeks of treatment and one patient dropped out). No adverse events were noted in mothers or infants. Patients who received UDCA had significant improvements in pruritis, serum bilirubin, and transaminases. In patients who received UDCA, deliveries occurred significantly closer to term compared with placebo. Larger and longer term studies are needed to draw more definite conclusions with regard to the efficacy of UDCA in IHCP and to delineate the long-term effects on mother and fetus. Preliminary results appear promising.

S-adenosyl-L-methionine therapy showed promise in early studies for symptomatic and laboratory improvement in IHCP. This drug was thought to inactivate estrogen metabolites, increase membrane fluidity, and alter bile acid metabolism. However, in a subsequent double-blind, placebo-controlled trial, no benefit could be demonstrated. However, one more recently published small study by Nicastri described a benefit of the combination of S-adenosyl-L-methionine therapy and UDCA over placebo or either drug alone with regard to pruritis and laboratory parameters. No side effects were reported in mother and infant. Given the small size of the study (8 patients in each treatment arm) further studies are needed before definitive conclusions can be reached.

Dexamethasone has also shown promise as a potential therapy for IHCP. Through suppression of fetoplacental estrogen production, which may contribute to IHCP, dexamethasone therapy may lead to amelioration of symptoms. In one small series, 10 women with IHCP received open-label oral dexamethasone at a dose of 12 mg/day for 7 days with subsequent gradual taper over 3 days. After initiation of treatment pruritis was relieved, serum estrogen and total bile acid levels decreased, and liver function tests improved. No adverse reactions to the steroids were noted. In fact, the authors noted a potential beneficial effect on fetal lung maturity in those infants who may be at risk for prematurity on the basis of maternal IHCP. Enthusiasm for dexamethasone has been tempered by a case report of worsening of a patient's status after initiation of dexamethasone. Further clinical studies are needed before dexamethasone can be widely recommended for IHCP.

Case reports have shown that other agents such as epomeidol (a terpenoid compound), peroral activated charcoal, and guar gum have been beneficial in treating patients with IHCP, although none have been studied in a rigorous fashion.

ACUTE FATTY LIVER OF PREGNANCY (Table 73-5)
Epidemiology and Risk Factors

Acute fatty liver of pregnancy (AFLP) is a rare and potentially fatal disease generally occurring in the last trimester of pregnancy. Before 1980 the estimated incidence of AFLP was approximately 1 in 1 million pregnancies. More recent reports reveal an incidence of 1 in 13,328 deliveries. This increase in frequency is likely a result of increased awareness, as well as to recognition of mild cases. AFLP is more com-

Table 73-5
Acute Fatty Liver of Pregnancy

Onset	Symptoms/Signs	Laboratory Tests
26 weeks–postpartum	+Nonspecific systemic symptoms	+Transaminases increase (1-5X) +Alkaline phosphatase increase (1-2X) +Bilirubin increase (<10 mg/dl)
Usually after 32 weeks	+Right upper quadrant pain	+Uric acid increase +/−Platelet decrease +/−PT/PTT increase Increased echogenicity on ultrasound

PT, Prothrombin time; *PTT,* partial thromboplastin time.

monly associated with primipara, twin gestations, and male fetuses. Recurrences of AFLP in subsequent pregnancies are rare but may be more common in women with a history of offspring with enzymatic defects in fatty acid oxidation.

Pathogenesis and Etiology

Although its clinical manifestations are somewhat variable given the systemic nature of this disorder, histologically it is characterized by a microvesicular fatty infiltrate of the liver.

The cause of AFLP in all patients is unknown. Many studies have documented that women carrying fetuses with deficiencies of long-chain 3-hydroxyacyl-CoA dehydrogenase (LCHAD), a recessively inherited disorder of mitochondrial fatty acid oxidation, may be at increased risk for developing AFLP and HELLP. Little is known about the mechanism of disease in these women. In addition, hepatic carnitine palmitoyltransferase I deficiency was noted in two children born to a mother who had AFLP and hyperemesis gravidarum in both pregnancies. Neither the mother nor the children had LCHAD deficiency. This finding potentially broadens the spectrum of fatty acid oxidation defects associated with maternal liver disease in pregnancy. Many experts advocate molecular diagnostic testing with appropriate genetic counseling in women with a history of AFLP, HELLP, or recurrent liver disease in pregnancy as well as those women with offspring or a family history of LCHAD deficiency for the following reasons: (1) increased maternal morbidity and mortality, as well as increased perinatal mortality, is associated with AFLP and HELLP; (2) early diagnosis and treatment of LCHAD deficiency can lead to excellent fetal outcomes; and (3) women with AFLP and infants with LCHAD deficiency may be at increased risk for recurrent liver disease in subsequent pregnancies.

LCHAD deficiency, however, does not contribute to AFLP in all patients. Not all women with AFLP have infants with this enzyme deficiency. The cause of AFLP in these women remains unknown.

History and Physical Examination

AFLP generally occurs in the third trimester usually between 32 and 38 weeks of gestation, but it has been reported in the 26th week and in the postpartum period. Symptoms associated with AFLP may be general and include headache, fatigue, malaise, nausea, vomiting, or abdominal discomfort, either localized to the midepigastrium or right upper quadrant or more diffuse. These prodromal manifestations may soon be followed by jaundice. Later or more severe stages include progressive liver failure with coagulopathy and/or encephalopathy and renal dysfunction with oliguria or uremia. In 20% to 40% of cases, the onset of AFLP may be similar to the onset of preeclampsia with associated peripheral edema, hypertension, and proteinuria. The physical examination is rarely helpful diagnostically.

Diagnostic Tests
Laboratory Tests

Laboratory tests are notable for cholestasis with mild to moderate elevations in transaminases. Bilirubin may be normal early in the course and then rises if pregnancy is not terminated. Bilirubin elevation is rarely greater than 10 mg/dl. Alkaline phosphatase levels may be mildly elevated above those values found in normal pregnancies. Transaminases are almost always elevated but usually to values less than 500 U/L, thereby helping to distinguish AFLP from acute viral hepatitis. Hyperuricemia, principally owing to impaired renal clearance, has been observed in approximately 80% of patients. In the case of more severe or later stage of AFLP, abnormal laboratory values consistent with acute liver failure can be seen and include decreased platelets, elevated prothrombin time (PT) and partial thromboplastin time (PTT), microangiopathic changes on peripheral blood smear, leukocytosis, hypoglycemia, and an elevated serum ammonia level.

Radiographic Imaging

Radiographic imaging using ultrasound (US) or CT provides a noninvasive method for diagnosing AFLP, especially if coagulopathy precludes liver biopsy. The US finding consistent with fatty infiltration of the liver is increased echogenicity, whereas CT demonstrates decreased attenuation. Although US is less expensive than CT, it is also less sensitive. CT, unlike US, however, carries a risk of radiation exposure to the unborn fetus. MRI has recently been used to image fatty infiltration of the liver, but its role in diagnosis remains undetermined. These tests should be considered complementary to the clinical picture and should not delay treatment.

Liver Biopsy

Liver biopsy may be helpful in making the diagnosis. If done, a frozen section is mandatory. The biopsy is notable for microvesicular fatty infiltration detected only on frozen sections prepared with special fat stains such as oil-red-O. Fat is generally deposited in the cytoplasm of centrolobular hepatocytes. Inflammation and disarray of lobular hepatocytes, as well as patchy cellular necrosis, are commonly found, a finding seen in other diseases in the nonpregnant population. Although this pathology may make preeclampsia/eclampsia or viral hepatitis unlikely, these biopsy findings still remain nonspecific. For the nonpregnant population, they may be present in Reye's syndrome and in tetracycline or valproic acid toxicity. The transmission electron microscopic appearance of AFLP compared with that of Reye's syndrome is notable for subtle differences in hepatocyte mitochondria. If coagulation parameters are normal, liver biopsy may be useful in confirming the presence of AFLP in patients with atypical presentations. Given the risks associated with liver biopsy, it should not be performed to confirm a classic presentation of AFLP or to distinguish AFLP from severe preeclampsia, as both require the same treatment, supportive care, and delivery.

Maternal and Fetal Outcomes

Earlier studies showed a poor prognosis in AFLP with maternal and fetal mortality rates approximating 85%. At present early diagnosis, rapid delivery after recognition, and aggressive supportive care have decreased maternal and fetal mortality rates to 18% and 23%, respectively. Liver function tests improve soon after termination of pregnancy. If no aggressive action is taken, women may develop fulminant hepatic failure and death may result.

MANAGEMENT

Early delivery is the mainstay of therapy and has improved maternal and fetal survival dramatically compared with continuation of pregnancy and medical management. Most women experience rapid improvement after delivery. Successful orthotopic liver transplantations in women with AFLP manifesting fulminant hepatic failure despite delivery and intensive supportive care have been reported.

PREECLAMPSIA/ECLAMPSIA (Table 73-6)
Epidemiology and Risk Factors

Preeclampsia is a systemic disorder in which the liver is one of the many target organs. It occurs in the second half of gestation and is characterized by hypertension, proteinuria, and edema.

Preeclampsia occurs in approximately 5% to 10% of pregnancies. It is generally a disease of primigravidas. Diabetes mellitus, hypertension, extremes of age (<20 years or <45 years), and a family history of preeclampsia/eclampsia are all associated with an increased incidence of preeclampsia/eclampsia. Plural gestations, hydatiform mole, fetal hydrops, polyhydramnios, and inadequate prenatal care have also been shown to correlate with the occurrence of preeclampsia/eclampsia.

Chapter 69 discusses preeclampsia and eclampsia in detail. This discussion focuses on highlights, especially with respect to the liver abnormalities.

Pathogenesis and Etiology

The precise mechanism of preeclampsia/eclampsia is not understood. A variety of etiologies have been proposed to explain the occurrence of this multisystem disorder (see Chapter 69). Hypotheses have included placental ischemia, vasospasm, very low-density lipoproteins versus toxicity-preventing activity, immune maladaptation, genetic imprinting, abnormal endothelial reactivity, and activation of coagulation.

History and Physical Examination

Characteristic clinical features associated with preeclampsia include the triad of hypertension, proteinuria, and edema. It

Table 73-6
Preeclampsia

Onset	Symptoms/Signs	Laboratory Tests
20 weeks delivery	+Nonspecific systemic symptoms	+Transaminases increase (1-100X) +/−Alkaline phosphatase increase (1-2X) +/−Bilirubin increase (<5mg/dl)
Usually late 2nd or 3rd trimester	+Hypertension +Edema	+Uric acid increase +/−Platelet decrease +/−PT/PTT increase +Urine protein

PT, Prothrombin time; *PTT,* partial thromboplastin time.

traditionally occurs during the second half of gestation and usually during the third trimester. Symptoms, however, may occur in the postpartum period as well. Edema is not a rigid criterion, since it is subjective and complicates approximately 30% of normal pregnancies. Eclampsia includes the signs and symptoms of preeclampsia with convulsions or coma unrelated to other chronic cerebral conditions. The absence of pruritis and jaundice early in its course helps to distinguish preeclampsia from other liver disorders occurring during pregnancy.

Distinguishing mild from severe preeclampsia is based on the magnitude of blood pressure elevation, proteinuria, and systemic organ involvement. In the literature, this distinction has been somewhat muddled by controversies regarding terminology and definitions. Preeclampsia/eclampsia is generally viewed as a multisystem disorder and may include renal, hematologic, hepatic, central nervous system, and fetal-placental involvement. In severe cases, headaches, visual changes, abdominal pain, congestive heart failure, respiratory distress, or oliguria may occur. Although the liver may not be primarily involved in early preeclampsia, it may become a target as the disease progresses.

Diagnostic Tests

Abnormal liver function tests may be associated with preeclampsia. In early reports aspartate aminotransferase was abnormal in 84% of women with eclampsia, 50% with severe preeclampsia, and 24% with mild preeclampsia, whereas alanine aminotransferase was abnormal in 90% of women with eclampsia, 24% with severe preeclampsia, and 20% with mild preeclampsia. The magnitude of transaminase elevations may range from 5 to 100 times normal values. Bilirubin is commonly normal; if elevated, the value rarely exceeds 5 mg/dl. Abnormal hematologic parameters include thrombocytopenia, microangiopathic hemolytic anemia, and/or disseminated intravascular coagulation (DIC). Additionally, uric acid levels are frequently elevated.

The diagnosis of preeclampsia with liver involvement is primarily clinical. Care must be taken to exclude other liver diseases associated with pregnancy, viral illness, and drug toxicity. Liver biopsy, although not required for diagnosis, may demonstrate periportal deposition of fibrin with associated hemorrhage. In severe cases, hepatocellular injury may lead to necrosis.

Maternal and Fetal Outcomes

The major risks to the mother include cardiovascular, hepatic, respiratory or renal failure, neurologic impairment, and hepatic rupture. The risks to the fetus include prematurity, fetal growth retardation, abruptio placenta, and low birth weight. Increased perinatal morbidity and mortality for the mother and fetus correlate with preterm delivery, severity of preeclampsia, multiple gestations, and preexisting maternal medical conditions such as hypertension. Perinatal morbidity and mortality in mild preeclampsia at term approximates that of normal pregnancies. The prognostic significance of liver function test abnormalities in mild preeclampsia is unclear. Some would argue that the finding of even mildly abnormal liver function tests indicates the presence of a systemic illness and should therefore change the classification of preeclampsia from mild to severe. This has prognostic importance as severe preeclampsia has a higher associated morbidity and mortality compared with mild preeclampsia. However, there has never been a rigorous study showing a correlation between abnormal liver function tests and maternal or fetal outcome.

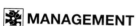 **MANAGEMENT**

The primary goals in managing preeclampsia are maternal health followed by delivery of a healthy newborn. The unequivocal therapy for eclampsia and term preeclampsia is delivery. The management of mild and severe preeclamptics remote from term is more controversial with regard to hospitalization, antihypertensive therapy, and timing of delivery as is outlined in Chapter 69. Hepatic dysfunction and associated liver function test abnormalities generally improve rapidly after delivery.

HELLP SYNDROME (Table 73-7)
Epidemiology and Risk Factors

HELLP, an acronym for Hemolytic anemia, Elevated Liver function tests, and Low Platelets, often occurs in the third trimester in association with preeclampsia/eclampsia but may occur independently.

HELLP occurs in approximately 0.1% to 0.6% of pregnancies and in 4% to 12% of women with severe preeclampsia. Although the majority of patients have hypertension, severe hypertension may be absent, leading to a delay in the clinical diagnosis of HELLP and in a subsequent therapeutic delivery. HELLP is more common in Caucasian multiparous women of older maternal age (mean age of 25 years) and generally occurs at approximately 32 weeks or later, although cases have been reported at or before 25 weeks. Onset occurs during the antepartum period in approximately two thirds of patients and in the postpartum period in approximately one third of patients. In cases occurring after parturition, onset may extend from hours to days after delivery, although the majority present within 48 hours. The recurrence rate for HELLP in subsequent pregnancies is in the range of 3% to 27%.

Pathogenesis and Etiology

The pathophysiology of HELLP has not been clearly delineated. Like preeclampsia/eclampsia, HELLP is a multisystem disease involving the liver and may be due to ab-

Table 73-7
HELLP Syndrome

Onset	Symptoms/Signs	Laboratory Tests
25 weeks immediate postpartum	+Nonspecific systemic symptoms	+Transaminases increase (1-100X)
		+/−Alkaline phosphatase increase (1-2X)
		+/−Bilirubin (<5 mg/dl)
Usually after 32 weeks	+Right upper quadrant pain	+Uric acid increase
		+/−Platelet decrease
		+/−PT/PTT increase
		+/−Urine protein

PT, Prothrombin time; *PTT,* partial thromboplastin time.

normal vascular tone, vasospasm, and/or coagulation. A more complete description of potential etiologies is included in Chapter 69.

History and Physical Examination

Symptoms associated with HELLP include epigastric pain, nausea, vomiting, headache, weight gain, and edema. Hypertension may be absent in as many as 15% of patients.

Diagnostic Tests

Laboratory tests include moderate proteinuria, microangiopathic hemolytic anemia with associated depression in haptoglobin, and elevations in lactose dehydrogenase and indirect bilirubin. Transaminases may be elevated to values as high as 4000 U/L, although milder elevations are more often the norm. Platelet counts may be depressed to values of 6000 to 100,000 around the time of delivery. Platelet counts tend to normalize 5 days postpartum. PT, PTT and fibrinogen may be abnormal in a minority of cases. Hypertension and proteinuria, if present, may take up to 3 months to resolve. Liver histology may demonstrate periportal or focal necrosis with hyaline deposits in sinusoids.

Maternal and Fetal Outcomes

Maternal and fetal outcomes do not correlate with the severity of liver involvement. Maternal mortality rate for women likely approaches 1.0% to 3.5%, although values up to 25% have been noted. Maternal morbidity has resulted from DIC, abruptio placenta, and renal, cardiopulmonary, or hepatic failure. Depending on the severity of the disease at the time of diagnosis, infant perinatal mortality has ranged from 10% to 60%. Infants are at increased risk for prematurity, intrauterine growth retardation, DIC, and thrombocytopenia.

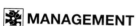 **MANAGEMENT**

Prompt recognition and management are critical to the survival of mother and infant. In cases with early signs of maternal and/or fetal distress, delivery is clearly recommended. For other less clear-cut cases, the optimal time of delivery is somewhat controversial. Liver function tests may return to normal soon after delivery without long-term sequelae as long as the patient's course is relatively uncomplicated. See Chapter 69 for further details on medical management.

HEPATIC RUPTURE (Table 73-8)
Epidemiology and Risk Factors

Hepatic rupture is a relatively rare complication of pregnancy. It is reported in 1 in 45,000 to 1 in 250,000 deliveries. It may occur spontaneously or may be associated with underlying hepatic pathology. Most cases reported have occurred in women with pregnancy-induced hypertension including preeclampsia/eclampsia and HELLP. Hepatic rupture in preeclamptic/eclamptic pregnancies occurs more commonly in older multigravidas. Hepatic rupture in pregnancy has more rarely been reported in association with hepatocellular carcinomas, adenomas, hemangiomas, hepatic abscesses, acute fatty liver of pregnancy, and HELLP. Recurrence of hepatic rupture in subsequent pregnancies is rare.

Pathogenesis and Etiology

The cause of spontaneous or secondary hepatic rupture in pregnancy is unknown. In cases with associated preeclampsia/eclampsia, DIC has been thought to play a role. Yet, rupture has been reported in pregnancies showing only minimal or early signs of DIC.

History and Physical Examination

Hepatic rupture generally presents with acute abdominal pain and associated nausea and vomiting occurring during the last trimester or less commonly in the first 24 hours after delivery. Signs and symptoms of preeclampsia/eclampsia may be present if rupture is secondary. Soon after, abdominal distention and hypovolemic shock ensue. Ruptures are generally limited to the right portion of the liver, although the left or both lobes may be involved.

Diagnostic Tests

Liver function tests are often elevated with an associated anemia and consumptive thrombocytopenia with or without DIC. Useful diagnostic tests include abdominal US, CT, magnetic resonance imaging (MRI), and angiography. These imaging tests may be performed in preparation for surgery or intraoperatively.

Maternal and Fetal Outcomes

Maternal and fetal mortality rates are high. Maternal rates are estimated at 50% to 75%, whereas fetal rates approximate 60%. Early recognition of hepatic rupture increases the chance of survival. The most frequent cause of maternal death after spontaneous rupture is hemorrhage. Mortality is lower in women with contained hematomas and in those who have prompt intervention. Fetal morbidity and mortality may be directly correlated with prematurity.

✳ MANAGEMENT

Survival depends on early recognition and prompt surgical attention. Most experts agree that a ruptured liver capsule mandates emergent surgery. In addition to delivery of the fetus, surgical options have included direct pressure, evacuation, packing or hemostatic wrapping, application of topical hemostatic agents, oversewing lacerations, hepatic artery ligation, and partial hepatectomy. Angiographic embolization has been reported but works best when the rupture is limited to only one lobe. Recent literature suggests that liver hematoma without rupture can be managed without immediate surgery if the patient is clinically stable or postpartum. In the setting of an intact liver capsule, if preeclampsia/eclampsia is present, early delivery is indicated given the significant maternal and fetal risks.

BIBLIOGRAPHY

Barq Y: Acute fatty liver of pregnancy, *Semin Perinatol* 22:134, 1998.

Barron WM: The syndrome of preeclampsia, *Gastroenterol Clin North Am* 21:851, 1992.

Barton JR, Sibai BM: Care of the pregnancy complicated by HELLP syndrome, *Gastroenterol Clin North Am* 21:937, 1992.

Barton JR et al: Recurrent acute fatty liver of pregnancy, *Am J Obstet Gynecol* 163:534, 1990.

Broussard CN, Richter JE: Nausea and vomiting of pregnancy, *Gastroenterol Clin North Am* 27:123, 1998.

Davidson KM: Intrahepatic cholestasis of pregnancy, *Semin Perinatol* 22:104, 1998.

Dekker G: Risk factors for preeclampsia, *Clin Obstet Gynecol* 42:422, 1999.

Dekker G, Sibai B: Etiology and pathogenesis of preeclampsia: current concepts, *Am J Obstet Gynecol* 179:1359, 1998.

Diaferia A et al: Ursodeoxycholic acid therapy in pregnant women with cholestasis, *Int J Gynaecol Obstet* 52:133, 1996.

Egerman R, Sibai B: HELLP syndrome, *Clin Obstet Gynecol* 42:3381, 1999.

Fisk NM, Storey GNB: Fetal outcome in obstetric cholestasis, *Br J Obstet Gynaecol* 95:1137, 1988.

Gitlin N: Liver disease in pregnancy. In Millward-Sadler GH, Wright R, Arthur MJP, editors: *Wright's liver and biliary disease: pathophysiology, diagnosis and management,* London, Philadelphia, 1992, WB Saunders.

Goodwin TM: Hyperemesis gravidarrum, *Clin Obstet Gynecol* 41:597, 1998.

Gylling H et al: Oral guar gum treatment of intrahepatic cholestasis and pruritis in pregnant women: effects on serum cholesterol and other non-cholesterol sterols, *Eur J Clin Invest* 28:359, 1998.

Hirvioja ML, Tuomala R, Vuori J: The treatment of intrahepatic cholestasis of pregnancy by dexamethasone, *Br J Obstet Gynaecol* 99:109, 1992.

Ibdah J et al: A fetal fatty acid oxidation disorder as a cause of liver disease in pregnant women, *N Engl J Med* 340:1723, 1999.

Innes AM et al: Hepatic carnitine palmitoyltransferase I deficiency presenting as amternal illness in pregnancy, *Pediatr Res* 47:43, 2000.

Johnson CD: Magnetic resonance imaging of the liver: current clinical applications, *Mayo Clin Proc* 68:147, 1993.

Kaaja RJ et al: Treatment of cholestasis of pregnancy with peroral activated charcoal, *Scand J Gastroenterol* 29:178, 1994.

Kaplan MM: Current concepts: acute fatty liver of pregnancy, *N Engl J Med* 313:367, 1985.

Knox T, Olans L: Liver disease in pregnancy, *N Engl J Med* 335:569, 1996.

•Loevinger EH et al: Hepatic rupture associated with pregnancy: treatment with transcatheter embolotherapy, *Obstet Gynecol* 65:281, 1985.

Table 73-8
Hepatic Rupture

Onset	Symptoms/Signs	Laboratory Tests
Late 2nd trimester; pain immediate postpartum	+Acute abdominal +/−Nausea +/−Vomiting	+Transaminases increase (2-100X) +Alkaline phosphatase increase +/−Bilirubin increase +/−Platelet decrease +/−PT/PTT increase
Usually 3rd trimester		

PT, Prothrombin time; *PTT,* partial thromboplastin time.

Nicastri PL et al: A randomized placebo-controlled trial of ursodeoxycholic acid S-adenosylmethionine in the treatment of intrahepatic cholestasis of pregnancy, *Br J Obstet Gynecol* 105:1205, 1998.

Palma J et al: Effects of ursodeoxycholic acid in patients with intrahepatic cholestasis of pregnancy, *Hepatology* 15:1043, 1992.

Palma J et al: Management of intrahepatic cholestasis in pregnancy, *Lancet* 339:1478, 1992.

Ralston SJ, Schwaitzberg SD: Liver hematoma and rupture in pregnancy, *Semin Perinatol* 22:141, 1998.

Reyes H: Review: intrahepatic cholestasis. A puzzling disorder of pregnancy, *J Gastroenterol Hepatol* 12:211, 1997.

Ribalta J et al: S-adenosyl-l-methionine in the treatment of patients with intrahepatic cholestasis of pregnancy: a randomized double-blind, placebo-controlled study with negative results, *Hepatology* 13:1084, 1991.

Saphier CJ, Repeke JT: Hemolysis, elevated liver enzymes, and low platelets (HELLP) syndrome: a review of diagnosis and management, *Semin Perinatol* 22:118, 1998.

Schorr-Lesnick B, Dworkin B, Rosenthal WS: Hemolysis, elevated liver enzymes, and low platelets in pregnancy (HELLP syndrome): a case report and literature review, *Dig Dis Sci* 36:1649, 1991.

Schorr-Lesnick B et al: Liver diseases unique to pregnancy, *Am J Gastroenterol* 86:659, 1991.

Sheikh FA, Yasmeen S, Pauly MP: Spontaneous intrahepatic hemorrhage and hepatic rupture in the HELLP syndrome, *J Clin Gastroenterol* 28:323, 1999.

Sibai BM: Management of pre-eclampsia remote from term, *Eur Obstet* 42:S96, 1991.

Sibai BM: Pitfalls in diagnosis and management of preeclampsia, *Am J Obstet Gynecol* 159:1, 1988.

Sibai BM: Preeclampsia-eclampsia: maternal and perinatal outcomes, *Contemp Obstet Gynecol* 32:109, 1988.

Sibai BM: The HELLP syndrome (hemolysis, elevated liver enzymes, and low platelets): much ado about nothing? *Am J Obstet Gynecol* 162:311, 1990.

Sibai BM et al: Pregnancy outcome in 303 cases with severe preeclampsia, *Obstet Gynecol* 64:319, 1984.

Smith LG et al: Spontaneous rupture of liver during pregnancy: current therapy, *Obstet Gynecol* 77:171, 1991.

Strauss A et al: Inherited long chain 3-hydroxyacyl-CoA dehydrogenase deficiency and a fetal-maternal interaction cause maternal liver disease and other pregnancy complications, *Semin Perinatol* 23:100, 1999.

CHAPTER 74

Nongynecologic Cancer in Pregnancy

Lawrence N. Shulman
Corey Stephen Cutler

Malignancy is not common in women of childbearing age, but it can occur, and when it does, it presents serious problems for both the mother and fetus. Malignancy complicating pregnancy is reported to occur in approximately 1/1000 pregnancies and is defined as any malignancy diagnosed during pregnancy or during the first year postpartum.

Symptoms associated with malignancy can be difficult to diagnose because they often mimic common symptoms experienced by the pregnant woman. Hormonal changes affecting the breast tissue during pregnancy may obscure a growing breast cancer. Fatigue and nonspecific constitutional complaints, which may be presenting signs of acute leukemia, are frequently seen in the healthy pregnant woman. Hodgkin's disease presenting in the mediastinum may manifest itself as cough and shortness of breath, the latter a common complaint, especially during the third trimester. Therefore identifying the rare pregnant woman with cancer may be difficult. Persistent complaints during pregnancy warrant further evaluation.

Once the diagnosis of cancer is made, there are special considerations during pregnancy (Box 74-1), which include the following:

1. Accurate staging of the malignancy at the time of diagnosis is critical. Most of the techniques used for staging pose low risk to the mother and fetus.
2. Assessment of the risk of the malignancy to the mother, both short- and long-term progression and prognosis, is important for treatment planning,
3. The risk of therapeutic intervention to both the mother and the fetus, including the immediate risk of maternal morbidity from treatment and fetal loss, and long-term implications such as fertility of mother, fetal malformation, and growth delay or subsequent risk of malignancy in child, must be identified.

Coordination of a multidisciplinary team composed of a high-risk obstetrician, neonatologist, hematologist-oncologist, primary care physician, other supporting physicians including surgeons, radiologists, and radiation oncologists, as well as a group of supporting staff composed of nutritionists, ethicists, and counselors is critical to optimizing outcome for both mother and fetus.

Although any malignancy can occur during pregnancy, those malignancies that affect young adults are most likely to coincide with pregnancy. Breast cancer, Hodgkin's and non-Hodgkin's-type malignant lymphomas, and the acute leukemias are some of the more common malignancies seen in this age group; however, virtually all forms of cancer have been reported to occur simultaneously with pregnancy. This chapter focuses on the three most common forms of nongynecologic cancer that occur in pregnant women.

BREAST CANCER

EPIDEMIOLOGY AND RISK FACTORS

Breast cancer arising during pregnancy or the year postpartum is reported to account for 0.2% to 3.8% of all cases of breast cancer. Although breast cancer incidence increases with age, it does occur in premenopausal women and therefore occasionally coincides with pregnancy. The majority of breast cancers occur in women with no family history of, and no identifiable risk factors for, breast cancer. The hereditary breast cancer genes, BRCA1 and BRCA2, may play a role in pregnancy-associated breast cancer, possibly because of the increased prevalence of breast cancer at a young age in the carriers of these mutations.

There are no data to suggest that pregnancy causes breast cancer. To the contrary, nulliparous women and women whose first pregnancy occurs late in life may be more likely to develop breast cancer.

Diagnosis

During pregnancy, the breasts become engorged owing to hormonal stimulation, which can make a breast cancer less obvious to a woman, even if she is accustomed to performing self-breast examination. The physician may also have difficulty detecting a mass in the breast of the pregnant patient or may ascribe changes caused by a carcinoma to effects of the pregnancy. The physician may be less likely to perform a mammogram and possibly less likely to perform a biopsy of a suspicious lesion. Although the sensitivity of mammography to identify a suspicious lesion may be less than for the nonpregnant female, it is considered a safe procedure for both mother and fetus, provided there is adequate shielding of the abdomen. Ultrasonography of the breast may help separate cystic lesions from solid tumors. If a cancer is suspected in a pregnant patient, techniques exist to diagnose the cancer without the need for general anesthesia. Percutaneous core needle biopsy can be safely performed and provides sufficient histologic information and the hormone receptor status of a breast tumor. If needle biopsy is unsuccessful, open biopsy under local anesthesia may be possible.

Once breast cancer has been diagnosed, staging studies, such as plain radiography and computed tomography (CT) scans can be performed safely with proper precautions. However, consideration of the impact of these results and how they may alter therapy must be weighed against the risk of fetal radiation exposure.

❀ MANAGEMENT

Once the diagnosis has been made, treatment decisions are difficult and need to be tailored for the individual, depending on the apparent extent of the cancer, the trimester of pregnancy, and the wishes of the mother and family. For the patient near term, it may be possible to deliver the fetus if it is sufficiently mature and then proceed with standard treatment. For the patient early in her pregnancy, therapeutic abortion is an option, and if rapidly performed, the physician can subsequently treat the patient in a manner similar to the nonpregnant breast cancer patient. There is no evidence that aborting a fetus alters the outcome of pregnancy-associated breast cancer. If the patient does not desire an abortion, or is too far advanced in her pregnancy for an abortion, then the decisions are particularly difficult. A patient diagnosed at 23 or 24 weeks of gestation is still 2 to 3 months from the time of preferred delivery, and during this period there may be substantial growth of the breast cancer if no treatment is instituted. If there are no apparent metastases and the cancer does not appear to be locally advanced, surgical options may be explored. A modified radical mastectomy is an option, although it will necessitate general anesthesia. If the tumor appears small and there is no obvious axillary nodal involve-

ment, simple excision with local anesthesia may be feasible. Although modest doses of radiation can be administered to the upper body with minimal "scatter" reaching the fetus, these doses are well below the usually acceptable antitumor doses used to control breast cancer. Therefore breast or chest wall radiation therapy should be deferred until after delivery if possible.

If the cancer is locally advanced (preventing surgical management) or if there is distant metastatic disease, then ideal therapy consists of systemic chemotherapy. One would prefer not to administer chemotherapy to the pregnant woman, although it is feasible when necessary. When possible, the fetus should be delivered and chemotherapy begun postpartum.

Two recent studies have documented the efficacy and safety of chemotherapy administered to patients while pregnant in second or third trimester. In a study from the M.D. Anderson Cancer Center, 24 patients were treated prospectively with standard chemotherapy with no adverse long-term maternal or fetal outcomes after treatment during pregnancy. In contrast, a national French study retrospectively documented 20 cases of pregnancy—associated breast cancer. Two first-trimester pregnancies with exposure to chemotherapy resulted in spontaneous abortions. Additionally, there was one neonatal death and one child born with intrauterine growth retardation.

Prognosis and Outcome

Even as early as 1880, it was suggested that breast cancers occurring in pregnancy had a particularly dire prognosis. In the 1940s, Haagensen described 20 pregnant women with breast cancer and commented on the advanced local and systemic manifestations of cancers in these patients compared with nonpregnant patients.

The hormonal milieu of the pregnant woman might lead to more rapid growth and dissemination of breast cancer, because breast cancer cells can have estrogen receptors on their cell surfaces and may proliferate under the influence of the high-estrogen state. Some have suggested that the poorer prognosis is due to a higher proportion of estrogen-receptor-negative tumors; however, false-negative assays for estrogen receptors using older immunohistochemical techniques may contribute to this perception.

As a result of delays in diagnosis, pregnant patients with breast cancer often present with larger tumors or advanced disease. In the Memorial Sloan Kettering series, patients who had their cancers diagnosed immediately postpartum had tumors that averaged 3.5 cm compared with nonpregnant patients whose tumors averaged 2.0 cm. The most predictive factor for the subsequent development of metastatic disease and ultimate death from breast cancer is axillary lymph node involvement. Of women reported from the Memorial series with postpartum diagnoses of breast cancer, 64% had involvement of axillary lymph nodes, compared with 38% for a group of nonpregnant women. Other series, including the recent M.D. Anderson experience, have confirmed the higher than expected incidence of axillary nodal involvement in breast cancer patients presenting during pregnancy. Of note was an unexpectedly high number (7 of 63) of patients who already had advanced breast cancer, with involvement of the skin, infraclavicular or supraclavicular nodes or with distant metastases found in the

Memorial series. This finding was not confirmed in the more recent series reported by investigators at M.D. Anderson, who reported that only one patient presented with Stage IV disease and two patients presented with recurrent disseminated disease during pregnancy.

Whether the hormonal milieu of pregnancy truly stimulates breast cancers to grow, disseminate, and negatively affect the prognosis of these patients remains controversial. These patients can clearly present at advanced stages, and even when clinical stage and lymph node involvement were controlled for, one recent study showed a poorer outcome for pregnant patients compared with nonpregnant control subjects.

HODGKIN'S DISEASE

EPIDEMIOLOGY

Hodgkin's disease is a common malignancy in women of childbearing age and is the most common hematologic malignancy diagnosed during pregnancy, complicating 1 in 6000 deliveries. Presentation of Hodgkin's disease is usually manifest by enlargement of the cervical, supraclavicular, or mediastinal lymph nodes; but retroperitoneal nodes, as well as extranodal organs can be involved. Fever, night sweats, and weight loss (so-called "B" symptoms) may be notable at diagnosis as well. Hodgkin's disease is a potentially curable disease even when disseminated, and management of the pregnant patient and the fetus should reflect this fact.

Diagnosis

Localized lymphadenopathy can be safely biopsied with local anesthesia alone. Once the diagnosis has been established, appropriate staging procedures must be undertaken, since the stage of disease influences eventual management. In the nonpregnant patient, CT scans of the thorax, abdomen, and pelvis are used to identify adenopathy; however, this approach is generally avoided in the pregnant patient since other modalities, such as magnetic resonance imaging (MRI), are available for adequate staging. If there is advanced mediastinal or retroperitoneal involvement, obstruction of major vessels, large airways, or ureters, MRI imaging of the mediastinum and retroperitoneum is warranted. Both staging laparotomy and bipedal lymphangiography, which have fallen out of favor for the diagnosis of the nonpregnant patient, are rarely used in the pregnant patient because of concerns of operative morbidity and fetal radiation exposure. In a large case-control study, pregnancy did not influence stage at the time of diagnosis, with 25% of patients presenting with Stage I disease, 46% with Stage II disease, 17% with Stage III disease, and 12% with Stage IV disease.

MANAGEMENT

The approach to the pregnant patient with Hodgkin's disease is determined by the trimester of pregnancy, the distribution and extent of the Hodgkin's disease, and the growth rate of the tumor. Hodgkin's disease can progress at extremely variable rates both in the pregnant and nonpregnant patient, and the rate of growth can often be assessed accurately after a week or two of observation. If the adenopathy is not rapidly growing and the patient is near term, treatment can be delayed until after delivery. If the disease is widespread, threatens vital structures (such as the heart, great vessels, major airways, or ureters), or progresses rapidly, some form of treatment is required.

In general, patients with localized disease often receive radiation therapy alone, whereas patients with more advanced or disseminated disease usually receive chemotherapy, with or without radiation therapy.

External beam radiotherapy with careful shielding and monitoring of fetal dose delivery is safe during the second and third trimesters for treatment of localized disease above the diaphragm. In a report of patients treated at the M.D. Anderson Cancer Center, definitive radiotherapy was delivered to 16 patients with Stage I to IIA (localized disease) Hodgkin's disease without adverse fetal effects. Twelve patients had long-term disease-free survival while four eventually relapsed. Because of this, therapeutic abortion is often recommended for patients during the first trimester of pregnancy who require radiotherapy-based treatment.

When disease is disseminated, bulky, or threatens vital structures, chemotherapy becomes necessary. Low doses of radiation can be used to provide temporary relief of compromised structures. Corticosteroids can significantly reduce bulky disease to remove immediate danger, and the response can be rapid. Unfortunately, the response to corticosteroids tends to be brief, although it may be long enough to allow safe and successful delivery of the fetus. Single agent cytotoxic chemotherapy using any one of the many active agents in this disease can be used until delivery. Generally, combination chemotherapy (ABVD regimen; Adriamycin, bleomycin, vincristine, dacarbazine) can be used after delivery, has minimal side effects, and low rates of resulting infertility. However, in the clinical situations where combination chemotherapy has been used during pregnancy, it has been reported to be safe and successful.

ACUTE LEUKEMIA

EPIDEMIOLOGY

Leukemia can be subdivided into two broad categories known as the acute and chronic leukemias, respectively. Both acute myelogenous leukemia (AML) and acute lymphoblastic leukemia (ALL) can complicate pregnancy. ALL is generally a disease of children and adolescents but may occasionally strike women in their 20s, 30s, and 40s. AML is a disease of young and elderly adults and is more common in women of childbearing age than ALL. Reynoso et al reported on 58 cases of acute leukemia; 35 were AML, 16 were ALL, 6 were acute leukemia not otherwise specified, and 1 was a case of the blast crisis phase of chronic myelogenous leukemia. Chronic leukemias are generally diseases of the elderly and are not dealt with here. There is no evidence that pregnancy causes acute leukemia, nor affects the prognosis.

The presenting characteristics of acute leukemia in the pregnant patient are similar to those found in the nonpregnant state. Typically, patients present with complications arising from pancytopenias: fatigue and weakness from anemia, bruising or bleeding from thrombocytopenia, and infection from leukopenia. Both AML and ALL can be associated with extremely elevated blast counts in the peripheral blood, which, if high enough, can result in leukostasis endangering both the mother and fetus.

Diagnosis of acute leukemia with bone marrow aspiration is a safe procedure during pregnancy, requiring only local anesthesia. In general, no other diagnostic tests are required, unless clinically warranted.

✳ MANAGEMENT

Acute leukemia can rapidly be fatal if treatment is delayed for even brief periods and therefore must be considered a medical emergency. Unless the fetus is sufficiently mature for delivery, the pregnant patient generally cannot delay therapy, because if infection occurs before the institution of antileukemic therapy, the risk of mortality to mother and fetus is very high.

Intensive chemotherapy is the standard of care for young pregnant patients with acute leukemia; however, every patient's care needs to be individualized. A consequence of intensive chemotherapy is a prolonged period of neutropenia during which the patient and her fetus are at great risk of life-threatening infection. Intravenous antibiotics are required as part of routine management. Complications from thrombocytopenia can generally be prevented by regular platelet transfusion. Anemia is treated with routine blood transfusions to prevent maternal and fetal tissue hypoxia. The fetus should be delivered at the earliest possible time when blood counts are adequate. Chemotherapeutic agents used in AML include daunorubicin and cytosine arabinoside. For treatment of acute promyelocytic leukemia, a subtype of AML, all-*trans* retinoic acid has been reported as safe for use in pregnancy in numerous case reports and represents an important part of the treatment regimen of this highly responsive form of leukemia. Treatment of ALL is more varied and may require regimen modification during pregnancy.

Outcome and Prognosis

Of the 58 patients reported by Reynoso, two suffered spontaneous abortions, three elected therapeutic abortion, and four patients had stillbirths. Of the remaining patients, about half delivered premature infants and the others carried to term. The major complications were related to neutropenia and infection, with severe maternal and fetal complications including sepsis, disseminated intravascular coagulation, and in one case, fetal death. The maternal prognosis from leukemia is generally no different than for the nonpregnant state.

EFFECTS OF THERAPY ON THE MOTHER AND FETUS
Chemotherapy

Many different chemotherapeutic agents are now available for use in the cancer patient, with many different mechanisms of action and toxicity profiles.

Chemotherapeutic drugs target rapidly proliferating cells, which, aside from malignant cells, can include both fetal and placental tissues, making their use potentially dangerous during pregnancy. Pregnancy can alter many of the drug's pharmacokinetic properties, including absorption, volume of distribution, protein-binding, half-life, and clearance.

The most serious potential toxicity of chemotherapy administered to pregnant women is bone marrow suppression with resultant neutropenia and thrombocytopenia. When the neutrophil count is less than $500/mm^3$, the patient is at high risk for serious bacterial or fungal infection. If fever develops with a neutrophil count below this level, prompt institution of broad-spectrum intravenous antibiotics is indicated, even if there is no apparent infection or source of fever. The longer the neutrophil count remains below $500/mm^3$, the greater the risk of serious bacterial infection; the longer the patient is treated with broad-spectrum antibiotics, the greater the risk of fungal infection. Even with prompt institution of intravenous antibiotics, infections can be lethal when the neutrophil count remains suppressed, and even if not lethal to the mother, they can result in sepsis, hypotension, and loss of the fetus. The use of recombinant human stem cell growth factors has been reported to be safe in pregnancy when used for neutropenia unrelated to chemotherapy.

Thrombocytopenia can lead to serious spontaneous (nontraumatic) hemorrhage when the platelet count is below $20,000/mm^3$, but hemorrhages are rare unless the platelet count falls below $10,000/mm^3$. Routine platelet transfusions are recommended for platelet counts below $10,000/mm^3$, but no guidelines exist for pregnancy, and therefore a more conservative value of $20,000/mm^3$ may be used as an indication for transfusion. Occasionally the patient will develop alloimmunization to platelets, and the platelet count will persist at dangerous levels in spite of transfusions. In this situation, the patient remains at risk for serious hemorrhage, including intracerebral, gastrointestinal, and peripartum bleeding.

Chemotherapeutic drugs are classified by their major modes of action. Extensive reviews of these drugs are beyond the scope of this chapter; only major modes of action, potential toxicities, and experience during pregnancy are discussed.

Alkylating Agents

Alkylating agents are prototypic chemotherapeutic agents and were among the first antineoplastic agents used. Cyclophosphamide is a commonly used agent and is active in breast cancer, Hodgkin's and non-Hodgkin's lymphomas, leukemias, and a variety of other malignancies. Alkylators bind to DNA bases, often at the N_7-guanine position, or the extracyclic oxygen, O_6-guanine. By binding at these and other sites on DNA, the alkylating agents can prevent DNA replication, either by blocking DNA polymerase directly, or by forming intrastrand or interstrand cross-links that prevent DNA polymerase from functioning normally. Cyclophosphamide can cross the placenta; however, the reduced oxidative capacity of the fetal liver limits the amount of active drug that is formed from the parent compound. Alkylators are known mutagens and several case reports document fetal malformations when cyclophosphamide was administered during the first trimester of pregnancy, often in conjunction with radiation.

Anthracyclines

The anthracyclines, including doxorubicin and daunorubicin, are used in the treatment of a wide variety of malignancies, including breast cancer, Hodgkin's disease and non-Hodgkin's lymphoma, and the acute leukemias. These agents work by intercalating DNA. They can cause significant, although transient, bone marrow suppression, particularly neutropenia. Congenital malformations caused by anthracyclines are rare even after treatment in the first trimester of pregnancy.

Large cumulative doses of anthracyclines may cause myocardial damage resulting in a cardiomyopathy that can be difficult to treat medically and has a high mortality rate. Although the elderly are particularly prone to this complication, possibly because of underlying heart disease, there is now evidence that children who receive anthracyclines may be at risk of developing cardiomyopathy later in life. Lipshultz et al reported that children treated with 228 mg/m^2 or more of doxorubicin had a 65% chance of developing either increased afterload or decreased contractility later in life, and that children under the age of 4 years were at greater risk. There is debate as to whether anthracyclines cross the placenta, but many feel they do; and the theoretical risk exists that their use could lead to cardiomyopathy in the child exposed *in utero*. Turchi reported the results of 28 pregnancies in patients treated with anthracyclines during pregnancy. In all 24 normal infants were born to these mothers, with bone marrow suppression seen in only an occasional infant, but cardiac disease was not reported.

Antimetabolites

Antimetabolite drugs include the nucleoside analogs, as well as the folic acid antagonists. Nucleoside analogs such as cytosine arabinoside (Ara-C) are used in the treatment of most hematologic malignancies. They act by being inserted into growing DNA strands during DNA replication and cause early termination of chain elongation. Ara-C has been used safely during the second and third trimesters of pregnancy, but fetal malformations have been reported with use in the first trimester, often associated with chromosomal abnormalities.

Methotrexate blocks the action of dihydrofolate reductase, an enzyme necessary to produce tetrahydrofolate, which is necessary, along with thymidylate synthetase, to produce thymidine nucleotides from uracil nucleotides. Without thymidine nucleotides, DNA cannot replicate. Methotrexate, when administered in high dose, suppresses the bone marrow, leading to pancytopenia, and can also cause mucositis and diarrhea. Methotrexate has been believed to be an abortifacient, possibly owing to effects on the placenta. In one study, when methotrexate was used in low doses in patients with rheumatic disease during the first trimester, of 10 pregnancies studied, 3 resulted in spontaneous abortion, 2 in therapeutic abortion, and 5 in full-term infants without obvious birth defects or delayed development. Because of these adverse fetal outcomes, methotrexate is used only rarely in pregnancy and never in the first trimester.

Radiation Therapy

Use of radiation therapy in a pregnant patient must take into account the anatomic location requiring radiation and its proximity to the fetus, the doses of radiation needed to control particular symptoms of the disease, and the trimester of pregnancy. As noted previously, in patients with Hodgkin's disease, radiation therapy could apparently be safely administered to the mediastinum in doses up to 4000 cGy, with beneficial effects to the mother and no apparent harmful effects to the fetus. Careful planning, adequate lead shielding of the gravid uterus, and simulated estimated fetal exposure should all be performed to limit fetal radiation dose. Aside from definitive treatment in Hodgkin's disease, radiation therapy is likely to be used to temporarily shrink a tumor that is compromising a vital structure or is causing unbearable local symptoms. In these circumstances, well-planned radiation therapy can be lifesaving for the mother and therefore for the fetus as well. Conversely, when radiation is administered to a woman who is unaware she may be pregnant, spontaneous abortion often occurs and therapeutic abortion is often recommended during the first trimester.

Fetal Outcome after Maternal Treatment for Cancer

Fetal outcome in the cancer patient depends on many factors, including the type of malignancy, the specific dangers posed to the mother and fetus by the malignancy, the trimester of pregnancy when the malignancy is discovered, fetal exposure to chemoradiotherapy in utero, and the amount of time required for safe delivery of the neonate. Perinatal complications of maternal treatment for malignancy can include spontaneous abortion and stillbirth, prematurity and low birth weight (a finding that may be influenced by attempts to deliver the fetus before term), fetal myelosuppression, and congenital malformation. Multiple reports suggest that the incidence of spontaneous abortion is increased in women treated for cancer during pregnancy. Methotrexate and other agents appear implicated in this complication. Myelosuppression of the fetus with neutropenia, thrombocytopenia, or both is seen in approximately 30% of patients receiving chemotherapy in the 4 weeks before delivery. In some cases neonatal sepsis has resulted from myelosuppression.

Congenital abnormalities may be increased in infants born to mothers who have received chemotherapy during pregnancy, particularly if administered in the first trimester. All chemotherapeutic agents are potentially mutagenic, but the alkylating agents are particularly so. In a series of 58 cases of leukemia monitored during pregnancy, there was only a single case of congenital malformation in one child of a twin pregnancy. This child later developed multiple malignancies as well. Similarly, there was one malformation noted in a series of infants born to mothers treated for Hodgkin's disease, but none were noted in a series of 85 live births after treatment for breast cancer.

◼ PREGNANCY IN THE CANCER SURVIVOR

The number of childhood, adolescent, and young adult cancer survivors in the United States continues to rise. It is estimated that by the year 2010, 1 in 250 young adults will be long-term survivors of childhood cancer. For the woman who has been previously treated for a malignancy, the decision to become pregnant is complicated and difficult. Many factors must be included in the discussion concerning a patient's desire to become pregnant. These factors include the patient's fertility after potentially sterilizing chemoradiotherapy, the risk of a poor neonatal outcome from prior chemotherapy, the risk of relapse during pregnancy or after childbirth, and the ability to carry a pregnancy to term after cardiac, pulmonary, or renal complications from cancer treatment.

Fertility after cancer treatment depends on the agents used in treatment, in addition to the age at which the patient was treated. Alkylating agents such as cyclophosphamide tend to be the most gonadotoxic drugs, whereas nonalkylators tend to be less sterilizing. When treatment occurs before puberty, sterility as a result of chemotherapy is less likely to occur because the prepubescent ovary may be resistant to chemotherapy induced damage. Despite this, attempts at preserving fertility by temporary suppression of ovarian function during chemotherapy have not been successful. Oocyte collection and preservation before cancer treatment may be an option for patients cycling before commencement of therapy.

The sterilizing effects of external beam radiotherapy are directly related to the proximity of the ovary to the treatment field and the radiation scatter delivered to the ovaries.

In general, women treated with chemotherapy and radiation more than a year before conception have no greater risk of a poor neonatal outcome than the general population. However, there have been recent reports of a higher incidence of perinatal mortality and low birth weight found in survivors of Wilms' tumor treated with abdominal radiotherapy and Hodgkin's disease survivors treated with combined chemoradiotherapy.

The prognosis for long-term remission varies with individual type of cancer and the stage at which the cancer was diagnosed before pregnancy. The probability of cancer recurrence is based on large groups of patients; therefore, an element of uncertainty always exists when counseling an individual patient contemplating pregnancy. Women with a high likelihood of relapse may find themselves dealing with recurrent cancer simultaneously with pregnancy or during the early years of a child's life and therefore are often counseled to defer pregnancy for 1 to 2 years after treatment. Relapses of cancer are rarely treated successfully (with the exception of Hodgkin's disease) and may be fatal to the mother, perhaps even before the fetus can safely be delivered. Later relapses may result in motherless children.

The issue of pregnancy after treatment for breast cancer is particularly complicated because of the concern that the high-estrogen state associated with pregnancy may stimulate an otherwise dormant breast cancer to grow. There is currently no evidence that pregnancy after treatment for breast cancer increases the chance of relapse from that cancer, or that these offspring are more likely to have birth defects than the general population.

Patients may be left with complications of either their diseases or therapies. Patients with Hodgkin's disease, for instance, have an inherent defect in T-cell immunity even before therapy, and this defect persists throughout life, even if they are cured of their disease. They may lose their previous immunity to infectious agents such as rubella and may respond poorly to currently administered immunizations. Patients may also have lung disease from bleomycin or radiation therapy, cardiac disease from doxorubicin or radiation therapy, or other complications of their previous treatment. All of these factors must be taken into account in counseling the woman who desires a pregnancy.

BIBLIOGRAPHY

Anselmo AP et al: Hodgkin's disease during pregnancy: diagnostic and therapeutic management, *Fetal Diagn Ther* 14:102, 1999.

Berry DL et al: Management of breast cancer during pregnancy using a standardized protocol, *J Clin Oncol* 17:855, 1999.

Blatt J: Pregnancy outcome in long-term survivors of childhood cancer, *Med Pediatr Oncol* 33:29, 1999.

Bonnier P et al: For the Société Française de Sénologie et de Pathologie: Chemotherapy in pregnancy, *Obstet Gynecol Clin North Am* 25:323, 1998.

Feliu J et al: Acute leukemia and pregnancy, *Cancer* 61:580, 1988.

Giacalone P-L, Laffargu F, Bénos P: Chemotherapy for breast carcinoma during pregnancy, *Cancer* 86:2266, 1999.

Haagensen CD, Stout AP: Carcinoma of the breast: criteria for operability, *Ann Surg* 118:859, 1943.

Incerpi MH, Miller DA, Posen R, Byrne JD: All-trans retinoic acid for the treatment of acute promyelocytic leukemia in pregnancy, *Obstet Gynecol* 89:826, 1997.

Johannsson O, Loman N, Borg Å, Olsson H: Pregnancy-associated breast cancer in BRCA1 and BRCA2 germline mutation carriers, *Lancet* 352:1359, 1988.

Kaufmann SJ, Sharif K, Sharma V, McVerry BA: Term delivery in a woman with severe congenital neutropenia, treated with growth colony stimulating factor, *Hum Reprod* 13:498, 1998.

King RM, Welch JS, Martin JK, Coulam CB: Carcinoma of the breast associated with pregnancy, *Surg Gynecol Obstet* 160:228, 1985.

Kozlowski RD et al: Outcome of first-trimester exposure to low-dose methotrexate in eight patients with rheumatic disease, *Am J Med* 88:589, 1990.

Lipshultz SE et al: Late cardiac effects of doxorubicin therapy for acute lymphoblastic leukemia in childhood, *N Engl J Med* 324:808, 1991.

Lishner M et al: Maternal and fetal outcome following Hodgkin's disease in pregnancy, *Br J Cancer* 65:114, 1992.

Mammaire Study Group: Influence of pregnancy on the outcome of breast cancer: a case-control study, *Int J Cancer* 72:720, 1997.

Mettlin C: Breast cancer risk factors: contributions to planning breast cancer control, *Cancer* 69:1904, 1992.

Nakamura K, Dan K, Iwakiri R, Gomi S, Nomura T: Successful treatment of acute promyelocytic leukemia in pregnancy with all-trans retinoic acid, *Ann Hematol* 71:263, 1995.

Nugent P, O'Connell TX: Breast cancer and pregnancy, *Arch Surg* 120:1221, 1985.

Ohba T et al: Aplastic anemia in pregnancy: treatment with cyclosporine and granulocyte-colony stimulating factor, *Acta Obstet Gynecol Scand* 78:458, 1999.

Petrek JA, Dukoff R, Rogatko A: Prognosis of pregnancy-associated breast cancer, *Cancer* 67:869, 1991.

Reynoso EE et al: Acute leukemia during pregnancy: the Toronto Leukemia Study Group experience with long-term follow-up of children exposed in utero to chemotherapeutic agents, *J Clin Oncol* 5:1098, 1987.

Trapido EJ: Age at first birth, parity and breast cancer risk, *Cancer* 51:946, 1983.

Treves H, Holleb AI: A report of 549 cases of breast cancer in women 35 years of age or younger, *Surg Gynecol Obstet* 107:271, 1958.

Turchi JJ, Villasis C: Anthracyclines in the treatment of malignancy in pregnancy, *Cancer* 61:435, 1988.

Velasquez WS et al: Radiotherapy during pregnancy for clinical stages IA-IIA Hodgkin's disease, *Int J Radiat Oncol Biol Phys* 23:407, 1992.

Wallack MK et al: Gestational carcinoma of the female breast, *Curr Probl Cancer* 7:1, 1983.

Woo SY et al: Pharmacology of antineoplastic agents in pregnancy, *Crit Rev Oncol/Hematol* 16:75, 1994.

Zemlickis D et al: Maternal and fetal outcome after breast cancer in pregnancy, *Am J Obstet Gynecol* 166:781, 1992.

Zuazu J et al: Pregnancy outcome in hematologic malignancies, *Cancer* 67:703, 1991.

CHAPTER 75

Seizures in Pregnancy

Phyllis Jen

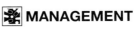 EPIDEMIOLOGY

Epilepsy is the most frequent neurologic problem encountered in pregnancy, occurring in 0.4% of all pregnancies. The majority (87%) of pregnant women with seizures during pregnancy have a history of seizure disorder, whereas 13% have a seizure for the first time during pregnancy. Pregnant women who have their first seizure during pregnancy should have eclampsia ruled out and should undergo immediate and thorough evaluation for underlying neurologic disease.

In pregnant women with a history of epilepsy, the frequency of seizures remains approximately the same in 50%, increases in 45%, and decreases in 5%. Increased seizure frequency can occur for many reasons: metabolic and hormonal changes that alter drug levels, noncompliance with medications, sleep deprivation, and possibly, hormonally mediated changes in seizure threshold.

RISK OF CONGENITAL MALFORMATIONS AND ADVERSE PERINATAL OUTCOME

Women with epilepsy have a two to three times increased incidence of infant congenital malformations compared with women without epilepsy. In addition, there is a two times increased risk of unfavorable perinatal outcome (stillbirth, low birth weight, mental retardation, microcephaly). Factors that contribute to the risk include maternal epilepsy, the occurrence of seizures during pregnancy, and the teratogenicity of antiepilepsy therapy. Maternal seizures can be associated with injury, postictal apnea and acidosis, and subsequent fetal hypoxia. In utero exposure to antiepilepsy drugs is associated with an adverse outcome incidence of 9% compared with a 3% incidence in infants with no drug exposure.

Congenital malformations, either from maternal epilepsy or from medications, can be major or minor anomalies. Major anomalies such as cardiac septal or neural tube defects, skeletal abnormalities, and mental retardation result from developmental derangements occurring in the first trimester. It is unclear which of the antiepilepsy drugs are the most teratogenic (all are in Food and Drug Administration category D); however, increased rate of congenital mal-

formations (especially neural tube defects) have been noted with valproate and primidone. Increased risk is also noted when drugs are used in high daily doses, in combination or with benzodiazepines (see Chapter 61).

MANAGEMENT
Goals

The goal of management of epilepsy in pregnancy is to prevent seizures while judiciously administering antiepilepsy medications at the lowest effective dose. Medication withdrawal before pregnancy should be considered if a woman has been seizure free for 2 years or has not had a grand mal seizure.

A woman who has an active seizure disorder should be counseled (preferably before conception) that she has a 90% chance of a normal child, but her risk of poor outcome or congenital anomalies is twice the normal rate, and that the occurrence of a seizure increases her risk. If antiepilepsy drug treatment is needed, monotherapy at the lowest effective dose should be used. Women on valproate or primidone should be taken off the medication unless all other agents have failed, and combinations using valproate or carbamazepine should be avoided, if possible. If seizures are controlled, there does not seem to be any benefit to switching to phenobarbital or any other medication. All women should be advised before conception to have adequate amounts of folic acid through diet or supplements. The combination of ultrasound and fetoprotein testing can identify 90% of neural tube anomalies.

Monitoring Levels and Treatment Changes

Frequent monitoring of drug levels during pregnancy is essential, preferably at trough levels. Increased clearance of medications during pregnancy requires an increase in the dosage, especially in the third trimester. If dosages are being adjusted, levels should be checked weekly. If levels are in therapeutic range, they should be rechecked monthly throughout pregnancy, then weekly after delivery. If seizures continue and compliance and sleep deprivation are not factors, a second drug may need to be added.

Treatment of Status Epilepticus

Treatment of status epilepticus requires aggressive in-hospital treatment. Blood samples should be taken for analysis of glucose level, drug levels, toxic screen, electrolyte levels, and blood gas; and intravenous glucose should be administered. Eclampsia should be ruled out. Adequate airway and oxygenation should be maintained, and precautions should be taken against aspiration. Lorazepam, 4 mg intravenously (IV), up to maximum of 8 mg; diazepam, 1 to 2 mg/min IV, up to a maximum of 20 mg IV; or phenytoin, up to 50 mg/min IV to a total of 18 mg/kg, can be used. If this fails to stop seizures, phenobarbital up to 100 mg/min IV can be given. Rarely, general anesthesia with halothane is required.

Bleeding Problems in the Newborn

Newborns of mothers on phenytoin or barbiturates may have decreased levels of vitamin K-dependent clotting factors and may experience bleeding problems soon after delivery. This can be prevented by giving oral vitamin K to the mother for 1 week before delivery and IV or intramuscular (IM) vitamin K to the newborn after delivery. This may need to be continued if results of clotting studies are persistently abnormal in the neonate. Mothers can safely breastfeed while taking all anticonvulsants, antiepilepsy medications except phenobarbital.

BIBLIOGRAPHY

Delgado-Escueta AV, Janz D: Consensus guidelines: preconception counseling, management and care of the pregnant woman with epilepsy, *Neurology* 42(4 suppl 5):149, 1992.

Kaneko S, Baltino D: Congenital malformations due to antiepileptic drugs, *Epilepsy Res* 33:145, 1999.

Samren EB, vanDuijn CM: Antiepileptic drug regimens and major congenital abnormalities in the offspring, *Ann Neurol* 46:739, 1999.

CHAPTER 76

Thyroid Disease in Pregnancy

Douglas S. Ross

ALTERATIONS IN MATERNAL THYROID FUNCTION DURING PREGNANCY

The most clinically significant change during pregnancy is a twofold to threefold increase in serum thyroxine binding globulin (TBG) levels. As a result total thyroxine (T_4) and triiodothyronine (T_3) concentrations in pregnant women are increased, whereas free thyroid hormone levels remain within the normal range (see Chapter 13). Serum thyroid-stimulating hormone (TSH) measurements are normal, although human chorionic gonadotropin (hCG) is a weak thyroid stimulator that may cause a slight rise in free thyroid hormone levels and a fall in serum TSH concentrations, usually within the normal range. In 10% to 20% of normal women, serum TSH concentrations are transiently low resulting in subclinical hyperthyroidism; these women do not require treatment. Hyperthyroidism may be more severe when very high hCG levels are associated with hyperemesis gravidarum. The thyroid enlarges slightly during pregnancy; however, in areas of borderline iodine intake, a substantial goiter may develop.

THYROID FUNCTION IN THE FETUS

The fetal thyroid begins to concentrate iodine and produce iodinated thyronines by 10 to 12 weeks. TSH is also detectable as early as 10 weeks; however, negative feedback may not fully develop until the third trimester. Iodine, propylthiouracil (PTU), methimazole, thyrotropin-releasing hormone (TRH), and thyroid-stimulating and blocking immunoglobulins cross the placenta well, whereas there is minimal transfer of thyroid hormones and no transfer of maternal TSH. The neonate experiences a surge in serum TSH concentrations that lasts 48 hours; fetal and neonatal T_3 levels are lower than those of children and adults.

MATERNAL HYPOTHYROIDISM

Fertility is impaired in hypothyroidism. However, studies using TSH measurements suggest that 0.4% to 2.5% of pregnant women may have mild or subclinical hypothyroidism. Maternal hypothyroidism is associated with an increased risk of spontaneous abortion (twofold), stillbirths, placental abruption, preeclampsia, and motor and mental retardation in the neonate. Children aged 7 to 9 years whose mothers had elevated serum TSH concentrations in the second trimester have a significant reduction in IQ scores. Therefore, unless there are serious cardiovascular contraindications, pregnant hypothyroid patients should be started on full replacement doses of thyroid hormone with titration of dose to obtain a normal serum TSH level. Some studies have suggested that the risk of miscarriage is better correlated with thyroid autoantibody titers than thyroid hormone levels.

Hypothyroid women on replacement levothyroxine may require an increased dose during pregnancy because hormone requirements are increased. TSH should be measured early during pregnancy and levothyroxine dose retitrated to normalize serum TSH level. At least one more TSH measurement should be made later in pregnancy.

MATERNAL HYPERTHYROIDISM

Thyrotoxicosis complicates about 0.2% of all pregnancies. Most patients have Graves' disease; however, other causes of hyperthyroidism may be present (see Chapter 13), and trophoblastic disease must be considered as the cause of the hyperthyroidism. It is difficult to confirm the diagnosis of subacute lymphocytic thyroiditis in pregnancy because determination of the radioiodine uptake is contraindicated. One can assume that hyperthyroidism that spontaneously resolves is due to thyroiditis; however, pregnancy also has an ameliorating effect on Graves' hyperthyroidism, and flares are commonly seen postpartum.

Hyperthyroidism complicating pregnancy is best prevented by treating Graves' disease with radioiodine or surgery before pregnancy (see Chapter 13). Poorly controlled hyperthyroidism is associated with spontaneous abortion, premature labor, low birth weight, preeclampsia, and congestive heart failure. Mild hyperthyroidism is generally well tolerated by mother and fetus, so the goal of therapy is to prevent overtreatment and accept mild hyperthyroidism. Beta-blockers can be given for symptoms. Older, poorly controlled studies reported rare growth retardation, hypoglycemia, and respiratory depression. More recent studies have disputed these findings, so these medications are considered safe to use during pregnancy. Radioiodine is absolutely contraindicated during pregnancy, and surgery is relatively contraindicated, so patients are managed with antithyroid drugs. Because of reports of a scalp defect, aplasia cutis, which occurs with methimazole therapy, propylthiouracil (PTU) is the antithyroid drug of choice. PTU should be given in the smallest doses necessary to control significant hyperthyroid symptoms to prevent fetal goiter and hypothyroidism. Pregnant women on PTU should have monthly thyroid function tests, as it can take 2 to 6 weeks to see any change in thyroid function. It is essential to appreciate the effects of TBG excess on total hormone values and to monitor free T_4 and T_3 concentrations, as TSH level may be subnormal throughout the pregnancy. Many patients can be weaned off PTU during the later stages of pregnancy as the hyperthyroidism becomes less severe. Levothyroxine should not be given with PTU, because it does not cross the placenta well and masks overtreatment.

FETAL AND NEONATAL HYPOTHYROIDISM

Excessive PTU therapy can lead to fetal hypothyroidism and goiter. Fetal goiter is rarely large enough to cause strangulation; however, this complication has been seen when pharmacologic iodine has been administered during pregnancy complicated by hyperthyroidism. Fetal thyroid size and fetal development should be monitored with ultrasound. Recently some have advocated percutaneous umbilical vein blood sampling for thyroid function tests. Intraamniotic or fetal intramuscular levothyroxine has been used to treat fetal hypothyroidism.

Congenital hypothyroidism complicates 1/4000 births and is now frequently assessed by neonatal screening. Children treated immediately after birth have normal development and usually have minimal neuropsychologic sequelae.

FETAL AND NEONATAL HYPERTHYROIDISM

Fetal and neonatal hyperthyroidism complicates about 2% of pregnancies in women with Graves' disease. The cause is transplacental transfer of thyroid-stimulating immunoglobulin (TSI). Mothers with a history of Graves' disease who have had their glands ablated (radioiodine or surgery) may still have significant TSI titers and give birth to children with thyrotoxicosis, even though they are euthyroid and are receiving levothyroxine replacement therapy. TSI should be measured early in the second trimester of such women; most cases of neonatal Graves' disease have occurred in mothers who have TSI titers that exceed 500% of normal.

Fetal thyrotoxicosis can lead to craniosynostosis and retarded growth and intellect. Fetal ultrasound can detect goiter, advanced bone age, and poor development. Fetal heart rates greater than 160 may suggest fetal hyperthyroidism. PTU may be given to a euthyroid mother to treat fetal hyperthyroidism, aiming for a fetal heart rate of 140. Percutaneous umbilical vein sampling may be used to monitor thyroid function. Neonatal hyperthyroidism may result 7 to 10 days after delivery as a result of persistent maternal TSI and falling PTU levels in the neonate.

THYROID NODULES DURING PREGNANCY

Thyroid scintigraphy is contraindicated during pregnancy. Fine needle aspiration can safely be done and will usually reassure patient and physician. Many small intrathyroidal papillary cancers can wait until after delivery for surgical excision with little risk to the patient. More aggressive neoplasms may require surgical intervention during pregnancy.

BIBLIOGRAPHY

Burrow GN: Thyroid function and hyperfunction during gestation, *Endocr Rev* 14:194, 1993.

Haddow JE et al: Maternal thyroid deficiency during pregnancy and subsequent neuropsychological development of the child, *N Engl J Med* 341:549, 1999.

Mandel SJ et al: Increased need for thyroxine during pregnancy in women with primary hypothyroidism, *N Engl J Med* 323:91, 1990.

McKenzie JM, Zakarija M: Fetal and neonatal hyperthyroidism due to maternal TSH receptor antibodies, *Thyroid* 2:155, 1992.

Moosa M, Mazzaferri EL: Outcome of differentiated thyroid cancer diagnosed in pregnant women, *J Clin Endocrinol Metab* 82:2862, 1997.

Roti E, Minelli R, Salvi M: Clinical review 80: Management of hyperthyroidism and hypothyroidism in the pregnant woman, *J Clin Endocrinol Metab* 81:1679, 1996.

Tan GH et al: Management of thyroid nodules in pregnancy, *Arch Intern Med* 156:2317, 1996.

Wassrstrum N, Anania CA: Perinatal consequences of maternal hypothyroidism in early pregnancy and inadequate replacement, *Clin Endocrinol* 42:353, 1995.

CHAPTER 77

Venous Thromboembolic Disease In Pregnancy

Samuel Z. Goldhaber

Pulmonary embolism (PE) is the leading cause of maternal death in the United Kingdom. It is gratifying that the number of cases has plummeted by two thirds since the mid 1950s. However, beginning in the 1980s, in the United States the number of fatal PEs has begun to increase, especially after vaginal delivery. In the mid 1990s, about two thirds of the fatal PEs occurred postpartum, with cesarean section accounting for approximately half of these catastrophic events (Fig. 77-1).

With respect to deep venous thrombosis (DVT), most occur in the left leg, probably because of disproportionate pressure on the left iliac vein by the gravid uterus. Two thirds of DVT occur during pregnancy, and the remainder occur postpartum. The risk of DVT is present throughout pregnancy, although it does increase during the third trimester. Of all antepartum DVT, about one fifth occur during the first trimester, one third during the second trimester, and almost one half during the third trimester. After delivery, two of the most important risk factors for DVT and PE are increased maternal age and cesarean section. Emergency cesarean section increases the venous thromboembolism (VTE) risk by about 50% compared with elective cesarean section (Fig. 77-2).

As expected, thrombophilia increases the risk of VTE during pregnancy and the puerperium. In one case-control study, the prevalence of factor V Leiden was 44% among women with a history of VTE during pregnancy or the puerperium, and the prevalence of the prothrombin gene mutation was 17%. Compared with controls, the Leiden mutation increased the risk of VTE ninefold, and the prothrombin gene mutation increased the risk by a factor of 15. The combination of the Leiden and prothrombin gene mutations virtually multiplied the risk, estimated to be 107 times greater than control. Fortunately, the absolute risk of VTE among carriers of each mutation was low: 0.2% for Leiden and 0.5% for the prothrombin gene. However, among those few women with both thrombophilic mutations, the absolute risk soared to 4.6%. The usually low absolute risk argues against routine screening for thrombophilia among healthy women who are considering pregnancy.

Thrombophilia has also been implicated in otherwise unexplained recurrent pregnancy loss. The factor V Leiden mutation appears to double the risk of fetal loss, possibly because of an increased frequency of placental vein thrombosis. In addition to fetal demise, genetic thrombophilia appears to be associated with obstetrical complications, such as preeclampsia, abruptio placentae, fetal growth retardation, and stillbirth.

DIAGNOSIS

During pregnancy, workup for DVT is generally confined to venous ultrasonography. Equivocal cases are referred for magnetic resonance venography. Standard contrast venography, which used to be the next step in the diagnostic workup, is rarely used unless catheter intervention is contemplated with catheter directed thrombolysis, suction catheter thrombectomy, or balloon angioplasty and stenting; however, the workup for PE during pregnancy can be more problematic. The D-dimer enzyme-linked immunosorbent assay, which has a high negative predictive value, will rule out PE in more than 90% of patients when the D-dimer level is normal. However, the D-dimer level rises above normal during pregnancy and many other conditions, such as pneumonia, myocardial infarction, sepsis, cancer, and the postoperative state. Therefore, the D-dimer is generally not useful after the first trimester of pregnancy because of its low specificity when positive.

Pregnant patients undergo lung perfusion scanning as the principal imaging test. To minimize radiation exposure, one third of the conventional dose of technetium-99m-labeled albumin is administered, and the patient is scanned for three times as long, on average 60 minutes rather than 20 minutes. Under the "worst case scenario," pregnant patients are exposed to a total of 0.5 rads if they require a chest x-ray study (<0.0001 rad), ventilation perfusion lung scanning (about 0.02 rads), chest CT scan (about 0.03 rads), and contrast pulmonary angiography (about 0.4 rads). Exposure to radiation of less than 5 rads has generally been considered safe.

PREVENTION

Prevention of VTE during pregnancy is more reliable than attempting early detection and treatment. Venous ultrasonography is unsatisfactory as a screening test for DVT during pregnancy because of its low sensitivity for asymptomatic

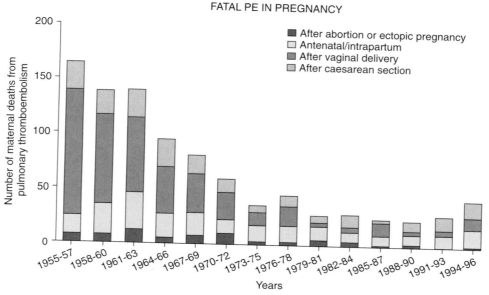

FIG. 77-1 Number of cases of fatal pulmonary embolism in pregnancy and the puerperium in England, 1955 to 1984, and in the United Kingdom, 1985 to 1996. (From the Confidential Enquiries into Maternal Deaths. Reprinted from Greer IA: *Lancet* 353:1258, 1999.)

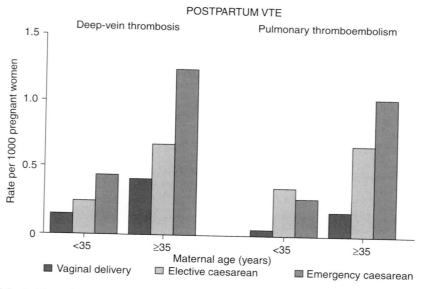

FIG. 77-2 Incidence of postpartum deep venous thrombosis and pulmonary embolism, according to maternal age and method of delivery. (From Greer IA: *Lancet* 353:1258, 1999.)

venous thrombosis. Therefore, preventive measures should be stressed during prepregnancy counseling sessions and throughout gestation. Mechanical prophylactic measures against VTE include vascular compression stockings and intermittent pneumatic compression devices. The principal pharmacologic preventive modality is low-dose unfractionated heparin or low-dose low-molecular-weight heparin. For patients at very high risk of VTE, combined mechanical and pharmacologic measures can be used.

Prolonged use of unfractionated heparin, even in "mini" doses of 5000 units twice daily, reduces bone density during

pregnancy, although fractures are uncommon. Warfarin cannot be used during the first trimester because it is teratogenic. In the United States, pregnant women rarely receive warfarin, even during the presumed "safe second trimester," except as a last resort. Warfarin embryopathy's clinical features can include short proximal limbs and phalanges, scoliosis, and a hypoplastic nose.

Neither unfractionated heparin nor low-molecular-weight heparin (LMWH) crosses the placenta. LMWH in prophylactic doses can be administered once daily and, for uncertain reasons, results in far less osteopenia and heparin-induced thrombocytopenia than unfractionated heparin. However, there are no rigorous randomized trials comparing unfractionated heparin and LMWH during pregnancy. Once daily doses of dalteparin (usually 5000 units) and enoxaparin (usually 40 mg) have been reported in case series to be safe and effective for VTE prophylaxis.

In an effort to prevent recurrent fetal loss in thrombophilic women, enoxaparin was administered in prophylactic doses of either 40 or 80 mg/day. Of 61 gestations prophylaxed with enoxaparin, 75% resulted in live births, compared with a live birth rate of 20% in these women before their being diagnosed with thrombophilia. Thus, enoxaparin appeared safe and effective in preventing pregnancy loss in thrombophilic women.

Case series of LMWH during pregnancy have identified fewer than 1000 women in whom LMWH was used. LMWH seems to be at least as safe and effective as unfractionated heparin. I wish there were a randomized clinical trial comparing LMWH with unfractionated heparin in the prevention and treatment of VTE during pregnancy; however, no such trial exists or is planned. Based on available data, I have switched to LMWH in my clinical practice. However, for women who have an uncertain delivery date because pharmacologic induction is not being planned, I revert to unfractionated heparin beginning about 3 weeks before the due date.

The excellent bioavailability and prolonged half-life of LMWH compared with unfractionated heparin prolong the anticoagulant effect, which, in turn, can complicate the administration of spinal or epidural anesthesia. Use of unfractionated heparin before delivery circumvents the tiny risk of epidural hematoma that has been reported in association with LMWH and epidural hematoma. Although exceedingly rare, epidural hematoma can result in permanent neurologic injury, even with emergency neurosurgical evacuation of the hematoma. LMWH has been implicated in about 50 cases reported to the Food and Drug Administration.

TASK FORCE RECOMMENDATIONS

The European Society of Cardiology's Task Force on PE has just released guidelines on diagnosis and treatment of PE during pregnancy. The Task Force endorsed the use of warfarin postpartum even in breastfeeding mothers. The guidelines state that "all diagnostic modalities, including CT scan and angiography, may be used without a significant risk to the fetus." Furthermore, the Task Force classified LMWHs as "probably safe" during pregnancy.

ANTICOAGULATION IN BREASTFEEDING WOMEN

Postpartum, oral anticoagulants such as warfarin and acenocoumarol are considered safe. However, the oral anticoagulant phenindione is contraindicated in breastfeeding women, according to the American Academy of Pediatrics. Both unfractionated heparin and LMWH are considered safe.

BIBLIOGRAPHY

Bloemenkamp KWM, Rosendaal FR, Helmerhorst FM, Vandenbroucke JP: Higher risk of venous thrombosis during early use of oral contraceptives in women with inherited clotting defects, *Arch Intern Med* 160:49, 2000.

Brandjes DPM et al: Randomised trial of effect of compression stockings in patients with symptomatic proximal-vein thrombosis, *Lancet* 349:759, 1997.

Brenner B et al: Gestational outcome in thrombophilic women with recurrent pregnancy loss treated by enoxaparin, *Thromb Haemost* 83:693, 2000.

Chan WS, Ray JG: Low molecular weight heparin use during pregnancy: issues of safety and practicality, *Obstet Gynecol* 54:649, 1999.

Chasan-Taber L, Stampfer MJ. Epidemiology of oral contraceptives and cardiovascular disease, *Ann Intern Med* 128:467, 1998.

Cummings SR et al: The effect of raloxifene on risk of breast cancer in postmenopausal women: results from the MORE randomized trial. Multiple Outcomes of Raloxifene Evaluation, *JAMA* 281:2189, 1999.

Daly E et al: Risk of venous thromboembolism in users of hormone replacement therapy, *Lancet* 348:977, 1996.

Douketis JD et al: The effects of long-term heparin therapy during pregnancy on bone density. A prospective matched cohort study, *Thromb Haemost* 75:254,1996.

Dulitzki M et al: Low-molecular-weight heparin during pregnancy and delivery. Preliminary experience with 41 pregnancies, *Obstet Gynecol* 87:380, 1996.

Fisher B et al: Tamoxifen for the prevention of breast cancer: report of the National Surgical Adjuvant Breast and Bowel Project P-1 Study, *J Natl Cancer Inst* 90:1371, 1998.

Gerhardt A et al: Prothrombin and factor V mutations in women with a history of thrombosis during pregnancy and the puerperium, *N Engl J Med* 342:374, 2000.

Goldhaber SZ, Visani L, De Rosa M: Acute pulmonary embolism: clinical outcomes in the International Cooperative Pulmonary Embolism Registry (ICOPER), *Lancet* 353:1386, 1999.

Goldhaber SZ et al: A prospective study of risk factors for pulmonary embolism in women, *JAMA* 277:642, 1997.

Grady D et al for the Heart and Estrogen/progestin Replacement Study Research Group: Postmenopausal hormone therapy increases risk for venous thromboembolic disease. The Heart and Estrogen/progestin Replacement Study, *Ann Intern Med* 132:689, 2000.

Greer IA: Thrombosis in pregnancy: maternal and fetal issues, *Lancet* 353:1258, 1999.

Grodstein F et al: Prospective study of exogenous hormones and risk of pulmonary embolism in Women, *Lancet* 348:983, 1996.

Hulley C et al: Randomized trial of estrogen plus progestin for secondary prevention of coronary heart disease in postmenopausal women. Heart and Estrogen/progestin Replacement Study (HERS) Research Group: *JAMA* 280:605,1998.

Hunt BJ et al: Thromboprophylaxis with low-molecular-weight heparin (Fragmin) in high risk pregnancies, *Thromb Haemost* 77:39, 1997.

Ito S: Drug therapy for breast-feeding women, *N Engl J Med* 343:118, 2000.

Jick H et al: Risk of hospital admission for idiopathic venous thromboembolism among users of postmenopausal oestrogens, *Lancet* 348:981, 1996.

Kupferminc MJ et al: Increased frequency of genetic thrombophilia in women with complications of pregnancy, *N Engl J Med* 340:9, 1999.

Lowe G et al: Thrombotic variables and risk of idiopathic venous thromboembolism in women aged 45-64 years. Relationships to hormone replacement therapy, *Thromb Haemost* 83:530, 2000.

Meinardi JR et al: Increased risk for fetal loss in carriers of the factor V Leiden mutation, *Ann Intern Med* 130:736, 1999.

Nelson-Piercy C, Letsky EA, de Swiet M: Low-molecular-weight heparin for obstetric thromboprophylaxis: experience of sixty-nine pregnancies in sixty-one women at high risk, *Am J Obstet Gynecol* 176:1062, 1997.

Parkin L et al: Oral contraceptives and fatal pulmonary embolism, *Lancet* 355:2133, 2000.

Ray JG, Chan WS: Deep vein thrombosis during pregnancy and the puerperium: a meta-analysis of the period of risk and the leg of presentation, *Obstet Gynecol Surv* 54:265, 1999.

Ridker PM et al: Factor V Leiden mutation as a risk factor for recurrent pregnancy loss, *Ann Intern Med* 128:1000, 1998.

Rosing J et al: Low-dose oral contraceptives and acquired resistance to activated protein C: a randomized cross-over study, *Lancet* 354:2036, 1999.

Sanson BJ et al: Safety of low-molecular-weight heparin in pregnancy: a systematic review, *Thromb Haemost* 81:668, 1999.

Task Force on Pulmonary Embolism, European Society of Cardiology: Guidelines on diagnosis and management of acute pulmonary embolism, *Eur Heart J* 21:1301, 2000.

Toglia MR, Weg JG: Venous thromboembolism during pregnancy, *N Engl J Med* 335:108, 1996.

Vandenbroucke JP et al: Increased risk of venous thrombosis in oral-contraceptive users who are carriers of factor V Leiden mutation, *Lancet* 344:1453, 1994.

Walrath K, Berkovitz P, Morrison R, Goldhaber SZ: Frequently asked questions of the Venous Thromboembolism Support Group. Brigham and Women's Hospital. 1999. Available at: http://web.mit.edu.karen/www/faq.html

Wellesley D, Moore I, Heard M, Keeton B: Two cases of warfarin embryopathy: a re-emergence of this condition? *Br J Obstet Gynaecol* 105:805, 1998.

CHAPTER 78

Urinary Tract Infections in Pregnancy

Stephanie A. Eisenstat

Urinary tract infections and acute pyelonephritis are common during pregnancy and pose a serious risk to the fetus. An association between urinary tract infections and increased risk of pyelonephritis development during pregnancy was reported in classic studies by Kass in 1960. Since that time multiple studies have confirmed that eradicating the urinary tract infection both decreases the risk of pyelonephritis and leads to improved fetal outcome. The relationship between bacteriuria and low birth weight was described by Kass in 1962. Data clearly demonstrate that screening for and then eradicating bacteriuria decrease the incidence of acute pyelonephritis and associated preterm birth.

This chapter summarizes the clinical recommendations regarding identification and treatment of bacteriuria, urinary tract infections, and pyelonephritis in pregnancy. A vast number of studies and books review this subject, with some key references listed at the end of this chapter. For more indepth discussion on evaluation and management of acute dysuria in women, see Chapter 23.

▦ EPIDEMIOLOGY

Multiple studies estimate that the prevalence of bacteriuria is similar in pregnant and nonpregnant women: 2% to 11%. Risk factors for persistent bacteriuria include lower socioeconomic status, sickle cell trait, and documented bacteriuria at the first prenatal visit. Early studies by Kunin suggested that the incidence of bacteriuria increased with age. However, age does not appear to be a factor if the woman is pregnant; rather bacteriuria appears to be correlated with parity. Women who have had more than three term pregnancies are at higher risk for bacteriuria.

Pyelonephritis occurs in 1% to 2% of all pregnancies and is one of the most serious infections in pregnancy. Preexisting bacteriuria is present in 60% of pregnant women.

DEFINITION

Bacteriuria, which can exist with or without symptoms of urinary tract infection, and is defined as the presence of more than 100,000 organisms/ml in a midstream clean-catch urine specimen. However, colony counts of less than 100,000/ml do not exclude infection; they may be low because of the timing of collection. If the urinary bacterial colony count is greater than 10,000 organisms/ml but less than 100,000 organisms/ml, a repeat urine culture should be obtained. *Repeat* urine culture results of less than 100,000 organisms/ml should be considered bacteriuria in the pregnant woman. Acute cystitis is defined as a positive urine culture and is associated with symptoms of frequency, dysuria, and urgency. Symptoms of fever, chills, nausea, and flank pain usually indicate acute pyelonephritis. Among women with acute pyelonephritis, urine cultures are invariably positive, and in 10% blood cultures are positive for this condition.

NORMAL PHYSIOLOGIC CHANGES DURING PREGNANCY

Various changes in the anatomy of the urinary tract during pregnancy predispose pregnant women to urinary tract infections and pyelonephritis. Dilation of the collecting system—renal calices, pelves, and ureters—begins during the first trimester and continues throughout pregnancy, probably a result of the dilating effect of progesterone on the smooth muscle of the tract. There is also an increase in renal length and compression of the bladder because of the enlarging of the uterus. These changes have been correlated with the increased risk of developing third-trimester pyelonephritis. Bacterial proliferation is promoted because of the urinary stasis, glycosuria, aminoaciduria, and incomplete emptying of the bladder.

PATHOGENS

The most common pathogens that cause bacteriuria and urinary tract infections in pregnancy are *Escherichia coli,* and *Klebsiella* and *Enterobacter* organisms. Other pathogens frequently isolated from women with bacteriuria include *Proteus mirabilis, Pseudomonas aeruginosa, Staphylococcus saphrophyticus,* enterococci, and group B beta-hemolytic streptococci. Group B beta-hemolytic streptococcal infection in the fetus can lead to severe morbidity and even death (see Chapter 67).

COMPLICATIONS OF BACTERIURIA

Acute pyelonephritis will develop during the pregnancy of 20% to 40% of pregnant women with bacteriuria. Bacteriuria is associated with acute pyelonephritis (usually occurring during the third trimester), anemia, toxemia, and chronic pyelonephritis in the mother. Acute pyelonephritis is more severe in pregnant women and has been associated with adult respiratory distress syndrome, hematologic abnormalities, renal insufficiency, and hypothalamic instability. For the infant there is an increased rate of prematurity and low birth weight, and some studies also suggest an increased rate of fetal infection, fetal wastage, and dorsal midline defects. Well-controlled studies have demonstrated that there is a marked reduction in the risk for pyelonephritis in women with bacteriuria who have been treated with antibiotics.

🏥 APPROACH TO THE PREGNANT PATIENT WITH URINARY TRACT INFECTION

Diagnostic Tests

Because up to 11% of pregnant women have asymptomatic bacteriuria, the recommendation of the American College of Obstetricians and Gynecologists is to obtain a urine culture in all pregnant women during the first prenatal visit (preferably before 16 weeks of gestation). Because fewer than 1% of pregnant women acquire asymptomatic bacteriuria during pregnancy, it is unnecessary to repeat screening. However, if symptoms (frequency, dysuria) of urinary tract infection occur, a repeat urine culture is indicated. Unfortunately more cost-effective testing measures—such as urine dipstick, urine for nitrates, urine for leukocytes, and rapid enzymatic urine screening tests—provide low sensitivity for identifying women with asymptomatic bacteriuria and therefore are not recommended as the initial screening measure. A Gram stain of the urine yields high results but is expensive.

The diagnosis of pyelonephritis is confirmed by positive urine culture and accompanying systemic symptoms (fever, rigors, chills, costovertebral angle-tenderness), or positive blood cultures or both.

🏥 MANAGEMENT

The goal of treatment is to eradicate the infection. The usual treatment is a complete course of antibiotics with follow-up cultures. Antibiotics cross the placenta; thus fetal safety needs to be considered. Standard therapies that are safe during pregnancy are noted in Table 78-1.

Choice of Therapy

Asymptomatic Bacteriuria or Urinary Tract Infection

Asymptomatic bacteriuria and urinary tract infection must be treated. Options for therapy appear in Table 78-1. Because of the emergence of resistance of *Eschericha coli* to Ampicillin, this is no longer considered the first line therapy. Rather, second and third-generation cephalosporins for acute urinary tract infections and nitrofurantoin, sulfixosazole or first generation cephalosporins for asymptomatic bacteriuria. The pregnant woman with acute symptomatic infection should be treated empirically until the results of urine culture are available. Traditionally 7- to 10-day courses have been used. Generally short course (1 or 3 day regimens) are

Table 78-1
Choice of Treatment for Urinary Tract Infections During Pregnancy

	Drug	Dosage
Asymptomatic bacteriuria or Acute cystourethritis	Nitrofurantoin	100 mg PO 7-10 days
	Cephalexin	250-500 mg PO qid 7-10 days
	Sulfisoxazole	500 mg PO qid 7-10 days
Pyelonephritis *Acute**	Cefazolin	1-2 g IV q6h 10-14 days and
	Tobramycin	3-5 mg/kg/day q8h
Chronic	Nitrofurantoin	50-100 mg PO qhs for duration of pregnancy
	Sulfisoxazole	500 mg PO bid for duration of pregnancy
Suppressive therapy†		
	Nitrofurantoin	100 mg qhs
	Sulfisoxazole	500 mg PO bid

* Intravenous until afebrile 48 hours, then consider oral therapy for total 10- to 14-day therapy. Follow-up urine culture; if positive, consider suppressive therapy.
† Complete 7-10 day course; if reinfected, then suppression for remainder of pregnancy.

not advised for pregnant women. Follow-up urine cultures 2 weeks after completion of treatment, are important to ensure that the infection is eradicated.

Pyelonephritis

Pregnant women with acute pyelonephritis should be treated with intravenous antibiotics. Because of the risk for severe complications with pyelonephritis during pregnancy, hospitalization is indicated. Fluid monitoring, rehydration, and fetal assessment are important. Because 30% of the women treated for pyelonephritis have persistent positive urine cultures, follow-up cultures and surveillance are important. If the urine culture remains positive for pyelonephritis and the patient's clinical condition is stable, suppressive therapy is indicated for the remainder of the pregnancy.

BIBLIOGRAPHY

Andriole VT, Patterson T: Epidemiology, natural history and management of urinary tract infections in pregnancy, *Med Clin North Am* 75:359, 1991.

Bachman J et al: A study of various tests to detect asymptomatic urinary tract infections in an obstetric population, *JAMA* 270:1971, 1993.

Cox S, Cunningham FG: Urinary tract infections. In Charles D, editor: *Obstetric and perinatal infections*, St Louis, 1993, Mosby.

Cunningham FG, Morris GB, Mickal A: Acute pyelonephritis in pregnancy: a clinical review, *Obstet Gynecol* 43:112, 1973.

Delzell JE, Lefevre ML: Urinary tract infections during pregnancy, *Am Fam Physician* 61:713, 2000.

Gilstrap et al: Renal infection and pregnancy outcome, *Am J Obstet Gynecol* 141:709, 1981.

Kass EH: Bacteriuria and pyelonephritis of pregnancy, *Arch Intern Med* 105:194, 1960.

Kass EH: Pyelonephritis and bacteriuria: a major problem in preventive medicine, *Ann Intern Med* 56:46, 1962.

Kass EH: The role of unsuspected infection in the etiology of prematurity, *Clin Obstet Gynecol* 16:134, 1973.

Kincaid-Smith P: Bacteriuria and urinary tract infection in pregnancy, *Lancet* 1:395, 1965.

Kreiger J: Complications and treatment of urinary tract infections in pregnancy, *Urol Clin North Am* 13:685, 1986.

Kunin CM: An overview of urinary tract infections. In *Detection, prevention and management of urinary tract infections,* ed, 3 Philadelphia, 1979, Lea & Febiger.

Lindheineir MD, Katz AI: The kidney in pregnancy, *N Engl J Med* 283:1095, 1970.

MacDonald P et al: Summary of a workshop on maternal genitourinary infections and the outcome of pregnancy, *J Infect Dis* 147:596, 1983.

McGregor JA, French JI: Prevention of preterm birth, *N Engl J Med* 339:1858, 1998.

McNeeley SG: Treatment of urinary tract infections during pregnancy, *Clin Obstet Gynecol* 31:480, 1988.

Naeye R: Causes of the excessive rates of perinatal mortality and prematurity in pregnancies complicated by maternal urinary tract infections, *N Engl J Med* 300:819, 1979.

Ovalle A, Levancini M: Urinary tract infections in pregnancy, *Curr Opin Urol* 11:55, 2001.

Pfau A, Sacks T: Effective prophylaxis for recurrent urinary tract infections during pregnancy, *Clin Infect Dis* 14:810, 1992.

Stamm WE et al: Diagnosis of coliform infection in acutely dysuric women, *N Engl J Med* 307:463, 1982.

Sweet RL: Bacteriuria and pyelonephritis during pregnancy, *Semin Perinatol* 1:25, 1977.

Waltzer W: The urinary tract in pregnancy, *Urol* 125:271, 1981.

Whalley P: Bacteriuria of pregnancy, *Am J Obstet Gynecol* 97:723, 1967.

Zinner H: Bacteriuria and babies revisited, *N Engl J Med* 300:853, 1979.

Zinner SH, Kass EH: Long term (10-14 years) follow-up of bacteriuria of pregnancy, *N Engl J Med* 285:820, 1971.

CHAPTER **79**

Breastfeeding and Mastitis

Ruth A. Lawrence

Breastfeeding is recommended for all infants under ordinary circumstances throughout the world. Even if the mother's diet is not perfect, it is still recommended, since the milk will be good. The health goals of the United States for the year 2010 include increasing the number of women who initiate breastfeeding to 75% and the number who are breastfeeding 6 months postpartum to at least 50% and at 1 year postpartum at least 25%. Early 2000 statistics indicate current rates of 59.7% and 21.6% at birth and at 6 months, respectively. The American Academy of Pediatrics has stated that some of the difficulty in increasing the number of breastfeeding mothers in Western countries is related to a lack of understanding among medical professionals about lactation.

ANATOMY AND PHYSIOLOGY OF LACTATION

Understanding the anatomy and physiology of lactation is important for any practitioner who cares for women. By understanding the physiologic characteristics of successful lactation, one can understand how to manage concurrent problems without interfering with the processing, as well as facilitate the process when it is faltering.

The first rudimentary breast tissues appear in both male and female embryos at about 8 weeks of gestation. Development of the breast in the fetus is used by neonatologists as one of the diagnostic landmarks to determine the gestational age of the infant at birth. After the development of a rudimentary duct system and the presence of a small areolar and nipple at birth, the breast is essentially dormant throughout early childhood until puberty (Fig. 79-1). In the female breast, development is one of the early signs of maturation. The nipple becomes more prominent and pigmented and is capable of becoming erect as the elastic tissue within it proliferates. The areolar increases in circumference and pigmentation. The presence of a significant breast bud at puberty is an important sign of female development. With each menstrual cycle the ductal system responds to the hormone milieu, slowly increasing in size and complexity in the next few years. With each menstrual cycle there is a microscopic increase in the breast ductal system until the age of 28, unless pregnancy ensues. At the onset of pregnancy, one of the early signs of conception that a woman perceives is the change in her breasts. The nipple and areolar increase in pigmentation and prominence. Montgomery's tubercles become visible and begin to secrete sebaceous material to protect the nipple and areola. The ductal system begins to proliferate and continues to do so for the first 16 weeks of gestation until the alveolar cells are capable of making milk.

The maternal body also builds up nutritional stores in the form of 8 to 10 pounds of body tissue intended to provide nutritional support for the production of milk. Milk is not actively produced until the placenta is removed, thus eliminating the source of prolactin-inhibiting hormone.

After birth the normal infant is prepared to nurse at the breast. The infant is born with the correct reflexes: the rooting reflex to "find" the breast and latch on and the coordinated suck and swallow reflex. Breastfeeding for the mother is not a reflex, and she needs to be taught how to position the infant on her breast and to trigger the infant's feeding reflexes.

Understanding the let-down reflex is basic to understanding human lactation (Fig. 79-2). When the infant suckles at the breast, a signal is sent to the brain via the nervous system, and the hypothalamus releases oxytocin and prolactin into the bloodstream. The oxytocin stimulates the myoepithelium cells surrounding the ductal system in the breast to contract and that results in the ejection of milk through the nipple. During the first week or two postpartum until the uterus totally involutes, the myoepithelial cells in the uterus also respond by contracting and tightening the uterine muscle (it may cause "after pains" for a day or so postpartum). As a result, a lactating woman does not need methylergonovine maleate (Methergine) to control uterine bleeding postpartum. The release of oxytocin can also be triggered through other sensory pathways such as hearing the infant cry, seeing the infant, or thinking about feeding time. The release of prolactin into the bloodstream, on the other hand, stimulates the lacteal cells to make milk. It triggers the Golgi apparatus and reticuloendothelium to move nutrients into the lumen of the alveolus. Prolactin levels are high during pregnancy and lactation. It is the surge of prolactin doubling baseline levels that initiate milk production. Prolactin is released only when the breast is stimulated by suckling or manual or mechanical pumping, but not by other sensory stimulus. Pain, stress, and anxiety interfere with let-down.

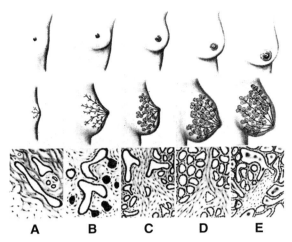

FIG. 79-1 Female breast from infancy to lactation with corresponding cross section and duct structure. **A, B,** and **C,** Gradual development of well-differentiated ductular and peripheral lobular-alveolar system. **D,** Ductular sprouting and intensified peripheral lobular-alveolar development in pregnancy. Glandular luminal cells begin actively synthesizing milk fat and proteins near term: only small amounts are released into lumen. **E,** With postpartum withdrawal of luteal and placental sex steroids and placental lactogen, prolactin is able to induce full secretory activity of alveolar cells and release of milk into alveoli and smaller ducts. (From Lawrence RA, Lawrence RM: *Breastfeeding: a guide for the medical profession,* ed 5, St Louis, 1999, Mosby.)

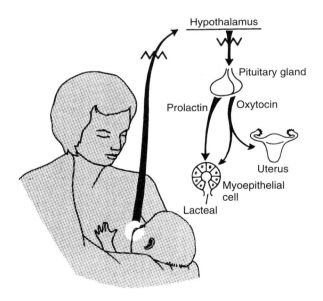

FIG. 79-2 Diagram of ejection reflex. When the infant suckles the breast, mechanoreceptors in nipple and alveola are stimulated and a stimulus along nerve pathways to the hypothalamus, which stimulates the posterior pituitary to release oxytocin. Oxytocin is carried via the bloodstream to breast and uterus. Oxytocin stimulates myoepithelial cells in the breast to contract and eject milk from the alveolus. Prolactin is secreted by the anterior pituitary gland in the let-down reflex. The sight or cry of an infant can stimulate the release of oxytocin but not of prolactin. (From Lawrence RA, Lawrence RM: *Breastfeeding: a guide for the medical profession,* ed 5, St Louis, 1999, Mosby.)

BENEFITS OF BREASTFEEDING

Nutrition and Growth

The human infant, who is born the most immature of all mammals (except the marsupials), has a particularly immature brain and nervous system at birth. Thus in the early days, weeks, and months of life the brain grows significantly. The brain doubles in size in the first year of life. This is reflected by the fact that the head circumference increases 4 inches in the first year and will only increase another 4 inches in the next 16 years. The constituents of human milk are specifically designed for optimal brain growth, as well as optimal physical growth. The nutritional benefits of human milk include the specific protein profile of ideal amino acids that are easily digested and completely absorbed. Also easily digested, absorbed, and essential for brain growth are special fat components, including polyunsaturated fats, cholesterol, and docosahexaenoic acid (DHA). Human milk contains cholesterol, whereas infant formula has not contained cholesterol for several decades. Cholesterol is a vital, basic constituent of brain tissue, myelin, and many enzymes in the human body. The microminerals such as copper and zinc are in perfect proportion to infant needs. Human milk contains dozens of enzymes that interact during the digestion of the milk itself, as well as interacting with the mucosal layer of the gut to enhance its development and improve its use and absorption of nutrients.

Immunologic Advantages

The infection protection provided by the immunoglobulins and other special constituents of human milk protect the newborn infant from gastrointestinal disease, as well as respiratory disease, ear infections, and other general infections. In developing nations this can be easily demonstrated by the fact that infants who are not breastfed have a 50% chance of dying from infection in the first year of life. The immunologic advantages of human milk are beginning to be recognized as science explores the intricacies of the immunologic protection provided. Epidemiologic studies have been published that reveal a protective effect of breastfeeding for at least 4 months against the childhood onset of diabetes, childhood cancers, Crohn's disease, and other gastrointestinal illnesses. An associated delayed onset of allergic symptoms, especially eczema and asthma, is also reported in infants who are exclusively breastfed.

Advantages to the Mother

Some of the advantages to the mother who breastfeeds are related to the physiologic features of the postpartum period. Breastfeeding immediately decreases the potential for uterine hemorrhage and enhances the involution of the uterus. The uterus of the lactating woman returns to its prepregnant state much more quickly than that of the woman who does not breastfeed. The weight loss in the postpartum period associated with lactation in most cases exceeds the weight loss of women who do not breastfeed. Long-range studies of women who breastfeed suggest that there is a lessened potential for obesity associated with childbirth for those women who breastfeed. Other long-term advantages include a decreased incidence of breast and ovarian cancers and a decreased incidence of long-term osteoporosis in women who breastfeed compared with those who bear children and do not breastfeed. In psychologic studies women who breastfed have higher self-esteem and mother their children differently. By understanding the tremendous benefits of breastfeeding to both the mother and infant, the clinician can better assess the risk/benefit ratio when confronted with a possible contraindication to breastfeeding, as the benefits usually far outweigh any risks.

DISADVANTAGES AND CONTRAINDICATIONS OF BREASTFEEDING

The only disadvantage of breastfeeding that has been documented is that only the mother can feed her infant. From the infant's standpoint, however, this means that the mother always gives the intimate attention the infant needs, and the important one-on-one relationship that was identified by Spitz many years ago in his studies of orphan children is protected by the mother's breastfeeding. A father who wishes to participate in his child's care has the important task of providing nonnutrient cuddling. Infants may often need to be cuddled when they do not need to be fed. When a breastfeeding mother cuddles her infant, the infant may root and nuzzle to be fed when feeding is not necessary. The infant smells the mother's milk. On the other hand, when the father cuddles the infant the infant is not fed and settles down quickly.

The most common reason for a woman not to breastfeed is a lack of desire to do so. From a medical standpoint there are a few clinical situations in which breastfeeding is not recommended. In industrialized countries today when there is an acceptable alternative, infants born to mothers who are human immunodeficiency virus (HIV)-positive should not be breastfed, according to the present understanding of the spread of the disease. Any infant born to a mother who is hepatitis B-positive should receive hepatitis immune globulin, as well as the first of the series of three hepatitis vaccine immunizations. The infant can be breastfed immediately if he will receive these two injections. When the mother has a medical disease that requires medications that might pass into the breast milk, it is important to know whether the drug might be contraindicated for the infant (Box 79-1). When a physician is concerned about a medication in a lactating woman, specific information should be obtained from

---

BOX 79-1
Drugs That Are Contraindicated During Breastfeeding

Cyclophosphamide
Cyclosporine
Doxorubicin
Ergotamine
Methotrexate
Phenindione
Drugs of Abuse
   Amphetamine
   Cocaine
   Heroin
   Marijuana
   Phencyclidine (PCP)

---

resources competent to provide information about lactation. Many resources that provide general information about medication do not give accurate information about the appearance of the compound in breast milk nor its risk to the infant.

The infant who has severe galactosemia at birth and is identified to have a deficiency of galactose-1-phosphate uridyl transferase does not tolerate lactose and thus cannot be breastfed. This infant must receive lactose-free formula.

MANAGEMENT IN THE IMMEDIATE POSTPARTUM PERIOD

Ensuring Good Milk Supply

The initiation of a good milk supply begins immediately after birth with the first feeding, which ideally takes place in the birthing area while the infant is alert and ready to suckle. After an hour or so of active, alert behavior, the infant will drift off to sleep and be difficult to arouse to feed for 4 to 6 hours. Infants best latch on to the breast when they are alert and hungry, not when they are sleeping or exhausted from crying hard.

The postpartum hospital staff is responsible for assisting the nursing dyad, but the physician may be called on to respond to maternal illness or concerns or to problems with the infant such as jaundice, excessive weight loss, or illness. An understanding of normal lactation is necessary to manage the problems without interfering with successful lactation. In general, the major cause of sore nipples and milk production problems can be solved by proper positioning at the breast and attention to suckling long enough to get the fat-laden hind milk. Introducing a bottle to the schedule in the first few weeks does not improve the milk production but diminishes it as the breast makes more milk in response to milk removal. The breast adapts to the infant's needs. As milk is taken by the infant, more is produced.

Illness and Breastfeeding

Minor illnesses in the mother such as a cold or flu, bladder infection, endometritis, or mild toxemia are not a contraindication to breastfeeding. The milk in fact will provide the infant with mother's antibodies and protect against infection. Hypothyroidism and its treatment with thyroid hormone are *not* contraindications. Hyperthyroidism treated with propylthiouracil is *not* a contraindication, but the use of thiouracil and iodine should be avoided. Asthma that is controlled with inhalants or with low-dose corticosteroids is not a contraindication. When a mother has persistent toxemia, hypertension, or cardiovascular disease, diuretics, antihypertensives, and sedatives should be prescribed that have the least tendency to get into the milk (nadolol rather than captopril, furosemide rather than chlorothiazide, magnesium sulfate or phenobarbital rather than morphine).

Poor Milk Supply

The most common causes of poor milk supply are inadequate information on breastfeeding and lack of support in the early initiation of lactation. Proper positioning at the breast with the infant facing the mother looking at the breast is fundamental to success: presenting the breast, supported by mother's hand, well back of the nipple and areolar. When the infant's lower lip is stimulated by the nipple, the infant opens the mouth wide and draws the breast into the mouth, elongating the areola into a teat that is compressed against the hard palate. The natural, undulating, or peristaltic motion of the tongue moves the milk from the ampulla of the ducts to be ejected through the nipple. Initially it takes 2 to 3 minutes for the reflex to start the flow of milk. After the first week it occurs more quickly. It also takes a few minutes for the fat to get into the milk, as the fat globules have to come together in the lacteal cells and pass into the lumen of the alveolus. The fat globule is enveloped by a membrane and suspended in the solution. The early milk at each feeding is low in fat, but the later or hind milk is rich in fat and thus in calories and fat-soluble vitamins. Infants who do not nurse long enough on one breast may not get this valuable nutrition and thus receive insufficient calories to gain weight. The physician's role is to rule out any true abnormality but also to instill confidence in the mother and see that the mother is provided with the necessary support and encouragement through the trained office staff or nurse practitioner, who will attend to details and assure that the mother is psychologically supported. Fatigue is a common cause of a failing milk supply. Assessing the mother's opportunities for adequate rest is an initial step. Mothers may need to be taught how to nap when the infant naps and how to set priorities for other activities in the early postpartum period. The infant's needs come first until the milk supply is well established.

When poor milk supply, resulting in failure to thrive in the infant, is not resolved by minor adjustments in positioning and timing, it requires a diagnostic evaluation to identify possible infant causes (Fig. 79-3) and possible maternal causes. A complete history of the pregnancy, delivery, diet,

and habits may identify a cause. The breasts should increase in size during pregnancy, and the nipples and areolae become more pigmented. Lack of breast changes suggests a fundamental organ failure. If the breasts do not become mildly to moderately engorged postpartum and especially if there is excessive vaginal bleeding there may be retained placenta. A small amount of placental tissue may produce enough prolactin-inhibiting hormone to suppress full lactation. If the mother had a severe hemorrhage or crisis during delivery, the pituitary gland could have been shocked, producing transient or permanent hypopituitarism known as Sheehan's syndrome. The classic diagnostic finding in Sheehan's syndrome is failure of breasts to become engorged. Transient hypopituitarism may respond to the use of nasal spray oxytocin to initiate lactation. A few drops are instilled on the mother's nasal mucous membranes just before she puts the infant to the breast for a feeding. This will stimulate letdown and, when administered with each feeding for 2 to 3 weeks, may lead to an increasing milk supply. Oxytocin is no longer available as Syntocin nasal spray. It must be prescribed as the intramuscular solution, placed in a nasal dropper bottle by the pharmacist. The dose of this more dilute preparation (10 units/ml) is now 4 drops in the nares just before putting the infant to the breast. The injectable form is one-fourth the concentration of the original Synotocin.

Analysis of the blood levels of prolactin is available through most hospital laboratories by radioimmunoassay. The baseline level of prolactin gradually decreases over time. Postpartum from levels well above 100 ng/ml drop to just under 100 ng/ml; the normal range for nonpregnant nonlactators is usually 10 to 25 ng/ml. It is not the baseline that is diagnostic but the surge of prolactin produced by

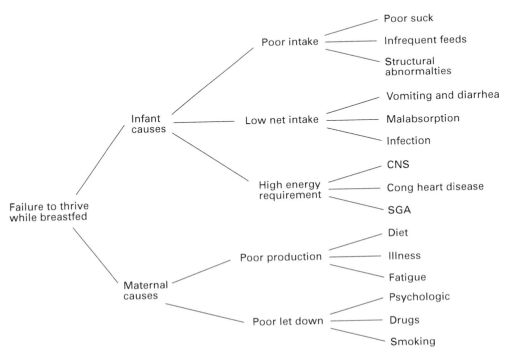

FIG. 79-3 Diagnostic flowchart for failure to thrive. (From Lawrence RA, Lawrence RM: *Breastfeeding: a guide for the medical profession*, ed 5, St Louis, 1999, Mosby.)

stimulus of the breast through infant suckling or mechanical breast pumping. The standard procedure is to insert an intravenous line with a heparin lock; allow the mother to recover from the needle stick, which can elevate prolactin level slightly; draw a baseline level; and then draw a second level after 10 minutes of full breast stimulus. The surge should double the baseline level. A failure to develop an adequate response to suckling suggests that prolactin insufficiency is responsible for the inadequate milk production.

Medical stimulus of prolactin has been demonstrated by maternal use of meclopromide (Reglan), 10 mg, three times a day. Published studies report use in women pumping to provide milk for their premature or ill infants who cannot nurse at the breast. It is also reported to be successful in women with faltering milk supply. Some medications, including bromocriptine and L-dopamine, suppress prolactin production, and their use could be the cause of the low prolactin levels. A complete history of all medications and ingestants may lead to the identification of a prolactin suppressant. This includes a review of natural foods, herbs, and teas, some of which may have potent pharmacologic action.

Other diagnostic procedures to evaluate the mother's ability to produce milk include thyroid function studies, since hypothyroidism may be associated with inability to lactate. Conversely abnormal galactorrhea may also be associated with either hypothyroidism or hyperthyroidism.

Several herbal remedies are said to increase milk supply including fenugreek, blessed thistle, and fennel. There are no placebo-controlled trials that confirm their effectiveness. Fenugreek smells like maple syrup and has the same allergic potential as peanuts and chickpeas. It is also recorded to lower blood sugar. Blessed thistle and fennel are not known to cause untoward symptoms.

Heavy smoking may interfere with the let-down reflex. Excessive exercise may also result in diminished milk supply. Reports of increased lactic acid level in the milk after exercise have been associated with infant refusal of the breast. It has been noted, however, that if the first few milliliters of milk are expressed and discarded and the breast washed to remove any sweat, there is no milk refusal.

MATERNAL DISEASE AND BREASTFEEDING
Diabetes Mellitus

Diabetes mellitus is not a contraindication to breastfeeding. In fact a woman may experience some lowering of her insulin requirements during lactation. The woman with diabetes makes good milk, and lactose production, which drives milk production, appears normal. The key to successful lactation in the diabetic woman is adequate kilocalories. When insufficient calories are consumed (<2000 kcal for average weight women), milk production falters. Careful dietary guidance is essential to the diabetic; associated adjustment (usually lowering) of insulin level usually provides a feeling of well-being. Breastfeeding is an opportunity for the diabetic woman to do something special for her infant when she has been led to believe her disease is a liability to the fetus in utero.

Seizure Disorders

Women with seizure disorders may breastfeed their infants if their maintenance medications are compatible with lacta-

tion. At birth the infant has some medication in the system, especially if a bolus was given during labor, and it may be necessary to supplement breastfeeding for a few days, pumping the breasts and discarding the milk. Levels of phenytoin (Dilantin), phenobarbital, and valproic acid can be easily measured in the neonate. If not fully feeding the infant, the mother should pump and discard her milk to continue to develop her milk supply. The infant will require some substitute feeding of formula, preferably given by small medicine cup or dropper, to prevent confusing the infant, because use of an artificial nipple may make it difficult for the infant to adjust to normal physiologic suckling at the breast. Usually after 2 to 3 days the infant can be fully breastfed. The small amount of medication that appears in the milk does not affect the infant. Valproic acid has milk/plasma ratios of 0.01 to 0.07 and is considered compatible with breastfeeding. If the infant is depressed and significant levels of phenobarbital or phenytoin are measurable in the infant, breast and formula feedings can be alternated. This will allow the mother to provide some of the great benefits of her milk while maintaining her own self-esteem. The important goal of maternal medication is to keep her seizure-free.

Thromboembolic Disease

A common postpartum complication is thromboembolic disease (see Chapter 77). When it occurs in the lactating woman, there are some important considerations. Heparin, because of its large molecular size, does not pass into the milk. Because it must be given parenterally, it is impractical in most cases for home use. Coumarin or warfarin does not usually pass into milk and can be used. A check at one month of the infant's prothrombin time can confirm this. A dose of vitamin K will improve any lowered levels. Studies have found no anticoagulant effect in infants whose mothers received coumarin. On the other hand, other anticoagulants, especially the synthetics, have been associated with problems in the infants and are not recommended for the lactating woman.

POSTPARTUM MASTITIS
Acute Mastitis

The acute onset of mastitis can occur anytime postpartum but is more common after 10 days and peaks in incidence at about 28 days. On rare occasions, it occurs before delivery in association with nipple exercises and manipulations that some recommend to prepare the nipple for lactation. Table 79-1 illustrates the important features of mastitis compared with those of engorgement and plugged ducts.

Engorgement

Engorgement occurs early, is bilateral, and is not associated with systemic disease. Maternal temperature is 101° F (38° C) or less. It can be treated with hot and cold compresses, warm showers that allow milk to drip freely, and, when all else fails, use of cabbage leaves. This historical remedy is carried out by placing cool fresh cabbage leaves on the breast until they fully wilt, replacing with fresh ones if necessary. Its effect has no scientific explanation. Engorgement is a self-limited discomfort that peaks on the fifth to the seventh day postpartum and then resolves. It is worse

Table 79-1
Comparison of Findings of Engorgement, Plugged Duct, and Mastitis

Characteristics	Engorgement	Plugged Duct	Mastitis
Onset	Gradual, immediately	Gradual, after feedings	Sudden, after 10 days postpartum
Site	Bilateral	Unilateral	Usually unilateral
Swelling and heat	Generalized	May shift/little or not heat	Localized, red hot, and swollen
Body temperature	<38.4° C	<38.4° C	>38.4° C
Systemic symptoms	Feels well	Feels well	Flulike symptoms

From Lawrence RA, Lawrence RM: *Breastfeeding: a guide for the medical profession*, ed 5, St Louis, 1999, Mosby.

in primiparas and in hospitalized or immobilized patients. It is important for the breasts to be gently massaged before a feeding to express a little milk to soften the areola. If this is not done, the infant cannot get a proper grasp and may clamp down on the nipple, causing considerable pain.

Plugged Ducts

A plugged duct is a unilateral lump in the breast that is not hot, red, or very painful. It is usually treated with warm compresses and massage sufficient to remove the plug and allow the drainage of lobule involved. A patient with recurrent plugs should be evaluated for underlying disease.

Clinical Presentation of Acute Mastitis

Acute mastitis is usually unilateral, but if it is bilateral streptococcal infection should be considered and aggressive treatment for mother and infant undertaken. A wedged-shaped area of the breast is reddened, hot, swollen, and painful. The mother usually has a temperature >101° F (>38° C) and feels ill. The common causes are *Staphylococcus* spp. *Escherichia coli.*

Choice of Therapy

Treatment is first to continue breastfeeding on both breasts, taking care to "empty" the involved breast. Antibiotics such as dicloxacillin, 500 mg every 6 hours, should be given for a minimum of 10 days, preferably 14 days. Following strict instructions to continue the medication even though the patient feels better is important. A small amount of most antibiotics gets into the milk, so a medication that can also be given directly to the infant is appropriate (avoid chloramphenicol and tetracycline).

Exhaustion is often the trigger point for mastitis so that complete care for mastitis is bed rest for the mother with feeding the infant her only responsibility until there is improvement. Local treatment includes hot or cold compresses, whichever gives the more relief of pain. Acetaminophen or ibuprofen safely provides relief of the local pain and generalized myalgia.

Recurrent and Chronic Mastitis

Inadequately treated mastitis can result in recurrent mastitis, which will continue to flare up every time antibiotics are discontinued. Early aggressive treatment of the initial bout of mastitis is the only way to prevent this. Recurrent mastitis quickly becomes chronic mastitis, which usually does not clear until the infant is weaned. In most cases, however, it is preferable to maintain the mother on low-dose antibiotics for the remainder of the lactation period. Erythromycin, 250 mg twice a day, is one treatment option.

Abscess

Abscess formation occurs when the initial mastitis is untreated or in some cases is inadequately treated. An abscess can be incised and drained without interfering with lactation. Milk may drain from the incision if a duct is cut in the procedure. It will heal while the infant continues to feed from the involved breast. The mother should press firmly over the incision with a sterile gauze square to minimize the flow of milk during a feeding.

Development of Candidal Infection of the Breast

Women who frequently harbor *Candida albicans* organisms vaginally are often subject to flare-ups of vaginal infection when taking antibiotics. Inflammation of the breast with *C. albicans* organisms can occur, usually after a treated breast infection. The common description is burning pain when the infant suckles likened to being stabbed to the chest wall with a hot poker. A course of antifungal cream combined with cortisone rubbed into the nipples and areola after each feeding will usually clear the symptoms. Because the source may well have been the baby, the infant should also be treated with nystatin orally, whether or not the child has oral evidence of the disease or monilial diaper rash. This may require a call to the pediatrician.

Candida infections of the breast are being over diagnosed. Not all shooting and burning pain of the breast is due to *Candida.* Candidiasis of the breast rarely occurs unless the mother has a history of vaginal moniliasis or the infant has oral lesions. Diflucan should be reserved for confirmed disease when local treatment has failed.

LACTATION AFTER BREAST SURGERY

Augmentation mammoplasty as a surgical procedure is not a contraindication to breastfeeding. The procedure does not interrupt vital nerves or ducts. The presence of silicone implants has become a point of concern. The U.S. Food and Drug Administration (FDA) has not recommended removal of an implant unless it has ruptured or there are serious symptoms (pain or tissue contractions). That silicone is in many products other than implants has led to further investigations. The present position of the FDA does not limit breastfeeding. The underlying reason augmentation was necessary for a given woman may be inadequate glandular tissue; however, that possibility can be identified only by initiating breast-feeding and measuring the ability to produce milk.

Reduction mammoplasty can be performed so that lactation can proceed without difficulty if the ducts are not cut and the nipple not removed and reimplanted. That information should be given to the woman before surgery while explaining the impact of the surgery, but if not then, at any time when requested by the patient. Women should be encouraged to ask questions before the procedure.

The removal of solitary lumps or cysts does not preclude breastfeeding. Fibrocystic disease is not a contraindication to breastfeeding. Breastfeeding after breast cancer is an individual matter that needs to be discussed with the woman's oncologist. The answer depends on the diagnosis and the pathologic characteristics of the tumor, as well as of the lymph nodes and the need for additional treatment with irradiation or chemotherapy and length of time since surgery. Usually, pregnancy is not recommended for at least 5 years posttreatment. Breastfeeding on the remaining breast has been successful. It is possible to nourish an infant fully with one breast, as it has been done for many other reasons including the preference of the infant. Whether lactation changes the probability of recurrence of the disease is not known, although 5-year survival rates in disease that was controlled for lactation are not reported to be different from those of women without pregnancy and lactation. As noted earlier, breastfeeding appears to have a protective affect against cancer of the breast in large series, especially premenopausal cancer.

BIBLIOGRAPHY

Academy of Breastfeeding Medicine: Guidelines for glucose monitoring and treatment of hypoglycemia in term breastfed neonates, *ABM News Views* 5:4, 1999.

Bryant CA: The impact of kin, friend and neighbor networks on infant feeding practices, *Soc Sci Med* 16:1757, 1982.

Cornblath M et al: Controversies regarding definition of neonatal hypoglycemia: suggested operational thresholds, *Pediatrics* 105:1141, 2000.

Cross NA et al: Calcium homeostasis and bone metabolism during pregnancy, lactation, and postweaning: a longitudinal study, *Am J Clin Nutr* 61:514, 1995.

Cross NA et al: Changes in bone mineral density and markers of bone remodeling during lactation and postweaning in women consuming high amounts of calcium, *J Bone Miner Res* 10:1312, 1995.

Dermer A: Smoking, tobacco exposure through breast milk, and SIDS, *JAMA* 274:214, 1995.

Ferris AM et al: Lactation outcome in insulin-dependent diabetic women, *J Am Diet Assoc* 88:317, 1988.

Furberg H et. al: Lactation and breast cancer risk, *Int J Epidemiol* 28:396, 1999.

Joseph KS, Kramer MS: Review of the evidence on fetal and early childhood antecedents of adult chronic disease, *Epidemiol Rev* 18:158, 1996.

Kalkwarf HJ et al: The effect of calcium supplementation on bone density during lactation and after weaning, *N Engl J Med* 337:523, 1997.

Kramer M et al: The promotion of breastfeeding intervention trial (probit): a cluster randomized trial in the Republic of Belarus, *JAMA* 285:463, 2001.

Lawrence RA: Herbs and breastfeeding [Online]. www.breastfeeding.com, http://216.167.14.128/reading_room/herbs.html. Fall 2000.

Lawrence RA: The pediatrician's role in infant feeding decision-making, *Pediatr Rev* 14:265, 1993.

Lawrence RA, Lawrence RM: *Breastfeeding: a guide for the medical profession,* ed 5, St Louis, 1998, Mosby.

Mascola MA et al: Exposure of young infants to environmental tobacco smoke: breast-feeding among smoking mothers, *Am J Public Health* 88:893, 1998.

Murtaugh MA et al: Energy intake and glycemia in lactating women with type 1 diabetes, *J Am Diet Assoc* 98:642, 1998.

Nafstad P et al: Weight gain during the first year of life in relation to maternal smoking and breast feeding in Norway, *J Epidemiol Comm Health* 51:261, 1997.

Nafstad P et al: Breastfeeding, maternal smoking and lower respiratory tract infections, *Eur Respir J* 9:2623, 1996.

Newton N: Psychologic differences between breast and bottle feeding, *Am J Clin Nutr* 24:993, 1971.

Report of the Surgeon General's workshop on breastfeeding and human lactation, Pub No HRS-D-MC 84-2, Department of Health and Human Services, 1984.

Ritchie LD et al: A longitudinal study of calcium homeostasis during human pregnancy and lactation and after resumption of menses, *Am J Clin Nutr* 67:693, 1998.

Ryan AS: The resurgence of breastfeeding in the United States, *Pediatrics* 99:12, 1997.

Sowers M: Pregnancy and lactation as risk factors for subsequent bone loss and osteoporosis, *J Bone Miner Res* 11:1052, 1996.

Subcommittee on nutrition during lactation: *Nutrition during lactation,* Institute of Medicine, National Academy of Sciences, 1991.

Wallace JP, Inbar G, Ernsthausen K: Infant acceptance of postexercise milk, *Pediatrics* 89:1245, 1992.

WHO/UNICEF: Protecting, promoting and supporting breastfeeding: the special role of maternity services. A Joint WHO/UNICEF Statement, Geneva, World Health Organization, 1989.

WHO/UNICEF: Innocenti declaration on the protection, promotion and support of breastfeeding, August, 1990, Florence, Italy.

Yoo K-Y et al: Independent protective effect of lactation against breast cancer: a case-control study in Japan, *Am J Epidemiol* 135:726, 1992.

CHAPTER 80

Postpartum Psychiatric Disorders

Adele C. Viguera

Psychiatric mood disorders complicate 8% to 10% of all deliveries, rivaling the prevalence of any complication seen in obstetrics. Postpartum psychiatric disorders are common and are often missed clinically. For many clinicians and their patients, confusion about distinguishing between normal postpartum emotional adjustment and postpartum psychiatric illness remains. The associated morbidity of failing to recognize postpartum depression is high, with significant potential long-term sequelae for the woman, infant, and her family. In more severe forms of postpartum depression, suicide and infanticide may occur. Thus, rapid diagnosis and treatment are imperative.

This chapter reviews the diagnosis and management of mood and anxiety disorders associated with childbirth.

EPIDEMIOLOGY

Mood and anxiety disorders are two to three times more common in women compared with men. Typically mood and anxiety disorders peak during the childbearing years. A recent epidemiologic study by Evans found that rates of depression *during* pregnancy were high (9%) but not significantly different from rates of depression in nonpregnant populations. These data suggest that pregnancy is not protective against occurrence of major depression as has been traditionally accepted.

Although it was initially thought that the postpartum period was a time of increased risk for major depression, data from epidemiologically derived populations suggest that the incidence rate of major depression is no different from the incidence rate of major depression at other times in a woman's life. The literature on the epidemiology of postpartum depression is difficult to interpret because of inconsistencies in the time frame used to delineate the postpartum period. The largest and most carefully controlled studies report rates of depression of 10% to 15% during the 6 to 12 weeks after delivery. A growing literature also suggests that while the postpartum period may not be a time of risk for all women, it clearly is a period of heightened risk in certain subgroups of women. In particular, women with a prior history of mood and/or anxiety disorders such as major depression, bipolar disorder, panic disorder, obsessive-compulsive disorder, and previous history of postpartum depression appear to be at the greatest risk.

ETIOLOGY

The postpartum period is a time during which significant physiologic changes occur. Within the first 48 hours after delivery, rapid shifts in the hormonal environment occur and are associated with a dramatic fall in estrogen and progesterone to hypogonadal levels within days of delivery. Gonadal steroids exert both direct and indirect effects on neuromodulation in multiple monoaminergic systems implicated in the pathogenesis of depressive disorders. Some investigators have proposed a role of these hormones in the pathophysiology of postpartum mood disturbance. However, no consistent hormonal differences have been found in postpartum women with and without depression, suggesting that women with postpartum depression have normal endocrine function.

Investigators have hypothesized that a possible underlying mechanism is that there are specific subpopulations of women who display a differential behavioral sensitivity to normal fluctuations in gonadal steroid levels. For example, a recent study by Bloch and colleagues at the National Institute of Mental Health investigated the possible role of changes in gonadal steroids levels in postpartum depression. They simulated the hormonal conditions related to pregnancy and the postpartum period in women with and without a history of postpartum depression under double-blind conditions. First, they administered supraphysiologic levels of gonadal steroids to the study subjects in an effort to simulate pregnancy. Then they simulated the postpartum period by withdrawing both estrogen and progesterone to hypogonadal levels. Over half the women with a history of postpartum depression and none of the women without a history of postpartum depression developed significant mood symptoms during the withdrawal period. The investigators concluded that women with a history of postpartum depression may have a differential sensitivity to changing gonadal steroids and that this sensitivity appears to be a trait vulnerability that is not present in women without a history of postpartum depression.

Interestingly, a similar finding has also been found in women suffering from premenstrual syndrome (PMS). Schmidt and Rubinow showed that women with PMS similarly have normal gonadal steroid levels, but exhibit a differential sensitivity to cyclic fluctuations in steroid levels. The mood of women with, but not without, PMS, is destabilized by normal changes in estrogen and progesterone levels.

Factors that may cause this differential responsivity to gonadal steroids in women with PMS and/or postpartum depression are unknown and require further study.

CLASSIFICATION AND DIAGNOSIS

Although the obstetric postpartum period ends at 6 weeks with uterine involution, the psychiatric postpartum period is defined, according to the Diagnostic and Statistical Manual of Mental Disorders, fourth edition (DSM-IV) by any mood disturbance occurring within the first 4 weeks after delivery. This time frame is fairly narrow, and others have defined a broader period of risk ranging from the first 3 months after delivery to any episode occurring within the first year after childbirth.

Postpartum (or puerperal) psychiatric illness is typically divided into three categories: postpartum blues, postpartum depression, and postpartum psychosis (Table 80-1). It is helpful to conceptualize these disorders, as existing along a continuum, where postpartum blues is the mildest and postpartum psychosis is the most severe form of puerperal illness. These two entities at either extreme of the continuum are presented first, followed by a discussion of the presentation and treatment of postpartum depression.

Postpartum Blues

Postpartum blues or "baby blues" affects 50% to 80% of new mothers. These symptoms typically start on the second or third day after delivery, peak on the fifth to seventh day, and generally remit by the second week. The blues are generally characterized by mood swings with times of feeling tearful, anxious, or irritable, interspersed with times of feeling well. Suicidality is not a symptom of the blues. The most important clinical characteristic of the blues is that these symptoms resolve spontaneously and they are considered nonpathologic.

Although the symptoms may be distressing, they typically do not interfere with the mother's ability to function and care for her infant. Psychiatric consultation is generally not required; however, the patient should be instructed to contact her obstetrician or primary care provider if the symptoms persist longer than 2 weeks, as the likelihood of an evolving postpartum depression is high. Approximately 20% of women with postpartum blues develop postpartum major depression. For those women with a prior history of psychiatric illness (e.g., recurrent major depression or previous postpartum depression), the blues may herald the development of a more significant postpartum mood disorder.

Postpartum Psychosis

Postpartum (puerperal) psychosis is the most severe form of postpartum psychiatric illness and should be considered a psychiatric emergency. In contrast to postpartum blues and depression, puerperal psychosis is rare. It occurs in approximately 1 to 2 per 1000 women after childbirth. Making the diagnosis of this disorder is relatively easy because its presentation is often dramatic with onset of symptoms as early as 48 to 72 hours after delivery. The full-blown illness usually appears with the first 2 weeks after delivery. Symptoms are characterized by agitation, pressured speech, confusion, poor appetite, and inability to sleep, as well as psychotic symptoms including hallucinations (auditory, command, visual, tactile, olfactory) and delusions (either grandiose or paranoid). Some investigators have described a waxing and waning course with lucid periods characteristic of acute delirium. Diagnostically, postpartum psychosis shares features of a manic psychosis, and many researchers believe that it is a subtype of bipolar disorder (manic-depressive illness). Follow-up of women with postpartum psychosis reveals that the majority eventually are diagnosed as having bipolar disorder.

Postpartum psychosis is a dangerous illness, associated with a high risk for suicide and infanticide. It must be aggressively treated within an inpatient setting. Rates of infanticide associated with untreated puerperal psychosis have been estimated to be as high as 4%. Acute treatment with mood stabilizers and antipsychotic medications is recommended. Electroconvulsive therapy is also useful for rapid relief of symptoms.

Postpartum psychosis also carries the highest risk of recurrence after future pregnancies. Risk for recurrence with a subsequent pregnancy is estimated to be as high as 90%.

Table 80-1
Classification of Postpartum Mood and Anxiety Disorders

Postpartum Mood Disorders	Incidence	Onset	Characteristic Symptoms
Postpartum blues	50% to 85%	Within first week to 10 days	Fluctuating mood, tearfulness, anxiety
Postpartum depression	10% to 15%	Usually within first 3 months	Insidious depressed mood, insomnia, excessive anxiety
Puerperal psychosis	0.1% to 0.2%	Within first 2 weeks	Dramatic confusion, agitation, depressed or elated mood; delusions, hallucinations; disorganized behavior; sleeplessness

Postpartum Anxiety Disorders	Incidence	Onset	Characteristic Symptoms
Panic disorder	Unknown	1-6 weeks	Chest tightness, hyperventilation, shortness of breath, fear of losing control, feeling of impending doom
Obsessive compulsive disorder	Unknown	1-6 weeks	Checking behaviors/contamination fears, recurrent intrusive thoughts

Because of this high rate of recurrence, some researchers have advocated the prophylactic use of mood stabilizers such as lithium either immediately before or after deliver. Studies have shown a clear reduction in risk of relapse with this therapeutic intervention.

Postpartum Depression

Symptom Presentation

The onset of symptoms may be acute (i.e., within the first 1 to 2 weeks) or may follow a period of relative well-being and appear later at 6 or 8 weeks postpartum or even later in the puerperium. Signs and symptoms of postpartum depression are generally indistinguishable from that characteristic of major depression occurring in women at other times. As with nonpuerperal depression, the diagnosis cannot be made unless a woman has at least 2 weeks of either depressed mood most of the day, nearly everyday, or loss of interest or pleasure in activities once enjoyed. Other characteristic symptoms of postpartum depression include agitation, mood liability, tearfulness, irritability, and hostility and anger, which are often directed at spouse or partner. Women suffering from postpartum depression may express no desire to hold the baby, care for the baby, or be left alone with the baby. Some women also develop a marked sleep disturbance. Typically, they describe difficulty falling asleep or they complain of an inability to stay asleep and wake even though the baby may be asleep.

A distinguishing feature of postpartum depression from nonpuerperal depression, however, is excessive anxiety. Women may present with different forms of anxiety including generalized anxiety, panic attacks, hypochondriasis, or obsessional thinking. Women may be overly preoccupied with the baby's health, or they may describe unwanted intrusive thoughts of harming the baby consisting of violent images such as stabbing or throwing the baby. These thoughts tend to be more obsessive than infanticidal. They are very frightening for the patient and can be a source of shame. Such thoughts are unlikely to be volunteered and they must be asked directly in a nonthreatening and nonjudgmental way. Often prefacing the inquiry by stating that such thoughts are not uncommon with postpartum depression will help put the patient at ease and allow her to disclose such information. Box 80-1 lists the characteristic symptoms of postpartum depression.

Who Is at Risk for Postpartum Depression?

The risk factors for postpartum depression frequently are present even before pregnancy. In fact, most of the time, if a comprehensive prepregnancy assessment is done, one can predict who might become ill postpartum by history alone. Therefore elucidating psychiatric risk factors antenatally is good clinical practice. For example, one of the most important risk factors for postpartum depression is having had a previous similar episode (Table 80-2). More than 50% of women who have had a previous postpartum depression will become depressed again with a subsequent delivery. If a woman has been depressed at *any* other time in her life, her risk of developing a postpartum depression also increases to about 30%. Women who have bipolar disorder (manic-depressive illness) are also at high risk, and their risk for postpartum depression has been estimated to be greater than

50%. As mentioned earlier, women with a history of postpartum psychosis represent a high-risk group, with estimated rates of relapse as high as 90% with a subsequent delivery.

In addition, depression *during pregnancy* has been demonstrated to be one of the most important predictors of postpartum relapse. Also women appear to be more vulnerable to postpartum relapse if they have a family history of postpartum depression, or experience mood changes premenstrually or with the use of oral contraceptive pills. If a woman presents with any of these risk factors, she must be monitored closely.

Psychosocial risk factors have also been identified and appear to play an important role in determining vulnerability to affective illness during the postpartum period. One of the most consistent findings is that among women who report marital dissatisfaction or inadequate social supports, postpartum depression is more common. In addition, several investigators have shown that stressful life events during pregnancy or near the time of delivery appear to increase the likelihood of postpartum depressive illness. Other investigators have focused on various demographic variables that may affect risk for postpartum depression including age, marital status, parity, education level, and socioeconomic status. However, there is little consistent evidence to suggest that any particular demographic factor significantly increases risk for postpartum depression.

Table 80-2
History of Psychiatric Illness and Risk for Postpartum Relapse

Prior History	Risk of Relapse
Major depression	30%
Postpartum depression	50%
Manic-depressive illness (ie, bipolar disorder)	50%
Postpartum psychosis	70%-90%

BOX 80-1
Characteristic Symptoms of Postpartum Depression

Mood liability
Anxiety
Irritability, hostility
Tearfulness
Obsessional, intrusive thoughts of harming infant
Poor concentration
Recurrent thoughts of guilt or self-blame for situation
Agitation, fidgetiness, inability to sit still
Feelings of hopelessness, helplessness
No desire to hold or care for the baby
No desire to be left alone with the baby
Inability to fall asleep
Inability to stay asleep, waking even though the baby may be asleep, and inability to fall asleep again
Poor appetite or excessive eating
Suicidal feelings or suicide plan

Impact of Postpartum Mood Disturbance

Research into postpartum disorders has highlighted important long-term sequelae of untreated disorder on the mother and on infant development. For the mother, postpartum mood and anxiety disorders may not be short-term illnesses. In one study, more than half the women were depressed 4 years later. Often failure to treat contributes to the emergence of a chronic and more treatment-refractory form of depressive illness.

In addition, a growing literature suggests the detrimental effect of maternal depression on child development. Attachment difficulties may be quite severe in women with postpartum depression or psychosis. Long-term follow-up studies have also shown that behavioral difficulties and cognitive deficits were more common in the children of mothers who suffered from postpartum depression. Moreover, child abuse and neglect are more common among women who suffer from postpartum psychiatric illness. Although infanticide is relatively uncommon, it is more likely to occur in women who present with psychotic symptoms.

EVALUATION

As in depressive episodes occurring outside the postpartum period, postpartum depressive disorders present along a continuum. Patients may experience mild to moderate depressive symptoms, as well as more severe depression characterized by prominent neurovegetative symptoms and marked impairment of functioning. Treatment of postpartum depression begins with an evaluation of severity of symptoms including psychotic symptoms (e.g., delusions, hallucinations) and safety considerations such as assessing the mother's suicidal risk and any thoughts she may have of harming her infant. Patients should also be carefully evaluated for any previous history of bipolar disorder (i.e., manic-depressive illness) since treatment with an antidepressant alone during the depressive phase of bipolar disorder may precipitate a worsening course of illness. Other medical causes of depression such as hypothyroidism or anemia should be ruled out as well. Some prospective studies have revealed a 2% to 4% incidence of hypothyroidism in postpartum depression.

There are no data to suggest that postpartum depression should be managed differently from nonpuerperal major depression. Therefore postpartum depression demands the same intensity of treatment as depression occurring at other times with standard antidepressant doses for an adequate duration of time. For mild symptoms that do not interfere significantly with a woman's ability to function, a patient may benefit from skilled psychotherapy alone. However, for more severe and persistent symptoms, antidepressant medications in addition to counseling and support are recommended.

MANAGEMENT

Pharmacologic Treatment

The goal of pharmacotherapy is rapid stabilization. Antidepressants should be started immediately once an accurate diagnosis has been made, and treatment should be continued for at least 6 months to 1 year. To date, only a small number of studies have assessed the efficacy of antidepressant medica-tions in the treatment of postpartum mood disturbance. Conventional antidepressant medications including the selective serotonin reuptake inhibitors (fluoxetine, paroxetine, sertraline, citalopram), tricyclic antidepressants (e.g., nortriptyline, desipramine), and serotonin-noradrenaline reuptake inhibitors (e.g., venlafaxine) have been shown to be effective in the treatment of postpartum depression.

There appears to be no one antidepressant better than another for the treatment of postpartum depression. Therefore the choice of antidepressant should be guided by the patient's prior response to antidepressant medication and a given medication's side effect profile. Selective serotonin reuptake inhibitors are ideal first-line agents, since they are anxiolytic, nonsedating, and well tolerated. However, they should be used with caution initially since they can occasionally produce agitation or worsening anxiety at the initiation of treatment. Tricyclic antidepressants such as nortriptyline and desipramine are frequently used and, because they tend to be more sedating, may be appropriate for women who present with prominent sleep disturbance, as well as excessive anxiety.

Using a benzodiazepine such as lorazepam or clonazepam in conjunction with an antidepressant may be helpful in providing immediate relief from anxiety symptoms or insomnia until the antidepressant dose is titrated to a therapeutic dose.

Hormonal Therapies

Some investigators have explored the role of hormonal manipulation in women who suffer from postpartum depression. Early reports suggested that progesterone might be helpful, but there are no systematically derived data to support its use in this setting. In a recent study, Gregoire and colleagues described the potential benefit of transdermal estrogen therapy as an adjunct to antidepressant treatment in women with postpartum depression. These women had a more rapid response to treatment than those using receiving antidepressant alone. At present, however, the use of estrogen or progesterone in the treatment of postpartum disorders is not considered standard of care given the limited data on efficacy and the health risks associated with hormonal treatments.

Nonpharmacologic Treatment

Nonpharmacologic therapies such as structured, time-limited psychotherapies including cognitive behavior therapy and interpersonal psychotherapy (IPT), are effective treatments and may be particularly useful for patients who are reluctant to use psychotropic medications or for patients with milder forms depressive illness. Several preliminary studies have yielded encouraging results. Appleby and colleagues have recently shown in a randomized, placebo-controlled study that short-term CBT was as effective as treatment with an antidepressant for the woman with mild postpartum depression. IPT was shown to be effective as well for the treatment of women with mild to moderate postpartum depression. IPT is also a time-limited treatment with a focus on interpersonal relationships, as well as issues related to being a new mother such as role transition, disruption of relationships with the spouse and other social supports, and interactions with the infant.

Other Treatment Strategies

Clinicians can help dispel the guilt associated with postpartum depression by assuring women that the phenomenon is common and manageable and not the mother's fault or the result of a "weak" or unstable personality. It is also helpful to involve family members such as the patient's partner in therapy to help them understand the symptoms of postpartum depression and cope with the increased stress of the family.

If depression is severe, it is important for a relative, friend, or paid helper to stay with and assist the mother at all times. Having the spouse or partner help with evening feedings will help the patient receive an uninterrupted period of sleep, which can further help stabilize mood. Patients should be urged to attend to their personal needs and to get adequate sleep, nutrition, and exercise.

Psychosocial interventions such as psychoeducational, supportive groups and community services are frequently included in the care of women during the postpartum period. Self-help groups such as Depression After Delivery (DAD) or Postpartum Support International (PSI) provide support for women with postpartum mood disorder and help decrease the isolation and stigma women may experience (Box 80-2). Community services such as home help, child care and self-help groups can also be an important adjunct to care.

SCREENING FOR POSTPARTUM MOOD AND ANXIETY DISORDERS

The greatest obstacle to the diagnosis of postpartum depression is the extent to which clinicians fail to inquire about mood/anxiety symptoms both *during* pregnancy and the postpartum period. Despite multiple contacts with the medical profession during the postpartum period, women with postpartum depression or postpartum anxiety disorders are often overlooked or misdiagnosed. Screening and patient education about the potential risk for postpartum depression should begin *during pregnancy* at routine prenatal care visits. A brief set of questions at the prenatal visits can help detect individuals at risk (Box 80-3). An affirmative answer to any of these questions places a woman in a higher risk group for developing postpartum depression, and such patients should be monitored closely during their entire pregnancy and in the weeks after childbirth for emergence of any anxiety or mood disorders.

Several rating scales are also available to screen for depression in the general population (Beck Depression Inventory, Center for Epidemiologic Studies Depression Scale). Although these scales have not been validated in postpartum populations, they may be useful in identifying women who need further evaluation. The Edinburgh Postnatal Depression Scale (EPDS) has been validated in postpartum populations and may also be used as a screening tool for depression in pregnancy. This scale is a 10-item, self-rated questionnaire that takes 10 minutes to complete and has been translated into several languages. It has been used extensively in many countries and cultures for the detection of depression in pregnancy and during the postpartum period. The EPDS could be easily integrated into the routine evaluation of women in both obstetric and pediatric settings and would alert the clinician to women who are in need of further evaluation and treatment. Incorporating such a scale in the second or third trimester as well as the 6-week postpartum visit would help facilitate a discussion between clinician and patient of this important issue.

BREASTFEEDING AND PSYCHIATRIC MEDICATIONS

Women with postpartum psychiatric disorders often face the dilemma of whether or not to use psychiatric medications while continuing to breastfeed their infants. All psychotropic medications including antidepressants are secreted in the breast milk at varying concentrations. However, infants are exposed to much less medication through breast milk than through placental circulation. Many mothers often forgo treatment rather than stop breastfeeding or expose their infant to medication through breast milk. The position of the American Academy of Pediatrics Committee on Drugs is weighed toward continuing breastfeeding when medications are necessary, because the multiple benefits of breastfeeding outweigh risks associated with the antidepressant exposure.

There are no controlled studies on the safety of psychotropic medications in nursing mothers. The literature consists mainly of case series and case reports and has recently been thoroughly reviewed by Burt and colleagues. To date, the available information across the serotonin reuptake inhibitors (including fluoxetine, sertraline, citalopram, paroxetine) and the tricyclic antidepressants (including nortriptyline, imipramine, desipramine), suggest *no acute adverse effects* to the infant, and antidepressant levels are either undetectable or at minimal levels in infants when breastfed by mothers taking these medications.

There is also limited information on the safety of benzodiazepines and breastfeeding. There have been only four published cases of adverse effects noted in the infants exposed to benzodiazepines in breast milk including sedation, lethargy, decreased tone, and decreased respiratory rate; in the majority of published cases (>40 cases), no adverse effects were noted. Because benzodiazepines can be useful and effective as an adjunctive treatment for postpartum mood and anxiety disorders, they should not be avoided or considered a contraindication to breastfeeding. For example, in clinical practice, one could consider the use of low-dose clonazepam or lorazepam (e.g., 0.5 to 1 mg twice or three times a day) with careful monitoring of the infant for any change in behavior.

Issues to address in the risk/benefit assessment of psychotropic medication use during breastfeeding include documented benefits of breastfeeding and the effects of untreated mental illness on the mother. Another risk to consider are the unknown long-term neurobehavioral effects of exposure to psychiatric medications via breast milk. In light of the well-established data on the adverse impact of untreated maternal illness on infant attachment and development; however, it is probably safer to err on the side of treating maternal mood and anxiety symptoms aggressively with medication and allowing the mother to continue to breastfeed.

Safeguarding the mental health of the mother, however, is of paramount importance and should be considered priority. Patients should be reminded of this, given the guilt associated with either discontinuing breastfeeding because of illness or deciding to use medications while breastfeeding. Patients and their clinicians should arrive at the best possible treatment decision at a given point in time, combining the available information about the safety of a particular medication and breastfeeding, the severity of the patient's symptoms, and the patient's wishes.

Overall, breastfeeding is not contraindicated when taking antidepressants and/or benzodiazepines and should not be discouraged. It is recommended that if the mother chooses to breastfeed while on medication, the infant should be observed for side effects such as sedation, sleep problems, agitation, or weight loss. If the baby develops health problems, the pediatrician can obtain an infant serum level to determine if the antidepressant and/or benzodiazepine is present in the baby in a significant amount and might be contributing to the problem.

POSTPARTUM ANXIETY DISORDERS

Although the traditional understanding of postpartum illness has focused on the mood disorders, more recent reports show that anxiety disorders such as panic disorder and obsessive-compulsive disorder also appear in the postpartum period and are often complicated by the onset of comorbid major depressive disorder. Although data are limited, the current literature suggests that postpartum patients may be at risk for *new onset* panic attacks or obsessive-compulsive symptoms. These illnesses can be frightening for the patient who has no prior history of these disorders. It is helpful to reassure patients that this is not an uncommon phenomenon postpartum, and symptoms are generally responsive to treatment.

For those patients with a preexisting history of anxiety disorders, the postpartum period represents a vulnerable time of worsening of their usual symptoms of anxiety. Clinically, it is helpful to inform the patient with such a prior history of their high risk for relapse. Close monitoring for any early sign of relapse and intervening quickly with anxiolytic medications and/or antidepressants will significantly help to reduce the high morbidity associated with these untreated disorders. In some cases, a preventive measure such as postpartum prophylaxis with an antidepressant or benzodiazepine (i.e., reintroducing medication either a few weeks before or immediately after delivery) may be indicated depending on the severity of the illness and the patient's wishes.

BIBLIOGRAPHY

Altshuler LL et al: The expert consensus guideline series: treatment of depression in women 2001, Special report. *Postgrad Med* March:1-116, 2001.

Appleby L et al: A controlled study of fluoxetine and cognitive-behavioral counseling in the treatment of postnatal depression, *BMJ* 314:932, 1997.

Bloch M et al: Effects of gonadal steroids in women with a history of postpartum depression, *Am J Psychiatry* 157:924, 2000.

Burt VK et al: The use of psychotropic medications during breastfeeding, *Am J Psychiatry 158:10001, 2001.*

Cogill SR et al: Impact of maternal depression on cognitive development of young children, *BMJ* 292:1165, 1986.

Cox JL, Holden JM, Sagovsky R: Detection of postnatal depression: development of the 10 item Edinburgh Postnatal Depression Scale, *Br J Psychiatry* 150:782, 1987.

Evans J et al: Cohort study of depressed mood during pregnancy and after childbirth, *BMJ* 323:257, 2001.

Gregoire AJ et al: Transdermal *oestrogen* for treatment of severe postnatal depression, *Lancet* 347(9006):930, 1996.

Murray L: The impact of postnatal depression on infant development, *J Child Psychol Psychiatry* 33:543, 1992.

Nonacs R, Cohen LS: Postpartum mood disorders: diagnosis and treatment guidelines, *J Clin Psychiatry* 59 (suppl 2):34, 1998.

O'Hara MW: Social support, life events, and depression during pregnancy and the puerperium, *Arch Gen Psychiatry* 43:569, 1986.

O'Hara MW, Swain AM: Rates and risk of postpartum depression—a meta-analysis, *Int Rev Psychiatry* 8:37, 1996.

O'Hara MW, Neunaber DJ, Zekowski EM: Prospective study of postpartum depression: prevalence, course, and predictive factors, *J Abnorm Psychol* 93:158, 1984.

Schmidt PJ et al: Differential behavioral effects of gonadal steroids in women with and in those without premenstrual syndrome, *N Engl J Med* 338:209, 1998.

Stuart S, O'Hara MW: Interpersonal psychotherapy for postpartum depression: a treatment program, *J Psychother Pract Res* 4:18, 1995.

PART III
Psychology and Behavioral Medicine

CHAPTER **81**

Depressive Disorders

Carol Landau
Iris Shuey
Felise B. Milan

The depressive disorders are among the most prevalent psychiatric conditions in women. Depression is the second most common diagnosis overall seen in primary care, second only to hypertension. Depression has been shown to increase the risk of morbidity and mortality in patients with coronary heart disease and is also associated with a higher health care cost than other common disorders in primary care. Major depression is one of the 15 leading causes of disability in industrialized countries. It is predicted that it will be the second leading cause of disability by the year 2020. Estimates are that 15% of people diagnosed with severe depression will die by suicide.

Because twice as many people turn to their primary care physician, rather than a psychiatrist with their mental health problem, the screening, identification, and treatment of women who suffer from depression is crucial to primary care clinicians. The literature, however, tells us that depression often goes underrecognized and undertreated in medical settings. Less than half of the depressed patients seen in a primary care practice are properly diagnosed and treated.

DIAGNOSTIC CRITERIA

Major depressive disorder is an acute condition in which frequent and severe symptoms are present on a daily basis and interfere with functioning. The two major symptoms are depressed mood and loss of interest (anhedonia). The full diagnostic criteria are listed in Box 81-1. Major depressive episodes may occur at any time. The differential diagnoses includes the other DSM-IV depressive disorders, including Dysthymia and Depressive Disorder Not Otherwise Specified. Dysthymia includes at least two of the signs or symptoms of major depressive episode and a lifelong tendency toward depressed mood. Thus, by definition it is a chronic condition. Such life crises as bereavement or divorce can produce Adjustment Disorders with Depressed Mood. Depressive Disorder Not Otherwise Specified includes women who have some symptoms of depression but do not meet the full criteria for one of the disorders. The continuum in Fig. 81-1 may be useful in diagnosis.

EPIDEMIOLOGY
Prevalence and Risk Factors

Epidemiologic research worldwide reveals that major depression is approximately twice as common in women as in men; the lifetime prevalence is 21% for women and 13% for men. In terms of current point prevalence for females, the rate of depression is 13%, whereas for males it is 8%. The average age of onset for men is in the late 20s and 30s, but for women may be in mid-adolescence. Other risk factors for depression include a family history of mood disorder, a previous history of major depression, age between 20 and 40 years, living in an urban environment, previous trauma, marital discord or divorce, and having young children at home.

A history of childhood abuse or sexual abuse is associated with adult-onset depression. Some research suggests that a disruption of the hypothalamic-pituitary-adrenal axis and subsequent hormonal dysregulation may predispose survivors of childhood abuse to depression. Because the ratio of male to female victims can be estimated as high as 12:1, this risk factor is obviously much more common in women.

Comorbidity

The national Comorbidity Survey revealed that depressed women have higher rates of psychiatric comorbidity, more often than men, especially with anxiety disorders, eating disorders, and somatization. In the Epidemiologic Catchment Area Study, more than 51% of the women with major depressive episode had a comorbid anxiety disorder. These included panic disorder, phobias, and general anxiety disorder.

Smoking is also associated with depression in women. Some research suggests that women smoke to improve mood and control weight. Major depressive disorder is more common among smokers than nonsmokers. Smokers who have a history of depression are less likely to be able to quit smoking successfully. This may be due either to the fact that nicotine withdrawal can produce depressive symptoms or that the smokers are using the nicotine to treat a mood disorder.

All women with depression should be screened for alcohol and other substance abuse and vice versa. Many women use alcohol specifically to reduce stress. This has the unfortunate result of alleviating anxiety short term but also the potential for alcohol abuse or addiction. Therefore it is important to carefully assess the possibility of substance abuse. In one study depression was the strongest predictor of alcohol dependence. In addition, clinical evidence suggests that use of alcohol in women has earlier and more severe medical complications. Multiple substance abuse is also common. A study of Alcoholics Anonymous members found that 40% of the females were addicted to another drug as well, and for women below age 30 the rate was 60%. Alcohol and substance abuse are discussed in detail in Chapter 90.

Special attention should be given to patients who have chronic medical comorbidity. One study found that these patients were less likely to have depression discussed with them as a possible diagnosis by their physician. Women's vulnerability to thyroid disorders, rheumatologic conditions, and migraine headaches also can make the diagnosis and treatment of depression complicated. It is likely that competing demands interfere with a physician's ability to correctly identify, evaluate, and discuss treatment options with patients who have chronic medical problems.

ETIOLOGY

Three types of theories have been proposed to account for the gender differences in depression: the artifact theory, biologic theories, and psychosocial theories. The artifact theory, as the name suggests, proposes that men are depressed as often as women, but that they are socialized not to express their depressive symptoms directly. Thus, women seek health care more often and reveal more depressive symptomology. It should be noted, however, that community-based research also reveals the gender difference. Others have suggested that men tend to self-medicate with alcohol and other drugs. This point of view does not argue that depression is overdiagnosed in women but rather that it is underdiagnosed in men.

Biologic theories acknowledge the genetic predisposition to the depressive disorders. In addition, the sex differences in prevalence of depression are attributed to shifts in reproductive hormones and the relative changes in serotonergic functioning. Research in reproductive psychiatry has now documented that a subgroup of women is particularly sensitive to hormonal changes that occur during the menstrual cycle. These women may be prone to premenstrual mood disorder, postpartum depression, and depression during the perimenopausal period (see Chapters 56 and 80).

Psychologic theories of depression, including the learned helplessness theory, as well as the cognitive theory, may well apply more to women than to men. With respect to relationships, Weissman and her associates have documented the interpersonal nature of depression. Recent reviews re-

---

BOX 81-1
Symptoms of Major Depressive Episode

Have you had at least *five* of the following symptoms during the same 2-week period, and is this a *change* from your usual functioning?

1. Depressed mood most of the day, nearly every day

-or-

2. Markedly diminished interest or pleasure in all, or almost all activities most of the day, nearly every day.

-and-

3. Significant weight loss or weight gain when not dieting (e.g., more than 5% of body weight in a month), or decrease or increase in appetite nearly every day.
4. Insomnia or hypersomnia nearly every day.
5. Psychomotor agitation or retardation nearly every day.
6. Fatigue or loss of energy nearly every day.
7. Feelings of worthlessness or excessive or inappropriate guilt nearly every day.
8. Diminished ability to think or concentrate, or indecisiveness, nearly every day.
9. Recurrent thoughts of death (not just fear of dying), recurrent suicidal ideation without a specific plan, or a suicide attempt or a specific plan.

Modified from *The Diagnostic and Statistical Manual of Mental Disorders,* ed 4, Washington, DC, 1994, American Psychiatric Association.
*If you answered YES to 1 or 2 and YES to four items from 3-9, you may be suffering from a major depressive episode.

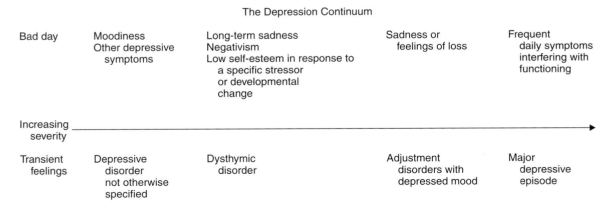

The Depression Continuum

| Bad day | Moodiness
Other depressive
symptoms | Long-term sadness
Negativism
Low self-esteem in response to
a specific stressor
or developmental
change | Sadness or
feelings of loss | Frequent
daily symptoms
interfering with
functioning |

Increasing severity ⟶

| Transient
feelings | Depressive
disorder
not otherwise
specified | Dysthymic
disorder | Adjustment
disorders with
depressed mood | Major
depressive
episode |

FIG. 81-1 The continuum of depressive disorders.

veal that when stressed, women tend to brood about problems and internalize them. Men, on the other hand, often turn to external sources of distraction including sports and other activities. Nolen-Hoeksema suggested that this brooding and rumination tend to make depression worse.

With respect to sociodemographics, women are more likely to experience poverty, physical and sexual abuse, lack of education, and job discrimination. These stressors can precipitate depression. Primary care clinicians' access to psychosocial information cast them in a unique role in patients' lives. By exploring stressful life events from a developmental perspective, the primary care clinician may be better able to detect all forms of depression and to make a therapeutic intervention.

DEVELOPMENTAL STRESSORS
Marriage

The role of marital happiness is critical to the understanding depression in women. The average age in the United States for first marriages for men is 27 years and women is 25 years. Several studies suggest that some of the risk factors for depression are related to family stressors including being unhappily married or divorced, the absence of a confidant, and having children under the age of 5 at home. The highest rates for major depression occur in women between the ages of 18 and 44. Finally, many depressed women are married to depressed men.

Weissman details the relationship issues in depression more clearly. She reported that rates of depression are lowest for men and women who are married and getting along well with their spouses. Although women have higher rates of depression overall, the increased risk for major depression in unhappy marriage is nearly the same for men and women and about 25-fold higher than those in happy marriages. When examining rates of depression, the only category in which men outnumber women is that of unemployment. Even given recent economic and social changes, it is not surprising that a loss of or major problem in a job for a man might well have the same emotional impact as the loss of or a major problem in a marriage or significant relationship for a woman. The social stigma of unemployment can lead a man to feel as devalued as a woman who is divorced or in an unhappy marriage.

An assessment of the patient's family life is critical in caring for a depressed patient. Difficulties in a relationship are often cited as a precipitant to a major depressive episode. Conversely, depression interferes with a woman's functioning in her marriage and other relationships. Many women feel ashamed, not only of their depression, but of marital problems. The negative cognitive set often associated with depression may well influence the woman's view of her marriage, so it is important to explore all the related issues with objectivity and sensitivity. Mothers of young children often find it extremely difficult to admit to depression because of their caretaking roles. They feel guilty, as if the depression somehow negates the value of their mothering.

Lesbian Relationships

Interactions between lesbianism, depression, and intimate relationships are complex and not fully understood. Lesbian and gay young people report greater victimization and depression than heterosexual counterparts. A pilot study of relationship commitment revealed that depression had a negative effect on commitment.

One study found that up to 40% of lesbian, gay, bisexual, or transgendered young people either attempted or considered suicide. An active coping style and social support have been associated with lower levels of depression of lesbians in the Latino community. Lesbians may have access to fewer social supports to help them in their relationships and to cope with life stressors. Moreover, many lesbians fail to confide in their health care professionals for fear of negative reactions. Further large scale research is necessary in this area to elucidate these issues.

Family Issues

The trend toward two career families has steadily increased since the 1970s. By 1995, 91% of fathers and 67% of mothers in married households with children under the age of 18 were employed. Many studies suggest that couples with young children feel more stress and pressure than any other group in the family life cycle. Ratings of life satisfaction tend to drop from high to average and remain there until the children leave home. Not surprisingly, the couples who are most satisfied are those who have been married the longest, who want children a great deal, and who have outside resources including time, money, and social support.

The stress of dual roles as caretakers of children and as full-time employees can precipitate depression. Some women may feel overwhelmed and conflicted about family responsibilities and work. Although much progress has occurred, working mothers still absorb the majority of household and childcare responsibilities. Reviewing the daily schedule of many such women reveals a long history of sleep deprivation, excessive consumption of caffeine, and virtually no personal time. It should be noted, however, that despite these stresses there is a slightly greater risk of depression in women who are at home full-time than in those who work outside the home. This may be a result of greater access to social support at work and the wider range of sources of gratification.

Single Parenting

According to recent census figures, almost 28% of all children under the age of 18 live with only one of their parents. The vast majority of these children (85%) live with their mothers, and 40% of these mothers have never been married. Thus single parent families are quite prevalent. Unfortunately, being a single parent mother is often highly correlated with poverty. Thus many single mothers who are employed struggle with even greater problems of stress, financial concerns, conflicting responsibilities, and lack of time. Although many single mothers have strong social support networks among their family members, others are socially isolated, thereby putting them at even greater risk for depression.

Miscarriage and Infertility

The most common psychologic issues associated with miscarriage or infertility include a feeling of lack of control, a feeling of helplessness, and problems in sexuality. Miscarriage may precipitate a feeling of loss and sadness and repeated miscarriages can be traumatic. Infertility is a major stress on the couple's relationship. In addition, negotiating the health care system itself may well have a negative impact on the couple. Psychologic support and guidance from the primary care clinician directed at coping with numerous specialists, understanding all the information, laboratory tests, and procedures involved can be quite helpful to infertile couples. Women bear the brunt of the medical procedures and may feel the stigma of infertility more deeply than their male partners. The issue of potential loss and marital stress can precipitate a depression at this time. Social isolation is another related problem. Attention should be paid to the couple's relationship and their access to social support. Individual or couples psychotherapy and such self-help groups as RESOLVE can be extremely helpful. In addition to breaking the cycle of social isolation and feelings of secrecy, RESOLVE can help couples explore the practical alternatives in coping with infertility.

Divorce

Divorce not only is a risk factor for depression but has other implications for health care use. The growing population of separated and divorced individuals includes every age group. The single point prevalence of divorced individuals is approximately 10%. Lifetime prevalence of divorce in first marriages approximates 50%. Divorce is most likely to occur during the early years of marriage, in childless marriages, among those who marry young, and among people who have unhappy marriages in their family of origin. People going through a divorce or separation are high users of health care services including office visits to primary care physicians, more emergency room visits, and increased rates of substance abuse.

Many women worry not only about their own future after divorce but about their children's futures as well. Wallerstein's work documented that, even 10 years after a divorce, up to 30% of children are suffering from psychologic problems. In the end, the responsibility for these children remains with their mothers more than 85% of the time. On average, divorced mothers experience a significant drop in their standard of living within the first year after divorce. It is particularly important, therefore, to ask female patients about the well-being of their children during and after a divorce and to suggest any available resources.

Midlife and Menopause

The association between the menopausal transition and depressive symptoms is both complex and controversial. In fact, after natural menopause, mood symptoms in all women tend to decrease, regardless of their previous psychiatric history. Although epidemiologic studies suggest that natural menopause in and of itself is not associated with depression in women, there are exceptions. Some women have a vulnerability to hormonal changes. Women who have previous histories of premenstrual mood disorder have a higher probability of a recurrence at this time. Women whose family lives show a great amount of social stress or who have worries about their partners and children also show an increase risk of depression. Finally, those women who have a long perimenopause with resulting symptoms may fall victim to depression. Preliminary small studies have found that estrogen improves mood in these women (see Chapter 48).

Older Women

Elderly women are the fastest growing segment of our population. Estimates indicate that between 5% and 20% of the elderly are in need of mental health services. Factors that have been identified as causal in the development of psychiatric problems include stress, losses, maladaptive personality styles, and histories of psychiatric and physical illness. Depression continues throughout the life cycle to be the most common psychologic problem for older women. Elderly women are at greater risk for having a drug-drug interaction or a chronic medical illness. Many of them have masked depressions. Rather than presenting with depressed mood, they are preoccupied with physical symptoms or even somatic delusions when depression itself may be the primary diagnosis. Conversely, some evidence indicates that positive perceptions about health are protective and positively correlated with adjustment to the death of a spouse or divorce.

A potential barrier to appropriate diagnosis and treatment is the widespread myth that depression is normal or expected with aging. A study of widows aged 54 or older revealed that during the first 2 years after being widowed, 30% of them experienced significant clinical depression. In contrast to the belief that depression during bereavement is acceptable, most clinicians believe that if the criteria for major depressive episode are met, treatment should be initiated.

Some small studies found that the addition of estrogen enhanced the effect of antidepressants in older women. Other research also reveals an interaction between estrogen and antidepressant medication. One study of elderly women found that unopposed estrogen, but not estrogen combined with a progestin, was associated with fewer depressive symptoms.

Occupational Stress

Employed women are buffered from depression if they have a supportive spouse and financial and social resources; however, many women are not in this situation. For them the work-family conflict can be extremely stressful. In addition, employed women can experience job stress, irrespective of their marital status. "Pink collar" workers, secretaries, and administrative assistants, for example, often are exposed to high levels of responsibility but lower levels of power and salary.

Berndt's study of early onset depression examined sex differences and income. Patients with onset of a major depressive episode before age 22 were compared with those with later onset. There were no overall differences in gender, employment, educational achievement, or annual earnings. However, among women, early onset depression was statistically significantly related to lower annual earnings. A 21-year-old woman with early onset depression would earn 12% less than her counterpart who was not depressed or who became depressed after the age of 22 years. In addition, women with early onset depression were more than twice as likely to abuse alcohol or drugs. Even when the investigators controlled for alcohol and drug use, the negative financial impact remained.

EVALUATION AND MANAGEMENT
Screening

A variety of screening instruments are available to detect depression. The most common inventory for depression is the Beck Depression Inventory (BDI). This questionnaire for patients is easy to administer in the office and takes only 5 to 10 minutes to complete. Other scales include the Zung Depression Scale and the PRIME MD. It is important to use these instruments consistently and to develop a follow-up mechanism for early identification and treatment.

Screening of the elderly is even more important than at earlier ages. The Geriatric Depression Scale (GDS) reflects the understanding that depressive symptoms in the elderly may differ than those of younger patients. This 30-question self-administered scale also uses a "yes/no" format, which may be more acceptable to elderly patients and easier to do and understand. This scale was also validated in inpatient/outpatient and partial hospital settings. A shorter form, 15-item scale was also developed and can be completed in an average of 5 to 7 minutes.

Careful consideration of the potential differential diagnoses is essential in the evaluation of the depressed patient. Boxes 81-2 and 81-3 list the possible medical conditions that include depression as a symptom and the major medications that cause depressive symptoms. When patients experience depression it is important to consider the possibility that one of these conditions could be involved.

Indications for Referral

Every patient with depression should be evaluated for suicidality. Patients who have suicidal ideation with specific plans should immediately be referred for evaluation and treatment by a mental health professional to assess whether hospitalization is necessary. Lack of social support, absence of a spouse, and medical illness are all risk factors for suicide. In addition, a family history of suicide and prominent feelings of hopelessness are red flags.

Other depressed patients who should be referred quickly for further evaluation and treatment include those with a psychotic depression, those with a history of treatment failures, those with a history of suicide attempts in the past, and those who have severe vegetative symptoms. Additionally, postpartum women who meet the DSM-IV criteria for postpartum depression should be considered for early referral to a psychiatrist.

Choice of Therapy

The primary care physician can play a unique role in treating depression in women. With early identification and treatment, depressive symptoms and morbidity can be reduced substantially. The first step is to determine whether the patient suffers from depressive symptoms, an adjustment disorder, dysthymic disorder, or major depressive disorder.

Women who have a major depressive *episode* should be evaluated for medication. Treatments for depressive *symptoms* or dysthymia that do not involve medication include increased exercise, increased light exposure, individual or marital psychotherapy, and St. John's wort (hypericum perforatum). Patient education materials such as *Feeling Good: The New Mood Therapy* by David D. Burns, MD, are also helpful.

Psychotherapy

Depressed patients can benefit from psychotherapy, whether or not they are prescribed an antidepressant. Studies of cognitive behavior therapy for depression have documented effectiveness comparable to antidepressant medication with fewer treatment dropouts. The psychotherapist should be someone who is familiar with women's health and should specialize in one of the psychotherapies that have been shown to be effective with depression, including cognitive therapy, behavioral therapy, or interpersonal psychotherapy. Psychodynamic therapy, because it usually does not focus on immediate symptom relief, has not been shown to be effective as a short-term treatment. Collaboration among primary care clinicians, psychiatrists, psychologists, or other psychotherapists produces optimal treatment and cost-effective results.

BOX 81-2
Medical Conditions Associated with Depression

Acquired immunodeficiency syndrome (AIDS)
Cancer
Coronary artery disease
Chronic fatigue
Chronic renal failure
Dementia
Diabetes
Fibromyalgia
Lyme disease
Stroke
Substance abuse
Thyroid disease

Modified from Depression Guideline Panel, Depression in Primary Care: Detection and Diagnosis, Vol. 1 Rockville, MD, 1993, U.S. Department of Health and Human Services.

BOX 81-3
Medications Possibly Associated with Depression

Cardiovascular Drugs	Hormones	Psychotropics
Alpha-methyldopa	Oral contraceptives	Benzodiazepines
Propranolol	ACTH (corticotropin)	Neuroleptics
Clonidine	and glucocorticoids	
Thiazide diuretics	Anabolic steroids	
Digitalis		

Anticancer Agents	Antiinflammatory/ Antiinfective Agents	Others
Cycloserine	Nonsteroidal anti-inflammatory agents	Cocaine (withdrawal)
	Ethambutol	Amphetamines (withdrawal)
	Disulfiram	L-dopa
	Sulfonamides	Cimetidine
	Baclofen	Ranitidine
	Metoclopramide	

Adapted from Popkin MK. Secondary syndromes in DSM-IV: a review of the literature. In Frances AJ, Widiger T, editors: *DSM-IV Sourcebook*. Washington, DC, 1994 American Psychiatric Press.
Note: These medications have been reported to induce depression in some cases. Not everyone receiving one of these will necessarily be depressed. The cause of depression in a depressed person receiving treatment is not necessarily the medication. This list indicates some medications that should be evaluated as possible causes of depression in particular patients.

Marital Psychotherapy

Marital therapy is recommended for depressed women with relationship problems. The relationship between marital problems and depression was explored in a study by Leff et al that compared couple's therapy with antidepressant medication. This study randomized subjects to either 1 year of couple's therapy when it was identified as the primary issue, or 1 year of either a tricyclic antidepressant or an selective serotonin reuptake inhibitors (SSRI). At the end of the year treatment ended and the subjects were followed for another year. Results indicated that depression scores were reduced significantly in the group that received antidepressant medication, but even more so with those who received couple's therapy. Follow-up data indicated that these results were maintained over the year. With respect to cost, the author suggested that although couple's therapy was originally more expensive, overall the costs were similar. In addition, the dropout rate was significantly higher for those who received antidepressant medication.

Antidepressant Medication

If a major depressive episode is diagnosed and symptoms are causing considerable distress and impairment in any sphere of a patient's life but not so severe as to necessitate hospitalization, antidepressant medication is generally indicated. Medication should always be recommended as an option when the patient's symptoms are severe, when there is a family history of depression, if the patient has had a previous disabling depressive episode, and if the patient is experiencing symptoms of psychosis. Short-term psychotherapy is another alternative, and a combination of pharmacotherapy and psychotherapy is often ideal.

Choice of Medication

Studies have shown that all prescription antidepressants available have statistically equal effectiveness in treating depression (Box 81-4). When patients are active in the decision to start medication and its selection, and when patients have been educated about side effects, compliance rates are higher. Therefore, in choosing an antidepressant the primary care physician needs to consider the individual patient's concerns, the cost, side effect profile, and medication interactions. The SSRIs (Box 81-4) have a more favorable side effect profile than the older tricyclic antidepressants (TCAs).

Medication interactions are determined by the sites of action of each drug. Potential for unwanted interactions is increased by the number of sites of actions involved. Because of their multiple site effects, significant TCA interactions can occur. Among the many potentially dangerous side effects are increased sedation with alcohol and hypnotics, increased antihypertensive effects of blood pressure medications and increased cardiac slowing with antiarrhythmic medication.

The most common drug-drug interactions are cytochrome P450 (CYP) enzyme-mediated. The more sites a drug inhibits, the more types of CYP enzyme-induced interactions are possible. Functionally, starting, changing, or stopping a dose of SSRIs translates into altering the dose of all other medications metabolized at the same site as the SSRI. Fluoxetine, paroxetine, and fluvoxamine substantially inhibit CYP enzymes, making it more likely for them to cause drug-drug interactions, and fluoxetine substantially inhibits multiple CYP enzymes. Because of its long half-

---

BOX 81-4

Classification of Antidepressants by Putative Mechanism(s) of Action Responsible for Antidepressant Efficacy:* Generic/(Trade) Names by Drug Class

Mixed Reuptake and Neuroreceptor Antagonists
- Amitriptyline (Elavil)
- Amoxapine (Ascendin)
- Clomipramine (Anafranil)
- Doxepin (Sinequan)
- Imipramine (Tofranil-PM)
- Trimipramine (Surmontil)

Norepinephrine Selective Reuptake Inhibitors (NSRIs)
- Desipramine (Norpramin)
- Maprotiline (Ludiomil)
- Nortriptyline (Pamelor, Aventyl)
- Protriptyline (Vivactil)

Serotonin and Norepinephrine Reuptake Inhibitor (SNRI)
- Venlafaxine (Effexor)

Serotonin-2A (5-HT2A) Receptor Blocker and Weak Serotonin Uptake Inhibitor
- Nefazodone (Serzone)
- Trazodone (Desyrel)

Serotonin (5-HT2A and 2C) and β-2 Norepinephrine Receptor Blocker
- Mirtazapine (Remeron)

Dopamine and Norepinephrine Reuptake Inhibitors
- Bupropion (Wellbutrin, Wellbutrin SR, Zyban Sustained-Release)

Monoamine Oxidase Inhibitors (MAOs)
- Phenelzine (Nardil)
- Tranylcypromine (Parnate)

Adapted from: Preskorn SH: *Clinical pharmacology of selective serotonin reuptake inhibitors,* Caddo, OK, 1996, Professional Communications.
5-HT, 5-Hydroxytryptamine (serotonin).
*The presumptive mechanism of action for each drug is based on the preclinical pharmacology of the drug and the fact that it and/or its active metabolites reach sufficient concentration in vivo to affect this site of action, given its in vitro potency.

---

life, fluoxetine can cause drug-drug interactions weeks after it has been discontinued. For each medication a patient takes, consideration must be given to the possibility of same-site metabolism, and patients must be aware to remind multiple physicians of their antidepressant medication if new medications are to be added (Table 81-1).

Recent analyses seem to show that the choice of pharmacologic treatment requires special consideration with regard to gender. Women may experience higher plasma levels, longer half-lives, and greater sensitivity to side effects than men. Some studies show that both premenopausal and postmenopausal women may respond less to TCAs, but more to SSRIs than men. Women may have more side effects with the TCAs.

The tricyclics also have significant anticholinergic side effects, and many have a sedative effect. Antidepressant choice should minimize sleep disturbances. Most of the antidepressants, including the sedating TCAs, have a negative effect on normal sleep architecture. The 5-HT2 antagonists (nefazodone and trazodone) are less disruptive of sleep stages but can cause incapacitating somnolence at therapeu-

Table 81-1
Effect of Cytochrome P450 Enzymes on Specific Drugs (Metabolism)

CYP 1A2	
Antidepressants	Amitriptyline, clomipramine, imipramine
Antipsychotics	Clozapine,* olanzapine,* thioridazine*
Beta-blockers	Propanolol
Opiates	Methadone*
Miscellaneous	Caffeine,* paracetamol, tacrine,* theophylline,* R-warfarin*
CYP 2C9/10	
Miscellaneous	Phenytoin,* S-warfarin,* tolbutamide*
CYP 2C19	
Antidepressants	Citalopram,* clomipramine, imipramine
Barbiturates	Hexobarbital, mephobarbital, S-mephenytoin*
Beta-blockers	Propranolol
Benzodiazepines	Diazepam
CYP 2D6	
Antiarrhythmics	Encainide,* flecainide,* mexiletine, propafenone
Antipsychotics thioridazine (minor)	Haloperidol (minor), molindone, perphenazine,* risperidone,*
Beta-blockers	Alprenolol, bufuralol, metoprolol,* propranolol, timolol
Miscellaneous phenformin, sparteine*	Debrisoquine,* 4-hydroxyamphetamine, perhexiline,*
Opiates	Codeine,* dextromethorphan,* ethylmorphine
SSRIs	Fluoxetine, N-desmethylcitalopram, paroxetine*
TCAs	Amitriptyline,* clomipramine,* desipramine,* imipramine,*
	N-desmethylclomipramine
Other antidepressants	Venlafaxine,* mCPP metabolite of nefazodone* and trazodone*
CYP 3A3/4	
Analgesics	Acetaminophen, alfentanil
Antiarrhythmics	Amiodarone, disopyramide, lidocaine, propafenone, quinidine
Anticonvulsants	Carbamazepine,* ethosuximide
Antidepressants	Amitriptyline, clomipramine, imipramine, nefazodone,* sertraline,*
	O-desmethylvenlafaxine*
Antiestrogens	Docetaxel, paclitaxel, tamoxifen*
Antihistamines	Astemizole,* loratadine,* terfenadine*
Antipsychotics	Quetiapine,* clozapine
Benzodiazepines	Alprazolam,* clonazepam, diazepam, midazolam,* triazolam*
Calcium channel blockers	Diltiazem,* felodipine,* minodipine, nicardipine, nifedipine,* niludipine,
	nisoldipine, nitrendipine, verapamil*
Immunosuppressants	Cyclosporine,* tacrolimus (FK506-macrolide)
Local anesthetics	Cocaine, lidocaine
Macrolide antibiotics	Clarithromycin, erythromycin, triacetyloleandomycin
Steroids	Androstenedione, cortisol,* dehydro-3 epiandrosterone, dexamethasone,
	estrogen,* testosterone,* estradiol,* ethinylestradiol, progesterone
Miscellaneous (sulfonation)	Benzphetamine, cisapride,* dapsone,* lovastatin, omeprazole

CYP, Cytochrome P450 enzyme; *SSRI,* selective serotonin reuptake inhibitor; *TCA,* tricyclic antidepressants; *mCPP,* meta-chlorophenylpiperazine.
*Principal CYP enzyme.
NOTE: Such lists are not comprehensive since the CYP enzyme(s) responsible for biotransformation is known for only approximately 20% of marketed drugs. The reason is that many drugs were developed before the necessary knowledge and technology existed. Some drugs are listed under more than one CYP enzyme. That does not necessarily mean that each of these enzymes contributes equally to the elimination of the drug. One enzyme may be principally responsible based on substrate affinity and capacity and abundance of the enzyme.

tic levels. Therefore, if insomnia is a main target symptom, a small dose of a serotonin receptor blocker (e.g., trazodone) may be added at bedtime to a SSRI. Of depressed women, 70% to 80% report decreased libido. However, many medications, especially the antidepressants, cause sexual dysfunction.

Many women will refuse to take or discontinue taking a medication that will cause increased appetite or weight gain. TCAs and monoamine oxidase inhibitors (MAOIs) have long been implicated with weight gain as has mirtazapine. Substantial weight gains have also been reported in SSRI-medicated women. Nefazodone, bupropion, and venlafaxine have not been reported to increase appetite or increase weight significantly.

Suicidality must be carefully considered when prescribing the tricyclics because ingestion of as little as a 10-day supply could be lethal. The SSRIs and venlafaxine, on the other hand, have little to no potential for lethal overdose. If bupropion is taken in amounts above its recommended dose range, patients are at greater risk for seizures.

The MAOIs have been suggested for women whose depression has been refractory to treatment with other antidepressants. Given the interactions of the MAOIs with foods that are rich in the amino acid tyramine and with certain cold remedies, it is suggested that patients be referred to a psychiatrist for this treatment.

The Food and Drug Administration has not approved any antidepressant medication as safe during pregnancy. Because many depressed women are in their childbearing years, this is a special risk. However, recent studies seem to suggest that the SSRIs throughout pregnancy do not increase risk of fetal deformity. Detectable levels of medication are found in breast milk, so special consideration for pregnant and nursing mothers needs to be given. Therefore, the severity of the risk of depression needs to be weighed against exposure (see Chapter 80).

Menopausal women present a complicated situation. Women with mild depressive symptoms and prominent vasomotor symptoms may well respond to a trial of estrogen therapy. However, for those women who have not had a hysterectomy, the addition of a progestin may be problematic because of the association with depressed mood (medroxyprogesterone) or somnolence (micronized progesterone). If the alleviation of vasomotor symptoms does not result in a decrease in mood symptoms, then antidepressant therapy should be considered. Women with moderate or severe symptoms of depression should receive antidepressant medication because estrogen alone is not indicated for the primary treatment of major depressive episodes.

Compliance can be increased by a careful discussion of potential side effects. Many of the side effects of the antidepressants are time-limited, falling away rapidly after the first week. It is important to exhort patients not to be discouraged and to emphasize that depression is a treatable disease and that treatment more than likely will be time limited. It should be made clear that the antidepressants are not addictive in contrast with the anxiolytics.

For patients with mild symptoms of anxiety and depression, prescribing anxiolytics should be avoided because of the lack of effectiveness in treating depression and because of the long-term addictive potential. Optimally single drug treatment is preferable. Choosing an antidepressant with known anxiety-reducing abilities is a good first choice. Sertraline, paroxetine, and venlafaxine, are FDA-approved for panic disorder or generalized anxiety disorder. Because anxious patients with depression may be more vulnerable to the nervousness that some antidepressants may cause, starting with a low dose of antidepressant is advisable. If anxiety increases and is difficult for the patient to tolerate, augmenting with an anxiolytic is possible. After 2 to 3 weeks, when the antidepressant is beginning to reach therapeutic levels, slow tapering of the anxiolytic can be tried.

Monitoring

During the initial stage of pharmacologic treatment (approximately 1 month) patients should be seen every week to foster compliance, to adjust dosages, and to monitor side effects. After a 4-week trial at therapeutic dose, if there has been a partial response but not full remission in the patient's symptoms, increasing the dose may increase the response. After 4 weeks at this higher dose, if there is not full or very substantial improvement, an alternative antidepressant may be tried. One of the most common reasons for treatment failure is an inadequate dose. Therefore, it is important to try to reach a therapeutic dose before concluding that a medication trial failed. Close attention should be paid to dosage and side effects because of the effects of age, body weight, and body composition in women. After the acute phase, monthly or 6-week visits are adequate.

Perhaps the most important issue in monitoring is follow-up care. Because hopelessness and lethargy are part of depression, up to one third of patients may not follow through with a medication trial. The primary care clinician who is treating a depressed patient needs to take an active, educational approach to engage the patient in the process. It may be necessary to change the antidepressant to another, possibly of another family, if side effects begin to undermine the benefit of the medication.

Duration of Treatment

The primary care physician is often confronted with the issue of when to discontinue antidepressant medication. After one episode of major depression, the traditional recommendation has been that antidepressant medication can be discontinued after 6 to 9 months. There is some evidence supporting use for 1 to 2 years.

Many experts feel that maintenance treatment will prevent a new episode of depression. Patients with three or more previous episodes of major depression should be considered for long-term antidepressant medication. Others suggest that this is also true for people who have had two episodes and one of the following: a positive family history of bipolar disorder, a history of recurrence within 1 year after previously effective medication was discontinued, onset of the first episode before age 20, or severe, sudden, or life-threatening episodes.

The decision of whether to discontinue use of antidepressants should be made in collaboration with the patient. Medications (including the SSRIs) should be tapered. It is possible that patients will experience some mild flulike disturbances during the discontinuation of the SSRI. It is important to discuss with patients their own ability to monitor their depression so that they will be able to seek treatment again if they see that depression is recurring.

Hypericum Perforatum

Another treatment option is the herb, hypericum perforatum, popularly known as St. John's wort. Several reviews and meta-analyses have concluded that hypericum perforatum is more effective at treating mild depression than placebo and equally as effective as low doses of tricyclics with fewer side effects. The average dose was 350 mg three times a day. Although more data are necessary from methodologically rigorous research, there is promise for this herbal remedy. Recently a smaller trial, not yet published, has shown St. John's wort to be as effective as 40 mg of fluoxetine a day. However, there remains a lack of standardization and regulation of herbal preparations, which needs to be communicated to the patient. There may also be interactions with medications as those documented with antidepressants.

BIBLIOGRAPHY

American Psychiatric Association: *Diagnostic and statistical manual of mental disorders,* ed 4, Washington DC, 1994, American Psychiatric Association.

Berndt ER et al: Lost human capital from early-onset chronic depression, *Am J Psychiatry* 157:6, 2000.

Carmin CN, Klocek JW: To screen or not to screen: symptoms identifying primary care medical patients in need of screening for depression, *Int J Psychiatr Med* 28:293, 1998.

Clayton AH, Holroyd S, Sheldon KA: Geriatric Depression Scale vs Hamilton Rating Scale for depression in a sample of anxiety patients, *Clin Gerontologist* 17:3, 1997.

Dell DL, Stewart DE: Menopause and mood, *Postgrad Med* 108:34, 2000.

Gaster B, Holroyd J: St. John's wort for depression: a systematic review, *Arch Intern Med* 160:152, 2000.

Heim C et al: Pituitary-adrenal and autonomic responses to stress in women after sexual and physical abuse in childhood, *JAMA* 284:592, 2000.

Holroyd S, Clayton AH: Measuring depression in the elderly: which scale is best?, *Medscape Mental Health* 5, 2000.

Ingram DM: Same gender sexually active Black/African women: sexual identities, sexual orientations, coping styles, and depression, Dissertation-Abstracts-International: Section B, *The Sciences and Engineering* 60(2B):0831, 1999.

Johnson J, Weissman MM, Klerman GL: Service utilization and social morbidity associated with depressive symptoms in the community, *JAMA* 267:1478, 1992.

Katon W et al: Collaborative management to achieve depression treatment guidelines, *J Clin Psychiatry* 58(suppl 1):20, 1997.

Kessler RC et al: Lifetime and 12-month prevalence of DSM-III-R psychiatric disorders in the United States: results from the National Comorbidity Survey, *Arch Gen Psychiatry* 51:8, 1994.

Kessler RC et al: Sex and depression in the National Comorbidity Survey, I: Lifetime prevalence, chronicity and recurrence, *J Affect Disord* 29:85, 1993.

Kornstein SG et al Gender differences in treatment response to sertraline versus imipramine in chronic depression, *Am J Psychiatry* 157:1445, 2000.

Kornstein SG, McEnany G: Enhancing pharmacologic effects in the treatment of depression in women, *J Clin Psychiatry* 61:18, 2000.

Lasa L et al: The use of the Beck Depression Inventory to screen for depression in the general population: a preliminary analysis, *J Affect Disord* 57:261, 2000.

Lehmann JB, Lehmann CU, Kelly PJ: Development and health care needs of lesbians, *J Womens Health* 7:379, 1998.

Leung KK et al: Screening of depression in patients with chronic medical diseases in a primary care setting, *Family Practice* 15:67, 1998.

McKinlay JB, McKinlay SM, Brambilla DJ: The relative contributions of endocrine changes and social circumstances to depression in mid-aged women, *J Health Soc Behav* 28:345, 1987.

Miller NB et al: Stressful life events, social support and the distress of widowed and divorced women: a counteractive model, *J Family Issues* 19:181, 1998.

Rost K et al: The role of competing demands in the treatment provided primary care patients with major depression, *Arch Family Med* 9:150, 2000.

Schmidt PJ et al: Estrogen replacement effectively treats perimenopausal depression, *Am J Obstet Gynecol* 183:414, 2000.

Smock PJ, Manning WD, Gupta S: The effect of marriage and divorce on women's economic well-being, *Am Sociological Review* 64:794, 1999.

Wallerstein JS, Lewis J: The long-term impact of divorce on children: a first report from a 25-year study, *Family and Conciliation Courts Review* 36:368, 1998.

Wells KB et al: The functioning and well-being of depressed patients: results from the medical outcomes study, *JAMA* 262:914, 1989.

Whooley MA, Grady D, Cauley JA: Postmenopausal estrogen therapy and depressive symptoms in older women, *J Gen Intern Med* 15:535, 2000.

World Health Organization: International classification of diseases, Draft 10th revision, Geneva, Switzerland, 1991.

Zea MC, Reisen CA, Poppen PJ: Psychological well-being among Latino lesbians and gay men. Cultural-Diversity and Ethnic Minority *Psychology* 5:371, 1999.

CHAPTER 82

Somatoform Disorders

Felise B. Milan
Carol Landau

Patients with somatoform disorders can be among the most frustrating in primary care. Lipowski has defined the concept of somatization as "a tendency to experience and communicate somatic distress and somatic symptoms unaccounted for by relevant pathological findings and to attribute them to physical illness and to seek medical help for them." Kaplan defines it as "the patient's experience of sensory bodily complaints when psychological or social problems are present and when there is no presently measurable pathophysiologic disturbance sufficient to explain the symptoms."

Many authors who have written about somatization in primary care have expressed the view that somatization should not be conceptualized as a distinct diagnostic entity. They suggest that it is an illness-focused behavior style with multiple causes that may be associated with a number of different disorders. It can occur in a wide spectrum of patients, from those with severe psychiatric comorbidity to those who only somatize in response to extreme emotional distress.

Transient somatization and hypochondriasis are often seen in medical and other health professional students who have gained a limited understanding of pathophysiology during a period of emotional and physical stress. In such students symptoms that previously had been dismissed are then attributed to some dreaded disease discussed in class. Individuals undergoing an acute grief reaction may also experience transient somatization or hypochondriasis. Somatization can also occur in the presence of disease or be precipitated by the diagnosis of a serious or chronic illness, which then produces a heightened concern about bodily processes and physical sensations. Whereas for some, somatization is transient behavior present only in times of distress, for others it is a deeply ingrained way of dealing with the world.

Although the data vary somewhat with setting (primary care versus psychiatric), it has been clearly shown that somatizing patients are extraordinarily high utilizers of medical services. They have higher rates of outpatient visits, laboratory investigations, hospitalizations and overall medical costs. Not surprisingly, these patients have disproportionately high rates of iatrogenic illness. Patients with somatization disorder use more medical services than patients with major depression and have a level of disability that is comparable. In addition, somatizing patients consistently rate their health as poor significantly more often and to a greater extent than patients with mood and anxiety disorders.

In an attempt to standardize the identification of these patients within psychiatric research settings, the Diagnostic & Statistical Manual, 4th Edition *(DSM-IV)* has divided the somatoform disorders into categories with distinct diagnostic criteria. The somatoform disorders outlined by *DSM-IV* include body dysmorphic disorder, conversion disorder, hypochondriasis, somatization disorder (formerly Briquet's syndrome), pain disorder (formerly somatoform pain disorder), and undifferentiated somatoform disorder. The terms *somatization* and *hypochondriasis* are often used interchangeably and, although the two processes may often occur together, the concepts are somewhat different. Both disorders involve patients who may amplify physical signs or sensations, who may seek medical care for these concerns, and who are without any clinical evidence of disease. Hypochondriacs, however, are preoccupied with the belief or fear that they have a serious illness. This belief persists despite medical reassurance. Another distinguishing feature of hypochondriasis is a relatively equal distribution over both genders, whereas somatization disorder is seen almost exclusively in women.

Body dysmorphic disorder and conversion disorder are rarely seen in the primary care setting and are not discussed here. Box 82-1 presents the *DSM-IV* criteria for hypochondriasis. There is a considerable amount of overlap among the other somatoform disorders (somatization disorder, pain disorder, and undifferentiated somatoform disorder) (Boxes 82-2 through 82-4). This chapter focuses on somatization disorder and pain disorder because of their prevalence in the primary care setting and their overwhelming predominance among women.

SOMATIZATION
Defining Somatization Disorder

The *DSM* criteria have always been based on exclusively psychiatric patient populations. For years there has been a strong and frequently expressed opinion that the *DSM* criteria for somatization disorder is too exclusive for use in primary care settings. Undifferentiated somatoform disorder,

BOX 82-1

Diagnostic Criteria for Hypochondriasis

A. Preoccupation with fears of having, or the idea that one has, a serious disease, based on the person's misinterpretation of bodily symptoms.

B. The preoccupation persists despite appropriate medical evaluation and reassurance.

C. The belief in Criterion A is not of delusional intensity (as in Delusional Disorder, Somatic Type) and is not restricted to a circumscribed concern about appearance (as in Body Dysmorphic Disorder).

D. The preoccupation causes clinically significant distress or impairment in social, occupational, or other important areas of functioning.

E. The duration of the disturbance is at least 6 months.

F. The preoccupation is not better accounted for by Generalized Anxiety Disorder, Obsessive-Compulsive Disorder, Panic Disorder, a Major Depressive Episode, Separation Anxiety, or another Somatoform Disorder.

From the *Diagnostic and statistical manual of mental disorders*, ed 4, Washington DC, 1994, American Psychiatric Association.

BOX 82-2

Diagnostic Criteria or Pain Disorder

A. Pain in one or more anatomic sites is the predominant focus of the clinical presentation and is of sufficient severity to warrant clinical attention.

B. The pain causes clinically significant distress or impairment in social, occupational, or other important areas of functioning.

C. Psychologic factors are judged to have an important role in the onset, severity, exacerbation, or maintenance of the pain.

D. The symptom or deficit is not intentionally produced or feigned (as in Factitious Disorder or Malingering).

E. The pain is not better accounted for by a Mood, Anxiety, or Psychotic Disorder and does not meet criteria for Dyspareunia.

From the *Diagnostic and statistical manual of mental disorders*, ed 4, Washington DC, 1994, American Psychiatric Association.

BOX 82-3

Diagnostic Criteria for Undifferentiated Somatoform Disorder

A. One or more physical complaints (e.g., fatigue, loss of appetite, gastrointestinal or urinary complaints).

B. Either **(1)** or **(2)**:

(1) after appropriate investigation, the symptoms cannot be fully explained by a known general medical condition or the direct effects of a substance (e.g., a drug of abuse, a medication)

(2) when there is a related general medical condition, the physical complaints or resulting social or occupational impairment is in excess of what would be expected from the history, physical examination, or laboratory findings

C. The symptoms cause clinically significant distress or impairment in social, occupational, or other important areas of functioning.

D. The duration of the disturbance is at least 6 months.

E. The disturbance is not better accounted for by another mental disorder (e.g., another Somatoform Disorder, Sexual Dysfunction, Mood Disorder, Anxiety Disorder, Sleep Disorder, or Psychotic Disorder).

F. The symptom is not intentionally produced or feigned (as in Factitious Disorder or Malingering).

From the *Diagnostic and statistical manual of mental disorders*, ed 4, Washington DC, 1994, American Psychiatric Association.

index and extremely high rates of comorbid depression and disability across diagnostic categories.

Another recent study (Kroenke) has assessed the validity of a similar newly proposed diagnostic criteria for "multisomatoform disorder." They found that 8.2% of a population of 1000 primary care patients met these criteria. They also found that this diagnosis was associated with a significant level of disability and a greater number of clinic and emergency room visits, all significantly greater than that seen for other psychiatric diagnoses.

Clinical Features

The essential features of somatization disorder are the chronicity of the illness and the multiplicity of the somatic complaints. The disorder begins before the age of 30, often in the teen years. The lifetime prevalence rates based on *DSM* criteria have been reported to range from 0.2% to 2.0% among women; the disorder is rarely diagnosed in men. As noted previously, prevalence rates ranging from 8% to 19% with equal distribution across genders have been seen using more inclusive diagnostic criteria. Female first-degree biologic relatives of women with somatization disorder have a higher than expected incidence of the disorder (10% to 20%). Male relatives of these women show an increased risk of substance abuse and antisocial personality disorders. Results from adoption studies have indicated that both genetic and environmental factors contribute to the development of this disorder. Frequently patients with this disorder have taken or are taking multiple psychoactive prescription medications and are at risk for psychoactive substance abuse disorders. The course of somatization disorder tends to be chronic, with some fluctuation in severity; spontaneous remission is rare.

although much more inclusive, is considered too vague and has never been validated. Until recently, what we knew about the prevalence demographics, prognosis, and natural history of this disorder came from studies using the *DSM* criteria.

A recent large international study involving more than 25,000 patients in 14 countries used WHO data to compare the prevalence of somatization in the primary care setting using DSM (III-R and IV) criteria, ICD criteria, and the Somatic Symptom Index (also referred to as abridged somatization disorder) (Box 82-5). Results showed poor agreement between which patients were identified by the *DSM IV* and *DSM III-R* criteria, and a much higher prevalence of somatization using the Somatic Symptom Index than using ICD-10 or DSM III-R criteria (19.7% versus 2.8% versus 0.9%, respectively). They also reported an equal distribution among males and females only when using the somatic symptom

---

BOX 82-4
Diagnostic Criteria for Somatization Disorder

A. A history of many physical complaints beginning before age 30 years that occur over several years and result in treatment being sought or significant impairment in social, occupational, or other important areas of functioning.

B. Each of the following criteria must have been met, with individual symptoms occurring at any time during the course of the disturbance:

(1) *four pain symptoms:* a history of pain related to at least four different sites or functions (e.g., head, abdomen, back, joints, extremities, chest, rectum, during menstruation, during sexual intercourse, or during urination)

(2) *two gastrointestinal symptoms:* a history of at least two gastrointestinal symptoms other than pain (e.g., nausea, bloating, vomiting other than during pregnancy, diarrhea, or intolerance of several different foods)

(3) *one sexual symptom:* a history of at least one sexual or reproductive symptom other than pain (e.g., sexual indifference, erectile or ejaculatory dysfunction, irregular menses, excessive menstrual bleeding, vomiting throughout pregnancy)

(4) *one pseudoneurologic symptom:* a history of at least one symptom or deficit suggesting a neurologic condition not limited to pain (conversion symptoms such as impaired coordination or balance, paralysis or localized weakness, difficulty swallowing or lump in throat, aphonia, urinary retention, hallucinations, loss of touch or pain sensation, double vision, blindness, deafness, seizures; dissociative symptoms such as amnesia; or loss of consciousness other than fainting)

C. Either (1) or (2):

(1) after appropriate investigation, each of the symptoms in B cannot be fully explained by a known general medical condition or the direct effects of a substance (e.g., a drug of abuse, a medication)

(2) when there is a related general medical condition, the physical complaints or resulting social or occupational impairment are in excess of what would be expected from the history, physical examination, or laboratory findings

D. The symptoms are not intentionally produced or feigned (as in Factitious Disorder or Malingering).

From the *Diagnostic and statistical manual of mental disorders*, ed 4, Washington DC, 1994, American Psychiatric Association.

BOX 82-5
Alternative Diagnostic Criteria for Somatization Disorder

I. Somatic Symptom Index (SSI) or Abridged Somatization Disorder: Patients are required to have some number of medically unexplained somatic symptoms
  Males > 4
  Females > 6

II. Multisomatoform Disorder
  1. Three or more medically unexplained symptoms which are currently present OR symptoms which result in greater than expected impairment
  2. Symptoms cause significant level of dysfunction
  3. Symptom(s) are present for more days than not for 2 years or more
  4. Patient does not have a factitious disorder
  5. Symptoms are not felt to be due to comorbid psychiatric disorder

III. ICD—10 (as defined by WHO)
  1. 6 or more medically unexplained symptoms from 2 of 4 designated organ systems (pain, gastrointestinal, cardiorespiratory, genitourinary)
  2. Symptoms have lasted 2 or more years
  3. 3 or more medical consultations or investigations for these symptoms
  4. Refusal to accept the opinion of physicians that there is no physical disease

---

PSYCHIATRIC COMORBIDITIES

Depression

The overlap between depression and the somatoform disorders, which are also diagnosed more often in women than in men, are difficult for the primary care provider to manage. Studies show that from 40% to 60% of people who are diagnosed with somatoform disorders have a coexisting mood disorder. The reported frequency varies depending on the studies clinical setting (primary care versus psychiatric clinic) and the diagnostic criteria used. On the other hand, 50% to 70% of primary care patients ultimately diagnosed with a psychiatric disorder initially presented with a somatic complaint. Up to 75% of patients diagnosed with major depression or panic disorder present to their primary care providers with exclusively somatic complaints.

In an attempt to understand the atypical presentation of these patients, some have referred to somatic symptoms as depressive equivalents and have used such terms as masked depression and atypical depression to describe this clinical picture. Masked depression is defined as a depressive illness in which somatic symptoms mask the mood and cognitive components of the disorder. The low rate of recognition of depression in primary care settings may be at least partially explained by the fact that some of the patients do not exhibit the expected symptoms of mood disturbance. There are many other explanations for why depressed patients may have somatic symptoms. Patients who are aware of their depressed moods may choose to focus on somatic symptoms to avoid a discussion of their underlying problems, which may be felt to be stigmatizing. Other patients are convinced that their somatic symptoms represent a primary physical illness to which their depression is secondary. There are also patients who may lack the ability to identify and express emotions (alexithymia) and therefore rely on physical symptoms to express feelings.

A number of studies have attempted to identify which characteristics make patients with depression more likely to somatize. When gender and sex were examined, depressed older women appear to have an increased tendency to somatize.

Anxiety

Patients with somatization disorder have been found to have high rates of comorbid generalized anxiety disorder (35%) and panic disorder (25%). The overlap between somatization and anxiety is complicated. As with depressed patients, anxious patients may experience any number of somatic symptoms. These symptoms are usually secondary to autonomic hyperactivity such as palpitations, diarrhea, flushing, and diaphoresis. In addition anxiety and emotional arousal seem to increase patients' sensitivity to bodily sensations. Several studies have found anxious patients to have a decreased tolerance for pain. Patients with panic disorder may focus on their somatic complaints and deny feelings of anxiety. One study of patients with panic disorder referred from a primary care service found their presenting complaints to be epigastric pain (28%), tachycardia (25%), chest pain (22%), dizziness or vertigo (18%), shortness of breath (13%), headache (11%), and syncope (9%). Other comorbid psychiatric disorders that are also prevalent in the somatizing population and need to be considered are obsessive-compulsive disorder, personality disorder, and substance abuse.

Pain Disorder

Formerly known as psychogenic or somatoform pain disorder, this disorder has as its essential feature chronic preoccupation (>6 months) with pain that is inconsistent with or out of proportion to physical findings. There is sometimes evidence of a temporal relationship between initiation and exacerbation of symptoms and psychosocial stressors. For some patients the pain has symbolic significance or may serve as unconscious punishment. For example, a patient with unresolved guilt over placing her mother in a nursing home may begin to experience chest pain after her mother dies of a myocardial infarction.

Onset can occur at any age but most frequently is in midlife. In almost half the cases the pain develops immediately after a physical trauma. The pain then may increase in severity over weeks or months, often resulting in a decreasing level of functioning. Patients will often stop working, seek disability compensation, and increasingly take on the sick role. These patients are also at risk for dependence on narcotic analgesics and often undergo numerous invasive surgical procedures.

Comorbid depression is so frequent that some have suggested that pain disorder is a variant of depressive disorder and that it can be successfully treated with antidepressant medication. Although the overall prevalence of the disorder is unclear; the ratio of females to males is 2:1.

CAUSES OF SOMATOFORM DISORDERS

Many different theoretic explanations for somatization have been proposed. We will consider four theories of cause: psychodynamic, personality-based, neurobiologic, and behavioral.

Engel has eloquently described psychodynamic theories of somatization. The basic premise of these theories is that patients' symptoms are symbolic, expressing an underlying conflict. As an example, a common clinical scenario is a patient whose symptom represents punishment that serves to ease unconscious feelings of guilt.

As evidence for the role of personality in somatization, Smith found that somatizers had frequent concurrent personality disorders. Barsky has described the somatizing personality and discussed three different personality styles and the role that somatizing may play within these different personality styles. There are the masochistic patients whose symptoms fulfill their need for suffering and self-sacrifice. The passive-aggressive personality style is often indirectly hostile, and their illness is consistent with their feelings of having been deprived and wronged by the world. Finally, patients with dependent personality style often use illness behavior to maneuver themselves into the position of needing care and their health care provider into the role of caregiver.

Patients with borderline personality disorders sometimes appear in the primary care setting with severe somatization disorder. They frequently have seen multiple practitioners and have often been dismissed by some. The patient with borderline personality disorder and somatization disorder is probably one of the most difficult for the primary care physician to treat. Neurobiologic theories of somatization basically posit that some individuals may have a constitutional predisposition to misinterpret and amplify bodily sensations. The proposed mechanism for this is an underlying abnormality of the central nervous system within the sensory pathways that alters patient's perceptions and cognitions of bodily symptoms.

Behavioral theories maintain that all behaviors evolve and are perpetuated by environmental factors. Somatization can be conceptualized as abnormal illness behavior that is learned during childhood and reinforced throughout life. In fact, in some dysfunctional families somatization is the only behavior that receives positive reinforcement. Women with one of the somatoform disorders often report a positive family history for somatization. They describe families in which a family members illness behavior was a significant ingredient in the family system or a family that used expression of somatic complaints as a means of communicating.

This family dynamic is frequently a function of cultural beliefs and attitudes. Many cultures discourage the direct expression of emotion or attach stigma to particular psychiatric disorders such as depression and anxiety. The tendency to generalize and dramatize somatic complaints has been shown to be related to one's cultural background. Many cultures attribute different meanings to symptoms that may be a cause of concern for the patient.

Both familial and cultural factors may play a role in situations in which symptoms are being reinforced and perpetuated by the patient's secondary gain. These secondary gains may include increased support and caring from one or more family members, relief from certain responsibilities including work inside or outside the home, and monetary gain such as disability compensation or anticipated compensation from litigation. The more chronic the disability becomes the more maladaptive behaviors the patient and her family have acquired and the greater the investment in continuing the symptom.

A history of childhood physical or sexual abuse is one environmental factor that may be particularly important in women with somatization disorders. Among some populations of patients seen for the treatment of chronic pain, the frequency of past abuse has been as high as 50%. Several studies have documented associations of chronic pelvic pain and functional gastrointestinal disorders in women with a history of abuse. Chapters 87 and 88 consider these subjects in greater detail.

EVALUATION

The diagnosis of somatization involves more than just ruling out physical disorders that would explain patient's symptoms. By obtaining a thorough history and listening carefully for the signs of somatization, the diagnosis of somatization can be made concurrently with the appropriate medical evaluation. Recognizing the diagnosis early may also prevent many unnecessary diagnostic tests and procedures.

The central issues in somatization are the complaint of multiple unexplained symptoms or unexplained pain coupled with overwhelming concern about the underlying cause of the symptom(s). One clue to somatization is the expression of a great deal of concern regarding the authenticity of symptoms. Women with somatization disorders have usually undergone many medical evaluations in the past by physicians who they felt did not take their symptoms seriously. Many will vehemently insist on finding a physical cause for their symptoms and deny the influence of any psychosocial factors despite what seem to be related life events and situational stressors.

Their medical history is often characterized by accounts of multiple inconclusive tests and unsuccessful therapies or much doctoring and little curing. Women with somatization have often undergone one or more of the following surgical procedures: laparoscopy, hysterectomy, laminectomy, or cholecystectomy.

The quantity and nature of the symptoms reported may offer a clue to the diagnosis of somatization. Women who somatize will list many symptoms involving multiple organ systems. The symptoms may also be vaguely described (I feel weak all over), bizarre in nature (the pain starts in my hair), or inconsistent (I have had this headache 24 hours a day, every day for the last 10 years). Despite a rather dramatic style of presentation these women may deny any emotional disturbance. (If not for this pain my life would be absolutely perfect.)

Another clue to the diagnosis has been described in patients with somatization as disease syndrome—illness behavior discrepancy. These patients' reactions to being told that they are healthy are not one of relief but of displeasure. They seem happiest when informed of a real or medical diagnosis regardless of the consequences.

It is helpful for clinicians to recognize the emotional reactions they may have to somatizing patients. Groves noted that somatizing patients can stimulate feelings of aversion, fear, guilt, inadequacy, and malice in their physicians. It is common to feel overwhelmed early in a patient encounter by the number of the complaints and the extensive medical history, frustrated by the vague descriptions, and angry with patients themselves. Anger may be felt in response to the patient's anger and to the constant demands for a diagnosis before an adequate assessment can be completed. There is often a struggle for control of the interview with feelings of dissatisfaction in both patient and clinician.

Several strategies are usually helpful when the diagnosis of somatization is suspected:

1. Explore the patient's beliefs about the illness or beliefs about both cause and treatment.
2. Start at the beginning. Find out what was going on in the patient's life when the symptoms first started and when she last felt well.
3. Assess how the symptom or symptoms have interfered with the patient's life.
4. Elicit what the patient hopes you will do for her, making sure to distinguish the goals of symptom management from cure or diagnosis.

Although asking these questions is always important in the evaluation of any patient's complaints, answers to these questions can be especially useful in uncovering the psychogenic origin of symptoms in patients with somatization.

DIFFERENTIAL DIAGNOSIS

Once somatization has been recognized it is always important to evaluate the patient for associated affective disorders. Other disorders that need to be considered in the differential diagnosis of the somatoform disorders are malingering, factitious illness, and Munchausen syndrome (Table 82-1). Malingerers are knowingly faking their symptoms for some clear benefit such as avoidance of imprisonment. In factitious illness the patient creates physical evidence of illness (such as a false reading on a thermometer) in order to adopt the sick role. These patients are often women in the health care field. Munchausen syndrome is quite rare and occurs primarily in men. These patients typically go from hospital

Table 82-1
Differential Diagnosis

Syndrome	Malingering	Factitious Disorder	Munchausen's Syndrome
Clinical description	Feigns illness for clear primary benefit (avoid army, jail, etc.)	Creates false evidence disease (i.e., heating thermometer)	Creates detailed story consistent with serious illness—history of many surgeries, many MDs in many locations
Risk factors	Males > females	Females >>> males; health care workers	Male >> female
Underlying psychopathology	Possible sociopathy	Major psychopathology	Major pathology
Treatment	Nonjudgmental confrontation, open discussion of issues	Psychiatric referral	Psychiatric referral

to hospital feigning serious illness that often requires invasive procedures or surgical intervention. Their stories are well rehearsed and often quite believable. Patients with Munchausen syndrome and those with factitious illness often have severe psychopathologic conditions and require psychiatric evaluation.

MANAGEMENT

The major determinant of management and prognosis is the time course of the patient's disorder. Women who have recently experienced a somatoform disorder in response to a major life stressor have a good prognosis and often respond to reassurance and education about the somatization process. The most important objective of treatment is to prevent the acute disorder from becoming a more chronic problem. The physician should help the patient identify how these symptoms are affecting her life, the stressors that precipitated the symptoms, and ways to handle the emotions associated with those stressors.

Women who have a history of a lifelong pattern of somatization have a much worse prognosis and are much more difficult to treat. The key principle of treatment involves setting realistic goals for both the patient and provider (Box 82-6).

Goals of Management

The most important goal for the physician and patient to discuss and agree on is symptom management rather than symptom cure. These patients and often their physicians are frequently frustrated and disappointed by unrealistic expectations of complete symptom resolution. With improved management of their symptoms, improved coping and socialization skills, and increased insight into their problems, these patients may achieve improved domestic and occupational functioning. In addition the physician may be able to help the patient avoid unnecessary surgical procedures,

---

avoid dependence on addicting medications, and use the medical system more appropriately. Patients who have regularly scheduled visits with their primary care provider will not need to use the emergency room or call their provider as frequently.

While helping the patient to achieve these goals it is important that the physician set firm limits and negotiate an arrangement with the patient with which he or she is comfortable. The physician should also increase awareness of and ability to manage many of the negative emotions that may be elicited by the patient.

Initial Management

The initial tasks are explaining the diagnosis to the patient and reassuring her that she does not have a serious or life-threatening disease. Empathic communication of this information is essential, with all patients recognizing that in all likelihood the patient's prior contact with the medical field has been filled with extensive negative workups and dismissive comments by physicians, often leaving them feeling misunderstood and resentful. Approaches that may be especially useful with somatizing patients include these:

- Legitimizing the seriousness of the symptom to the patient ("It is clear how incapacitating this pain has been for you").
- Expressing respect for whatever adaptive behavior the patient has exhibited ("I'm impressed that you've been able to continue working considering how uncomfortable you are").
- Reflecting the emotions the patient expresses about their situation ("You are clearly very upset about how these headaches are affecting your marriage").
- Expressing support and partnership in helping the patient address her concerns ("I want you to know that I will work with you and do what I can to help make things better for you").

When attempting to reassure these patients, it is important not to dispute the presence or severity of their symptoms. Rather than saying "Your symptoms are not serious and there's nothing wrong with you," it may be more effective to say, "I understand how serious these symptoms are to you but the good news is that I don't think they represent a progressive or life-threatening illness."

For reassurance to be effective it is also important that it comes after the patient feels that the physician has all the necessary information. It is better to postpone giving reassurance until after a full history and physical examination have been completed even when patients ask for it early in an evaluation.

When discussing the formulation, the message should depend on how ready the patient is to accept a psychologic diagnosis. For patients who seem ready to accept this idea, it is useful to explain the connection between emotions and physical symptoms sensitively using examples from everyday life, such as the sweaty palms and dry mouth that may accompany stage fright, the role of stress in the development of gastric ulcers, and the common understanding of tension as a cause of headaches.

To those who are more resistant to these ideas it is useful to explain their problems in more scientific terms, emphasizing the physiologic nature of the mind-body connection. One approach that has been successful involves explaining

---

BOX 82-6
Goals of Management

For the Patient
- Achieve better management of symptom(s) (not cure)
- Improve occupational and domestic functioning
- Avoid unnecessary surgery and procedures
- Avoid dependence on potentially addicting medications, i.e., narcotics and benzodiazepines
- Improve overall health status through improvement of healthy behaviors
- Improve coping and socialization skills
- Decrease medical overutilization
- Gain insight into the connection between emotions and symptoms

For the Physician
- Help patient to achieve goals above
- Use limit setting to achieve an arrangement that is comfortable (office visits, phone calls, etc.)
- Improve awareness and handling of emotional reactions to patient such as anger, frustration, and feelings of inadequacy

how the chemicals in the brain (referring to neurotransmitters) are altered by our emotions and in turn affect the functioning of the entire body. This oversimplified but not untrue concept can provide a framework acceptable to both the physician and patient.

There are somatizing patients who will resist all attempts at making any connection between emotions and somatic complaints. These patients may benefit from receiving a descriptive diagnosis soon that describes their symptoms but does not carry with it unwarranted implications. It is possible to satisfy some patients needs for a diagnostic label with descriptions such as abnormal gastrointestinal motility, muscle contraction headaches, and hyperventilation syndrome.

Long-Term Management

Once a relationship with the somatizing patient has been established, it is important for the physician to recognize that it is tremendously therapeutic for the patient to have an objective, caring individual listen empathically to her problems. To quote Barsky, "The most powerful therapeutic tool is the physician; his or her attention, concern, interest and careful listening: don't just do something, stand there." In the context of this relationship it is important to reinforce the discussion of emotions and psychosocial stressors positively with active listening and questioning, while negatively reinforcing the expression of somatic complaints.

Frequent but time-limited visits that are regularly scheduled independent of changes in symptoms can change the patient's orientation toward physician utilization. Ideally patients will feel that they do not need to have new complaints in order to see their physicians. Strictly limiting the time available for each visit is important. If there are long lists of symptoms and concerns, it is useful to begin each visit by negotiating which one or two symptoms the patient wishes to discuss in the time available.

Although each symptom should be taken seriously and possible organic diseases ruled out when indicated, laboratory studies should be ordered in the same manner as for any other patient. Limits should be set with regard to referrals to specialists. Physicians need to decide what arrangement is acceptable to them and communicate that to the patient. Many physicians will make it clear to their patients that frequent self-referral could lead to termination from their practice.

Pharmacologic Therapy

In general somatoform disorders are not effectively treated with medication. It may be beneficial, however, to treat specific target symptoms or clearly defined affective disorders such as major depression, generalized anxiety disorder, and panic disorder. Although many patients with somatization disorder may complain of nonspecific feelings of anxiety, treatment with benzodiazepines should be avoided, as these symptoms of anxiety are almost always chronic and may provide the patient with some stimulus to deal with the emotional component of their problem.

There are two exceptions to this general principle. The first exception is chronic pain disorder. Chronic pain, as mentioned previously, has been approached by some as an indication of depression and has been successfully treated with tricyclic antidepressants. Narcotic analgesics should be avoided.

The other exception is monosymptomatic hypochondriasis, which some consider a variant of obsessive-compulsive disorder. Therefore the selective serotonergic receptor uptake inhibitors (SSRIs) (fluoxetine, sertraline, and paroxetine) and clomipramine (the tricyclic with the greatest amount of serotonergic activity) have been used to treat this disorder.

Psychotherapy

The patient may gradually come to accept the association between her emotional reactions and physical complaints. At that time the primary care provider may consider referring the patient for psychotherapy. Headaches, chronic back pain, and other forms of chronic pain can be effectively treated with behavioral methods (such as relaxation techniques and biofeedback) and cognitive psychotherapy.

Although data are limited by lack of consistent diagnostic criteria, psychotherapy has shown some benefit for somatization disorder. In randomized controlled trials, cognitive behavioral therapy for medically unexplained physical symptoms has been shown to produce a significant decrease in the frequency of symptoms and illness behavior with improved social functioning. These effects were maintained after 12 months of follow-up monitoring.

SUMMARY

Somatization disorder, pain disorder, and the more general illness behavior of somatization are frequently seen in women in the primary care setting. The overlap of these disorders with the affective disorders and several of the personality disorders makes their recognition and management difficult. There are definite signs of somatization in these patients' histories. The most important clue is a history of multiple complaints with multiple evaluations and few explanations. Obtaining a family history of somatization and a history of physical or sexual abuse can also be helpful in making the diagnosis. Once the diagnosis is made and empathically communicated to the patient the physician-patient relationship may be tremendously therapeutic. With frequent, time-limited, regularly scheduled visits the physician can often redirect the patient's focus from her somatic symptoms to her emotional distress. It is important to avoid pharmacologic therapy in these patients unless there is a clearly defined disorder or target symptom to be treated. Physicians can reduce much of the frustration felt by both the patients and themselves by setting realistic goals, aiming for management of symptoms and not cure.

BIBLIOGRAPHY

American Psychiatric Association: *Diagnostic and statistical manual of mental disorders,* ed 4, Washington DC, 1994, American Psychiatric Association.

Barsky AJ III: Patients who amplify bodily sensations, *Ann Intern Med* 91:63, 1979.

Barsky AJ III: A 37-year-old man with multiple somatic complaints, *JAMA* 278:673, 1997.

Berry J, Storandt M, Coyne A: Age and sex differences in somatic complaints associated with depression, *J Gerontol* 39:465, 1984.

Engel GL: Psychogenic pain and the pain prone patient, *Am J Med* 26:899, 1959.

Groves JE: Taking care of the hateful patient, *N Engl J Med* 298:883, 1978.

Gureje O et al: Somatization in cross-cultural perspective: a World Health Organization study in primary care, *Am J Psychiatry* 154:989, 1997.

Kaplan C, Lipkin M Jr, Gordon G: Somatization in primary care: patients with unexplained and vexing medical complaints, *J Gen Intern Med* 3:177, 1988.

Katon W: Panic disorder and somatization, *Am J Med* 77:101, 1984.

Kroenke K et al: Multisomatiform disorder, *Arch Gen Psychiatry* 54:352, 1997.

Lipowski Z: Somatization and depression, *Psychosomatics* 31:13, 1990.

Simon GE et al: An international study of the relation between somatic symptoms and depression, *N Engl J Med* 341:1329, 1999.

Smith RG, Monson R, Ray D: Patients with multiple unexplained symptoms: their characteristics, functional health, and health care utilization, *Arch Intern Med* 146:69,1986.

Speckens AEM et al: Cognitive behavioral therapy for medically unexplained physical symptoms, *BMJ* 311:1328, 1999.

CHAPTER 83

Anxiety Disorders

Naomi N. Simon
Nicole B. Korbly

Anxiety disorders are common and disabling conditions that are frequently underdiagnosed and significantly affect quality of life. Women with anxiety disorders frequently present to their primary care physicians, or in other medical settings, reflecting their fear of and sensitization to symptoms of physiologic arousal and other bodily symptoms. Research examining the cost of undiagnosed anxiety disorders has clearly demonstrated an excessive use of medical services, including emergency room visits, tests, and procedures, as well as lost productivity by these patients. This chapter focuses on panic disorder (PD), with or without agoraphobia, generalized anxiety disorder (GAD), and social anxiety disorder (SAD). Anxiety disorders also include post-traumatic stress disorder (PTSD) and obsessive compulsive disorder. The epidemiology, presentation and management of PD, SAD, and GAD are reviewed, with special reference to any data regarding gender differences. Finally, anxiety symptomatology and treatment considerations for women in the context of pregnancy, post-partum, menstrual fluctuations (including premenstrual symptoms), and menopause are discussed.

PANIC DISORDER WITH OR WITHOUT AGORAPHOBIA

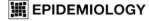 EPIDEMIOLOGY

PD with or without agoraphobia has a lifetime prevalence of 3.5%, and the rate of panic disorder in primary care populations is between 8% and 13%. Rates of panic worldwide are twice as common for women. Lifetime prevalence of panic disorder in women has been reported as 5%. The Epidemiologic Catchment Area (ECA) study reported the highest prevalence for women between the ages of 25 and 44 and found an even greater elevation of agoraphobia in women at two to four times the rate in men.

Presentation and Course

Panic attacks, the hallmark of panic disorder, consist of an acute onset of anxiety reaching a peak within 10 minutes with at least four associated cognitive and somatic symptoms such as palpitations, chest tightness, shortness of breath, dizziness, sweating, nausea, tremulousness, and fear of dying or losing control. Although many people without panic disorder experience panic attacks in response to stressful or

feared situations, patients with panic disorder must also have unexpected attacks and develop fear or concern about attacks, which may consist of a sense of anticipatory anxiety or dread. Panic attacks may become associated with common agoraphobic situations such as places where escape may be difficult, airplanes, far travel, shopping malls, bridges, tunnels, driving, public transportation, open spaces, or being home alone. Patients who develop anxiety about these situations may develop avoidance, leading to job loss and social isolation in cases of agoraphobia where patients are fearful of leaving the house. Further, patients with panic attacks have a significantly elevated risk of major depression and should be screened and monitored for the development of depressive symptomatology. For all patients with PD, there is a significant deleterious effect on quality of life and functioning, making diagnosis and treatment imperative. However, medical problems that may cause PD symptoms (Box 83-1) should be considered before making a diagnosis of PD.

In addition to a higher prevalence of PD in women, differences in symptom characteristics and course have been noted. Women have been reported to have greater agoraphobic avoidance when facing situations alone and thus a greater likelihood to require a companion to leave the home. Women appear to have more catastrophic thoughts and a greater fear of physical sensations. Women also have higher rates of comorbid SAD and PTSD, although no specific gender differences for depression or panic attacks themselves have emerged. Finally, Yonkers and colleagues examined the course of PD by gender and found equivalent rates of remission at 5 years (39%), but a greater rate of relapse in women (82%) than men (51%) during the 5-year period, independent of the presence of agoraphobia. For both men and women, PD commonly has a chronic and recurrent course.

GENERALIZED ANXIETY DISORDER

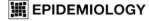 EPIDEMIOLOGY

GAD has a lifetime prevalence of 5% according to the National Comorbidity Survey (NCS), with 12-month prevalence rates of 3%. GAD, however, may be the most common anxiety disorder in primary care settings. Higher rates of GAD for women than men have been consistently reported,

BOX 83-1
Medical Differential Diagnosis of Anxiety

Cardiovascular and Respiratory
Arrhythmia
Cardiac ischemia
Congestive heart failure
Hypoxia (i.e., in COPD)
Pulmonary embolus

Endocrine and Metabolic
Adrenal dysfunction
Acute intermittent porphyria
Electrolyte abnormalities
Hyperparathyroidism
Hypoglycemia
Pheochromocytoma
Thyroid dysfunction

Neurologic
Brain tumor
Cerebral anoxia
Delirium (toxic, metabolic, infectious)
Epilepsy (especially complex partial seizures)
Migraines
Vestibular dysfunction

Substance Intoxication
Amphetamines
Antidepressants
Antiparkinsonian agents
Caffeine
Chemotherapy
Cocaine
Corticosteroids
Digitalis
Neuroleptics
Sympathomimetics
Theophylline
Thyroid hormone

Substance Withdrawal
Alcohol
Narcotics
Sedative-hypnotics

with twice the prevalence for women as men in the NCS. The reported age of presentation has varied; although many patients report symptoms since childhood, GAD can present throughout the lifespan.

Presentation and Course

GAD is characterized by excessive anxiety and worry about numerous events or activities. Although symptoms may fluctuate in response to situational life stressors, patients with GAD are described as persistent "worriers," and at least three associated symptoms must be present along with anxiety more days than not for at least 6 months by DSM-IV diagnostic criteria. Associated symptoms include insomnia, fatigue, an inability to relax, restlessness, poor concentra-

tion, irritability, and muscle tension. Patients may also describe numerous associated physical complaints such as headaches, diarrhea or gastrointestinal distress, tremulousness, and dizziness. Although patients with GAD may occasionally have panic attacks triggered by their worries, their anxiety is not primarily caused by a fear of panic attacks, and should be persistent and generalized. Comorbidity with GAD is very common; if GAD is detected, patients should be carefully screened for depression and other anxiety disorders, particularly PD and SAD. The presence of depression directs treatment away from benzodiazepines toward an antidepressant. GAD appears to be a chronic illness that may wax and wane in response to life stressors, with a significant impact on quality of life measures. Clearly, medical problems that may cause GAD symptoms (Table 83-1) should be considered before making a diagnosis of GAD.

There are currently no data available assessing gender differences in presentation or treatment response.

SOCIAL ANXIETY DISORDER
EPIDEMIOLOGY

SAD has been reported with a prevalence of 3% to 12% depending on the threshold used for diagnosis, with more stringent criteria requiring multiple areas of fear and avoidance. Patients frequently report SAD symptoms as present since early childhood, and the age of onset peaks at age 11 to 15 in the ECA data. The ECA also found women with twice the risk of social phobia as men. However, clinical samples have reported equal rates for men and women.

Presentation and Course

SAD is characterized by fears of embarrassment, humiliation, criticism, or scrutiny in a number of social and performance situations. Generalized SAD is differentiated from the more common type of social phobia limited to performance situations such as public speaking. Situations that commonly induce fear and/or avoidance for patients with SAD include meeting new people, attending parties, participating in group meetings or social gatherings, being the center of attention, interacting with authority figures, confrontations, and eating or drinking in public, in addition to public speaking. Although many people have some difficulty with some of these situations, people with SAD have excessive fear and/or avoidance of multiple situations, and often experience associated physical symptomatology such as blushing, sweating, tremulousness, and palpitations. The presence of physical symptoms serves to heighten already present fears of showing anxiety or drawing attention, and may confuse the diagnosis. Clearly, medical problems that may cause SAD symptoms (Table 83-1) should be considered before making a diagnosis of SAD. In addition, it is important to differentiate patients who are embarrassed in public due to body image concerns, including those with eating disorders, as well as those who are obsessed with a part of their body being ugly or distorted as part of body dysmorphic disorder.

As with PD and GAD, SAD significantly impairs quality of life, and may interfere with educational attainment, job advancement, and the ability to have a family or social life. SAD has also been associated with an increase in health care utilization. Reported lifetime rates of comorbid major de-

Table 83-1
Medication Treatment and Dosing for Anxiety Disorders

Medication	Initial Dose (mg)	Dose Range (mg)	Dosing Schedule	Main Limitations	Indication
SSRIs					
Citalopram (Celexa)	10	20-60	QD	Sedation, SSRI side effects	
Fluoxetine (Prozac)	5-10	10-80	QD	SSRI side effects	PD, SAD, GAD
Fluvoxamine (Luvox)	50	50-300	QD	SSRI side effects	
Paroxetine (Paxil)	10	10-50	QHS	Sedation, SSRI side effects	
Sertraline (Zoloft)	25	25-200	QD	SSRI side effects	
TCAs					
Clomipramine (Anafranil)	25	25-250	QHS	Weight gain, sedation, TCA side effects	PD, GAD
e.g., Desipramine (Norpramin)	10-25	150-300	QHS	Jitteriness, TCA side effects	
Novel Antidepressants					
Venlafaxine (Effexor)	37.5	75-300	BID-TID XR: QD	Jitteriness, GI distress	PD, GAD, ?SAD
Nefazodone	50	300-550	BID	Sedation, GI distress	?PD, ?GAD, ?SAD
MAOIs					
e.g., Phenelzine (Nardil)	15-30	45-90	BID	Drug and diet interactions, MAOI side effects	PD, SAD, ?GAD
Buspirone (Buspar)	5-10	15-60/day	BID-TID	Dysphoria	GAD
Beta-blockers					
e.g., Propranolol (Inderal)	10-20	10-160	1 hour prior	Depression, sedation	SAD esp. performance PD and GAD (adjunctive)
Benzodiazepines					
Alprazolam (Xanax)	0.25	2-10/day	QID	Memory impairment, abuse risk, sedation,	
Clonazepam (Klonopin)	0.25 QHS	1-5/day	BID-TID	Discontinuation difficulties, interdose	PD, SAD, GAD
Lorazepam (Ativan)	0.5 TID	3-12/day	TID-QID	Anxiety (shorter-acting agents)	

GAD, Generalized anxiety disorder; *PD,* panic disorder; *SAD,* social anxiety disorder; *BDZ,* benzodiazepine; *MAOI,* monoamine oxidase inhibitor; *SSRI,* serotonin reuptake inhibitor; *TCA,* tricyclic antidepressant.

pression have been reported as high as 70%. Thus detection of SAD should trigger careful screening and education of the patients about the risk of depression to aid in early detection and treatment. In addition, this significantly elevated risk of depression may argue for the use of medications with antidepressant efficacy (i.e., SSRIs) first-line over anxiolytics alone (i.e., benzodiazepines). In addition to comorbid mood and anxiety disorders, alcohol abuse is common and should be assessed.

Although epidemiologic studies support a higher prevalence of SAD in women than men, more men appear to seek treatment for the disorder. Societal expectations and gender roles may play a role in this difference, with possibly diminished acceptance of shyness and inhibition as traits for men

and boys. Although some situations may be more feared by women than men (and vice-versa), there do not appear to be significant gender differences in the level of impairment, or in comorbidity with SAD. There are no currently available data examining gender differences in treatment response (Table 83-1).

TREATMENT APPROACHES TO PANIC DISORDER, GENERALIZED ANXIETY DISORDER, AND SOCIAL ANXIETY DISORDER

First-line treatment interventions for PD, GAD, and SAD include **cognitive-behavioral therapy** (CBT) and pharmacotherapy. CBT therapy usually consists of a 12-week program focused on specific elements. For PD, these elements include education about PD and the identification of cognitive distortions (e.g., "If I have another panic attack, my heart will stop."), fears of bodily symptoms, and the "fear of fear" cycle that leads to anticipatory anxiety and avoidance. Patients learn anxiety management skills and undergo relaxation training. However, exposure to feared symptoms (e.g., shortness of breath) and situations (e.g., crowded stores, trains) through interoceptive (imaginative) and in vivo (actual) graded exposure programs is thought to be the most critical aspect of return to normal functioning. CBT techniques are similar for SAD, but focus on catastrophic cognitions about social and performance situations (e.g., "if my voice quavers, everyone will notice and think I am incompetent") with consideration of fears of embarrassment, humiliation, and criticism and exposure to avoided situations. CBT for GAD applies similar techniques, focusing on patient's excessive worries, unrealistic fears, and the frequent focus on physical symptomatology. CBT is an excellent option for patients averse to taking medications, intolerant of or nonresponsive to pharmacotherapy, or those for whom pharmacotherapy is relatively contraindicated (e.g., pregnant women), but is limited by the availability of trained therapists in some areas.

First-line pharmacotherapy for all three anxiety disorders currently consists of **serotonin-selective reuptake inhibitors (SSRIs),** which include citalopram, fluoxetine, fluvoxamine, paroxetine, and sertraline. Although the amount of double-blind data available for specific SSRIs are variable, there is no evidence of significant differences in efficacy and which SSRI selected is generally based on side effect profile (e.g., paroxetine is relatively more sedating and may avoid the need for additional medication for insomnia), concern regarding drug interactions (e.g., relatively less for sertraline and citalopram), and patient preference. In addition, an important issue for young women considering pregnancy in the near future is the relatively greater safety data available for fluoxetine demonstrating a lack of increase in rates of miscarriage or congenital malformations. Although a number of studies have identified gender differences in the absorption, distribution, and metabolism of drugs in general, there are no clinically useful data available delineating differences in dosing of psychotropic agents by gender.

Because of the increased sensitivity to physical sensations of patients with anxiety disorders, initiation side effects of SSRIs such as jitteriness, insomnia, nausea, and anxiety can be quite troubling. Thus all anxiety patients should be started at low doses (i.e., 5 to 10 mg fluoxetine, 25 mg sertraline, 10 mg paroxetine or citalopram) and titrated slowly as tolerated; however, a frequent error resulting in undertreatment is the failure to raise the dose in response to residual symptomatology. Although optimal dosing has not been worked out specifically for any of the anxiety disorders, some data and clinical experience suggest higher doses may be necessary than for depression (i.e., 40 mg paroxetine). Patients frequently stop medication on their own once their symptoms resolve, but current recommendations based on panic disorder data are to continue medication at least 1 year after anxiety symptomatology resolves before attempting a slow taper of the SSRI to reduce the risk of relapse. A total of 50% to 75% of patients with PD eventually experience relapse after discontinuing pharmacotherapy and are then restarted on medication and treated indefinitely.

Benzodiazepines (BZDs) are also effective for the treatment of PD, SAD and GAD. The majority of data for PD is for the **high potency benzodiazepines** (e.g., alprazolam, clonazepam). Although benefiting from a rapid onset of action without the initiation difficulties associated with the SSRIs, BZDs carry the risk of psychologic and physiologic dependence and should be avoided if possible for patients with alcohol or substance abuse histories. Alprazolam, a shorter acting BZD, carries a greater risk of "interdose rebound anxiety" symptoms and may be more difficult to discontinue, resulting in a preference for clonazepam among some clinicians. If benzodiazepines are prescribed, clinician or patient moralistic beliefs that "less is better," or excessive concerns about abuse can result in undertreatment. Available data for PD suggest 6 mg is more effective than 2 mg for alprazolam, and that target dosing for clonazepam is 1 to 2 mg, although some patients may require higher doses. As needed use instead of regular dosing in patients with daily anxiety symptoms as a method of limiting dosing can also be detrimental, resulting in greater psychologic dependence on "the bottle" and supporting patients' catastrophic beliefs that acute anxiety or panic attacks are dangerous and must be stopped abruptly. Finally, the lack of antidepressant efficacy of the benzodiazepines should be considered given the high rates of comorbid depression with anxiety disorders.

Buspirone, a partial serotonergic agonist at the $5\text{-}HT_{1A}$ receptor, is indicated for the treatment of GAD and lacks the abuse potential of the benzodiazepines. However, although used adjunctively for some patients with partial response to other agents such as the SSRIs, buspirone has not proven effective for SAD or PD as monotherapy. In addition, buspirone has been used clinically for adjunctive treatment of SSRI-induced sexual dysfunction, as well as anxious depression. Buspirone is well tolerated; potential side effects include insomnia, fatigue, headache, and dizziness that may be minimized, as with the SSRIs, by gradual upward dose titration. Buspirone may be initiated at 5 mg two to three times per day with a dose range typically from 30 to 60 mg/day distributed on a BID or TID basis. As with the antidepressants, anxiolytic effects usually do not manifest for a few weeks after buspirone initiation.

Tricyclic antidepressants (TCAs) (e.g., imipramine, nortriptyline) are also effective for the treatment of panic disorder and have been studied extensively; however, TCAs have not proven effective for the treatment of SAD. Even for PD the relatively more benign safety and side effect profile of the SSRIs have resulted in TCAs becoming second-line pharmacotherapy. **Monoamine oxidase inhibitors (MAOIs)** also have efficacy for anxiety disorders, but are reserved for refractory patients because of their associated risks, drug interactions, and dietary prohibitions.

Many **new antidepressants** have been developed and show promise for the treatment of anxiety disorders. **Venlafaxine** is indicated for use in GAD and shows promise for both PD and SAD. Venlafaxine does not have significant effects on cardiac conduction. The side effect profile has been notable for dose-related increases in diastolic blood pressure, but this is less of a concern with the extended release (XR) formulation. Venlafaxine is generally well tolerated; nausea, sweating, dizziness, insomnia, nervousness, and constipation may occur, but are less common when venlafaxine is initiated at low doses (i.e., 37.5 mg/day). **Nefa-**

zodone and **mirtazapine** appear to have anxiolytic properties, but have not been widely studied for patients with primary anxiety disorders.

Beta-blockers such as propranolol and atenolol have been used to treat the autonomic arousal associated with anxiety, but do not appear effective for the cognitive components. Beta-blockers should be used as monotherapy only for the treatment of performance anxiety alone (defined in DSM-IV as Social Phobia, Performance Type); they are not effective as primary therapy for PD, GAD, or the generalized form of SAD.

Valproate is an anticonvulsant commonly used in psychiatry for the treatment of bipolar disorder. There have been open studies of valproate efficacy for panic disorder including for patients refractory to other medications, but no double-blind data are available. Valproate, however, is not first-line pharmacotherapy for anxiety disorders because of the drug's side effect profile, including weight gain, hair loss, and hepatic and hematologic abnormalities, as well as concern regarding potential drug interactions and the need for serum monitoring. In addition, the well-described risks of fetal malformations in pregnancy limit the use of valproate for young women with anxiety disorders. **Gabapentin** is an anticonvulsant that has shown promise as an anxiolytic both in clinical practice, open series, and in recent double-blind trials of PD and SAD. It also appears to be useful as an alternative to BZDs for GAD. The ease of use of gabapentin, which is renally excreted, is free of drug interactions, and does not require serum monitoring, has resulted in a greater level of use in psychiatry, either as monotherapy or to augment other medications such as the SSRIs. However, there is limited experience or data regarding the safety of gabapentin in pregnancy (Table 83-1).

SPECIFIC ISSUES FOR WOMEN WITH ANXIETY DISORDERS
Menstrual Fluctuations and Premenstrual Syndrome

The menstrual cycle, which is characterized by fluctuations in estrogen and progesterone levels, may influence the onset and course of anxiety disorders. Some women report a worsening of anxiety symptoms during the premenstrual period, but available reports examining this issue are equivocal. Although an increase of PD symptoms during the premenstrual phase has been suggested, hypothesized as due to a decrease in endogenous anxiolytic progesterone metabolites, more recent studies using prospective evaluations have not supported a premenstrual exacerbation.

Premenstrual syndrome (PMS), which is characterized by a variety of emotional, behavioral, and somatic symptoms, can include anxiety symptomatology, which may explain some reports of increased anxiety by patients with primary anxiety disorders. For example, women with both GAD and PMS report an increase in anxiety symptoms compared to women with GAD alone. Nonetheless, screening for PMS (see Chapter 56) is important in the assessment of anxiety symptoms, and cyclic changes should be considered when evaluating the effectiveness of anxiety treatment. Finally, primary mood and anxiety disorders should be ruled out for patients presenting for evaluation of PMS.

PREGNANCY AND POST-PARTUM

There is little research about the effect of pregnancy on the risk for, and course of, anxiety disorders. Available data regarding anxiety disorders during pregnancy and the postpartum period focus mainly on PD, which appears to have a variable course during pregnancy. Some patients report a reduction of panic symptoms during pregnancy, whereas others report persistence or worsening of their symptoms. An important decision needs to be made regarding the psychopharmacologic treatment of anxiety disorders during pregnancy. Medication discontinuation may increase the risk of relapse and untreated anxiety disorders may pose a risk to the mother and the fetus; consequently the risk of psychotropic drug use during pregnancy must be weighed against the risk of the untreated anxiety disorder. Currently available data, including concern regarding a possible increased risk of oral clefts with first trimester benzodiazepine exposure, support the preferred use of TCAs and fluoxetine in pregnancy. Women who wish to conceive or women who have an unplanned conception may want to discontinue medications, in which case a slow taper is recommended. Adjunctive CBT may facilitate medication discontinuation. However if relapse occurs, pharmacotherapy may be indicated to protect both mother and fetus.

Although PD appears to have a variable course during pregnancy, the postpartum period appears to be a time of heightened vulnerability to onset, relapse, and exacerbation of PD, suggesting that treatment is indicated. Of note, all psychotropics pass into breast milk and counseling regarding the specific medication and lactation is recommended. For a more detailed discussion of postpartum psychiatric disorders, see Chapter 80.

Menopause

There are minimal data examining the course of anxiety disorders in menopause. However, anxiety symptoms have been well described during the perimenopausal period. In addition, this period may be associated with a significant increased risk of recurrence of anxiety symptomatology for patients with previously remitted disorders. Patients with anxiety disorders entering the perimenopausal period should be carefully screened and monitored.

BIBLIOGRAPHY

American Psychiatric Association: *Diagnostic and statistical manual of mental disorders,* ed 4, Washington DC, 1994, American Psychiatric Association.

American Psychiatric Association: Practice guidelines for the treatment of patients with panic disorder, *Am J Psychiatry* 155:1, 1998.

Andrade L, Eaton WW, Chilcoat HD: Lifetime co-morbidity of panic attacks and major depression in a population-based study: age of onset, *Psychol Med* 26:991, 1996.

Altshuler LL, Hendrick V, Cohen LS: Course of mood and anxiety disorders during pregnancy and the postpartum period, *J Clin Psychiatry* 59(suppl 2): 29, 1998.

Bailey JW, Cohen LS: Prevalence of mood and anxiety disorders in women who seek treatment for premenstrual syndrome, *J Womens Health Gender Based Med* 8: 1181, 1999.

Ballenger J: Panic disorder in primary care and general medicine. In Rosenbaum JF, Pollack MH, editors: *Panic disorder and its treatment,* New York, 1998, Marcel Dekker.

Ballenger J et al: Alprazolam in panic disorder and agoraphobia: results from a multicenter trial: I. efficacy in short-term treatment, *Arch Gen Psychiatry* 45:413, 1988.

Chambers CD: Birth outcomes in pregnant women taking fluoxetine, *N Engl J Med* 335:1010, 1996.

Cohen LS, Rosenbaum JF: Psychotropic drug use during pregnancy: weighing the risks, *J Clin Psychiatry* 59(suppl 2):18, 1998.

Cohen LS et al: Course of panic disorder during pregnancy and the puerperium: a preliminary study, *Biol Psychiatry* 39:950, 1996.

Cohen LS: Personal communication, April 2000.

Cook BL et al: Anxiety and the menstrual cycle in panic disorder, *J Affect Disord* 19:221, 1990.

Gater R et al: Sex differences in the prevalence and detection of depressive and anxiety disorders in general health care settings: report from the World Health Organization Collaborative Study on Psychological Problems in General Health Care, *Arch Gen Psychiatry* 55:405, 1998.

Fisch R: Postpartum anxiety disorder, *J Clin Psychiatry* 50:268, 1989.

Hertzberg T, Wahlbeck K: The impact of pregnancy and puerperium on panic disorder: a review, *J Psychosom Obstet Gynaecol* 20:59, 1999.

Katon W et al: Panic disorder: epidemiology in primary care, *J Fam Pract* 23:233, 1986.

Kessler R, McGonagle K, Zhao S: Lifetime and twelve-month prevalence of DSM III-R psychiatric disorders in the United States: results from the National Comorbidity Survey, *Arch Gen Psychiatry* 51: 8, 1994.

McLeod DR, Hoehn-Saric R, Foster GV, Hipsley PA: The influence of premenstrual syndrome on ratings of anxiety in women with generalized anxiety disorder, *Acta Psychiatr Scand* 88:248, 1993.

Metz A, Sichel D, Goff D: Postpartum panic disorder, *J Clin Psychiatry* 49:278, 1988.

Pande AC et al: Treatment of social phobia with gabapentin: a placebo-controlled study, *J Clin Psychopharmacol* 19:341, 1999.

Pande AC et al: Placebo-controlled study of gabapentin treatment in panic disorder, *J Clin Psychopharmacol,* 20:467, 2000.

Pastuszak A: Pregnancy outcome following first-trimester exposure to fluoxetine, *JAMA* 269:2246, 1993.

Pedersen CA: Postpartum mood and anxiety disorders: a guide for the nonpsychiatric clinician with an aside on thyroid associations with postpartum mood, *Thyroid* 9:691, 1999.

Pigott TA: Gender differences in the epidemiology and treatment of anxiety disorders, *J Clin Psychiatry* 60(suppl 18): 4, 1999.

Pollack MH, Otto M: Long-term pharmacologic treatment of panic disorder, *Psychiatr Ann* 24:291, 1994.

Regier DA et al: The de facto US mental and addictive disorders service system. Epidemiologic catchment area prospective 1-year prevalence rates of disorders and services, *Arch Gen Psychiatry* 50:85, 1993.

Rosenbaum J, Moroz G, Bowden C: Clonazepam in the treatment of panic disorder with or without agoraphobia: a dose-response study of efficacy, safety, and discontinuance, *J Clin Psychopharmacol* 17:390, 1997.

Schneier FR et al: Social phobia. Comorbidity and morbidity in an epidemiologic sample, *Arch Gen Psychiatry* 49:282, 1992.

Simon NM, Pollack MH: Current status and future prospects for anxiolytic drug therapy, *Prim Care Psychiatry* 4:157, 1998.

Simon NM, Pollack MH: Treatment-refractory panic disorder, *Psychiatr Clin North Am* 6:115, 1999.

Simpson HB et al: Imipramine in the treatment of social phobia, *J Clin Psychopharmacol* 18:132, 1998.

Starcevic V et al: Characteristics of agoraphobia in women and men with panic disorder with agoraphobia, *Depress Anxiety* 8:8, 1998.

Stein MB et al: Panic disorder and the menstrual cycle: panic disorder patients, healthy control subjects, and patients with premenstrual syndrome, *Am J Psychiatry* 146:1299, 1989.

Turgeon L, Marchand A, Dupuis G: Clinical features in panic disorder with agoraphobia: a comparison of men and women, *J Anxiety Disord* 12:539, 1998.

Turk CL et al: An investigation of gender differences in social phobia, *J Anxiety Disord* 12:209, 1998.

Van Ameringen M, Mancini C, Styan G, Donison D: Relationship of social phobia with other psychiatric illness, *J Affect Disord* 21:93, 1991.

Villeponteaux VA et al: The effects of pregnancy on preexisting panic disorder, *J Clin Psychiatry* 53:201, 1992.

Weinstock LS: Gender differences in the presentation and management of social anxiety disorder, *J Clin Psychiatry* 60:9, 1999.

Weissman MM, Merikangas KR: The epidemiology of anxiety and panic disorders: an update, *J Clin Psychiatry* 46:11, 1986.

Wittchen HU et al: DSM-III-R generalized anxiety disorder in the National Comorbidity Survey, *Arch Gen Psychiatry* 51:355, 1994.

Yonkers KA et al: Is the course of panic disorder the same in women and men? *Am J Psychiatry* 155:596, 1998.

Yonkers KA: Panic disorder in women, *J Womens Health Gender Based Med* 3:481, 1994.

CHAPTER 84

Eating Disorders

Nancy A. Rigotti

Anorexia nervosa and bulimia nervosa are psychiatric disorders of disturbed eating behavior that have serious medical consequences. More than 90% of cases occur in women. The task of the primary care physician is to recognize the syndromes, evaluate patients for medical complications, assist in ambulatory management, and determine when a patient requires hospitalization.

EPIDEMIOLOGY AND CLINICAL PRESENTATION

Anorexia nervosa is a syndrome of severe weight loss that results from inadequate food intake by individuals with no medical reason to lose weight. Instead an intense fear of becoming fat and a disturbance in body image lead to a refusal to maintain weight within a normal, healthy range for age and height. The American Psychiatric Association has developed criteria to guide diagnosis (Box 84-1).

Weight loss can occur in two ways. About half of patients severely limit food intake (restricting subtype); a second group purges after eating, usually by vomiting or taking laxatives, and may also have eating binges (binge-eating/purging subtype). Both groups may exercise vigorously. Restricting anorexics are also likely to have obsessive-compulsive symptoms, whereas those who binge may have other impulse control problems, including substance abuse. Patients with the purging subtype of anorexia nervosa have more medical problems and a worse prognosis than individuals with the restricting subtype.

Bulimia nervosa is an illness characterized by repeated episodes of binge eating, during which an individual rapidly consumes a large amount of food and feels unable to stop. To prevent weight gain after a binge, the bulimic patient either purges by inducing vomiting or taking laxatives or diuretics (purging subtype) or fasts or exercises for a prolonged period (nonpurging subtype). Bulimic patients fear losing control of their eating behavior and are ashamed when it happens. Binges must occur at least twice weekly for 3 months to meet diagnostic criteria for bulimia nervosa, but they may be repeated as often as several times daily. In severe cases there may be no regular eating pattern. The result of this behavior is frequent weight fluctuations but *not* severe weight loss.

There is considerable overlap between anorexia nervosa and bulimia nervosa. Preoccupation with food and body weight, a disturbed body image, poor self-esteem, and a fear of loss of control are hallmarks of both disorders. Symptoms of depression occur at a high rate in both conditions. Individuals may alternate between diagnoses during the course of the illness. Approximately half of anorexic patients have bulimic symptoms, and about half of patients with bulimia nervosa have a history of anorexia nervosa or have the symptoms during the illness. Nonetheless, the syndromes do differ in presentation. The emaciation of an anorexic patient often leads others to get her medical attention, even though she denies that she is ill. The physician then has the task of convincing the patient of the seriousness of her condition. In contrast, bulimics are aware that their behavior is abnormal, but shame leads them to conceal the problem. The bulimic's near-normal weight permits the illness to be hidden. Detection of surreptitious vomiting or laxative abuse is a challenge for the primary care physician.

Eating disorders start early in life. Anorexia nervosa usually begins during adolescence, with peaks occurring at ages 14 and 18, but it can appear before puberty or in adulthood. The onset frequently coincides with a stressful life event such as separation from home or the loss of a loved one by illness, death, or divorce. Once considered a disorder of upper socioeconomic groups, it is now more evenly distributed across social strata. Bulimia nervosa begins in adolescence or young adulthood, with a peak incidence at age 18. Typically it begins during or after a diet.

Eating disorders appear to be increasing in prevalence. Approximately 0.5% to 1% of women between the ages of 15 and 30 have anorexia nervosa. Bulimia is more common, affecting 1% to 3% of adolescent and college-aged women. Many more women are preoccupied with food and weight, diet unnecessarily, and may even binge eat and purge occasionally without meeting the strict diagnostic criteria of anorexia nervosa or bulimia nervosa.

CAUSES AND PATHOGENESIS

The cause of anorexia nervosa and bulimia nervosa appears to be multifactorial, arising from an interplay of sociocultural, genetic, psychologic, and familial factors. Whatever

BOX 84-1
Diagnostic Criteria for Anorexia Nervosa and Bulimia Nervosa

Anorexia Nervosa

1. Refusal to maintain a minimal normal body weight for age and height, resulting in weight below 85% of that expected.
2. Intense fear of gaining weight or becoming fat, even though underweight.
3. Disturbance in the way in which body weight or shape is experienced, undue influence of body weight or shape in self-evaluation, or denial of the seriousness of current low weight.
4. Amenorrhea of ≥3 months.

Bulimia Nervosa

1. Recurrent episodes of binge eating, characterized by:
   a. Eating a large amount of food within a discrete period of time, and
   b. Feeling a lack of control over eating during the episode.
2. Recurrent inappropriate compensatory behavior to avoid weight gain (e.g., self-induced vomiting, laxative or diuretic use, fasting, or excessive exercise).
3. Binge eating and compensatory behaviors occur an average of twice a week for 3 months.
4. Self-evaluation is unduly influenced by body shape and weight.
5. Symptoms occur when body weight is at least 85% of normal for age and height (e.g., patient does not have concurrent anorexia nervosa).

Modified from *Diagnostic and statistical manual of mental disorders*, ed 4, Washington, DC, 1994, American Psychiatric Association.

the predisposing cause, the immediate precipitant is usually a dissatisfaction with body shape that leads to dieting that has gotten out of control. The physical and psychologic consequences of starvation help to perpetuate the illness. Even normal individuals who are experimentally starved develop food preoccupations, social withdrawal, loss of libido, symptoms of depression, and when they are refed, temporary bingeing.

The cultural pressure on women to be slender presumably explains the higher prevalence of eating disorders in Western societies and the female predominance of the disorders. Eating disorders rarely occur in societies that lack abundant food and do not value leanness in females. In US culture, eating disorders appear to be more prevalent in individuals for whom thinness is associated with professional success (e.g., dancers, gymnasts, figure skaters, long-distance runners, jockeys, models, and actors). However, cultural norms cannot explain why only some women have the illness.

Genetic, biologic, psychologic, or familial factors may contribute to an individual's vulnerability to development of an eating disorder. Twin studies suggest that anorexia nervosa may have an inherited component. Anorexic patients have well-documented neuroendocrine abnormalities, but the fact that these reverse with weight gain suggests that they are the consequence and not the cause of the illness. The early age of onset of these disorders suggests that difficulties in emotional development or disturbed family dynamics are involved.

There is a strong association between eating disorders and mood disorders. Patients with eating disorders have a high rate of comorbid depression, which may abate with weight gain. Affective disorders are more common in family members of individuals with eating disorders. Whether depression is a predisposing factor or a consequence of eating disorders is debated. Other psychiatric illnesses are also associated with eating disorders. Obsessive-compulsive disorder occurs in approximately 10% of anorexic patients. Bulimic patients have an increased rate of anxiety disorders, chemical dependency, and impulsive behavior such as overspending, shoplifting, sexual promiscuity, substance abuse, and self-mutilation. A history of sexual abuse has been reported in as many as one half of patients with anorexia and bulimia.

CLINICAL MANIFESTATIONS AND MEDICAL COMPLICATIONS
Anorexia Nervosa

The physical consequences of anorexia nervosa are those of starvation. Inadequate nutrient intake results in a **loss of fat stores** and then **atrophy of skeletal and cardiac muscle.** Weight loss is accompanied by a compensatory slowing of metabolism mediated by thyroid hormone. This reduces energy expenditure and conserves body mass. In prepubertal patients skeletal growth, physical development, and sexual maturation stop. The signs and symptoms of anorexia nervosa reflect both the starvation and homeostatic response. Anorexic patients who purge suffer additional physical consequences. Nearly all physical consequences are reversible with refeeding, but prepubertal patients may never grow to previously anticipated height.

The most serious medical consequences are **cardiac arrhythmias,** which may lead to sudden death. Prolonged QT intervals preceded death in one case series. A variety of other supraventricular and ventricular arrhythmias occur; as bradycardia is most common. Electrocardiographic changes include low voltage ST-segment depression and T-wave flattening. Cardiac muscle mass atrophies with starvation, but cardiac output is preserved and congestive heart failure does not occur. Echocardiography reveals mitral valve prolapse in up to one third of cases; it disappears with weight gain and is of little clinical significance.

Weight loss is also accompanied by widespread alterations in endocrine function. Thyroid hormone metabolism changes to slow metabolism and conserve body mass, a condition known as the **euthyroid sick syndrome.** Thyroxine is preferentially converted to the inactive reverse-triiodothyronine (reverse-T_3) rather than to the more potent triiodothyronine, as normally occurs. Thyroxine levels are in the low-normal range, but triiodothyronine levels are reduced, and anorexics have some clinical features suggesting hypothyroidism (such as bradycardia, hypothermia, dry skin, cold intolerance, and constipation). However, there is no compensatory rise in the level of thyroid-stimulating hormone. Patients are euthyroid and no treatment other than refeeding is necessary.

Starvation also leads to a reversible dysfunction of the hypothalamic-pituitary axis. A critical amount of body fat is necessary to initiate the cyclic gonadotropin release required for ovulation. Reduced gonadotropin secretion leads to **anovulation, hypothalamic amenorrhea,** and **estrogen deficiency.** Weight loss does not entirely explain the amenorrhea, because up to 25% of anorexics lose menses before losing much weight, and amenorrhea may persist after weight is regained. The hypothalamic-pituitary-adrenal axis is overactive, leading to elevated plasma cortisol levels and elevation in urinary free cortisol, but there are no clinical signs of Cushing's syndrome. Persistently elevated cortisol levels probably contribute to amenorrhea. Reduced vasopressin secretion from the posterior pituitary may occur and account for **polyuria.** The anorexic's hypothalamus defends core temperature poorly in the face of changes in environmental temperature, resulting in **hypothermia.**

Anorexic women have a reduced skeletal mass and an increased risk of fracture. The **osteoporosis** is multifactorial; estrogen deficiency, low dietary calcium intake, inadequate nutrition, and excess cortisol probably all contribute. Bone density reductions have not been shown to reverse with refeeding, raising concerns that an episode of anorexia nervosa will predispose to osteoporosis later in life.

Anorexics' diets are deficient in carbohydrates and total calories but, because protein and vitamin intake is relatively preserved, vitamin deficiencies and hypoalbuminemia are unusual. The metabolic slowing of anorexia nervosa is accompanied by characteristic changes. **Gastrointestinal motility** is slowed, explaining symptoms of abdominal bloating and constipation. A reversible **bone marrow depression** occurs, characterized by mild anemia (rarely caused by iron, folate, or vitamin B_{12} deficiency) and leukopenia (without immunosuppression). **Cholesterol** and **carotene levels** increase, reflecting alteration in lipoprotein metabolism rather than excess dietary intake. Blood levels of glucose are normal or mildly reduced. However, when starvation is very advanced, severe hypoglycemia leading to coma and death has been reported. Mild elevations in **liver enzyme** levels and low serum zinc levels also occur in some patients. Electrolyte abnormalities are unusual in restricting anorexic patients. **Hyponatremia** can be seen, possibly reflecting excess water drinking or altered regulation of vasopressin. Other electrolyte abnormalities generally indicate purging behavior.

Bulimia Nervosa

The medical consequences of bulimia nervosa are largely the consequence of the patient's purging, not binge eating. Binge eating has few sequelae other than abdominal distention and discomfort and increased dental caries. The complications of purging depend on the patient's specific behavior. Chronic vomiting can cause **gastric and esophageal irritation and bleeding** and, rarely, Mallory-Weiss tears. Repeated regurgitation of stomach contents produces **volume depletion** and a **hypochloremic metabolic alkalosis. Dizziness, syncope,** and **orthostatic hypotension** occur in the volume-depleted patient. Renal compensation for the alkalosis and volume depletion leads to potassium depletion and **hypokalemia,** accompanied by low serum and urine chloride levels. Symptoms of hypokalemia are nonspecific: muscle cramps and weakness, paresthesias, polyuria, constipation. Reversible painless **parotid gland swelling,** often accompanied by hyperamylasemia, can occur with chronic vomiting. Repeated exposure of the teeth to stomach acid decalcifies enamel and leads to irreversible **dental erosion.** Abuse of emetine (ipecac) to induce vomiting causes a re-

versible **myopathy** of proximal skeletal muscle and a potentially fatal cardiomyopathy.

The **abuse of laxatives** may begin as a response to constipation and continue because of the weight loss it causes. Weight loss is transient and secondary to fluid depletion rather than to reduced absorption of calories. Stimulant laxatives are often used. They increase colonic motility, producing abdominal cramps, watery diarrhea, and electrolyte loss. Volume depletion, hyponatremia, hypokalemia, and either metabolic acidosis or alkalosis may result. Hypocalcemia and hypomagnesemia have also been reported. Rapid fecal transit may irritate intestinal mucosa or hemorrhoids, causing rectal bleeding and even rectal prolapse. Rarely, chronic laxative abuse results in an immotile "cathartic colon" unable to produce bowel movements without stimulation. Usually, however, bowel function returns when laxative use stops.

Patients use **diuretics** more often to prevent fluid retention than to induce weight loss. Chronic use leads to a hypochloremic metabolic alkalosis, hypokalemia, volume depletion, and dilutional hyponatremia. In contrast to vomiters and laxative abusers, diuretic users do not have low urine sodium and chloride levels.

Even though bulimic women are not underweight, they may have **menstrual irregularity** or even a **hypothalamic amenorrhea.** The cause is not known, but elevations in serum cortisol level may contribute.

⬛ EVALUATION
Anorexia Nervosa

The presentation of the anorexic patient is remarkable for the lack of complaints despite emaciation. In contrast to patients who lose weight because of medical illness, the patient with anorexia nervosa is often unconcerned about, or even proud of, her weight loss. Unlike other starving individuals anorexics are usually not fatigued until malnutrition is advanced. Most are restless and physically active, and some exercise to excess. Patients may report difficulty sleeping, abdominal discomfort and bloating after eating, constipation, cold intolerance, and polyuria. Amenorrhea is uniformly present in females.

Anorexia nervosa should be suspected when patients experience unexplained weight loss. A careful history usually suggests the diagnosis (Box 84-2). The history should explore the patient's attitude toward her body shape, her weight loss, her desired weight, and her eating habits. A 24-hour dietary recall is more revealing than general questions about diet. Detailed weight and menstrual histories should be obtained, including the date and circumstances at the onset of weight loss, minimum and maximum weights, and recent weight changes. All patients should be asked about binge eating, vomiting, and use of laxatives, diuretics, diet pills, and emetics. The amount of daily exercise should be quantified. Patients should be asked about symptoms of malnutrition (fatigue), dehydration (light-headedness, syncope), and hypokalemia (cramps, weakness, paresthesias, polyuria, palpitations). Inquiry should also include questions about depressive symptoms, substance use, and suicidal ideation.

Physical examination, supplemented by laboratory studies, excludes other causes of weight loss and quantifies the

---

BOX 84-2
Evaluation of Anorexia Nervosa

History	Attitude Toward Body Shape
	Weight loss history
	Desired weight
	Eating habits: 24-hour dietary recall
	Menstrual history
	Bingeing/purging history
	Exercise level
	Depression, substance use
Physical Examination	Height, weight without stress cloths
	Temperature, orthostatic vital signs
	Skin: color, hair
Laboratory Tests	Complete blood count
	Blood urea nitrogen, creatinine, electrolytes
	Liver function
	Thyroid-stimulating hormone
	Calcium, magnesium, phosphorus, albumin
	Electrocardiogram
	Bone densitometry

BOX 84-3
Evaluation of Bulimia Nervosa

History	Screening: "Are You Satisfied with Your Eating Pattern?"
	"Do you ever eat in secret?"
	Weight fluctuations
	Bingeing/purging behaviors
Physical Examination	Orthostatic signs, weight
	Parotid enlargement
	Dental enamel erosion
Laboratory Tests	Serum and urine electrolytes
	Blood urea nitrogen, creatinine
	Magnesium, calcium
	Electrocardiogram

---

severity of malnutrition and dehydration. A careful physical examination should include measurement of height, weight (without street clothing), temperature, and orthostatic vital signs. The patient is typically emaciated and bundled in clothing. Skin is dry and may be pale due to anemia or yellow-tinged due to carotenemia. Fine downy hair, termed *lanugo,* may cover face and arms. Acrocyanosis may be present. Bradycardia, hypotension, and hypothermia are seen with very low weight. The female pattern of fat distribution disappears, but axillary and pubic hair are preserved.

Laboratory investigation should include a complete blood count; blood urea nitrogen (BUN); levels of serum electrolytes, creatinine, and glucose; liver and thyroid function tests; and an electrocardiogram. If weight loss is severe, calcium, phosphorus, magnesium, and albumin levels should be measured. Mild abdominal discomfort and distention are common and do not require further evaluation; if symptoms are severe or accompanied by diarrhea, abdominal radio-

graphs, barium studies, and stool examination may be indicated to exclude occult bowel disease. Bone densitometry should be considered for women who have been underweight and amenorrheic for 12 months.

Extensive evaluation of symptoms or laboratory or endocrinologic abnormalities common to anorexia is not necessary. However, if the clinical picture is atypical the physician must consider other causes of weight loss, including malignancy, chronic infection, intestinal disorders (malabsorption, inflammatory bowel disease, or hepatitis), and endocrinopathies (hyperthyroidism, panhypopituitarism, adrenal insufficiency, diabetes mellitus). Rarely, central nervous system tumors or seizure disorders mimic anorexia nervosa or bulimia; computed tomography or electroencephalography can exclude these diagnoses in patients with neurologic signs or symptoms. Psychiatric illnesses that can be confused with anorexia include depression and obsessive-compulsive disorder.

Bulimia Nervosa

Making the diagnosis of bulimia requires maintaining a high index of suspicion, because binge eating and purging are easily concealed by a normal-weight woman (Box 84-3). Clues include a preoccupation with weight and food, a history of frequent weight fluctuations, and complaints common to patients who purge and become dehydrated (dizziness, thirst, syncope) or hypokalemic (muscle cramps or weakness, paresthesias, polyuria). Vomiters may also have hematemesis or heartburn; laxative abusers may complain of constipation, rectal bleeding, and fluid retention. Two questions can screen for bulimia: (1) Are you satisfied with your eating patterns? and (2) Do you ever eat in secret? When the diagnosis is suspected the physician should ask directly and nonjudgmentally about bingeing and purging and assess serum electrolyte levels. A direct inquiry may elicit the history from a patient seeking help but ashamed to volunteer the information. Patients suspected of bulimia should also be asked about alcohol and substance use, depressive symptoms, and suicidal ideation.

Physical examination is often unrevealing, especially in patients with milder degrees of illness. The examination should include measurement of postural signs for evidence of volume depletion. Enlarged parotid glands, erosion of dental enamel, and scars on the dorsum of the hand used to induce vomiting (Russell's sign) are signs of chronic self-induced vomiting. Laboratory studies should include tests of serum and urine electrolytes, serum creatinine and BUN, and an electrocardiogram. Electrolyte levels are often normal early in the disease or in those who purge less often. The pattern of serum and urine electrolytes helps to determine the mode of purging. Calcium and magnesium levels should be measured in laxative abusers. Some patients who vomit deny that it is voluntary. Organic causes of chronic vomiting should be excluded in these cases with barium studies. The combination of unexplained hypochloremic alkalosis, concern about weight gain, and absence of other abnormality strongly suggests bulimia.

CHOICE OF THERAPY

The goals of treatment are (1) to restore weight to correct the physical and psychologic sequelae of malnutrition, (2) to control abnormal eating behavior, and (3) to prevent relapse by addressing the associated psychologic and family problems. Because the illness is multidimensional a multidisciplinary treatment approach, combining medical, nutritional, psychologic, and pharmacologic therapies, is the standard of care for eating disorders.

Anorexia Nervosa

Weight restoration is the first goal of treatment for patients with anorexia nervosa. Achieving this goal may require hospitalization, ideally in a psychiatric unit experienced in treating eating disorders. Refeeding can usually be accomplished with a normal diet. Nasogastric tube feeding or parenteral nutrition is rarely necessary and best avoided because of the risk of complications. Inpatient treatment also includes medical monitoring, behavioral therapy that links desired activities to achievement of weight goals, supervised exercise, psychotherapy, and family therapy. This approach generally produces weight gain, but relapse is common. Outcome is best if the patient remains hospitalized until she has reached a normal weight. Some anorexic patients can gain weight as outpatients; they are less underweight, medically stable, highly motivated to change, and have a supportive environment. Close medical monitoring is necessary. If the patient does not gain weight within a few weeks, hospitalization is indicated. A variety of medications, including antidepressants, antipsychotics, and appetite stimulants, have been tried for anorexia nervosa. No drug is dramatically effective in controlled trials. Even though anorexic patients are often depressed, there is little evidence of benefit from the use of antidepressants, although fluoxetine may help stabilize weight gain once it has occurred.

Bulimia Nervosa

Most patients with bulimia nervosa can be treated as outpatients. The best evidence supports **cognitive-behavioral therapy,** which helps patients monitor their behavior and alter their attitudes about weight and eating. Individual or group psychotherapy and family therapy are also commonly used. Treatment may be supplemented with support groups (e.g., Overeaters Anonymous). Substance abuse, if present, must be treated concurrently.

In contrast to their role in anorexia nervosa, **antidepressants** are effective in reducing the symptoms of bulimia nervosa, even in patients without coexistent depression. Placebo-controlled trials have demonstrated the efficacy of tricyclic agents (imipramine and desipramine used at doses of up to 300 mg/day), fluoxetine (60 mg/day), trazodone, and monoamine oxidase inhibitors (phenelzine and isocarboxazid) in decreasing the frequency of binge eating and purging in bulimic patients. Drug treatment should supplement, not replace, psychologic treatment of bulimic patients.

NATURAL HISTORY AND PROGNOSIS

Anorexia nervosa has a variable course. Women may recover after a single episode, repeatedly gain and lose weight, or remain chronically underweight. More than half experience relapse after an initial hospitalization for weight gain. In studies monitoring anorexic patients for at least 4 years, approximately half of anorexic patients have a complete recovery of weight and menses, 30% have a partial recovery, and 20%

develop chronic illness. Factors associated with poor outcome are lower weight, older age at presentation, longer duration of symptoms before treatment, and coexisting bulimia. Weight preoccupation, unusual eating behavior, and psychosocial problems often persist after weight gain. Up to 40% of anorexic women develop bulimia. Because of the early age of onset of anorexia nervosa, physicians caring for adults are more likely to see women with a chronic syndrome.

The mortality rate is 0.56% per year. Most deaths are sudden, apparently caused by cardiac arrhythmias. Prolonged QT intervals may be a harbinger. Fatal hypoglycemic coma has also been reported. Suicide is also a cause of death in anorexic patients. The risk of death increases with greater weight loss, especially when weight loss exceeds 30% of premorbid weight. Bulimic anorexics with metabolic abnormalities are probably also at higher risk.

The natural history of bulimia nervosa appears to be similar to anorexia nervosa, but the mortality rate is lower. The disorder can persist for years before and after it is discovered. Short-term prognosis is good: 70% of patients completing outpatient treatment programs achieve substantial symptom reduction, but 25% have a relapse within 6 months. The course is most often episodic with gradual improvement.

✳ MANAGEMENT

Treating the patient with an eating disorder requires attention to both medical and psychosocial problems. For outpatient treatment the primary care physician usually works with a psychiatrist or psychologist to develop a coordinated treatment plan in which the primary care physician assumes responsibility for the patient's physical care while the psychiatrist coordinates psychosocial treatment. A dietitian is usually involved to address eating behaviors and diet composition and to help the patient learn to eat regular, small meals. The team approach eases the physician's burden when treating a patient who may deny the seriousness of the illness; can be deceptive, manipulative, and angry; and has difficulty trusting the physician. All caretakers must agree on overall goals and maintain contact with each other during the treatment.

The first challenge may be to convince an indifferent patient that treatment is necessary. The physician should inform the patient of the nature of the illness, its seriousness, and its potential complications. The patient with anorexia nervosa should understand that she has a life-threatening illness and that the first priority is to protect her life so that psychiatric treatment can proceed. The necessity of weight gain to prevent long-term sequelae such as osteoporosis must be emphasized. Bulimics should be educated about the consequences of their behavior, especially the irreversible dental damage associated with chronic vomiting. The ineffectiveness of laxative or diuretic use for real weight loss should be explained. The connection between the eating disorder and any symptoms or laboratory abnormalities present should be pointed out.

The physician should set explicit guidelines for outpatient management (Box 84-4). It is helpful to make these explicit in a written contract signed by the physician and patient and shared with other caretakers. It should specify the conditions that must be met for outpatient medical treatment to continue; these usually include a minimum acceptable weight, maintenance of normal electrolyte levels, and regular psychologic and nutritional therapy. It should be understood that hospitalization will be required if these conditions are not met. The minimum weight is usually set at 30% below premorbid or ideal body weight. The weight goal is more difficult to determine and can be a point of disagreement between physician and patient. An estimate of desirable weight for height can be derived from standard tables. The weight goal should be at least 85% of this value and be a weight at which the patient has menstruated. It is often close to the patient's premorbid weight. During treatment the patient's weight, vital signs, and serum electrolyte levels (if abnormal) should be monitored regularly—weekly if the patient is very underweight, less often as the condition stabilizes.

To minimize potential complications of refeeding (gastric dilation, fluid retention, dependent edema) and to prevent the development of binge eating, patients should regain weight slowly, at a rate of 1 to 2 pounds a week. A dietitian can formulate and monitor an eating plan. Nutritional supplements can be added if the patient is unable to gain weight at an acceptable rate. Although vitamin deficiencies are uncommon in anorexia nervosa, it is prudent to recommend a daily multivitamin. Complications of refeeding and rehydration should be anticipated and explained. Patients with pedal edema can be aided by support stockings, leg elevation, mild salt restriction, and reassurance that the condition is temporary. Diuretics should be avoided because of their potential for abuse.

There is no evidence that treatment with estrogen or calcium can prevent or reverse the bone loss associated with anorexia nervosa. However, it is reasonable to ensure that dietary calcium intake is adequate by prescribing supplements so that intake reaches 1500 mg/day and to prescribe a multivitamin to ensure adequate vitamin D intake. Women who have been amenorrheic for at least 12 months warrant consideration of bone densitometry. The decision about estrogen replacement should be individualized. If estrogen replacement is used, the regimen used for postmenopausal patients is better tolerated than oral contraceptives, which have a higher estrogen dose. Bone loss can persist even during estrogen treatment, and weight gain appears to be necessary for osteoporosis prevention.

A trial of antidepressants to control symptoms should be tried in bulimics. Serum potassium levels and orthostatic vital signs must be monitored, and the patient instructed to eat potassium-rich foods. Serum sodium should be monitored in anorexics with excess water intake. Maintaining normal electrolyte levels should be a condition of continued outpatient treatment. If the potassium level falls below normal despite dietary measures, supplemental potassium is indicated. This must be given as potassium chloride to correct the metabolic alkalosis that maintains the hypokalemia. Patients should be told to take the supplement at a time when purging does not occur; often this is at bedtime. Patients who vomit should be referred for dental evaluation and informed about the irreversibility of enamel loss. Those using laxatives should be informed of the ineffectiveness of these agents for real weight loss and urged to stop, either abruptly or by gradual tapering. When laxative abuse stops, transient constipation, fluid retention, dependent edema, and weight gain are common. The reequilibration period may last several weeks. Fluid retention and edema also occur temporarily when diuretic use stops. To prevent constipation patients should increase dietary fiber intake and may benefit from fiber supplements or stool softeners. Physicians caring for bulimics should be alert to the possibility of drug and alcohol abuse, which is more common in these patients.

INDICATIONS FOR HOSPITAL ADMISSION

The primary care physician should assess and then monitor the patient's physical state to determine whether hospitalization is necessary. Patients with severe degrees of weight loss, dehydration, metabolic derangement, and depression require hospital admission (Box 84-5).

BOX 84-4
Guidelines for Medical Management

1. Assist in diagnosis by excluding other causes of weight loss or purging.
2. Assess the degree of malnutrition, dehydration, and electrolyte disturbance to determine whether hospitalization is necessary (see Box 84-3).
3. Coordinate management with psychologist or psychiatrist and dietitian.
4. Educate the patient about the medical complications of the illness.
5. Set guidelines for outpatient management:
   a. Minimum acceptable weight
   b. Weight goal (underweight patients)
   c. Rate of weight gain (1-2 lb/wk) for underweight patients
   d. Maintenance of normal electrolyte levels
   e. Compliance with psychiatric and dietary therapy
6. Monitor weight, vital signs, and electrolyte levels regularly during treatment.
7. Treat hypokalemia with potassium chloride.
8. Prescribe a daily multivitamin.
9. Prescribe calcium supplements (1500 mg/day) for amenorrheic patients.
10. Consider bone densitometry and estrogen replacement therapy for patient underweight and amenorrheic for 12 months.
11. Consider a trial of antidepressants to control symptoms in bulimics.

BOX 84-5
Indications for Hospital Admission

Weight loss >30% of premorbid or ideal weight
Rapidly progressing weight loss
Cardiac arrhythmias
Persistent hypokalemia unresponsive to outpatient treatment
Severe depression or suicidal ideation
Behavior out of the patient's control (e.g., purging or exercise)

BIBLIOGRAPHY

American Psychiatric Association: Practice guideline for eating disorder, *Am J Psychiatry* 150:212, 1993.

American Psychiatric Association: Eating disorders. In *Diagnostic and statistical manual of mental disorders,* ed 4, Washington DC, American Psychiatric Association.

Becker AE, Grinspoon SK, Klibanski A, Herzog DB. Eating disorders. *N Engl J Med* 340:1092, 1999.

Beumont PJV, Russell JD, Touyz SW: Treatment of anorexia nervosa. *Lancet* 341:1635, 1993.

Bo-Linn GW et al: Purging and calorie absorption in bulimic patients and normal women, *Ann Intern Med* 99:14, 1983.

Freund KM et al: Detection of bulimia in a primary care setting, *J Gen Intern Med* 8:236, 1993.

Garner DM: Pathogenesis of anorexia nervosa, *Lancet* 341:1631, 1993.

Gold PW et al: Abnormal hypothalamic-pituitary-adrenal function in anorexia nervosa, *N Engl J Med* 314:1335, 1986.

Grinspoon S, Thomas E, Pitts S et al. Prevalence and predictive factors for regional osteopenia in women with anorexia nervosa. *Ann Intern Med* 133:790, 2000.

Humphries LL et al: Hyperamylasemia in patients with eating disorders, *Ann Intern Med* 106:50, 1987.

Isner JM et al: Anorexia nervosa and sudden death, *Ann Intern Med* 102:49, 1985.

Klibanski A, Biller BMK, Schoenfeld DA et al. The effects of estrogen administration on trabecular bone loss in young women with anorexia nervosa. *J Clin Endocrinol Metab* 80:898, 1995.

Meyers DG et al: Mitral valve prolapse in anorexia nervosa, *Ann Intern Med* 105:384, 1986.

Palmer EP, Guay AT: Reversible myopathy secondary to abuse of Ipecac in patients with major eating disorders, *N Engl J Med* 313:1457, 1985.

Rich LM et al: Hypoglycemic coma in anorexia nervosa: case report and review of the literature. *Arch Intern Med* 150:891, 1990.

Rigotti NA et al: The clinical course of osteoporosis in anorexia nervosa: a longitudinal study of cortical bone mass, *JAMA* 265:1133, 1991.

Salisbury JJ, Mitchell JE: Bone mineral density and anorexia nervosa in women, *Am J Psychiatry* 148:768, 1991.

CHAPTER 85

Evaluation and Management of Obesity

Susan M. Cummings

Janey S.A. Pratt

Lee M. Kaplan

Few issues generate more concern among patients than excess body weight. In the United States and many other parts of the world, cultural ideals stress thinness, particularly for women. These ideals lead many women to pursue popular weight loss diets and other, sometimes questionable, strategies for weight loss. The drive for thinness makes women vulnerable to unrealistic claims for weight loss strategies and willing—perhaps too willing—to try unproven weight loss potions and programs. Despite these cultural pressures, the average body weight of women in the United States has risen dramatically and steadily during the last 25 years. Using standard definitions (described later), approximately 25% of white women and 60% of African-American women are obese by middle age. At best, the dichotomy between the idealized image and the reality experienced by most women leads to frustration and anxiety, and in many cases, it predisposes to depression. Worse, this conflict may promote a distorted body image and a variety of eating disorders, including binge eating and bulimia.

Notwithstanding these cultural considerations, we must also recognize the significant negative impact that excess body weight has on physical and mental health. As the overall population has become heavier and heavier, the number of women who meet the criteria for obesity has risen dramatically. The number of these women who experience debilitating or life-threatening complications of their obesity has risen even faster, and simple reassurance, or encouragement to accept their body size, inadequately addresses their medical issues.

There are several reasons why the primary care physician needs expertise in the management of obesity. First, women frequently have serious concerns about being overweight that affect their overall quality of life. In addition, as described later, obesity causes, exacerbates, or substantially increases the risk of nearly 40 different medical conditions. Both morbidity from these disorders and overall mortality are directly related to excess body fat. With increasing weight and obesity, these risks increase exponentially.

This chapter outlines an approach to weight disorders in the primary care setting. Most important, it aims to help primary care physicians to differentiate between high-risk obesity, which mandates intensive, occasionally invasive treatment, and the less severe (but more common) weight disorders for which more incremental and graded approaches are most appropriate. Knowing how to define and measure obesity and understanding the associated health consequences will help identify and effectively treat those patients who need intervention. Familiarity with the range of available treatments, their appropriate use, and their effectiveness are a prerequisite to optimal management of obesity and weight disorders in the practice setting.

DEFINITIONS

Obesity is defined as excess body fat. In most clinical settings, **body mass index (BMI)** correlates well with total body fat. BMI is a ratio between an individual's weight and the square of her height and is reported as kg/m^2. The following formula can be used to convert from English to metric units:

$$\text{BMI (in kg/m}^2) = \frac{\text{Weight (lbs.)}}{[\text{height (in)}]^2} \times 703$$

The normal BMI for adults (that BMI associated with the lowest morbidity and mortality) ranges from approximately 18 to 25. According to 1998 standards established by the U.S. Public Health Service and the World Health Organization, *overweight* is defined as a BMI between 25 and 30, and *obesity* is defined as a BMI greater than 30. Obesity is further subdivided by severity and risk of medical complications into **class I** (BMI = 30-35), **class II** (BMI = 35-40), and **class III** (BMI > 40). Because of the rising prevalence of severe obesity, some practitioners and investigators have further segregated class III obesity to reflect the particular challenges of "super-obesity" (BMI > 50) and beyond. Recognizing that the term *obesity* as defined in this medical context differs from its colloquial use, many health professionals prefer to use the terms *clinically overweight* and *medical obesity* or *clinical obesity* to avoid confusing or inadvertently insulting their patients.

EPIDEMIOLOGY

The average BMI of U.S. adults is now approximately 27 kg/m^2; thus, more than half of American adults are overweight. Approximately one fourth (27%) have obesity, up from 16% as recently as 1980. Obesity is particularly prevalent in selected population subgroups. More than 60% of African-American and Mexican-American women have this disorder. According to data from the U.S. Centers for Disease Control and Prevention, the prevalence of obesity among U.S. adults increased *every year* between 1985 and 1999 and shows no indication of abating in the first decade of the twenty-first century. Obesity in children and adolescents, which strongly correlates with obesity in adulthood, is also on the rise. Recent studies indicate that approximately 15% of US children have obesity, up from 7% as recently as 1980. These rapid changes show that despite the importance of genetics in determining predisposition to obesity, development of obesity itself is strongly influenced by environmental factors. Such factors likely include (1) the overall decrease in physical activity; (2) the increased availability, caloric density, fat and carbohydrate content, homogeneity, and processing of consumed foods; (3) the increasing speed and chaotic patterns of eating; and (4) the increased stress and pace of life (including eating). The increasing prevalence of obesity in children supports the prediction that this epidemic has not nearly reached its peak.

Obesity is the second leading cause of premature death in the United States after tobacco use. Medical complications of obesity affect a wide variety of organs and physiologic systems (Box 85-1). A group of these disorders known as *metabolic syndrome* or "syndrome X," including type 2 diabetes mellitus, hypertension, hypercholesterolemia, and atherosclerotic cardiovascular disease, is responsible for a large portion of obesity-associated morbidity and mortality.

Metabolic complications are those that reflect the direct metabolic, hormonal, or biochemical consequences of excess body fat. They include diabetes mellitus, hyperlipidemia, fatty liver disease, coagulation disorders, and central sleep apnea (Pickwickian syndrome caused by respiratory insensitivity to elevated circulating CO_2 levels). In most cases, the metabolic consequences of obesity are more prominent in individuals with a predominantly abdominal (versus gluteal) and visceral (versus subcutaneous) distribution of excess body fat.

Anatomic complications arise as a result of changes in body and tissue shape. They include the results of anatomic distortion (e.g., obstructive sleep apnea or intertriginous fungal infections) and alterations in normal thoracoabdominal pressure relationships (e.g., gastroesophageal reflux disease, stress incontinence, and pseudotumor cerebri). **Degenerative complications** include the predictable effects of chronic obesity on the musculoskeletal system (e.g., vertebral disk disease and osteoarthritis), as well as the long-term consequences of obesity-associated metabolic diseases, such as atherosclerosis, the other complications of diabetes, and hepatic fibrosis and cirrhosis. **Neoplastic complications** also appear to result from the long-term effects of the metabolic and anatomic consequences of obesity. Most of the neoplastic complications affect reproductive organs, suggesting a role for obesity-associated hormonal changes. For adenocarcinoma of the esophagus, however, the etiologic pathway appears to be obesity-associated gastroesophageal reflux disease (GERD), leading to Barrett's esophagus, dysplasia, and ultimately, neoplasia. During the last 20 years, the incidence of adenocarcinoma of the esophagus in the United States has risen more quickly than for any other solid

---

BOX 85-1
Complications of Obesity

Metabolic
Diabetes mellitus, type 2
Hypertriglyceridemia
Hypercholesterolemia
Hypertension
Gallstones
Fatty liver disease
Pancreatitis
Central sleep apnea
Platelet dysfunction (hypercoagulability)

Anatomic
Obstructive sleep apnea
Gastroesophageal reflux disease (GERD)
GERD-associated asthma
Stress incontinence
Pseudotumor cerebri
Venous stasis
Stasis-associated cellulitis
Deep venous thrombosis
Pulmonary embolism from deep vein thrombosis
Fungal skin infections (intertrigo)
Decubitus ulcers
Accidental injuries

Degenerative
Atherosclerotic cardiovascular disease
Complications of diabetes (neurologic, ophthalmologic, renal)
Heart failure
Degenerative joint disease
Vertebral disc disease
NASH (nonalcoholic steatohepatitis)-related cirrhosis

Neoplastic
Breast carcinoma
Ovarian carcinoma
Endometrial carcinoma
Prostate carcinoma
Colorectal carcinoma
Gallbladder carcinoma
Esophageal adenocarcinoma
Renal cell carcinoma

Psychologic
Anxiety disorders
Depression
Binge eating disorder
Reactive bulimia

---

tumor. It has been estimated that as much as 75% of the recent *increase* in incidence of esophageal adenocarcinoma is directly attributable to the rising prevalence of obesity in this country.

The **psychologic complications** of obesity form a distinct category. They appear to result from several different causes, including cultural pressures, prejudice, frustration with the physical and social limitations imposed by excess body weight, and frustration with the inability to substantially reverse obesity once it has developed. While psychologic factors can contribute to the generation of obesity (setting up a vicious circle as described previously), it is important to recognize that in most cases the psychologic *consequences* of weight disorders are far more common and usually account for the predominance of psychologic symptoms experienced by women with obesity.

BIOLOGIC REGULATION OF BODY WEIGHT

Body weight is tightly regulated, with caloric intake and energy expenditure normally matched to within a tolerance of 0.15%. Obesity results from the failure of this sophisticated regulatory system, with an imbalance between total energy intake and expenditure. Given the total amount of food consumed on a daily basis, even a small imbalance between energy ingested and expended, over time, can result in significant alterations in body weight. An unopposed 10% increase in calorie intake would cause a *yearly* weight gain of 14 pounds, which if sustained would cause severe obesity. More typically, day-to-day variations in energy intake are matched by commensurate changes in basal energy expenditure. In our current environment, however, something occurs to disrupt this fine balance, whether it is an alteration of natural regulatory mechanisms or simply that the degree of excess food intake overwhelms the body's ability to compensate metabolically.

What causes the normally well-regulated balance between energy intake and energy expenditure to go even mildly awry? Obesity is induced by some combination of genetic, environmental, and psychologic influences. Regulation of body weight appears to be coordinated primarily by the hypothalamus, which receives afferent input from several sources. Circulating levels of the adipocyte-derived hormone leptin signal body energy stores. Through neurohumoral mechanisms, the gastrointestinal tract provides information about recent food ingestion, and the cerebral cortex provides input about environmental conditions and behavior. Most people appear to maintain their weight around a physiologic setpoint, and it is thought that obesity results in part from an innate or environmentally induced disturbance in this control system (the mechanisms of which are not yet known). Significant deviation from the setpoint leads to appropriate compensatory responses: thus acute weight loss generates a simultaneous drive for energy conservation (decreased metabolic rate) and increased caloric intake (increased hunger). The body goes into a "starvation response" mode, even as it remains overweight with increased energy stores. Forced overeating generates the opposite effects.

The effector arm of hypothalamic control of body weight includes the regulation of food intake, metabolic activity, and energy expenditure (primarily in muscle and fat tissue). Among the dozens of mediators of these regulatory systems are melanocyte-stimulating hormone, neuropeptide Y, melanin-concentrating hormone, insulin, and the sympathetic nervous system. It is likely that obesity represents the common outcome of a spectrum of different disorders, each arising from distinct defects (or groups of defects) in the cortical (including psychologic), hypothalamic, gastrointestinal, endocrine, and metabolic components of the weight regulatory system.

GENETICS OF BODY WEIGHT REGULATION

Several lines of epidemiologic evidence suggest that genetic factors account for up to 80% of an individual's *predisposition* to developing obesity. The discovery during the last 5 years of specific genetic defects that lead to or provide protection against obesity in animals and humans has increased our understanding of the important role of genes in this disorder. Evidence for a strong genetic contribution to human obesity comes from a variety of sources, including twin and family studies. Several such studies have calculated the correlation between BMIs of related pairs of individuals. For genetically unrelated spouses, the BMI correlation is approximately 10%. For first cousins it is about 15%. For parent-child pairs and siblings, the correlation is approximately 25%, and for monozygotic twins, it is between 80% and 90%.

Other support for the genetic basis of obesity comes from animal studies. There are several naturally occurring models of weight dysregulation in mice and rats, including single-gene defects that lead inexorably to obesity and polygenic traits that affect the susceptibility of these animals to diet-induced obesity. The defect in one of these strains, the *obese (ob/ob)* mouse, was shown by Friedman and colleagues to reside in the gene encoding **leptin,** a circulating hormone secreted by fat cells that signals the level of energy reserves (body fat) to the hypothalamus. The *obese* mice fail to synthesize leptin. The hypothalamus interprets the absence of leptin as severely diminished energy stores and generates a coordinated response that includes increased appetite and food ingestion and decreased energy expenditure. Replacement of the missing leptin reverses these effects.

Although a few individuals with severe obesity have been shown to lack leptin, nearly all obese individuals exhibit an *excess* of circulating leptin in direct proportion to their BMI. Thus, human obesity appears to result from functional *resistance* to the effects of leptin, much as type 2 diabetes reflects resistance to the physiologic effects of insulin.

MEDICAL CAUSES OF WEIGHT DISORDERS

Specific, identifiable, medical causes of obesity and weight gain are relatively rare. Some, such as hypothyroidism and Cushing's syndrome are generally correctable, so they should be considered in all patients presenting for obesity evaluation. Polycystic ovary syndrome (PCOS) is commonly associated with obesity in women; however, there is currently no specific therapy for PCOS that improves the associated weight disorder. Several medications are associated with weight gain (Box 85-2), most notably steroids, insulin, and several classes of psychotropic agents.

Environmental Contributors

Although genetic mechanisms strongly influence body weight regulation, recent history shows clearly the important role of the environment. Several environmental factors have been proposed to explain the recent rise in the prevalence of obesity. There is a decreased requirement for physical activity at school, home, or work, or for short-distance travel. Work and leisure time activities are less and less likely to require physical exertion. Remote controls, computers, escalators, and automobiles are integral parts of modern life that contribute to this phenomenon. Food has never been more

---

BOX 85-2
Medications Commonly Associated with Weight Gain

Corticosteroids
Estrogens
Hormone-replacement therapy
Olanzapine (Zyprexa)
Valproic acid (Depakote and others)
Antidepressants
Serotonin-selective reuptake inhibitors (SSRIs)
Insulin
Sulfonylureas
Thiazolidinediones (Rosiglitazone, Pioglitazone)

---

abundant or accessible. Moreover, our appetite and weight regulatory mechanisms may be fooled by highly processed, homogeneous and/or calorie-dense foods, leading to excess calorie intake. The marginal economic cost of additional calories has plummeted with the trend toward "supersizing" in fast food restaurants and outsized quantities of food available through wholesale outlets. There has been an average 200 to 250 kcal/day increase in adult food consumption over the last 25 years, despite a decrease in the *proportion* of fat in the diet. The consumption of carbohydrates, particularly simple sugars and starches, has risen profoundly during this time. Other potential environmental contributors are the chaotic patterns of food consumption, with rapid eating, snacking, "grazing," and steady consumption of high-calorie soft drinks the norm. These patterns have largely replaced the regular, slow-paced meals that remain in parts of the world where obesity is less prevalent (although U.S. habits have spread rapidly elsewhere). The increasing stress and speed of modern life may also play a role; their specific effect on the weight regulatory machinery is not known. Finally, weight regulation may be heavily affected by eating and exercise patterns established during childhood. If so, the increasing portion of the diet from carbohydrate-rich snack foods, the increasing use of fast food restaurants, and the use of food as a reward in time-pressed households, along with decreased physical activity in school and at play, may conspire to set patterns that are impossible to reverse later in life.

Psychologic Factors

Some overweight women appear to increase food intake in response to emotional stress. The degree to which psychologic factors are the *primary* cause of obesity is unclear. Several studies have reported an association between previous psychologic trauma (sexual, physical and/or emotional) and the development of obesity. Others, however, suggest that people with weight disorders are no more likely to have experienced such trauma than people without excess weight or obesity. They would conclude that the eating disorders associated with obesity reflect an innate predisposition or conditioned response to stressful experiences.

Although the precise role of psychologic factors is debated, there is little question that they contribute significantly to weight disorders. Nonetheless, care must be exercised to avoid stigmatization of women with obesity. Psychologic issues must be addressed directly, but over-

emphasis on the causative role of these factors has often led to the characterization of obesity as resulting from a character flaw or even a moral lapse.

EVALUATION OF THE PATIENT WITH OBESITY

As with other disorders, the history is the first step in gathering data relevant to obesity. It should be conducted with sensitivity to the patient's possible embarrassment and lifetime struggle with her weight. When the history is obtained in this way, it elicits crucial clinical information and facilitates the development of rapport that will enhance the patient's long-term satisfaction and success.

The primary goals of the initial evaluation are to identify specific causes of the weight disorder, to detect existing and looming medical and psychologic complications, and to assess the degree to which genetic, psychologic, and nutritional factors contribute to the patient's obesity and may affect the approach to treatment. Evaluation of the patient with obesity is often divided into medical, nutritional, and psychologic assessment. The components of these assessments are listed in Tables 85-1 and 85-2 and Boxes 85-3 and 85-4.

✴ MANAGEMENT OF OBESITY
Goals of Management

Should all women who consult the primary care physician wanting to lose weight be encouraged to do so? The advisability of dieting should be questioned for women who are in early adolescence, have little weight to lose, or have a history of weight cycling. **Adolescence** is a critical time for growth and development, both physically and psychosocially. Overemphasis on thinness and dieting may lead to eating disorders or a lifetime of poor self-image and weight cycling. It is important for the mildly overweight adolescent to be educated about the expected weight changes during this time. Emphasis should be placed on healthy food choices and increased activity rather than dieting per se. For the severely overweight adolescent, modification of eating and exercise behaviors may require more intensive intervention such as individual counseling or family therapy. Of these, family-based therapies in which both the adolescent and her parents are counseled about healthy eating and exercise habits have been shown to be most effective. Such approaches presumably help the parents create a healthier environment for the overweight adolescent.

The **adult woman who has little weight to lose (BMI < 30)** is at a higher risk of losing muscle mass with aggressive dieting and should be dissuaded from this approach. Some women who have been weight cycling for many years find that dieting becomes a way of life, marked by little success at maintaining a lower weight and a rebound to a successively higher weight after each episode of dieting. These women are often extremely sensitive about their weight and have a low sense of self-esteem and self-efficacy. If there are no medical problems associated with the excess weight, education about healthy eating and increased activity is appropriate regardless of the weight.

For the **woman with major complications of obesity or a heightened risk** of any of those complications, more intensive treatment may be indicated. There is strong evidence that significant health benefits of weight loss occur with reduction

Table 85-1
Medical Evaluation of the Woman with Obesity

Goal	Assessment
A. Identify potential causes of obesity	
1. Endocrine/Neurologic	
Hypothyroidism	Serum TSH
Cushing's syndrome	Fasting serum cortisol
	Provocative testing
Pituitary tumors	Serum prolactin
Traumatic brain injury	History
2. Medications (see Box 85-2)	History
3. Genetic	History: Age of onset
	Family weight history
B. Identify obesity-associated disorders	
Polycystic ovary syndrome	History and examination
	Laboratory evaluation to exclude hyperandrogenism (see Chapter 46)
C. Identify past and current medical complications of obesity (see Box 85-1)	History
	Physical examination
	Neck circumference (for sleep apnea)
	Laboratory evaluation:
	Fasting glucose
	HbA1c
	Lipid profile
	Liver enzymes
D. Determine extent of physical disability	Physical examination
E. Assess risk of future complications of obesity (see Box 85-1)	Control of metabolic complications
	Control of anatomic complications
1. Cardiovascular risk	History: Cigarette smoking
	Physical examination: Waist circumference
	Exercise capacity
	Laboratory studies: Elevated fasting glucose
	Lipid profile
	ECG
2. Cancer risk	Ensure adequate screening (mammograms, rectal and pelvic exams may be more difficult than usual)
	Careful assessment for GERD and its complications
3. Risk of physical disability	Careful social history: Living conditions
	Accident risk
	Physical examination: Mobility
	Accident risk

of as little as 5% to 10% of initial body weight. In fact, one large study showed that mere prevention of continued weight gain improved women's morbidity and mortality compared with the control group. Sharing this information with the patient may relieve her of the overwhelming feeling of having to achieve an ideal body weight and may provide a motivation for modest weight loss achieved slowly and steadily.

Attention should be given to the patient's goals, whether or not she desires weight loss, and whether she is ready, motivated, and willing to make the commitments required for success. The stages-of-change paradigm described by Prochaska and DiClemente (Box 85-5) is a valuable model for behavior modification that can be used to assess a patient's readiness for making lifestyle changes and to provide guidelines for professional intervention.

For the patient who is ready to take action, defining appropriate short- and long-term **goals** is important. These goals should be affirmative, feasible, and specific. Often the patient may need the physician's guidance in setting appropriate goals. Current recommendations are that treatment of obesity should set an initial goal of no more than 10% weight loss. Once this weight loss has been achieved and maintained for 1 year, a goal of an additional 10% weight loss, if clinically indicated, is then feasible. A weight loss of 10% has been shown to significantly reduce the risk of complications such as hypertension, coronary artery disease, diabetes, and degenerative arthritis. It is also likely to reduce the severity of most complications of obesity that have already developed. Depending on the clinical needs and patient readiness, appropriate goals may focus on preventing further weight gains acutely or stabilizing weight over the long term, a particularly valuable outcome for the chronic weight cycler.

Most studies indicate that more than 95% of individuals who lose weight in physician-supervised or other formal

Table 85-2
Psychologic Assessment of the Woman with Obesity

Goal	Assessment
A. Identify potential psychologic causes of obesity	History
1. Psychotropic medications	Mental status examination
2. Depression	History
	Survey instrument (e.g., Beck's Depression Inventory II)
3. Post-traumatic stress disorder	
4. Addictive behavior	
B. Identify psychologic disorders potentially associated with obesity	History
	Mental status examination
1. Bipolar disorder	
2. Bulimia nervosa	
C. Identify past and current psychologic complications of obesity (see Box 85-1)	History
	Mental status examination
D. Assess risk of future psychologic complications of obesity (see Box 85-1)	Psychiatric history: Self-mutilation
	Suicidal ideation
	Social history: Support systems
	Communication with mental health providers (requires special permission from patient)
E. Identify need for further interventions	Psychologic or psychiatric evaluation
	Psychopharmacology evaluation
	Cognitive-behavioral therapy

weight loss programs regain *all* of the lost weight by the end of 5 years. Although these are discouraging statistics, they fail to account for the observation that people who undertake weight loss on their own or who have not previously tried to lose weight are more likely to succeed. In developing a plan for the management of obesity and weight disorders, it is important to recognize that several benefits of intervention do not depend on sustained weight loss. Although exercise alone does not typically generate significant weight loss, it has been shown to increase the likelihood of maintaining lost weight. This effect is thought to result primarily from preservation of muscle mass during exercise. Since muscle mass correlates with resting energy expenditure, its preservation helps to avoid some of the decreased energy expenditure that typically accompanies weight loss. In addition, several studies have shown that improved physical fitness reduces risk of cardiovascular disease at any weight. Thus, "fit-and-fat" is healthier than "unfit-and-fat." Adoption of a long-term exercise program improves cardiovascular fitness irrespective of its effect on weight.

Similarly, diminished mental health is common among women with weight disorders. Both exercise and behavioral counseling can improve "mental fitness" independent of long-term weight loss. Obviously, women who stably reduce their weight can obtain enhanced physical and mental health benefits. Recognition of the benefits of exercise and other lifestyle interventions, however, allows both physician and patient to be more optimistic and can avoid the cycle of perceived futility, frustration, and relapse that often complicates obesity.

Self-Guided Weight Loss

For the otherwise healthy patient with adult onset obesity for whom weight gain can be attributed primarily to environmental factors, an appropriate first step would be to de-

velop realistic exercise and nutritional goals. An emphasis on an adequate caloric intake (no fewer than 1000 kcal/day) should be coupled with an exercise program that may include both aerobic activity for fat burning and strength training to increase lean body mass. By using the visual aid of the Food Guide Pyramid (U.S. Department of Agriculture; www.usda.gov), the clinician can teach the patient how to build a healthy diet using starches, fruits, and vegetables as a foundation, meeting calcium needs by incorporating low-fat or nonfat milk and/or yogurt, and complementing these foods with protein (15% to 20% of total calories). Simple sugars and fats are at the top of the pyramid and should be consumed less frequently in a healthy, low-calorie meal plan. For effective weight management, no more than 25% of total calories should be derived from fat. For a 1200- to 1500-calorie plan, this approach would include 33 to 42 grams of fat per day; on an 1800 calorie meal plan, it would include approximately 50 grams of fat per day.

For women who pursue a self-guided weight loss program, periodic visits to the primary care clinician may be important for monitoring progress and providing valuable external reinforcement for initial weight loss and continued maintenance. Regardless of the specific therapies used, it is important that the clinician provide ongoing support and guidance. This can be done most effectively by:

- Forming a partnership with the patient based on shared responsibility. Whenever possible, assemble and use a patient-care team that includes a physician, dietitian, physical or exercise therapist, and psychologist.
- Providing structure to help the patient contemplate, analyze, decide, and apply her knowledge and skills. Be careful not to do the work for the patient, however.
- Recommending small changes that allow for early success and thus facilitate larger, sustainable changes in

---

BOX 85-3
Nutritional Assessment of the Woman with Obesity

Weight History
Age of onset
Highest and lowest adult weights
Patterns of weight gain and loss
Triggers of weight gain
Triggers of excessive or abnormal eating

Diet History
Numbers and types of diets
Other weight loss programs
Weight loss medications
Vitamins and minerals
Other dietary supplements
Complementary and alternative approaches for weight loss
Success of previous weight loss efforts

Current Eating Patterns
- Temporal eating patterns
  Meals, snacks
- 24-hour food recall
  Nutrient distribution
  Nutrient density
- Abnormal eating patterns
  Compulsive; binge eating
- Triggers of normal and abnormal eating

Environmental Factors
Consumption of ethnic food
Person in household who is responsible for cooking and shopping
Use of prepared foods
Primary location of meals

Exercise History
Previous exercise patterns
Current lifestyle
Current structured exercise activities
Barriers to exercise

Motivation and Readiness for Change
Rationale for addressing weight disorder
Goals of weight loss
Readiness for lifestyle change
Willingness to undertake effort
Availability for time commitment

BOX 85-4
Ongoing Primary Care Screening for Weight Disorders

A. Risk assessment
  1. Personal weight history
  2. Family history of weight disorders
  3. Review of medications: institute preventive measures against drug-induced obesity
B. Height measurement (every 5-10 years)
C. Weight measurement (every 3 years)
D. Waist circumference (every 3 years)

BOX 85-5
Stages of Readiness for Behavioral Change

1. **Precontemplation**
   Unaware of, denies, or minimizes the problem
   Needs: confrontation and information
2. **Contemplation**
   Aware of problem, but weighing costs and benefits of change
   Needs: gentle confrontation, information and rationale for change, clarification of any misinformation
3. **Motivation/preparation**
   Has decided to make change, plans to do so within next month, or has limited action to data collection or information gathering
   Needs: strategies for making change, goal setting
4. **Action**
   Plan is in progress; attitudinal and behavioral changes have begun
   Needs: tools and techniques to implement goals, positive reinforcement
5. **Maintenance/relapse**
   Action maintained over 6 months (maintenance) or return to old habits (relapse)
   Maintenance is most difficult stage; if maintained for 6 months prognosis good (note that "a lapse does not a relapse make")
   Needs: tools for successful maintenance, feedback and encouragement
         self-monitoring: checklist for each day (food intake, exercise)
         coping skills and stress management
         support systems
         cognitive restructuring

Modified from Prochaska J, DiClemente C, Norcross J: *Am Psychol* 47:1102, 1992.

---

lifestyle and weight. Remember to start from "where the patient is."

Individual and Group-Based Programs

Many practitioners believe that matching patients to an appropriate program may increase their chances for success and minimize risks that can be associated with the weight loss process. Women should be encouraged to choose a program that focuses on nutritious food choices, exercise, activities of daily living, reversal of cognitive distortions around eating behavior, and ongoing support. For the woman who has weight cycled throughout her adolescent or adult life, treatment should focus on halting the weight cycling and stabiliz-

ing her weight. If there are obesity-related health problems, deemphasizing weight and focusing on healthy eating and physical activity may be most beneficial. Counseling about exercise and providing an appropriate exercise prescription are particularly important. There is accumulating evidence that overweight women who are physically active have lower rates of morbidity and mortality than those with similar BMIs who are sedentary.

There is a continuum of philosophy and clinical practice that ranges from complete reliance on internal control mechanisms to formal structural supports provided by prescribed diets. Programs that emphasize internal regulation of food intake are described as "non-dieting," "normalized eating" or "intuitive eating" approaches. These programs urge that food intake be guided by internal cues of hunger and satiety. They require lengthy interventions and can be compromised by emotional associations with food and eating. To the extent that obesity results from a failure of the internal regulatory systems that control hunger and satiety, as described previously, these approaches will likely be inadequate for long-term control of weight. Approaches that promote both improved internal controls on food intake and external guidance systems appear more likely to provide long-term benefit. They provide structure and support while counseling individuals on how to respond to their endogenous signals of hunger and satiety most effectively.

For women referred to any individual or group program, close monitoring in a primary care setting is often necessary for assessment of the clinical effects of weight loss, adjustment of medications, and screening for potential complications of weight loss, including gallbladder and fatty liver diseases. To reduce the risk of gallbladder disease, weight loss diets should include adequate amounts of protein and fat (14 g of protein and 10 g of fat at one meal daily) to ensure adequate gallbladder contraction). Weight loss should be limited to an average of 2 pounds or less per week, and the diet limited to 12 weeks or fewer in duration.

Diets

Weight loss diets come in all varieties, from "fad" diets to medically supervised very low calorie diets to balanced deficit diets (BDD), which are designed to cause a calorie deficit that will induce weight loss without strongly biasing the distribution of calories among carbohydrates, fat, and protein. See Table 85-3 for a comparison of several of the more popular diets.

Balanced deficit diets are considered to be generally safe for individuals who are up to 40% overweight (BMI, 26

to 35). For women, an appropriate daily caloric intake for weight loss will typically range between 1000 and 1500 calories. The calorie intake should be adjusted to produce a deficit of 300 to 750 kcal/day compared with baseline total energy expenditure. This degree of calorie deficit will lead to an initial weight loss of 1 to 2 pounds per week. The baseline total energy expenditure (TEE) for normoactive, ambulatory women can be estimated by a modification of the Harris-Benedict equation, as follows:

$$\text{TEE (kcal/day)} = 852 + [5.7 \times \text{weight (pounds)} + 5.6 \times \text{height (inches)} - 6.1 \times \text{age (years)}]$$

The most popular diets in the 1990s were diets that were low in fat. Low-fat diets may be appropriate for women with weight disorders at high risk for atherosclerotic cardiovascular disease. However, it is important to note that as Americans have adopted diets lower in fat and the food industry has endorsed a "low-fat" craze, daily caloric intake has increased. Thus, the substitution of simple carbohydrates for fat has been associated with progressively more obesity and its complications.

In recent years, high protein diets have made their way back to the popular diets list. These diets (Atkins, The Zone, SugarBusters and others), which are high in protein and low in carbohydrates, fiber, and many essential nutrients, frequently yield good short-term weight loss; but long-term adherence and effectiveness is poor. Moreover, these diets can generate ketosis with associated metabolic and cardiovascular disturbances. If these diets are followed over time, the elevated fat intake may also increase the risk of atherosclerotic cardiovascular disease. Overall, in the absence of evidence that nutrient-biased diets provide significant advantage, most authorities agree that successful weight management for adults requires a life-long commitment to healthy lifestyle behaviors, emphasizing eating

Table 85-3
Summary of Popular Diets

Type of Diet	Very Low Fat	Moderate Fat	Low Carbohydrate	Other
Examples	Ornish Diet Pritikin Diet	USDA Food Guide Pyramid NIH DASH Diet Weight Watchers Jenny Craig Nutri-Systems	Atkins Diet *Protein Power* *Life without Bread* *The Carbohydrate Addicts Diet*	The Zone Diet *SugarBusters*
% kcal from carbohydrate	75	60	<20	40
% kcal from fat	10	20-30	55	30
% kcal from protein	10-15	15	30	30
Total kcal/day	1450	1450	1450	1000
Notes	Vitamin B_{12} may need to be supplemented (Ornish)	Calculated to provide a deficit of 500-1000 kcal/day without limiting required nutrients	High in saturated fat and cholesterol, low in fruits, vegetables and fiber, low in vitamin A, calcium, iron and potassium	Restricts simple sugars and refined carbohydrates, although not low in carbohydrates overall; allows most fruits and vegetables; low in whole grains and calcium

practices and daily physical activity that are sustainable and enjoyable.

Very-Low-Calorie Diets

Very-low-calorie diets (VLCDs) were developed to provide larger and more rapid short-term weight loss than the standard low-calorie diets, while avoiding the dangers and adverse effects of total fasting. A VLCD is a hypocaloric diet providing 800 calories or fewer per day and including 0.8 to 1.5 g/day of protein of lean body weight daily. VLCDs are often given in a form that completely replaces usual food intake (e.g., liquid formulations) or as food-based, protein-sparing modified fasts using lean meat, fish, and fowl. The liquid formulations contain all of the necessary nutrients, but the food-based diets must be supplemented with daily vitamins and minerals. These diets are typically used for 12 to 16 weeks to achieve rapid, short-term weight loss necessary for specific goals (e.g., to allow surgery or other diagnostic or therapeutic procedures). For long-term weight control, VLCDs have not been shown to be any more effective than other, less radical diet-based approaches. Given their associated risks of dehydration, essential nutrient deficiencies, and renal and cardiac disturbances, VLCDs should be used only if specifically indicated and always under the guidance of an experienced physician.

Pharmacologic Therapy

The role of medications in the management of obesity is evolving. In the past, the potential for abuse and the risk of complications have limited the use of appetite-suppressant agents. The introduction of dexfenfluramine (Redux) and the "phen-fen" combination of fenfluramine (Pondimin and others) and phentermine in the mid-1990s led to renewed excitement and hope among physicians and their patients with obesity. The availability of these apparently effective pharmaceutical agents and the associated marketing efforts substantially increased public understanding of obesity as a serious medical disorder. This initial optimism was short-lived, however. The recognition of associated cardiac valvular abnormalities and rare but life-threatening pulmonary hypertension led to withdrawal of fenfluramine from the market in 1997. Although the withdrawal of these agents was met with disappointment and considerable disillusionment, enhanced appreciation of the medical consequences of obesity has remained, providing further support for ongoing drug development efforts.

Several agents are currently available that enhance the short-term effectiveness of multidisciplinary approaches to weight loss. In each case, however, maximum efficacy is observed in the first year of treatment, with weight *gain* observed in most patients with continued treatment thereafter. Moreover, none of the currently available agents have been approved by the U.S. Food and Drug Administration (FDA) for use beyond 1 year. They are best considered as short-term interventions. In all cases, these agents are recommended for use as part of a comprehensive weight management program (i.e., as an *adjunct* to dietary, exercise, and lifestyle modification approaches).

Pharmacologic therapies for obesity may be particularly helpful for women who have an urgent need to lose weight acutely, such as to permit a diagnostic or therapeutic procedure. Some clinicians have used them to "jump-start" the weight loss process and provide reinforcement for patients unable to lose weight with conventional therapies. Dexfenfluramine and the phen-fen combination were particularly effective for this use, but currently available agents are far less potent. Medications have also been used on an intermittent basis in an attempt to facilitate better weight loss maintenance, but controlled studies demonstrating efficacy of this approach are not yet available. The following are the most commonly used weight loss medications in the United States.

Sibutramine (Meridia)

Sibutramine is a centrally acting, monoamine reuptake inhibitor. It increases the concentration of neurotransmitters at serotonergic, adrenergic, and to a lesser extent, dopaminergic synapses. The overall effects of sibutramine are to depress appetite and increase resting energy expenditure, thus acting somewhat like a weak version of the phen-fen combination. In contrast to phen-fen, however, sibutramine has not been associated with cardiac or pulmonary abnormalities. Common side effects of sibutramine are hypertension and dry mouth. It is contraindicated in patients who have uncontrolled hypertension, and individuals taking sibutramine should have careful blood pressure monitoring. Sibutramine typically leads to weight loss of approximately 10 to 25 pounds in 3 to 12 months. Weight loss after 2 years of treatment is usually less than that after 1 year, suggesting progressive resistance to its effects. Studies to examine efficacy at 5 years are in progress. Dosing is 10 or 15 mg/day, and this agent is currently FDA-approved for up to 1 year of use. Weight loss should be monitored monthly. Failure to lose 4 pounds per month after 1 or 2 months is an indication to stop treatment.

Orlistat (Xenical)

Orlistat is an inhibitor of pancreatic lipase that blocks absorption of up to 30% of ingested fat. Like sibutramine, it has been shown to induce weight loss of approximately 10 to 25 pounds in 12 months. The effectiveness of this agent appears to correlate with diet. Patients consuming a high-fat diet are more likely to experience weight loss than those who consume a high-calorie, predominantly carbohydrate diet. Unfortunately, consumption of a high-fat diet while on orlistat also appears associated with an increased rate of complications, including steatorrhea and fat-soluble vitamin deficiencies. To avoid steatorrhea, patients frequently adapt to a diet higher in carbohydrates, limiting the long-term effectiveness of this drug. Like sibutramine, orlistat is FDA-approved for short-term (1-year) use.

Phentermine

The weaker (and safe) component of the phen-fen combination, phentermine, is an adrenergic agent that modestly decreases food intake and enhances energy expenditure. It is a generic drug that has been on the market for more than 30 years, and few controlled studies of its effects on weight loss are available. Side effects may include tachycardia and hypertension. It is FDA-approved for short-term (3 months) treatment of obesity.

Surgical Treatment of Obesity

The absence of effective, long-term behavioral or pharmacologic treatments for most patients with obesity has led to renewed appreciation of the utility of surgical approaches. The most common surgical procedure to induce weight loss, Roux-en-Y gastric bypass, is now the most common upper gastrointestinal surgical procedure performed in the United States and the fastest growing of all general surgical procedures. Surgical therapy should be considered for patients with major medical complications of their obesity, whose need to lose weight and *maintain* the weight loss is paramount, and who have not been successful with more conservative approaches.

Gastric surgery is currently the most effective way to achieve sustained weight loss in women with moderate to severe obesity. Approximately 85% to 90% of patients undergoing Roux-en-Y gastric bypass achieve significant short-term weight loss (measured as loss of 50% of excess body weight), and 70% to 80% experience significant weight loss over 5 years. Sustained weight loss after gastric surgery is strongly facilitated by postoperative behavior modification therapy. With surgery alone, 5-year success is approximately 50%; addition of an intensive postoperative lifestyle change program increases the success rate to 80%. More than 95% of patients who maintain weight loss for 5 years subsequently maintain it for an additional 10 years. Of importance, the long-term effectiveness of gastric surgery has provided strong evidence that several obesity-related disorders are reversible with significant weight loss (Table 85-4). Thus, although surgery is invasive and associated with substantial risks, for many women the risks of continued obesity and its associated diseases far outweigh the risks of surgery.

Women with class II or III obesity (BMI > 35) with major medical complications (e.g., diabetes, atherosclerotic cardiovascular disease, sleep apnea, steatohepatitis, debilitating arthritis, or intractable gastroesophageal reflux with asthma) are likely to benefit substantially from surgical therapy. Because of the major psychologic complications and medical risks associated with severe obesity, women with class III obesity without active complications may also be considered for weight loss surgery. Contraindications to surgery include untreated major depression, untreated eating disorder, ongoing alcohol or drug abuse, and inability of the patient to comply with postoperative medical, nutritional, and psychologic management. Optimal long-term outcome is dependent on the patient's ability to participate in and comply with a postoperative lifestyle modification program that includes nutritional, eating, psychologic, and exercise counseling. Most reputable obesity surgery centers now require both preoperative and postoperative education and support programs. It is also important that each patient undergoing weight loss surgery have strong support from family, friends, and/or significant others; and it may be necessary for physicians to counsel family members (with the patient's permission) before surgery is undertaken.

Several gastrointestinal procedures have been shown to induce weight loss. Most of them include restriction of caloric intake by reducing the size of the gastric reservoir. The most effective procedures include a bypass of a portion of the gastrointestinal tract. Although these procedures were originally thought to work by physical restriction of food intake and/or malabsorption, it is now felt that they exert their major effect by altering gastrointestinal regulation of hunger and satiety. Distention of the small stomach pouch creates a sensation of early satiety by activation of vagal afferent neurons that project from the stomach to the satiety centers in

Table 85-4
Improvement in Obesity Complications After Gastric Bypass Surgery*

Co-Morbidity	Percent Experiencing Significant Improvement or Complete Resolution of Condition*
Diabetes mellitus	92-98
Obstructive sleep apnea	90-98
Hypercholesterolemia	87-93
Hypertension	80-92
Hypertriglyceridemia	99-100
Gastroesophageal reflux	77-98
Urinary incontinence	81-97
Osteoarthritis	72-97

* Information synthesized from several published and unpublished series of more than 1000 patients with 2-year follow-up after laparoscopic and open gastric bypass procedures.

the brain. For procedures that include gastric bypass, early passage of nutrients into the jejunum appears to provide a second stimulus to satiety. For patients who fail to experience the satiety-inducing effects of gastric surgery, the small pouch reinforces the need to limit food intake.

Gastrointestinal surgery for weight loss can be divided into procedures that are primarily restrictive (e.g., vertical banded gastroplasty and adjustable gastric banding) and those that include a rerouting of the food stream (gastric bypass) to achieve increased satiety and in some cases cause mild protein-calorie malabsorption.

Vertical Banded Gastroplasty

The most common "restrictive" procedure performed in the United States is the vertical banded gastroplasty, which is colloquially called "stomach stapling" (Fig. 85-1, *A*). This procedure involves stapling through the proximal stomach to create a small pouch and then placing a fixed band around the outlet to delay transit of food from the pouch to the distal stomach. Although popular in the 1980s, this procedure accounts for fewer than 10% of weight loss procedures currently performed in the United States.

Adjustable Gastric Banding

The most common weight loss procedure performed in Europe is adjustable gastric banding (Fig. 85-1, *B*). This laparoscopic procedure creates a small proximal gastric pouch by placing an adjustable Silastic ring around the cardia of the stomach. Recent US trials of one such device (Lap-Band) have revealed it to be substantially less effective than gastric bypass surgery and predisposed to significant complications, including band slippage, erosion into the stomach lumen, and esophageal dilation. In all, 25% of patients in these clinical trials had the band removed because of mechanical complications, inability to tolerate the device, or lack of therapeutic effect. This device was approved by the FDA in 2001 for use in patients who would otherwise qualify for gastric weight loss surgery. Its long-term efficacy and appropriate use have not yet been determined with certainty, however.

Strictly restrictive procedures can lead to long-term loss of 30% to 60% of excess body weight. Although this degree

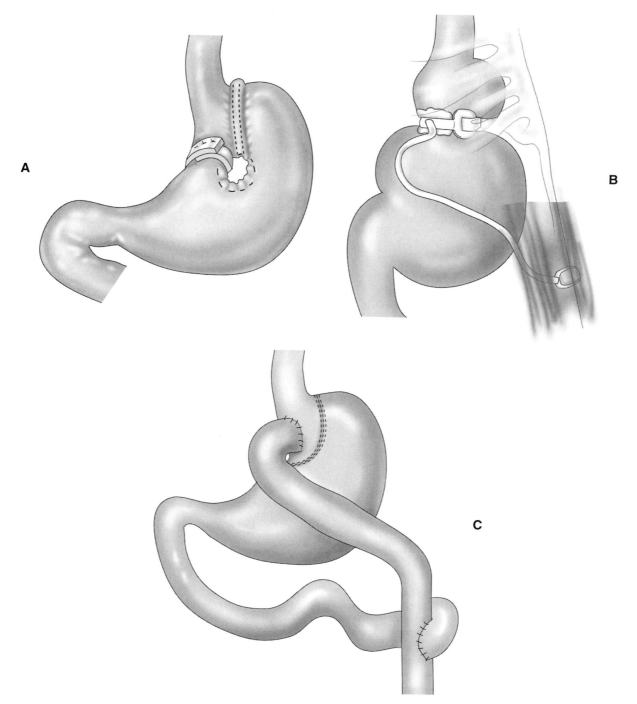

FIG. 85-1   Surgical weight loss procedures. **A,** Vertical banded gastroplasty; **B,** adjustable gastric banding; **C,** Roux-en-Y gastric bypass.

of weight loss is impressive, bypass procedures are even more effective. Moreover, vertical banded gastroplasty and adjustable gastric banding are less effective at inducing early satiety. As a result, some patients tend to overeat despite the gastric restriction by adjusting to a high-calorie liquid diet. Other potential complications of banded gastroplasty include outlet obstruction leading to persistent vomiting and severe gastroesophageal reflux, which can often be improved by endoscopic balloon dilation of the pouch outlet.

Roux-en-Y Gastric Bypass

The most common surgical weight loss procedure performed in the United States overall is the Roux-en-Y gastric bypass (Fig. 85-1, *C*). This procedure involves creating a small proximal gastric pouch, which limits food intake, and then connecting this pouch to a limb of jejunum brought up to bypass the stomach and duodenum. Long-term studies have shown sustained weight loss averaging 65% of excess body weight. In recent years, laparoscopic techniques for gastric bypass surgery have been developed, and several centers now use this approach extensively. Advantages to the laparoscopic approach include generally faster postoperative recovery and a decreased risk of wound infections and postoperative hernias. Laparoscopic gastric bypass is a technically difficult procedure, however, with longer operative (and anesthesia) times and a possibly higher risk of anastomotic stricture. There is a significant learning curve, and centers with extensive experience and high patient volumes have the best outcomes.

Mortality associated with each of these weight loss procedures is less than 0.5% and the major morbidity is 5% to 10%. Revisional surgery is required in approximately 5% to 10% of patients. Major early complications include wound infection (5% to 15%), pneumonia (2% to 10%), anastomotic leak (1% to 5%), and deep venous thrombosis and pulmonary embolus (<0.5%). Late complications include stomal stenosis (4% to 20%), marginal ulcer and/or staple line breakdown (5% to 15%), incisional hernia (10% to 20%), transient dumping syndrome (5% to 10%), and deficiencies of iron, calcium, vitamin D, or vitamin B_{12} (up to 30%).

Most of these complications can be avoided with careful monitoring and/or nutritional management. Postoperative management of patients undergoing weight loss surgery includes vitamin and mineral supplements, nutritional counseling, and a comprehensive behavior modification program. Dumping syndrome, which may include food-induced lightheadedness, fatigue, and nausea and diarrhea, can usually be minimized by avoiding concentrated carbohydrates and beginning each meal with protein. In severe cases, dumping can be treated effectively with octreotide (Sandostatin).

As noted previously, severe obesity may be associated with reproductive dysfunction. Many women who were unable to become pregnant previously are able to do so after surgically induced weight loss. It is important to note, however, that pregnancy should be deferred for at least 18 months after weight loss surgery, when weight has largely stabilized. Before this time, there is an increased risk of birth defects, presumably from the metabolic effects of rapid weight loss.

BIBLIOGRAPHY

Allison DB et al: Annual deaths attributable to obesity in the United States, *JAMA* 282:1530, 1999.

Barsh GS, Farooqi IS, O'Rahilly S: Genetics of body-weight regulation, *Nature* 404:644, 2000.

Bray GA, Greenway FL: Current and potential drugs for treatment of obesity, *Endocr Rev* 20:805, 1999.

Bray GA, Tartaglia LA: Medicinal strategies in the treatment of obesity, *Nature* 404:672, 2000.

Colditz GA: Economic costs of obesity and inactivity, *Med Sci Sports Exerc* 31:S663, 1999.

Cummings SM, Goodrick KG, Foreyt JP: Position of the American Dietetic Association: weight management, *J Am Dietet Assoc* 99:71, 1997.

Epstein LH, Valoski A, Wing RR, McCurley J: Ten-year follow-up of behavioral, family-based treatment of obese children, *JAMA* 264:2519, 1990.

Friedman JM, Halaas JL: Leptin and the regulation of body weight in mammals, *Nature* 395:763, 1998.

Halsted CH: Obesity: effects on the liver and gastrointestinal system, *Curr Opin Nutr Metab Care* 2:425, 1999.

Kaplan LM: Genetics of obesity and body weight regulation, *Curr Opin Endocrin Diabetes* 7:218, 2000.

Kaplan LM: Leptin, obesity and liver disease, *Gastroenterology* 115:997, 1998.

Kellum JM, DeMaria EJ, Sugerman HJ: The surgical treatment of morbid obesity, *Curr Prob Surg* 35:791, 1998.

Kopelman PG: Obesity as a medical problem, *Nature* 404:635, 2000.

Leibel RL, Rosenbaum M, Hirsch J: Changes in energy expenditure resulting from altered body weight, *N Engl J Med* 332:621, 1995.

MacLean LD, Rhode BM, Nohr CW: Late outcome of isolated gastric bypass, *Ann Surg* 231:524-528, 2000.

National Institutes of Health: Clinical guidelines on the identification, evaluation and treatment of overweight and obesity in adults—the evidence report, *Obesity Res* 6 (Suppl 2):51S, 1998.

National Institutes of Health: Gastrointestinal surgery for morbid obesity. Consensus development conference statement, *Am J Clin Nutr* 55:615S, 1992.

Rissanen A, Fogelholm M: Physical activity in the prevention and treatment of other morbid conditions and impairments associated with obesity: current evidence and research issues, *Med Sci Sports Exerc* 31:S635, 1999.

Rosenbaum M, Leibel RL, Hirsch J: Obesity, *N Engl J Med* 337:396, 1997.

Sachs GS, Guille CH: Weight gain associated with the use of psychotropic medications, *Clin Psychiatry* 60 (suppl. 21):16, 1999.

Schwartz MW et al: Central nervous system control of food intake, *Nature* 404:661, 2000.

Solomon CG, Manson JE: Obesity and mortality: a review of the epidemiologic data, *Am J Clin Nutr* 66:1044S, 1997.

Sugerman HJ: The epidemic of severe obesity: the value of surgical treatment, *Mayo Clin Proc* 75:669, 2000.

Willett WC, Dietz WH, Colditz GA: Guidelines for a healthy weight, *N Engl J Med* 341:427, 1999.

CHAPTER 86

Fatigue and Chronic Fatigue Syndrome

Anthony L. Komaroff

CHRONIC FATIGUE

Nearly 15 million office visits per year in the United States are for the complaint of fatigue, and most of the patients seeking care are women. Indeed, many persons experience fatigue much of the time. In one British survey, 20% of adults said that they had "always felt tired" during the preceding month. The pace of life in the twenty-first century is fast. Far from evolving toward a "leisure society," we are working increasingly longer hours, with less time for relaxation. Moreover, some sleep physiologists believe that many citizens of the developed nations suffer from a chronic state of sleep deprivation.

Fatigue is one of those presenting complaints that physicians do not like to deal with. For one thing, the complaint of "fatigue" is imprecise, meaning different things to different patients: an unusual urge to sleep during the day, trouble finding the energy to start new tasks, difficulty concentrating, muscle weakness, or fatigability. Also, because many patients seen in a primary care practice are the anxious "worried well," a physician is likely to be skeptical that the patient's degree of fatigue is really beyond the normal life experience of every human being. In addition, attempts at treatment often are unsuccessful; thus, the physician is likely to feel a failure. Because patients seeking medical care for fatigue often have remarkable degrees of functional impairment, the physician is likely to feel even more discouraged at his or her inability to help the patient. Physicians often underestimate the severity of fatigue and its importance to the patient, even when the cause of the fatigue is a serious, organic disease, such as cancer.

Causative Factors

There are a variety of causes of fatigue, many of which are summarized in Box 86-1. Lifestyle factors (e.g., the pace of life, substance abuse) are at the top of the list, along with primary psychiatric disorders. Various well-characterized organic illnesses, as well as a few poorly understood illnesses, also can cause fatigue.

In the patient whose presenting complaint is chronic fatigue, the first question to consider is whether lifestyle factors are likely to explain the fatigue. The second question

to consider is whether the patient is depressed; depression (often with associated anxiety or somatization disorder, or both) is a common cause of chronic fatigue. The depression may be "masked" and therefore difficult to diagnose. Because depression is a stigmatizing diagnosis in our society, patients may refrain from expressing feelings of sadness; rather, they may offer physical symptoms as the "ticket of entry" into the physician's office. If and when the physician makes the diagnosis of depression, the stigma attached to this illness may cause patients to have trouble accepting it. The diagnosis and treatment of depression, anxiety disorders, and somatization disorder in a primary care practice are discussed in Chapters 81 through 83.

According to careful studies, well-characterized organic diseases of any type explain the complaint of fatigue in fewer than 10% of patients. Clinically, thyroid disease, various autoimmune disorders, and the chronic fatigue syndrome (CFS) are the most common organic causes of chronic fatigue in women (CFS probably is an organic disease). They also can be difficult to diagnose. The physician thus is faced with a troublesome problem. Although there appears to be no organic disease present in most cases, a large number of diseases, each of which requires a number of different diagnostic tests to help establish the diagnosis, may need to be excluded. The question of when to order various diagnostic tests in the patient with fatigue is considered later in this chapter.

Unlike the autoimmune diseases and CFS, most of the other organic diseases listed in Box 86-1 usually are readily recognizable from findings of the history, physical examination, or laboratory testing. One is unlikely to miss fatigue caused by cardiac or respiratory insufficiency. The history indicates that the fatigue is worsened by physical challenge and becomes progressively more severe, and physical signs usually are present. Weight loss, fever, pallor, and lymphadenopathy usually accompany the infectious, neoplastic, and hematologic diseases that produce fatigue. Chronic anemia usually is severe before it produces fatigue. Fortunately, many of these conditions can be suggested or diagnosed by inexpensive, routine blood tests.

A substantial fraction of patients do not have evidence of either organic or psychiatric causes of fatigue. Some

BOX 86-1
Some Causes of Fatigue*

Physiologic
Increased physical exertion
Inadequate rest
Sedentary lifestyle
Environmental stress (noise, vibration, heat)
New physical disability, recent illness, surgery, trauma

Habit Patterns
Caffeine habituation
Alcoholism
Other substance abuse

Psychosocial
Depression
Dysthymia and grief
Anxiety-related disorders
Stress reaction

Pregnancy

Autoimmune Disorders
Systemic lupus erythematosus
Multiple sclerosis
Thyroiditis (with or without thyroid dysfunction)
Rheumatoid arthritis
Myasthenia gravis

Sleep Disorders
Sleep apnea
Narcolepsy

Infectious Diseases
Mononucleosis
Human immunodeficiency virus infection
Chronic hepatitis B or C virus infection
Lyme disease
Fungal disease
Chronic parasitic infection
Tuberculosis
Subacute bacterial endocarditis

Endocrine Disorders
Hyperparathyroidism
Hypothyroidism

Apathetic "hyperthyroidism"
Adrenal insufficiency
Cushing's syndrome
Hypopituitarism
Diabetes mellitus

Syndromes of Uncertain Etiology
Chronic fatigue syndrome
Fibromyalgia (fibrositis)
Sarcoidosis
Wegener's granulomatosis

Occult Malignant Disease

Hematologic Problems
Anemia
Myeloproliferative syndromes

Hepatic Disease
Alcoholic hepatitis or cirrhosis

Cardiovascular Disease
Low output states
"Silent" myocardial infarction
Bradycardias
Mitral valve dysfunction

Metabolic Disorders
Hyponatremia
Hypokalemia
Hypercalcemia

Renal Disease
Chronic renal failure

Respiratory Disorders
Chronic obstructive pulmonary disease

Miscellaneous
Medications
Autonomic overactivity
Reactive hypoglycemia

Modified from Komaroff AL. In Branch WT Jr, editor, *Office practice of medicine*, ed 3, Philadelphia, 1994, WB Saunders.
* This list is not meant to be an exhaustive catalogue of every illness that can cause chronic fatigue; rather, it is intended to highlight some of the illnesses that most commonly do so.

organic illnesses that commonly produce fatigue may manifest initially in a less than full-blown form. Multiple sclerosis (MS) (see Chapter 27) and systemic lupus erythematosus (lupus) (see Chapter 38) are prime examples. Indeed, in many patients with mild MS or lupus, the predominant symptom for which they seek medical care is fatigue rather than a focal neurologic deficit, a malar rash, or other characteristic manifestation of the illness.

APPROACH TO THE WOMAN WITH CHRONIC FATIGUE

History

Assessment of Underlying Psychiatric Disorders

The assessment of underlying psychiatric disorders is detailed in the section on psychology and behavioral medicine and is discussed only briefly here. When the patient with fatigue or other somatic symptoms is suffering from depression or anxiety, the interview serves as both a diagnostic and a therapeutic tool. The taking of the medical history, by exploring both organic and psychiatric issues, can make the patient aware of how his or her feelings relate to the symp-

---

BOX 86-2

**Recommended Laboratory Tests
(National Institutes of Health)**

Complete blood cell count
Manual differential white blood cell count (unless automated counts
    accurately determine atypical lymphocytes)
Erythrocyte sedimentation rate (Westergren method)
Chemistry panel, including assessment of renal and hepatic function and
    levels of glucose, electrolytes, calcium, phosphate, total cholesterol,
    albumin, and globulin
Thyroid function tests (highly sensitive TSH [thyroid-stimulating
    hormone] is sufficient)
Antinuclear antibodies and rheumatoid factor, if there are prominent
    arthralgias and myalgias
Urinalysis

Modified from Schluederberg A et al: *Ann Intern Med* 117:325, 1992.

toms, an essential first step in management. In attempting to elicit submerged information, it is important to remember that occult alcohol abuse (and other forms of substance abuse) often produces chronic fatigue, either directly as a result of chronic intoxication or indirectly through its disruptive effects on sleep or its production of inflammatory disease of the liver (see Chapters 90 and 91). Also, domestic violence, either in childhood or currently, can lead women to seek medical care for "unrelated" symptoms, such as fatigue (see Chapter 87). A simple interviewing technique can be based on the biopsychosocial approach developed by Engel.

Assessment of Underlying Organic Disorders

Although underlying psychiatric disorders are common in patients with fatigue—and even though the interview may suggest that the patient has a current or lifetime psychiatric diagnosis—it is nevertheless important to assess the possible presence of concomitant organic illness. The depression itself can result from the patient's awareness of an impending or actual change in health status.

Diagnostic Tests

Laboratory Testing

In the patient with fatigue of modest severity and relatively short duration (e.g., 1 to 3 months) who probably is most typical of patients seeking medical care for fatigue, no laboratory testing may be necessary. This is particularly true when the patient clearly has enough lifestyle features to explain fatigue, when a psychologic disorder is deemed likely, and when no other symptoms suggest an organic abnormality.

When the fatigue has lasted 6 months or more or is significantly interfering with a patient's ability to work or maintain her primary responsibilities at work or at home, a modest screening evaluation is warranted to look for evidence of an underlying organic disorder. A panel of tests recommended by a National Institutes of Health conference is shown in Box 86-2. Not all of these tests are highly sensitive for organic disease (e.g., erythrocyte sedimentation rate) or highly specific for any particular disease; however, they serve as a useful screen for organic illness as a cause of the chronic fatigue.

MANAGEMENT

There are no specific treatments for chronic fatigue. Instead, treatment follows from the differential diagnosis of fatigue. Thus treatment could include antidepressant therapy, immunosuppressive therapy of an underlying connective tissue disorder, a prescription to get more sleep, or other therapies.

CHRONIC FATIGUE SYNDROME
Definition

Chronic fatigue syndrome (CFS) is a syndrome, defined by a group of symptoms and signs, of uncertain etiology. Very few patients (perhaps fewer than 5%) of all patients who seek medical care for the complaint of chronic fatigue meet criteria for CFS.

CFS was first defined in 1988; the Centers for Disease Control and Prevention (CDC) led the development of a working case definition (Fig. 86-1). The CDC case definition relies entirely on a combination of symptoms (not signs or laboratory data) and on the exclusion of chronic active organic or psychiatric illnesses that can produce chronic fatigue.

Recent epidemiologic data from private investigators and from the CDC indicate that 200 to 800 of every 100,000 Americans have CFS. Among women 40 to 49 years old, more than 800 per 100,000 have CFS.

Although CFS has been defined only recently, similar syndromes with different names have long been described in the medical literature. These include neurasthenia (or neurocirculatory asthenia), first described in the mid-nineteenth century; myalgic encephalomyelitis (ME), a similar chronic fatiguing illness, typically occurring in epidemic form; fibromyalgia, originally called fibrositis, an illness characterized by fatigue and chronic musculoskeletal pain, as well as tenderness at specific sites known as *tender points;* and chronic mononucleosis, a form of CFS that follows in the wake of classic acute infectious mononucleosis.

Causes

CFS probably is a heterogeneous collection of related disorders that all share certain pathogenic features and symptoms. It is unlikely to be, as is the acquired immunodeficiency syndrome (AIDS), a novel syndrome caused by a single new infectious agent. In recent years, research laboratories have reported a variety of abnormalities in patients with CFS, in contrast to healthy control subjects. In general, these studies indicate abnormalities in the central nervous system, a state of chronic activation of the immune system, and an association with a variety of infectious agents. At the same time, it is fair to say that no clear model of the pathogenesis of the symptoms of CFS has yet emerged: the abnormalities seen in CFS are generally not specific for CFS and have not been shown to actually account for the suffering experienced by patients.

A Model for the Pathogenesis of Chronic Fatigue Syndrome

Many view CFS as primarily an immunologic disturbance, one that allows reactivation of latent and ineradicable infectious agents, particularly viruses. Reactivation of these viruses may only be an epiphenomenon. Alternatively, once

Severe fatigue that persists or relapses for ≥ 6 months.

▶ Exclude if patient found to have:

1. Active medical condition that may explain the chronic fatigue, such as untreated hypothyroidism, sleep apnea, narcolepsy

2. Previously diagnosed medical conditions that have not clearly fully resolved, such as previously treated malignancies or unresolved cases of hepatitis B or C virus infection

3. Any past or current major depressive disorder with psychotic or melancholic features; bipolar affective disorders, schizophrenia, delusional disorders, dementias, anorexia nervosa, or bulimia nervosa

4. Alcohol or other substance abuse within two years before the onset of chronic fatigue and at any time afterward

▶ Classify as **chronic fatigue syndrome** if:

Sufficiently severe: of new or definite onset (not lifelong), not substantially alleviated by rest, and results in substantial reduction in previous levels of occupational, educational, social or personal activities; **and**

Four or more of the following symptoms are concurrently present for ≥ 6 months:

1. Impaired memory or concentration
2. Sore throat
3. Tender cervical or axillary lymph nodes
4. Muscle pain
5. Multijoint pain
6. New headaches
7. Unrefreshing sleep
8. Post-exertional malaise

▶ Classify as **idiopathic chronic fatigue** if fatigue severity or symptom criteria for chronic fatigue syndrome are not met

FIG. 86-1 Case definition and evaluation of chronic fatigue syndrome and idiopathic chronic fatigue. (From Fukuda K et al: *Ann Intern Med* 121:953, 1994.)

secondarily reactivated, these viruses may contribute to the morbidity of CFS—directly, by damaging certain tissues (e.g., the pharyngeal mucosa) and indirectly, by eliciting an ongoing immunologic response in which a variety of cytokines are chronically elaborated, producing symptoms and signs such as fever, adenopathy, myalgias, arthralgias, mood and cognitive disorders, and sleep disorders, as already discussed.

What triggers the immune dysfunction in the first place? Many factors could do so: atopic disorders, new infection with lymphotropic infectious agents, environmental toxins, stress, and even the biology of an underlying affective disorder. A recently described neuraxis abnormality that results in a basal hypocortisolism in CFS also could render the immune system "hyperresponsive" to antigenic stimulation, contributing to a state of chronic activation and partial exhaustion described in a later discussion. Clearly, like most illnesses, CFS seems likely to have multifactorial etiologic factors.

Why Chronic Fatigue Syndrome Especially Affects Women

In most studies of patients seeking medical care for chronic fatigue, and of that fraction that meets criteria for CFS, most patients are women. To put this observation in context, adult women more frequently seek medical care than do adult men for many medical conditions, although this is not true in childhood. There are many theories as to why women seek care more often for fatigue and for CFS, but none has been proved.

Proponents of the idea that fatigue and CFS are the somatic expression of psychic distress argue that the stresses of a woman's role in contemporary society are the explanation. They argue that women have an exhausting lifestyle that often requires major responsibilities both at work and at home. In addition, women remain subordinated and undervalued. Finally, women may be more likely than men to seek help for "nonemergent" conditions because in Western society, giving and receiving interpersonal support come more easily to women than to men.

Proponents of the idea that CFS represents primarily an organic illness—one that involves immune dysregulation—note that many immunologically mediated diseases occur predominantly in women. This is especially true of three diseases that can be confused with CFS: multiple sclerosis, lupus erythematosus, and thyroiditis. Moreover, in animal models of autoimmune diseases it is typically the females of the species that become ill. Thus endocrinologic or other factors associated with female gender may predispose women to CFS.

Table 86-1
Frequency of Symptoms and Signs in Chronic Fatigue Syndrome*

Symptom/Sign	Frequency	Symptom/Sign	Frequency
Fatigue	100%	**Neuropsychologic Symptoms**	
Intermittently bedridden/shut-in	50%	Awaken most mornings unrested	87%
Regularly bedridden/shut-in	19%	Difficulty concentrating, frequent and recurrent	83%
Systemic Symptoms		Headaches, new or different in character, frequent and recurrent	76%
Night sweats, frequent and recurrent	50%	Unusually forgetful, frequent and recurrent	71%
Unintentional weight loss (Median, 10 pounds)	49%	Depression, by self-report	
Unintentional weight gain (Median, 15 pounds)	63%	Following onset of CFS	68%
Low-grade fever (by self-report), frequent and recurrent	36%	Before onset of CFS	6%
Temperature >99.3° F, by examination[†]	30%	Anxiety, by self-report	
Temperature <97.0° F, by examination[†]	20%	Following onset of CFS	65%
		Before onset of CFS	12%
Respiratory Tract Symptoms		Alcohol regularly makes symptoms worse	59%
Sudden onset with "flulike" illness	85%	Tingling/numbness in extremities, frequent and recurrent	57%
Swollen lymph glands in neck, frequent and recurrent	58%	Bright lights hurt eyes, frequent and recurrent	56%
Sore throat, frequent and recurrent	51%	Dizzy when move head suddenly	51%
Cough, frequent and recurrent	27%	Visual blurring, frequent and recurrent	50%
Palpable posterior cervical nodes[†]	54%	Impaired tandem gait, by examination[†]	23%
		Abnormal Romberg test, by examination[†]	22%
Musculoskeletal Symptoms		Impaired serial 7s test, by examination[†]	40%
Muscles hurt, frequent and recurrent	89%		
Postexertional malaise, frequent and recurrent	88%	**Miscellaneous Symptoms**	
Joints painful but not red/swollen, frequent and recurrent	75%	Premenstrual exacerbation of fatigue, frequent and recurrent	61%
Generalized muscle weakness, frequent and recurrent	70%	Nocturia, frequent and recurrent	46%
Morning stiffness, frequent and recurrent	58%	Nausea, frequent and recurrent	44%
Gelling, after sitting for hours, frequent and recurrent	56%	Sudden rapid heartbeat, frequent and recurrent	44%
Digits turn blue/white with cold, then red when warm	21%		

* Summarized from formal studies of 320 patients as of April 1992. From Komaroff AL: In Straus SE, editor: *Chronic fatigue syndrome*, New York, 1994, Marcel Dekker.
† As detected on at least one physical examination.

Clinical Presentation

History and Symptoms

CFS is characterized by varying degrees of chronic fatigue and chronic or recurring fever, pharyngitis, myalgias, headache, arthralgias, paresthesias, depression, cognitive problems, and other symptoms. Table 86-1 presents a list of current experience with the presence of symptoms in more than 300 systematically studied patients.

Typically the chronic illness begins abruptly with an acute infectious-like syndrome that includes respiratory or gastrointestinal symptoms, or both, with associated fever, myalgias, and arthralgias. The chronic symptoms that are experienced regularly in the years *after* the acute onset of the illness clearly were not experienced regularly by these patients in the years *before* the onset of the illness. Virtually all patients perceive themselves to be impaired in some way. Some patients are completely disabled by the fatigue, muscular weakness, and pain.

Three features of CFS are particularly remarkable. The first is the sudden onset, typically with a **flulike illness.**

The patient had been functioning very well, and then one day became acutely ill (patients often can remember the exact day and date). From that day forward, their lives change. The fact that the onset is so sudden, that it includes objective indicators of organic illness (e.g., fever, adenopathy), and that the change in a patient's functional status is so dramatic—all are in striking contrast to the much more common condition in which patients seek medical care for fatigue secondary to depression, describing symptoms that have occurred so gradually that it is difficult to pinpoint the time of onset.

A second remarkable feature of CFS is **postexertional malaise.** This is characterized not only by symptoms that could simply represent deconditioning—pain and weakness of the muscles involved in the exertion—but also by exacerbation of "systemic" symptoms, for example, fatigue, fevers, pharyngitis, adenopathy, and impaired cognition. Recent studies have confirmed that patients with CFS develop impairments in cognition after physical exertion.

The third remarkable symptom is **night sweats.** These are recurring problems in nearly 50% of the patients studied.

The night sweats are drenching, requiring changes of bed-clothes and sheets. The night sweats are every bit as dramatic as can be seen with chronic infections (e.g., tuberculosis) or lymphoproliferative disorders. On those occasions when patients take their temperatures, they are sometimes febrile but often have unusually low body temperatures (see following discussion).

A few patients with this disorder have had transient acute neurologic events, typically in the first 6 months of the illness: primary seizures, acute, profound ataxia, focal weakness, transient blindness, and unilateral paresthesias (not in a dermatomal distribution). Similar acute and transient neurologic events occasionally have been reported in outbreaks of myalgic encephalomyelitis as well.

The onset of the syndrome typically seems to be in young adulthood, although it also may begin in childhood or later in life. By definition (see Fig. 86-1), there is no evidence of rheumatologic, endocrinologic, infectious, malignant, or other chronic diseases. The diagnosis has been made about twice as often in women as in men.

Most elements of the medical history are unremarkable in patients with CFS. However, a strikingly high percentage of patients (60% to 80%) report long-standing atopic disorders compared with only 20% of the general population.

Physical Examination

A few physical examination findings may be seen more often in persons with CFS than in healthy persons, although this remains to be determined from controlled studies with blinded observers: fevers, unusually low basal body temperature (below 97° F), posterior cervical adenopathy, and abnormal findings on tests of balance (Romberg and tandem gait). Patients have detectable tender points with a frequency approaching that seen in fibromyalgia, and they occur much more often than in healthy control subjects. Therefore the finding of a significant number of tender points, along with the absence of tenderness at control sites, is evidence in favor of the diagnosis of CFS, although the absence of tender points does not rule out the diagnosis of CFS.

Diagnostic Tests

Standard Laboratory Testing. Results of standard laboratory testing can be unremarkable. However, controlled studies have demonstrated that a few abnormalities may occur more frequently in CFS than in healthy control subjects of similar age and sex: atypical lymphocytosis, elevated alkaline phosphatase, lower levels of lactic dehydrogenase, and elevated total cholesterol values. None of these abnormalities is seen in more than 50% of patients with CFS; thus none constitutes a sufficiently sensitive diagnostic test. Moreover, each can be seen in other disorders; thus none is a sufficiently specific test.

Differential Diagnosis. The differential diagnosis of CFS generally is the same as the differential diagnosis for chronic fatigue, as already discussed. Because patients with CFS typically have been more debilitated for a longer time than patients with chronic fatigue, the physician perceives a greater sense of urgency about making the proper diagnosis.

Immunologic Testing. A large and growing literature reports immunologic abnormalities in patients with CFS. In some, it appears that the immune system is chronically waging a battle against antigens that it perceives as foreign.

Although not all reports of immune function in CFS reach consistent conclusions, a few immunologic abnormalities have been found by multiple investigators studying different groups of patients with CFS. First, the function of natural killer (NK) cells is impaired. NK cells play a central role in the immunologic containment of viral infections; thus their impairment of function in CFS is of particular interest. Second, about 30% to 45% of patients with CFS have circulating immune complexes, a much higher frequency than is seen in healthy patients of the same age and sex. The immune complexes are present in low levels and without evidence of immune-complex-mediated disease. Third, there appears to be a higher number of B and T cells in an activated state in CFS, as manifested by the discovery of activation antigens on the cell surface. Finally, several studies have found that an antiviral enzyme system within lymphocytes, called the 2-5A system, is upregulated in patients with CFS. A widely held hypothesis is that the state of chronic immune activation leads to most of the symptoms of CFS by causing a chronic "overproduction" of various proinflammatory immune system mediators. The evidence is strongest for tumor necrosis factor-α, and interleukin-1 family of molecules. These cytokines can produce most of the symptoms characteristic of CFS: fatigue, fevers, adenopathy, myalgias, arthralgias, sleep disorders, cognitive impairment, and mood disorders.

Neurologic Studies. Several neuroimaging studies have compared findings in patients with CFS to those in healthy control subjects and to patients in various disease comparison groups, including AIDS encephalopathy and major depression. Areas of abnormal signal in the subcortical white matter and deeper structures have been found by magnetic resonance imaging (MRI). The use of single photon emission computed tomography (SPECT) has shown diffuse impairment of perfusion and/or of central nervous system cellular function.

Many studies have found abnormalities of the autonomic nervous system (ANS) in pediatric and adult patients with CFS, primarily orthostatic intolerance and neurally mediated hypotension seen on tilt table tests. However, the value of ANS testing remains uncertain.

Many studies also have found abnormalities of cognition on formal psychometric testing. Although the results are not entirely consistent across all studies, in general, deficits of attention, concentration, processing, speed, and hand-eye coordination have been reported.

Neuroendocrine Studies. Several abnormalities of hypothalamic-pituitary axes have been demonstrated in CFS. The data indicate that in CFS there is diminished secretion by the hypothalamus of corticotropin-releasing hormone (CRH), leading to diminished secretion of adrenocorticotropic hormone (ACTH) by the pituitary, which results in diminished production of cortisol by the adrenal glands. This abnormality of the HPA axis is the opposite of what is seen in patients suffering from major depression. A recent study, using computed tomography, found that the adrenal glands of patients with CFS were half the size of adrenals from healthy control subjects. Abnormalities of vasopressin and of prolactin secretion also have been reported. Finally, circulating immune system cells seem to be poorly responsive to neuroendocrine signals, such as glucocorticoids or beta-2 adrenergic stimuli.

Infectious Disease Studies. CFS typically begins suddenly with an infectious-like illness, although it apparently can begin after a variety of stressful noninfectious events (e.g., major surgery, accidents, and severe allergic reactions). CFS has been shown in some cases to follow in the wake of well-documented infection with Epstein-Barr virus infection, influenza virus infection, parvovirus infection, Lyme disease (in patients who have received adequate antibacterial treatment), and other infections. The aforementioned cases are important because they document that an acute infection can trigger CFS. They also demonstrate that CFS probably is not caused by a single infectious agent. However, these observations leave unexplained the pathogenetic mechanisms by which the *triggering* agent initiates the disease process, as well as the question of whether the infectious agent is necessary for the *perpetuation* of the process.

Human herpesvirus–6 (HHV-6) has been found to be actively replicating more often in patients with CFS than in matched healthy control subjects. The evidence indicates that reactivation of a long dormant infection with HHV-6, rather than new infection with HHV-6, is present in CFS. Thus the active HHV-6 infection most likely represents a secondary phenomenon in CFS. As such, it could be an epiphenomenon having nothing to do with the illness. Alternatively, even if the reactivation of HHV-6 is a secondary phenomenon, the reactivated virus could contribute to the symptoms of the illness: HHV-6 infects many target tissues that are affected in CFS: lymphocytes, pharyngeal cells, intestinal cells, glial cells, and probably neurons.

Several studies have incriminated the enteroviruses (coxsackieviruses, echoviruses, polioviruses) in some cases of CFS. Enteroviral nucleic acid has been found much more often in the muscle of patients with CFS than in healthy control subjects, and enteroviral antigen has been found more frequently in the stool and serum of patients with CFS. Enteroviruses can produce chronic, persistent infection and are both lymphotropic and neurotropic. They can be transmitted casually.

Psychologic Studies. Most studies find that many patients with CFS *become* depressed and anxious *after* the onset (usually sudden) of their disorder. For many patients the depression and anxiety become the most debilitating parts of their illness. At the same time, these studies also indicate that a substantial fraction of patients with CFS (25% to 50%) have no evidence of any active psychiatric disorder since the onset of CFS. By and large the studies also find a higher frequency of psychiatric disorders in patients *before* they developed CFS than in the population at large: the average across all studies is approximately 30% (range, 20% to 50%) of CFS patients. On one hand, this past history of psychiatric disorders is greater than is found in the population at large (range, 5% to 10%); on the other hand, despite extensive psychiatric evaluation, no evidence of a preexisting psychiatric disorder can be found in most patients with CFS.

Although psychologic illness is not found in a substantial fraction of patients with CFS, it could well be playing a dominant role in the suffering of some patients with CFS. Even if CFS is triggered by an organic illness, such as an in-

fection, the chronic illness that ensues could, in some patients, reflect the reemergence of an underlying depression. Or it could indicate that the biologic underpinnings of depression somehow render one vulnerable to the "organic" abnormalities (e.g., the immunologic and virologic findings) seen in CFS. Or, in the individual patient, more than one of these factors may be operative.

✵ MANAGEMENT

Choice of Therapy

Low-Dose Tricyclic Agents. Randomized, controlled trials have shown that low-dose tricyclic drugs reduce the level of fatigue, musculoskeletal pain, and objectively demonstrable tender points in patients with fibromyalgia. Because CFS and fibromyalgia are similar, many physicians have tried the same therapy in CFS. No controlled trial of low-dose tricyclic agents has been mounted in CFS. However, it is the general anecdotal experience of most physicians that such treatment clearly improves the quality of sleep; as a consequence, perhaps, many patients state that their fatigue, myalgias, arthralgias, and cognitive problems also improve. The alpha-wave intrusion on delta wave–sleep disorder that has been found in both fibromyalgia and CFS improves with low-dose tricyclic therapy; thus there is objective confirmation of the experience reported by patients.

Amitriptyline or **doxepin** are the tricyclic drugs most often used for CFS; a typical regimen is 10 to 20 mg taken orally before bedtime. Of interest is that most patients with CFS cannot tolerate doses of tricyclic drugs usually used for depression (e.g., amitriptyline, 100 to 300 mg/day). Even with these very low doses, for about the first week of therapy, most patients with CFS report increased somnolence and fatigue in the morning. Patients should be warned of this transient adverse effect and urged to continue for at least 1 to 2 months before drawing any conclusions about the efficacy of the therapy.

In patients with concomitant depression and a sleep disorder, **sertraline,** 25 mg, **fluoxetine,** 5 to 20 mg, or another SSRI each morning often is coupled with low-dose tricyclic drugs at bedtime. Low doses are achieved by cutting the capsules or tablets or suspending them in measured amounts of liquid, or both. As with tricyclic agents and all other central nervous system–active substances, patients with CFS often cannot tolerate usual doses of fluoxetine. Also, the sleep-disruptive potential of fluoxetine may be greater in CFS, leading to the recommendation that this medication be taken in the morning. Having said this, one randomized controlled trial of fluoxetine in patients with CFS, some of whom also suffered from concurrent depression, found no benefit in treating either fatigue or depression.

Treatment of a concomitant depression by psychotherapy or pharmacotherapy in patients with CFS often reduces the mood disorder; however, it rarely eliminates the fatigue, cognitive problems, myalgias, arthralgias, postexertional malaise, respiratory tract symptoms, fevers, and adenopathy. Cognitive behavior therapy has helped improve the level of function in many patients, but is not a cure for the illness.

Other Treatments. One antiviral agent, acyclovir, has been shown to be ineffective in CFS; however, it also has little in vitro effect on the viruses that have been associated with

CFS. Controlled trials of gamma globulin have come to conflicting conclusions; at best, gamma globulin may offer a very brief and transient benefit, except in the unusual patients with CFS who also have a concomitant hypogammaglobulinemia and associated recurrent infections with encapsulated bacteria. Low-dose replacement therapy with corticosteroids or fludrocortisone have not been shown to be beneficial.

One randomized study reported a magnesium deficiency in CFS and a benefit from magnesium therapy; that study subsequently received much criticism. Although many patients take vitamins, there is no evidence that vitamins are helpful in CFS; one controlled trial found no evidence of benefit from vitamin B_{12} therapy. On the other hand, one study has found low levels of several B vitamins (particularly pyridoxine, riboflavin, and thiamine), and a small randomized controlled trial has reported improvement with a polynutrient supplement containing these B vitamins. A large number of treatments, some of which have a reasonable conceptual basis, have been proposed but not studied. As with any illness for which no definitive therapy exists, a variety of unconventional therapies have been used. Also, frankly exploitative "quack" remedies are being promoted.

Nonpharmaceutical Treatments. Patients should be encouraged to be as active as possible but to avoid activities that involve intensive physical or emotional stress. Limbering exercises are recommended for all patients. Several studies have found that the average patient benefits from a slowly graduated program of aerobic exercise, although in some patients this leads to relapses, including recurrence of fevers and adenopathy.

Gynecologic Conditions, Pregnancy, and Chronic Fatigue Syndrome

One case control study has found that women with CFS report a higher frequency of gynecologic complications—irregular cycles, periods of amenorrhea, and intermenstrual bleeding—than healthy control subjects. They also more often reported factors suggesting abnormal ovarian function, such as a history of polycystic ovarian syndrome, hirsutism, and ovarian cysts. Interestingly, they reported a *lower* incidence of premenstrual symptomatology.

There is no evidence that CFS adversely affects either the pregnant woman or the fetus. No anecdotal or published data reveal any increase in the rate of fetal abnormalities or in the subsequent health, growth, and development of the children. Most women with CFS seem to feel somewhat better during the course of the pregnancy, although some clearly feel worse. In the first 6 to 9 months of the postpartum period, most women with CFS (like those without CFS) feel more fatigued, but they usually do not feel more ill. That is, the energy required to deal with the needs of a new baby may be exhausting for the patient with CFS, just as it may be for a healthy person. However, the other symptoms of CFS—myalgias, arthralgias, sore throat, fevers—do not seem to regularly worsen. Indeed, many patients seem to receive a psychologic lift from childbearing because it demonstrates that they can be successful at one of life's most important challenges.

As has been discussed, the most commonly prescribed treatment in CFS is low-dose tricyclic therapy. Although

teratogenic effects from tricyclic agents (in doses that are equivalent to those used in human beings) have not been reported in animals, many tricyclic drugs cross the placenta, and occasional case reports of fetal abnormalities have led the Food and Drug Administration (FDA) to recommend caution in the use of tricyclic drugs during pregnancy. These agents also can be excreted into breast milk, and the FDA cautions against tricyclic therapy in nursing mothers.

BIBLIOGRAPHY

Ahmed SA, Talal N: Sex hormones and autoimmune rheumatic disorders, *Scand J Rheumatol* 18:69, 1989.

Bakheit AMO et al: Possible upregulation of hypothalamic 5-hydroxytryptamine receptors in patients with postviral fatigue syndrome, *Br Med J* 304:1010, 1992.

Bates DW et al: Clinical laboratory test findings in patients with the chronic fatigue syndrome, *Arch Intern Med* 155:97, 1995.

Blackwood SK et al: Effects of exercise on cognitive and motor function in chronic fatigue syndrome and depression, *J Neurol Neurosurg Psychiatry* 65:541, 1998.

Bou-Holaigah I, Rowe PC, Kan J, Calkins H: The relationship between neurally mediated hypotension and the chronic fatigue syndrome, *JAMA* 274:961, 1995.

Buchwald D et al: A chronic illness characterized by fatigue, neurologic and immunologic disorders, and active human herpesvirus type 6 infection, *Ann Intern Med* 116:103, 1992.

Cannon JG et al: Interleukin-1β, interleukin-1 receptor antagonist and soluble interleukin-1 receptor type II secretion in chronic fatigue syndrome, *J Clin Immunol* 17:253, 1997.

Centers for Disease Control and Prevention: Chronic Fatigue Syndrome Program Review; Objective 1: Surveillance. November 1999.

Cleare AJ et al: Contrasting neuroendocrine responses in depression and chronic fatigue syndrome, *J Affect Disord* 35:283, 1995.

Cleare AJ et al: Low-dose hydrocortisone in chronic fatigue syndrome: a randomized crossover trial, *Lancet* 353:455, 1999.

De Meirleir K et al: A 37kDa 2-5A binding protein as a potential biochemical marker for chronic fatigue syndrome, *Am J Med* 108:99, 2000.

Demitrack MA et al: Evidence for impaired activation of the hypothalamic-pituitary-adrenal axis in patients with chronic fatigue syndrome, *J Clin Endocrinol Metab* 73:1224, 1991.

Engel GL: The need for a new medical model: a challenge for biomedicine, *Science* 196:129, 1977.

Freeman R, Komaroff AL: Does the chronic fatigue syndrome involve the autonomic nervous system? *Am J Med* 102:357, 1997.

Fukuda K et al: The chronic fatigue syndrome: a comprehensive approach to its definition and study, *Ann Intern Med* 121:953, 1994.

Goldenberg DL, Felson DT, Dinerman H: A randomized, controlled trial of amitriptyline and naproxen in the treatment of patients with fibromyalgia, *Arthritis Rheum* 29:1371, 1986.

Gow JW et al: Enteroviral RNA sequences detected by polymerase chain reaction in muscle of patients with postviral fatigue syndrome, *Br Med J* 302:692, 1991.

Harlow BL et al: Reproductive correlates of chronic fatigue syndrome, *Am J Med* 105:94S, 1998.

Heap LC, Peters TJ, Wessely S: Vitamin B status in patients with chronic fatigue syndrome, *J R Soc Med* 92:183, 1999.

Hickie I et al: The psychiatric status of patients with the chronic fatigue syndrome, *Br J Psychiatry* 156:534, 1990.

Jason LA et al: A community-based study of chronic fatigue syndrome, *Arch Intern Med* 159:2129, 1999.

Kavelaars A et al: Disturbed neuroendocrine-immune interactions in chronic fatigue syndrome, *J Clin Endocrinol Metab* 85:692, 2000.

Klimas NG et al: Immunologic abnormalities in chronic fatigue syndrome, *J Clin Microbiol* 28:1403, 1990.

Komaroff AL et al: Health status in patients with chronic fatigue syndrome and in general population and disease comparison groups, *Am J Med* 101:281, 1996.

Kroenke K et al: Chronic fatigue in primary care: prevalence, patient characteristics, and outcome, *JAMA* 260:929, 1988.

Landay AL et al: Chronic fatigue syndrome: clinical condition associated with immune activation, *Lancet* 338:707, 1991.

Marcel B et al: Cognitive deficits in patients with chronic fatigue syndrome, *Biol Psychiatry* 40:535, 1996.

McKenzie R et al: Low-dose hydrocortisone for treatment of chronic fatigue syndrome. A randomized controlled trial, *JAMA* 280:1061, 1998.

Moss RB, Mercandetti A, Vojdani A: TNF-α and chronic fatigue syndrome, *J Clin Immunol* 19:314, 1999.

Patarca R et al: Dysregulated expression of tumor necrosis factor in chronic fatigue syndrome: interrelations with cellular sources and patterns of soluble immune mediator expression, *Clin Infect Dis* 18:S147, 1994.

Peterson PK et al: A preliminary placebo-controlled crossover trial of fludrocortisone for chronic fatigue syndrome, *Arch Intern Med* 158:908, 1998.

Schluederberg A et al: Chronic fatigue syndrome research: definition and medical outcome assessment, *Ann Intern Med* 117:325, 1992.

Schor JB: *The overworked American: the unexpected decline of leisure,* New York, 1992, Basic Books.

Schwartz RB et al: SPECT imaging of the brain: comparison of findings in patients with chronic fatigue syndrome, AIDS dementia complex, and major unipolar depression, *Am J Roentgen* 162:943, 1994.

Scott LV et al: Small adrenal glands in chronic fatigue syndrome: a preliminary computer tomography study, *Psychoneuroendo* 24:759, 1999.

Sharpe M et al: Increased prolactin response to buspirone in chronic fatigue syndrome, *J Affect Disord* 41:71, 1996.

Sharpe M et al: Cognitive behaviour therapy for the chronic fatigue syndrome: a randomised controlled trial, *Br Med J* 312:22, 1996.

Stewart JM et al: Orthostatic intolerance in adolescent chronic fatigue syndrome, *Pediatrics* 103:116, 1999.

Suhadolnik RJ et al: Upregulation of the 2-5A synthetase/RNase L antiviral pathway associated with chronic fatigue syndrome, *Clin Infect Dis* 18(Suppl 1):S96, 1994.

Suhadolnik RJ et al: Biochemical evidence for a novel low molecular weight 2-5A-dependent RNase L in chronic fatigue syndrome, *J Interferon Cytokine Res* 17:377, 1997.

Tiersky LA et al: Neuropsychology of chronic fatigue syndrome: a critical review, *J Clin Exp Neuropsychol* 19:560, 1997.

Verbrugge LM, Wingard DL: Sex differentials in health and mortality, *Women Health* 12:103, 1987.

Vercoulen JHMM et al: Randomized, double-blind, placebo-controlled study of fluoxetine in chronic fatigue syndrome, *Lancet* 347:858, 1996.

Vogelzang NJ et al: Patient, caregiver, and oncologist perceptions of cancer-related fatigue: results of a tripart assessment survey, *Semin Hematol* 34:4, 1997.

White PD et al: The validity and reliability of the fatigue syndrome that follows glandular fever, *Psychol Med* 25:917, 1995.

White PD et al: The existence of a fatigue syndrome after glandular fever, *Psychol Med* 25:907, 1995.

CHAPTER **87**

Domestic Violence

Stephanie A. Eisenstat

One in seven women who comes to the physician's office for general medical care has a history of domestic abuse; yet this history rarely is obtained during the office visit. Under diagnosis of domestic abuse is a critical problem because the health consequences of domestic abuse are then under treated. Significant morbidity, and sometimes mortality, ensues because of clinicians' failure to identify domestic abuse.

This chapter reviews the clinical presentation of domestic violence in the primary care setting, considers reasons for the difficulty in identification of clinical cases, and outlines strategies for evaluation and intervention for identified cases of domestic abuse.

A variety of guides has been developed by physician groups and professional organizations to help assist in the identification and evaluation of cases of domestic abuse. The available guides are listed at the end of this chapter.

EPIDEMIOLOGY

Domestic abuse is a leading cause of morbidity and mortality in women. It is a social problem that has serious and far-reaching public health consequences including the potential for injury and death. On the basis of national crime statistics, an estimated 2 million women are battered each year in the United States. Because of underreporting the actual numbers probably are closer to 4 million. One in five women is the victim of a completed rape during her lifetime. Male perpetrators are four times more likely to use lethal violence than females. According to a report issued by the Council on Scientific Affairs of the American Medical Association homicidal deaths resulting from one partner killing the other approached 40,000 from 1976 through 1986. More than half of these victims were women. In McLeer and Anwar's study of patients seeking emergency room treatment, one in three women was found to have a history of partner violence. One in six pregnant women was battered in a study by McFarlane and others of almost 700 pregnant women (Box 87-1).

DEFINITION AND CAUSE

Domestic violence (also referred to as battering or partner abuse) is a pattern of psychologic, economic, and sexual coercion of one partner in a relationship by the other that is punctuated by physical assaults or credible threats of bodily harm.

The aim of violence is to assert control and power. Fig. 87-1, which illustrates the relationship between physical assaults, sexual assault, and other types of abusive and controlling behavior, was developed by the Duluth Domestic Abuse Intervention Project on the basis of discussions with more than 200 women.

In a 1985 survey by Gelles and Straus, 1 of every 100 men (1.8 million) severely assaulted a female partner or cohabitant during the preceding 12 months and included punching, kicking, choking, threats with a knife or gun, or use of a knife or gun. Often economic threats, emotional abuse, intimidation, isolation, and threats against the children occur along with the physical and sexual violence. Neither victim nor batterer fit a distinct personality or socioeconomic profile. Battering is seen as a set of learned, controlling behaviors and attitudes of entitlement that are culturally supported and produce a relationship of entrapment (Box 87-2).

Many batterers have neither a diagnosable mental health condition nor criminal history. Generally the severity, intensity, and frequency of the violent episodes increases as the abuser loses control and power over the targets of the abuse, usually a woman and her children. The physical abuse becomes recurrent and escalates in frequency and severity as illustrated in Fig. 87-2. The violent partner often refuses to help the victim when she is sick, and his behavior interferes with her obtaining proper medical treatment.

Psychologic abuse includes threats of harm, jealousy, possessiveness, and intimidation. Sexual abuse is any form of forced sex or sexual degradation. Most batterers are verbally abusive between violent episodes, and this alone can be an indicator of domestic violence.

RISK FACTORS

Although all women are at risk for domestic abuse, studies by Flitcraft and others have shown that some subgroups of women appear to be at higher risk (Box 87-3). Race is not indicative of who is at risk for domestic violence. Generally women who are single, young, and recently separated or divorced are at high risk. A history of alcohol or substance

BOX 87-1
Statistics on Battering

2 to 4 million women are battered per year
1 in 5 *women is* the victim of completed rape
1 in 4 *women is* physically abused
1 in 3 women seeking emergency room care has a history of partner violence
1 in 7 women coming to physicians' office for general medical care has a history of domestic abuse
1 in 6 pregnant women are battered every year
1 in 4 women who attempt *suicide* is a victim of abuse
Fifty to seventy percent of the mothers of abused children are also being abused by their partners

BOX 87-2
Characteristics of Batterer

That Are Consistently True
Controlling
Entitled/self-centered
Believes he is the victim
Manipulative/good public image
Skillfully dishonest
Good early in relationships
Disrespectful, superior, depersonalizing
Externalizes responsibility
Punished, retaliates
Batterers serially
Danger increases postseparation
That may be present, but not consistently true
Substance abuse
Psychopathology
Male-on-male violence
"Traditional" attitudes
Controlling personality type

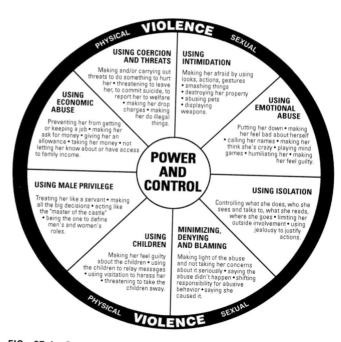

FIG. 87-1 Power and control wheel. (From Domestic Abuse Intervention Project, Duluth, Minn.)

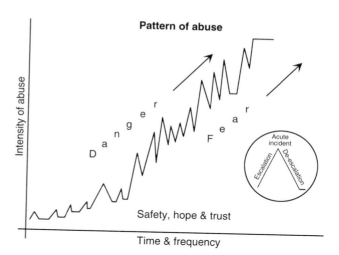

FIG. 87-2 Pattern of abuse. (From the New York State Office for the Prevention of Domestic Violence, 1990.)

abuse and mental illness in the patient or partner has been correlated with increased risk of domestic violence. Health status has been shown to be a risk factor. Studies have shown those with chronic debilitating medical conditions and disabilities to be at higher risk for abuse.

Pregnancy

A major risk factor is pregnancy. The incidence of domestic violence in pregnant patients was 8% in a study of a random sample at both private and public prenatal obstetric clinics by Helton et al and 7% to 11% in studies by Hilliard and Amaro of nonrandom, university-based obstetric practices. According to Strauss and Gelles' review of the Second National Family Violence Survey, 15% of women in the first trimester of pregnancy and 17% of pregnant women during the second and third trimester pregnancy reported acts of domestic violence. For many women, the abuse starts during pregnancy, and according to McFarlane et al, for those with a prior his-tory of partner abuse, the violence often escalates during pregnancy. The frequency, severity, and potential danger of homicide increase as well. A study of pregnant women by Bullock showed a higher rate of miscarriage and increased risk for low-birth-weight infants in pregnant women who were in abusive relationships. Other complications associated with battering during pregnancy are shown in Box 87-4.

History of Childhood Abuse

Studies by Flitcraft revealed that women with a history of childhood physical or sexual abuse were at increased risk of experiencing domestic violence as adults. In addition, a correlation exists between child and wife abuse in the same family. In those families in which child abuse has been identified, outreach services should be offered to the wife as well.

Immigration Status

Domestic violence does appear to be more prevalent among immigrants to the United States compared with US citizens. This may be because they come from cultures that accept domestic violence or because they have less access to legal and social services than US citizens. Often, immigrant batterers and victims believe that the penalties and protections of the US legal system do not apply to them. Although a victim may be in the country legally by virtue of her marriage to the batterer, her status may be conditional. It is common for a batterer to exert his control over his wife's immigration status to force her to remain in the relationship. Undocumented women may be reported to immigration and naturalization services by law enforcement or social service from whom they may seek assistance.

Economic Factors

Financial instability is the most common reason why women cannot leave the abuser. A total of 15% to 50% of abused women report interference from their partner with education, training, or work. It also appears to be a risk factor for domestic violence. A study by Raphael showed that the majority of welfare recipients had experienced domestic violence in their adult lives.

BARRIERS TO IDENTIFICATION

For the clinician, dealing with cases of domestic abuse involves confronting difficult and ambiguous emotional circumstances. Sources of support and referral are not always readily available, and a number of barriers make the accurate identification of domestic violence particularly difficult.

Patient Barriers

Patients have misconceptions that interfere with their ability to tell the clinician about incidences of violence. The woman may think that the clinician is neither interested in her situation nor has the time to deal with it. Shame, guilt, and embarrassment can be overwhelming for the patient. Survivors of domestic violence report fear of the partner's reprisals, fear of threats to the children, and fear for their own safety. The battering of the woman's self-esteem results in the patient's perception that she deserves the abuse. Often there are financial threats, as well as threats to the children.

Physician Barriers

Physicians also face a number of barriers in dealing with cases of domestic abuse. Many clinicians hold deep-seated myths about abused patients (Box 87-5) that interfere with identification of these cases in the clinical setting. The reality for most of these women is that they are living in an environment of "terrorism" and because of the fear and manipulation on the part of the abuser are unable to escape from the relationship. The patient does not provoke the violence. The abuser has a lack of impulse control and a need to control the partner. Cases of domestic abuse are seen in all socioeconomic and racial groups.

In addition to myths about these patients and intervention, the physician faces other barriers to identification. These include the following:

1. Lack of education on strategies for identification and intervention.
2. Discomfort with dealing with the emotional aspects of the problem.
3. Lack of proper resources and referral networks.

In a small study of primary care physicians, Sugg and Inui explored the experience and attitudes of physicians with cases of domestic violence. The physicians identified lack of comfort with the problem, lack of time to deal with the problem, lack of resources and education, and a fear of offending the patient as barriers in diagnosis and treatment of the problem. Although clinicians are under time constraints, with proper training and access to resources, domestic violence cases can be identified and addressed in an efficient and effective manner.

BOX 87-3
Women at Risk

Single women
Women who have been recently separated or divorced from their husband
Ages 17-28 years
History of alcohol or substance abuse; mental illness in patient or partner
Pregnant woman
History of childhood abuse
Women with disabilities
Immigrants

Modified From Alpert E et al: *Partner violence: how to recognize and treat victims of abuse—a guide for physicians,* Waltham, Mass, 1992, Massachusetts Medical Society.

BOX 87-4
Adverse Pregnancy and Birth Outcomes in Abusive Relationships

Miscarriage
Low birth weight
Fetal fractures
Abruptio placentae
Uterine rupture
Premature rupture of membranes
Antepartum hemorrhage

BOX 87-5
Myths About Abused Patients

Violence is private
Patient can leave
Patient provokes violence
Problem of poor patients
Takes time to diagnose and intervene
Nothing can be done to prevent

Modified from Sugg NK, Inui T: *JAMA* 267:3157, 1992.

HEALTH EFFECTS OF BATTERING

Although domestic violence happens in the home, the health and psychologic consequences of battering make it a priority for the primary care clinician. Battering has severe effects on the victim's health, well-being, and self-esteem. Obvious effects of domestic abuse are the physical trauma and potential risk of homicide. Abused women constitute 20% to 35% of all women who seek emergency room treatment for physical injuries. In addition to the physical trauma, continuous domestic abuse is associated with an increased risk for mental illness, alcoholism, substance abuse, and somatoform and eating disorders (Box 87-6).

There is evidence that domestic violence is associated with increased rates of physical and psychologic symptoms, hospitalizations, and substance abuse. Bergman and Brismar's controlled study of 117 women indicated higher rates of hospital utilization (Table 87-1) for trauma and for medical and gynecologic problems. The increased rates were particularly pronounced for inpatient hospitalizations for suicide attempts, gynecologic disorders, and observation (undefined disorders). The rates of mental illness, especially for depression, alcoholism, and substance abuse, were all increased in this study group as compared with the control group of women without a history of domestic violence (Table 87-2). The same correlation between prior sexual abuse and subsequent medical problems is suggested in a study by Springs and Friedrich as well.

In a study of 206 women seeking care at a gastroenterology practice for functional or organic disorders, 44% of women reported sexual and physical abuse during childhood or adulthood. Half of the abused women stated that some form of abuse was continuing into adulthood. Only about a third of these women told their physicians about the actual incidents of abuse. The group with a history of functional gastrointestinal complaints and physical abuse was four times more likely to have associated complaints such as diffuse pelvic pain, backaches, shortness of breath, and an increased rate of lifetime surgery. Despite multiple visits to the physician's office, fewer than 20% of the physicians were aware that the patients had experienced abuse. These findings are consistent with other clinical studies and reemphasize the need to suspect and identify cases of domestic violence, especially if the woman manifests the particular spectrum of complaints in the next section.

CLINICAL PRESENTATION
History and Symptoms
The Interview

The first step in case identification is to ask the woman questions that will elicit a history of domestic violence. Box 87-7 lists common examples of such questions. In a study of 322 women by Feldhaus, these simple screening questions were found to be accurate in detecting domestic abuse, with a sensitivity of 71% and a specificity of 85%. Generally, written questionnaires screening for abuse have not been as successful as asking the questions directly. It is important *not* to ask the question "Are you abused?" Studies have found that these women do not see themselves as "abused" and often will answer "no" to such a question but "yes" if the clinician asks "Has your partner ever hit you?" Any patient encounter is an opportunity for screening, and may be the only opportunity. However, routine medical, gynecologic, obstetric, and pediatric visits provide unique opportunities for screening

---

BOX 87-6
Health Effects of Abuse

Physical trauma
Mental illness
Increased risk for alcoholism and substance abuse
Somatoform disorder
Eating disorders

Table 87-1
Use of Somatic Hospital Care During a 15-Year Period (1973-1988) by Battered Women and Age-Matched Control Subjects

Reason for Care	BATTERED WOMEN (n = 117)		CONTROLS (n = 117)	
	No. of Women	No. of Admissions	No. of Women	No. of Admissions
Surgical disorders (not trauma)	25	40*	19	22
Trauma	47†	70†	15	18
Gynecologic disorders	48†	91†	24	41
Induced abortion	20‡	22‡	7	8
Medical disorders	40†	71†	14	17
Suicide attempts	23†	55†	2	2
Observation	28†	71†	9	11
Total	90†	420†	58	119

From Bergman B, Brismar B: *Am J Public Health* 81:1486, 1991.
*$p < 0.05$.
†$p < 0.01$.
‡$p < 0.001$.

Table 87-2
Diagnosis in Psychiatric Inpatient Care of Battered Women and Control Subjects During a 15-Year Period (1973-1988)

Diagnoses	BATTERED WOMEN (n = 117)		Control Subjects (n = 117)
	No.	%	
Depression	19	6*	0
Psychoses	10	9†	1
Alcoholism	27	23*	0
Drug addiction	10	9†	0
Suicide attempt	18	15*	0
Other and unspecified diagnosis	13	11†	0
Total number of psychiatric inpatients	69	59	1

From Bergman B, Brismar B: *Am J Public Health* 81:1486, 1991.
*$p < 0.01$.
†$p < 0.001$.

BOX 87-7

Diagnosis and Identification of Domestic Violence: Questions to Ask*

Do you ever feel unsafe at home?[†]
Has anyone at home hit you or tried to injure you in any way?[†]
Has anyone ever threatened you or tried to control you?
Have you ever felt afraid of your partner?

---

*Any positive response to any of the questions constitutes a positive disclosure for abuse.
[†]Study by Feldhaus, 1997 demonstrated sensitivity of 71% in detecting domestic violence and a specificity of almost 85%.

---

and early prevention. The American Medical Association and other professional organizations recommend screening all female patients from adolescent to the elderly for a history of past or present abuse. Screening of men is not recommended unless the indicators of abuse are present (Box 87-8). Many practitioners ask the domestic violence screening questions along with other preventive care inquiries or during the social history to reinforce the routine nature of the questions. In practice, clinicians should perform routine screening whenever a patient starts a new intimate relationship or presents with any of the clinical indicators of domestic violence, even if previously screened.

It is important to make the patient feel comfortable, safe, and reassured. To promote this environment, it is important to interview the patient alone without the partner present and in a confidential manner. To avoid conflict, partners, family members, and friends should be told that practitioners routinely need at least 5 to 10 minutes alone with each patient during each visit. If the patient is non-English speaking, an interpreter with training in domestic violence interviewing should be used. Family members or friends should never be used as interpreters because they may be in collusion with the abuser. Begin the screening interview by emphasizing the routine nature of the questions and an explicit assurance of confidentiality. A common statement that can be used to preface the screening questions is, "We care about the health consequences of partner abuse/domestic violence and have begun asking all our female patients a few questions." The clinician should not break confidentiality by discussing the allegations with the patient's partner or other family members. Words such as *domestic violence, abuse,* or *battered* should not be used during interviews with patients. Because of their own perceptions of their situation, they will not necessary identify themselves as abused or in a relationship of domestic violence (Box 87-9). It also is important not to ask what the victim did to bring on the violence or why she has not left the relationship. Both statements are inappropriate and self-defeating.

The screening questions should assess for the hallmarks of domestic violence: lack of safety, fear of the abuser, and control and harm by the abuser. Easily phrased, all four questions should be asked simply and with direct eye contact (Box 87-7).

The clinical presentation of the battered woman is *repeated physical injuries, medical complaints,* and *mental health problems.*

BOX 87-8

Diagnosis and Identification of the Abused Patient

Physical Trauma
Dental, head and neck injury common
Any death
Central distribution of injuries
Multiple areas of injuries
Bruises at different stages of healing
Sexual assault
Injury during pregnancy
Delay of treatment for injury
Inconsistent explanation for injuries

Medical Presentations (Alone or In Combination)
Chronic somatic complaints without documented etiology:
Headaches, abdominal pain, pelvic pain, back and joint pain
Irritable bowel syndrome
Fatigue and insomnia
Palpitations
Hyperventilation and choking sensation
Sexually transmitted disease
Noncompliance with medical recommendations

Common Associated Psychologic Disorders
Eating disorders
Substance abuse
Depression and suicidal ideation
Anxiety symptoms and panic disorder
Hyperventilation
Post-traumatic stress disorder

Other Possible Indicators
No prenatal care or unwanted pregnancy
Pregnancy complications
Stroke in young woman
Physical/sexual abuse of children in the home

Common Behaviors
Evasiveness
Repeated emergency/office visits
Fear
Aggressive partner
Social isolation
Jumpiness
Passivity
Crying

Modified from Eisenstat S, Bancroft L: *N Engl J Med* 341:886, 1999.

Physical Trauma

The presenting complaints may clearly suggest battering with obvious physical trauma or they may be more obscure. Obvious clues to abuse include bilateral distribution of trauma in multiple areas, central distribution of injuries, bruises at different stages of healing, sexual assault, and trauma during pregnancy (Box 87-8). Another clue to diagnosis is that the patient's *explanation* for the injury is often inconsistent with the *extent* of injury, and there may be a delay between the onset of the injury and presentation to the physician for treatment. The most common area of in-

BOX 87-9

Guidelines for Interviewing the Patient in Suspected Cases of Domestic Violence

Interview the patient alone.
Assure confidentiality.
Reassure patient that environment is safe.
Do not disclose allegations to partner.
Use interpreter services if non-English speaking, not family members.

BOX 87-10

Helpful Responses to a Disclosure of Abuse

I know about this issue and am not shocked by your disclosure.
I am glad you trusted me with this information.
I am sorry that this happened to you.
I can offer you help and connect you to others who can provide resources for you.
No one has the right to abuse anyone else.
You did not cause the abuse.

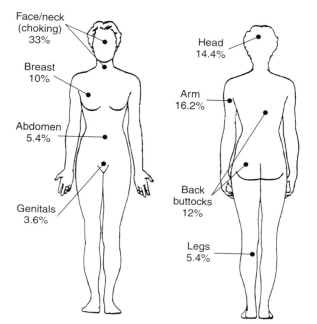

FIG. 87-3 Sites and percentages of abuse injuries. (From Helton A, Anderson E, McFarlane J: *Protocol of care for the battered woman*, White Plains, NY, 1986, March of Dimes Birth Defects Foundation.)

jury usually is the head and neck region as illustrated in Fig. 87-3, followed by the upper extremities, breast, back, and buttocks.

Somatic Complaints and Associated Psychological Disorders

More subtle presentations include somatic complaints such as headaches, insomnia, fatigue, hyperventilation, and back or pelvic pain to list a few examples. A complaint of choking should prompt concern about the possibility of physical or sexual abuse. Eating disorders and other mental health problems such as depression, anxiety disorders, and post-traumatic stress disorder are more common in women with a history of abuse.

A rare presentation is stroke in a young woman, and unexplained stroke in a young woman warrants further evaluation for suspected abuse. Lack of prenatal care and the physical or sexual abuse of the woman's children are other clues.

Common Behaviors

Often women experiencing domestic violence are mistrustful of the primary care provider and fearful of reprisal from the abusive partner. This reaction is not totally unfounded inasmuch as studies have shown that violence by the partner may escalate after identification of the abuser and when the woman decides to leave the abuser. Dealing with this aspect of the problem is addressed in the next section. Because of fear and distrust, the profile of a woman who has a history of abuse may include evasive behavior, vague historic recollection, and anxious behavior during the interview. Frequent visits to the emergency room or outpatient office and an overly aggressive or attentive partner accompanying the woman should raise the clinician's suspicion for abuse. Box 87-8 lists these and other common behaviors seen in the battered woman.

Physical Examination

A thorough documentation of the patient's account and complaints should be completed and a complete physical examination performed, with special attention to the areas of the patient's complaints. Any possible injuries should be photographed after informed consent. This can be helpful in any future legal proceedings. If domestic abuse is suspected, it is a good idea to contact a social worker, if one is available, as soon as possible to expedite the process of intervention.

Responding to a Disclosure

It can be difficult to know how to help when the patient has made a disclosure of domestic violence or when one of the team members has identified a history of violence through routine screening. This is particularly the case when the abuser is present in the office or emergency room setting.

A positive response to *any* of the questions constitutes a disclosure of domestic violence and should be followed by brief exploratory questions. Patients have reported that validation of their ability to disclose has often given them the confidence to consider options. Helpful responses are listed in Box 87-10.

Documentation

Appropriate documentation may be tricky, but is very important, both to decrease medical liability and also to help the victim in future legal action against the perpetrator. It is important to document the history and physical clearly in the medical record, using body maps and photographs if necessary. Maintaining confidentiality is paramount. Never divulge a patient's revelations of abuse to a partner. When domestic violence is suspected but the patient denies the history, record "injury inconsistent with explanation" in the medical record. Although it is important to document that referral has been completed, if she ultimately requires shelter for protection, do not document or disclose the hiding place. Do not record a mother's disclosures in a pediatric chart and do not list domestic violence as a discharge diagnosis, since the billing and insurance may be managed by the batterer.

MANAGEMENT
Goals of Management

The primary care clinician does not have to be an expert in the psychosocial aspects of domestic violence to effectively prevent future trauma and the development of associated medical disorders. The clinician's role is to diagnose and identify the problem, then to provide the appropriate referral network. It is important to investigate the various options available before facing a case of domestic violence and to have a general strategy and referral network in place. A more public campaign can support the efforts of individual providers (i.e., having resource cards in the female bathrooms, support group numbers, posters on the wall, etc). If available, ideal intervention is interdisciplinary and involves social services and nursing. The primary care physician's role is important in supporting the patient and validating the patient's experiences (Box 87-11).

Referral

Building on the work of the 25-year-old grass roots Battered Women's Advocacy Movement, health care and medicine have recently begun to assume an increasing role in the coordinated community response to end domestic violence. In the late 1980s, the first hospital-based advocacy programs were developed in the United States (WomanKind, Minnesota and AWAKE [Advocacy for Women and Kids in Emergencies], Children's Hospital, Boston). More recently, with the development of the Family Violence Prevention Fund, a national organization focusing on the health care response to domestic violence, these programs have been replicated across the United States.

Various options for action are available to the woman who has been subjected to domestic abuse (Box 87-12). Services are voluntary aimed at rebuilding the victim's self-esteem and autonomy. The patient retains the right to make a personal decision regarding choice of intervention or no intervention. As a competent adult, the patient has the right to make her own decisions and as such the right to refuse intervention, which is a difficult clinical situation for the medical provider. "Refusal for intervention" should not be interpreted as a rejection of medical treatment. It is crucial for clinicians to understand that she may not be able to act at

the time of presentation. However, if the door is kept open for these patients and the woman at least understands her options (such as appropriate phone numbers to use to contact help when she is ready, your concern for her safety, and your interest in her well-being), she may be able to decide to take action. Often this occurs after she has had some time to think about the danger and the physical and psychologic trauma she has already endured. To maintain supportive contact it is helpful to arrange follow-up appointments with the primary care physician and any other social service advocates.

Every practitioner should be aware of the National Domestic Violence Hotline at 1-800-799-SAFE (7233) and use this resource to identify hospital- and community-based resources for any patient interested in accessing services.

Restraining Orders and Shelters

The patient needs to be aware of the existence of shelters, the availability of law enforcement, and the method for obtaining legal restraining orders. Providing this information requires each physician to contact local agencies to determine local available resources. Many states now have strict laws and guidelines that protect all women in a familial or dating relationship, providing them the option to obtain an emergency, temporary, and/or permanent restraining order against the abuser. A permanent restraining order, which is valid up to 1 year, may be obtained through superior, probate, and family district or municipal court. In most states, if the batterer violates the restraining order or stalks the woman, the police must arrest him. It is important to remember that although legal restraining orders have been shown to decrease physical violence in the short run, they do not eliminate the risk of continuing abuse or homicide. In a study by Buzawa, 60% of women reported acts of abuse after the entry of a protection order and 30% reported acts of severe violence. Those batterers with prior criminal histories are more likely to violate an order than those who do not. In addition, many victims face other legal issues, such as difficult child custody battles. Some courts mistakenly penalize the victim in custody cases by assuming that the victim is emotionally unstable because of the violence or because the victim was in

---

BOX 87-11
Support for the Patient

Reinforce that patient is not alone.
Reinforce that patient is not to blame.
State that help is available.
Validate the patient's experiences.
Give options to patient and assess safety.
Offer advocacy services if available.

BOX 87-12
Role of the Physician: Management and Referral

Document history and physical examination clearly in medical record
History
Following a disclosure of abuse, proceed with brief historical questions (when, where, how, nature of the incident, associated trauma, worst incident and appropriate medical history)
Physical examination
After examining the injuries, note specifically the character, appearance, depth, location and direction of the injuries
Use body map and photography if necessary
Provide primary medical care.
Contact social worker.
Assess patient's safety.
Coordinate access to:
  Shelters
  Law enforcement
  Legal restraining orders

some way responsible for the abuse. In many states, custody statutes now recognize that domestic violence is relevant to the abuser's parental fitness.

From 1970 to 1990 more than 1200 shelters were established in the United States. It is important to realize that most women do not use shelters. Bed availability can vary and often many shelters are ill-equipped to care for those women with severe medical problems, who are pregnant, have a history of substance abuse, or are in same sex battering relationships. Many local groups for battered women have available information on shelters and state laws, as well as volunteers who serve as patient advocates.

Mandatory Reporting

If violence is perpetrated against an elderly person, a child younger than 18 years old, or a disabled person, or if there is a sexual assault, the incident *must* be reported to state authorities (Box 87-13).

Assessment of Safety

Determining safety can be challenging, but is crucial. After identification of domestic abuse, the episodes of abuse may escalate, making leaving the abuser the most dangerous time. Although it is not common for the abuser to be violent with clinical staff members, he may be more abusive to the patient. The responsibility of the clinician is to evaluate whether the patient is safe to leave the premises and understands the risks/benefits of the options offered. With the help of a social worker or domestic violence victim advocate (if available), one should assess the *abuser's threats about homicide and suicide, depression, weapons possession, obsession with his partner, drug and alcohol consumption, access to the battered woman,* and the *degree of escalation of threats and violence.* The woman needs to understand her potential risk. Most women want to accept help, but the process of ending the relationship (however bad it is) is painful and difficult. If the woman is not ready to leave the abusive situation, even temporarily, every effort should be made to keep her options open and contact with the medical and social service system readily available.

Domestic Violence Victim Advocates: The New Health Care Professionals

Many health care institutions and community practitioners have come to recognize domestic abuse as a public health care problem, yet the medical setting is still not fully equipped to respond adequately to the needs of battered women.

Domestic violence victim advocates are commonly found in battered women's shelters, police departments, district at-

torneys offices, and courthouses around the country. The role is new within the health care system. Advocates, who may or may not be survivors themselves, have training and experience in the complex problems associated with domestic violence and have a link to community services. They help the survivor understand their legal and safety options and, if ready to leave the abuser, strategies for providing safe exit. This may include obtaining a restraining order, finding an available bed in a shelter, putting the children in a different school, or even moving out of the area. For those women not ready to leave, they can counsel them on strategies for increasing safety at home, such as hiding weapons from the abuser, ensuring access to a phone, hiding money and important papers for emergencies, and having a list of people to call for help. They also conduct support groups that help improve the woman's self-esteem and confidence and recovery from the trauma. They link women to services that help them achieve financial independence, such as employment opportunities, transitional assistance, and education.

For Men Who Batter

When confronted with a batterer in the office or emergency room setting who is threatening to the staff or the patient, it is best to contact office or hospital security personnel or local law enforcement. If possible, do not try to manage aggressive behavior alone. To further promote victim and staff safety, try to avoid aggressive or verbal confrontation, do not reveal to the batterer anything you have learned from the victim, be careful not to accept the batterer's word as fact, and be careful about documenting domestic violence in a pediatric medical record, regardless of who discloses, since the batterer can legally obtain it and retaliate against the mother or child.

Programs are available to provide counseling and intervention for the batterer. Many batterers go only because mandated by the court. Unfortunately, the success of these programs is controversial, and more research data are needed to establish their efficacy. Short-term (6 to 12 weeks) psychoeducational batterer intervention programs have helped some batterers stop the immediate physical violence but have been found to be inadequate in stopping abuse over time. Even more concerning, some batterers become more sophisticated in their psychologic abuse and intimidation after attending such programs. The initial intervention is to separate the patient from the violent situation and ensure that the woman (and her children) are in a safe environment.

BOX 87-13
Mandatory Reporting of Abuse

Children younger than 18 years old
Elderly persons aged 60 years or older
Disabled persons
Sexual assault (without name identification)
Gunshot and stab wounds

BOX 87-14
RADAR

R *R*emember to ask routinely about partner violence.
A *A*sk directly about violence with questions such as "At any time has your partner hit you?" *Interview in private.*
D *D*ocument your findings.
A *A*ssess your patient's safety.
R *R*eview options with your patient.

From Alpert E et al: *Partner violence: how to recognize and treat victims of abuse— a guide for physicians,* Waltham, Mass, 1992, Massachusetts Medical Society.

Alpert et al developed the acronym RADAR, which summarizes the important aspects in identification and intervention (Box 87-14).

BIBLIOGRAPHY

Policy Statements and Recommendations from Professional Medical Organizations

American Academy of Pediatrics. Committee on Child Abuse and Neglect: The role of the pediatrician in recognizing and intervening on behalf of abused women (RE9748), *Pediatrics* 101:1091, 1998.

American College of Obstetricians and Gynecologists (ACOG): Washington, DC, *The battered woman* (Tech Bull 209), 1995, The College.

American College of Emergency Physicians: Emergency medicine and domestic violence, *Ann Emerg Med* 25:442, 1995.

American College of Surgeons: Statement on Domestic Violence. *Bull Am Coll Surgeons* 85: 2000.

Cornwell E et al: National Medical Association Surgical Section Position Paper on Violence Prevention. A Resolution of Trauma Surgeons Caring for Victims of Violence, *JAMA* 273:1788, 1995.

Council on Scientific Affairs, American Medical Association: Violence against women: relevance for medical practitioners, *JAMA* 267:3184, 1992.

Flitcraft A et al: American Medical Association Diagnostic and Treatment Guidelines on Domestic Violence, *Arch Fam Med* 1:39, 1992.

General Bibliography

Alpert E et al: *Partner violence: how to recognize and treat victims of abuse—a guide for physicians*, Waltham, Mass, 1992, Massachusetts Medical Society.

Amaro H et al: Violence during pregnancy and substance abuse, *Am J Public Health*, 80:575, 1990.

Atwood JD: Domestic violence: the role of alcohol, *JAMA* 265:460, 1991 (letter).

Bergman B, Brismar B: A five year follow up study of 117 battered women, *Am J Public Health* 81:1486, 1991.

Buzawa E, Buzawa C: *Domestic violence. The criminal justice response,* Thousand Oaks, CA, 1996, Sage Publications.

Carmen E, Rieker P, Mills T: Victims of violence and psychiatric illness, *Am J Psychiatry* 141:378, 1984.

Davies J: *Safety planning with battered women: complex lives/difficult choices,* Thousand Oaks, CA, 1998, Sage Publications.

Diaz-Olavarrieta C et al: Domestic violence against patients with chronic neurological disorders, *Arch Neurol* 56:681, 1999.

Drossman D et al: Sexual and physical abuse in women with functional or organic gastrointestinal disorders, *Ann Intern Med* 113:828, 1990.

Eisenstat S, Bancroft L: Domestic violence, *N Engl J Med* 341:886, 1999.

Eisenstat S, Zimmer B: Providing medical care and advocacy for survivors of domestic Abuse, *J Clin Outcomes Mngmt* 5:54, 1998.

Feldhaus KM et al: Accuracy of 3 brief screening questions for detecting partner violence in the emergency department, *JAMA* 277:1357, 1997.

Freund KM, Blackhall LJ: Detection of domestic violence in a primary care setting, *Clin Res* 38:738A, 1990.

Gazmararian JA et al: Prevalence of violence against pregnant women, *JAMA* 277;1125, 1997.

Haber JD, Roos C: Effects of spousal abuse and/or sexual abuse in the development and maintenance of chronic pain in women, *Adv Pain Res Ther* 9:889, 1985.

Haydon S, Barton E, Hatden M: Domestic violence in the emergency department: how do women prefer to disclose and discuss the issues? *J Emerg Med* 15:447, 1997.

Jacobson A, Richardson B: Assault experiences of 100 psychiatric inpatients: evidence of the need for routine inquiry, *Am J Psychiatry* 144:908, 1987.

Kyriacou DN et al. Risk factors for injury to women from domestic violence against women, *N Engl J Med* 341:1892, 1999.

Larkin GL et al: Universal screening for intimate partner violence in the Emergency Department. Importance of patient and provider factors, *Ann Emerg Med* 33:669, 1999.

Malek AM et al: Patient presentation, angiographic features, and treatment of strongulation-induced bilateral dissection of the cervical internal carotid artery. Report of three cases, *J Neurosurg* 92:481, 2000.

Massey J: Domestic violence in neurologic practice, *Arch Neurol* 56:659, 1999.

McFarlane J et al: Assessing for abuse during pregnancy: severity and frequency of injuries and associated entry into prenatal care, *JAMA* 267: 3176, 1992.

McGrath M, Hogan J, Peipert J: A prevalence survey of abuse and screening for abuse in urgent care patients, *Obstet Gynecol* 91:511, 1998.

McKibben L, De Vos E, Newberger E: Victimization of mothers of abused children: a controlled study, *Pediatrics* 84:531, 1989.

McLeer SV, Anwar R: A study of battered women presenting in an emergency department, *Am J Public Health* 79:65, 1989.

Muelleman R, Lenaghan P, Pakieser R: Battered women: injury locations and types, *Ann Emerg Med* 28:486, 1996.

Newberger E et al: Abuse of pregnant women and adverse birth outcome: current knowledge and implications for practice, *JAMA* 267:2370, 1992.

Raphael J: Prisoners of abuse. In *Domestic violence and welfare receipt,* Chicago, 1996, Taylor Institute.

Reiter RC, Gambone JC: Demographic and historic variables in women with idiopathic chronic pelvic pain, *Obstet Gynecol* 75:428, 1990.

Reiter RC et al: Correlation between sexual abuse and somatization in women with somatic and nonsomatic chronic pelvic pain, *Am J Obstet Gynecol* 165:104, 1991.

Rodriguez MA et al: Mandatory reporting of intimate partner violence to police: views of physicians in California, *Am J Public Health* 89:575, 1999.

Rodriguez R, Bauer H, McLoughlin E: Screening and intervention for intimate partner abuse: practices and attitudes of primary care physicians, *JAMA* 282:468, 1999.

Schecter S: *Interviewing battered women: guidelines for the mental health practitioner in domestic violence cases,* Washington, DC, 1987, NCAV.

Shumway J et al: Preterm labor, placental abruption, and premature rupture of membrane in relation to maternal violence or verbal abuse, *J Matern Fetal Med* 8:76, 1999.

Straus MA, Gelles RJ, editors: *Physical violence in American families: risk factors and adaptions to violence in 8145 families,* New Brunswick, NJ, 1990, Transaction Books.

Sugg N, Inui T: Primary care physicians' response to domestic violence: opening Pandora's box, *JAMA* 297:3157, 1992.

Tjaden P, Thoennes N: Prevalence, incidence and consequences of violence against women: findings from the National Violence Against Women Survey. National Institute of Justice. Centers for Disease Control and Prevention, November 1998 (NCJ-172837).

Zierler S et al: Violence victimization after HIV infection in a US probability sample of adult patients in primary care, *Am J Public Health* 90:208, 2000.

CHAPTER **88**

Sexual Assault

Stephanie A. Eisenstat

Sexual assault against women is common, with one in six women reporting a history of sexual assault. It carries both short-term and long-term physical and psychologic effects. The term *rape* is a legal term, not a medical one. The trauma inflicted brings the patient in contact with the health care system, and for the clinician it is important to know how to evaluate victims of a rape and to develop strategies for dealing with both the short- and long-term consequences of sexual assault. This chapter addresses the physician's role and responsibility in dealing with a woman who has experienced sexual assault and outlines protocol for evaluation and management. Acute evaluation should be done by providers specifically trained to care for victims of sexual assault when possible. Many institutions have established SANE (Sexual Assault Nurse Evaluation) models or related programs for acute care because of the skill and procedures required to adequately collect forensic evidence and provide the necessary psychologic support for the victim.

Reviews have been published on management of the victim of sexual assault, and they are listed in the bibliography at the end of this chapter. The following discussion highlights the important principles in evaluation and management and draws on the information in these reviews.

DEFINITION

Rape is a legal term, the definition of which has changed over the years and varies from state to state. Rape is now defined as the "nonconsensual sexual penetration of an adolescent or adult obtained by physical force, by threat of bodily harm, or when the victim is incapable of giving consent by virtue of mental illness, mental retardation or intoxication." This crime of violence is often motivated by aggression and rage, with the perpetrator using sexual contact as a weapon for power and control.

EPIDEMIOLOGY

Sexual assault is one of the most common crimes against women. One in five adult women, one in six college women, and one in eight adolescent girls have been sexually assaulted over their lifetime, as reported from national crime statistics from the U.S. Department of Justice. These numbers are likely underestimated because of the hesitancy of rape victims to report the sexual assault; 39% of rape victims report having sustained physical injury, and only 54% of these women receive medical care for the injuries. Fatalities occur in about 0.1% of all sexual assault cases.

HEALTH CONSEQUENCES
Rape Trauma Syndrome

Rape trauma syndrome is the psychologic reaction of the rape trauma victim, which is characterized by two major phases after sexual assault (Box 88-1). The first phase of shock and disbelief can last from 6 weeks to a few months, with the woman displaying either intense fear and anxiety and crying episodes or the opposite, with little display of emotion. Frightening recollections of the assault may be associated with generalized hypersensitivity to environmental stimuli. The second phase is delayed and involves a psychologic reorganization, a long-term process that can last a few months or indefinitely. The woman develops various coping strategies to deal with activities of daily living and to integrate the experience and thus achieve psychologic recovery. Flashbacks, phobias, and depression still may occur, in addition to gynecologic and somatic complaints. Sexual dysfunction is common. There appears to be a time in between these two phases when the woman enters a phase of denial and gives the outward appearance of coping. During this period, medical symptoms may develop or intensify, causing the woman to seek medical attention, but she may not inform the clinician of the sexual assault because of intense shame and guilt. It is important for clinicians to ask patients directly during the interview about a history of sexual assault.

Medical Disorders

Nongenital physical injuries occur in approximately 40% of completed sexual assault cases, with 3% of these cases requiring overnight hospitalization.

Any sexual assault or trauma can lead to the development of chronic physical complaints and an increased risk for serious mental illness such as depression or suicidal impulses (Box 88-2). Somatic complaints include extreme fatigue, abdominal pain, nausea, headaches, and gynecologic and menstrual complaints. A constant concern is the development of sexually transmitted diseases (3.6% to 20% of all sexual assaults), pregnancy (4.7%), and human immunodeficiency virus (HIV) infection. HIV transmission risk rate from sexual assault is estimated at 1 in 500. Frequent utilization of primary medical care for up to 2 years after the assault is common.

Sexual Assault During Pregnancy

Sexual assault often occurs during pregnancy, although the exact incidence is difficult to estimate because of underreporting. Overall pregnancy outcome has been found to be normal in small retrospective studies of pregnant women who have been sexually assaulted; however, there is an increased risk for low–birth-weight infants and premature delivery. In these studies pregnant women had the same incidence of vulvar, oral, and anal penetration as matched nonpregnant sexual assault victims, but they experienced less truncal injuries if the assault occurred after 20 weeks of ges-

---

BOX 88-1
Rape Trauma Syndrome

Acute Phase (May Last Hours to Days)
Paralysis of patient's coping mechanisms
Shock, denial, disbelief
Classic triad:
 Haunting, intrusive recollections
 Numbing of feelings
 Generalized hypersensitivity to environmental stimuli
Body pain, insomnia
Vaginal discharge, pain or itching, and rectal pain
Depression, anxiety, and mood swings

Delayed (Organizational) Phase (May Occur Months to Years after Assault)
Flashbacks, nightmares
Phobias and depression
Gynecologic and menstrual complaints
Somatic complaints: extreme fatigue, abdominal pain, nausea, headaches
Sexual dysfunction
Serious psychosocial dysfunction with increased risk of suicide and substance abuse

From Burgess AW, Holmstrom LL: In Burgess AW, Holmstrom LL, editors: *Rape: victims of crisis,* Bowie, Md, 1974, Robert J Brady.

BOX 88-2
Medical Disorders Associated with Sexual Assault

Depression and suicidality
Substance abuse
Gastrointestinal complaints
Headaches
Insomnia
Gynecologic and menstrual complaints
Sexual dysfunction

---

tation. There was a higher incidence of sexually transmitted diseases, urinary tract infections, and vaginitis. It is important in the evaluation of sexual assault during pregnancy to remember that pregnancy and its effect on the vaginal flora do not preclude the collection or interpretation of clinical or forensic evidence, and every effort should be made to collect the appropriate specimens. Prophylaxis against sexually transmitted disease also is important (see Management).

EVALUATION
Goals

The physician's responsibility in evaluating a woman who has been sexually assaulted is to stabilize her medical condition and then to document the history and physical evidence clearly in the medical record, to assess the patient's psychologic state, and to provide prophylactic therapy to prevent sexually transmitted disease and pregnancy (Box 88-3). It is important to avoid judgmental statements to the patient. It is not the role of the physician to determine whether or not the rape has occurred.

History and Symptoms
The Interview

Ensuring confidentiality and privacy is important when the clinician interviews the victim of sexual assault. One needs to obtain informed consent before proceeding with the history, physical examination, and collection of specimens for physical evidence. A clear explanation for the process and protocol for evaluation is reassuring and helpful. An overt statement that the patient is safe is often necessary. It is helpful if a rape counselor is present during the history and physical examination (Box 88-4).

History

The key events in the history are summarized in Box 88-5. Reassuring the patient and explaining the reasoning behind the questions can be helpful. Often the woman feels shame and humiliation because she may think she caused the as-

---

BOX 88-3
Physicians' Responsibilities in Dealing with a Woman Who Is a Victim of Sexual Assault

Medical
Obtain accurate gynecologic history
Assess and treat physical injuries
Obtain appropriate cultures and treat any existing infections
Provide therapy to prevent unwanted conception
Provide counseling
Arrange for follow-up medical care and counseling

Legal
Provide accurate recording of events
Document injuries
Obtain consent for evidence collection kit and collect samples
Report to authorities as required

From American College of Obstetricians and Gynecologists: *Int J Gynecol Obstet* 42:67, 1993.

sault. Assurance and support help the victim. It is important to document the age of the patient, date and time of assault, circumstance of the assault, and details of the contact. The activities of the victim after the assault and a general medical and gynecologic history should be ascertained. It also is important to assess the patient's psychologic status, coping strategies, and support systems. The history should be clearly documented, and judgmental statements should be avoided (Box 88-6). Most emergency room settings have rape evaluation kits to help in the appropriate documentation, or these can be obtained from the local crime forensics laboratories.

Physical Examination

A complete physical examination should be performed with particular focus on the area of injury. The woman is asked to disrobe over paper sheets on which any debris or fibers can be collected. Her clothes are then placed in labeled paper bags to avoid contamination. Careful collection of specimens for evidence should be performed as listed in Box 88-7. After collection the specimens should be locked in a safe place until the police can remove them. Photographs should be taken if necessary and with informed consent. Because as many as 67% of victims have external extragenital trauma, a careful examination for lacerations, abrasions, and bruising should then be completed. Common sites for external trauma include the mouth, throat, wrist, arms, breast, and thighs. Bite marks also are common and should be examined for.

Gynecologic Examination

A complete gynecologic examination, including a rectal examination, should be performed, and the use of lubri-

cants, which can be spermicidal, should be avoided. The presence of genital trauma should be ascertained by visual examination. Staining with toluidine can help in the detection of subtle tears. Because determining subtle genital trauma can be difficult, some clinicians have advocated the use of colposcopy to determine genital trauma in rape victims, if available. Given the potential psychologic trauma of a colposcopic examination, more controlled studies of its use should be undertaken. Aspiration of the posterior vaginal fornices after normal saline wash should be performed if no obvious secretions can be identified and collected. After collection, the aspirate should be suspended in warm normal saline and examined for the presence of sperm, documenting both the number and motility per high-power field. The rest of the aspirate is then sent to a forensics laboratory to be tested for acid phosphatase. High concentrations of the enzyme is associated with recent coitus. The sample also should be assayed for the glycoprotein p30, which is present in seminal fluid, and for genetic testing. A few studies have

---

BOX 88-6
Medical Documentation

Do not use *rape* or *sexual assault* because these are legal terms
Use terms such as *consistent with the use of force*
Collect physical evidence as soon as possible
Document physical and emotional condition
Document thorough history and physical examination

BOX 88-4
Initial Interview

Ensure confidentiality
Ensure safety
Obtain informed consent
Obtain rape counselor
Explain protocol and procedures

BOX 88-5
Key Factors in the History

Accurate account of events: include date, time, description or identification of perpetrator, assault history (penetration, weapons, threats, physical violence), known or suspected substance abuse, and subsequent activities
Objective description for documentation
Thorough sexual and gynecologic history:
  Pregnancy history
  Use of contraception
  Date of last menstrual period
  History of sexually transmitted diseases
Assessment of emotional status, coping strategies, and support

---

BOX 88-7
Key Factors in Physical Examination

Collect clothing
Complete physical examination
To include photographs and drawings of injured areas
Skin examination
Cuts, bruises, bite marks
Head and neck examination
Oral secretions for acid phosphatase
Injuries as a result of oral penetration
Culture for gonorrhea
Genitourinary examination
Pubic hair combing and sampling
Vaginal secretions and cervical mucus:
  Motile sperm
  Acid phosphatase
  Glycoprotein p30
  DNA fingerprinting by wet or dry swab
Pap smear
Cultures for gonorrhea and chlamydia
Complete pelvic examination for gynecologic injury, trauma, and foreign objects with colposcopy if available
Rectal examination
Examination for trauma
Culture for gonorrhea
Collect secretion for motile sperm and acid phosphatase if indicated

used prostate specific antigen (PSA) as a marker, but further studies are needed before its use can be recommended.

If there is a delay in transport of the specimens, they should be kept refrigerated. In addition to the complete gynecologic examination, a particular emphasis should be placed on the examination of the perineal and inner thigh area. This is accomplished with a Wood's lamp to detect semen stains. Areas of fluorescence should then be swabbed with saline-moistened cotton swabs and smeared on a slide to examine for the presence of sperm. Culture specimens for *Neisseria gonorrhoeae* and *Chlamydia trachomatis* should be obtained from all sites of entry. Pap smear and pubic hair sampling should be completed. Combing of the pubic hair increases the yield of the assailant's hair samples. Samples of the patient's hair should be clipped and stored.

Diagnostic Tests

In addition to cultures (pharyngeal swabs for gonorrhea and chlamydia, vaginal/cervical swabs for gonorrhea, chlamydia, *Trichomonas vaginalis,* and herpes simplex virus and rectal swabs for gonorrhea, chlamydia, and herpes simplex), certain blood tests should be obtained (Box 88-8). These include pregnancy test (serum human chorionic gonadotropin) and a baseline VDRL (or rapid plasma reagin [RPR]) for

---

BOX 88-8
Key Diagnostic Tests

Cultures
Pharyngeal
Gonorrhea
Chlamydia
Vaginal/cervical
Gonorrhea
Chlamydia
Trichomonas
Herpes simplex
Rectal
Gonorrhea
Chlamydia
Herpes simplex
Fingernail scrapings

Other tests
Pregnancy test: urine or serum
Baseline VDRL for syphilis
Serologic tests:
   Herpes simplex virus
   Hepatitis B: HbcAB, HBSAb, HBSAg
   HIV
Cytomegalovirus
Saliva for major blood group antigen
Toxicology screen for rape drugs if patient meets the following criteria:
   History of amnesia or lack of motor control
   Patient presents within 72 hours of assault
   Patient's suspicion that she was drugged before sexual assault
   Patient consent obtained

---

syphilis. Many clinicians also obtain serologic data for herpes simplex virus, hepatitis B, cytomegalovirus, and, with consent, baseline HIV testing. Seroconversion for HIV infection can occur up to 1 year after exposure and therefore is repeated at 3-month intervals for 1 year. It also is necessary to collect (1) saliva for the major blood group antigen and (2) scrapings from the woman's fingernails.

MANAGEMENT
Choice of Therapy
Prophylaxis for Sexually Transmitted Diseases and HIV

According to the Centers for Disease Control and Prevention (CDC), up to 6% to 12% of victims contract gonorrhea and chlamydial infection, and 3% of victims contract syphilis. Trichomonal infection and bacterial vaginosis also are frequently contracted. Therefore prophylaxis for gonorrhea and chlamydia and testing for syphilis are indicated for all victims of sexual assault. Treatment for trichomonal infection and bacterial vaginosis has been recommended by the CDC as well. The standard treatment protocols are listed in Table 88-1. Recommendations for the pregnant woman are included.

The CDC recommends postexposure hepatitis B vaccination without HB immunoglobulin as adequate protection against hepatitis B virus, but little data exists regarding the efficacy of this recommendation except for HB immunoglobulin. Many institutions continue to use HB immunoglobulin as prophylaxis in addition to vaccination. If primary vaccination is administered, follow-up doses of hepatitis B vaccine should be administered 1 and 6 months after the first dose. Vaccination is not necessary if the person has had previous hepatitis B vaccine and documented immunity.

Prophylactic treatment with antiviral agents for HIV following sexual assault remains controversial. The risk of contracting HIV after a sexual assault is estimated at 1 in 500. Present recommendations are based on data from occupational exposure to HIV, which suggests that antivirals are most effective at preventing HIV transmission if given within 4 hours of the assault (Box 88-9). Women should be counseled regarding HIV transmission and safe sex practices. If the woman desires testing for HIV, it should be done at the time of the assault, then every 3 to 4 months up to 1 year before assurance can be given regarding seroconversion. Generally, seroconversion occurs within 6 months after exposure to HIV. For more details regarding HIV, see Chapter 21.

Prevention of Pregnancy

Pregnancy occurs in 5% of all fertile female victims. The patient should be offered the "morning-after pill" for prevention of pregnancy, unless by history the woman is menstruating or is known to be pregnant. It should be offered regardless of the woman's cycle phase at the time of the assault. Standard regimen is two orally administered combination contraceptive pills, usually 50 mg estrogen each (such as Ovral) immediately and again 12 hours later. The "morning-after pill" is effective within 72 hours of the assault. This and other options for pregnancy prevention appear in Box 88-10. For a more detailed discussion on the morning-after pill, see Chapter 58.

Counseling and Follow-up

Rape counseling is important for the victim and should be arranged at the time of evaluation (Box 88-11). Follow-up medical evaluation should be arranged within 72 hours of the initial assault to assess bruising and the woman's psychologic state, followed by another evaluation within 2 weeks. Often the victim of sexual assault develops symptoms such as gastrointestinal complaints, headaches, insomnia, nightmares, eating disorders, and irritability, which are not directly related to the physical injuries but are a result of the severe psychologic trauma. Characteristics of posttraumatic stress syndrome may develop, such as flashbacks, sensitivity to certain stimuli, hypersensitivity, and difficulty with concentration.

A VDRL for syphilis and other serologic tests (Box 88-11) should be repeated after 4 to 6 weeks. HIV testing should be completed with informed consent every 3 months for the first year after the assault. Pregnancy counseling and safe sex practices should be completed at the time of the assault and readdressed at each follow-up visit.

Table 88-1
Management of Sexual Assault: Treatment Guidelines for Sexually Transmitted Diseases

| Disease | PROPHYLACTIC ANTIBIOTICS | |
	Recommended Treatment	Alternatives
Gonorrhea	Ceftriaxone 125 mg IM once	Cefixime 400 mg PO once* OR
Vaginitis, urethritis, cervicitis, proctitis, and pharyngitis (NOT pelvic inflammatory disease)		Ciprofloxacin 500 mg po OR† Spectinomycin 2 g IM once*‡
Pregnancy	Same	Same except for Ciprofloxacin
Chlamydia Urethral, cervical, rectal	Doxycycline 100 mg PO bid	Azithromycin 1 g PO × 7 days once§ OR Erythromycin 500 mg PO qid 7 days
Pregnancy	Erythromycin 500 mg PO qid 7 days	Erythromycin ethylsuccinate 800 mg PO qid 7 days¶ OR Amoxicillin 500 mg PO tid 7 days
Trichomonas	Metronidazole (Flagyl) 2 g PO once bid 7 days	Flagyl 500 mg PO
Pregnancy First trimester Wait until after first trimester, then treat with Flagyl Second and third trimesters Oral Flagyl		
Bacterial vaginosis	Flagyl 500 mg PO bid 7 days OR Flagyl 2 gm orally single dose	Clindamycin cream 2%, 1 vaginal application qhs 7 days OR Clindamycin 300 mg PO bid 7 days OR Flagyl 2 g PO once
Pregnancy First trimester Clindamycin cream Second and third trimesters Oral or vaginal Flagyl		
Hepatitis B immune globulin**	0.06 ml/kg single IM dose within 14 days of exposure	
Vaccination**	Three doses, each 1 ml IM in the deltoid muscle at 0, 1, 6 mo	

Modified from Centers for Disease Control and Prevention: *MMWR* 47:108, 1998.
* Not effective against pharyngeal gonorrhea nor against incubating syphilis.
† Contraindicated in pregnancy and does not treat syphilis.
‡ Use for patients with penicillin allergy. May not treat incubating syphilis and pharyngeal gonorrhea.
§ Safety during pregnancy not been established.
¶ Can switch to 250 mg PO qid for 14 days if not tolerated; erythromycin estolate is contraindicated during pregnancy.
** Both safe in pregnancy.

BOX 88-9
Other Prophylactic Interventions

HIV Prophylaxis in consultation with ID specialist:
Combivir (AZT 300 mg and 3TC 150 mg), 1 tablet BID
For those with high risk exposures add: Nelfinavir (Viracept) 1250 mg BID (5 × 250 mg tabs)
Hepatitis B vaccine for those meeting the following criteria:
Unimmunized patients
If history is suggestive of vaginal or rectal penetration and victim's immune status is negative or unknown
Dosage of Vaccine:
Age 11-19: Recombivax 5 μg or Engerix B 10 μg IM
Age > 19 years: Recombivax 10 μg or Engerix B 20 μg IM
Note: First dose of Hepatitis B vaccine without HBIG should adequately protect against HBV. Patient should be informed of need for follow-up doses at 1 and 6 months tetanus vaccine

BOX 88-10
Options for Pregnancy Prophylaxis

No immediate therapy; wait until next menses before performing repeat pregnancy test
No immediate therapy; repeat serum pregnancy test in 1 week
Prescribe: "Morning-after" pill
Ethinyl estradiol–norgestrel (Ovral) (50 mg estrogen)
2 tablets at time victim is seen, then 2 tablets in 12 hr
with Compazine 10 mg po 30 minutes before Ovral administration*
or
Ethinyl estradiol 5 mg PO 5 days
or
Conjugated equine estrogen 20-30 mg PO qd 5 days
or
Diethylstilbestrol 25 mg PO bid 5 days

Modified from American College of Obstetricians and Gynecologists: *Int J Gynecol Obstet* 42:67, 1993; Beebe D: *Am Fam Physician* 43:2041, 1991.
*Menstrual period may be early or delayed. Repeat pregnancy test in 1 month.

BOX 88-11
Sexual Assault Follow-up

Provide rape counseling
See patient within 72 hours to assess delayed bruising and coping
See patient again in 1-2 weeks for counseling and follow-up
Provide pregnancy counseling
Repeat cervical cultures and serologic tests for hepatitis B, RPR (syphilis) and HIV in 6 weeks
Repeat RPR (syphilis testing) and HIV testing again at 3 and 6 months
Advise condom use until completion of serologic testing
To complete the primary vaccination for Hepatitis B, vaccination should be given at 1 month and 6 months after initial dose

BIBLIOGRAPHY

American College of Obstetricians and Gynecologists: Sexual assault (ACOG Tech Bull No 172), *Int J Gynecol Obstet* 42:67, 1993.

American College of Obstetricians and Gynecologists: Adolescent victims of sexual assault (ACOG Tech Bull No 252), *Int J Gynecol Obstet* 64:195, 1999.

Anglin D, Spears KL, Hutson R: Flunitrazepam and its involvement in acquaintance rape, *Acad Emerg Med* 4:323, 1997.

Association of Genitourinary Medicine and the Medical Society for the Study of Venereal Diseases: National guideline for the management of adult victims of sexual assault, *Sex Trans Infect* 75:S82, 1999.

Bachman R, Saltzman L: Violence against women: estimates from the redesigned survey. Washington, DC, 1995, US Department of Justice, Office of Justice Programs, (Bureau of Justice Statistics Special Report, no. NCJ-154348).

Beebe D: Emergency management of the adult female rape victim, *Am Fam Physician* 43:2041, 1991.

Burgess AW, Holmstrom LL: Rape trauma syndrome. In Burgess AW, Holmstrom LL, editors: *Rape: victims of crisis,* Bowie, MD, 1974, Robert J Brady.

Calhoun K, Atkeson B: *Treatment of rape victims. Facilitating psychosocial adjustment,* New York, 1991, Pergamon Press.

Centers for Disease Control and Prevention: 1998 sexually transmitted diseases treatment guidelines, *MMWR* 47:108, 1998.

Committee on Adolescence: Sexual assault and the adolescent, *Pediatrics* 94:761, 1994.

Council on Scientific Affairs: Violence against women: relevance for medical practitioners, *JAMA* 267:3184, 1992.

Department of Justice, Federal Bureau of Investigation: *Uniform crime reports for the United States,* Washington, DC, 1997, US Government Printing Office.

Elam AL, Ray VG: Sexually related trauma: a review, *Ann Emerg Med* 15:576, 1986.

Glaser A: Emergency postcoital contraception, *N Engl J Med* 337:1058, 1997.

Gostin A: HIV testing, counseling and prophylaxis after sexual assault, *JAMA* 271:1436, 1994.

Hamptom HL: Care of the woman who has been raped, *N Engl J Med* 332:324, 1995.

Harlow CW: *Injuries from crime,* Washington, DC, 1989, Department of Justice, Bureau of Justice Statistics.

Hicks DJ: Sexual battery: management of the rape victim. In Sciarra JJ, editor: *Gynecology and obstetrics,* vol 6, Philadelphia, 1990, Harper & Row.

Holmes MM et al: Rape-related pregnancy: estimates and characteristics from a national sample of women, *Am J Obstet Gynecol* 175:320, 1996.

Jenny C et al: Sexually transmitted diseases in victims of rape, *N Engl J Med* 322:713, 1990.

Koss MP, Harvey M: *The rape victim: clinical and community approaches to treatment,* Beverly Hills, Calif, 1991, Sage Publications.

Koss MP, Koss, PG, Woodruff WJ: Relation of criminal victimization to health perceptions among women medical patients, *J Consult Clin Psychol* 58:147, 1990.

Koss MP, Woodruff WJ, Koss PG: Deleterious effects of criminal victimization on women's health and medical utilization, *Arch Intern Med* 151:342, 1991.

Lenehan LC, Ernst A, Johnson B: Colposcopy in evaluation of the adult sexual assault victim, *Am J Emerg Med* 16:183, 1998.

Linden J: Sexual assault, *Emerg Clin North Am* 17:685, 1999.

Patel HC: Colposcopy and rape, *Am J Obstet Gynecol* 168:1334, 1993.

Rambow B et al: Female sexual assault: medical and legal implications, *Ann Emerg Med* 21:727, 1992.

Resick P et al: Adjustment in victims of sexual assault, *J Consult Clin Psychol* 49:705, 1981.

Satin A et al: Sexual assault in pregnancy, *Obstet Gynecol* 77:710, 1991.

Satin A et al: The prevalence of sexual assault: a survey of 2404 puerperal women, *Am J Obstet Gynecol* 167:973, 1992.

1998 Guidelines for Treatment of Sexually Transmitted Diseases. *MMWR* 47(RR1):108, 1998.

Slaughter L et al: Patterns of genital injury in the female sexual assault victims, *Am J Obstet Gynecol* 176:609, 1997.

Slaughter L, Brown C: Colposcopy to establish physical findings in rape victims, *Am J Obstet Gyncol* 166:83, 1992.

Young W et al and the New Hampshire Sexual Assault Medical Examination Protocol Project Committee: Sexual assault: review of a national model protocol for forensic and medical evaluation, *Obstet Gynecol* 80:878, 1992.

CHAPTER 89

Tobacco Use

Nancy A. Rigotti

Cigarette smoking is a major health hazard for women. It is the leading preventable cause of death for both women and men in the United States and is responsible for more than 400,000 deaths each year, or one in every five deaths. Primary care physicians take care of the health consequences of their patients' tobacco use. It is equally important for them to prevent smoking-related disease by addressing their patients' tobacco use.

▦ EPIDEMIOLOGY
Patterns of Tobacco Use

Cigarette smoking in the United States was uncommon before 1900, rose rapidly in the first half of the century, and peaked in 1965, when 40% of adult Americans smoked cigarettes. Since then smoking rates have declined as the public became aware of the health risks of tobacco use. By 1998, 24% of adult Americans smoked. This decline is primarily attributable to smoking cessation. In both sexes smoking starts during childhood and adolescence; 90% of smokers begin to smoke before the age of 18, and smoking initiation rates increased during the 1990s.

These aggregate data conceal dramatic differences in the smoking patterns of men and women. American women did not take up smoking in large numbers until World War II, three decades later than men. When smoking prevalence peaked in 1965, only 32% of adult women smoked, compared with 50% of men. After 1965 smoking rates fell four times faster in men than in women. The result was a convergence in the smoking rates of men and women. By 1998, 22% of adult women and 26% of men smoked cigarettes. The gender gap in tobacco use is expected to narrow further because adolescent males and females now start to smoke cigarettes at the same rates.

Smoking is inversely related to educational attainment in both women and men in the United States. Educational attainment is a marker for socioeconomic status, and smoking is a problem becoming concentrated in lower socioeconomic groups. Young adults, aged 18 to 44, have the highest smoking rates; 28% of them smoked in 1998. Racial differences in smoking are smaller in women than in men. In 1998 the prevalence of smoking was 13% in Hispanic women, 21% in black women, and 24% in white women.

Health Consequences of Tobacco Use

Epidemiologic studies of the health consequences of tobacco use were first conducted in men because of their higher smoking rates. Subsequent studies in women have confirmed that the relationships identified for male smokers hold for female smokers. In short, women who smoke like men get sick and die like men. In addition, smoking poses health risks for women that are not shared by men.

Cigarette smoking increases the overall mortality and morbidity rates of both women and men. In both sexes smoking is a cause of cardiovascular disease (including myocardial infarction and sudden death), cerebrovascular disease, peripheral vascular disease, chronic obstructive pulmonary disease, and cancers of the lung, larynx, oral cavity, and esophagus. Middle-aged women who smoke are three times more likely to die of coronary artery disease and five times more likely to die of a stroke than are nonsmoking women. Women who smoke are more than 10 times more likely to die of lung cancer, laryngeal cancer, esophageal cancer, and chronic obstructive pulmonary disease than are nonsmoking women.

Lung cancer, once a rare disease in women, has increased dramatically since 1950. In 1986 lung cancer surpassed breast cancer to become the leading cause of cancer death in women. Cigarette smokers also have higher rates of cancers of the bladder, pancreas, kidney, and stomach. Smoking interacts with alcohol to increase the risk of laryngeal, oral cavity, and esophageal cancers in both sexes. Tobacco interacts with asbestos and other occupational exposures to greatly increase cancer risk.

Smokers have higher rates of peptic ulcer disease, poorer ulcer healing, and higher recurrence rates than nonsmokers. They are more susceptible to respiratory infections and have higher rates of cataracts, macular degeneration, and sensorineural hearing loss than nonsmokers. The majority of residential fire deaths are caused by smoking.

There is no safe level of tobacco use. Smoking as few as 1 to 4 cigarettes per day doubles a woman's risk of myocardial infarction and cardiovascular mortality. Smoking cigarettes with reduced tar and nicotine delivery does not reduce the health hazards of smoking.

The health hazards of smoking are not limited to those suffered by smokers. Nonsmokers are harmed by chronic exposure to environmental tobacco smoke (ETS). The children of parents who smoke have more serious respiratory infections during infancy and childhood, more respiratory symptoms, and a higher rate of chronic otitis media and asthma than the children of nonsmokers. Nonsmoking women whose husbands smoke have a higher lung cancer risk than nonsmoking women whose husbands do not smoke. A 1993 Environmental Protection Agency report summarized the evidence regarding the health effects of passive smoking and identified ETS as a carcinogen, responsible for approximately 3000 lung cancer deaths each year in U.S. nonsmokers. Passive smoke exposure also increases nonsmokers' risk of coronary heart disease.

Special Health Concerns for Women

Women who smoke have health risks not shared with male smokers. These relate to pregnancy, oral contraceptives, cervical cancer, and osteoporosis.

Smoking is associated with many **pregnancy complications.** It is a cause of low–birth-weight (<2500 g) infants. Infants born to smokers weigh, on average, 200 g (7 oz) less than infants of nonsmoking mothers. This lower weight is primarily attributable to intrauterine growth retardation (IUGR), although smoking in pregnancy also increases the risk of preterm delivery. Smoking is the major known cause of IUGR in the developed world, responsible for an estimated 30% of cases. Other adverse pregnancy outcomes linked to smoking are miscarriage (spontaneous abortion), stillbirth, and neonatal death. Placenta previa, abruptio placentae, and bleeding occur more often in smokers than nonsmokers, suggesting that smoking impairs placental function.

Smoking during pregnancy affects children even after birth. Sudden infant death syndrome is two to four times more common in infants born to mothers who smoked during pregnancy. Cognitive deficits and developmental problems in childhood have also been linked to maternal smoking during pregnancy. The adverse health effects of smoking extend to reproductive function before pregnancy. Smoking has been associated with reduced fertility in both men and women.

Oral contraceptive use compounds a woman smoker's risk of serious cardiovascular disease. Women smokers who use the pill have a substantially increased risk of subarachnoid hemorrhage and stroke, and their risk of myocardial infarction rises 10-fold. The excess risk increases with age, especially after age 30.

Cervical cancer rates are higher in smokers than in nonsmokers. The excess risk conferred by smoking is independent of other factors known to increase cervical cancer risk. Adding biologic plausibility to this association is the discovery that components of tobacco smoke can be isolated from the cervical mucus of smokers. Cervical cancer rates are lower in ex-smokers than in current smokers, suggesting that risk is reversible after smoking cessation.

Female smokers also have an increased risk of postmenopausal **osteoporosis** and fracture than nonsmokers. This may be explained by the fact that women who smoke are thinner and go through menopause 1 to 2 years earlier than nonsmokers. Smoking may also have an antiestrogen effect. One large cohort study found that estrogen replacement protected nonsmokers but not smokers from osteoporotic hip fractures.

Smokers have more prominent **skin wrinkling** than nonsmokers, an association independent of sun exposure. Although this effect is not limited to women, it may be of greater concern to women, reflecting the stronger cultural emphasis for women to have a youthful appearance.

HEALTH BENEFITS OF SMOKING CESSATION

Epidemiologic data show that smoking cessation has health benefits for women and men of all ages, even those who stop smoking after the age of 65 or who quit after the development of a smoking-related disease. Smoking cessation decreases the risk of lung cancer and other cancers, heart attack, stroke, chronic lung disease, and peptic ulcer disease. After 10 to 15 years of abstinence, smokers' overall mortality rate approaches that of persons who never smoked. The cardiovascular risk reduction occurs more rapidly than the risk reduction for lung cancer or overall mortality. Half of the excess risk of cardiovascular mortality is eliminated in the first year of quitting, whereas for lung cancer 30% to 50% of the excess risk is still evident 10 years after quitting and some excess risk remains after 15 years.

The benefits of stopping smoking translate into a longer life expectancy for former smokers, as compared with continuing smokers. The degree to which former smokers benefit from cessation depends on their previous lifetime dose of tobacco, their health status at the time of quitting, and the elapsed time since quitting. Smokers who benefit the most are those who quit when they are younger, have fewer years of tobacco exposure, and are free of smoking-related disease. The health benefits of smoking cessation far exceed any risks from the small weight gain that occurs with cessation.

Women benefit as much as men from quitting smoking. In the Nurses' Health Study, which followed a cohort of more than 100,000 female nurses, former smokers had a 24% reduction in cardiovascular death rates within 2 years of quitting. The risks of total mortality, cardiovascular mortality, and total cancer mortality among former smokers approached the level of that for persons who had never smoked after 10 to 14 years of abstinence. Benefits of cessation were present regardless of daily cigarette consumption or the age at which smoking started.

Smoking cessation also diminishes the hazards of smoking to the fetus. Women who stop smoking before pregnancy or during the first 3 to 4 months of gestation have infants who weigh the same as those born to women who never smoked. Pregnant smokers who stop smoking at any time up to the 30th week of gestation have infants with higher birth weights than women who smoke throughout pregnancy.

SMOKING BEHAVIOR AND CESSATION

More than 90% of current smokers know that smoking is harmful to health yet they continue to smoke. They do so because tobacco use is both an addiction and a learned behavior. Cigarettes and other tobacco products contain nicotine, a drug that creates tolerance, physical dependence, and a withdrawal syndrome in habitual users who abstain. Nicotine withdrawal symptoms include cigarette craving, irritability, impatience, restlessness, difficulty concentrating, depressed mood, anxiety, increased appetite, and sleep disturbance. These symptoms begin within a few hours of the last cigarette, peak 48 to 72 hours later, diminish rapidly during the first week of abstinence, and wane further in subsequent weeks. Other than craving for a cigarette, the symptoms are nonspecific, and many smokers fail to recognize them as nicotine withdrawal. Nevertheless, the discomfort of nicotine withdrawal is a major reason why smokers fail in their efforts to stop.

The severity of nicotine withdrawal varies, reflecting the severity of a smoker's nicotine dependence. Heavy smokers (>1 pack per day) and those who have their first cigarette within 30 minutes of awakening have stronger nicotine dependence and more severe nicotine withdrawal. Gender differences in nicotine withdrawal have not been identified. Nicotine withdrawal symptoms may be more severe during the luteal phase of a woman's menstrual cycle, but there is no evidence that quitting smoking is more likely to succeed at any particular point in the menstrual cycle.

Tobacco use is maintained not only because of nicotine dependence but also because smoking is a habit, a behavior that has become an integral part of a daily routine. Smokers come to associate cigarettes with recurring activities, such as finishing a meal or having a cup of coffee. These actions trigger the desire for a cigarette in smokers who are trying to quit. Smokers also use cigarettes to cope with stress and negative emotions such as anger, anxiety, loneliness, or boredom. Quitting smoking represents the loss of a valuable coping tool, one that may be especially important for women, for whom the direct expression of anger is less socially sanctioned. To stop smoking, a smoker must identify and break the cues to smoking, learn to anticipate and handle urges to smoke that do occur, and learn alternative coping strategies for handling negative emotions.

Approximately half of living Americans who ever smoked have quit smoking. According to surveys, a majority of the remaining smokers would like to stop smoking and nearly one third make an attempt to stop each year. Earlier studies suggested that female smokers have more difficulty quitting smoking than male smokers do, but recent data indicate that men and women are equally likely to try to quit and to succeed in quitting. However, the process of quitting differs in men and women because of gender differences in weight concerns, social support, and mood disorders.

The majority of former smokers did not succeed in stopping on their first try. Behavioral scientists regard smoking cessation as a learning process rather than the result of willpower. In this model, smokers are attempting to learn a behavior and temporary setbacks (e.g., relapse to smoking) are expected. Smokers who learn from mistakes made during a prior attempt to quit increase the likelihood that the next attempt will succeed.

TOBACCO TREATMENT METHODS

Clinical guidelines for treating tobacco use were released by the U.S. Public Health Service in 2000, based on a systematic review of evidence about the efficacy of smoking cessation treatment methods. The most effective treatments generate cessation rates of 30% to 40% at 1-year follow-up, compared with a 5% to 10% success rate for an unaided effort. The efficacy of treatment increases with its intensity,

Table 89-1
Drugs Used to Treat Tobacco Use

Product	Availability	Recommended Daily Dose
Nicotine Replacement Therapy		
Transdermal nicotine patch		
Nicoderm (21 mg, 14 mg, 7 mg)	OTC	1 patch for 24 hrs
Nicotrol (15 mg)	OTC	1 patch for 16 hrs
Generic	OTC	1 patch for 24 hrs
Nicotine gum (Nicorette) (2 mg, 4 mg)	OTC	1 piece/hour 12 pieces/day
Nicotine vapor inhaler (Nicotrol inhaler)	Rx	6-16 cartridges/day
Nicotine nasal spray (Nicotrol NS)	Rx	1-2 doses/hr 12-24 doses/day
Non-Nicotine Drug Therapy		
Bupropion SR (Zyban, Wellbutrin SR)	Rx	150 mg bid
Nortriptyline	Rx	75 mg qd
Clonidine		
Oral	Rx	0.1 mg bid
Transdermal patch	Rx	0.1-0.2 mg qd

OTC, Over the counter (nonprescription sale); *Rx*, prescription only sale.

but even brief interventions of the type feasible for use in office practice are effective. Two effective treatment methods were identified: pharmacotherapy and behavioral counseling. These methods are synergistic such that combining the two produces higher quit rates than either one alone. First-line pharmacologic treatment includes nicotine replacement (gum, patch, oral inhaler, and nasal spray) and bupropion, an antidepressant (Table 89-1). Each has been approved by the U.S. Food and Drug Administration for treatment of tobacco use. Second-line drugs with evidence of efficacy for smoking cessation include nortriptyline and clonidine. There is no evidence to support the efficacy of any other antidepressant or any anxiolytic agent for treating tobacco use.

Counseling methods that are effective for treating tobacco use teach practical skills training and problem solving techniques, increase social support, and build a smoker's confidence in the ability to quit. These methods can be delivered in formal group programs, individual treatment, or even over the telephone. In contrast, no evidence supports the efficacy of hypnosis for smoking cessation, and acupuncture is ineffective for this indication.

Pharmacologic Treatment

Nicotine Replacement Therapy

The rationale of nicotine replacement is to prevent nicotine withdrawal symptoms in smokers attempting to quit by supplying nicotine in a form other than tobacco. Four nicotine replacement products are approved for use in the United States: a gum, skin patch, an oral inhaler, and a nasal spray. Each produces a substantially different pattern of nicotine exposure from the fluctuating blood levels of nicotine produced by cigarette smoking.

Randomized placebo-controlled trials show that each nicotine replacement product reduces nicotine withdrawal symptoms and increases smoking cessation rates. Meta-analyses have found that the patch more than doubles smoking cessation rates compared with placebo, and the nicotine gum increases smoking cessation rates by 50% to 60%. Individual trials of the nasal spray and vapor inhaler have found that these products double quit rates compared with placebo. The four nicotine replacement products showed similar efficacy in the one trial that directly compared them. Combinations of the nicotine patch with the gum or nasal spray are safe and more effective than single products. The effectiveness of each product also depends on the amount of behavioral counseling that accompanies it. The intensity of the behavioral program sets the baseline cessation rate, which is doubled by the addition of nicotine replacement therapy. Side effects differ, depending on the method of nicotine administration. Side effects are fewest with the patch and inhaler and greatest with the nasal spray.

Contraindications to nicotine replacement include unstable angina, myocardial infarction in the last 2 weeks, and life-threatening arrhythmias. Nicotine replacement is safe to use in smokers with stable coronary artery disease. The safety of nicotine replacement in pregnancy is not established. Using nicotine replacement is safer than smoking cigarettes, which exposes the fetus to a wide array of toxic compounds and a higher nicotine dose, but nicotine does cross the placenta. Clinicians generally reserve nicotine replacement therapy for use in pregnant patients who have failed a behavioral stop-smoking program, use the lowest dose possible, and prescribe it after documenting a risk-benefit discussion with the patient. Nicotine gum may be preferable to nicotine patch in pregnancy because it is used intermittently and exposes the user to a lower daily dose of nicotine than the patch.

The **transdermal nicotine patch** continuously releases a fixed dose of nicotine that is absorbed through the skin. Several different nicotine patches are available, and all are sold without prescription. Each is more effective than placebo in relieving withdrawal symptoms and promoting smoking cessation. No studies have directly compared different patches; therefore data are insufficient to recommend any one patch as most effective. The most common side effect is local skin irritation, which rarely requires discontinuation of treatment and can be minimized by rotating patch sites and using topical steroids. Vivid dreams, insomnia, and nervousness have also been reported. They can be managed by removing the patch at bedtime or using a lower-dose patch.

The smoker applies the first patch on the morning of her quit day, removes it 16 to 24 hours later, and applies a fresh patch to a new skin site each morning afterward; 8 weeks of treatment is sufficient. Lower starting doses are recommended for patients who weigh less than 100 lb or who smoke fewer than 10 cigarettes each day. Long-term dependence on the nicotine patch is uncommon.

Nicotine gum is sold without prescription in 2- and 4-mg strengths. Careful instruction in proper chewing technique is essential to ensure that the nicotine reaches the bloodstream and to prevent side effects. The gum should not be chewed like regular gum. A "chew and park" method is recommended. A piece is chewed only long enough to release nicotine, producing a peppery taste, then placed between the gums and buccal mucosa ("parked") to allow nicotine absorption through the oral mucosa. When the nicotine taste disappears, the user chews it just enough to release more nicotine, then "parks" it again. After 30 minutes it is discarded. No liquid should be drunk while the gum is in the mouth, and acidic beverages (e.g., coffee) avoided for 1 to 2 hours before gum use because they reduce nicotine absorption. Side effects are common but minor; they include those related to nicotine (nausea, dyspepsia, hiccups, dizziness) and to chewing (sore jaw, mouth ulcers).

The gum is approved for use as needed to handle urges to smoke; however, most smokers underuse it. Consequently, many clinicians use fixed-dose schedules (e.g., chewing one piece for the first 30 minutes of every hour) to achieve adequate blood nicotine levels to prevent withdrawal. Approximately 5% to 10% of gum users develop long-term dependence on the gum.

The **nicotine inhaler** delivers nicotine vapor through a tube into the smoker's mouth and throat each time the smoker inhales. The inhaled nicotine is absorbed through the mouth and throat, not in the lungs as cigarette smoke is. The inhaler also provides an oral substitute for smoking. Smokers using the inhaler receive much less nicotine per inhalation than they obtain from puffing on a cigarette and need to use multiple cartridges daily. The recommended dose is 6 cartridges daily for up to 12 weeks. Side effects are few (mouth and throat irritation and cough). It is available only by prescription.

The **nicotine nasal spray** delivers a nicotine solution onto the nasal mucosa, where it is absorbed into the bloodstream. Because nicotine absorption occurs more rapidly through the nasal mucosa than through the mouth or skin, the nicotine nasal spray generates a peak nicotine level faster than the gum, inhaler, and patch do. This provides faster withdrawal relief but also a greater potential for development of dependence to the inhaler. Its use is limited by side effects. Spraying nicotine into the nasal mucosa is irritating, producing sneezing, cough, runny nose, and watery eyes. The product, sold only by prescription, may be best suited for smokers with high levels of nicotine dependence.

Bupropion (Zyban, Wellbutrin SR)

Bupropion is an antidepressant with dopaminergic activity. Clinical trials in nondepressed smokers have shown that the drug doubles smoking cessation rates compared with placebo, as well as reducing nicotine withdrawal symptoms and craving. It was superior to the nicotine patch in the one trial in which the two products were compared directly. In that study, the combination of bupropion and nicotine gum was safe but not significantly better than bupropion alone. The major concern with bupropion is the risk of seizure, because the drug, like all antidepressants, lowers the seizure threshold. The risk of seizure in clinical trials is below 0.1%, but the drug is contraindicated in patients with a seizure history or predisposition. Prominent side effects are insomnia, agitation, and anxiety. The dose, 150 mg to 300 mg daily, is started 1 week before the day on which the smoker plans to quit and continued for 3 to 6 months.

PHYSICIAN'S ROLE

Physicians have the opportunity to intervene with smokers, because each year they see an estimated 70% of the 23 million American women who smoke. Physicians have the additional opportunity of seeing smokers at times when symptoms have made them concerned about their health and therefore more likely to change their smoking behavior. Many smokers rationalize that they are immune to the health risks of smoking until these risks become personally salient. Current symptoms (e.g., cough, breathlessness, chest pain) stimulate change in smoking behavior more powerfully than does fear of future disease. Pregnancy or illness in a family member may also motivate smoking cessation. Other smoking-related conditions may also provide "teachable moments" when smokers are more receptive to advice to stop smoking.

Randomized controlled trials conducted in primary care practices have shown that providing brief advice to stop smoking to all patients increases patients' smoking cessation rates. Supplementing this advice with brief smoking counseling is even more effective. Programs shown to be effective consist of brief structured counseling during which the physician advises cessation, assesses a smoker's readiness to quit, assists the smoker in making an attempt to quit smoking, and provides follow-up monitoring. Cost-effectiveness analyses show that counseling smokers in office practice is highly cost-effective compared with other accepted medical practices and that counseling smokers as part of prenatal care is cost-saving. However, physicians should understand that many of the smokers they encounter are not ready to quit. Tobacco use is analogous to a chronic disease. It requires long-term management rather than a quick solution.

Smoking Counseling in Office Practice

The primary care of adult women should include a routine assessment of smoking status in all patients, strong advice to all smokers to quit, and assistance for those smokers who are ready to stop. The elements of effective smoking cessation counseling consists of five steps (Box 89-1).

Ask

Physicians should routinely ask all patients at every visit whether they smoke cigarettes.

Advise

The second step is to deliver clear advice to each smoker about the importance of stopping smoking. The message should be strong and unequivocal. If appropriate, advice should be tailored to the clinical situation, either current symptoms or family history. For example, the smoker can be informed that she will have fewer colds, less asthma or angina, or a healthier baby if she stops smoking. Advice is more effective when phrased in a positive way (e.g., emphasizing the benefits to be gained from quitting rather than the harms of continuing to smoke).

Assess

Smokers should be asked whether they are interested in quitting smoking. This permits the physician to determine the smoker's readiness to change. Smokers pass through a series of cognitive stages as they move toward nonsmoking: (1) initial lack of interest in quitting, (2) thinking about health risks and contemplating quitting, (3) actively preparing to quit within the next month, and (4) taking action to stop smoking. Current smoking cessation methods are most effective for the 20% to 30% of smokers who are ready to make a quit attempt. Most smokers are at earlier stages in the progression toward quitting and need a different approach. Categorizing smokers in this way is a clinically useful approach that helps the physician to determine what counseling strategy is appropriate and to set achievable goals for that encounter. Although the clinician's overall goal is to assist the smoker to stop permanently, a realistic goal for a single office visit is to move the smoker to the next stage of readiness to stop smoking.

Assist

The fourth step is to assist the smoker in quitting smoking. The physician's approach should be tailored to the smoker's readiness to stop smoking.

BOX 89-1

Smoking Cessation Counseling Strategy for Office Practice

- **Ask** about smoking at every visit.
  "Do you smoke?"
- **Advise** every smoker to stop.
  "Stopping smoking now is the most important action you can take to stay healthy."
  Tailor advice to the patient's clinical situation (symptoms or family history).
- **Assess** the smoker's readiness to quit.
  "Are you interested in quitting at this time?"
- **Assist** the smoker in stopping smoking.
  For smokers ready to quit:
  Ask smoker to set a "quit date."
  Provide behavioral treatment (e.g., self-help material to take home).
  Offer pharmacotherapy
  Consider referral to a formal cessation program.
  For smokers not ready to quit:
  Elicit patient's view of benefits and harms of smoking.
  Identify barriers to attempting cessation.
  Advise smoker to avoid exposing family members to passive smoke.
  Indicate willingness to help when the smoker is ready.
  Ask again about smoking at the next visit.
- **Arrange** follow-up visits.
  Make follow-up appointment 1 week after quit date.
  For smokers who have quit:
  Congratulate!
  Ask smoker to identify future high-risk situations.
  Rehearse coping strategies for future high-risk situations.
  For smokers who have not quit:
  Ask, "What were you doing when you had that first cigarette?"
  Ask, "What did you learn from the experience?"
  Ask smoker to set a new "quit date."

If the smoker is interested in quitting smoking, the physician should ask her whether she is ready to set a "quit date," a date within the next 4 weeks when she will stop smoking. If she is ready, the date should be recorded in the chart and on material given to the patient to take home. The physician should ask about the patient's previous attempts to quit to identify what approach is most likely to be successful. The physician should offer both behavioral counseling and pharmacotherapy. Behavioral strategies can be provided in a take-home booklet containing standard behavioral strategies. Alternatively, smokers can be referred to formal cessation programs, telephone counseling services provided in many states, or to web-based programs.

More intensive treatment is indicated for smokers who lack confidence in their ability to quit, who have been unsuccessful in previous attempts to quit, who lack social support for nonsmoking, or who have comorbid depression or substance abuse. Formal smoking cessation programs provide intensive training in behavioral smoking cessation skills combined with social support from the counselor and other group members.

For the smoker not interested in quitting or not ready to set a quit date, the physician should ask questions to elicit the patient's view of the benefits and harms of continuing to smoke. From an understanding of the patients' perspective, the physician can correct gaps in knowledge about health risks and correct misconceptions about the process of smoking cessation. The discussion should focus on short-term benefits rather than distant risks, and the physician should be prepared to discuss common barriers to smoking cessation. The clinician should advise the smoker not to expose family members to passive smoke (e.g., not smoke inside her home if nonsmokers are present) and indicate his or her future availability to help the smoker when she is ready to quit.

Follow-up

Offering follow-up visits increases the success of physician counseling. The smoker should be contacted by telephone or seen in the office shortly after her quit date to monitor progress.

If the smoker has stopped smoking at the follow-up visit she should be congratulated but warned that continued vigilance is necessary to maintain abstinence. The level of nicotine withdrawal symptoms should be assessed and, if indicated, treated pharmacologically. To prevent relapse to smoking, the patient should be asked to identify future situations in which she anticipates difficulty remaining abstinent. The physician can help her to plan and rehearse coping strategies for these times. Further follow-up visits or telephone calls should be offered.

If the smoker has not been able to remain abstinent since the quit date, the physician's role is to redefine an experience that the smoker considers to have been a failure into a partial success. The smokers can be told that even one day without cigarettes is the first step toward quitting and reminded that it takes time to learn to quit just as it took time to learn to smoke. To help the smoker learn from the experience, the physician should ask in detail about the circumstances surrounding the first cigarette smoked after the quit date. The smoker should be asked what she learned from the experi-

ence that can be used for her next attempt to quit. Finally, she should be asked whether she is ready to set a new quit date.

Office Environment

Smoking counseling need not and should not be limited to the physician's actions. An office-wide approach reduces the burden on a busy physician. In this model the physician's primary role is to provide advice to stop smoking and discuss the setting of a quit date. The patient's smoking status is assessed by a staff member before the physician sees the patient. The assistant asks each patient about smoking status and records the information in the chart to remind the physician to discuss smoking. Simple reminder systems such as this increase the amount of time physicians spend counseling smokers. Office personnel can also supplement physician advice to provide counseling, medication instruction, or referrals to outside programs.

MANAGEMENT OF BARRIERS TO SMOKING CESSATION (Box 89-2)

Fear of Failure

When smokers view cessation as a test of willpower, they fear failure. It is helpful to reinterpret quitting smoking as a learning process in which setbacks are expected. It may help the smoker to know that former smokers usually need to make several quit attempts before succeeding.

BOX 89-2
Barriers to Smoking Cessation

- **Fear of Failure**
  Quitting smoking is a learning process, not a test of will power.
  Relapse is part of the process. Most smokers require several attempts before succeeding.
  Learn from past mistakes made in previous quit attempts.
- **Nicotine Withdrawal Symptoms**
  Intensify pharmacotherapy, combining products as needed.
- **Weight Gain**
  Counter fears about amount of weight gain.
  Do not diet simultaneously.
  Start aerobic exercise program.
  Nicotine gum or bupropion SR may reduce and delay weight gain.
- **Poor Social Support for Nonsmoking**
  Ask other smokers in household to smoke outside or only in restricted areas.
  Find a "buddy" (a former smoker who can provide help).
  Recommend a formal group treatment program.
- **Mood Disorders**
  Temporary sadness at losing cigarettes is normal.
  Watch for symptoms of depression, especially those with a history of depression.
  Consider more intensive treatment (e.g., formal group program or mental health referral).
- **Alcohol and Other Substance Abuse**
  Be alert to this possibility in smokers who repeatedly try to quit without success.
  If present, refer for simultaneous treatment of substance abuse.

Nicotine Withdrawal Symptoms

Many smokers do not recognize that the discomfort they experience on quitting is nicotine withdrawal. Nicotine withdrawal symptoms can be controlled by drugs, combining products as necessary.

Weight Gain

Smokers weigh 5 to 10 lb less than nonsmokers of comparable age and height. When smokers quit 80% of them gain weight. The average weight gain of 10 to 12 lb poses a minimal health risk, especially when compared with the benefits of smoking cessation. Women gain more weight than men. Though many women fear large weight gains, only about 10% gain more than 25 lb after cessation. Heavier smokers (>25 cigarettes/day) gain more than lighter smokers. The mechanism is incompletely understood, but a nicotine-related decrease in metabolic rate and an increase in food intake appear to be responsible. Weight gain occurs in both sexes, but it concerns female smokers more than male smokers, presumably because women experience greater cultural pressure to be slender. Although weight gain has been considered a trigger to relapse, some studies show that successful abstainers gain more weight than relapsers. Smokers who quit using nicotine gum or bupropion gain less weight than those who quit with a placebo, although the weight gain is just delayed until after the drug is stopped. The effect of the nicotine patch on weight gain is contradictory across studies. Vigorous aerobic exercise reduces postcessation weight gain and increases the success of cessation efforts.

The best approach to the problem weight-concerned smoker is to encourage adoption of an exercise program, supplemented by nicotine gum or bupropion. It may reassure some smokers to learn that the amount of weight gain is less than they fear. Accepting a small increase in weight until smoking cessation is secure is a better strategy than attempting to stop smoking and lose weight simultaneously.

Lack of Social Support

Women with nonsmoking spouses are more likely to quit than women whose partners smoke. Smokers, especially female smokers, whose efforts to stop are supported by partners, family, and friends are more likely to succeed than smokers without this support. Those who live with smokers can ask them to restrict smoking to outdoor areas or to limited areas of the home, in order to provide a smoke-free area in the home. The social support provided by a formal cessation is also helpful for smokers with little nonsmoking support in their environment.

Mood Disorders

Stopping smoking represents a loss for many smokers. Cigarettes have been reliable "companions," as well as coping tools. Transient sadness is common and requires no special treatment. Acknowledgment that this is normal can be helpful.

There is an association between smoking and mood disorders. Smokers have more depressive symptoms than nonsmokers and are more likely to have a history of major depression. Smokers with depression are less likely to stop smoking than nondepressed smokers. These observations suggest that some smokers use nicotine to regulate mood. Clinicians should be alert to the possibility of depression in smokers. If present it should be treated before cessation is attempted. Smokers with a history of depression should be watched for the reemergence of symptoms during smoking cessation. Close attention to the possibility of mood disorders may be particularly important for women smokers, because depression is a more common diagnosis in women than in men.

Substance Abuse

Smokers of both sexes use more drugs—including coffee and alcohol—than nonsmokers. Because alcohol is frequently an ingredient in relapse situations, smokers attempting to quit are commonly advised to avoid alcohol temporarily after quitting. Smoking increases caffeine excretion. Smokers who stop should be advised to reduce caffeine intake to avoid increased blood levels and jitteriness. There is a high rate of smoking among abusers of alcohol, cocaine, and heroin. Depression and substance abuse should be considered as potential comorbid disorders in smokers who repeatedly try and fail to quit.

BIBLIOGRAPHY

Benowitz NL: Nicotine replacement therapy during pregnancy, *JAMA* 266:3174, 3177, 1991.

Cromwell J et al: Cost-effectiveness of the clinical practice recommendations in the AHCPR Guideline for Smoking Cessation, *JAMA* 278:1759, 1997.

Curry SJ, Grothaus LC, McAfee T, Pabiniak C: Use and cost-effectiveness of smoking cessation services under four insurance plans in a health maintenance organization, *N Engl J Med* 339:673, 1998.

Fiore MC et al: The effectiveness of the nicotine patch for smoking cessation: a meta-analysis, *JAMA* 271:1940, 1994.

Fiore MC et al: Tobacco dependence and the nicotine patch: guidelines for effective use, *JAMA* 268:2687, 1992.

Fiscella K, Franks P: Cost-effectiveness of the transdermal nicotine patch as an adjunct to physicians' smoking cessation counseling, *JAMA* 275:1247, 1996.

Fontham ETH et al: Environmental tobacco smoke and lung cancer in nonsmoking women: a multicenter study, *JAMA* 271:1752, 1994.

Glassman A: Cigarette smoking: implications for psychiatric illness, *Am J Psychiatry* 150:546, 1993.

Glynn TJ, Manley MW: *How to help your patients stop smoking: a National Cancer Institute manual for physicians,* Bethesda, 1989, US Department of Health and Human Services, Public Health Service, National Institutes of Health, National Cancer Institute, Division of Cancer Prevention and Control. NIH Publication No. 89-3064.

Hall SM et al: A randomized trial of nortriptyline for smoking cessation, *Arch Gen Psychiatry* 55:683, 1998.

Hollis JF et al: Nurse-assisted counseling for smokers in primary care, *Ann Intern Med* 118:521, 1993.

Hughes JR, Goldstein MG, Hurt RD, Schiffman S: Recent advances in the pharmacotherapy of smoking cessation, *JAMA* 281:72, 1999.

Hurt RD et al: A comparison of sustained-release bupropion and placebo for smoking cessation, *N Engl J Med* 337:1195, 1997.

Jorenby DE et al: A controlled trial of sustained-release bupropion, a nicotine patch, or both for smoking cessation, *N Engl J Med* 340:685, 1999.

Joseph A et al: The safety of transdermal nicotine as an aid to smoking cessation in patients with cardiac disease, *N Engl J Med* 335:1790, 1996.

Kawachi I et al: Smoking cessation in relation to total mortality rates in women: a prospective cohort study, *Ann Intern Med* 119:992, 1993.

Kiel DP et al: Smoking eliminates the protective effect of oral estrogens on the risk for hip fracture among women, *Ann Intern Med* 116:716, 1992.

Lancaster T, Stead L, Silagy C, Sowden A: Effectiveness of interventions to help people stop smoking: findings from the Cochrane Library, *Br Med J* 321:355, 2000.

Lasser K et al: Smoking and mental illness: a population-based prevalence study, *JAMA* 284:2606, 2000.

Marcus BH et al: The efficacy of exercise as an aid for smoking cessation in women, *Arch Intern Med* 159:1229, 1999.

Prochazka AV et al: A randomized trial of nortriptyline for smoking cessation, *Arch Intern Med* 158:2035, 1998.

Rigotti NA: Clinical crossroads: a 36-year-old woman who smokes cigarettes, *JAMA* 284:741, 2000.

Sutherland G et al: Randomized controlled trial of nicotine nasal spray in smoking cessation, *Lancet* 34:324, 1992.

Tobacco Use and Dependence Clinical Practice Guideline Panel: A clinical practice guideline for treating tobacco use and dependence, *JAMA* 283:3244, 2000. [www.surgeongeneral.gov/tobacco]

Tonnesen P et al: A double-blind trial of a nicotine inhaler for smoking cessation, *JAMA* 269:1268, 1993.

Williamson DF et al: Smoking cessation and severity of weight gain in a national cohort, *N Engl J Med* 324:739, 1991.

CHAPTER 90

Alcohol Abuse

Michele G. Cyr
Kelly A. McGarry

Alcohol use disorders have increasingly been recognized as a significant problem among female patients seen by primary care physicians. Several aspects of this disorder are specific to women, including the epidemiology, physiologic effects, psychosocial and medical consequences, and detection and management. This chapter concentrates on these issues.

Alcohol abuse is used as a generic term in this chapter to describe abuse of and dependence on alcohol. Abuse of any substance is characterized as repetitive, chronic pattern of use associated with impairment of psychosocial functioning and health. Dependence is characterized by loss of control of the use of a substance with evidence of tolerance (requiring increasing amounts of the substance to achieve the desired effects) or addiction (evidence of withdrawal when use of a substance decreases or ceases).

EPIDEMIOLOGY

Women compose an estimated one third of all those having alcohol abuse or dependence (alcoholism) disorders in the United States, or approximately 2.7 million women, according to statistics from the 1998 National Household Survey on Drug Abuse. The percentage of women who reported heavy drinking (five or more drinks on one occasion on each of 5 or more days in the past month) was 2% compared with 8% of women who reported "binge" drinking (5 or more drinks on one occasion on at least 1 day in the past 30 days). These percentages have been steady throughout the 1990s. Women ages 18 to 25 years reported the highest prevalence of both heavy and "binge" drinking (8% and 20%, respectively).

Use of alcohol varies according to race and ethnicity as well as level of education. African-American and Hispanic women are more likely to abstain from alcohol than white women, although recent data suggest that alcohol use is increasing among Hispanic adolescents. The 1998 National Household Survey on Drug Abuse demonstrated that African-American women were least likely to report "binge" drinking; however, Hispanic women reported the highest rates of heavy alcohol use (6.2% compared with 5.8% for white women). Women who are college graduates are more likely to drink than high school graduates; however, they are less likely to report heavy alcohol use than are less educated women. Single, divorced, or separated women are more

likely to drink heavily and experience alcohol-related problems than married or widowed women. In addition, 30% to 70% of female alcoholics are codependent on other drugs, including sedatives and minor tranquilizers. Recent evidence suggests that concurrent use of alcohol and illicit drugs may be increasingly common among younger women.

The prevalence of substance abuse problems among women who consult medical care providers varies, depending on the setting. Specifically, 21% of women attending a clinic for the treatment of premenstrual disorders, 10% to 17% attending internal medicine or family medicine clinics, and 12% of those attending a private gynecology practice were substance abusers. The percentage of women with alcohol-related problems on inpatient services ranges from 8% to 12%, depending on the specialty.

Physicians frequently miss the diagnosis of alcohol abuse in patients and, even when they do recognize it, do not recommend treatment. A recent survey of primary care physicians found that only 65% reported screening 80% to 100% of their patients for alcohol abuse on the initial visit, with only 34% screening their patients annually; 72% of the physicians preferred not to counsel patients themselves. Additionally, Moore and colleagues found that only 30% to 60% of patients with substance abuse were identified through surgical, medical, and psychiatric services. The rate of recognition was 0% to 7% on the gynecology service. Physicians have been less likely to diagnose women than men with active drinking problems. In a study by Buchsbaum and others, 24% of women with drinking problems were recognized compared with 67% of men. Women may be more likely to seek or be referred for care in non–alcohol-specific settings such as mental health treatment centers.

CONSEQUENCES OF ALCOHOL ABUSE
Pathophysiology

There are significant differences in the way women and men metabolize alcohol. After a given dose of alcohol adjusted according to body weight, women have higher blood alcohol levels than men. The higher proportion of body fat in women, changes in the absorption of alcohol with the menstrual cycle, and differences in the relative amounts of gastric alcohol dehydrogenase found in men and women account for this observation. These differences may explain the "telescoping" phenomenon of alcohol use in women, that is, the earlier appearance and increased severity of complications from drinking seen in women compared with men. Despite lower levels of consumption and later onset of problem drinking for women, cirrhosis develops over a shorter period and women die at an earlier age. Both Native American and African-American women have particularly high rates of cirrhosis and death from cirrhosis.

Psychosocial Consequences

Women are more likely to begin problem drinking in response to a specific trauma such as divorce, death of a family member, children leaving home, and health problems, even with no prior history of alcohol abuse. In addition, once problem drinking has begun, women continue to suffer important psychosocial consequences. Family and marital problems are more common among women, whereas job and legal problems are more commonly reported consequences in men. Women are more likely to be divorced after entering treatment (9 of 10 marriages in which the woman is alcoholic end in divorce compared with 1 of 10 in which the male is alcoholic) and report a fear of losing custody of their children as an important motivating factor for treatment.

Women who drink heavily or who are alcoholic are more likely to be victims of alcohol-related aggression such as rape. Women with alcohol problems often have male partners with alcohol problems, and male alcohol use is highly associated with spousal abuse. Younger women with substance abuse report particularly high rates of violence—48% report episodes of violence and 32% report rape or coerced sexual intercourse.

Psychiatric Disorders

All psychiatric diagnoses are more prevalent in alcohol-abusing women than in both female nonalcoholics and alcohol-abusing men. Only antisocial personality disorder is more prevalent in male alcoholics. Studies have shown the prevalence of comorbid depression, the most common psychiatric comorbidity among alcohol-abusing women, to be between 30% and 70%. Many women cite worsening depressive symptoms as their main reason for entering treatment. Interestingly, women with alcohol problems may have a much higher rate of "dual diagnoses" in which a primary affective disorder predated their chemical dependence. The Epidemiologic Catchment Area Study revealed that for 66% of alcohol-abusing women, depression was primary and alcoholism secondary in contrast to 78% of the men in which alcoholism was primary and depression secondary.

Alcohol-abusing women appear to be more vulnerable to suicidality than nonalcoholic women, attempting suicide at four times the rate seen in nonalcoholic women. Among adult alcoholics, the suicide rate for women equals that of men; however, women have more suicide attempts than men. Comorbid eating disorders are also more prevalent in alcohol-abusing women ranging from 15% to 32%. This is significantly higher than the prevalence in the general population, which is estimated at 1.5% for anorexia and 7% for bulimia.

Mortality

Although there is substantial evidence that moderate alcohol consumption can reduce the risk for coronary heart disease and all-cause mortality among women, for alcohol-abusing women life expectancy is decreased an average of 15 years compared with non–alcohol-abusing women owing to cirrhosis, alcohol-related accidents, and suicide/homicide. Additionally, female alcoholics have death rates 50% to 100% higher than male alcoholics.

Cardiovascular Disease

Moderate alcohol consumption has been shown to reduce cardiovascular mortality among men, women and, recently, among women with type 2 diabetes mellitus. For women, alcohol has a narrow therapeutic window between benefit and harm. Thus, counseling women on alcohol's benefits and risks can be difficult. Recent data support the narrow margin of safety for alcohol use in women. When compared with nondrinkers, women who consumed 1 to 7 drinks per week had the greatest reduction in 10-year cardiovascular risk; women consuming more than 15 drinks per week had an increased prevalence of hypertension. A second study, which evaluated more than 58,000 US female nurses for 4 years found that compared with nondrinkers, women drinking approximately two to three drinks per day had a significantly elevated relative risk of 1.4 for hypertension. For women consuming more than three drinks per day, the relative risk for hypertension was 1.9 after adjustment for smoking and dietary factors, suggesting that the risk for hypertension may increase progressively with increasing alcohol intake. In addition to hypertension, alcohol-abusing women are at risk for alcohol-induced cardiomyopathy at lower levels of alcohol intake than men. Furthermore, the risk of hemorrhagic stroke is increased in women drinking more than two drinks per day.

Breast Cancer

A recent meta-analysis of six, large prospective cohort studies showed a positive association between alcohol use and the risk of breast cancer. Women who consumed, on average, 30 to 60 g/day of alcohol (about 2.5 to 5 drinks/day) had a relative risk of breast cancer of 1.41 compared with nondrinkers. Of importance, this study also found a dose-response relationship between alcohol consumption and breast cancer risk: Breast cancer risk was elevated by 9% for each 10 g/day (approximately 0.75 to 1 drink per day) increase in alcohol intake for intakes up to 60 g/day.

Gynecologic Consequences

Alcohol and other drug problems are more prevalent among women consulting gynecologic practices than in the general population. Higher rates of amenorrhea, dysfunctional uterine bleeding, dysmenorrhea, infertility, premenstrual syndrome, and sexual dysfunction have been described among women who are heavy drinkers.

Obstetric Issues

Results from an ongoing national survey reveal an increasing prevalence of alcohol use among pregnant women between 1992 and 1995, from 9.5% to 15.3%. In addition, frequent alcohol use increased from 0.9% in 1991 to 3.5% by 1995. Maternal alcohol consumption is a leading preventable cause of birth defects and childhood disabilities in the United States. Although alcohol crosses the placenta, its effects on the fetus vary with the degree and timing of exposure, maternal metabolism, and interaction with other drugs. Women who drink two or more drinks per day during pregnancy are at higher risk for spontaneous abortions, low–birth-weight infants, preterm deliveries (threefold increase), and perinatal mortality. Infants born to alcohol-abusing mothers are at risk for full-blown fetal alcohol syndrome characterized by severe physical, behavioral, and cognitive abnormalities. Affected infants are also at risk for other alcohol-related neurodevelopmental disorders and birth defects, including cardiac, skeletal, renal, ocular, and auditory defects.

Hip Fractures

Alcohol consumption influences the incidence of hip fractures among women. Women less than 65 years old who consumed 2 to 6 oz of alcohol each week had an increased risk of hip fracture. This increased risk may be due to an increased incidence of falling and to alcohol's inhibitory effect on bone remodeling, which has been demonstrated in men. However, several large studies have suggested that moderate alcohol consumption may be associated with increased bone mineral density in postmenopausal women.

Human Immunodeficiency Virus Disease

There is considerable evidence that both women and men expect drinking to have positive effects of sexual experience despite the fact that, physiologically, alcohol decreases sexual arousal. Despite these expectations, most women do not report significant effects of drinking on their sexual behavior. Several recent studies, however, have found associations between heavier or more frequent drinking and higher levels of sexual risk taking among female adolescents and adults, which may place these individuals at risk for human immunodeficiency virus and other sexually transmitted diseases.

SCREENING AND IDENTIFICATION
Screening
History and Physical Examination

Primary care physicians are in a unique position to educate women about the health effects of alcohol and other drugs, to identify women with alcohol problems, and to make appropriate referrals for treatment. Routine screening for alcohol abuse and dependence in women is easily justified by the high prevalence of alcohol-related problems, the susceptibility of women to the medical and psychosocial consequences of drinking, the availability of effective screening tools, and the efficacy of primary care interventions. Buchsbaum and others reported that lifetime rates for alcohol abuse and dependence for women in primary care settings are as high as 25%. Yet, women are much less likely to be identified as having alcohol-related problems than are men.

It is true that there are significant obstacles to diagnosing alcohol problems in women. Women may be more likely to deny a drinking problem than men, because of the social stigma specifically attached to female alcoholism. Even at low levels of consumption, women can experience alcohol-related problems that may not be suspected as such by the patient, her family, or her primary care provider. Further compounding the difficulty of detection is the fact that women are less likely to experience the stereotypical alcohol-related problems, such as driving while intoxicated, than men. In fact, many of the original screening tools depended largely on more male-oriented drinking problems and therefore performed less well in women.

Routine screening is critical to identify patients at risk for, and those with a diagnosis of, alcohol abuse. While questions about the quantity and frequency of alcohol use are both insensitive and unreliable in identifying alcoholism, they do provide an entree to a discussion about the patient's use of alcohol. The National Institute of Alcohol Abuse and Alcoholism (NIAAA) defines "at risk drinking" for women to be >7 drinks/week or >3 drinks/occasion. Spandorfer et al. surveyed primary care physicians and found that of the 65% who reported screening patients, 95% used quantity–frequency questions; only 35% used other screeners often. Because polydrug use is so prevalent among women, it is important that physicians additionally ask about use of prescription and illicit drugs.

An excellent review of screening tests by Bradley et al. revealed that three questionnaires are considered optimal for women: the CAGE, AUDIT, and TWEAK (Boxes 90-1 to 90-3). Not only does the performance of these depend significantly on gender, but also greatly on ethnicity and race. In general, all three screening questionnaires are more sensitive for alcohol abuse and dependence in black women than in white women. If the recommended cut-offs are used, the CAGE and AUDIT miss between 41% and 62% of white women with problems. The TWEAK performs better in white women than either the CAGE or the AUDIT.

Overall, the TWEAK is the recommended screening test for mixed populations of women. The AUDIT has the advantage of acquiring more information about drinking pat-

---

BOX 90-1
CAGE

Have you ever tried to **cut** down on your drinking?
Have you ever been **annoyed** by criticism of your drinking?
Have you ever felt **guilty** about your drinking?
Have you ever had an **eye** opener?

* One point for each "yes" answer.

BOX 90-2
TWEAK

Tolerance: How many drinks does it take before you begin to feel the effects of the alcohol? (>2 indicates tolerance)
Worry: Have close friends or relatives worried or complained about your drinking?
Eye-Opener: Have you ever taken a drink to steady your nerves or get over a hangover?
Amnesia: Has a close friend or relative ever told you about things you said or did when drinking that you could not remember?
"Kut" down: Have you ever felt the need to cut down on your use of alcohol?

* Two points each for tolerance and worry, 1 point each for others.

BOX 90-3
AUDIT
(Alcohol Use Disorders Test)

How often do you drink containing alcohol?
    (0) Never (1) Monthly or less (2) 2 to 4 times a month (3) 2 to 3 times a week (4) 4 times a week
How many drinks containing alcohol do you have on a typical day when you are drinking?
    (0) 1 or 2 (1) 3 or 4 (2) 5 or 6 (3) 7 or 9 (4) 10 or more
How often do you have 6 drinks on one occasion?
    (0) Never (1) Less than monthly (2) Monthly (3) Weekly (4) Daily or almost daily
How often during the last year have you found that you were not able to stop drinking once you had started?
    (0) Never (1) Less than monthly (2) Monthly (3) Weekly (4) Daily or almost daily
How often during the last year have you failed to do what was normally expected from you because of drinking?
    (0) Never (1) Less than monthly (2) Monthly (3) Weekly (4) Daily or almost daily
How often during the last year have you needed a first drink in the morning to get yourself going after a heavy drinking session?
    (0) Never (1) Less than monthly (2) Monthly (3) Weekly (4) Daily or almost daily
How often during the last year have you had a feeling of guilt or remorse after drinking?
    (0) Never (1) Less than monthly (2) Monthly (3) Weekly (4) Daily or almost daily
How often during the last year have you been unable to remember what happened the night before because you had been drinking?
    (0) Never (1) Less than monthly (2) Monthly (3) Weekly (4) Daily or almost daily
Have you or someone else been injured as a result of your drinking?
    (0) No (2) Yes, but not in the last year (4) Yes, during the last year
Has a relative, friend, or a physician or other health care worker been concerned about your drinking or suggested to you to cut down?
    (0) No (2) Yes, but not in the last year (4) Yes, during the last year

*Numbers in parenthesis are scoring weights. AUDIT total score is the sum of scoring weights.

---

terns and dependence and has been validated as a self-administered screener. For predominantly black populations of women, the CAGE is a reasonable tool for alcohol dependence, but not for heavy drinking alone. It is recommended that for all three tests, lower cut-offs be used for women, that is, ≥ 2 for the TWEAK, ≥ 4 for the AUDIT, and ≥ 1 for the CAGE.

In a university-based family practice clinic, Steinbauer and others evaluated the AUDIT, CAGE, and SAAST (Self-Administered Alcohol Screening Test) for accuracy among patients of varied ethnic backgrounds. The CAGE and SAAST, using standard cut-offs, performed least well for Mexican-American women. Overall, the AUDIT was least affected by sex and ethnic biases compared with the CAGE and the SAAST. Further study is needed, however, to identify optimal cut-offs and compare performance among varied populations of women.

Clues to the Diagnosis

Specific risk factors for alcohol abuse in women include a family history of alcoholism, history of physical or sexual abuse, other substance use, and young age at first intoxication. Other factors in the history, although not considered risk factors, raise concern for an alcohol problem, including eating disorders, history of depression or anxiety disorders, reproductive difficulties, divorce, and a partner with heavy alcohol or drug use.

Symptoms that may serve as clues to a potential problem may be nonspecific, or the more specific complaints of sleep disturbance, fatigue, gastrointestinal complaints, premen-

---

BOX 90-4
Historical Clues to a Diagnosis of Alcohol Abuse

Symptoms
Nonspecific complaints
Insomnia
Depressive symptoms
Anxiety
Gastrointestinal symptoms
Sexual dysfunction
Severe PMS

Past Medical History
Trauma
Eating disorders
Depression
Anxiety disorders
Sexual or physical abuse
Gynecologic disorders

Family History
Alcohol or other substance abuse

Social History
Other drug use
Divorce
Family problems
Legal problems
Job problems

strual syndrome, sexual dysfunction, and depressive symptoms (Box 90-4). For the most part, the physical findings related to alcohol abuse occur late in the course of the disease, but hypertension may be a relatively early indication of heavy drinking. Likewise, laboratory abnormalities, including elevated liver function tests and mean corpuscular volume (MCV), are often late findings and have very low sensitivity as screening tools. If they are abnormal, however, they provide important evidence that there may be a diagnosis of alcohol abuse.

Making the Diagnosis

Establishing the diagnosis of alcohol abuse requires additional data gathering regarding the adverse consequences of the patient's drinking. Specific questions can identify the relationship between alcohol use and family problems, problems with a spouse or significant other, job problems, legal and financial problems, and medical problems. For example, if a patient is having problems at home, expresses concern about a child's behavior, or mentions difficulty with a spouse, ask how drinking affects the problem. "How do you feel your son's behavior is affected by your drinking?" "How do you and your husband get along when you are drinking?" Open-ended, general questions such as "Tell me more about your drinking?" can be revealing, but some patients may offer specific information only when asked directly.

Even after gathering more data about the patient's alcohol use, the physician may still be unsure about the diagnosis. Still, it is important to share that concern with the patient and elicit their reaction. Together, the physician and patient can develop a plan for follow-up and reevaluation. This might include a trial of controlled drinking. Specific recommendations are most effective, both for patient adherence and future evaluation (e.g., "Limit your drinking to no more than 7 drinks per week and we will discuss it at your next appointment in 4 weeks."). The physician should reassure the patient of her or his willingness to continue to work with her whether or not she is able to follow the agreed upon plan. The patient's concerns and reactions should be solicited and will often reveal more information about the role alcohol plays in her life. When she returns, the success or failure of the trial can provide further understanding of her drinking. If she was able to follow through with the recommendations, she should continue to be evaluated to monitor her alcohol use. If she demonstrates an inability to cut down or stop, this provides ample evidence of a problem. At this point, the patient may be willing to accept that she has a problem.

✚ MANAGEMENT

Once the Diagnosis Is Established

Patients who are at risk for alcohol abuse or who are drinking in a hazardous fashion can benefit greatly from education about the consequences of drinking. Many women are uninformed about the consumption levels that put them at risk for the medical consequences of drinking. Breast cancer, osteoporosis, and gynecologic risks are of particular concern to most women. Women who are contemplating pregnancy and those who are pregnant should be informed specifically about the effects of cigarettes, alcohol, and other drugs on the fetus. Because no level of alcohol use has been definitely shown to be safe in pregnancy, abstention is generally recommended.

Once alcohol abuse has been identified as a diagnosis, it is important that the physician express her or his concerns to the patient. It is best to avoid labeling the patient as an alcoholic, in favor of simply linking the negative consequences to her alcohol use, "I am concerned that your problems at work, your difficulties with your husband, and your sleeping problem point to a problem with alcohol." Furthermore, it is essential to inform the patient that there is help available for her problems.

Brief physician advice has been shown to be an effective intervention in primary care settings. In fact, Fleming and colleagues demonstrated superior results in women problem drinkers versus men (31% versus 14% reduction in alcohol use at 1 year) using a physician advice intervention in community-based primary care practices. One example of a brief intervention is summarized by the mnemonic FRAMES.

Feedback about the adverse effects of alcohol. "Even though it seems that the alcohol helps you get to sleep, in fact, you're tired during the day because the alcohol is waking you up in the middle of the night."

Responsibility for the change in drinking behavior. "Only you can decide that you want to stop drinking and see what happens to your fatigue."

Advice about alcohol consumption. "For the next 2 weeks, stop drinking and let's see how you feel."

Menu of options. "If you find that not drinking for the next 2 weeks is impossible, then we should consider other options like group or individual counseling or Alcoholics Anonymous."

Empathy for patients. "I know that this may be difficult for you, since it seems that drinking helps your anxiety and you've had a lot of stressful situations lately."

Self-efficacy "I am impressed that you are considering making this change. Your strong determination is going to help you succeed in this."

Treatment

Depending on the results of the trial, the physician and patient may need to identify a treatment plan tailored to the patient's individual situation. Men and women with comparable demographic characteristics at comparable stages of disease do equally well in treatment. However, for women additional issues may need to be addressed in treatment including self-esteem, sexual abuse, sexism, and interpersonal relationships. It may also be necessary to find treatment alternatives that address specific child care and other family responsibilities. Box 90-5 lists the various treatment plan components.

Referral to a 12-step program such as Alcoholics Anonymous and follow-up treatment with the primary care physician may be appropriate first steps for the woman who has a stable social situation and no impending social disaster such as threat of lost custody, job loss, or divorce. In general, women respond better to self-help programs and to all-female groups. Physicians are most effective if they familiarize themselves with the process of 12-step programs and refer their patients to meetings that are appropriate for them (e.g., an all-women's meeting, appropriate socioeconomic group, nonsmoking, gay). During follow-up visits, the

---

BOX 90-5
Treatment Components

Alcohol Specific
- Brief intervention
- Self-help (patient and family)
- Alcohol counseling
- Residential treatment

Support Services
- Child care
- Family therapy
- Legal services
- Psychiatric services
- Vocational skills training

---

physician can work with the patient to help her learn new behaviors to deal with stress, anxiety, anger, and other potential triggers for drinking and to identify specific ways to maintain sobriety.

Individuals with significant medical problems, abusive home situations, legal problems, and partners with substance abuse should be referred for intense outpatient, inpatient, or residential treatment. Additionally, family therapy can help a family learn more about the disease, deal with anger and anxiety, and participate in the recovery process. Referrals of family members to self-help programs (e.g., AlAnon, AlAteen) can be particularly helpful for families dealing with alcohol problems.

BIBLIOGRAPHY

American Academy of Pediatrics. Committee on Substance Abuse and Committee on Children With Disabilities: Fetal alcohol syndrome and alcohol-related neurodevelopmental disorders, *Pediatrics* 106(2 Pt 1): 358, 2000.

Ashley MJ et al: Morbidity in alcoholics: evidence for accelerated development of physical disease in women, *Arch Intern Med* 137:883, 1977.

Bohn MJ, Babor TF, Kranzler HR: The alcohol use disorders identification test (AUDIT): validation of a screening instrument for use in medical settings, *J Stud Alcohol* 56:423, 1995.

Bradley KA et al: Alcohol screening in women: a critical review, *JAMA* 280:166, 1998.

Bradley KA et al: Medical risks for women who drink alcohol, *J Gen Intern Med* 13:627, 1998.

Buchsbaum DG et al: Physician detection of drinking problems in patients attending a general medicine practice, *J Gen Intern Med* 7:517, 1992.

Buchsbaum DG et al: Screening for alcohol abuse using CAGE scores and likelihood ratios, *Ann Intern Med* 115:774, 1991.

Bush BT et al: Screening for alcohol abuse using the CAGE questionnaire, *Am J Med* 82:231, 1987.

Chasnoff IJ, Landress HJ, Barrett ME: The prevalence of illicit-drug or alcohol use during pregnancy and discrepancies in mandatory reporting in Pinellas County, Florida, *N Engl J Med* 322:1202, 1990.

Daeppen JB et al: Reliability and validity of the Alcohol Use Disorders Identification Test (AUDIT) imbedded within a general health risk screening questionnaire: results of a survey in 332 primary care patients, *Alcohol Clin Exp Res* 24:659, 2000.

Dixit AR, Crum RM: Prospective study of depression and the risk of heavy alcohol use in women, *Am J Psychiatry* 157:751, 2000.

Ebrahim SH et al: Alcohol consumption by pregnant women in the United States during 1988-1995, *Obstet Gynecol* 92:187, 1998.

Epstein JA, Botvin GJ, Diaz T: Etiology of alcohol use among Hispanic adolescents: sex-specific effects of social influences to drink and problems behaviors, *Arch Pediatr Adolesc Med* 153:1077, 1999.

Fiellin DA, Reid MC, O'Connor PG: Outpatient management of patients with alcohol problems, *Ann Intern Med,* 133:815, 2000.

Fiellin DA, Reid MC, O'Connor PG: Screening for alcohol problems in primary care: a systematic review, *Arch Intern Med* 160:1977, 2000.

Fleming MF et al: Brief physician advice for problem alcohol drinkers. A randomized controlled trial in community-based primary care practices, *JAMA* 277:1039, 1997.

Ganry O, Baudoin C, Fardellone P: Effect of alcohol intake on bone mineral density in elderly women: The EPIDOS Study. Epidemiologie de l'Osteoporose, *Am J Epidemiol* 151:773, 2000.

Gronbaek M et al: Type of alcohol consumed and mortality from all causes, coronary heart disease, and cancer, *Ann Intern Med* 133:411, 2000.

Liebschutz JM, Mulvey KP, Samet JH: Victimization among substance-abusing women. Worse health outcomes, *Arch Intern Med* 157:1093, 1997.

Moore RD et al: Prevalence, detection, and treatment of alcoholism in hospitalized patients, *JAMA* 261:403, 1989.

Morse BA, Hutchins E: Reducing complications from alcohol use during pregnancy through screening, *J Am Med Womens Assoc* 55:225, 240, 2000.

Nanchahal K, Ashton WD, Wood DA: Alcohol consumption, metabolic cardiovascular risk factors and hypertension in women, *Int J Epidemiol* 29: 57, 2000.

National Institute on Drug Abuse: Sample size and U.S. population size tables. In *National household survey on drug abuse: population estimates 1998,* Rockville, 2001, Department of Health and Human Services.

Parker DA, Harford TC, Rosenstock IM: Alcohol, other drugs, and sexual risk-taking among young adults, *J Subst Abuse* 6:87, 1994.

Piazza NJ, Vrbka JL, Yeager RD: Telescoping of alcoholism in women alcoholics, *Int J Addict* 24:19, 1989.

Ray WA et al: Psychotropic drug use and the risk of hip fracture, *N Engl J Med* 316:363, 1987.

Russell M et al: Detecting risk drinking during pregnancy: a comparison of four screening questionnaires, *Am J Public Health* 86:1435, 1996.

Russell M et al: Screening for pregnancy risk-drinking, *Alcohol Clin Exp Res* 18:1156, 1994.

Samet JH, Rollnick S, Barnes H: A brief clinical approach after detection of substance abuse, *Arch Intern Med* 156:2287, 1996.

Smith-Warner et al: Alcohol and breast cancer in women: a pooled analysis of cohort studies, *JAMA* 279:535, 1998.

Solomon et al: Moderate alcohol consumption and risk of coronary heart disease among women with type 2 diabetes mellitus, *Circulation* 102: 494, 2000.

Spandorfer JM, Israel Y, Turner BJ: Primary Care Physicians' views on screening and management of alcohol abuse: inconsistencies with national guidelines, *J Fam Pract* 48:899, 1999.

Steinbauer JR et al: Ethnic and sex bias in primary care screening tests for alcohol use disorders, *Ann Intern Med* 129:353, 1998.

Svarstad BL et al: Gender differences in the acquisition of prescribed drugs: an epidemiological study, *Med Care* 25:1089, 1987.

Thun MJ et al: Alcohol consumption and mortality among middle-aged and elderly U.S. adults, *N Engl J Med* 337:1705, 1997.

Weisner C, Schmidt L: Gender disparities in treatment for alcohol problems, *JAMA* 268:1872, 1992.

Wilsnack RW, Wilsnack SC, Klassen AD: Women's drinking and drinking problems: patterns from a 1981 national survey, *Am J Public Health* 74:1231, 1984.

Wilsnack SC et al: Predicting onset and chronicity of women's problem drinking: a five-year longitudinal analysis, *Am J Public Health* 81:305, 1991.

Witteman JC et al: Relation of moderate alcohol consumption and risk of systemic hypertension in women, *Am J Cardiol* 65:633, 1990.

CHAPTER 91

Substance Abuse

Grace Chang

Drug use and dependence are highly prevalent in the general population. Data from the National Comorbidity Survey indicate that 18% of noninstitutionalized civilian women aged 15 to 54 will satisfy diagnostic criteria for any lifetime substance abuse or dependence, and 6.6% will have any substance abuse or dependence diagnosis within the last 12 months. However, the majority of individuals with substance abuse and dependence do not receive professional treatment. The lack of professional treatment is particularly true for women, who experience more stigma and shame for their use of substances. Because women are more likely to receive primary care than substance abuse treatment, clinicians in primary care settings have an opportunity to identify, diagnose, and refer their patients.

Substance disorders are costly, even when treated. Between 1988 and 1995, Americans spent $58 billion on drugs: $38 billion on cocaine, $10 billion on heroin, $7 billion on marijuana, and $3 billion on other illegal drugs and the misuse of legal drugs. A study prepared by the Lewin Group for the National Institute on Drug Abuse estimated the total economic cost of drug abuse (excluding nicotine) in 1992 to be $98 billion, which would include costs associated with substance abuse treatment and prevention, health care costs, costs associated with reduced job productivity or lost earnings, and costs to society, such as crime and social welfare.

This chapter focuses on the major substances of abuse and dependence. Substance abuse and substance dependence are not interchangeable terms, and both differ from the substance-induced disorders (e.g., intoxication, withdrawal, or delirium).

The essential feature of substance abuse is a maladaptive pattern of substance use manifested by recurrent and significant adverse consequences related to the use of substances in a 12-month period. Examples of adverse consequences include repeated failure to fulfill major role obligations, multiple legal problems, repeated substance use in situations in which it is physically hazardous, and recurrent social and interpersonal problems.

The essential feature of substance dependence is a cluster of cognitive, behavioral, and physiologic symptoms, indicating that the individual continues substance use, despite significant, drug-related problems. There is a pattern of repeated self-administration that usually results in tolerance, withdrawal, and compulsive drug-taking behavior.

ANABOLIC-ANDROGENIC STEROIDS

Anabolic-androgenic steroids can be used to enhance athletic performance and to improve physical appearance. Hundreds of thousands of people aged at least 18 abuse anabolic steroids at least once a year. Taken orally or injected, typically in cycles of weeks or months, steroid abuse is higher among male than among female adolescents and adults. However, steroid abuse is growing most rapidly among young women.

Gender-specific side effects in women include growth of facial hair, male-pattern baldness, changes in the menstrual cycle, clitoral enlargement, and a deepened voice. Women who abuse steroids are also at risk for developing liver tumors and cancer, jaundice, fluid retention, high blood pressure, adverse changes in the cholesterol profile, kidney tumors, severe acne, and trembling. As steroids may be injected, with nonsterile technique or after illegal manufacture under nonsterile conditions, abusers are at risk for developing viral infections, such as human immunodeficiency virus (HIV) or hepatitis B or C, or bacterial infections, such as endocarditis or skin abscess.

Finally, psychiatric side effects have been reported to result from steroid abuse. Mood swings, irritability, jealousy, delusions, and maniclike symptoms culminating in violence have been described.

COCAINE AND STIMULANTS

Cocaine is a sympathomimetic substance that elicits states of heightened awareness, elevated mood, and increased psychomotor activity. Cocaine may be taken intranasally, injected intravenously, or smoked. High doses may result in acute medical problems such as agitation, psychosis, hyperthermia, seizures, hypertension, and tachycardia. Central nervous system depression follows stimulation and may be characterized by paralysis of motor activity, hyperreflexia followed by eventual areflexia, stupor progressing to coma, loss of vital functions, and even death.

Results from the 1996 National Household Survey on Drug Abuse indicate that crack cocaine dominates America's illicit drug problem. In 1996, there were 1.75 million current cocaine users. Although more men use cocaine than women, female crack users in their 30s and with no prior drug history constitute a fast-growing group of new users.

The putative consequences of prenatal cocaine exposure have been described in hundreds of articles. Unfortunately, many of the studies are limited by methodologic shortcomings. The few studies with controls for cocaine dose and time of exposure indicate that cocaine effects are dose-related and related to the stage of pregnancy when the drug was used. Sequelae linked to high-dose prenatal cocaine exposure include abruptio placenta, preterm labor, decreased uterine blood flow, intrauterine growth retardation, preterm birth, spontaneous abortion, and fetal death.

ECSTASY (Methylenedioxymetamphetamine)

Methylenedioxymethamphetamine (MDMA) is similar to the stimulant amphetamine and the hallucinogen mescaline. It can produce both stimulant and psychedelic effects. MDMA is the fastest growing drug of abuse in the United States, no longer limited to "club kids," but with increased use by older groups.

MDMA is taken orally and its effects last for about 3 to 6 hours. It is popularly described to lower inhibitions and foster feelings of well-being and closeness to others, in addition to an increase in heart rate, blood pressure, and a sense of alertness. The stimulant effects may encourage frenetic activity, which could lead to dehydration. At high doses, MDMA has been associated with malignant hyperthermia. Some users have experienced confusion, depression, anxiety, sleep disturbance, and paranoia for many weeks after their last MDMA exposure.

MDMA is not physically addicting. It is neurotoxic and impairs the function and long-term production of serotonin. Although few deaths have been attributed to MDMA, the full extent of the consequences of MDMA use remains to be determined.

HEROIN

Since 1992, heroin use has increased. With abundant supplies and price reduction, heroin has attracted many new users who smoke, snort, or sniff it. There is a high incidence of new users in the younger age groups, often among women. Heroin snorters tend to shift to injection because of increased tolerance or nasal soreness, thereby exposing themselves to increased risk of HIV infection. There are at least 500,000 people addicted to heroin, one quarter of whom are women. Latest figures show nearly 1,000,000.

Most opiate-dependent women are untreated. In contrast to opiate-dependent men, these women have higher rates of unemployment, medical problems, depression, and negative self-images and are generally perceived by society to be more deviant. Opiate-dependent women are frequently involved in heroin-oriented relationships, which have been shown to have an adverse effect on successful treatment outcome. Finally, the course of female opiate addiction is telescoped, thereby allowing less time for identification, intervention, and treatment.

Although patients rarely seek medical attention for opiate intoxication, overdose, or withdrawal, medical complications frequently catalyze treatment. At analgesic doses, opiates produce changes in mood and feeling. Opioid drugs have diverse actions on many organ systems, but the most prominent effects are on the central nervous system and the gastrointestinal tract. Disturbed menstrual function results from the inhibition of gonadotropin-releasing hormone by opiate effects on the neuroendocrine system.

Medical problems frequently prompt women struggling with opiates into treatment. Medical complications resulting from the injection of heroin include serious infectious diseases (e.g., HIV), liver disease (e.g., chronic hepatitis), renal disease (e.g., nephrotic syndrome), and immunologic abnormalities even in the absence of HIV infection (e.g., generalized lymphadenopathy).

About three fourths of opiate-dependent women are of child-bearing age. The medical and social costs of opiate dependence during pregnancy are great. Opiate-addicted pregnant women experience significant increases in maternal obstetric and neonatal complications. Pregnancy complications include low birth weight, toxemia, third trimester bleeding, malpresentation, puerperal morbidity, fetal distress, and meconium. Neonatal complications include narcotic withdrawal, postnatal growth deficiency, microcephaly, neurobehavioral problems, and sudden infant death syndrome.

Methadone maintenance has been recommended for the treatment of opiate addiction during pregnancy because it eliminates the need for illicit opiate use and may confer other benefits such as stabilization of maternal drug levels and of her social circumstances such that the patient may initiate evaluation and treatment of associated health problems. However, the use of methadone during pregnancy remains controversial because it does not prevent the use of other drugs during pregnancy, and it can result in neonatal withdrawal.

MARIJUANA

Marijuana is the most widely used illicit substance in the United States; more than 65 million Americans have used it, and there were 2.4 million new users in 1995 alone. Marijuana use is growing in popularity, to the extent that the rate of female use is achieving parity with male use in the younger (18- to 25-year-old) age groups. Results from a study of 1934 individual female twins, including both members of 485 monozygotic and of 335 dizygotic pairs, suggest that genetic factors have a moderate effect on the probability of ever using cannabis and a strong impact on the liability of women to develop cannabis use, abuse, and dependence.

Sometimes classified as an hallucinogen because it can produce many of the effects associated with lysergic acid diethylamide (or LSD), tolerance and withdrawal are not typically associated with marijuana use. The adverse medical consequences of marijuana use have not been well documented, but are likely to be associated with the impact of smoking. Marijuana use in a prepaid health care-based study cohort of 65,171 enrollees between 15 and 49 years old had little effect on non-AIDS mortality in men and on total mortality in women. Nonetheless, cannabis may act as a gateway drug that encourages other forms of illicit drug use, a hypothesis with empirical support.

Marijuana is the most commonly used illicit substance during pregnancy. Prenatal marijuana use may vary by age, racial or ethnic differences, and socioeconomic status. The impact of prenatal marijuana use on the infant is not clearly known. A retrospective analysis of 8350 births at Johns Hopkins Hospital found that 5% of the mothers used only marijuana, and there was no association between marijuana use and prematurity or congenital anomalies. On the other hand, a longitudinal study of 3-year-old children exposed to marijuana in the first and second trimesters of lower socioeconomic women found that they had significantly reduced performance on the Stanford-Binet intelligence scale, which was moderated in Caucasian children attending preschool or daycare.

PRESCRIPTION DRUGS

Compared with male patients, female patients receive disproportionately more psychotropic medications from physicians. A recent study of data from the 1987 National Medical Expenditures Survey of approximately 14,000 households and 38,446 noninstitutionalized civilian individuals demonstrates that women are more likely to use an abusable prescription drug, and in particular, narcotics and anxiolytics.

Being female, however, was not a statistically significant predictor of sedative-hypnotic or stimulant use. Although these findings are not necessarily synonymous with abuse or dependence of the narcotics or anxiolytics by women and might reflect valid clinical needs, they highlight the need for clinicians to be cognizant of the potential that their female patients are receiving a disproportionate number of habit-forming prescriptions.

PSYCHIATRIC COMORBIDITY

Coexisting mental illness is common among people with alcohol or other drug disorders. And, as in the general population, the rate of depression in female alcoholic adults is twice the rate in males. Moreover, there is a link between eating disorders, especially bulimia, and alcohol and drug problems in women. In all 15% to 32% of women with alcohol or drug use disorders will satisfy lifetime diagnostic criteria for an eating disorder. Conversely, high percentages of female bulimics have alcohol abuse or dependence (14% to 49%) or other drug abuse or dependence (8% to 36%).

More generally, nearly one third of people with mental disorders have a substance abuse disorder. These comorbid conditions can complicate treatment, particularly if one or the other is overlooked. Finally a history of alcohol or drug use disorders is a well-known risk factor for suicide and domestic violence.

IDENTIFICATION AND TREATMENT

Routinely asking patients about the quantity and frequency of drug and alcohol use can be effective. Alcohol screening instruments such as the TWEAK and the T-ACE have been shown to be particularly effective for female patients. Unfortunately, there are no comparable screening instruments for drug abuse or dependence. However, neutrally worded questions about cigarette smoking and then questions about the use of other drugs can be helpful.

Of course, the patient must not only be able to communicate the necessary information, but also willing to disclose accurate descriptions of the amount and type of substance ingested, especially in settings where there are concerns about self-incrimination. Because patients are not aware of the exact nature of additives, the adulteration of many illicit substances may obscure the clinical history. Inquiries about an acute episode of intoxication may allow the clinician to learn more about chronic patterns of dysfunctional substances use and select appropriate treatment referrals.

Analysis of biologic samples is another way to identify substance use. There is no agreement among research groups about the methods of choice when analyzing biologic samples. For example, urine is the best choice for analysis of marijuana, because of its long half-life. In contrast, analysis of hair may be best for cocaine and opiates. Moreover, the value of blood markers for identification of significant prenatal alcohol exposure is being examined. Yet, patient acceptability and cost of these analyses may limit their routine implementation.

Patients who screen positive for alcohol or drug use should then be assessed for the significance of their use of substances. Individuals with moderate to severe problems should be referred to professional treatment. Brief interventions, offered by the primary care physician, for alcohol use have been effective when the severity of the alcohol problem is mild to moderate.

Three decades of scientific research and clinical practice have yielded a variety of effective treatment approaches to drug addiction treatment. Drug addiction treatment can include behavioral therapy, medications, or their combination. Treatment of addiction is as successful as treatment of other chronic diseases such as diabetes, hypertension, and asthma, resulting in benefits to the patient, her family, and community.

BIBLIOGRAPHY

American Psychiatric Association: *Diagnostic and statistical manual of mental disorders,* ed 4, Washington, DC, 1994, American Psychiatric Association.

Brown HL et al: Methadone maintenance in pregnancy: a reappraisal, *Am J Obstet Gynecol* 179:459, 1998.

Chang G: Tobacco, alcohol, and drugs during pregnancy, *Zero to Three* 19:9, 1999.

Dattel BJ: Substance use in pregnancy, *Semin Perinatol* 14:179, 1990.

Day NL, Richard GA: Prenatal marijuana use: epidemiology, methodologic issues, and infant outcome, *Clin Perinatol* 18:77, 1991.

Day NL et al: Effect of prenatal marijuana exposure on the cognitive development of offspring at age three, *Neurotoxicol Teratol* 16:169, 1994.

Fergusson DM, Horwood JL: Does cannabis use encourage other forms of illicit drug use? *Addiction* 95:505, 2000.

Finnegan LP, Wapner RJ: Narcotic addiction in pregnancy. In Neiby JR, editor: *Drug use in pregnancy.* Philadelphia, Lea & Febiger.

Fleming MF, Manwell LB: Brief intervention in primary care settings, *Alcohol Res Health* 23:128, 1999.

Gruber AJ, Pope HG: Psychiatric and medical effects of anabolic-androgenic steroid use in women, *Psychother Psychosom* 69:19, 2000.

Jaffe JH, Knapp CM, Ciraulo DA: Opiates: clinical aspects. In Lowinson JH, Ruiz PR, Millman RB, Langrod JG, editors: *Substance abuse, a comprehensive textbook,* ed 3, Baltimore, 1997, Williams & Wilkins.

Kendler KS, Prescott CA: Cannabis use, abuse, and dependence in a population-based sample of female twins, *Am J Psychiatry* 155:1016, 1998.

Kessler RC et al: Lifetime and 12 month prevalence of DSM-III-R psychiatric disorders in the United States, *Arch Gen Psychiatry* 51:8, 1994.

Kosten TR, Kleber HD: *Clinician's guide to cocaine addiction,* New York, 1992, Guilford Press.

Lilienfeld LR, Kaye WH: The link between alcoholism and eating disorders, *Alcohol Health Res World* 20:94, 1996.

National Institute on Drug Abuse. Club Drugs. http://165.112.78.61/ClubAlert/Clubdrugalert.html. 18 June 2000.

National Institute on Drug Abuse. Costs to Society. www.nida.nih.gov/infofax/costs.html. 5 November 1999.

National Institute on Drug Abuse. Nationwide Trends. www.nida.nih.gov/infofax/nationtrends.html. 29 March 2000.

National Institute on Drug Abuse. Principles of Drug Addiction Treatment, A Research Based Guide. www.nida.nih.gov/PODAT/PODAT.html. 15 December 99.

Regier DA et al: Comorbidity of mental disorders with alcohol and other drug abuse: results from the Epidemiological Catchment Area (ECA) Study, *JAMA* 21:2511, 1990.

Russell M et al: Screening for pregnancy risk-drinking, *Alcohol Clin Exp Res* 18:1156, 1994.

Sidney S et al: Marijuana use and mortality, *Am J Public Health* 87:585, 1997.

Simoni-Wastila L: The use of abusable prescription drugs: the role of gender, *J Health Women's Health Genderbased Med* 9:289, 2000.

Sokol RJ, Martier SS, Ager JW: The T-ACE questions: practical prenatal detection of risk drinking, *Am J Obstet Gynecol* 160:863, 1989.

Stoller JM et al: The prenatal detection of significant alcohol exposure with maternal blood markers, *J Pediatr* 133:346. 1998.

Strano-Rossi S: Methods used to detect drug abuse in pregnancy: a brief review, *Drug Alcohol Dependence* 53:257, 1999.

Wagner LA et al: Prevalence and correlates of drug use and dependence in the United States, *Arch Gen Psychiatry* 52:219, 1995.

CHAPTER 92

Stress Management

Kathleen Hubbs Ulman

In recent years the role of stress in the development and course of illness has been increasingly recognized and integrated into the overall understanding of health in our culture. Experts define stress in several ways: (1) as a stimulus, acute or chronic, that requires adaptation or (2) as the altered state that is the result of inadequate adaptation to a life event.

Recent studies of the relationship between stress and health suggest that the increase in risk of illness for an individual is mediated by several psychosocial factors. The key factors are the meaning of an individual's life situation, adaptation to stress as determined by an individual's personality and coping style, and the influence of an individual's characteristic psychologic reactions on general physiologic functioning and, in particular, the immune system.

As with much medical and psychologic research, men were the subjects of the majority of the initial studies of stress. Only in the last few decades have women been included as subjects in studies concerning the effects of work, personal life, personality, coping style, and emotional functioning on health. This research has shown that the circumstances under which women experience psychologic and physical distress are sometimes different from those that influence men. In addition, psycholinguistic theory and research have shown gender differences in the ways in which men and women present and discuss physical and emotional symptoms with their physicians.

The primary care physician can increase the recognition of the role of stress in the symptoms of women patients by learning about the role of stress in illness in general and understanding the risk factors associated with increased illness in women, in particular. In addition, the primary care physician can increase the likelihood of diagnosing a stress-related illness in female patients by listening carefully to a woman's description of symptoms and asking for information regarding the context of her life, general mood, and sense of satisfaction with her life. During the information-gathering portion of the examination it is important for the physician to convey to the patient a sense of understanding and acceptance of her situation. Women in particular respond more positively to a physician's recommendations if they feel understood and listened to rather than labeled.

Once the stress in a woman's life is diagnosed and acknowledged by both patient and physician, the primary care physician can provide basic counseling in methods to reduce stress. All suggested changes should be carefully outlined in detail. The physician's prescription for stress-reducing lifestyle changes such as exercise, recreation, or increased social contact has great power for women who have been socialized to put others' needs first. Some women will be able to initiate stress-reducing changes and set limits on demands of family and work only by invoking the authority of their physician. For patients with more complicated situations, the primary care physician can supplement the basic counseling with an appropriate psychiatric referral (Box 92-1).

EPIDEMIOLOGY AND RISK FACTORS FOR STRESS
Prevalence

It is well established in the medical literature that at a given age men have increased rates of mortality and life-threatening illness, whereas women have increased rates of morbidity and nonfatal chronic conditions. Thus men die at a younger age, and women have more chronic illness that interferes with everyday functioning and impairs their quality of life. Women are twice as likely as men to suffer from depression, another risk factor for increased morbidity rate. Women also have increased rates of symptom reporting and increased use of medication and medical services.

Epidemiologic studies suggest that biologic factors play a primary role in the sex differences in mortality rate, whereas social factors play a major role in the sex differences in morbidity rate. In U.S. society women are more vulnerable to the social factors associated with increased risk of nonfatal chronic conditions. These risk factors are discussed in the following section.

Risk Factors for Stress
Men and Women

Psychosocial factors that compromise health can be divided into acute and chronic categories (Box 92-2). The acute stressors may be external events such as loss of employment, sudden illness, death of a loved one, rape, or a natural disaster.

BOX 92-1
Order of Psychosocial Interventions

Diagnose stress
Suggest appropriate environmental and behavior change
Schedule follow-up visit to evaluate change
With appropriate change:
   Reinforce change
   Consider referral to counseling for further exploration and change
   Refer cases of incest and rape for counseling
No appropriate change:
   Refer for counseling with follow-up evaluation

BOX 92-2
Risk Factors for Health Impairment: Men and Women

Acute
Loss of employment
Assault
Natural disaster

Chronic
Personal:
   Marital conflict
   Recent separation
   Bereavement
   Loneliness
   Dissatisfaction with one's life
   Type A personality
   History of incest
   History of physical abuse
Work-related:
   Job with little control
   Dissatisfaction with one's job
Work and personal:
   Roles with irregular schedules
   Roles with little time pressure
   Roles with great time pressure
   Roles with decreased responsibility
   Roles with decreased activity

Chronic stressors may be any ongoing aversive situation that requires adaptation such as marital problems, divorce, conflict at work, job insecurity, economic pressure, a history of childhood trauma, a chronic medical problem in a family member or oneself, or an emotional problem such as anxiety or depression.

Research on the impact of acute stressors such as natural disasters and unexpected events shows that most people recover and do well after such events. Recovery depends in part on how the acute stressor fits into the worldview of the individual and how it meshes with her history. If the individual feels that the event can be understood within her expectations for her life, the event is less likely to cause prolonged distress. However, if the event drastically challenges the individual's view of the world and interferes with the individual's sense of control, the experience can be traumatic and have psychologic and physical consequences. For example, if a woman believes that death is part of a greater scheme and that she will see her loved one after her death, she may move from a state of shock and distress caused by the unexpected death of her husband to a state of acceptance and adaptation more quickly and completely than someone who feels that death is random. If a woman is raped in her own home, her general sense of where she is safe in the world has been violated. For a while she may feel in constant danger and will remain in a continual state of arousal and distress. The longer she stays in this state of arousal and distress, the more likely it is that her health may suffer. The length of time in which she remains in a state of physical arousal will depend in part on her history, her style of coping, and the psychosocial context of her life.

There are some areas of similarity in the effects of chronic stress on health risk for both sexes. For men and women alike dissatisfaction with one's life and roles is associated with ill health. It is the individual's subjective reactions to his or her roles that have impact on health rather than the exact job or life position. Roles associated with less responsibility and less activity are associated with ill health. In addition roles that include either great or little time pressure are associated with increased health risk. In contrast, increased role involvements or responsibilities for men and women are not associated with increased health risks. Rather, involvement in an activity that has value and meaning for the individual at a level of responsibility that matches his or her temperament and physical and emotional capacity is associated with decreased health risk.

Personality and coping style are thought to play a role in the impact of stressful events or roles on health. For many years a type A personality style has been associated with increased risk for heart disease in men. This personality style includes a chronic sense of time urgency. Thought patterns can also influence health. A pattern of critical and negative thoughts about oneself and others is associated with an increased risk of depression and ill health. Kobasa found that individuals who shared three characteristics she called stress-hardiness had a decreased risk of ill health when subjected to stress. These characteristics are (1) a strong sense of commitment to life and work, (2) a sense of control over one's life, and (3) a perception of life changes as a challenge.

Women
Roles

The type and variety of roles a woman enjoys have an influence on her health. Married employed parents have the best health profiles. Employment contributes the most health protection to married women. In contrast, marriage contributes the most protection to men. Unemployed married women above age 40 have the poorest health.

As stated previously, women's increased risk of morbidity has been attributed to social factors related in part to women's roles. Many women tend to be dissatisfied with their primary roles, which they often see as having low status. They also tend to have fewer roles and thus decreased opportunities to derive gratification and enjoyment from a number of sources. Women's traditional roles include characteristics associated with increased morbidity rate such as low income, irregular time schedules, and low or high time pressure. Women who pursue advanced career opportunities of their choice may enjoy some protection from these health risks. However, career women with children often have irregular time schedules and high time pressure. These women are at risk for the development of stress-related illness when their multiple roles involve excessive demands. Brisson et al. found that women with both high job strain and significant family responsibilities had greater increases in blood pressure than those women who had only one of these factors.

Social Context

The generality of the increased health protection afforded by roles is influenced by the context of a woman's life at home and at work. The amount of physical help a married woman receives at home and the amount of emotional support and validation she receives in her marriage influence her health. In addition, the degree to which others depend on her for care and nurturance influences a woman's vulnerability to ill health. Too few or too many demands from others increase a woman's health risk. Depression in mothers increases as the number of children increases and the age of the youngest child decreases. Luecken et al. reported that working women with children at home excreted more cortisol and reported higher levels of strain at home than working women without children at home. When an elderly parent needs care, women usually take on these responsibilities in addition to work and care for their own children. Primary caregivers of Alzheimer's patients have been found to have decreased immune function.

The quality of a woman's relationships at home and at work is an important factor related to her health and her satisfaction with her roles. For a woman, a supportive relationship must be one in which she can confide her feelings as well as provide caring. Depression in women is often associated with unequal relationships in which women provide much care and nurturance and receive little affirmation and support in return. Thus involvement in large social networks where many individuals depend on a woman for help and give little in return increases her health risk.

The impact of employment on a woman's health depends on the conditions of her work and her feelings about her work. A woman who works out of economic necessity in a clerical job with little control or satisfaction enjoys much less health protection than a woman who has chosen to work, who finds work relationships supportive, or who is in a career of her choice.

Women are also vulnerable to particular stressors in our culture such as violence, rape, incest, sexual objectification, and economic problems that increase risk of morbidity. Hamilton reported that young women who have been sexually objectified and treated as adornments demonstrate symptoms of stress and have an increased vulnerability to depression. Goldenhar et al. found that women construction workers exposed to sexual harassment and gender discrimination reported increased levels of nausea and headaches. Often stressors such as rape and incest are accompanied by shame, which promotes isolation, impedes the use of social and medical resources, and thus increases health risk. Women with histories of childhood sexual abuse are particularly susceptible to the effects of daily stress and often have increased reporting of physical symptoms. Pennebaker found that women who had experienced childhood trauma and had not confided in anyone saw physicians more often than those who had discussed the trauma with someone.

Sex Role Socialization and Psychologic Development of Women

Women's psychologic development is profoundly affected by our culture's definition of a desirable woman as being attractive, nurturing, selfless, and peace-making. The development of self-esteem is impaired in young females as they become aware of the devaluation and categorization of women as second-class citizens by virtue of their biologic characteristics. Socialization encourages women to be compliant with social expectations and to neglect their own sensations and perceptions of events in favor of responding to others' needs. As a consequence many adult women today derive self-esteem from and organize their identity around pleasing and caring for others. They are encouraged to locate the control of their lives in others' needs and are thus disconnected from their own perceptions and needs. This difficulty in separating herself from the needs and distress of those around her makes it difficult for a woman to set limits on others to attend to her own emotional or physical needs and puts her at risk for ill health.

Difficulty in setting limits occurs for many women both at home with their families and at work. Women in professional careers are not immune from this difficulty of setting limits. Yet according to Lawler and Schmidt, the ability to see oneself, rather than external events, as the source of decisions and control of one's life is the very aspect of "stress-hardiness" that appears to be most protective of women's health. Thus women's tendency in our culture to see themselves and their lives as determined by external forces contributes to an increased health risk.

Personality Style and Identity

The degree to which a woman's roles fit with her views of herself as a woman influences her health. As stated previously the personality traits associated with stress-hardiness are incompatible with the ways women are socialized in our society. In addition the direct and strong expression of anger is discouraged in women. Direct expression of anger is associated with decreased heart rate and blood pressure in women as well as men. Thomas and Williams report that the more a woman can discuss anger directly at work or at home rather than suppress it or use it to blame others, the better her health. Women with less traditional sex role norms are better able to negotiate for themselves and to express anger than women who identify with a traditional female sex role.

Roles, social context, and sex role norms can come together to provide increased health risk for women. Clerical workers have almost twice the rate of coronary heart disease (CHD) of women who work in the home. The factors associated with CHD for clerical workers are suppressed hostility, a nonsupportive boss, and decreased job mobility. The highest rate of CHD is in clerical workers with children who are married to blue-collar workers. Women with traditional sex role norms whose spouses offer only minimal task sharing and who do not have a supportive confidante are at the greatest risk for health problems.

A list of risk factors for health impairment in women is shown in Box 92-3.

BOX 92-3
Risk Factors for Health Impairment: Women

Acute
Rape

Chronic
Personal:
   Intimate relationship with unsupportive mate
   Friendships that are not supportive
   Family relationships that are not supportive
   Family relationships that require extra help and support
   Sick spouse, child, or parent
   Personality that suppresses anger
   Several young children
   Lack of sharing of domestic chores
Work:
   Unsupportive boss
   Work in clerical job out of economic necessity
   Decreased job mobility
Overall:
   Unemployed, married, and more than 40 years old
   Clerical worker with children and married to blue-collar worker

PATHOPHYSIOLOGY

The belief that psychologic experiences influence risk of ill health and course of disease has been part of everyday folklore for centuries. However, it wasn't until the twentieth century that scientists were able to describe the physiologic association between stress and emotion and illness. Cannon and Selye demonstrated that stress and emotions activate the sympathetic adrenal-medullary system and the hypothalamic-pituitary-adrenocortical system as well as other endocrine systems. Each of these systems affects immunity.

The sympathetic adrenal-medullary system is usually stimulated by the emotions of fear, anger, and excitement. When activated this system releases epinephrine, norepinephrine, and other catecholamines. The release of catecholamines has been shown to reduce the functional efficacy of lymphocytes while at the same time moving them out of storage. The hypothalamic-pituitary-adrenocortical system is associated with chronic stress and depression. The activation of this system results in the release of adrenocorticotropic hormone and corticosteroids, which in turn has been shown to result in suppression of T-cell and natural killer cell activity. Additionally, stress stimulates the release of endogenous opioids. In animal studies opioids have been associated with suppressed immune function.

Life situations that include loss or conflict are often associated with decreased immune system functioning and with increased symptoms of ill health or with a more severe course of an illness. According to Kiecolt-Glaser, individuals in a distressed marital relationship or those recently separated have decreased immune function as measured by percentage of natural killer cells. The degree of decreased immune function is related to the amount of attachment to the spouse and to the length of separation. The longer the individual has been separated, the more likely the immune function will return to normal. Other studies have indicated that loneliness and bereavement are related to poor immune functioning. Finding a new partner is associated with increased immune function for separated and divorced people.

It appears that having a supportive social network in which a woman can express her feelings and experience a sense of understanding and respect promotes good immune functioning and may interact with other physiologic factors to influence the course of an illness. The act of putting feelings into symbolic expression, particularly words, relieves distress and diminishes risk of ill health. Pennebaker has found that writing about feelings associated with current stressful situations or past traumas improves immune function, decreases physician visits, and decreases subjective distress. Individuals who have not discussed their feelings about unpleasant situations or traumas demonstrate the largest increases in immune functioning as a result of writing about feelings. Holding back feelings may heighten autonomic system activity, which, over time, leads to changes in immune functioning. Individuals with a medical illness who participate in individual or group psychotherapy demonstrate decreased use of medication, decreased number of medical office visits, and increased immune functioning.

DIFFERENTIAL DIAGNOSIS

The diagnosis of either acute or ongoing stress in a medical patient is complex and often not definitive. Yet a timely diagnosis and appropriate interventions are important parts of a patient's overall care and may increase the rate of recovery from an acute illness, prevent the development of an ongoing chronic condition, or stabilize a chronic disease, thereby significantly improving the quality of life and decreasing physician office visits and medication use. The cost of interventions such as a stress management group is offset by fewer office visits to the primary care physician and decreased use of medication. The primary care clinician may be the only person in contact with the patient who is in a position to make the diagnosis and initiate the appropriate intervention. When evaluating a patient for stress-related problems, the possibility of a depression or anxiety disorder should always be considered. Often these can be diagnosed and treated concurrently with the evaluation and treatment of stress.

Stress can influence any system and aggravate any chronic disease. Thus the diagnosis cannot be made on the basis of a specific constellation of symptoms. The process of diagnosing stress-related problems is further complicated by the fact that patients often do not recognize that they are stressed, and if they do recognize the stress, they are not aware that the physician can offer interventions that will decrease their level of stress. The presence of symptoms that may be related to stress can be suspected when the total picture does not make sense: when for example an infection persists or reappears repeatedly despite recommended treatment, or a chronic disease has an unexpected flare-up. The diagnosis is often made by using a combination of knowledge of known risk factors and knowledge of the particular patient's medical history and life situation.

In addition to evaluating the presence of known risk factors, the clinician can look for the presence of behaviors associated with emotional distress such as sleep disturbance, changes in eating, increased alcohol consumption, changes in balance of time spent in work or recreation, changes in amount of time spent with others, and increases in negative critical thoughts. When such changes are present the possibility of a depression or anxiety disorder should be considered. The clinician should also inquire about factors known to be protective of health such as the ability to devote some time to work or hobbies that are meaningful, time spent relaxing, and availability of a supportive network of friends. Such questions as "How many people depend on you?" "Whom do you talk to?" "Do you have someone to confide in?" and "Whom can you ask to take over when you need help?" often provide important information.

Clinical Presentation

Women whose lives involve the level of distress that might compromise their health present themselves in the physician's office in several ways. The presentation depends, in part, on the woman's personality, her understanding of her symptoms, and her situation.

The Insightful Patient

A woman who recognizes the connection between symptoms and stress will often start her visit with the statement that some physical symptoms are bothering her and she is also going through a difficult time in her life. She often wants reassurance that the symptoms are connected to stress and not a more serious illness. She may also want assistance in the form of listening or a referral for stress management or counseling. The difficulty with such patients is that in spite of the stress there also may be more serious physical problems that need to be evaluated and treated. Thus the physician should not be too easily swayed by the patient's self-diagnosis of stress.

The Naive Patient

Another common presentation is that of a woman who has a list of physical complaints such as tiredness, stiff neck, and stomach pains that have developed in the past year. In response to questioning, she states that a relative is dying and her husband recently lost his job. She has not connected her symptoms with her life situation but does acknowledge she is experiencing psychologic distress. Her ability to experience and acknowledge psychologic distress will make it easier for the physician to make the diagnosis and for the patient to assume some responsibility to initiate new behaviors to take care of herself.

The Stoical Patient

One of the more difficult presentations is that of a woman who describes a variety of symptoms that are causing her significant physical distress. All physical and laboratory findings are normal. On questioning she maintains that emotionally she is fine although she has had significant losses or changes in her life in the past year. It is in relation to this type of patient that knowledge of the known risk factors associated with ill health in women is important. This woman is not able to perceive or acknowledge that the circumstances of her life are putting her at risk. Often some of these women are opposed to acknowledging the influence of the overall context of their lives on their health because they need to see themselves as being invulnerable to stress and as having the capacity to weather any life circumstance with no emotional or physical sequelae. Chapter 82 provides a more detailed discussion of somatization.

The Denying Patient

Another type of presentation is given by a woman who does not expect much out of her life. This woman's identity is derived from taking care of others. She has little or no appreciation of her own needs. Her personality and view of herself do not allow for active assessment of the situation or interventions to ameliorate the condition for herself. Often this type of patient just wants her symptoms treated and does not want to embark on any exploration of her life situation because she fears any disruption of her sense of self or of close relationships.

A complicated situation in which the contribution of stress is often not recognized is that of a woman who has an acute life-threatening illness such as a myocardial infarction or a serious exacerbation of a chronic illness such as diabetes or asthma. The patient's medical condition is so serious that the initial focus must be on stabilization and treatment of symptoms. However, even when medical treatment is instituted, her condition may remain unstable or she may not return to her previous level of health. This lack of expected progress or relapse should be a red flag to the physician to explore the role of stress in the patient's recuperation and adjustment to her illness. For such a patient the diagnosis of the contribution of stress to her serious medical condition is essential to the outcome of her disease. The woman's life situation may include several risk factors associated with diminished health, such as an abusive marriage, single parenthood, inability to enlist the help of her husband in order to decrease her responsibilities at home, absence of a confidante, and presence of a history of childhood sexual trauma.

For such patients two types of psychosocial interventions may be useful. The first is an overall evaluation of her day-to-day life with consideration of whether there is anyone to help her and whether she continues to care for others such as her husband, children, and other relatives in spite of her serious medical difficulties. This is often particularly characteristic of older couples with traditional lifestyles. Women with serious medical conditions may continue to take total responsibility for their own and their husband's care and may not mention this to their physician unless directly asked. In such cases some form of counseling that includes the spouse and other family members may be useful.

The second type of intervention is to provide the opportunity for the woman to talk about previously unexpressed feelings with a confidante, a therapist, a support group, or a stress management group. Such a process can bring about increased self-esteem, an increase in an internal sense of control, and an increase in options that provide a woman with a sense that she can exert control over her day-to-day life by asking others for help and initiating activities that are gratifying and rewarding for her. As stated previously, having a supportive network and talking to a confidante increase immune function and thus may contribute to the stabilization of a serious chronic medical condition. Individuals with a medical illness who participate in individual or group psychotherapy demonstrate decreased use of medication, decreased number of office visits, increased immune functioning, and in some studies, increased longevity.

THERAPY AND MANAGEMENT

Once the physician has determined that a woman's symptoms are in part stress-related, several types of intervention are available. The particular intervention or combination of interventions chosen will depend on the symptom pattern, the patient's life circumstances, and the patient's personality (Box 92-4).

One of the most useful treatment strategies is to change the individual's environment when possible. Areas that can be changed include increasing the amount of help with physical responsibilities, decreasing the burden of responsibilities involved in caring for others, rearranging the daily schedule to make it less stressful, increasing opportunities for care for the patient, and arranging changes in the physical environment if appropriate.

The second type of useful treatment strategy is to change the patient's behavior and psychologic functioning. One major mode of behavior change is to stop behavior that perpetuates the stressful experience. This might include improved nutrition, changes in sleep routine, improved time management, decrease in alcohol use, decreased negative thinking, and decreased exposure to stressful relationships or tasks. Another behavioral intervention is to introduce behavior that produces a state of relaxation such as training in relaxation, meditation, self-hypnosis, or introduction of exercise in the appropriate amount.

The introduction of opportunities to change psychologic functioning and self-esteem is the third form of intervention to reduce stress. Examples include encouragement of increased time spent in validating and supportive relationships, increase in meaningful responsibilities, and expression of emotion in writing or in person to the appropriate people.

One result of a discussion of possible behavioral and psychologic changes is to increase the patient's awareness of the possibility of change and the existence of alternatives. Such a discussion also conveys to the patient that her physician sees her as worthy of having her needs taken seriously and as being able to take active control over some aspects of her life.

The degree to which the clinician will be able to discuss these possible changes with a patient will depend on available time and severity of illness. However, the time spent in discussing these options for lifestyle changes and stress reduction will be offset by the decreased number of office visits. It is important for the clinician to remember that direct advice from the physician or from other clinicians in authoritative roles can be effective in empowering a woman to make changes that have a positive influence on her health. Many women who experience stress-related health problems have low self-esteem, have been socialized to derive their self-esteem from caring for others, and may be in a personal or work relationship that continues to encourage them to neglect themselves. Often they have become disconnected from their own perceptions and lack the belief that they can take their needs into account and still be valued.

Straightforward prescriptions for lifestyle changes are important. The physician's authority gives the patient permission and validation to set limits on the demands of others and to engage in stress-reducing behaviors. Although statements such as "You must find time to exercise each week" may seem simple, the physician may be the first person or at least the only person in her current life that conveys to her a sense of worthiness and entitlement to self-care.

The final option for behavior and psychologic change is to refer for stress management or counseling. Stress management will provide an opportunity for the patient to reflect on the relationship between her internal experience, external events and her physical symptoms. Counseling will provide an opportunity for the patient to receive validation, to organize her thoughts and feelings into words, to discuss feelings and memories of events that may never before have been shared, and to become aware of options for change—all factors that have been demonstrated to reduce health risks and improve immune function. Domar and Dreher have outlined in great detail the positive health benefits for women of stress management programs, particularly for premenstrual syndrome, hot flashes, and infertility.

Indications for Referral

The primary care clinician can help the woman initiate changes to reduce her level of stress. Initially the clinician can suggest behavior changes (e.g., exercise, recreation, alcohol intake, family care responsibilities) with a return visit in a month. The return visit will give the clinician an opportunity to assess the ability of the patient to initiate changes in her life. If the appropriate behavior changes have been made, the clinician and patient can assess the degree of symptom relief that the patient has obtained from these changes. If the degree of relief is satisfactory, the patient can be encouraged to continue the new behavior and return for follow-up evaluation in several months.

If the degree of relief is not satisfactory, in spite of the behavior changes the patient may be referred for further help such as relaxation training, hypnosis, or a stress management

---

BOX 92-4
Stress-Reducing Interventions

Change Environment
Reducing external stress such as noise, pollution
Reducing stimulation at home
When possible reducing stimulation at work
Reducing threats to physical safety
Ensuring fulfillment of basic physical needs

Change Behavior
Nutrition
Exercise
Alcohol consumption
Sleep
Relaxation, meditation, or hypnosis
Reduced exposure to conflicted situations
Time management

Change Psychologic Functioning
Increasing awareness of options
Increasing awareness of possibility of internal change
Increasing sense of validity of limit setting
Increasing awareness of feelings
Increasing verbal expression of feelings
Increasing confidence in one's perceptions

group. If the patient is interested in exploring the role of her psychologic functioning and feelings in the development of the stress-related symptoms a referral for psychotherapy can be considered. The possibility of an unrecognized depression or anxiety disorder should also be evaluated. The diagnosis of depression or anxiety does not exclude further recommendations for stress reduction. Referrals for stress management or psychotherapy are cost-effective in the long run. Most managed care programs will cover such referrals.

If at the follow-up visit it is determined that behavior changes have not been initiated, the clinician should gently explore the reasons why. Often underlying issues that may prevent the implementation of such changes will become evident. For example, a woman may be so out of touch with signals from her body that the word *relaxation* has no meaning to her; a patient may have used excessive activity as a means of distracting herself from intolerable feelings and may not be able to relax until she begins to address the intolerable feelings; or a woman may be so dependent on her husband or others for approval that she may be unable to set limits in order to care for herself. Again the possibility of an underlying depression must be considered. When a patient is unable to initiate behavior changes a referral for psychotherapy is appropriate for the exploration and treatment of obstacles to change. A referral for behavior therapy or relaxation training may fail until the underlying obstacles to change are identified and changed. If the patient feels she might be able to initiate behavior changes in the context of increased support, a referral to a support group or stress management group could be made. However, with a patient who has demonstrated difficulty with initiation a follow-up to the referral is recommended.

Women are vulnerable to diminished health and are at risk for illness in our society because of their vulnerability to violence and because of their focus on providing nurturance for others as a source of self-esteem in a society that does not value that role. Visiting a physician for ill health is acceptable to women in their roles as nurturers. Thus physicians need to understand the importance to female patients of their suggestions and prescriptions for change and use them to help women care for themselves and set limits on others. It is vital that physicians who treat women appreciate the value of indicating to female patients in a variety of ways that the balance of rewards and demands in their lives has an impact on their physical and psychologic well-being.

BIBLIOGRAPHY

Abel JL, Larkin KT, Edens JL: Women, anger, and cardiovascular responses to stress, *J Psychosom Res* 39:251, 1995.

Belle D: Gender differences in the social moderators of stress. In Barnett RC, Biener L, Baruch GK, editors: *Gender and stress,* New York, 1987, The Free Press.

Brisson C et al: Effect of family responsibilities and job strain on ambulatory blood pressure among white-collar women, *Psychosom Med* 61:205, 1999.

Domar, AD, Benson, H: Application of behavioral medicine techniques to the treatment of infertility. In Seibel M, editor: *Technology and infertility,* New York, 1993, Springer.

Domar AD, Dreher H: *Healing mind, healthy woman.* New York, 1996, Henry Holt.

Domar AD, Irvin JH, Mills D: Use of relaxation training to reduce the frequency and intensity of tamoxifen induced hot flashes, *Mind Body Medicine* 2:82, 1997.

Ferrie JE et al: An uncertain future: the health effects of threats to employment security in white-collar men and women, *Am J Public Health* 88:1030, 1998.

Frankenhauser M, Lundberg U, Chesney M, editors: *Women, work, and health: stress and opportunities,* New York, 1991, Plenum Press.

Goldenhar LM et al: Stressors and adverse outcomes for female construction workers, *J Occup Health Psychol* 3:19, 1997.

Goodale I, Domar AD, Benson H: Alleviation of premenstrual symptoms with the relaxation response, *Obstet Gynecol* 75:649, 1990.

Hamilton JA: Objectification experiences in relational orientation predict depression in women. Unpublished paper presented at American Psychological Association meeting Psychosocial Factors in Women's Health: Creating an Agenda for the 21st Century, Washington, DC, May 1994.

Haynes SG, Feinlieb M: Women, work, and coronary heart disease: findings from the Framingham heart study, *Am J Public Health* 70:133, 1980.

Kiecolt-Glaser JK et al: Marital quality, marital disruption, and immune function, *Psychosom Med* 49:13, 1987.

Kiecolt-Glaser JK et al: Negative behavior during marital conflict is associated with immunological down-regulation, *Psychosom Med* 55:395, 1993.

Kiecolt-Glaser JK et al: Spousal caregivers of dementia victims: longitudinal changes in immunity and health, *Psychosom Med* 53:345, 1991.

Kobasa SCO: Stress responses and personality. In Barnett RC, Biener L, Baruch GK, editors: *Gender and stress,* New York, 1987, The Free Press.

Lawler KA, Schmidt LA: A prospective study of women's health: the effects of stress, hardiness, locus of control, type A behavior, and physiological reactivity, *Women Health* 19:27, 1992.

Luecken LJ et al: Stress in employed women: impact of marital status and children at home on neurohormone output and home strain, *Psychosom Med* 59:352, 1997.

O'Leary A: Stress, emotion, and human immune function, *Psychol Bull* 108:363, 1990.

Pennebaker JW: Putting stress into words: health, linguistic, and therapeutic implications, *Behav Res Ther* 31:539, 1993.

Peterson C, Seligman MEP, Vaillant GE: Pessimistic explanatory style is a risk factor for physical illness: a thirty-five-year longitudinal study, *J Personality Social Psychol* 55:23, 1988.

Spiegel D, Bloom JR, Kraemer HC, Gottheil E: Effect of psychosocial treatment on survival of patients with metastatic breast cancer, *Lancet* ii:888, 1989.

Thakkar RR, McCanne TR: The effects of daily stressors on physical health in women with and without a childhood history of sexual abuse, *Child Abuse Neglect* 24:209, 2000.

Thomas SP, Williams R: Relationships among perceived stress, trait anger, modes of anger expression, and health status of college men and women, *Nurs Res* 40:303, 1991.

Ulman KH: Group psychotherapy with the medically ill. In Kaplan HI, Sadock BJ, editors: *Comprehensive group psychotherapy,* Baltimore, 1993, Williams & Wilkins.

Vanfossen BE: Sex differences in the mental health effects of spouse support and equity, *J Health Soc Behav* 22:130, 1981.

Verbrugge LM: Role burdens and physical health of women and men, *Women Health* 11:47, 1986.

Woods NF: Women's lives: pressure and pleasure, conflict and support. *Health Care Women Int* 8:109, 1987.

Wortman CB et al: Stress, coping, and health: conceptual issues and directions for future research. In Friedman HS, editor: *Hostility, coping and health,* Washington, DC, 1992, American Psychological Association.

CHAPTER 93

Care of the Homeless Woman

Roseanna H. Means

EPIDEMIOLOGY

Despite a public perception of robust economic prosperity at the turn of the millennium, homelessness is on the rise in the United States as a result of increased poverty and a lack of affordable housing. Additional factors in the increasing numbers of homeless are the rising numbers of uninsured and the explosion in domestic violence, with few safe options available for the fleeing victims, the majority of whom are women. Battered women's shelters are often filled, leaving women and often, their children, choosing between an unsafe home and the street or a less safe shelter.

DEMOGRAPHIC FEATURES

Most recent point-prevalence estimates put the total of homeless at 1 to 3 million. The U.S. Conference of Mayors estimates that, among the urban homeless, single men account for 45%, single women 14%, and families the rest. Families headed by single women are the fastest growing subgroup, representing more than 40% of all homeless. Children under 18 make up 25% of the urban homeless population.

The racial/ethnic composition of homeless persons is 49% African-American, 32% Caucasian, 12% Hispanic, 4% Native American, and 3% Asian.

The rising numbers of homeless place an additional financial burden on a strained health care system in longer lengths of stay and increased costs of care. This chapter focuses on the scope of the care of women without homes: risk factors, screening, the pathophysiology of homelessness, clinical aspects, how to perform an evaluation of the homeless woman patient using a history-taking tool and finally, strategies to engage homeless women in the health care system.

RISK FACTORS

Risk factors for homelessness in women are a history of violence, especially childhood sexual assault, foster home placement, or any prolonged, unrelenting psychologic, and physical or emotional trauma. All of these factors can produce emotional developmental paralysis, which leads to indecisiveness, disorganized thinking, impulsive behavior, unrealistic expectations, and an inability to cope with every-

day life stresses. Trauma and abuse lead to post-traumatic stress disorder (PTSD). Women who use alcohol or drugs to escape trauma memories, guilt, or shame complicate their lives further, and put their children at risk of public custody. Mental illness is not thought to be a major independent cause of homelessness in women, but becomes a risk factor when accompanied by poverty and lack of social support.

SCREENING

The majority of homeless women are found in cities. Homelessness exists in the suburbs and countryside, but fewer shelters are established in those locations. Some readily report their status and where they are staying, or it will be obvious to the provider because the address given is a shelter address. However, many women report feeling profoundly humiliated by their homelessness. Society views women as nurturers and caretakers. They report feeling numb, embarrassed, and ashamed. Because of the perceived stigma of homelessness, these women will not readily reveal this fact about themselves in health care settings. The caregiver needs to look for "warning signs" in the patient's history or behavior to open the door to a line of questioning about homelessness.

Impoverished women who demonstrate "warning signs" in their histories or behaviors should be considered at risk of homelessness (Box 93-1).

PATHOPHYSIOLOGY
Paths to Homelessness

The paths to homelessness are both acute and chronic. It can start with an acute devastating loss such as a natural disaster (fire, flood) or financial burden such as an unforeseen medical crisis. Or, it can happen over time, with a gradual slide into poverty without affordable housing alternatives. Acutely homeless women are often helped by private relief organizations such as the Red Cross, Salvation Army, or the United Way when a natural disaster occurs. These women are not usually at risk of chronic homelessness because they have family and social supports to carry them through the crisis period. But women who are impoverished financially, emotionally, mentally, cognitively, or behaviorally, or who are

BOX 93-1
History Indicative of Possible Homelessness

- Chronic and persistent noncompliance with treatment regimens or appointments
- Poor judgment or high-risk behaviors, especially for situations where the choices are clearly detrimental to their health
- Poor hygiene manifested as profound body odor, unkempt appearance, or serious or resistant lice or scabies infections
- Secretive or inconsistent responses to questions about address
- Chronic alcoholism and/or substance abuse
- Mental illness with inadequate social support
- Victim of repeated and/or profoundly threatening physical, sexual, and/or emotional abuse
- Chronic somatization of underlying abuse such as refractory gastrointestinal illness, psychologic illness, or chronic pain

victims of battery or chronic medical conditions are at much greater risk of slipping through the safety net and ending up on the streets or in the shelters. The task of obtaining food, clothing, shelter, and safety each day becomes progressively harder, impairing the ability to end the homelessness. To avail oneself of public benefits requires navigating a confusing array of bureaucratic agencies, each with its own rules and regulations. Lacking a stable address or phone number impedes this application process as well as securing employment. Eligibility requirements are determined through state and federal policies, many of which are confusing. Nevertheless, for health coverage, Medicaid benefits can improve health care access for homeless persons, so every effort should be made to help with enrollment.

THE IMPACT OF HOMELESSNESS ON WOMEN AND THEIR FAMILIES

Women on the cusp of homelessness use short-term solutions: family and friends, or private relief. When those solutions end, women are faced with the daunting prospect of finding shelter, often a process of trial and error.

The first burden faced by each homeless woman is that the ability to secure a shelter is contingent on available facilities and daily availability of a shelter bed. Many states categorize homeless persons by age, gender, family status, mental health status, or whether fleeing from a batterer. Pregnant women and single women with families are eligible for family shelters, single women can go to teen or adult women's shelters, and women who qualify for Department of Mental Health (DMH) assistance can go to a DMH shelter. Even if shelter beds are available, women are forced to make difficult choices to be sheltered. The shelter may be distant from her known community. Her teenage male children may not be allowed. She may not be able to sleep with her partner. The shelter may not be in a safe area, close to her source of medical care, or she might not qualify through the state's eligibility rules.

To function successfully, many shelters have rules that hinder personal autonomy, often with strict curfews, set hours for services, and level of services dependent on the shelter's budget. For instance, one might get housing help at one location but will need to go elsewhere for a midday meal or for medical care. In shelters located in the city, one must line up outside and wait often for several hours to secure a bed for the evening, risking outdoor exposure and precluding regular employment.

Safety is a significant problem. Often shelters are in unsafe areas of the city with many single women from urban shelters reporting suffering physical and sexual assault, gun shot, or knife injuries. The nature of the population—gang members, ex-convicts, drug addicts and dealers, and those with severe personality disorders and mental illness—contributes to the lack of safety. Nationally, there are too few shelters for battered women, so that some women fleeing a batterer end up in an adult shelter where they face further assault on the streets. The constant need to be hypervigilant and the transient lifestyle contribute to chronic sleep deprivation and its consequences.

BARRIERS TO CARE

The extraordinary number of individuals who have fallen below society's safety nets are not always able to access appropriate health care because of a multitude of barriers, both intrinsic and extrinsic. Intrinsic barriers include an overwhelming sense of hopelessness, prior negative experiences with multiple governmental bureaucracies, past emotional and psychologic insults, or from coexisting mental illness or substance abuse. Homeless pregnant women and immigrants fear exposing themselves to authorities out of perceived concerns that they will be vulnerable to punitive action.

The extrinsic factors are generated from the social reality of homelessness, from the medical profession, and from the government and insurance agencies. Being homeless poses challenges of distance, poverty, lack of insurance, transience, exhaustion and sleep deprivation, trauma, and violence.

As a result of the relentless assaults on one's autonomy, safety, nutrition, and health, many suffer from permanent psychologic harm. Chronically homeless women may exhibit signs of emotional numbing, dissociation, illogical reasoning, poor judgment, self-harm, and inconsistency.

Homeless patients often report being reprimanded or mislabeled as "psych patients" by practitioners for their adaptive behaviors, without knowing why the patient was making poor choices. Clinics and emergency departments often are uneducated about available community services. Follow-up and compliance with medical treatment are difficult for the homeless and frustrating for the clinician.

Finally, government and public agencies present extraordinary challenges for women who are homeless. Each agency has its own eligibility, application, and enrollment process. Women requiring multiple services are required to apply at multiple sites, many of which require documentation such as W-2 forms, birth certificates, or Social Security cards, and all of these are easily stolen if one is attacked on the street. Under Medicaid, one must prove eligibility for initial and continued access. The rules change with the political winds and bear little reality to the exigencies of life on the streets. Without a fixed address or telephone, many women who go through the process of applying can lose their benefits simply because they cannot be adequately tracked.

BOX 93-2

Unique Influences of Homelessness on Health

- Outdoor exposure
- Violence/crime
- Prolonged standing, walking
- Infectious disease exposure in crowded shelters
- Limited access to showers for personal hygiene or treatment
- Sexually transmitted diseases from rape, sex for drugs or protection
- HIV exposure from rape, injection drug use, sex partners
- Isolation
- Inability to store medications; must carry
- Home care interventions impossible
- Irrevocable psychologic deterioration over time
- Death

GENDER DIFFERENCES

Some of the gender differences noted in the literature between homeless men and women are that more men than women tend to have prior and current histories of alcoholism and criminal behavior, that lone men will be homeless longer than women with families, and that men will more often than women lose touch with their children after becoming homeless. More homeless women than men have been married but also report more instances of prior physical and sexual abuse. A higher rate of mental illness is reported in homeless women compared with homeless men, but many studies are flawed by methodologic and sampling errors. Homeless women do experience more PTSD than men, with many having the diagnosis of PTSD before becoming homeless because of antecedent physical, sexual, or emotional abuse. Homeless women are uniquely at risk of sexually transmitted diseases and the health risks of pregnancy.

More than simply the challenges of poverty, women without safe or stable homes face unique aspects of the homeless lifestyle that seriously affect their health. Some of the common influences are listed in Box 93-2.

MEDICAL PROBLEMS OF HOMELESS WOMEN

Prolonged outdoor exposure increases the risk of frostbite and hypothermia, especially in colder climates. In the summer and warmer climates, women risk sunburn and dehydration.

The elevated rates of trauma and violence both preceding homelessness and caused by it have serious physical, emotional, and cognitive consequences. Homeless women may experience the classic symptoms of PTSD, such as nightmares, flashbacks, or intrusive thoughts or more subtle manifestations such as dissociation, anxiety disorders, medication-resistant depression, chronic pain syndromes, and even frank psychosis. Drug and/or alcohol abuse may be a source of self-medication for painful memories. This must be kept in mind for women drug addiction recidivists.

The prolonged gravitational pull of many hours of standing, walking, and waiting in line can cause venous stasis, skin breakdown, ulcers, and cellulitis. Many women experience chronic foot problems including pain, bunions, cal-luses from walking in poorly fitting shoes, and from trauma or exposure.

Infectious diseases from close contact in crowded shelters include airborne illnesses such as tuberculosis, pneumococcal pneumonia, and meningococcal meningitis. In Boston, in 1994, there was a rubella outbreak among the homeless population. Skin infestations such as scabies and lice are contracted by contact with other infected individuals or fomites. Sporadic access to showers means that treatment cannot always be done in a timely manner. Although many of the reported studies were conducted a decade ago, the increased risks of infectious diseases among the homeless have not decreased. Indeed, recent reports in the literature demonstrate a resurgence of "trench fever" in homeless populations. All homeless women are candidates for the flu vaccine, Pneumovax, and tuberculin testing by PPD.

Homeless women who are victims of sexual assault or who have male sex partners that are intravenous drug users are at higher risk of sexually transmitted diseases including human immunodeficiency virus/acquired immunodeficiency syndrome (HIV/AIDS). This includes women who exchange sex to support a drug habit or for perceived protection. Many sexual assaults go unreported because the women feel unprotected by the criminal justice system, and they lack safe shelter. Many women who are victims of sexual assault and live on the street are reluctant to use publicly funded homeless clinics because they fear exposure to past and potential street batterers.

Many chronic conditions are not tended to until an emergency occurs. Food, clothing, shelter, and protection are the first priorities. Common chronic conditions seen in the homeless include chronic obstructive pulmonary disease, poorly treated hypertension, and advanced stages of congestive heart failure, arthritis, coronary artery disease, diabetes, alcoholic liver disease, asthma, cancer, seizure disorders, HIV/AIDS, and a range of skin conditions. As a result of homelessness, the complications of these diseases occur earlier than in a housed population.

Pregnant homeless women are at high risk for poor birth outcomes from poor nutrition, inadequate prenatal care, smoking, and substance abuse. Cocaine and heroin abuse during pregnancy are associated with lower gestational age at delivery, lower birth weights, stillbirths, and perinatal neurologic impairment. In some states, positive urine screens for drugs in the third trimester or at delivery will result in state custody of the child. Some homeless women avoid all prenatal care under the misperception that a drug screen at any time can risk custody. Therefore it is important to know your state's laws, so that diagnosis early in the pregnancy can be used to motivate the patient to work toward sobriety. In a study by Racine et al. of close to 8000 cocaine addicts, even four prenatal visits by cocaine addicts was shown to positively affect birth outcomes compared with none.

The rates of chronic alcoholism and substance abuse differ between homeless men and women: 45% of men and 15% of women. A majority of homeless men have alcoholism or substance abuse issues before becoming homeless, but these illnesses in homeless women are often seen as a response to the trauma and terror of their lives. With the welfare reform changes initiated in 1996, Supplemental Security Income and Social Security Disability Insurance are no longer available for a primary diagnosis of alcoholism or

Health Care Provider History/Contact Form for Homeless Women

1) NAME: _____

2) SOCIAL SECURITY NUMBER: _____

3) WHERE STAYING: _____

4) DATE OF BIRTH: _____

5) CONTACT PERSON AT SHELTER (ie, Nurse, Counselor): _____

6) BENEFITS:
   (Medicaid/Emergency Aid; SSI; SSDI; TANF; WIC; Medicare; Hospital Free Care; food stamps;
   public transportation pass; VA; Other; None)
   CARD NUMBERS:

7) SOCIAL HISTORY:
   Married/Divorced (Why?)/Separated(Why?)/Single/Gay/Straight/Bisexual Parents/Sibs/Children/
   Any contact? _____

   IF YOUR CHILDREN ARE NOT WITH YOU, WHERE ARE THEY AND WHY? _____
   _____

8) VETERAN STATUS:
   Branch of Service/Years served?/Combat? _____
   Honorable/General/Dishonorable Discharge? _____
   Any Service-Connected Disabilities? _____

9) HOW DID YOU BECOME HOMELESS? _____
   How long homeless? _____

10) MENSTRUAL/REPRODUCTIVE HISTORY:
    Last Pap? _____ Ever abnormal? _____
    How many pregnancies?/Live births?/Abortions?: _____
    Birth control? _____

11) EVER HAD A MAMMOGRAM? _____ WHY? _____ RESULT: _____

12) HAVE YOU EVER HAD A SEXUALLY TRANSMITTED DISEASE? (GC, Syphilis, Herpes, Hepatitis,
    etc.) _____ TREATED? _____ DO YOU PRACTICE SAFE SEX? _____

13) LAST PPD/HISTORY OF TB — WHERE? _____ WHEN? _____
    RESULT: _____ CONTROLS? _____

    LAST CHEST X-RAY/RESULT: _____ PRIOR TREATMENT FOR TB? _____

14) ALCOHOL HISTORY:
    At what age did you start? _____ Why? _____
    COMPLICATIONS? (Seizure, Pancreatitis, GI bleed, Blackouts, DTs, Trauma, Job Loss,
         Relationship Loss, etc)
    EVER BEEN IN DETOX? _____ HOW MANY? _____
    HOW LONG? (5d, 28d). HALFWAY HOUSE? _____
    NAMES OF DETOXES: _____
    LONGEST SOBRIETY? _____ HOW DID IT FEEL? _____
    REASON FOR RELAPSE? _____

FIG. 93-1 Health Care Provider History/Contact Form for Homeless Women: A Tool for Primary Care. (From Roseanna H. Means, MD MSC)

substance abuse, making it more difficult for homeless individuals to avail themselves of treatment programs.

The prevalence rates of mental illness in homeless women are difficult to ascertain. Studies differ on definitions, the population studied, severity of illness, and coexisting conditions such as substance abuse. In general, about 30% of homeless women reportedly qualify for a diagnosis of major mental illness. That figure is tempered by the women's individual histories, both before and after becoming homeless, whether they are victims of violence (reported in more than 90% of homeless women), whether the symptoms of mental illness were present and documented before homelessness, and how much the symptoms are reactions to life on the streets: paranoia, hypervigilance, mistrust, anxi-

15) DRUG HISTORY:
    At what age did you start?_____ Why? _____
    WHICH DRUGS? (pot, cocaine, heroin, amphetamines, narcotic analgesics, anxiolytics, other)
         ROUTE? (oral/snort/IV/smoke)
    COMPLICATIONS? (OD, Skin infections, Endocarditis, Hepatitis A/B/or C, Cardiac, Muscle, Nasal,
        HIV/AIDS, etc)
    EVER BEEN IN DETOX?_____ NAMES: _____
    EVER BEEN IN A METHADONE PROGRAM? _____
    HOW LONG? _____ HOW MANY MG/DAY? _____

16) EVER BEEN HIV TESTED? _____
    WHERE? _____ WHEN? _____
    RESULT: _____ CD4: _____ VIRAL LOAD: _____

17) VACCINATIONS:
    FLU/PNEUMOVAX/Td/MMR/HEPATITIS A or B. WHEN? _____

18) PSYCHIATRIC HISTORY:
    EVER BEEN TREATED FOR DEPRESSION, NERVOUS BREAKDOWN, ANXIETY, VOICES (AH),
    WANTING TO KILL YOURSELF (SI) OR SOMEONE ELSE (HI)? ANY SYMPTOMS (describe) BEFORE
    YOU BECAME HOMELESS? _____

    NAMES/DATES OF PSYCH HOSPITALIZATIONS, COUNSELORS/THERAPISTS _____
    _____
    _____

    HAVE YOU EVER BEEN PHYSICALLY OR SEXUALLY HURT?_____ BY SOMEONE YOU LOVED?_____
    WERE YOU ABLE TO GET ANY HELP? _____ DO YOU WORRY ABOUT IT HAPPENING AGAIN? _____
    DO YOU HAVE BAD DREAMS, FLASHBACKS OR DISTRACTING/INTRUSIVE THOUGHTS ABOUT IT?____
    DO YOU KNOW HOW TO GET HELP IF IT HAPPENS AGAIN? _____ DO YOU HAVE A SAFE PLACE? _____

19) HOW MANY TIMES DO YOU REMEMBER MOVING AS A CHILD? _____

20) LIST YOUR CLOSEST FRIENDS, ANYONE YOU CAN COUNT ON FOR SUPPORT, WHO TO CALL IN AN
    EMERGENCY. _____

21) TELL ME WHO YOU WOULD WANT TO BE NOTIFIED IF YOU DIED. _____
    _____

> Key:
> SSI: Supplemental Security Income
> SSDI: Social Security Disability Insurance
> TANF: Temporary Assistance to Needy Families
> WIC: Women, Infants and Children
> VA: Veterans Administration
> GC: Gonorrhea
> PPD: Purified protein derivative
> TB: Tuberculosis
> DTs: Delirium Tremens
> OD: overdose
> HIV: Human immunodeficiency virus
> tD: Tetanus/Diptheria
> AH: Auditory hallucinations
> SI: Suicidal ideation
> HI: Homicidal ideation

FIG. 93-1, cont'd   For legend see opposite page.

ety, and emotional numbing. Overriding all these things is the profound sense of loss that homeless women face each day: the loss of identity, autonomy, safety, health, and especially their families and their children, if they are estranged or if the state has taken custody. Even though the true rates are not clearly established in the literature, what is clear is that the longer women are homeless, the more they suffer irrevocable psychologic, emotional, and physical deterioration. Over time, the relentless assault on every aspect of one's life can cause permanent psychologic and psychiatric impairment leading to the "homeless persona," the "crazy people" one sees wandering in the streets, talking to invisible voices, and refusing all help except the most basic outreach. These women represent our greatest challenge.

BOX 93-3
Strategies for Treating Homeless Women

Build Trust
- Offer praise, even for small steps forward like showing up for appointments or partially following through with treatment, even when the patient has not fulfilled all your expectations
- Set predictable, consistent limits on inappropriate behavior
- In extreme cases of noncompliance, use contracts to reinforce mutual expectations

Be Predictable
- Be there when you say you will. (But don't create unrealistic expectations. You are not "the only one who understands," and you will not "always be there for them.")

Listen
- Listen to what they are asking for
- If you aren't sure they are homeless, ask "Where are you staying?" not "Where do you live?"
- Discern whether they are sober, safe, and sheltered

Recognize the Trauma in their Lives
- Respect their psychologic space
- Don't touch anyone's bags without permission
- Try not to rush. Speak calmly and listen first. Avoid the temptation to start the examination before hearing the whole history
- Don't do invasive bodily examinations without explaining why and getting permission
- Explain every step of what you are going to do before you do it, particularly for gynecologic and breast examinations

Show Concern
- Don't be afraid to ask when they need to get to the shelter to get a bed.
- Call the shelter and ask them to hold a bed if it is late in the day.
- Ask if they can handle their medications. Will they be able to do simple interventions (ice, elevation, bed rest)?
- Speak to the shelter nurse if there are special instructions.

Don't Try to Do Too Much in One Visit
- Prioritize health issues
- Treat the most important conditions first
- Empower the patient by offering options and choosing what can be accomplished together

Simplify Medical Regimens
- Choose medicines with proven track records and minimal side effects
- Use once daily dosing, if possible

Use Creative Solutions
- Combine insulin with oral agents
- Keep the welfare form until the laboratory work needed for eligibility has been completed
- Use meal vouchers to reward completion of therapy
- Use your local network of shelter nurses to give medications
- Consider giving homeless battered women a brief, portable health record in case they must go to multiple care sites to stay safe

Refer Judiciously
- Pick colleagues sensitive to the special needs of complex patients
- Arrange referral dates soon after appointment dates. (Waiting increases the no-show rate.)

Arrange Frequent Visits
- Homeless people don't have watches or calendars, so it's hard for them to stick to long-term schedules
- Frequent visits provide an opportunity to show consistent concern and establish the habit of following through, and have been shown to improve outcomes. Brief once or twice weekly visits are especially important during vulnerable periods
- Spread clinical contact among the treatment team to broaden the clients' base of support and minimize staff burnout

Don't Judge or Scold for Failure to Follow Through or to Stay Sober/Clean
- Always praise first for showing up
- Acknowledge the failed behavior as evidence of the many barriers that can only be overcome with the help of the treatment team

Learn How to Enroll Patients in Medicaid
- Most homeless individuals qualify but need help with the enrollment process. Medicaid enrollment increases the use of services

Practice Comprehensive Discharge Planning from Inpatient Care
- Ensure that all clinicians involved in patient's care get a copy of the discharge summary as soon as possible
- Document the social, medical, and behavioral health services that will be needed by the patient and communicate them to the patient's primary provider
- Do not discharge a patient to a shelter without shelter staff permission or without the staff understanding the degree of care and follow-up required

Know Your Resources
- Create a file of local resources including shelters, advocacy groups, outreach workers, and public benefit agencies
- Know the hours of operation of your area's shelters, whether they have clinics, and what degree of follow-up care can be provided, if any
- Maintain a dialogue with these resources and with area emergency departments and urgent care centers so that the lines of communication stay open

Know Your Limits: Indications for Intense Case Management
- Homeless women who are relentless recidivists, at risk of mortality from chronic substance abuse, trauma, and poor judgment may be candidates for intense case management under Homeless At Risk of Mortality (H.A.R.M.) guidelines: chronic organic brain disease, uncontrollable social behavior, multiple injuries, documented impaired mental status or competence, inability to recognize dangerous situations, loss of social supports, and massive treatment resistance.
- Women who qualify can receive multidisciplinary treatment through the collaborative efforts of all their caregivers, including the state supported mental health team, shelter workers, the primary care clinicians and emergency department personnel. In extreme cases, this treatment may result in guardianship proceedings.
- Women with severe mental illness alone can benefit from Intensive Case Management (ICM) or Assertive Community Treatment (ACT) that not only improves health outcomes but reduces overall health care costs.

Homeless persons are at least four times more likely to die than their housed counterparts. In a 5-year study of homeless adults conducted in Boston from 1988 to 1993, AIDS was the leading cause of death in women 25 to 44 years old. Heart disease and cancer were the leading cause of death in homeless women over age 45.

EVALUATION

To properly evaluate homeless women requires understanding the cultural context. Clinics that serve homeless individuals need to know what shelter, clinical, advocacy, outreach, and public benefit resources exist in one's community and the individuals who staff these services. A file or directory of these resources should be developed and maintained in all medical facilities that serve the homeless. Clinicians who provide a calm, safe clinical environment where the women are treated with dignity and respect will have higher return rates. This can be done in one's own office, or by providing outreach care in a woman's shelter or drop-in center. Consistent, predictable availability help to bring down barriers of mistrust.

One is also encouraged to develop a demographic and baseline clinical database for the homeless clients to further maintain continuity. Figure 93-1 is an example of the Health Care Provider History/Contact Form to use when interviewing homeless women. These questions can be asked over a series of visits as one builds trust and an ongoing relationship.

Finally, providers who care for homeless women should make every effort to communicate their clinical interventions not only in the patient's office or emergency room record, but, with the patient's consent, to all the clinicians and shelter/outreach contacts involved in the life of that individual in order to maximize clinical continuity.

MANAGEMENT STRATEGIES FOR HOMELESS WOMEN

Caring for homeless women requires a balance of responses. It requires knowing how to gain her trust so that she will feel safe enough to return. It requires patience and sensitivity but also an appreciation of maladaptive and manipulative behavior and using therapeutic boundaries. They must be supportive but not enabling. Providers must refrain from actions or expectations in pursuit of a diagnosis or treatment goal that might be perceived as threatening to someone responding out of fear. They must not self-direct hateful comments that reflect years of anger at someone else or some other system. Box 93-3 summarizes strategies to use when treating homeless women.

BIBLIOGRAPHY

Bassuk EL et al: Homelessness in female-headed families: childhood and adult risk and protective factors, *Am J Public Health* 87:241, 1997.

Bassuk El et al: The characteristics and needs of sheltered homeless and low-income housed mothers, *JAMA* 276:640, 1996.

Browne A: Family violence and homelessness: the relevance of trauma histories in the lives of homeless women, *Am J Orthopsychiatry* 63:370, 1993.

Calsyn RJ, Morse G: Homeless men and women: commonalities and a service gender gap, *Am J Commun Psychiatry* 18:597, 1990.

Centers for Disease Control: Tuberculosis among homeless shelter residents, *MMWR* 40:869, 1991.

Child J, Bierer MF, Eagle K: Unexpected factors predict control of hypertension in hospital-based homeless clinic, *Mt Sinai J Med* 65:304, 1998.

DeMaria A et al: An outbreak of type 1 pneumococcal pneumonia in a men's shelter, *JAMA* 244:1446, 1980.

Drossman DA et al: Sexual and physical abuse and gastrointestinal illness, review and recommendations, *Ann Intern Med* 123:782, 1995.

Ferguson A: Discharge planning from A & E: Part 1, *Accid Emerg Nurs* 5:210, 1997.

Ferguson MA, Ragosta CW: Homeless at risk of mortality: a proactive approach to vulnerable "repeaters," *J Emerg Nurs* 24:546, 1998.

Filice GA et al: Group A meningococcal disease in skid rows: epidemiology and implications for control, *Am J Public Health* 74:253, 1984.

Fischer PJ: Victimization and homelessness—cause and effect, *N Engl J Public Policy* 8:229, 1992.

Fleischman S: Trauma and victimization. In Wood D, editor: *Delivering health care to homeless persons,* New York, 1992, Springer Publishing.

Gelberg L et al: Health, homelessness and poverty. A study of clinic users, *Arch Intern Med* 150:2325, 1990.

Glied S et al: Medicaid and service use among homeless adults, *Inquiry* 35:380, 1998.

Herman DB et al: Adverse childhood experiences: are they risk factors for adult homelessness? *Am J Public Health* 87:249, 1997.

Herman JL: *Trauma and recovery,* New York, 1992, Basic Books.

Hibbs JR et al: Mortality in a cohort of homeless adults in Philadelphia, *N Engl J Med* 331:304, 1994.

Hodnicki D, Horner SD, Boyle S: Women's perspectives on homelessness, *Public Health Nurs* 9:257, 1992.

Hwang SW et al: Causes of death in homeless adults in Boston, *Ann Intern Med* 126:625, 1997.

Johnson AK, Kreuger LW: Toward a better understanding of homeless women, *Social Work* 34:537, 1989.

Koegel P, Burnham MA: Traditional and non-traditional homeless alcoholics, *Alcohol Health Res World* 11:28, 1987.

Koegel P et al: Childhood risk factors for homelessness and homeless adults, *Am J Public Health* 85:1642, 1995.

Koegel P, Sherman D: Assessment and treatment of homeless mentally ill adults. In Wood D, editor: *Delivering health care to homeless persons,* New York, 1992, Springer Publishing.

Lehman AF et al: Cost-effectiveness of assertive community treatment for homeless persons with severe mental illness, *Br J Psychiatry* 174:346, 1999.

Lindenberg CS et al: A review of the literature on cocaine abuse in pregnancy, *Nurs Res* 40:69, 1991.

Link BG et al: Lifetime and five-year prevalence of homelessness in the United States, *Am J Public Health* 84:1907, 1994.

Lockyer JR: Hypothermia and exposure among homeless persons. In Wood D, editor: *Delivering health care to homeless persons,* New York, 1992, Springer Publishing.

Long HL et al: Cancer screening in homeless women: attitudes and behaviors, *J Health Care Poor Underserved* 9:276, 1998.

McBride K, Mulcare RJ: Peripheral vascular disease in the homeless. In Brickner PW et al, editors: *Health care of homeless people,* New York, 1985, Springer Publishing.

McCauley J et al: Relation of low-severity violence to women's health, *J Gen Intern Med* 13:687, 1998.

Means RH: Health care for homeless women. In Carr PL, Freund KM, Somani S, editors: *The medical care of women,* New York, 1995, WB Saunders.

National Coalition for the Homeless: Why are people homeless? Fact Sheet #1, June 1999.

National Coalition for the Homeless: How many people experience homelessness? Fact Sheet #2, February 1999.

National Coalition for the Homeless: Who is homeless? Fact Sheet #3, February 1999.

National Coalition for the Homeless: Employment and homelessness, Fact Sheet #4, February 1999.

National Coalition for the Homeless: Homeless families with children, Fact Sheet #7, June 1999.

National Coalition for the Homeless: Domestic violence and homelessness, Fact Sheet #8, April 1999.

North CS, Smith EM: Posttraumatic stress disorder among homeless men and women, *Hosp Commun Psych* 43:1010, 1992.

Nyamathi A, Flaskerud J, Leake B: HIV-risk behaviors and mental health characteristics among homeless or drug-recovering women and their closest sources of social support, *Nurs Res* 46:133, 1997.

Padgett DK, Struening EL: Victimization and traumatic injuries: associations with alcohol, drug, and mental problems, *Am J Orthopsychiatry* 62:525, 1992.

Racine A, Joyce T, Anderson R: The association between prenatal care and birth weight among women exposed to cocaine in New York City, *JAMA* 270:1581, 1993.

Robrecht LC, Anderson DG: Interpersonal violence and the pregnant homeless woman, *J Obstet Gynecol Neonatal Nurs* 27:684, 1998.

Salit SA et al: Hospitalization costs associated with homelessness in New York City, *N Engl J Med* 338:1734, 1998.

Shlay JC et al: Human immunodeficiency virus seroprevalence and risk assessment of a homeless population in Denver, *Sex Transm Dis* 23:304, 1996.

Spach DH et al: Bartonella (rochalimaea) quintana bacteremia in inner-city patients with chronic alcoholism, *N Engl J Med* 332:424, 1995.

Tull J: Homelessness: an overview, *N Engl J Public Policy* 8:25, 1992.

Usatine RP: Skin diseases of the homeless. In Wood D, editor: *Delivering health care to homeless persons,* New York, 1992, Springer Publishing.

Weinreb L et al: Health characteristics and medical service use patterns of sheltered and low-income housed mothers, *J Gen Intern Med* 13:389, 1998.

Wrenn K: Foot problems in homeless persons, *Ann Intern Med* 113:567, 1990.

Wright JD et al: Ailments and alcohol. Health status among drinking homeless, *Alcohol Health Res World* 11:22, 1987.

Zolopa AR et al: HIV and tuberculosis infection in San Francisco's homeless adults: prevalence and risk factors in a representative sample, *JAMA* 272:455, 1994.

Zuckerman B et al: Effects of maternal marijuana and cocaine use on fetal growth, *N Engl J Med* 320:762, 1989.

CHAPTER 94

Disability in Women

Susan E. Herz

EPIDEMIOLOGY

Disability has a profound effect on women's health; approximately 28 million women in America live with disabilities. There are multiple sociomedical, legal, and treatment issues. Medical definitions of disability abound. Unless otherwise indicated, the term means a physical or mental impairment that substantially limits one or more major life activities, such as walking, seeing, hearing, speaking, breathing, learning, caring for one's self, and working.

In light of the many definitions used in surveys and studies, counting and describing women with disabilities are challenging at best. According to a subsample of the 1990 US census, which collected comprehensive data about disability, nearly one fifth (19.4%) of the US population aged 15 or older has a disability.

In the United States, female disability rates are somewhat similar among Native Americans (22%), African Americans (22%), and whites (20%), while Hispanic women (16%) and Asian/Pacific Islanders (11%) have significantly lower rates. However, "severe disability"—an inability to perform a functional activity—affects African Americans (12%) at a significantly higher rate than Native Americans (10%), whites (9%), and people of Hispanic origin (8%). Once again Asians and Pacific Islanders have a rate (5%) roughly half that of the general population. Recognition of the cultural context of patients' conditions may be critical to successful treatment.

More women than men have disabilities, and some disabling conditions are more prevalent among women. Women's greater longevity may account for the majority of these disparities (e.g., vision impairment), although in some instances, age-adjusted measures show significantly higher prevalence among women (e.g., arthritis).

Working women with disabilities earn less than working women without disabilities, and less than working men with disabilities. Women with disabilities who are African or Hispanic experience disproportionately higher rates of unemployment than other women with disabilities. These socioeconomic factors may combine with cultural barriers to hinder routine medical care.

BACKGROUND

Paradoxically, although people with disabilities constitute a medically defined minority group, the medical community has only recently begun to systematically address the needs of this diverse subpopulation. Historically, a relative handful of physicians specialized in treatment of particular institutionalized populations. More primary care physicians are treating more patients with disabilities for a number of reasons:

- Many people with severe physical disabilities and/or mental retardation have left institutions for community living;
- Increased longevity among the general population is associated with late onset disabling conditions;
- Increasing numbers of people with disabilities are receiving care covered by managed care plans offered through Medicaid, Medicare, and/or other public or private insurance;
- People with disabilities tend to use more health services than do those without disabilities, in part due to secondary conditions that could have been averted by appropriate medical intervention,
- The law now requires disability-accessible office practice in most instances.

SOCIOMEDICAL ISSUES

Among the general population, women with disabilities are seen as passive, damaged, either asexual or inactively heterosexual, helpless, dependent, lacking in self-direction, burdensome, pitiable, and either weak or courageous. In addition, research shows that most people tend to react to those with disabilities either extremely positively or extremely negatively. Such myths and messages may affect attitudes and body image differently for patients depending on whether their disabilities are late onset or lifelong.

For many practitioners, a patient's disability sends a signal that the medical system has failed. This perception may prevail even where the disability requires no particular medical services (e.g., congenital blindness). The patient's disability may also lead to provider discomfort associated with lack of training or knowledge about treating the patient. Difficulty may be encountered seeing past the disability to note the complete human being.

Associated misapprehensions about the significance of disability may place patients at risk for developing preventable secondary conditions. For example, it may be assumed that because of her disability, a woman is asexual or abstinent. Such assumptions may contribute to the significantly decreased rate of Pap smears and mammograms among patients with disabilities compared with patients without disabilities. Similarly, women with major mobility impairments experience significantly decreased rates of alcohol and tobacco use screening, even though the presence of disability has been shown to increase the risk for abusing alcohol, drugs, and, in some instances, tobacco. Some researchers speculate that this disparity may result from physicians' beliefs that patients with pronounced disabilities live intolerable lives, and that it would be inappropriate to deprive them of the few pleasures available to them. Others suggest that when focusing on the disability and seeing only "the cerebral palsy patient," important signs and symptoms unrelated to the individual's disability may be overlooked.

Physical and mental functional disabilities may be associated with childhood physical, sexual, or emotional maltreatment histories. Women with such histories are more likely to engage in health risk behaviors such as probable alcoholism, driving while intoxicated, and having sexual relations without knowing their partner's sexual history. They are also more likely to have eating disorders and somatic complaints and are less likely to either obtain medical care or act on medical advice.

Studies show that compared with younger women without disabilities, younger women with disabilities are more likely to delay medical care or to encounter barriers associated with finances and insurance. Younger women with more severe disabilities have particular difficulty obtaining mental health care, dental care, prescription medicine, and eyeglasses. They are also at risk for experiencing depression or anxiety, and twice as likely to smoke as younger women without disabilities.

Disability is highly correlated with age, with 40% of women 65 years and older having at least one functional limitation. Those who become deaf or hard of hearing late in life are at notable risk for social isolation; many resist acknowledging the hearing loss and refrain from using hearing aids. In addition, some patients experience secondary conditions during aging. These secondary functional losses may be associated with significant emotional adjustment issues for individuals who already have disabling impairments. For example, changing from a crutches to a wheelchair may alter interaction with the environment and with other persons, or developing blindness after lifelong epilepsy can lead to the perception of control again lost.

Estimates of prevalence of mental illness among adults with learning disabilities and mental retardation vary from 10% to 60%. Substantial underdiagnosis of psychiatric disabilities among patients with intellectual disabilities results from atypical clinical presentations and the common belief that psychiatric symptoms are an inherent part of cognitive dysfunction. Further, the pharmacokinetics, pharmacodynamics, and side-effect profiles of psychotropic medications among people with learning disabilities and mental retardation have received limited study.

Many women with complex or lifelong disabilities have learned to advocate for themselves in the medical environment, directing their own care. Labeling such patients as self-directing rather than difficult may lead to productive partnerships with the physician.

Whether or not the patient presents as a self-advocate, her opinions should be considered when selecting a treatment's outcome measures and acceptable side effects. She is often the best estimator of her overall quality of life. Although a patient's assessments of physical disability may correlate with the clinician's assessments, measures of overall health related quality of life show wide disparity. For example, in one study, Rothwell showed that whereas functional abilities of patients with multiple sclerosis rank high in physicians' quality of life assessments, vitality, mental health, and general physical well-being take precedence for the patients.

The majority of people with disabilities rate their lives as somewhat or very satisfying. Those dissatisfied with their lives associate their dissatisfaction with social and economic concerns, not their medical conditions. Although disabling conditions vary widely in pathology and comorbidities, people with disparate conditions tend to encounter socially constructed barriers rooted in common limiting assumptions. Whether the barriers take form in negative attitudes among prospective employers, a shortage of sign language interpreters, or inaccessible public transportation, they ultimately lead to limited opportunities for employment, education, recreation, health care, public services, and participation in and contribution to the larger community. The combined effect of unequal treatment and stereotypic assumptions have led to identification of this subpopulation as a minority group. Significantly, many deaf people expressly reject disability status. Instead, those who are prelingually deaf may see themselves as members of a cultural minority with its own language, values, and mores. Appreciating the distinction between the patient's medical condition and her minority group status as a deaf or disabled woman may lead to an enhanced physician-patient relationship.

LAW AND ACCESS

Until relatively recently, many physicians were legally free to turn away patients based on the presence of disability. In 1990, the enactment of the Americans with Disabilities Act (ADA) altered the landscape by designating the "professional offices of health care providers" to be places of public accommodation enjoined from disability-based discrimination. Some states and municipalities have patterned similar laws and interpretations on the ADA, seeking to ensure that people with and without disabilities enjoy equally effective opportunities to enter medical settings and receive services. Accordingly an appreciation of the legal framework defining programmatic and structural requirements may help inform a plan to treat women with disabilities.

ELIGIBILITY FOR SERVICE

Every practitioner need not serve every woman for every health condition. In the eyes of the law, criteria may establish whether a woman is "qualified" to receive medical services, as long as these criteria are applied equally to those with and without disabilities. For example, a legitimate criterion might be that the individual's treatment not increase the practitioner's active caseload beyond a particular number.

Evaluation of whether a woman is "qualified" to receive health care should include consideration of whether accommodations need to be made to her disability. Such accommodations may include changes in rules, policies, or practices; removal of physical barriers; and/or provision of aids and services to assist in communication.

Eligibility criteria may not screen out women with disabilities unless such requirements are necessary for operation of the medical service provided. Eligibility criteria that screen out all people with a particular disability may be unlawful, as this would require showing that every person with that disability should be excluded. For example, a rule that no mentally retarded person can receive an office's medical services or that patients must have a driver's license to pay by check would violate the law.

Physicians routinely referring nondisabled patients based on their need for a particular treatment or service may appropriately refer similarly situated patients with disabilities. Similarly, practitioners specializing in treating patients with particular conditions may not refer out a woman with a disability solely on the basis of that disability.

In addition to excluding women who are not qualified for service or treatment, practitioners may exclude those who pose a direct threat to the health or safety of others. To exclude an individual with a disability based on the perception of a direct threat, the physician must identify a significant risk of harm that cannot be eliminated or mitigated by an accommodation. A determination that someone poses a direct threat must find root in "an individualized assessment based on reasonable judgment that relies on current medical knowledge or on the best objective evidence." For example, it would be unlawful to refuse to provide medical services to a woman with a psychiatric diagnosis solely out of concern that psychiatric impairment can lead to harming others. The fact that the physician fears the threat in good faith does not pass legal muster. An objective assessment is crucial.

PROGRAMMATIC ACCESS
Services

Medical offices are required to make reasonable modifications in rules, policies, and practices where necessary to accommodate women with disabilities. Modifications that would fundamentally alter the nature of the programs or services offered are not required. An example of an appropriate—albeit not necessarily required—modification might involve allowing a patient to bring a guide dog or other service animal despite a policy prohibiting patients from bringing pets.

Women with severe disabilities who require assistance with such activities as dressing, bathing, or toileting often hire personal care attendants (commonly known as PCAs). The provider may need to modify policies regarding outsiders attending a medical examination with respect to PCAs. For the woman without a PCA, the ADA does not appear to require physicians to assist persons with physical disabilities with services of a personal nature (assistance in lifting, dressing, or toileting).

Communications

Effective communication represents the new legal "gold standard." Women with cognitive impairments may need information explained repeatedly and/or in a rudimentary fashion. Policies may be modified to allow her more time to communicate, and/or to provide an office assistant to explain, and/or to provide written advice, as appropriate.

Those with vision impairments may require modifications such as readers, braille materials, large-print materials, audio recordings, or computer diskettes.

Women who are deaf or hard of hearing may require Sign language interpreters, or, in some instances, note-writing or printed materials. Because the ADA prohibits either imposing a surcharge on hearing impaired patients or billing a third-party payer for interpreter services, the office may plan ahead by, for example, setting aside a "communication fund" and/or making arrangements with a nearby hospital for procuring services of their on-staff qualified interpreter. When providing services to a deaf person, the health care professional pays for the interpreter, enjoys certain tax relief for this, and makes the final decision regarding use of an interpreter or another alternative. At the same time, under the ADA, the patient's preference about whether to use a qualified interpreter should be given primary consideration. The presence of a certified sign language interpreter (rather than a friend or family member) will help ensure the confidentiality of communications, and the effective, accurate, and impartial interpretation of both signed and voiced communications, using any necessary specialized vocabulary. It should be noted that when unaccompanied by residual hearing, lip reading is inherently unreliable because 60% to 70% of English speech is not visible externally.

Structural Access

Architectural access is a means to programmatic access. Specific requirements may be amended from time to time and, in any event, may vary from state to state. Nonetheless, the following general rules may be useful.

Not every existing building or part of every existing building needs to be accessible. The general rule is that when viewed in its entirety, the physician's full array of services should be readily accessible to people with disabilities.

The ADA requires private medical offices to remove architectural barriers in existing facilities, including communication barriers that are structural in nature, where such removal is readily achievable—that is, if removal will not incur much difficulty or expense. Some "readily achievable" steps may include ensuring designated accessible parking spaces, making curb cuts in sidewalks and entrances, adding raised markings on elevator control buttons, installing flashing alarm lights, widening doorways, installing accessible door hardware, rearranging furniture in the waiting room, rearranging toilet partitions, installing raised toilet seats, repositioning paper towel dispensers, and arranging examination rooms so that people in wheelchairs have adequate turn-around space.

When renovations are made to existing buildings, the renovated portions should be accessible to the maximum extent feasible, featuring a wheelchair-accessible entrance, a wheelchair accessible restroom, telephone, and water fountain. When remodeling, a continuous, unobstructed pedestrian path from the outside entrance of the building should lead to the altered, accessible area.

BOX 94-1
Key Accessibility Features at a Glance

*1. Handicapped parking spaces reasonably close to entrances; ramps; curb cuts
*2. Doors interior and exterior wide, easy to open
*3. Accessible route to and throughout the facility and service areas
*4. Waiting room: clear floor space so women who are short or using wheelchairs can reach amenities such as magazine racks and can navigate
*5. Examination room: ensure that women who are short or using wheelchairs can reach controls and storage facilities
6. Equipment: adjustable height treatment and examination tables
*7. Accessible toilet and dressing rooms
8. Sensitivity training for all staff on interacting with people with disabilities: include information about using the telephone relay system, procuring qualified sign language interpreters, referring women to facilities with accessible mammograms, and identifying accessible battered women's shelters

* Required if readily achievable, meaning easily accomplishable and able to be carried out without much difficulty or expense.

If the physician is building a new facility or buying or renting space in a new building, the entire building is required to be accessible to people with disabilities. Detailed state and federal accessibility codes spell out construction requirements. In any event, providers are not required to take any action that would result in a fundamental alteration of their programs or activities or in undue financial or administrative burdens.

The ADA and Code of Federal Regulations currently contain no accessibility standards for furniture and equipment. Making offices fully appropriate for patients with physical disabilities involves going beyond the ADA. While a padded or adjustable-height examination table and a sitting scale meet the law's spirit, courts have not been asked to determine whether they are required by the law's letter. Box 94-1 includes a list of key accessibility features.

Costs

A surcharge may not be imposed on women with disabilities to cover the costs of accommodations. If the physician can show that providing a certain accommodation would require an undue financial or administrative burden or would fundamentally alter the nature of the medical office, the accommodation need not be provided. In such a case, providing another less costly or burdensome accommodation or seeking funding for the accommodation from another source satisfies the law. The law gives the clinician the responsibility of proving the existence of an undue burden or fundamental alteration of the program.

CLINICAL EVALUATION
History
Taking a History

The core skills of both history-taking and performing a physical examination remain critical to a good practice. Studies show that the information obtained during a skilled

medical interview may provide sufficient information to make a diagnosis, even before the physical examination and additional testing. In addition, the act of history taking may function as a key component of the therapeutic aspect of the physician-patient relationship. Moreover, patient satisfaction and compliance have been shown to be associated with physician behavior, including friendliness, empathy, openness, and nonjudgmental attitude.

Sending all women a checklist to fill out in advance of the appointment may be good general practice. In the alternative, the patient may fill out the checklist in the office with assistance from staff as needed. This approach saves time during the office visit, facilitates key information gathering, and can lead to more focused discussions.

A functional history of a woman with a mobility impairment will indicate whether her home features stairs, whether she needs them for initial entry and/or for access to the bedroom or bathroom, and for what other purposes she uses stairs. Asking whether and when the patient has been assessed for mobility aids (walker, cane, crutches) may lead to appropriate use of durable medical equipment. An appropriate match between the individual and assistive technology can increase functional capacity substantially.

For some cognitively impaired patients, a case manager may assist in providing information, facilitating communication, ensuring informed consent, and later implementing a treatment regime.

It is estimated that nearly half of all Americans with major psychiatric disorders fail to seek treatment. Inquiring about the patient's management of her psychiatric disability and, as appropriate, the perceived effects of medication may assist medical diagnosis and treatment, relieve the indignity and embarrassment associated with stigma, and remind the patient that her whole being is acknowledged.

As stated previously, artful communication with the patient may enhance the physician-patient partnership. The clinician should talk directly to the deaf person, even as the patient faces the interpreter to learn what is being said to her. Phrases such as "Please tell her that . . ." should be omitted. The physician should face the hard-of-hearing person, with hands open and away from the mouth, and, as a courtesy, should face the light source. A person with a speech disability should receive complete, unhurried attention. When a statement is not understood, it is good practice to repeat the part that was clear, and to ask for assistance in understanding the rest. A blind patient should be given verbal descriptions of activities and procedures. A patient with a mental retardation may best comprehend concrete terms, sometimes repeated, other times creatively communicated—for example by drawing a picture of a pill and a dish of food.

Respectful language describes patients by using the active rather than passive voice, for example, *wheelchair user* rather than *wheelchair bound, woman with mobility impairment* rather than *crippled female*. The terms *deaf* and *hard of hearing* may be acceptable, while *deaf-mute* and *deaf and dumb* are not.

Physical Examination
Breast Examination

Breast cancer is the second most common cancer in women, and nulliparity increases the risk for women over 40.

When a woman's disability affects manual dexterity or upper extremity range of motion, she may be unable to perform an adequate self-examination. Inaccessible examination tables may impede if not prohibit adequate clinical examinations. Standard mammography screenings do not accommodate women who cannot stand or raise their arms and turn their bodies. No guidelines ensure optimal breast examinations for women with mobility impairments.

Pelvic Examination

A number of barriers typically decrease the likelihood of giving pelvic examinations to women with disabilities: cervical cancer is associated with sexual activity, and assumptions may be made about abstinence; the procedure may be declined by some women with psychiatric disabilities; inaccessible examination tables may be daunting if not prohibitive; and an examination may be terminated in the face of symptoms such as pain, spasticity, or autonomic dysreflexia for which the physician is unprepared.

Welner has written extensively about pelvic examinations for women with mobility impairments, and this subsection draws on her published experiences, observations, and recommendations. She recommends asking each woman what would make the examination comfortable. She points out that examination tables with handrails and adjustable boots that support the entire leg in various positions may ease pelvic examinations greatly. Absent such equipment, women may choose to forego a Pap smear. Women with impaired leg function or hip joint flexibility may experience pain getting on the table and positioning appropriately. To examine women with range of motion restriction and spasticity of the lower extremities, extra personnel should be available to assist in transferring and in stabilizing lower extremities during the examination. The need to have extra staff hold legs apart may be demeaning and uncomfortable. Increased spasticity may be associated with neurologic conditions affecting the lower extremities, and this may be managed by gently stretching the lower extremities during positioning and applying 2% lidocaine gel.

Patients with neurologic disabilities should be instructed to first empty the bladder and lower colon to help avoid bladder and bowel accidents and to minimize the risk of autonomic dysreflexia. Also known as autonomic hyperreflexia, this autonomic nervous system condition can be stimulated by discomfort in the visceral organs, including the bowel, bladder, uterus, and cervix. Women with spinal cord injury above the T6 level may develop this potentially life-threatening condition during the pelvic examination. Signs include rapid heart beat, irregular pulse, increased blood pressure, facial flushing, spasms, chills, and headache. Precautions include application of lidocaine gel, careful blood pressure monitoring, semisupine positioning, avoidance of digital rectal examination, and availability of extra staff to monitor and manage the process. If staff is unfamiliar with management of autonomic dysreflexia, the presence of a physiatrist or anesthesiologist during the examination will help prevent serious complications.

Welner also notes the significance of physical findings. Vaginal infections are extremely common in wheelchair users because of poor ventilation and accumulation of moisture in the perineum. Yeast infection, bacterial vaginosis, and sexually transmitted diseases should be considered.

Women with sensory impairments may not experience pain, a common sign of pelvic impairment. Women with visual disabilities may not note the presence of perineal lesions such as herpes, syphilitic chancres, rashes, or condyloma. Accordingly, tests for all STDs should be considered.

Management Issues

Making Appointments

All employees should know that the office is a place of public accommodation, and beginning with telephone appointments, should avoid any act or practice that might bar a woman's access.

Employees responsible for answering telephones should be familiar with relay operator services and with TTYs (also known as TDDs, a telecommunication keyboard device used by deaf people that permits visual display of typed communications using the telephone lines). Particularly with new patients, inquiry should be made about the caller's communication needs. Responses should be duly noted, and office procedures followed for determining whether and how to procure qualified interpreters. State offices and the Registry of Interpreters for the Deaf in Silver Spring, Maryland may serve as useful resources.

Many adults with mental retardation may evade the medical system because of actual or perceived difficulties in using standard appointment systems. Working cooperatively with case managers may facilitate treatment, beginning at the point of scheduling and keeping an appointment.

A list of locations of mammogram machines that are accessible for women with mobility impairments should be available to all staff who facilitate referrals. State public health departments may be able to assist in this compilation.

Preconception Counseling

Some medications commonly taken by members of this subpopulation may inhibit libido: diuretics, serotonin uptake inhibitors, phenothiazines, baclofen, phenytoin, lithium, digoxin, reserpine, and naproxen. Some of these are contraindicated in pregnancy (see Chapter 61). Patients may be unaware of this potential side effect. Moreover, some women with disabilities may lack essential information about sexuality, contraception, and pregnancy. For example, in one study of people with spinal cord injuries, women were twice as likely as men to report having received no sex education or counseling during their rehabilitation. In addition many women may lack the confidence to ask questions about such matters. Routine, nonjudgmental questions about sexual activity may help counter this reluctance.

Various risk factors limit contraceptive options for women with different disabilities. For example, women with conditions such as multiple sclerosis, paralysis, and cerebral palsy may encounter risks with pregnancy. Women with diabetes, renal failure, myocardial infarction, or compromised lower extremity muscle tone, mobility, or circulation may encounter particular risks with oral contraception. Women with recurrent bladder or vaginal infections, with weakened pelvic muscles, or with limited manual dexterity may be poor candidates for a diaphragm and in some instances, for a cervical cap. Limited manual dexterity may also make an intrauterine device (IUD) a poor choice, to the extent that inability to locate the string would prevent ascertaining whether the device is in place. In addition, those with inability to feel the pain that would warn them about dislocation or infection may be poor candidates for the IUD.

Secondary Prevention

Women with certain disabilities may be at greater risk for common health conditions than those in the general population. Nonetheless, evidence indicates that in many instances, such secondary health conditions are preventable through health maintenance strategies and timely interventions. Coordinated care with specialists may assure optimal outcomes. To ensure baseline support, referral to an Independent Living Center for PCA services may ensure that day-to-day needs are met.

To avoid compromising the patient's health, weight control and substance abuse reduction should be considered. For many people with a variety of disabilities, adapted swim classes may be appropriate. Others may be better served by a physiatrist's development of a therapeutic exercise prescription for cardiovascular endurance, peripheral muscle strength, coordination, flexibility, pain reduction, and/or pelvic rehabilitation.

Every woman with a disability should be routinely screened for violence. She is particularly vulnerable to abuse by family members, caretakers, and service providers. At least for a few minutes, every patient should be seen outside the presence of her caretaker, PCA, caseworker, friend, or family member. If a qualified sign language interpreter is facilitating communications, reminding the patient about the confidentiality of communications may be particularly important.

Implementation of Alpert's RADAR protocol (see Chapter 87) should include information about shelters that are accessible, noting whether the accessibility is limited to women with physical, cognitive, psychiatric, and/or communication disabilities.

BIBLIOGRAPHY

Americans with Disabilities Act of 1990, 42 U.S.C. 12101 et seq.

Asch A: Distracted by disability, *Camb Q H Care Eth* 7:77, 1998.

Aspray TJ et al: Patients with learning disability in the community, *Br Med J* 318:476, 1999.

Becker H, Stuifbergen A, Tinkle M: Reproductive health care experiences of women with physical disabilities: a qualitative study, *Arch Phys Med Rehabil* 78:S-26, 1997.

Bragdon v. Abbott, 118 S.Ct. 2196 (1998).

CDC: Use of cervical and breast cancer screening among women with and without functional limitations—United States, 1994-1995, *MMWR Weekly* 47:853, 1998.

CDC: Current trends: prevalence of disabilities and associated health conditions—United States, 1991-92, *MMWR Weekly* 43:730, 1994.

Code of Federal Regulations, Ti. 28, Sec. 36.208(c).

DeJong G: An overview of the problem I, *Am J Phys Med Rehabil* 76:2, 1997.

Gledhill J, Rangel L, Gerralda E: Surviving chronic physical illness: psychological outcome in adult life, *Arch Dis Child* 83:104, 2000.

Iezzoni LI et al: Mobility impairment and use of screening and preventive services, *Am J Public Health* 90:955, 2000.

National Organization on Disability: *NOD/Harris Survey of Disabled Americans,* New York, 1994, National Organization on Disability.

Rothwell PM et al: Doctors and patients don't agree: cross sectional study of patients' and doctors' perceptions and assessments of disability in multiple sclerosis, *Br Med J* 314:1580, 1997.

Santosh PJ, Baird G: Psychopharmacotherapy in children and adults with intellectual disability, *Lancet* 354:233, 1999.

Walker DA et al: Adult health status of women with histories of childhood abused and neglect, *Am J Med* 107:332, 1999.

Welner SL et al: Practical considerations in the performance of physical examinations on women with disabilities, *Obstet Gynecol Surv* 54:457, 1999.

Welner S: *A Providers Guide for the Care of Women with Physical Disabilities and Chronic Medical Conditions,* Raleigh, 1999, North Carolina Office on Disability and Health.

PART IV
Prevention

CHAPTER **95**

Breast Cancer Screening

Susan E. Bennett

Women and their physicians are more worried about breast cancer than at any time in the past, learning about the "breast cancer epidemic" from the media and popular culture. Most women are more frightened of breast cancer than other more common and lethal conditions such as heart disease. There is the false perception that breast cancer can be conquered— even prevented by regular screening examinations. Thus many women believe screening tests are powerful tools with perfect sensitivity and specificity. They expect to have breast cancer detected at an early stage with certain survival if they follow screening recommendations.

Health providers, however, know that screening is limited, although many are unsure about the efficacy of various screening tests. Many clinicians harbor doubts about their ability to palpate breast abnormalities, and this can result in risky dependence on mammography and ultrasound. Finally, physicians know that many women hold unrealistic hopes for breast cancer screening and fear that patients will be angry and possibly litigious if screening fails to detect cancer in the earliest stages. Much will be accomplished if physicians better understand the goals and limitations of screening for breast cancer and convey these facts to women.

▦ EPIDEMIOLOGY

Breast cancer is the most common malignancy for women in North America and Europe. The incidence of breast cancer is increasing in South America, Australia, and Asia; second-generation immigrants to high-incidence countries are acquiring breast cancer at higher rates than women in their parents' countries of origin. Although increased detection of breast cancer accounts for some of the rising incidence, it does not account for all of the increase. In North America (and most populations studied worldwide) the incidence of breast cancer is increasing by 1% to 2% each year. As a result the estimated lifetime risk of development of breast cancer has increased from 1:11 to 1:8; this estimate, however, presumes that women will live to age 110 and predicts that roughly one third cancers will occur after age 75.

Table 95-1 shows that absolute risk is age-dependent and is perhaps a less threatening way to predict risk. According to this model the risk of acquiring breast cancer in the forties is

1:1000, whereas the risk for a woman in her 50s is 1:500. The risk of dying of breast cancer before age 75 is only 2.5%.

Breast cancer risk is race-dependent as well as age-dependent: the cumulative probability of a white woman's having breast cancer by age 75 is 8%, whereas that for African-American women is 7% and that for Hispanic-American women is 5%. The cumulative breast cancer risk among Japanese-American women is 5%.

It is important for women and their physicians to understand that all women are at risk for breast cancer. Three fourths of women with breast cancer have no identifiable risk factor. Understanding this concept and some basic facts about the pathophysiologic characteristics of breast cancer helps the clinician to make decisions about screening frequency and tests.

PATHOPHYSIOLOGY

It has been well established that survival of breast cancer is inversely proportional to the size of the primary tumor and to the number of axillary lymph nodes involved with metastases. The mastectomy originated on the basis of this evidence and the belief that breast cancer did not undergo hematogenous dissemination until local lymph nodes were invaded. The American surgeon, William Stewart Halsted (1852-1922), popularized the mastectomy, and wrote that "breast cancer in the broad sense is a local affection . . . invariably [spreading] by process of lymphatic permeation, and not embolic by way of the blood." However, later studies proved this hypothesis wrong, documenting that breast cancer recurred in a substantial proportion of women who had stage 1 breast cancer at radical mastectomy. Evidence evolved that breast cancer is a heterogeneous disease, with marked variability in biologic behavior.

An aggressive subset of tumors were identified in a study of the natural history of breast cancer. Approximately 40% of breast cancers appears to be aggressive, with a relative mortality rate of 25% each year. Lead time bias based on the existence of an aggressive subset of breast cancers confounds the results of screening studies, in that early detection lengthens the time between diagnosis and death without altering the outcome.

Table 95-1
Probability of Eventually Developing and Dying of Breast Cancer*

Age Interval	Risk of Developing Breast Cancer (%)	Risk of Developing Invasive Breast Cancer (%)	Risk of Dying of Cancer (%)
Birth-110	10.2	9.8	3.6
20-30	0.04	0.04	0.00
20-40	0.49	0.42	0.09
20-110	10.34	9.94	3.05
35-45	0.88	0.83	0.14
35-55	2.53	2.37	0.56
35-110	10.27	9.82	3.56
50-60	1.95	1.86	0.33
50-70	4.67	4.48	1.04
50-110	8.96	8.66	2.75
65-75	3.17	3.08	0.43
65-85	5.48	5.29	1.01
65-110	6.53	6.29	1.53

Seidman H et al: *Ca-A Journal for Clinicians* 35:36, 1985.
*White females.

Approximately 60% of breast cancers appear to be indolent, with a relative mortality rate of 2.5% each year. These malignancies either grow very slowly, undergoing late hematogenous dissemination, or appear histologically malignant while behaving clinically benignly. Ductal carcinoma in situ (DCIS) is an example of a histologic entity that progresses to invasive carcinoma only sometimes. Autopsy series suggest that the reservoir of DCIS may be quite large in the general population, as it is found at autopsy in 6% to 18% of women with no history of breast cancer. Length bias based on the existence of an indolent subset also confounds studies of screening by detecting preclinical tumors that would have remained undetected and, perhaps, harmless. There is evidence that breast cancers detected by mammography have better prognoses than those found by other means because they are biologically more indolent.

Randomized trials of screening for breast cancer have been ongoing for the past four decades with long follow-up periods; lead time and length bias become less important as study groups are followed over many years.

EARLY DETECTION BY MAMMOGRAPHY

Table 95-2 displays the results of the randomized clinical trials of screening mammography. Most trials found that women screened by mammography alone, or mammography with clinical breast examination (CBE) had significantly lower breast cancer mortality than women not screened. Women who entered the trials in their 40s benefited less than women who were over 50 years old at entry, and the benefit did not emerge until the second decade after screening commenced. A very influential meta-analysis of the Swedish trials reported a 29% mortality reduction attributed to screening mammography for women age 50 to 69 years old, and a

significant 18% mortality reduction for women who entered the trial in their 40s.

Two large, well-designed randomized trials, Malmo and the Canadian National Breast Screening Study failed to show screening efficacy in any age group. When Danish biostatisticians Gotzsche and Olsen analyzed data from the randomized trials shown in Table 95-2, they found evidence for methodologic problems that could invalidate the results. They focused their analysis on whether there was randomization bias, masking of screening outcomes, or subject exclusion after randomization. The only two trials that did not have evidence for one or more of these problems were the Malmo and Canadian trials. Gotzsche and Olsen concluded that "screening for breast cancer with mammography is unjustified."

Although many screening advocates have criticized the analysis of Gotzsche and Olsen, it is noteworthy that after nearly 40 years of screening trials involving hundreds of thousands of women, there is still controversy about whether mammography reduces breast cancer mortality. Indeed, the researchers who argued against the proof of screening efficacy were inspired by the fact that there has been no reduction in breast cancer mortality in Sweden after 15 years of mass screening. Based on the assumption that screening mammography lowers breast cancer mortality by 29%, there should have been an 11% decline in mortality over 15 years, but only an insignificant 0.8% was reported.

EARLY DETECTION BY CLINICAL BREAST EXAMINATION

Does CBE make an independent contribution to screening? In the Health Insurance Plan of Greater New York (HIP) study a large proportion of cancers found at screening were detected by CBE alone. In the Breast Cancer Detection Demonstration Project (BCDDP), however, with improved mammographic technique, less than 10% of cancers were palpable but invisible on mammography. This was among the reasons that Swedish investigators commenced studies of screening with mammography only. It was an appealing concept that clinicians could defer to mammography rather than depend on an often-inconclusive breast examination, especially in premenopausal women whose breasts are more nodular and thus more difficult to examine.

Researchers pooled data from the randomized trials of screening with both CBE and mammography, and reported that CBE has a sensitivity of 54% and a specificity of 94%. The likelihood that a positive CBE resulted in a cancer diagnosis was quite good at 10.6 (95% C.I. 5.8-19.2) and the likelihood ratio of a negative CBE was excellent at 0.47 (95% C.I. 0.4-0.56). In a separate analysis, the overall sensitivity of a first screening mammogram was 90% (increasing with age), and the overall specificity ranged from 93% to 95% (no variation with age). The likelihood ratio of a positive mammogram was 14.0 (95% C.I. 13.1-14.9) and decreased with age. The likelihood ratio of a negative mammogram did not change with age and was 0.11 (95% C.I. 0.07-0.16).

Although CBE has a lower sensitivity than mammography, sensitivity improves with experience and search time. In the Canadian National Breast Screening Study where CBE sensitivity approached that of mammography, clinicians esti-

Table 95-2
Randomized Trials and Results*

Study	Dates	NUMBER RANDOMIZED		NUMBER OF DEATHS FROM BREAST CANCER		Relative Risk (95% CI)
		Screening	Control	Screening	Control	
HIP	63-69	30,131	30,565	153	196	0.79(0.64-0.98)
Malmö	76-86	21,088	21,195	63	66	0.96(0.68-1.35)
Kopparberg	77-85	38,589	18,582	126	104	0.58(0.45-0.76)
Östergötland	77-85	38,491	37,403	135	173	0.76(0.61-0.95)
Edinburgh	79-88	22,926	21,342	156	167	0.87(0.70-1.08)
Canada	80-87	44,925	44,910	120	111	1.08(0.84-1.40)
Stockholm	81-85	40,318	19,943	66	45	0.73(0.50-1.06)
Göthenburg	82-88	11,724	14,217	18	40	0.55(0.31-0.95)

*Table abstracted and modified from paper by Gotzsche and Olsen, *Lancet* 355:129, 2000.

mated that search time averaged 10 minutes per CBE. In another study, clinicians trained to detect small lumps in silicone breast models improved their sensitivity from a mean of 57% to 63%.

Despite these findings, there is no evidence that CBE alone lowers breast cancer mortality. In a meta-analysis of the non-Swedish randomized trials of screening mammography and CBE, CBE had no independent effect on relative risk.

EARLY DETECTION BY BREAST SELF-EXAMINATION

Is there a role for breast self-examination (BSE) in screening for breast cancer? After 9 years of follow-up in the St. Petersburg/WHO Program for the Evaluation of the Effectiveness of BSE involving 122,471 women, there was no difference in breast cancer mortality between women instructed in BSE and the control group.

A randomized trial of BSE has been ongoing in China since 1989. This study enrolled 267,040 employees associated with the Shanghai Textile Industry Bureau. Subjects were randomly assigned to either a BSE instruction group or a control group that received training sessions on the prevention of low back pain. Although women trained in BSE demonstrated improved proficiency in detecting lumps in silicone breast models compared with women in the control group, the breast cancers detected in the BSE group were not diagnosed at smaller sizes or at earlier stages than those detected in the control group. Cumulative breast cancer mortality was the same in both the BSE and control groups 5 years after entry into the study. There is hope that differences will emerge between the two groups with longer follow-up times, although this seems unlikely given that the stages of breast cancers detected were equivalent. The primary difference between the BSE and control group was that many more benign breast lesions were detected in the instruction group than in the control group.

OTHER SCREENING TESTS

Digital and scintimammography, magnetic resonance imaging, and positron emission tomography are imaging techniques that hold promise for screening. Ultrasound is an

important diagnostic tool and has a role in augmenting screening mammography. None of these tests, however, have been demonstrated to lower breast cancer mortality in a randomized trial of screening.

RISKS AND DRAWBACKS OF SCREENING

What are the drawbacks to screening? The potential hazard attributable to radiation exposure from a modern mammogram is presumed to be negligible by clinicians and screening advocates. Radiation hazard is greatest among women in the second and third decades of life and should be avoided whenever possible. Howe and McLaughlin estimated that, assuming a 30% reduction in breast cancer mortality, biennial mammography at 2 mGy per view would prevent 242 deaths among women 50 to 69 for every death induced by the ionizing effect of radiation on breast tissue. Making the same assumptions for women in their 40s, screening would prevent 97 deaths for every death resulting from radiation-induced breast cancer.

The primary drawback of screening mammography is its low positive predictive value, estimated to be 8.6% in the Canadian National Breast Screening Study. Kerlikowske reported that there were 71 abnormal mammograms for every 1000 women 50 years of age and older screened for the first time. These abnormal tests resulted in 132 procedures, including 25 biopsies to diagnose 7.5 invasive cancers and 2.5 cases of DCIS. There were 53 abnormal mammograms among women screened for the first time in their 30s and 40s; this lead to 102 procedures including 13 biopsies to diagnose one invasive breast cancer and one case of DCIS. Thus there were 50 tests for every cancer diagnosed under 50 years of age, and 15 tests for every cancer diagnosed in women 50 years of age and older.

The cumulative false-positive rate after five mammograms is 30% among women under 50, and 24% among women 50 years of age and older. Lerman reported that 47% of women continued to have mammography-related anxiety and 41% continued to be worried about breast cancer 3 months after a false-positive mammogram.

The false negative rate of mammography is 20% to 25% among women in their 40s and 10% among women 50 years

Table 95-3
Recommendations for Screening Mammography

Age Group (years)	FREQUENCY OF MAMMOGRAPHY (years)				Evidence from RCT's*
	ACS	USPSTF	Sweden	UK	
<40	once	0	0	0	No evidence of benefit
40-49	1-2	0	1.5	0	Benefit controversial
50-69	1	1	2	3	Benefit controversial
>69	1	1	2	0	Benefit controversial

ACS, American Cancer Society; *USPSTF*, United States Preventive Services Task Force; Sweden, Swedish Board of Welfare; *UK*, United Kingdom.
*See Table 95-2 for results of randomized controlled trials (RCTs).

of age and older. False-negative mammogram results may falsely reassure women and their doctors, so that they ignore breast lumps that become palpable in the months after screening. In a study by the Physician Insurers Association, women with palpable breast lumps who had false-negative mammograms were the most likely to experience a delayed diagnosis of breast cancer.

Screening CBE and BSE lack the sensitivity needed to detect breast cancer early enough to affect breast cancer mortality. Like screening mammography, CBE and BSE increase the detection of benign breast lumps and thus increase the emotional and material cost of screening. Does the benefit of screening outweigh the drawbacks? Investigators used computer models to perform a cost-effectiveness analysis assuming the mortality reduction reported from the randomized trials and meta-analyses. They predict that screening mammography extends life 12 days at $704 per woman in the 50 to 69 age group. Among women in their 40s, screening mammography extends life 2.5 days at $676 per woman. The cost-effectiveness ratio was $21,400/year/ life saved for older women, and $150,000/year/life saved for women in their 40s.

Despite this cost and the other drawbacks described previously, most organizations recommend regular screening with mammography and CBE. Table 95-3 compares screening recommendations of the American Cancer Society (ACS), United States Preventive Services Task Force, Sweden, and the United Kingdom. Because screening efficacy remains controversial, society takes a leap of faith that benefits outweigh risks. It is not controversial, however, that better screening tests are needed, such as a biologic marker detectable by blood assay. Primary prevention of breast cancer may be the best hope for reducing the burden of this common and feared disease.

SUMMARY RECOMMENDATIONS

To comply with the standard of care established by panels of experts and organizations that publish screening guidelines, clinicians should offer screening to their patients. Given the lack of certainty about the efficacy of screening for breast cancer, however, clinicians should inform patients about the limitations and drawbacks of mammography, CBE, and BSE.

1. All women over 40 years of age should be offered mammography at least every 2 years. Although randomized trials of screening excluded women over 70 years old, active and healthy elderly women should be offered screening.
2. Average-risk women should have CBE at the time of their periodic health examination at all ages.
3. BSE should not be encouraged as a regular screening exercise. Because a large proportion of breast cancer is self-discovered, women should not be discouraged from being familiar with their breast texture.
4. High-risk women should have annual mammography and CBE commencing at age 35, or 5 years earlier than the age at which their first-degree relative acquired breast cancer. Such women should also be offered genetic testing to see whether they could benefit from preventive therapy with a selective estrogen receptor modulator or preventive surgery.

BIBLIOGRAPHY

Alexander FE et al: Fourteen years of follow-up from the Edinburgh randomised trial of breast-cancer screening, *Lancet* 353:1903, 1999.

Anderson I et al: Mammographic screening and mortality from breast cancer: the Malmo mammographic screening trial, *Br Med J* 297:943, 1988.

Baker LH: Breast cancer detection demonstration project: five year summary report, *Cancer* 32:194, 1982.

Beemsterboer PM, Warmerdam PG, Boer R, de Koning HJ: Radiation risk of mammography related to benefit in screening programs: a favourable balance? *J Med Screen* 5:81, 1998.

Bjurstam N et al: The Gothenburg breast screening trial: first results on mortality, incidence and mode of detection for women ages 39-49 years at randomization, *Cancer* 80:2091, 1997.

Chu KC, Smart CR, Tarone RE: Analysis of breast cancer mortality and stage distribution by age for the Health Insurance Plan clinical trial, *J Natl Cancer Inst* 80:1125, 1988.

Elmore JG et al: Ten year risk of false positive screening mammography and clinical breast examination, *N Engl J Med* 338:1089, 1998.

Fisher B, Slack NH: Number of lymph nodes examined and the prognosis of breast carcinoma, *Surg Gynecol Obstet* 131:79, 1970.

Fox M: On the diagnosis and treatment of breast cancer, *JAMA* 24:489, 1979.

Frisell J, Lidbrink E, Hellstrom L, Rutqvist LE: Follow-up after 11 years: update of mortality results in the Stockholm mammographic screening trial. *Breast Cancer Res Treat* 45:263, 1997.

Gotzsche PC, Olsen, O: Is screening for breast cancer with mammography justifiable? *Lancet* 355:129, 2000.

Harris JR et al, editor: *Breast diseases,* ed 2, Philadelphia, 1991, JB Lippincott.

Kerlikowske K: Efficacy of screening mammography: a meta-analysis. *JAMA* 273:149,1995.

Kerlikowske K et al: Likelihood ratios for modern screening mammography: risk of breast cancer based on age and mammographic interpretation, *JAMA* 276:39, 1996.

Kerlikowske K et al: Positive predictive value of screening mammography by age and family history of breast cancer, *JAMA* 270:2444, 1993.

Miller AB, Baines CJ, To T, Wall C: Canadian National Breast Screening Study: 1-breast cancer detection and death rates among women aged 40-49 years, *Can Med Assoc J* 147:1459, 1992.

Miller AB, Baines CJ, To T, Wall C: Canadian National Breast Screening Study: 2-breast cancer detection and death rates among women aged 50-59 years, *Can Med Assoc J* 147:1477, 1992.

Moody-Ayers SY, Wells CK, Feinstein AR: Benign tumors and early detection in mammography-screened patients of a natural cohort with breast cancer, *Arch Intern Med* 160:1109, 2000.

Nystrom L et al: Breast cancer screening with mammography: overview of Swedish randomized trials, *Lancet* 341:973, 1993.

Salzmann P, Kerlikowske K, Phillips K: Cost-effectiveness of extending screening mammography guidelines to include women 40-49 years of age, *Ann Intern Med* 128:878, 1998.

Semiglazov VF, Sagaidak VN, Moiseyenko VM, Mikhailov EA: Study of the role of breast self-examination in the reduction of mortality from breast cancer. The Russian Federation/World Health Organization Study, *Eur J Cancer* 29:2039, 1993.

Tabar L et al: Efficacy of breast cancer screening by age: new resuots from the Swedish Two-country Trial, *Cancer* 75:2507, 1995.

Thomas DB et al: Randomized trial of breast self-examination in Shanghai: methodology and preliminary results, *J Natl Cancer Inst* 89:355, 1997.

Welch HG, Black WC: Using autopsy series to estimate the disease "reservoir" for ductal carcinoma in situ of the breast: how much more breast cancer can we find? *Ann Intern Med* 127:1023, 1997.

Wells J: Mammography and the politics of randomised controlled trials, *Br Med J* 317:1224, 1998.

CHAPTER 96

Cervical Cancer and Human Papillomavirus

Ellen E. Sheets

▦ EPIDEMIOLOGY

Because of the natural history of invasive cervical cancer, which includes a lengthy preinvasive stage and an easy-to-perform, readily available screening test, it has long been thought that this disease is preventable. In the United States approximately 12,800 new cases and 4600 deaths will occur in the year 2000 as a result of this disease. However, worldwide approximately 400,000 new cases occur yearly, making it second only to breast cancer as the documented cause of cancer death among women. Every study that evaluates the role of cervical cytologic screening shows a significant decrease in the occurrence and mortality rates of cervical cancer.

The incidence of cervical cancer varies according to race. In the United States the incidence rate for African Americans, Hispanics, and Native Americans is approximately twice that of whites. The risk for Asians is similar to that of whites. Interestingly, results from the 1987 U.S. National Health Interview Survey indicate that African Americans are screened at rates comparable to or higher than those for whites through age 69. Hispanics have a lower screening rate than whites. Why African Americans have a higher incidence rate is unknown.

Age appears to alter the incidence of invasive cervical cancer worldwide. Studies show that the age-related pattern is for women to decrease their use of cervical cytologic screening as their age increases. This coincides with an age-related increase in the incidence of invasive cervical cancer. Most studies grouped patients by age, before 65 and after 65, but the greatest difference occurred between those women 44 years old or younger and those 65 years old or older.

Geography also appears to play a role in incidence of this disease. High rates of cervical cancer are found in the Caribbean and Latin America. Annual incidence rates are greater than 20/100,000 women in Latin America compared with 2 to 5/100,000 in the United States. Other regions with high incidences are Hong Kong, parts of India, Denmark, Romania, and the Northwest Territories of Canada. Whether these differences represent deficiencies of screening or general health care, artifact, or areas with higher rates of causal factors is not clear. Further, it is possible that the causative factors involved in cervical cancer affect the population in these areas differently.

RISK FACTORS FOR CERVICAL CANCER
Sexual Factors

It is not a recent idea that cervical cancer is sexually transmitted. One of the first reports supporting this idea was the 1842 report of Rigoni-Stern, who noted that married (i.e., sexually active) women had a greater risk of development of cervical cancer than cloistered women. Since then there have been numerous accounts of sexually related risk factors. These factors have been pared down to early sexual activity (before age 17) and numerous sexual partners (greater than 5). Other factors, such as associated sexually transmitted diseases, poor sexual hygiene, and contact with a high-risk male, have variably been related to cervical cancer development. Not all studies support these other factors, and their importance is most probably a reflection of the primary risk factors. The role of the high-risk male was suggested by studies of men whose consorts had cervical cancer, whose subsequent consorts were at higher risk of development of cervical cancer.

Smoking

When trying to assess the risk of nonsexual factors, studies must be controlled for the major sexual risk factors. Epidemiologic studies reveal a twofold increased risk for preinvasive and invasive cervical cancer for smokers. In addition the risk appears to increase the longer one smokes, the more one smokes, and with use of unfiltered cigarettes. Several factors have been implicated as the potential cause of this increased disease risk. Reports have indicated a decrease in local cervical immune function, constituents of smoke in cervical mucus, and alterations of cellular DNA.

Diet

Although dietary factors have not been studied as extensively as other risk factors, there appears to be a general trend. When confounding factors are controlled for it appears that those women whose diet is deficient in vitamin A or C are at greater risk for cervical cancer. Less solid are data implicating folic acid deficiency as a risk factor. These factors may help explain the regional variation in cervical cancer incidence.

Oral Contraceptives

As a result of confounding factors, the role of contraceptive method in cervical carcinogenesis is difficult to evaluate. Traditional risk factors require controls as well as the contraceptive method. Women who use barrier contraceptives may have more protection than those who do not. Studies that control for all of these factors indicate that the longer a woman uses the pill, the greater her risk of cervical cancer becomes. Overall relative adjusted risk from the World Health Organization (WHO) Collaborative Study of Neoplasia and Steroid Contraceptives for pill users was 1.2. The same group found a 1.5 relative adjusted risk when the pill was used for 5 years or more.

Role of Human Papillomavirus

An association between human papillomavirus (HPV)-induced lesions and preinvasive disease of the female lower reproductive tract was first noted in 1976. Then exophytic and flat condylomata were seen in conjunction with cervical intraepithelial neoplasia (CIN) and some cases of invasive cervical cancer. Immunochemical studies using antibodies that reacted to exophytic condylomata antigens revealed proteins associated with HPV in preinvasive cervical lesions. This finding has only been strengthened with the isolation first of HPV 6 DNA and subsequent DNA types. Using DNA hybridization techniques a strong association has been found between the presence of HPV DNA and preinvasive and invasive cervical disease. Case control studies comparing the rate of invasive cervical cancer between groups known to be infected with HPV to noninfected individuals reveals an odds ratio of 10 to 15 and in a few studies greater than 15. Late in the 1980s it became apparent that HPV DNA can integrate into host cell DNA. Integration seems to correlate strongly with increasing grades of CIN and with invasive cervical cancer. No final step between HPV infection and development of invasive cervical cancer has been determined.

PATHOPHYSIOLOGY

Transition from Normal Epithelium to Precancerous to Cancerous Lesions

Cervical neoplasia develops from normal cervical epithelium. It is initiated at the transformation zone by an HPV infection. HPV causes a vegetative infection that creates histologic changes interpreted as low-grade CIN. Some of these lesions will evolve to encompass the full epithelial thickness and thus are called high grade CIN or carcinoma in situ (CIS). A small fraction of the high-grade CIN will over time become invasive cervical cancer. The development of high-grade CIN (often designated CIN2/CIN3/CIS) and invasive cancer is associated with integration of HPV into the host cell DNA.

HPV

Historical Aspects

Descriptions of clinical lesions that we now know were caused by HPV have been in the literature since antiquity. These lesions even then were thought to be transmitted sexually. Since the isolation of HPV 6 DNA in 1980 an explosion of knowledge about HPV has occurred. The vast majority of these data were accumulated by using molecular biologic techniques. The reason such sophisticated science is needed is that HPV will not grow in cell culture. Although advances in DNA techniques have helped, the lack of a culture system for HPV has certainly constrained the limits of our knowledge.

Definition of HPV Type

HPV will only grow within human epithelium; however, different viral types appear to have preferences for certain regions of epithelium. A type is defined by the extent of its DNA homology with other, previously isolated HPV DNA types. To be a new type it must have less than 90% homology within the L1 gene in comparison to known types. This homology is measured in a standard liquid hybridization assay. Classification is then based on DNA analysis and predilection for certain epithelium. There are now more than 100 known HPV types. In general the important ones in the human reproductive tract are HPV 6, 11, 16, 18, 31, 33, 35, 39, 42, 43, 44, 45, 50, and 51 to 60. If HPV-related lesions are separated into two groups, low-risk (condylomata, low-grade CIN) versus high-risk (high-grade CIN, invasive cancer), certain HPV types are associated with each group. Types 6, 11, and 42 are found in low-risk lesions, and 16, 18, 33, 35, and 39 in high-risk lesions.

Methods of HPV Detection

Methods that detect the presence of HPV can be divided into two groups: those that will detect only clinically evident infection and those that will detect both clinical and subclinical diseases. For the clinically evident infection, Pap smears and histologic examination detect the presence of HPV-related lesions. Any other proof that HPV is indeed present thus far relies on DNA analysis. Until HPV can be grown in a culture system some type of DNA analysis will be necessary to detect subclinical disease and to confirm its presence in clinically evident infection.

Thus far, the methods of clinical detection rely on characteristic findings on cytologic or histologic review. These methods, although documented as highly reliable for the presence of HPV DNA, will not reveal the HPV type that is associated with the lesion. Cytologic evidence is defined as the presence of koilocytic changes through tissue associated with preinvasive or invasive disease. Histologic counterparts exist for koilocytic changes and preinvasive disease. Some progress has been made in defining morphologic changes that can be associated with HPV 16, which is commonly thought to be strongly associated with high-grade CIN.

Categories of DNA studies can be made by using the sensitivity of the assay as the basis for distinction. In order of increasing sensitivity there is in situ hybridization (detects 10 to 50 HPV gene copies per cell), southern blot hybridization (detects less than one HPV gene copy per cell), and polymerase chain reaction (detects one HPV gene per 100,000 cells). Even such sophisticated techniques cannot be viewed as 100% accurate. This is due to variations in any given laboratory's ability to perform and interpret these techniques, and detection is subject to sampling error. HPV DNA is not equally distributed within the lower reproductive tract epithelium, and it is possible to obtain different results from different epithelial areas within the same patient. Most investigators try to use at least two different DNA techniques for any study.

Natural History of HPV Infection

The risk of developing a HPV-related genital tract lesion starts at the time of initial sexual contact. Such contact does not require intercourse, as skin to skin contact is sufficient for passage of the virus. Initial infections generally occur in the late teens to early 20s; most are infected with high-risk HPV types. The majority who are exposed will spontaneously resolve their HPV infection over the next 2 years. Persistence of a HPV infection or a HPV-related preinvasive lesion greater than 2 years is a significant risk factor for the development of a high-grade CIN or invasive cancer. The next significant peak of HPV activity is in the late 30s to early 40s and generally present as high-grade CIN. These women are at significant risk for the development of invasive cervical cancer.

Factors Involved in Prevalence of HPV

Determining the prevalence of HPV is fraught with many problems. These problems range from the characteristics of the group being screened to the method of detection and the age of the patient group. Every study looking at the issue of prevalence must define these parameters.

It would be helpful to determine the background rate of HPV infection in humans. This has been approached by evaluating low-risk women, that is, those who do not have risk factors for cervical cancer. The problem with this approach is that it is not entirely clear that the risks for HPV infection mirror those for cervical cancer. Studies have focused on women who do not have any clinical evidence of HPV infection. Unfortunately these studies were not always controlled for cervical cancer risk factors. Also it is difficult to screen large asymptomatic groups through methods that require tissue or even cytologic specimens. Some progress has been made with serologic techniques, but these methods are extremely time consuming and labor intensive.

Once the characteristics of the study group have been defined, the method of detection becomes a factor. The lack of standardization of these methods has hampered the ability to compare studies and subsequent rates of infection. Generally the overall rate of asymptomatic infection detected by clinical methods ranges from 3% to 30%.

Most studies have indicated that the peak infection rate occurs at about 20 years of age, with about 15% to 30% being infected. Although there appears to be a stabilization of the rate at about 10% after the age of 40, these values may change as the population ages. This infection rate most likely will vary if risk factors for cervical cancer are applied to each group; however, large prospective studies have not yet addressed both issues.

A significant factor in the prevalence and persistence of HPV is the woman's immune system. Those who suffer from autoimmune disorders, are taking immunosuppressive drugs for organ transplants, have had other malignancies, or are infected with human immunodeficiency virus are at greater risk for contracting a HPV infection and having it persist. These findings indicate that the ability to spontaneously resolve a HPV infection is dependent on the woman mounting an adequate immune response to the virus.

Role of HPV Types in Cervical Cancer Development

There is no doubt that worldwide data support a strong causal role between HPV infection and the development of preinvasive and invasive cervical disease. Common factors associated with HPV infections and cervical cancer can be summarized as follows:

1. HPV is a sexually transmitted disease and has the same associated risk factors as those known to predispose women to cervical cancer.
2. HPV is involved in all facets of benign, preinvasive, and invasive disease.
3. HPV infection shares the same natural history as that of CIN (potential to progress to invasive disease if left untreated).
4. Data support a long latency period for HPV infection in both sexes.
5. HPV type and physical state of the virus (i.e., integration versus episomal state) appear to be related to the malignant potential of the virus.
6. HPV probably does not act alone in cervical carcinogenesis but requires some form of cofactor.
7. HPV infections appear to vary in their clinical course if the immunologic status of the host is altered.

Of all the HPV types, type 16 has had the strongest association. Its presence in high-grade CIN and invasive squamous cervical cancer is generally reported as 80% to 95%. Further, it has been found that HPV 16 becomes integrated into the host cell DNA. It is believed that integration represents a significant step in the subsequent development of high-grade preinvasive and invasive disease. Obviously the viral DNA's ability to affect host cell function will be markedly changed with this development.

The mechanism by which HPV causes cellular transformation on a molecular level is well defined. Expression of the viral DNA within the host cell occurs and HPV has two major regions of DNA: the late reading frames that give rise to the viral capsule and the early reading frames that cause alterations in the host cell function. Specifically two of the early reading frames, E6 and E7, produce proteins that bind to cell tumor suppressor genes, p53 and pRB, respectively. It is this event that allows for host cell transformation, and the persistence of expression of E6/E7 is required for malignant transformation.

SCREENING
History of the Papanicolaou Smear

The Papanicolaou smear was developed by Dr. George Papanicolaou in the 1930s. Widespread usage for screening started in the 1940s. It was initially used as a tool to identify those patients who had asymptomatic cervical cancer. Since the 1960s when the concept of preinvasive disease became widely accepted, there has been an explosion of detection of preinvasive disease and a significant decrease in incidence of invasive cancer and related death.

The Pap smear process depends on collecting exfoliated cervical cells by scraping the cervical epithelium. False-negative Pap smear results can be caused by improper scraping technique and lack of exfoliation of the cervical cells. Marked improvement occurs when the clinician uses an endocervical brush in addition to an Ayer's wooden or plastic spatula. Other reasons for false-negative Pap smear results are improper fixation or staining of the cells and incorrect interpretation. False-negative rates of 20% to 57% have been reported.

Significance of Screening

Factors that affect the mortality rate of cervical cancer include the population's natural incidence of the disease, the preclinical stage duration, the sensitivity and specificity of the screening process, and the quality of treatment available for preinvasive and invasive diagnoses. Studies have evaluated the age at which screening should start, the frequency with which it should be done, the age when screening should cease, and the appropriate personnel to perform the screening examination.

There seems to be little debate as to when a woman should start to undergo periodic screening. Most would agree that once regular intercourse has started the risk for development of preinvasive disease is present. How often a Pap smear should be done after initiation of periodic screening is not clear (Table 96-1). The American College of Obstetricians and Gynecologists in conjunction with several other major cancer organizations have recommended that every woman should have a yearly Pap smear and pelvic examination starting at age 18 or at the onset of sexual activity. Screening should occur yearly for 3 years. If the results are normal the physician can recommend that the screening interval be extended. One concern clinically is that if women do not have annual Pap smears they also will not have annual bimanual examinations. Therefore, screening

for other gynecologic problems as well as ovarian cancer (for which there is no other adequate screening protocol) will not be completed. There are no consistent recommendations for how often to perform the bimanual examination or whether the bimanual examination is a sensitive screening procedure.

Studies have retrospectively looked at the interval between diagnosis of cervical cancer and the previous Pap smear. Uncontrolled data from New York State assessed the interval from the last Pap smear and the onset of cervical cancer in 261 women diagnosed from 1983 to 1985. Data indicated that 54% had an interval of greater than 3 years between the last Pap smear and diagnosis of disease. When case-controlled studies were evaluated it was found that the overall number of Pap smears was inversely related to the risk of disease. Although the exact number varied, most patients received significant protection from cervical cancer when the interval of screening was 4 or fewer years. Compared with those patients who were never screened, those who had at least three Pap smears had a 90% decreased risk of development of cervical cancer. Interestingly, those patients whose Pap smears were done by an obstetrician-gynecologist had significantly less chance of development of invasive cancer over any specific interval evaluated. This finding may be related to the introduction of the cervical brush.

Unfortunately large retrospective studies show that screening decreases as age increases. Estimates of never-screened women age 65 years or older are as high as 63%.

Table 96-1
Recommendations for Routine Papanicolaou's Smear Screening for Cervical Cancer

Group	Age to Start	Interval to Repeat	Age to Stop	Other Comments
National Institute's Health Consensus Conference on Cervical Cancer Screening, 1980	18 or onset of sexual activity	1-3 years after 2 normal, consecutive annual results	60 if previous screening adequate and Pap smears negative findings	
Canadian Task Force on Cervical Cancer, 1991	18 or onset of sexual activity	1-3 years after 2 normal, consecutive annual results	69 and stop if all previous screen results were normal	
American College of Obstetricians and Gynecologists, 1989	18 or onset of sexual activity	Annually for 3 consecutive years then at physician recommend interval	No recommendation	Annual bimanual pelvic examination
United States Preventive Health Task Force, 1989	Onset of sexual activity	1-3 years on physician recommendation based on risk factors	65 if physician can document consistently normal previous Pap smear results	
National Cancer Institute, 1990	18 or onset of sexual activity	After 3 normal consecutive annual results, repeat less frequently	No recommendation	

American College of Obstetrics and Gynecology Committee Opinion: *Report of the task force on routine cancer screening*, Washington, DC, 1989, American College of Obstetrics and Gynecology;
Report of a national workshop on screening for cancer of the cervix, *Can Med Assoc J* 145:1301, 1991.
Fink DJ: *Cancer* 38:127, 1988.
Guide to clinical preventive services: an assessment of the effectiveness of 169 interventions: report of the U.S. Preventive Services Task Force, Baltimore, 1989, William & Wilkins.
McPhee SJ, Bird JA: *J Gen Int Med (Suppl):* 116, 1990.
HIV, Human immunodeficiency virus.

Even more unfortunate are the retrospective data indicating that close to 80% of these unscreened women had seen a medical practitioner within the last 2 years, with greater than 90% reporting visits within the last 5 years. These data, along with data indicating that only 11% of women realize that Pap smears are done to prevent cervical cancer, indicate how important it is to educate women and primary care providers. When a mathematical model is used to predict reductions in mortality rate by instituting triennial screening in women over 65 years old, approximately a 74% reduction in cervical cancer mortality could be achieved. Still there is no consensus when a patient should stop having routine Pap smear screening. Although there is a documented increased risk of development of cervical cancer as age increases, a patient who has had frequent, negative Pap smear results before the age of 65 benefits less from routine screening after age 65. Since a large percentage of patients in this age group have not been either screened or screened regularly, it seems prudent to extend periodic testing beyond age 65. Again a physician should make such a decision.

New Screening Methods

Owing to the inherent false-negative rate of the Pap smear, other cytologic methods of cervical cancer screening have been developed in the last decade. These methods depend on the rinsing of collection devices into a preservative fluid rather than smearing the collected cells onto a slide. This liquid method of preparation increases the number of evaluable cells taken from the cervix thus statistically increasing the chance that abnormal cells could be detected. The liquid cell preparation is then sent to the cytology laboratory where a representative slide of the cells is prepared creating a thin, uniform layer of cells. Two different thin-layer systems have been approved to replace the Pap smear by the Food and Drug Administration (FDA), the ThinPrep Pap Test and the AutoCyte Pap. Whether either of these methods is more cost-effective than the conventional Pap smear is under evaluation.

In addition to thin-layer cytology preparations, the FDA approved a test for the detection of HPV in exfoliated cervical cells, either as a separate sample from the cervix or from residual cells in the thin-layer specimens. The test, known as the Digene Hybrid capture, sorts HPV into high and low risk categories for reporting the presence or absence of HPV DNA in a given patient sample. Several different scenarios for use of this test are currently under trial and include using it to triage women for colposcopy to increase the detection of cervical histologic abnormalities, or for the primary detection of cervical preinvasive or invasive disease. More clinical studies will be required to define the role of such HPV DNA detection in the management of HPV-related disease.

Cost-effectiveness of Screening

Given the contracted medical resources of the 1990s and beyond, cost-effective screening plans are essential. Much discussion has been given to the appropriate interval of cervical cytology screening, and most screening models agree that intervals of less than 3 years between Pap smear screening are increasingly costly without a major impact on the rate of invasive disease. The problem is that patient compliance always lags behind recommended screening intervals.

Thus the recommended screening interval for women in the United States has been 1 year, unless the interval is extended at the advice of a physician.

The use of yearly conventional Pap smear screening versus thin-layer cytology preparations on a yearly or greater interval has led to even more discussion on the cost-effectiveness of using new screening methods and their interval of use compared with the Pap smear. Such debate is based on the relative superior screening results of thin-layer tests, and such data are used in cost-effectiveness medical models. There is as yet no consensus regarding which method will be ultimately most cost-effective.

Recommendations for Routine Pap Smear Screening

The current recommendations for when to perform screening Pap smears appear in Table 96-1. The standard of care generally adheres to the recommendations by the American College of Obstetricians and Gynecologists and the United States Preventive Health Task Force.

APPROACH TO WOMEN WITH ABNORMAL PAP SMEAR RESULTS
Follow-up of Abnormal Pap Smear Results

All Pap smear results in the United States are reported according to the criteria of the Bethesda System. This system of cervical cytology diagnoses was developed to decrease the variability between cytology examiners for a given type of disease noted on a Pap smear. The system splits results into no evidence of malignant disease, atypical cells of undetermined significance (both squamous and glandular), low-grade squamous intraepithelial lesions (LSIL), high-grade squamous intraepithelial lesions (HSIL), and invasive cancers. The recommendations for evaluation follow the guidelines set up by the NIH/NCI for the Bethesda System results.

The results of the screening Pap smear will determine the recommendations and advice the clinician gives to the woman. Table 96-2 summarizes current recommendations for follow-up evaluation of an abnormal Pap smear result.

If the Pap smear result is **negative for malignant cells** and is an adequate sample (judged by the presence of endocervical cells) then the clinician should follow the guidelines for routine Pap smear screening outlined in Table 96-1. It is important to know that endocervical cells are present to ensure an adequate sampling. If the **endocervical cells are not present** then the clinician should schedule the repeat Pap smear on the basis of the risk of development of disease for the particular woman. For instance if the woman has multiple risk factors and therefore is at increased risk for the development of cervical dysplasia and cancer, one generally repeats the Pap smear not less than 6 weeks or more than 3 months after the inadequate sample. If the patient is at low risk, then it is appropriate to recommend that the Pap smear be repeated at the annual visit.

Some results on Pap smears, such as **squamous metaplasia,** are considered normal and require no intervention other than following the guidelines for routine Pap smear screening.

The finding of **atypical cells of undetermined significance** is abnormal. If the cells are noted to be squamous, the

Table 96-2
Follow-up of Abnormal Pap Smear Results

Pap Smear Result	Recommendation for Follow-up
Negative for malignant cells No endocervical cells	See guidelines for routine Pap smear If high risk, repeat within 1 month If low risk, repeat at annual check-up Use cervical brush technique for improved sampling Normal result
Squamous metaplasia Atypical cells of undetermined significance	
Squamous	Consider treatment for underlying infection Repeat in 4-6 months for 2 years. If abnormal again, refer for colposcopy If HIV-positive, refer directly for colposcopy
Glandular	First atypical glandular pap requires colposcopy Refer for colposcopy
Squamous intraepithelial lesions Low or high grade	
Invasive cancer squamous or adenocarcinoma	Refer for colposcopy

current recommendation is to repeat the Pap smear every 4 to 6 months for 2 years. If any abnormality is detected in that interval, evaluation by colposcopy is indicated. Women with excessive high risk factors such as human immunodeficiency virus (HIV) seropositivity or immune disorders should move on to colposcopy with the first abnormal smear. If the smear is atypical on the basis of glandular cells, colposcopy is mandatory with the first abnormal smear.

For findings of a **squamous intraepithelial lesion,** low or high grade, colposcopy is indicated. Because of the crossover of the risk factors (i.e., sexual activity) between HPV and HIV exposure, women with dysplasia should be screened for all HIV risk factors. Testing should be considered when appropriate or on the request of the patient.

BIBLIOGRAPHY

American College of Obstetrics and Gynecology Committee Opinion: *Recommendations on frequency of pap test screening,* Washington DC, 1995, American College of Obstetrics and Gynecology.

Arends MJ, Buckley CH, Wells M: Aetiology, pathogenesis, and pathology of cervical neoplasia, *J Clin Pathol* 51:96, 1998.

Bishop JW et al: Multicenter masked evaluation of autocyte prep thin layers with matched conventional smears, *Acta Cytol* 42:189, 1998.

Fahs MC et al: Cost effectiveness of cervical cancer screening for the elderly, *Ann Intern Med* 117:520, 1992.

Fletcher A: Screening for cancer of the cervix in elderly women, *Lancet* 335:97, 1990.

Greenlee RT, Murray T, Bolden S, Wingo PA: Cancer statistics, 2000, *CA Cancer J Clin* 50:7, 2000.

Guide to clinical preventive services: an assessment of the effectiveness of 169 interventions: report of the U.S. Preventive Services Task Force, Baltimore, 1989, William & Wilkins.

Harlan LC, Bernstein AM, Kessler LG: Cervical cancer screening: who is not screened and why? *Am J Public Health* 81:885, 1991.

Ho GYF et al: HPV 16 and cigarette smoking as risk factor for high-grade cervical intraepithelial neoplasia, *Int J Cancer* 78:281, 1998.

Janerich DT et al: The screening histories of women with invasive cervical cancer, Connecticut, *Am J Public Health,* 85:791, 1995.

Kinney W et al: Missed opportunities for cervical cancer screening of HMO members developing invasive cervical cancer (ICC), *Gynecol Oncol* 71:428, 1998.

Klassen AC, Celentano DD, Brookmeyer R: Variation in the duration of protection given by screening using the pap test for cervical cancer, *J Clin Epidemiol* 42:1003, 1989.

Koutsky L: Epidemiology of genital human papillomavirus infection, *Am J Med* 102:3, 1997.

Kurman RJ, Henson DE, Herbst AL, Noller KL: Interim guidelines for management of abnormal cervical cytology, *JAMA* 271:1866, 1994.

Lacy JV et al: Oral contraceptives as risk factors for cervical adenocarcinomas and squamous cell carcinoma, *Cancer Biomark Prev* 8:1079, 1999.

Lee KR et al: Comparison of conventional papanicolaou smears and a fluid-based, thin-layer system for cervical cancer screening, *Obstet Gynecol* 90:278, 1997.

Manos MM et al: Identifying women with cervical neoplasia using human papillomavirus DNA testing for equivocal papanicolaou results, *JAMA* 281:1603, 1999.

National Cancer Institute Workshop: The 1988 Bethesda system for reporting cervical/vaginal cytological diagnoses, *JAMA* 262:932, 1989.

Parazzini F et al: Screening practices and invasive cervical cancer risk in different age strata, *Gynecol Oncol* 38:76, 1990.

Schwartz M et al: Woman's knowledge and experience of cervical screening: a failure of health education and medical organization, *Community Med* 11:279, 1989.

Stoler MH: Human papillomaviruses and cervical neoplasia: a model for carcinogenesis, *Int J Gynecol Pathol* 19:16, 2000.

Sun XW et al: Human papillomavirus infection in human immunodeficiency virus-seropositive women, *Obstet Gynecol* 85:680, 1995.

van Ballegooijen M et al: Diagnostic and treatment procedures induced by cervical cancer screening, *Eur J Cancer* 26:941, 1990.

van der Graaf Y et al: The effectiveness of cervical screening: a population-based case-control study, *J Clin Epidemiol* 41:21, 1988.

CHAPTER 97

Ovarian and Vulvar Cancer Screening

Karen J. Carlson

In the course of providing routine care, the primary care clinician has the opportunity to screen asymptomatic women for common gynecologic malignancies. The value of the Papanicolaou's (Pap) smear for early detection of cervical neoplasia is well supported by a body of indirect evidence (Chapter 96). There is less scientific information to document the benefit of screening for other malignancies of the female genital tract, including endometrial, ovarian, and vulvar cancers. This chapter provides an overview of the epidemiology and risk factors for these diseases, reviews screening procedures suitable for the primary care setting, and provides recommendations for screening based on the available evidence for its effectiveness. The focus of this chapter is screening of the asymptomatic woman. The approach to women with symptoms warranting evaluation of endometrial cancer (Chapter 52), ovarian cancer (Chapter 49), or vulvar cancer (Chapter 44) is discussed elsewhere.

ENDOMETRIAL CANCER
Epidemiology

Endometrial cancer is the most common gynecologic malignancy (Table 97-1). Its incidence has increased in the last two decades, probably as a result of the growth in use of estrogen replacement therapy as well as the aging of the population. The incidence of endometrial cancer increases with age (Fig. 97-1), with a median age at diagnosis of 66 years. The mortality rate from endometrial cancer has fallen slightly over the last 20 years, and it is a less important cause of cancer deaths than other gynecologic malignancies (Fig. 97-2). When endometrial cancer is still localized at the time of diagnosis, 5-year survival rate is 96%. The 5-year survival rate for all stages combined is approximately 80% for white women and 55% for African-American women.

The **risk factors** for endometrial cancer (Box 97-1) reflect a strong role for an excess of estrogen relative to progesterone in the biologic mechanism of some endometrial cancers. These factors include **unopposed estrogen therapy, obesity, chronic anovulation, nulliparity,** and **late menopause** (after age 55). Studies of unopposed

estrogens document a relative risk of endometrial cancer ranging from 4 to 8. Obesity is associated with a twofold to threefold increase in risk when weight is more than 200 pounds or body mass index more than 27. The remaining factors listed previously increase risk by roughly twofold. **Diabetes** increases risk independently of its association with obesity, perhaps reflecting underlying immune compromise. Hypertension does not have an effect on risk independent of obesity. **Tamoxifen** has a stimulatory effect on the endometrium and has been shown to increase endometrial cancer risk approximately twofold after 2 years of use.

The evidence for a **familial association** of endometrial cancer is relatively weak, except in rare kindreds with a hereditary syndrome of colon, endometrial, and ovarian cancer. Although familial syndromes are rare, identification of this risk factor is important as screening for endometrial cancer may be justified in such women. In families with hereditary nonpolyposis colorectal cancer (HPNCC), women carry a lifetime risk of developing endometrial cancer of 22% to 50%. These tumors occur on average 15 years earlier than do sporadic cases.

Two factors have been consistently shown to be associated with a **lower risk** of endometrial cancer: use of the **oral contraceptive pill** and **pregnancy.**

Screening Techniques

The **Pap smear** is a relatively insensitive technique for early detection of endometrial cancer. However, if benign endometrial cells are observed on a Pap smear in a postmenopausal woman, further evaluation with endometrial sampling is necessary.

Endometrial sampling has a high correlation with the results of formal dilatation and curettage for detection of endometrial cancer. A variety of sampling methods are available for use in the outpatient setting. Methods that provide tissue specimens are more accurate than those that yield cytologic specimens; however, the cytologic techniques produce less discomfort and are easier to use in the ambulatory setting. The sensitivity of cytologic sampling methods (measured in women with vaginal bleeding) ranges from 80% to 100% for detection of endometrial carcinoma and 35% to

45% for detection of endometrial hyperplasia. A single large cohort study of cytologic screening in asymptomatic women showed an apparent sensitivity of 80% for detection of cancer.

Transvaginal ultrasound is a noninvasive method for evaluating the endometrium. In postmenopausal women, the thickness and homogeneity of the endometrial stripe correlate highly with the presence of endometrial hyperplasia and carcinoma; cyclical variations in the endometrium of cycling women limit its accuracy in the premenopausal population. Studies comparing endometrial biopsy and transvaginal ultrasound for detection of endometrial abnormalities in postmenopausal women with abnormal bleeding indicate that the sensitivity of transvaginal ultrasound for detection of significant abnormalities is 95%—equivalent to endometrial biopsy—when the criterion for a normal result is a homogenous endometrial stripe less than or equal

to 4 mm. An endometrial thickness of 5 to 8 mm cannot distinguish proliferative endometrium from hyperplasia or carcinoma and requires endometrial biopsy for further investigation.

Effectiveness of Screening

There are sparse data to support routine screening of asymptomatic **average-risk women** for endometrial cancer. In the largest study of cytologic screening for endometrial cancer by Koss et al., in which the prevalence of cancer was 7/1000,

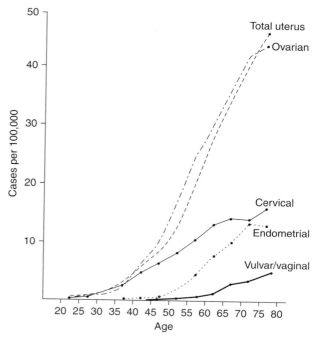

FIG. 97-2 Age-specific mortality rate of gynecologic cancers in women in the United States. (From Knapp RC, Berkowitz RS: *Gynecologic oncology*, New York, 1986, Macmillan.)

Table 97-1
Estimated Incidence and Deaths from Gynecologic Cancers in the United States, 2000

Site	New Cancer Cases	Deaths
Endometrium	36,100	6500
Cervix	12,800	4600
Ovary	23,100	14,000
Other genital sites	5300	1100

Estimates based on rates from Surveillance, Epidemiology, and End Results (SEER) Program, National Cancer Institute.

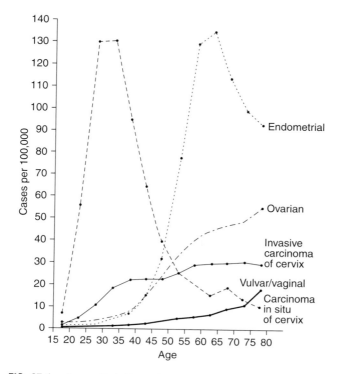

FIG. 97-1 Age-specific incidence of gynecologic cancers in women in the United States. (From Knapp RC, Berkowitz RS: *Gynecologic oncology*, New York, 1986, Macmillan.)

BOX 97-1
Risk Factors for Endometrial Cancer

Increased Risk
Increasing age
Unopposed estrogen
Obesity (weight >200 or body mass index >27)
Tamoxifen
Chronic anovulation
Late menopause
Nulliparity
Diabetes

Decreased Risk
Oral contraceptive pill
Pregnancy

Marked Increase in Risk
Hereditary nonpolyposis colorectal cancer

the positive predictive value of screening was 17% to 20%. Thus 80% of women with a positive screening test result would be free of cancer but would be required to undergo further evaluation (such as dilatation and curettage). There have been no randomized trials of screening using endometrial sampling or transvaginal ultrasound. Observational studies of screening with endometrial biopsy or transvaginal ultrasound in postmenopausal women on hormone replacement therapy have consistently shown unacceptably low yields of routine screening, and there is consensus that routine monitoring with either technique in this population is not warranted.

In **women with risk factors for endometrial cancer,** there is clinical consensus about the role of screening in specific populations of women. For women receiving **unopposed estrogen replacement therapy,** consensus supports performance of annual endometrial biopsy.

Because **tamoxifen** is in wider use for treatment and prevention of breast cancer, there has been great interest in identifying a screening technique for early detection of endometrial carcinoma in women taking tamoxifen, particularly women over 50 years old who are at risk for this complication. However, numerous studies have indicated that transvaginal ultrasound in this population has a high false-positive rate, and endometrial biopsy. For this reason, the American College of Obstetricians and Gynecologists issued a committee opinion in 2000 recommending the following for women taking tamoxifen:

- Annual pelvic examination.
- No routine endometrial monitoring in asymptomatic women.
- Education of the patient about prompt reporting of abnormal vaginal bleeding.

Women with **hereditary nonpolyposis colorectal carcinoma syndrome (HPNCC)** constitute about 5% of all endometrial cancer cases and have a lifetime risk of cancer of 22% to 50%. An expert committee of the American Cancer Society has recommended routine screening for endometrial cancer by transvaginal sonography for women with established or suspected HPNCC, beginning at age 35 years. Their recommendation acknowledges that scientific evidence for effectiveness of the recommendation is not available.

In women with other risk factors for endometrial cancer, the appropriate role for screening has not been defined. There has been a single study of cytologic screening in women at increased risk, which showed a prevalence of preinvasive endometrial abnormality in 6% of diabetic women ages 45 to 69 years compared with 1% of women with hypertension.

Recommendations

Routine screening for endometrial cancer in asymptomatic women is not recommended. Women receiving unopposed systemic estrogen replacement therapy should undergo periodic endometrial biopsy. In asymptomatic postmenopausal women with risk factors for endometrial cancer such as tamoxifen use, obesity, or diabetes, routine screening with endometrial sampling is not recommended. Expert opinion suggests that women with HPNCC undergo routine screening with transvaginal sonography and CA125 beginning at age 35 years.

OVARIAN CANCER
Epidemiology

Ovarian cancer is the most common cause of death from a gynecologic malignancy (Table 97-1). Mortality rate from the disease has increased slightly over the last two decades. The incidence of ovarian cancer increases with age; the average age at clinical presentation is 59 years.

Aside from age, the strongest risk factor for ovarian cancer identified to date is familial evidence of ovarian cancer (Table 97-2), which is present in about 7% of women with the disease. The two types of familial patterns of ovarian cancer are associated with different magnitudes of risk. The rare **hereditary ovarian cancer syndromes** account for less than 1% of ovarian cancer cases. The most common hereditary syndrome is the breast-ovarian cancer syndrome; most of these families have germ-line mutations in BRCA1 or BRCA2 genes. Estimates of the lifetime risk of ovarian cancer associated with a BRCA mutation range from 20% to 50%. Clues to a hereditary ovarian cancer syndrome include the occurrence of ovarian, breast, endometrial, or colorectal cancers in several members of two or more generations of the family and presentation of ovarian cancer at an early age (<50 years).

Much more common is a **family history of ovarian cancer** in a single first-degree or second-degree relative. Such a history is associated with a modest increase in absolute risk of the disease. One meta-analysis estimated that a family history of ovarian cancer in one relative increased the lifetime probability of ovarian cancer in a 35-year-old woman from 1.6% to 5%.

Two reproductive factors have been strongly associated with a substantially decreased risk of ovarian cancer in epidemiologic studies: **oral contraceptive pill use** and **parity** (Table 97-2). Studies of women with infertility indicate that infertility itself is a risk factor for the ovarian cancer, but infertility treatment does not independently increase risk.

Screening Techniques

The **pelvic examination** has been the traditional method of screening for ovarian cancer in the primary care setting; however, its value for the early detection of ovarian cancer has never been established. Some of the published studies of the pelvic examination for screening asymptomatic women

Table 97-2
Risk Factors for Ovarian Cancer

Risk Factor	Relative Risk	Lifetime Risk for Ovarian Cancer (%)*
No risk factors	1.0	1.2
Hereditary ovarian cancer syndrome	Unknown	Up to 50
One relative with ovarian cancer	3.1	3.7
Two or three relatives with ovarian cancer	4.6	5.5
Oral contraceptive pill use	0.65	0.8
Pregnancy	0.5	0.6

Modified from Carlson KJ et al: *Ann Intern Med* 121:124, 1994.
*Risk for cancer in a 50-year-old woman.

suggest that an examination by a highly skilled examiner may identify early-stage ovarian cancer.

Pelvic ultrasonography by the transabdominal or transvaginal route has been investigated as a screening technique for ovarian cancer. The sensitivity of ultrasound for the detection of ovarian cancer (all stages combined) is 80% in studies of asymptomatic women and its specificity is 94% to 99%.

The **CA125 radioimmunoassay** measures a tumor marker detectable in the serum of approximately 80% of women with ovarian cancer and in some with endometrial and pancreatic malignancies. Serum CA125 level may also be elevated in benign gynecologic conditions, including endometriosis, leiomyomas, benign ovarian cysts, and pelvic inflammatory disease. Levels of CA125 fluctuate during the menstrual cycle. Most studies of CA125 for ovarian cancer screening have focused on postmenopausal women. The sensitivity of CA125 for detecting preclinical disease (defining abnormal as 35 U/ml or greater) ranges from 70% to 80%; its specificity in postmenopausal women ranges from 98% to 99%.

Effectiveness of Screening

The feasibility of either ultrasonography or CA125 for screening has been limited by the relatively high false-positive rate of both tests. In studies of **average-risk populations** of women 50 years and older, the positive predictive value of CA125 or ultrasound screening alone has been less than 3%; that is, 100 women would be surgically evaluated to detect 3 cases of ovarian cancer. The adverse consequences of false-positive test results are considerable because of the need for invasive diagnostic tests (laparotomy or laparoscopy) to evaluate suspected ovarian cancer.

A recent prospective study of annual transvaginal sonography in 14,469 asymptomatic women over age 50 or over age 25 with a history of family history of ovarian cancer showed a more favorable positive predictive value of 9%, and the 5-year survival in the screened population was higher than that in the control group (87% vs. 50%). The finding that 57,000 scans were necessary to identify 17 cancers suggests that cost-effectiveness may be a limiting factor in the use of ultrasonography alone as a screening method.

Serial CA125 levels or CA125 combined with ultrasonography show promise as screening strategies with acceptable predictive value in average-risk postmenopausal women. A randomized trial of 22,000 women in England using a protocol of annual CA125 levels, ultrasound following an abnormal CA125 level (defined here as greater than 30 U/ml), and exploratory surgery following an abnormal ultrasound has achieved a positive predictive value of 27% (that is, surgery performed in four women for every case of ovarian cancer detected). After 7 years, median survival in women with ovarian cancer in the screened group was 73 months, vs. 42 in the unscreened control group; this trend toward improved survival was not associated with a significant difference in mortality rate. This trial and others currently in progress will better define the effectiveness of screening strategies in women at average risk.

In **women with a family history of ovarian cancer in one relative,** the prevalence of ovarian cancer is higher, and the predictive value of screening with a single annual CA125 is increased to approximately 10%. The predictive value of CA125 or ultrasonography in women with the **rare hereditary ovarian cancer syndromes** is unknown. In clinical practice a policy of screening female members of such families with CA125 and ultrasound is recommended because of the very high lifetime risk of malignancy.

Recommendations

The available scientific evidence does not support screening for ovarian cancer with ultrasound or CA125 in premenopausal and postmenopausal women without a family history of ovarian cancer. For women with a family history of ovarian cancer in one or more relatives without evidence of a hereditary cancer syndrome, routine screening is not recommended. Individualized decisions about screening can be made after such women are counseled about their individual risk (considering age, parity, and history of oral contraceptive pill use) and advised of the potential adverse effects of screening. Because of the high risk of ovarian cancer in women from families with the rare hereditary ovarian cancer syndromes, referral of such women to a gynecologic oncologist for surveillance, including CA125 and possibly other tumor markers and ultrasonography, is recommended.

VULVAR CANCER
Epidemiology

Vulvar cancer is a relatively rare cause of cancer death in women (Fig. 97-2). Invasive vulvar cancer largely occurs in older women; the average age at diagnosis is 70 years. Five-year survival rate for all stages combined is approximately 55%.

There is growing evidence that vulvar carcinoma may comprise two distinct clinical subsets. The first, occurring primarily in younger women, is related to sexually transmitted factors, principally human papillomavirus (HPV). A total of 20% to 30% of vulvar cancers subjected to histopathologic analysis contain HPV. HPV16 seropositivity increases the risk of vulvar cancer fourfold; concomitant smoking increases risk 18-fold.

The pathogenesis for the majority of vulvar carcinomas, which occur in older women, is less clear. A strong link between vulvar cancer and chronic vulvar inflammatory disease (also known as vulvar dystrophies) has been established. However, the risk of future vulvar carcinoma in women with hyperplastic or atrophic vulvar diseases has been reported at less than 5%, suggesting that in the great majority of women with these diseases, cancer will not develop. Epidemiologic evidence for an association with other diseases (such as diabetes) is inconclusive.

Screening Techniques

The most important screening technique for the primary care clinician is careful inspection of the vulva. Any white, reddened, ulcerated, nodular, fissured, or abnormal raised pigmented area should undergo biopsy.

Effectiveness of Screening

There are no studies to determine whether early detection of vulvar cancer by screening is associated with reduced mortality rate from the disease.

Recommendations

Careful inspection of the vulva should be part of a pelvic examination performed for other reasons, such as cervical cancer screening. The epidemiologic associations of vulvar cancer suggest that the vulvar examination is particularly important in women with HPV and those with chronic vulvar inflammatory diseases. The value of periodic vulvar examination in women without risk factors who are not undergoing pelvic examination for other reasons has not been established.

BIBLIOGRAPHY

Carlson KJ, Skates SJ, Singer DE: Screening for ovarian cancer, *Ann Intern Med* 121:124, 1994.

Creasman W et al: American Cancer Society guidelines for the early detection of cancer: update of early detection guidelines for prostate, colorectal, and endometrial cancer. *CA Cancer J Clin* 51:7, 2001.

Crum CP: Carcinoma of the vulva: epidemiology and pathogenesis, *Obstet Gynecol* 79:448, 1992.

Gronroos M et al: Mass screening for endometrial cancer directed in risk groups of patients with diabetes and patients with hypertension, *Cancer* 71:1279, 1993.

Gull B et al: Transvaginal ultrasonography of the endometrium in women with postmenopausal bleeding: Is it always necessary to perform an endometrial biopsy? *Am J Obstet Gynecol* 182:509, 2000.

Jacobs IJ et al: Screening for ovarian cancer: a pilot randomized controlled trial. *Lancet* 353:1207, 1999.

Kerlikowske K, Brown JS, Grady DG: Should women with familial ovarian cancer undergo prophylactic oophorectomy? *Obstet Gynecol* 80:700, 1992.

Koss LG et al: Detection of endometrial carcinoma and hyperplasia in asymptomatic women, *Obstet Gynecol* 64:1, 1984.

Madeleine MM et al: Cofactors with human papillomavirus in a population-based study of vulvar cancer, *J Natl Cancer Inst* 89:1516, 1997.

Pritchard KI: Screening for endometrial cancer: is it effective? *Ann Intern Med* 110:177, 1989.

Smith-Bindman R: U.S. Preventive Services Task Force: *Guide to clinical preventive services,* ed 2, Baltimore, 1996, Williams & Wilkins.

Van Nagell JR et al: The efficacy of transvaginal sonographic screening in asymptomatic women at risk of ovarian cancer, *Gynecol Oncol* 77:350, 2000.

CHAPTER **98**

Occupational Hazards

L. Christine Oliver
Carolyn S. Langer

On September 6, 1991, 25 workers were killed and 55 injured in an attempt to escape a fire that broke out in a chicken processing plant in Hamlet, North Carolina. Contributing to the high death toll were the lack of automatic heat-detection sprinkler systems and fire evacuation plan, as well as blocked fire doors that failed to meet national safety standards. The plant had not undergone a safety inspection in the 11 years of its existence. Many of those killed were women. This unnecessary tragedy was reminiscent of the fire at the Triangle Shirtwaist Company in New York City on March 25, 1911. That fire killed 145 employees trapped in the burning building. Most of them were women.

In 1970 the Occupational Safety and Health Act (OSHA) was signed into law. The purpose of the act was to ensure, insofar as possible, a safe and healthful workplace for every working American and to preserve human resources. Increasingly, working Americans are women and American women are working outside the home. In 2000, 68 million females were employed on nonfarm payrolls, constituting 48% of the civilian labor force and over 60% of the total female population in the United States.

Historically, women have been employed primarily in the service industries, in clerical jobs, and in semiskilled work in manufacturing industries. Currently 89% of working women are employed in service-producing industries, and the remaining 10% in goods-producing industries. Of those in the latter category, less than 1% are employed in mining or construction; the remainder are employed in manufacturing. In these industries, women occupy a larger proportion of low-paying unskilled jobs—jobs with high rates of injury, such as those in the poultry processing industry. In 1989 the U.S. Department of Labor's Bureau of Labor Statistics identified the poultry processing industry as second only to ship building/repair in the number of serious work-related illnesses and injuries. The service-producing sector includes eating and drinking establishments, retail grocery stores, hospitals, nursing facilities, department stores, and hotels and motels. These are industries in which female employees are likely to predominate.

Occupational disease is preventable. As a leading federal agency for prevention, the Centers for Disease Control and Prevention (CDC) has categorized its approaches to injury and disease prevention on the basis of (1) delivery of pre-vention technologies and (2) timing of intervention by stage of disease or injury. Both approaches rely heavily on the primary care physician (1) to detect and reduce causal risk factors, such as lead exposure or poorly designed computer work stations; (2) to detect and appropriately treat disease at an early stage; and (3) to organize and deliver relevant tertiary health care. In the case of occupational injury or disease the latter includes rehabilitative services that minimize morbidity and allow for return to work at the same job in a different capacity or at a different job altogether. In many cases accomplishment of these tasks requires a joint effort of the primary care physician and public health professionals, government and labor union officials, and employers.

This chapter discusses diagnosis of occupational disease, using a system-oriented approach to highlight occupational diseases for which women are at special risk. Legal and ethical issues are discussed in the context of the female worker and the attendant responsibilities of her primary care physician.

DIAGNOSIS OF OCCUPATIONAL DISEASE

Symptoms and physical findings in cases of occupational illness, disease, and injury are not unlike those seen in cases of disease and injury unrelated to work. Laboratory test results are rarely specific. For the clinician then the key to diagnosis is the *occupational history*. In addition to allowing correct diagnosis the occupational history promotes proper treatment, prevents worsening of disease or unnecessary development of iatrogenic disease, prevents the occurrence of disease in similarly exposed co-workers, and contributes to a database that allows a better understanding of the epidemiologic characteristics of occupational disease and injury.

Individuals may present clinical evidence of illness or disease or a history of work at a job that is potentially hazardous, on the basis of either an airborne or surface exposure or an ergonomic or physical hazard, such as heavy lifting or noise. In both cases the approach to the occupational history is the same. A chronologic lifetime work history is ideal and may be necessary in cases of known or suspected disease with long latency, such as asbestosis or asbestos-related lung cancer. In general a shorter and more focused history is sufficient for the primary care physician.

If occupational disease is diagnosed or strongly suspected on the basis of the history or laboratory findings, the physician may wish to refer the patient to an occupational physician in situations such as the following: (1) diagnosis depends on a more detailed evaluation of the workplace; (2) elimination of the causal exposure is possible only if the patient leaves her place of employment and a higher level of certainty regarding diagnosis is desired; or (3) the patient wishes to file a workers' compensation claim or suit against a third party and a medical opinion or legal testimony from the diagnosing physician will be required.

BOX 98-1
Occupational History: Key Questions

What is your present job?
What was your previous job?
What was the job you worked at the longest?

For Risk Assessment
Job title and job description
Tasks performed
Exposures (e.g., chemical, dust, gas, fumes): type and level
Adequacy of work area ventilation
Availability of personal protective equipment (e.g., gloves, respirators)

For Evaluation of Symptoms
Correlation between symptoms and known health effects of exposures
Temporal association of symptoms with work
Occurrence of symptoms or disease in co-workers

Principal components of the occupational history for the primary care clinician are shown in Box 98-1. For each job, years of hire and termination, as well as total duration of employment, are needed. Both job *title* and job *description* should be obtained. Estimates of level (e.g., mild, moderate, heavy) of exposure by the patient are useful in overall exposure assessment.

Of critical importance, particularly with regard to short-latency disease or illness such as asthma or angina, is an understanding of the temporal association of symptoms with work. Questions about severity of symptoms during the workday and workweek, at night and over the weekend, and on vacation will help elicit this information. Also important is information about occurrence of illness, disease, or injury among co-workers—particularly co-workers with the same job. Turnover rate may provide indirect information about the health and safety of the workplace.

In addition, Material Safety Data Sheets (MSDS) should be obtained where possible. Under the OSHA Hazards Communication Standard (29 Code of Federal Regulations 1910.1200), both employees and their physicians have a "right to know" what chemicals are in their workplace. This information exists in the form of MSDSs. These give both generic and brand names, chemical composition, reported acute and chronic health effects, and steps to be taken in the event of overexposure. Because MSDSs are required only for chemicals and because employers may resist providing MSDSs, it is useful to obtain additional information from other sources (see Resources). Information about exposures may be obtained on the basis of reported job and nature of work, and information about health effects, on the basis of exposures. Examples are shown in Table 98-1. When assess-

Table 98-1
Occupational Respiratory Hazards

Site of Effect	Causal Agents	Disease Process	Typical Exposures in Women
Lung parenchyma	Irritant gases (e.g., chlorine, nitrogen dioxide, ammonia)	Pulmonary edema Pneumonitis	Cleaning, laboratory work, welding
	Organic dusts (e.g., thermophilic actinomycetes)	Hypersensitivity pneumonitis (acute phase) Fibrosis, granulomatosis (chronic phase)	Farming, clerical work
	Inorganic dusts (e.g., asbestos, silica)	Pulmonary restriction	Textile manufacture, construction, household contact
	Metals (e.g., beryllium, cobalt)	Pulmonary restriction or obstruction; granuloma formation	Electronics, tool and die manufacture, ceramics manufacture
Airways	Irritants, gases, fumes, dust	Bronchitis	Laboratory work, construction, cleaning
	High-molecular-weight particles (e.g., wheat, rye flour, enzymes)	Asthma	Detergent manufacture, baking, shellfish processing
	Low-molecular-weight compounds (e.g., toluene diisocyanate)	Asthma	Paint, polyurethane, and plastics manufacture
	Irritants, gases, fumes (e.g., nitrogen oxides)	Asthma	Welding
	Metals (e.g., cobalt, platinum, nickel)	Asthma	Welding, tool and die manufacture
	Inadequate ventilation ("sick building syndrome")	Rhinitis, laryngitis, cough, bronchospasm	Clerical, service jobs

ing the potential for exposure to hazards, all routes of exposure should be considered, including transdermal, inhalation, and ingestion.

OCCUPATIONAL HEALTH HAZARDS FOR WOMEN BY SYSTEM

Respiratory

Occupational lung disease is one of the nation's 10 leading causes of work-related illness and disease. Although it does not preferentially affect women as a rule, it is a major cause of morbidity among female workers. Causes include inhaled organic and inorganic dusts, irritants, vapors, gases, and fumes, as well as work in inadequately ventilated buildings. Both upper and lower respiratory tracts may be affected. Latency may be short (e.g., asthma, rhinitis, acute pulmonary beryllium disease) or long (e.g., asbestosis, chronic pulmonary beryllium disease, exposure-related lung cancer). In the past dust-related interstitial fibrosis of the lung has been the major type of occupational lung disease seen in the clinical setting; it likely has been supplanted by occupational asthma, as exposure to such agents as asbestos and coal dust has diminished in the United States, and new chemicals with the potential to induce bronchospasm have been introduced into the workplace.

Categorization by Effect

The workplace exposures described may affect the lung interstitium, the airways, the pleura, and the nasal mucosa and sinuses. Effects on the lung parenchyma include inflammation, fibrosis, and granuloma formation. Causal agents and respiratory effects are summarized in Table 98-1. In the case of irritant gases such as NO_2, exposure may antedate the onset of pulmonary edema by 12 to 24 hours. The degree of penetration into the lung is inversely related to water solubility, so that gases with less solubility, such as NO_2, penetrate deeply into the lung, whereas those with greater solubility, such as ammonia, are deposited higher in the respiratory tract.

Hypersensitivity pneumonitis may present acutely, with symptoms of shortness of breath, cough, chest pain, and fever. If the illness is not diagnosed and exposure continues, a chronic form of the disease may develop, with granuloma formation and irreversible fibrosis. **Asbestosis, silicosis,** and **coal workers' pneumoconiosis** have characteristic radiographic and pathologic pictures. Latency is generally 10 years or more and may vary by level of exposure.

Work-related airways disease includes industrial bronchitis and reversible and irreversible airway obstruction. Industrial bronchitis is characterized by cough and sputum, which is worse at work. It is a nonspecific manifestation of airway irritation and inflammation and may occur in association with exposure to irritants, gases, fumes, and dusts. **Occupational asthma** is reversible airway obstruction related to a workplace exposure(s). It may be new in onset or the result of workplace aggravation of preexisting asthma **(occupationally-aggravated asthma).** In cases in which the causal exposure is to a potentially sensitizing agent such as latex or a diisocyanate, elimination of the exposure is necessary because of risk of a life-threatening attack of asthma with reexposure. **Reactive airways dysfunction syndrome** (RADS) is an example of reversible airway ob-

struction that may occur after a single or limited number of exposures to relatively high levels of irritant gases and fumes. Once considered a distinct entity, RADS is now considered to be asthma without latency, associated with exposure to airborne irritants usually at high levels. Symptoms of asthma often persist for years after exposure, with a direct relationship between persistence and duration of continued exposure once symptoms begin. Because of the variable nature of airway obstruction and the possibility of normal lung function when the patient is on optimal medication, clinical assessment of disability from work is particularly difficult with asthma. It may be that there is disability without demonstrable physiologic impairment at given points in time.

Among the first case reports of **pulmonary beryllium disease** were those from a group of women exposed to beryllium during the course of work in fluorescent light bulb manufacture. Beryllium disease is a T-cell mediated disorder resulting from sensitization to beryllium. Chronic pulmonary beryllium disease is characterized by granuloma formation in the lungs and, in more severe cases, fibrosis. Beryllium exposure may also result in formation of granulomas in the airways, producing an obstructive physiologic defect. Clinically and pathologically, pulmonary beryllium disease resembles sarcoidosis.

A constellation of respiratory health effects has been reported among workers in buildings with inadequate ventilation—so-called **sick building syndrome.** Symptoms include rhinitis, laryngitis, cough, and wheeze. Often associated with work in sick buildings is another entity known as **multiple chemical sensitivity** (MCS), which is also referred to by the World Health Organization as idiopathic environmental intolerance. The disease is characterized by multisystem involvement that may include respiratory symptoms. For both sick building syndrome and MCS, identified causal factors include formaldehyde and other volatile organic hydrocarbon vapors from carpeting, draperies, and upholstered furniture; fiberglass dust from ceiling tiles and insulation material; adhesives; diesel emissions entrained from outside traffic; vapors from cleaning agents, perfumes, and colognes; and environmental tobacco smoke. Other sources include equipment used in homes and offices such as copiers, printers, and facsimile and binding machines. Because women predominate in the service sector, they are at particular risk for development of these problems.

Musculoskeletal

Musculoskeletal disorders rank as the leading cause of disability in the United States for work-aged individuals. At least 50% of the workforce will be affected by musculoskeletal injuries at some point in their careers. These include "acute and chronic injuries to muscles, tendons, ligaments, nerves, joints, bones, and supporting vasculature." Injuries most commonly involve the back, cervical spine, and upper extremities and are usually characterized by the structure affected (e.g., tendonitis, synovitis, bursitis). Although women experience more than 30% of all work-related injuries and illnesses, they experience more than 60% of all repetitive motion injuries and account for 69% and 61% of lost work-time cases as a result of carpal tunnel syndrome and tendonitis, respectively.

Musculoskeletal injuries result from biomechanical stresses that exceed the worker's physical capabilities and limitations (Box 98-2). Primary risk factors include heavy lifting, repetitive motion, vibration, poor posture, and excessive bending, twisting, reaching, pushing, and pulling. Secondary factors include age, gender, strength, physical fitness, fatigue, trauma, emotional stress, and preexisting conditions such as degenerative changes. Women may be particularly prone to musculoskeletal injuries because many work stations, tools, and types of protective gear are designed for the average male body stature and physical capacity.

Despite indications that the *average* female tolerates lower maximum weights and forces than the *average* male, physical capacities vary widely among *individual* males and females. Therefore employers should use sound ergonomic principles that seek to fit specific jobs to individual workers, whether male or female. Mechanical aides and work station and tool redesign represent the most effective ways to reduce the risk of musculoskeletal injuries in the workplace. Examples include use of conveyor belts, hoists, lift tables, proper work-surface heights, and contoured hand grips on tools.

Employee selection by type of job is a less suitable method for prevention of musculoskeletal injuries in the workplace. Selection criteria may be discriminatory, unrelated to actual job demands, or poorly predictive of potential for injury. For example, radiographs of the lumbosacral region, once widely used as a screening tool, have been invalidated as a predictor for back injuries in workers.

Physicians who treat workers for musculoskeletal injuries should inquire beyond job titles into specific job tasks with particular emphasis on frequency, intensity, duration, and direction of biomechanical forces to which patients are exposed. Careful exploration of work station conditions and job demands not only will assist in identifying the cause of many work-related musculoskeletal disorders but may lead to useful insights into prevention and job modification through ergonomic interventions. Carpal tunnel syndrome, an occupational musculoskeletal disorder common in women, is discussed in detail in Chapter 35.

BOX 98-2
Risk Factors for Occupational Musculoskeletal Disorders

Primary Risk Factors
Heavy lifting
Repetitive motion
Vibration
Poor posture
Excessive bending, twisting, reaching, pushing, pulling

Secondary Risk Factors
Age
Gender
Strength and physical fitness
Fatigue
Trauma
Emotional stress
Preexisting conditions (e.g., degenerative arthritis)

Psychological

In a survey reported by the U.S. Department of Labor Women's Bureau in 1994, 60% of working women identified stress as the most important work-related health problem. Occupational stress occurs when coping mechanisms and resources are overwhelmed by conditions at the workplace. Effects are both psychologic and physical and include anxiety and depression, gastrointestinal and sleep disorders, and increased job absenteeism. An important factor contributing to work-related stress for men and women is discrepancy between decision latitude and psychologic demand (i.e., between degree of control and job demand: low control-high demand or high control-low demand). Women are more likely than men to work in subordinate jobs, with little control over their work or work environment. Low control-high demand jobs are associated with frustration, anxiety, and low self-esteem; those with low control-low demand are apt to be boring.

Other stressors likely to be greater for women than for men are work-family conflicts, financial and economic strain, and gender-specific stress related to sexual discrimination and sexual harassment. More than 80% of working married women report primary responsibility for household chores and more than 60% for paying bills. Women have primary responsibility for child and elder care. In 1997 women earned 79% as much as men earned. This discrepancy, together with the fact that women are more likely than men to be single parents, contributes to excessive financial strain on women. The salary and promotion barriers that exist for women add to the psychologic strain, but perhaps most important in terms of psychologic distress is sexual harassment in the workplace. It has been estimated that more than 50% of women will be subjected to this form of workplace stress during their working lifetime.

For primary care physicians, stress-related health problems may be difficult to recognize and even more difficult to treat. Symptoms are nonspecific and often not linked to the workplace by the patient, and there are likely to be other sources of stress that must be sorted out. Once recognized, stress management strategies in the workplace and/or individual psychotherapy may be helpful in alleviating symptoms, but it is also necessary to identify the source of the problem and treat that as well. Giving workers the opportunity to participate in decision making, job redesign, increasing opportunities for job promotion and career advancement, flexible schedules that allow time for child and elder care, and introduction of policies against sex discrimination and sexual harassment are "treatments" that might be prescribed.

Reproductive

The National Institute for Occupational Safety and Health (NIOSH) has ranked disorders of the reproductive system among the nation's 10 leading categories of work-related injuries and illnesses. Reproductive hazards include any chemical, physical, or biologic agent that can harm the reproductive system or a developing fetus or child. For women the effects of reproductive hazards can include one or more of the following: altered menstrual function, decreased libido, reduced fertility, adverse pregnancy outcomes (e.g., spontaneous abortion, preterm birth, low birth weight, structural abnormality, or functional deficiency), breast milk contamination, and childhood cancer in offspring.

Chemical Hazards

Table 98-2 lists some of the known or suspected reproductive hazards in the workplace, typical jobs in which these chemicals are used, and their potential reproductive effects. Although the table lists potential effects on the female reproductive system only, most reproductive hazards affect both the male and female reproductive systems.

The physician should use caution when comparing results of workplace monitoring to legal standards for occupational exposure. Most of the 60,000 chemicals in commercial use have not been thoroughly evaluated for reproductive or developmental toxicity. Only four agents have been regulated in part to prevent reproductive damage (lead, radiation, dibromochloropropane, ethylene oxide), and these regulations may not be sufficiently protective. NIOSH has issued Recommended Exposure Limits that, although not legally enforceable, provide guidelines for estimating safe exposure limits.

Physical Hazards

Exposure to several physical agents can result in adverse reproductive and developmental effects. Ionizing radiation is in widespread use in occupations in medicine, industry, government, and nuclear fuel operations. Depending on dose, exposure to ionizing radiation during pregnancy can result in birth defects, mental retardation, childhood leukemia, and other childhood cancers in offspring. Radiation exposure before implantation of the fetus is not likely to result in birth defects, however, because either the death of the conceptus or total effective repair will occur.

With the widespread use of computers in the past decade, there has been growing concern about the reproductive effects of video display terminals (VDTs). To date the majority of epidemiologic data, including those from a well-designed study by NIOSH, do not support a significant association between VDT use and spontaneous abortion. Although VDTs produce a minimal amount of

Table 98-2
Potential Reproductive Hazards in the Workplace

Occupational Hazard	Types of Jobs	Potential Effects on Female Reproductive System and Pregnancy
Arsenic and arsine	Jobs involving use of pesticides, herbicides, metal alloys, special glasses and enamels, antifouling paints, semiconductor devices, and printed circuits	Birth defects and low birth weight in offspring, breast milk contamination
Anesthetic gases	Dental workers, health care workers, chemical workers	Spontaneous abortion, stillbirths, birth defects
Benzene	Chemical manufacture, paint and varnish removal, laboratory workers	Mutagenesis. In animal studies: teratogenesis in offspring of exposed animals
Cadmium	Paint pigment making, artists, electrical workers, welding, metal machining	Menstrual irregularities, spontaneous abortion, stillbirth, breast milk contamination
Carbon disulfide	Electrical, hospital and health care, laboratory, refinery, pesticide, textile, and rubber workers	Menstrual irregularities, fetotoxicity, spontaneous abortion. In animal studies: birth defects, behavioral changes in offspring
Carbon monoxide	Tunnel workers, traffic police, auto repair, fork lift operators, truck drivers, firefighters, workers exposed to environmental tobacco smoke	Low birth weight and birth defects in offspring, increased fetal or infant death, decreased fertility
Chlordane, heptachlor	Manufacture and use of pesticides	Possible blood disorders and childhood cancer in offspring; in animal studies: mutagenesis, decreased fertility
Chlorpyrifox	Manufacture and use of pesticides	Decreased fertility
Cytotoxics, antineoplastics	Health care workers	Spontaneous abortion, birth defects in offspring of women treated with these drugs, mutagenesis, breast milk contamination
2,4 Dichlorophenoxy-acetic acid (2,4,D)	Manufacture and use of pesticides	In animal studies; birth defects
Ethylene oxide (ETO)	Hospital and health care workers, food workers, chemical workers, manufacture and use of pesticides	Mutagenesis; in animal studies: decreased fertility, birth defects, fetolethality
Formaldehyde	Pathology laboratory workers, cosmetic/plastic resin manufacture, textile workers, work involving use of particle board or adhesive	Menstrual irregularities, mutagenesis
Glycol ethers (e.g., 2-Methoxyethanol)	Electronic and semiconductor workers, auto workers, general manufacturing	Spontaneous abortion, decreased fertility; in animal studies: birth defects
Lindane	Manufacture and use of pesticides	Possible brain damage in offspring; in animal studies: possible death of offspring

Continued

Table 98-2
Potential Reproductive Hazards in the Workplace—cont'd

Occupational Hazard	Types of Jobs	Potential Effects on Female Reproductive System and Pregnancy
Lead	Bridge painters, house painters and deleaders, people who work with stained glass or ceramics, auto radiator repair workers, welders	Menstrual irregularities, decreased fertility, birth defects, stillbirth, brain defects in offspring (e.g., hyperactivity, learning disabilities)
Mercury	Dental and health care workers, electrical workers, pharmaceutical and chemical workers, manufacture and use of pesticides, thermometer manufacture	Menstrual irregularities, spontaneous abortion, breast milk contamination; in animal studies: decreased fertility, birth defects, damage to developing fetus, stillbirth
Methyethyl ketone (MEK, 2-butanone)	Many manufacturing jobs, including plastics, textiles, paints	Damage to developing fetus
Methylene chloride	Furniture stripping, chemical manufacturing	Breast milk contamination; in animal studies: birth defects, mutagenesis
Perchloroethylene (tetrachloroethylene)	Dry cleaners, degreasers	Breast milk contamination; in animal studies: fetotoxicity
Styrene	Plastics workers, paper workers	Menstrual irregularities, decreased fertility
Toluene	Chemical and general manufacturing, laboratory workers	Spontaneous abortion; in animal studies: fetotoxicity, fetolethality
1,1,1 trichloroethane (methyl chloroform)	Manufacturing	In animal studies: fetotoxicity, birth defects, mutagenesis
Trichloroethylene	Electronics	In animal studies: birth defects, impaired growth in offspring
Xylene	Laboratory workers, plastics manufacture, synthetic textiles, paints, lacquers, varnishes, adhesives, cements, pharmaceuticals	Menstrual irregularities; in animal studies: fetotoxicity

Modified from Massachusetts Coalition for Occupational Safety and Health: *Confronting reproductive health hazards on the job,* 1992.

ionizing radiation, they also emit very low-frequency and extremely low-frequency radiation, which have been shown in some experimental studies to cause biologic damage. Other characteristics of jobs involving prolonged use of VDTs include stress and ergonomic factors that may contribute to potential adverse reproductive outcome. Because little is known about the effects of low-frequency electromagnetic fields on humans, users of VDTs should minimize their exposure by taking the following precautions: (1) maintaining a minimum distance of 18 inches from the screen, (2) ensuring proper ergonomic design of the work station, and (3) taking periodic breaks to prevent eye and musculoskeletal strain.

Little information is available on human reproductive effects of occupational exposure to noise. In animal studies, pregnancy-rate reduction has been a consistently reported effect of noise, and noise exposure is associated with increased embryolethality and fetolethality.

Physically strenuous work may be safe until late in pregnancy for a healthy woman who receives adequate nutrition and prenatal care. There is growing evidence, however, that repetitive heavy lifting in the last trimester can cause uterine contractions. The American Medical Association has issued guidelines for continuation of various job tasks during pregnancy.

Biologic Hazards
Several infectious agents that may be acquired in the workplace can cause intrauterine infections, produce terato-

genic effects in an embryo or fetus, infect offspring through contamination of breast milk, or act as abortifacients. These agents include the rubella virus, cytomegalovirus, hepatitis B and C, human immunodeficiency virus, parvovirus B19 (fifth disease), and chickenpox. Workers exposed to infectious disease include health care workers, housekeepers, laundry workers, laboratory workers, day care workers, teachers, workers in contact with animals and animal products, and sanitation workers.

Counseling Women Regarding Pregnancy
Many reproductive hazards can exert teratogenic effects before a woman is aware of pregnancy (Fig. 98-1). For this reason it is desirable to identify and eliminate or reduce exposure to workplace reproductive hazards before conception. Because of increasing evidence of male-mediated effects on the fetus, a woman planning a pregnancy should be informed that her partner's exposure to chemicals in the workplace may result in adverse reproductive outcome.

The frequency, timing, duration, and intensity of exposure must all be taken into account in assessing potential reproductive outcome. For example, exposures that occur within the first 2 weeks of pregnancy are either likely to cause death of the conceptus or damage to only a few cells with full recovery. Exposures from 3 to 8 weeks are more likely to cause major morphologic abnormalities, whereas those that occur later are more likely to cause functional defects and minor congenital anomalies (Fig. 98-1). It is important that the primary care physician counsel women

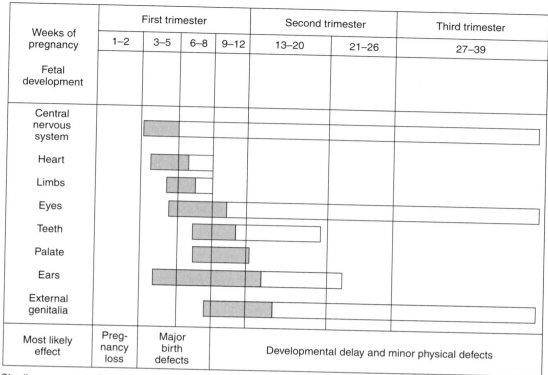

Shading represents time when major defects could occur; clear areas represent less sensitive times.

FIG. 98-1 Fetal development: times when a fetus can be most susceptible to defects. (From Massachusetts Coalition for Occupational Safety and Health: *Confronting reproductive health hazards on the job,* Boston, 1992, MassCosh.)

who are considering pregnancy about the potentially devastating effects of some exposures during the early stages of pregnancy and about the importance of an occupational and environmental exposure assessment before conception.

The physician may be asked to make suggestions for improvements in the work environment to protect worker health. The "hierarchy of controls" is applicable to reproductive hazards, like all workplace hazards. Elimination of the hazard or substitution (e.g., with a safer chemical) is the most effective control strategy. Engineering controls (e.g., well-maintained local exhaust ventilation or enclosure of the work process) are less effective but can significantly reduce exposure. Use of personal protective equipment (e.g., respirators, protective clothing) is the least effective control strategy but may be necessary on a short-term basis.

If exposure cannot be controlled satisfactorily, the physician may need to assist the patient in obtaining a temporary job transfer or leave. It is essential to be aware of the economic consequences of these options for the patient: how a leave or transfer will affect income, seniority, health insurance, and disability payments; and whether she is guaranteed a job on return from leave. With a few exceptions, employers are not typically required to provide special accommodations to pregnant workers. Experience has shown, though, that in many instances needed accommodations are minimal and can be worked out informally between the treating provider and employer. Finally by law the employer

may not treat requests by pregnant women for job transfers and leaves differently from requests by other nondisabled workers.

LEGAL ISSUES IN WOMEN'S OCCUPATIONAL HEALTH

As women continue to enter the workforce in unprecedented numbers and to assume broader roles in traditionally male occupations, it is important that primary care practitioners understand the statutory, regulatory, and judicial mechanisms that protect female workers from occupational exposures and gender-based employment discrimination. Such knowledge will allow appropriate counseling of patients and employers and appropriate referral of patients to outside resources for assistance when necessary.

OSHA and Regulatory Protection

OSHA was established in 1970 to "ensure so far as possible every working man and woman in the Nation safe and healthful working conditions." Under the general duty clause (Section 5(a)(1)) of the OSHA Act, employers must provide places of employment "which are free from recognized hazards that are causing or are likely to cause death or serious harm" to employees. The standard setting provision of Section 6(b) authorizes the Secretary of Labor to promulgate any occupational safety and health standard "dealing with toxic materials or harmful physical agents" and to "set the standard which most adequately assures . . .

that no employee will suffer material impairment of health or functional capacity." OSHA is empowered with the authority and responsibility for enforcement of the act.

The Hazards Communication Standard

OSHA promulgated the Hazards Communication Standard (HCS) in 1987 to provide for the transmission of information about the hazards of chemicals in the workplace to employers and employees. Under the HCS employers must (1) ensure that each container of hazardous chemicals is labeled with the identity and toxicity of the contained chemical, (2) "provide employees with information and training on hazardous chemicals in their work area" at the time of initial assignment and whenever a new chemical is introduced, and (3) maintain and ensure employee access to this information.

Antidiscrimination Legislation

Despite differences in male and female body stature, muscle strength, and childbearing capacity, there are few situations that justify different treatment of women in the workplace. The Civil Rights Act of 1964 (Title VII) explicitly prohibits sex-based discrimination with respect to hiring, discharge, compensation, terms, privileges, and other conditions of employment. This Act was further amended by the Pregnancy Discrimination Act of 1978 to prohibit sex-based discrimination on the basis of pregnancy, childbirth, or related medical conditions, except in those circumstances in which sex is a bona fide occupational qualification reasonably necessary to the normal operation of that particular business or enterprise. Such a job qualification must relate to the essence or the central mission of the employer's business. Thus an employer may legitimately refuse to hire females for jobs in which "male" attributes lie at the core of the job (e.g., as models for men's clothing). Otherwise, when individual women or the class of women possess the necessary job-related skills and aptitudes they must receive equal treatment in employment decisions.

Fetal Protection Policies

Despite the provisions of the Civil Rights Act of 1964 and the Pregnancy Discrimination Act of 1978, employers persisted throughout the 1980s in discriminating against female workers through the institution of fetal protection policies. These policies were in fact practices implemented by employers—typically through workplace exclusion policies—to minimize occupational exposures that potentially could result in adverse pregnancy outcomes. For example, in 1982 Johnson Controls, a lead battery manufacturer, instituted a fetal protection policy that excluded women of all ages from jobs that involved potential lead exposure—creating an exception only for those women who presented medical documentation of sterility.

In 1991 the U.S. Supreme Court invalidated fetal protection policies in a landmark decision called *International Union, UAW v. Johnson Controls, Inc.* The court declared these policies to be a form of gender discrimination because they did not apply equally to the reproductive capacity of male and female employees. The court further held that sex was not a bona fide occupational qualification because sex and childbearing capacity did not relate to the central mission of the employer's business. Thus, despite employers'

concerns about fetal safety (and potential tort liability), the court concluded that "decisions about the welfare of future children must be left to the parents who conceive, bear, support, and raise them rather than to the employers who hire those parents."

The Americans with Disabilities Act

Title I of the Americans with Disabilities Act (ADA) prohibits all employment practices that discriminate against the disabled. The act creates an exception when reasonable accommodation of disabled workers is not feasible and their disability poses a direct threat to others. The ADA applies to all employers with 15 or more employees.

The ADA defines *disability* as (1) a physical or mental impairment that limits one or more major life activities, (2) a history of such impairment, or (3) *being regarded as* having such an impairment. The ADA has little impact on gender discrimination because of the Act's interpretation of a physical impairment ("any physiological disorder, or condition, cosmetic disfigurement, or anatomical loss affecting one or more . . . body systems") and its emphasis on the nature, severity, and duration of impairment. For example, a pregnant woman is not protected under the ADA because pregnancy is not the result of a physiologic disorder and is only a temporary condition.

The primary care physician should be aware that the ADA prohibits (1) preoffer medical examinations and (2) except in limited circumstances divulgence of specific diagnoses or disabilities to the employer. Thus, although employers may administer preoffer nonmedical tests (such as agility testing) that are job-related, they may not require a medical examination until the applicant has been given a job offer that is contingent only on passing the medical examination. During the postoffer medical examination, the physician must determine whether the applicant meets the employer's health and safety requirements but should disclose to the employer only directly relevant information about functional ability and limitations (e.g., preferred disclosure: "Applicant should not work at heights"; improper disclosure: "Poorly controlled epilepsy"). The employer is then responsible for making determinations about feasibility of reasonable accommodation.

Legal Remedies Available to Workers

Government regulations proactively address health and safety issues by establishing safe standards for the workplace. In contrast, legal remedies provide compensation after an injury has occurred. In theory such compensation provides incentives for a safe and healthful workplace. Legal remedies available to workers include **workers' compensation** (WC) and remedy under the **tort system.** WC is a nofault system largely instituted in the United States in the 1920s and based on systems operative in Great Britain and the Republic of Germany at the time. It represents a compromise between labor and industry whereby the employee gives up her right to sue the employer, and the employer automatically accepts the employee's claim of a work-related injury or disease. Thus the employee is automatically entitled to certain benefits after incurring an occupational injury or disease, irrespective of fault. The employer on the other hand is protected from unpredictable jury awards that may be not only compensatory but also punitive.

Although WC may provide reasonable compensation in cases of work-related injury, the system fails to provide adequate restitution for occupational diseases—particularly those with long latencies and those without pathognomonic features, such as asthma and infertility. Contested cases typically center around causality and the existence or extent of disability from work. The worker must prove that the injury or illness "arose out of or in the course of employment." To be compensable, however, a disorder must not only be causally related to work but must also produce disability and, as a corollary, a reduction in earning capacity. For example, infertility, impotence, or miscarriage arising out of a workplace injury or exposure does not necessarily produce disability or diminish employment opportunities. Therefore some states may not adequately compensate workers for these conditions unless the WC laws make specific provisions for such effects as "loss of reproductive function/organs."

Tort Remedies

In cases in which employees are injured or disease results from action of a "third" party, remedy is available under the toxic torts system. Employees may sue the third party under negligence or strict liability doctrines. For example in many of the asbestos cases, affected workers alleged that asbestos manufacturers negligently failed to place warning labels on asbestos-containing products put into workplaces or used in the manufacture of end products. Workers exposed to asbestos in workplaces have successfully sued these manufacturers, even though they were barred by the exclusive remedy provisions of WC law from suing their employers. Tort cases are adjudicated in a court of law, where a jury determines the award and, in addition to wage replacement and medical costs typically allowed in WC cases, are more likely to take into account other damages, such as pain and suffering.

Role of the Health Care Provider

Primary care physicians who recognize the statutory, regulatory, and judicial avenues available to workers can significantly improve the occupational health of their patients. Because of the legal remedies available to workers, the physician caring for a patient with work-related disease or injury has responsibilities that extend beyond simple diagnosis and treatment. These duties include (1) determination of nature and extent of impairment/disability, (2) determination of causality, (3) provision of written opinion regarding diagnosis and causality, (4) provision of examining physician testimony at a deposition or in a court of law, and (5) facilitation of workplace evaluation in some cases. By definition *causality* in medical-legal terms means "more likely than not," or with greater than 50% certainty. For example, to diagnose occupational asthma in a patient with reversible airway obstruction, the primary care physician must believe that, more likely than not, exposure to a chemical or fume at work was causally related to the development or worsening of asthma.

Providing a written opinion is important because statutes of limitation begin to run under both WC and tort law at the time an injury occurred or the worker should have reasonably known that an injury occurred. Notice in writing to the patient prevents subsequent ambiguity regarding time of di-

---

> **BOX 98-3**
> **Resources**
>
> **Regulatory Agencies**
> Occupational Safety and Health Administration | Standard setting and enforcement, etc.
> NIOSH | Research and recommendations re: standards
> State Department of Labor | Worksite inspections by request
>
> **Hotlines**
> Pregnancy Environmental Hotline
> State Poison Control Networks
>
> **Computer Databases**
> Toxline | Contains >400,000 references
> Reprotox | Contains information on effects of >600 substances on reproductive health

---

agnosis. Such ambiguity may bar a worker from a remedy to which she is entitled.

Health care professionals must appreciate the limitations of regulatory and legal remedies in the prevention of workplace injuries and illnesses. A careful understanding of women's occupational health issues and early consultation with patients and their employers may avert the development of occupational disease or injury, thus obviating the need for regulatory enforcement action and legal remedies.

RESOURCES

Resources available to the primary care physician caring for a patient with known or suspected occupational illness, injury, or disease are summarized in Box 98-3. Enforcement and advisory agencies exist at both the federal and state levels, and depending on the mission of the agency may provide telephone consultations, workplace consultations, written materials, or training. The state committees on occupational safety and health, or COSH groups, are nonprofit organizations that have been formed in many states to educate workers and others, including health care providers, about occupational safety and health. These COSH groups are a valuable source of written material about the potential adverse health effects of specific jobs and exposures. Additionally they often provide safety and health training for workers.

BIBLIOGRAPHY

Massachusetts Coalition for Occupational Safety and Health: *Confronting reproductive health hazards on the job: a guide for workers.* Boston, 1992, Mass Cosh.

Messite J, Bond MB: Occupational health considerations for women at work. In Zenz C, editor: *Occupational medicine: principles and practical applications,* Chicago, 1988, Year Book Medical.

Office of Technology Assessment: *Reproductive hazards in the workplace,* OTA-BA-266, Washington, DC, 1985, Government Printing Office.

Oleinich A et al: Current methods of estimating severity for occupational injuries and illnesses: data from the 1986 Michigan comprehensive compensable injury and illness database, *Am J Industr Med* 23:231, 1993.

Oliver LC, Shackleton B: The indoor air we breathe: a public health problem for the 90's, *Public Health Reports* 113:398, 1998.

Oliver LC, Stoeckle JD: Prevention and evaluation of occupational respiratory disease. In Goroll AH, May LA, Mulley AC, editors: *Primary care medicine,* New York, 2000, Lippincott Williams & Wilkins.

Paul M, editor: *Occupational and environmental reproductive hazards,* Baltimore, 1993, Williams & Wilkins.

Paul M, Himmelstein J: Reproductive hazards in the workplace: what the practitioner needs to know about chemical exposures, *Obstet Gynecol* 71:921, 1988.

Proposed national strategy for the prevention of leading work-related diseases and injuries, DHHS (NIOSH) Publication No 89, 1986.

Rosenstock L, Lee LJ: Caution: Women at work, Editorial, *JAMWA* 55:67, 2000.

Swanson NG. Working women and stress, *JAMWA* 55:76, 2000.

Teutsch SM: A framework for assessing the effectiveness of disease and injury prevention, *MMWR* 41:1, 1992.

CHAPTER **99**

Screening and Immunization Guidelines

Barbara J. Woo

This chapter presents the current guidelines for screening interventions and immunizations in adult women. Principles of screening and the methods by which evidence-based authorities arrive at their recommendations are reviewed to provide a foundation for clinicians to devise their own recommendations for individual patients when discordance between authorities exists or when available data to support a preventive measure effectively are limited. Screening for cervical, ovarian, and breast cancer is considered in greater detail in Chapters 95, 96, and 97. Chapters 12 and 67 include material on screening for osteoporosis and immunizations during pregnancy. More extensive discussion regarding substance abuse, domestic violence, and safe sex counseling is presented in Chapters 22, 87, and 91.

SCREENING GUIDELINES

The concept of the periodic comprehensive physical examination was developed at the turn of the century and has remained one of the most common reasons for a visit to the doctor today. Many women still expect an annual check-up, complete with a comprehensive physical examination, Pap smear, and battery of blood tests. In the last 15 years, however, the rationale for this long-standing practice has been challenged. Physicians have gradually been convinced that many screening interventions are not beneficial, as these maneuvers have been subjected to more scientific scrutiny.

Principles of Screening

The objective of a screening maneuver is to reduce morbidity and mortality rates of a given disease in a defined population at a reasonable cost. For this to occur, the target disease and screening tool must meet the following criteria:

1. The disease must have a significant burden of suffering in terms of prevalence, morbidity, and mortality.
2. The disease must have an asymptomatic period during which detection and treatment can yield a therapeutic result superior to that obtained by delaying treatment until symptoms appear.
3. The screening test must be sufficiently sensitive, specific, safe, and acceptable to the patient and must be available at a reasonable cost.

Development of Screening Guidelines

In the last 25 years a concerted effort has taken place to develop screening guidelines that are more evidence-based. The Canadian Task Force (CTF) was one of the first authorities to rigorously outline and apply the screening principles just discussed to evaluate the usefulness of individual preventive maneuvers. For each preventive intervention the existing literature was reviewed and evaluated. The studies that were subject to less bias and misinterpretation were given more weight. For instance, randomized controlled trials were relied on more strongly than cohort studies or expert opinions. On the basis of their review of the available literature, the authorities then devised a quality-of-evidence profile for each intervention (Box 99-1). Using this assessment of the literature the CTF created a 5-point strength of recommendation scale in an attempt to translate the science into a clinical recommendation (Box 99-2). The A, B, D, and E recommendations reflect good evidence for the inclusion or exclusion of a screening tool in clinical practice. Unfortunately many screening tests are given C rankings, indicating that there is poor evidence for inclusion or exclusion of the procedure, but that recommendations can be made on other grounds. In some instances a "C" ranked maneuver may be described as clinically prudent despite the lack of convincing evidence of effectiveness if it is not associated with significant harm or cost. In other cases, a recommendation against a "C" ranked procedure is made even if the quality of evidence to exclude the procedure is poor, because of high cost, risk of the procedure, or a high false-positive rate. When the reviewers judge that there is inadequate evidence to make a recommendation for or against a procedure, each clinician then must use their own judgment and take into consideration the unique circumstances of each patient to decide whether to recommend the procedure or not. Finally, it is primarily in the "C" ranked category that authorities may differ in their recommendations. The American Cancer Society, which may be more aggressive toward cancer detection, may be more willing to recommend a test than those authorities that are primarily evidence-based.

In 1989, using the same criteria and process as the CTF, the United States Preventive Services Task Force (USPSTF) published the most comprehensive set of guidelines assessing the effectiveness of 169 screening interventions. These guidelines were subsequently updated and expanded in 1996. The following text summarizes some of the highlights of the USPSTF report and, when significantly different, compares and contrasts their recommendations to other authorities such as the American College of Physicians (ACP), the American College of Obstetrics and Gynecology (ACOG), and the American Cancer Society (ACS). Given the high cost of screening and the high cost of treating potentially preventable diseases, it is clear that much research still needs to be done to evaluate screening procedures and guide clinicians more effectively.

Screening Guidelines

A preventive care timeline of core clinical preventive services for normal-risk adults is presented in Fig. 99-1. This summary of preventive guidelines, put forth by the U.S. Department of Health and Human Services, displays in black bars services for which a strong consensus exists among U.S. authorities. The lighter bars in the figure indicate areas in which authorities differ in regard to the periodicity and age of onset of certain preventive services.

History and Physical Examination

Most authorities no longer recommend the annual comprehensive physical examination. Advocates of these examinations emphasize the benefits of establishment of the physician-patient relationship and opportunities for immunizations and counseling. Opponents argue that the annual health check-up is not cost-effective, has not been shown to reduce morbidity and mortality rates, and may convey a sense of false reassurance to patients. Most physicians, however, would not argue the utility of an initial *baseline* history and physical examination. Although there are no data to support this as a cost-effective screening procedure, knowledge of a patient's medications, allergies, current and past medical history, health habits, and social and family history is essential to the provision of preventive medical care.

Blood pressure measurements every 1 to 2 years and at each office visit is generally recommended. The ACP recommends that blood pressure should be checked at least yearly if a patient has a diastolic BP between 85 and 89, is African-American, has moderate or extreme obesity, has a first-degree relative with hypertension, or has a personal history of hypertension.

Height and weight measurement is recommended periodically in adults by most authorities as a routine screening test for obesity.

Thyroid Disease

The ACS and ACOG recommend periodic **thyroid palpation** for detection of thyroid cancer. The USPSTF states that there is insufficient evidence for or against performance of the examination, but that it may be warranted in high-risk patients with a history of irradiation. The ACP suggests routine periodic testing of **thyroid-stimulating hormone (TSH)** for women over the age of 50, given the high prevalence of subclinical hypothyroidism and hyperthyroidism. The American Thyroid Association recommends a TSH test every 5 years beginning at age 35. Most other authorities, however, do not recommend periodic TSH screening in asymptomatic patients. They state that even if subclinical thyroid disease is found, there is insufficient evidence that treatment is sufficiently useful to justify screening.

Cholesterol

Several studies have established that lowering cholesterol levels can reduce coronary heart disease; hence all authorities recommend screening for hyperlipidemia. Authorities differ, however, on the age to start and stop screening. The USPSTF and ACP recommend screening for all men age 35 to 65 years old and women 45 to 65 years old. There is insufficient evidence to recommend for or against screening of younger adults and adults 66 to 75 years old. The USPSTF does state that testing of these individuals may be based on other considerations such as the presence of cardiac risk factors and the potential long-term benefits of early lifestyle interventions. Screening of patients over age 75 is not recommended. The National Cholesterol Education Program

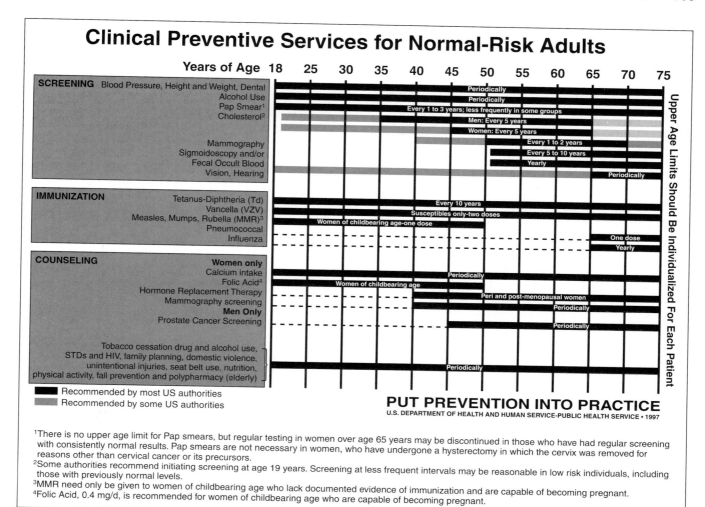

FIG. 99-1 Clinical preventive services for normal risk adults.

(NCEP) of the National Heart, Lung and Blood Institute recommends total cholesterol and high-density lipoprotein (HDL) cholesterol every 5 years for individuals 20 years of age or older. See Chapter 4 for further details regarding cholesterol screening and management.

Skin Cancer Screening

Nearly 900,000 cases of basal and squamous cell carcinoma, and 40,000 cases of malignant melanoma were diagnosed in 1997. Given that most skin cancers are curable if detected early, the ACS, the American Academy of Dermatology, and an NIH Consensus Panel recommends regular periodic skin examinations. The USPSTF states there is insufficient evidence to recommend for or against routine screening for skin cancer by primary care physicians, as no controlled studies thus far have demonstrated that screening for melanoma by primary care providers improves outcome. They caution that clinicians should remain alert for skin lesions with malignant features when examining patients for other reasons, especially patients with established risk factors such as dysplastic nevi, a large number of moles, a per-

sonal or family history of skin cancer, or significant sun exposure or severe burns as a child.

Breast Cancer Screening: Breast Self-Examination, Clinical Breast Examination, and Mammography

It is clear that breast cancer meets the criteria as a target disease for screening. It has a high prevalence, morbidity, and mortality; and there is convincing evidence that screening can reduce mortality from breast cancer. The magnitude of benefit from each of the three available screening methods, the frequency of testing, and the age range for screening are somewhat controversial.

The quality of evidence and strength of recommendation for clinical breast examination and mammography in women age 50 to 59 are very strong. For patients 60 and over the data and recommendation for screening are fairly strong. Controversy exists primarily for women ages 40 to 49, owing to inconsistency in results across studies and differences in individual interpretation of specific studies. For these reasons recommendations for patients in there 40s differ among authorities. Authorities such as the CTF and

ACP do not believe that the evidence shows a sufficient reduction in mortality, and that the cost, radiation exposure, and risks of false-positive results incurred by mammography are not justified for women ages 40 to 49. Other groups, such as the ACS, find the data persuasive enough to recommend mammography to these women. (See Chapter 95 for a more detailed discussion of breast cancer screening.)

The **self-breast examination (SBE)** is the least efficacious of the screening maneuvers; however, the procedure itself is inexpensive and not associated with any risks. The ACS and National Cancer Institute recommend monthly SBE despite the poor sensitivity and specificity of the test. The USPSTF and the CTF, however, do not make a recommendation for or against SBE. Because of the potential for false-positive results to cause unnecessary doctors visits, testing, and anxiety, their recommendations are less aggressive than those of the ACS.

The ACS recommends **the clinician breast examination** (CBE) every 3 years for ages 20 to 40 and then yearly thereafter. For women who have a family history of breast cancer, they recommend more frequent examinations starting at age 20. The ACP recommends yearly CBE beginning at age 40. The USPSTF states that there is insufficient evidence to recommend for or against CBE.

For women age 50 and older, all authorities recommend routine **mammogram** screening. The ACP, NCI, and USPSTF recommend a frequency of every 1 to 2 years. The ACS, ACOG, and the CTF recommend yearly screening.

The USPSTF found insufficient evidence to recommend screening of women 70 years of age and older, although recommendations for screening can be made on other grounds for such women when they have a reasonable life expectancy. The ACP states that the use of mammography after the age of 75 should be discouraged.

For women aged 40 to 49, the ACP and CTF do not recommend routine mammography. The USPSTF states there is insufficient evidence to recommend for or against screening in this age group, but screening high-risk women may be appropriate. The ACS recommends mammography every year for women 40 years of age and older. (Their previous recommendation of a baseline study between ages 35 and 39 was deleted in 1992.)

For high-risk women with a family history of premenopausal breast cancer, the CTF and ACOG recommend regular mammography beginning at age 35. The ACP and USPSTF state there is insufficient evidence in this area, and that recommendations should be made on other grounds.

Pelvic Examination for Ovarian CA Screening

The pelvic examination as a separate screening tool apart from the Papanicolaou's (Pap) smear is not considered by many authorities. The USPSTF and CTF do *not* recommend the pelvic examination as a screening tool for ovarian cancer, owing to the poor sensitivity and specificity of the examination and the lack of evidence that detection of an ovarian cancer by palpation is likely to improve overall survival. They do state, however, that it is clinically prudent to examine the uterine adnexa when performing gynecologic examinations for other reasons. The ACS and ACOG recommend a pelvic examination or bimanual examination every 1 to 3 years with the Pap smear for ages 18 to 40 and every year after age 40. The ACS recommends the pelvic examination

because "bimanual palpation of the ovaries is the only examination that currently meets the American Cancer Society's criteria of feasibility, practicality, reasonable cost, and low risk. (See Chapter 97 for further details on screening for ovarian cancer.)

Papanicolaou's Smear and Cervical Cancer

A large body of evidence supports the efficacy of the Pap smear in decreasing morbidity and mortality from cervical cancer. All authorities agree on the effectiveness of regular Pap smears; however, the frequency of the test and the age at which Pap smears can be discontinued are controversial.

The ACS and ACOG recommend that all women who are or who have been sexually active or who have reached age 18 should have an annual Pap smear and pelvic examination. After a woman has had three or more consecutive satisfactory normal test results, the Pap smear may be performed every 1 to 3 years at the discretion of her physician. The ACS does not stipulate an age to discontinue testing. The USPSTF recommends Pap smears every 1 to 3 years depending on patient risk factors, beginning at age 18 or when the woman becomes sexually active. At age 65, Pap smears may be discontinued if the physician can document consistently normal Pap smear results in the previous 10 years.

All groups recommend more frequent testing if high-risk conditions exist such as early onset of sexual activity, low socioeconomic status, or multiple sexual partners. Women who have undergone a hysterectomy in which the cervix was removed do not require PAP testing, unless the hysterectomy was performed because of cervical cancer or its precursors. (See Chapter 96 for further details on screening for cervical cancer.)

Colorectal Cancer: Rectal Examination, Stool for Occult Blood, Sigmoidoscopy, and Colonoscopy

Colorectal cancer is the third leading cause of cancer death in women in the United States. Although public awareness of colorectal cancer is growing, compliance with screening recommendations remains a major problem.

The **rectal examination** has little usefulness in screening for colorectal cancer, given that less than 10% of cancers are within reach on a digital examination. The ACS and ACOG recommend a rectal examination for colorectal cancer screening every 5 to 10 years for patients 50 and older. The USPSTF states there is insufficient evidence to recommend for or against the digital rectal examination for colon cancer screening.

The reported sensitivity and specificity for colorectal cancer with **fecal occult blood testing** (FOBT) are 26% to 92% and 90% to 99%, respectively. The reported positive predictive value among asymptomatic persons over age 50 is only about 2% to 11% for carcinoma. Hence, for every one case of cancer detected by FOBT, as many as 50 patients will undergo evaluations that will ultimately be negative. However; since 1993, several randomized-controlled trials have clearly demonstrated that FOBT can reduce mortality from colorectal cancer. A Minnesota study showed a 33% reduction in mortality using rehydrated stool samples collected yearly and a 21% reduction when collected every other year. Two European trials in 1996 using nonrehydrated FOBT every other year showed a 16% to 18% reduction in mortality.

Sigmoidoscopy with the 60-cm flexible sigmoidoscope can reach 50% to 60% of colorectal cancers. Several well-designed case-control studies have shown a decrease in colorectal cancer mortality by 59% to 79% in the part of the bowel examined. There is some evidence to support combined FOBT and sigmoidoscopy from a nonrandomized trial that found a 43% mortality reduction for the combination compared with sigmoidoscopy alone.

Colonoscopy, although theoretically the most sensitive method for detection of polyps and early cancers, has not traditionally been favored as a screening method because of cost, patient discomfort, and risk of perforation. Colonoscopy has been shown to reduce colon cancer deaths by 76% to 90% in patients with polyps. The effect of colonoscopic screening on mortality rates in asymptomatic persons is unknown. However, recent research indicates that colonoscopy detects a substantial number of asymptomatic colorectal cancers or polyps associated with a high risk of cancer that would be missed by sigmoidoscopy alone. In Imperiale's study of screening, 50 of 2000 asymptomatic persons had advanced proximal neoplasms that would have been missed by sigmoidoscopy. Future advances in technology such as virtual colonoscopy and changes in reimbursement and delivery systems may make colonoscopy more feasible for screening average risk patients. Screening for patients at average risk of colorectal cancer begins at age 50. The ACS recommends rectal examinations and FOBT annually and sigmoidoscopy every 5 years. Other alternatives include colonoscopy every 10 years or double contrast barium enema every 5 to 10 years. The ACP states that patients 50 to 70 years old should be offered sigmoidoscopy, colonoscopy or double-contrast barium enema every 10 years, with annual FOBT for those who decline these options. The USPSTF currently recommends screening for colorectal cancer in patients 50 and older with annual FOBT or sigmoidoscopy (periodicity unspecified) or both.

Most authorities consider the data adequate to recommend earlier screening in patients at higher risk, including those with a first-degree relative (parent, child or sibling) with colorectal cancer or adenomatous polyps (especially if diagnosed before age 55 or 60, respectively), or a previous diagnosis of inflammatory bowel disease. These patients can be offered the same screening options as those at average risk, starting at age 40. Periodic colonoscopy is recommended for all persons with a personal history of adenomatous polyps or colorectal cancer or a family history of familial polyposis.

Counseling

Poor health habits contribute to almost half the deaths attributable to the leading causes of mortality in adults. Even if counseling is successful at changing behavior in only a minority of patients, it is likely to have a significant impact on overall morbidity and mortality rates given the high prevalence of diseases with which poor health habits are associated. As clinicians, we should spend more time counseling about diet, exercise, seat belt use, safe sexual practices, smoking, and drug and alcohol abuse. Women should also be counseled on calcium intake and hormone replacement therapy. See individual chapters for further discussion on these subjects.

IMMUNIZATION RECOMMENDATIONS

Unlike the uncertainty of efficacy for many of the screening tools described here, the effectiveness of immunizations for the control of many infectious diseases has been clearly shown. Unfortunately immunizations are often a low priority for primary care physicians, with the result that only a minority of patients are properly immunized. Patients may also be unaware of the need for immunizations or be concerned about side effects. It is imperative therefore that all clinicians be aware of the recommendations and make certain that a thorough immunization history is completed. Information regarding risk factors related to lifestyle and occupational exposures and travel history should also be detailed.

Adverse reactions to immunizations are very rare. Contraindications to the routinely used adult vaccines include the following:

- Anaphylactic reactions to eggs: measles, mumps, and influenza vaccines are prepared from viruses grown in embryonated eggs and therefore have small quantities of egg proteins
- Anaphylactic reactions to neomycin (MMR-containing vaccines)
- Known hypersensitivity to preservatives or stabilizers in the vaccines
- Live vaccines (especially rubella) during pregnancy; inactive vaccines are considered safe
- Live vaccines in immunocompromised hosts (i.e., lymphoma, leukemia, chemotherapy, symptomatic human immunodeficiency virus [HIV] infection); low-dose steroids in any form are usually not immunosuppressive.

Misconceptions about contraindications deserve special mention, as they prevent clinicians from appropriately vaccinating their patients. As outlined by the Centers for Disease Control and Prevention, the following are *not* contraindications:

- Reaction to a previous vaccination that involved only localized soreness, redness, or swelling or temperature less than 40.5° C
- Mild acute upper respiratory or gastrointestinal illnesses with fever less than 38° C
- Current antibiotic therapy or convalescent phase of illness
- Pregnancy of a household contact
- Recent exposure to an infectious disease
- Breastfeeding
- History of nonspecific allergies or relatives with allergies
- Allergies to penicillin
- Family history of an adverse event after vaccination

General recommendations on Immunization in the United States are primarily those of the Immunization Practices Advisory Committee of the Center for Disease Control. A summary of recommendations for adult immunization is presented in Table 99-1. For specific, detailed IPAC recommendations, refer to the full statements published in the MMWR.

Specific Guidelines (Table 99-1)
Tetanus-diphtheria

Approximately 40% of patients above age 60 lack protection to tetanus and diphtheria. Correspondingly, most cases

Table 99-1
Routine Vaccines for Adults

Vaccine	Indicated for	Dosage	Contraindications	Adverse
Tetanus-diphtheria (toxoid)	All adults	Booster every 10 yrs of 0.5 m IM	Neurologic reaction or hypersensitivity to previous dose	Local pain and swelling can be more severe if boosters given <5 years apart
	Never immunized	Primary series 3 doses 0.5 ml IM at 0, 1-2 mo, then 6-12 mo		
Measles (live vaccine)	Unimmunized born after 1956	2 doses 0.5 ml SC at least 1 mo apart	Egg allergy; hypersensitivity to neomycin; pregnancy; immunocompromised patients	Low-grade fever; rash, local pain, and swelling in patients previously immunized
	Previously immunized with one dose, for college entry, health care workers, and foreign travel	1 dose 0.5 ml SC		
Rubella (attenuated live virus grown in human diploid cells)	Unimmunized young women and health care workers	1 dose 0.5 ml SC	Pregnancy; immunocompromised patients; hypersensitivity to neomycin	Arthralgias in 40% of non-immune adults
Hepatitis B (noninfectious recombinant hepatitis B surface antigen)	High-risk patients and health care workers	3 doses 1 ml IM in the deltoid, second dose after 1 month, third dose 6 months after first dose; higher dose for immunocompromised and dialysis patients	None	Local soreness
Influenza (inactivated whole or virus subunits, grown in chick embryo cells)	High-risk patients, health care workers, and all more than 65 years old	1 dose 0.5 ml IM annually	Egg allergy	Infrequent fevers, chills, myalgia lasting 1-2 weeks
Pneumococcal (Capsular polysaccharide from 23 types)	High-risk patients and more than 65 years old	1 dose 0.5 ml IM		Local soreness in approx. 50% of patients

Modified from *Med Lett* 32:54, 1990.

occur in elderly patients. One should ensure that all elderly patients have received a primary series of three shots.

If the primary vaccination schedule has been interrupted or delayed, there is no need to restart a series. An adequate level of immunity will still be reached on completion of the primary series.

For clean, minor wound management, patients should receive a tetanus booster if they have not had one in 10 years or have not completed a primary series. For more serious wounds patients should receive a booster if more than 5 years has passed since their last booster or primary series was completed. If they have not completed a primary series or their immunization status is unknown, they should also receive tetanus immune globulin.

Measles

All persons born before 1957 are considered immune. Because of recent outbreaks of measles, a second dose of live vaccine should be considered for young adults entering college, travelers to foreign countries, or health care work-

ers. It is recommended that women vaccinated for measles receive the combined measles, mumps, and rubella (MMR) vaccine if there is any uncertainty about immunity to any one of these diseases. Even if immunity exists already there is little risk to the combined vaccine.

Rubella

Approximately 10% to 15% of young adults are susceptible to rubella. Outbreaks have occurred in schools and hospitals. If infection occurs early in pregnancy, the sequelae may include fetal abnormalities, miscarriages, and stillbirths. All women of childbearing age and health care workers should be either empirically vaccinated if no documentation exists regarding previous immunization or tested serologically for rubella antibodies. Those who receive the vaccine should be counseled not to become pregnant for 3 months. Although studies have not shown fetal problems in women inadvertently vaccinated during pregnancy, the vaccine should be avoided in pregnant women. It is recommended that patients requiring rubella vaccination receive the combined MMR vaccine if any uncertainty exists about their immunity to measles or mumps, as there is little risk to the combined vaccine.

Hepatitis B

The three-dose vaccination series confers immunity to 90% to 95% of healthy young adults. Protection exists for at least 7 years despite the fact that antibody levels can fall or even become undetectable. Therefore routine serologic testing for antibody levels and booster shots are not currently recommended. More studies will be necessary to determine the duration of protection and when and whether boosters will be necessary.

Influenza

The influenza vaccine is 50% to 60% effective in preventing hospitalizations and pneumonia and 80% effective in preventing death in older adults. Because fear of side effects is a common barrier to patients' receiving the flu vaccine, one can reassure these patients that a randomized trial comparing a saline injection to a flu vaccination found no difference in rates of systemic side effects. Antiviral prophylaxis against influenza A virus with amantadine or rimantadine should also be considered as an adjunct to the vaccine when community outbreaks exist. It should be given for 2 weeks until antibodies from the vaccine appear.

Pneumococcus

Pneumococcal vaccination should be given to all candidates for the influenza vaccine. In addition, women with asplenia, chronic liver disease, or alcoholism should be vaccinated. Pregnant women at high risk may be vaccinated, although it is preferable to wait until after the first trimester. The current 23-valent pneumococcal vaccine represents 85% to 90% of serotypes in the United States that cause invasive disease.

The issue of revaccination has not been fully resolved. Routine revaccination of immunocompetent persons is not recommended. High-risk patients vaccinated before 1983, when only the 14-valent vaccine was available, should be considered for revaccination with the 23-valent vaccine for increased coverage of pneumococcal serotypes. Persons aged 65 and older should be administered a second dose of vaccine if they received the vaccine more than 5 years previously and were less than 65 at the time of the first vaccination. For patients at greatest risk (i.e., asplenic patients) revaccination once is recommended after 5 years. Revaccination should be considered for patients with serious cardiopulmonary or liver disease as well. Finally, for patients with nephrotic syndrome and renal failure, revaccination after 3 to 5 years is recommended because of rapidly declining antibody levels. Although early studies indicate that local reactions are more common with revaccination occurring within 2 years of the first dose, subsequent studies with revaccination 4 or more years later, have not shown an increased incidence of reactions.

Varicella

The varicella vaccine became available in the United States in 1995, and most children are now routinely vaccinated against chickenpox between the ages of 12 and 18 months. Because adults achieve poorer antibody responses, it is recommended that nonimmune adults at risk receive two doses of vaccine. Booster doses are currently not recommended until further data are available regarding the duration of immunity provided by the vaccine. The vaccine is effective in preventing chickenpox or reducing the severity of disease if used in susceptible adults within 3 days, and possibly up to 5 days after exposure.

Hepatitis A

In more than 96% of healthy young adults, seroconversion occurs within 30 days of the first dose and in essentially all recipients after the second dose. Efficacy rates of prevention of hepatitis A in children have been reported at 94% to 100%. No booster doses after the initial two doses are recommended.

Lyme Disease

The efficacy of the vaccine in clinical trials was 49% after two doses and 76% after three doses. The need for booster doses after the initial three series of injections has not been determined. (See Chapter 67 for further details on immunizations during pregnancy.)

BIBLIOGRAPHY

Byers T et al: American Cancer Society guidelines for screening and surveillance for early detection of colorectal polyps and cancer: update 1997. *CA Cancer J Clin* 47:154, 1997.

Canadian Task Force on the Periodic Health Examination: The periodic health examination, *Can Med Assoc J* 121:1193, 1979.

Centers for Disease Control and Prevention: Update on adult immunization: recommendations of the Immunization Practices Advisory Committee, *MMWR* 43(RR-1):1, 1994.

CDC: Prevention of pneumococcal disease, *MMWR* 46(RR-8):1, 1997.

CDC: Recommendations for the use of lyme disease vaccine, *MMWR* 48(RR-7):1, 1999.

CDC Website for updated immunization recommendations: www.cdc.gov/nip/publications/ACIP-list.htm

Hardcastle JD et al: Randomized controlled trial of faecal-occult-blood screening for colorectal cancer, *Lancet* 348:1472, 1996.

Helfand M et al: Screening for thyroid disease, *Ann Intern Med* 129:141, 1998.

Immunization Action Coalition: *Vaccinate adults bulletin* Vol 3, No 2, Fall/Winter 1999-2000.

Imperiale TF et al: Risk of advanced proximal neoplasms in asymptomatic adults according to the distal colorectal findings, *N Engl J Med* 343:169, 2000.

Kronborg O et al: Randomised study of screening for colorectal cancer with faecal-occult-blood test, *Lancet* 348:1267, 1996.

Landis SH et al: Cancer statistics, 1998, *CA Cancer J Clin* 48:6, 1998.

Lieberman DA et al: Use of colonoscopy to screen asymptomatic adults for colorectal cancer, *N Engl J Med* 343:162, 2000.

Mandel JS et al: Reducing mortality from colorectal cancer by screening for fecal occult blood, *N Engl J Med* 328:1365, 1993.

Mandel JS et al: Colorectal cancer mortality: effectiveness of biennial screening for fecal occult blood, *J Natl Cancer Inst* 91:434, 1999.

Margolis KL et al: Frequency of adverse reactions to influenza vaccine in the elderly: a randomized, placebo-controlled trial, *JAMA* 264:1139, 1990.

Selby JV et al: A case-control study of screening sigmoidoscopy and mortality from colorectal cancer, *N Engl J Med* 326:653, 1992.

Selby JV et al: Effect of fecal occult blood testing on mortality from colorectal cancer, *Ann Intern Med* 118:1, 1993.

U.S. Dept of Health and Human Services: *Clinician's handbook of preventive services,* ed 2, Washington, DC, 1998, US Government Printing Office.

U.S. Preventive Services Task Force: *Guide to clinical preventive services,* ed 2, Baltimore, 1996, Williams & Wilkins.

Winawer SJ et al: Screening for colorectal cancer with fecal occult blood testing and sigmoidoscopy, *J Natl Cancer Inst* 85:1311, 1993.

Summary of Drug Interactions with Oral Contraceptives

Drugs that interfere with oral contraceptive efficacy
  Drugs that reduce efficacy
    Anticonvulsants
      Phenytoin, phenobarbital, methylphenobarbital, primidone, carbamazepine, ethosuximide
    Antibiotics
      Rifampin (proven)
      Ampicillin, tetracycline, other broad-spectrum antibiotics (possibly)
      Griseofulvin (possibly)
  Drugs that increase plasma levels of contraceptive steroids
    Ascorbic acid
Oral contraceptives that interfere with the metabolism of other drugs
  Increase plasma levels of the following drugs:
    Benzodiazepines
    Theophylline and caffeine
    Cyclosporine
    Metaprolol
    Phenazone
    Prednisolone
    Ethanol (possibly)
  Decrease plasma levels of the following drugs:
    Aspirin
    Clofibric acid
    Morphine
    Paracetamol
    Temazepam

From Rayburn WF, Zuspan FP: *Drug therapy in obstetrics and gynecology,* ed 3, St Louis, 1993, Mosby. Data from Back O, Orme ML'E: *Clin Pharmacokinet* 18:472, 1990.

Possible Effects of Oral Contraceptives on Laboratory Tests*

Laboratory Test	Effects	Probable Mechanism
Serum, Plasma, Blood		
Albumin	Slightly decreased	Decreased hepatic synthesis
Aldosterone	Increased	Activates renin-angiotensin system
Amylase	Slightly increased (common)	Not established
	Markedly increased (rare)	Pancreatitis
Antinuclear antibodies	Become detectable	Not established
Bilirubin	Increased (rare)	Reduced secretion into bile
Ceruloplasmin	Increased	Increased hepatic synthesis
Cholinesterase	Decreased	Decreased hepatic synthesis
Coagulation factors	Increased II, VII, IX, X	Increased synthesis
Cortisol	Increased	Increased cortisol-binding globulin
Fibrinogen	Increased	Increased hepatic synthesis
Folate	Decreased or no change	Decreased folate absorption
Glucose tolerance tests	Small decrease in tolerance	Several mechanisms proposed
γ-Glutamyl transpeptidase	Increased	Altered secretion in bile
Haptoglobin	Decreased	Decreased hepatic synthesis
HDL cholesterol	Increased with estrogens and decreased with progestins	Not established
Iron-binding capacity	Increased	Increased transferrin levels
Magnesium	Decreased or no change	Decreased bone resorption
Phosphatase, alkaline	Increased (rare)	Altered secretion in bile
Plasminogen	Increased	Increased hepatic synthesis
Platelets	Slightly increased	Not established
Prolactin	Increased	Not established
Renin activity	Increased	Increased synthesis of renin substrate
Thyroxine (total)	Increased	Increased thyroxine-binding globulin
Transaminases	Slightly increased	Not established
Transferrin	Increased	Increased hepatic synthesis
Triglycerides	Increased	Increased synthesis
Triiodothyronine resin uptake	Decreased	Increased thyroxine-binding globulin
Vitamin A	Increased	Increased retinol-binding protein
Vitamin B_{12}	Decreased	Not established
Zinc	Decreased	Shift of zinc into erythrocyte
Urine		
δ-Aminolevulinic acid	Increased	Increased hepatic synthesis
Ascorbic acid	Decreased or no change	Not established
Bacteria	Increased incidence of bacteriuria	Not established
Calcium	Decreased	Decreased bone resorption
Cortisol (free)	Unchanged	
Porphyrins	Increased (may precipitate porphyria in susceptible patients)	Increased δ-aminolevulinic acid synthetase
17-Hydroxycorticosteroid	Slightly decreased or no change	Increased binding proteins
17-Ketosteroid	Slightly decreased or no change	Increased binding proteins

From Rayburn WF, Zuspan FP: *Drug therapy in obstetrics and gynecology,* ed 3, St Louis, 1993, Mosby.
*These effects are thought to be dose dependent and uncommon with the use of low-dose preparations.

Adult Weight for Height Tables

Metropolitan Weight* and Height† Tables (1983)

WEIGHT				HEIGHT	
Pounds		**Kilograms**			
Average	Range	Average	Range	Feet	Centimeters
117	102-131	53.2	46.4-59.5	4'9"	145
119	103-134	54.1	46.8-60.9	4'10"	147
121	104-137	55.0	47.3-62.3	4'11"	150
123	106-140	56.0	48.2-63.6	5'0"	152
126	108-143	57.3	49.1-65.0	5'1"	155
129	111-147	58.6	50.5-66.8	5'2"	158
133	114-151	60.5	51.8-68.6	5'3"	160
136	117-155	61.8	53.2-70.4	5'4"	163
140	120-159	63.6	54.5-72.3	5'5"	165
143	123-163	65.0	55.9-74.1	5'6"	168
147	126-167	66.8	57.3-75.9	5'7"	170
150	129-170	68.2	58.6-77.3	5'8"	173
153	132-173	69.5	60.0-78.6	5'9"	175
156	135-176	70.9	61.4-80.0	5'10"	178
159	138-179	72.3	62.7-81.4	5'11"	180
—	—	—	—	6'0"	183
—	—	—	—	6'1"	185
—	—	—	—	6'2"	188
—	—	—	—	6'3"	191

Modified from 1979 Build Study Society of Actuaries and Association of Life Insurance Medical Directors of America, 1980, Metropolitan Life Insurance Company.
*Weights are at ages 25 to 59 years based on lowest mortality. Weight is in pounds (indoor clothing weighing 3 lb).
†The table is adjusted to reflect subject *without shoes* for height measurement.

Human Chorionic Gonadotropin

Methods for Measurement of Human Chorionic Gonadotropin

Method	Type of Analysis	Principle	Use	Comments
Qualitative Assays				
Slide tests	Agglutination inhibition	Colored latex or other visible particles (red blood cells) coated with hCG, antibodies to hCG, and urine are mixed with particles. Negative urine results in visible agglutination; presence of hCG in urine inhibits agglutination (or protein flocculation).	Was frequently used as stat urinary pregnancy test; urine	Least sensitive of all hCG methods; most rapid (2-3 min)
Tube tests	Same as preceding method	Same as preceding method 1; reaction occurs in tube.	Was sometimes used for stat urine pregnancy tests; urine	More sensitive than slide; some approach upper limit of sensitivity of RIA methods; 45-120 min per assay
Immunoenzymatic concentration tests	Sandwich immunometric assay	Solid-phase, double-antibody sandwich ELISA in which hCG binds to antibody. Enzyme-labeled antibody added, and residual activity directly related to hCG concentration.	Has become assay of choice, has speed of "slide" and sensitivity of "tube" with a colored end point; urine and serum	Reported sensitivity 20-50 mU/ml, 5- to 5-min assay; many forms: membrane, bead, paddle, dipstick, coated tube.
Quantitative Assays—Serum and Urine				
Radioimmunoassay (RIA)	Competitive inhibition	Radiolabeled (radioactive iodine, ^{125}I) hCG competes with sample analyte for binding to anti-hCG. Increased hCG in sample, decreased bound radioactivity.	Infrequently used as stat procedure; serum or urine	Most sensitive hCG assay available; 40-60 min per assay
Enzyme-linked immunosorbent assay (ELISA)	Sandwich immunometric assay	Enzyme-labeled anti-hCG reacts with sample hCG bound to solid-phase anti-hCG. Amount of bound enzyme activity directly proportional to amount of hCG in sample.	Most frequently used assay; serum and urine	Reported sensitivity of 2-10 U/ml; assay time 1-3 hr

From Kaplan LA, Pesce AJ: *Clinical chemistry: theory, analysis, and correlation,* ed 2, St Louis, 1989, Mosby.

Values of Serum Human Chorionic Gonadotropin with Gestational Age

Gestational Age	hCG (mU/ml)
0.2-1 wk	5-50
1-2 wk	50-500
2-3 wk	100-5000
3-4 wk	500-10,000
4-5 wk	1000-50,000
5-6 wk	10,000-100,000
6-8 wk	15,000-200,000
2-3 mo	10,000-100,000

From Kaplan LA, Pesce AJ: *Clinical Chemistry: theory analysis, and correlation,* ed 2, St Louis, 1989, Mosby.

APPENDIX V

Laboratory Reference Values

Endocrinologic Normal Values

Hormone and Metabolite Normal Values

Adrenocorticotropin (ACTH), serum	15-100 pg/ml
Aldosterone (mean ± standard deviation)	
Serum	
210 mEq/day sodium diet	
Supine	48 ± 29 pg/ml
Upright (2 hr)	65 ± 23 pg/ml
110 mEq/day sodium diet	
Supine	107 ± 45 pg/ml
Upright (2 hr)	532 ± 228 pg/ml
Urine	5-19 μg/24 hr
Calcitonin, serum	
Basal	0.15-0.35 ng/ml
Stimulated	<0.6 ng/ml
Catecholamines, free urinary	<110 μg/24 hr
Chorionic gonadotropin, serum	
Pregnancy	
First month	10-10,000 mIU/ml
Second and third months	10,000-100,000 mIU/ml
Second trimester	10,000-30,000 mIU/ml
Third trimester	5000-15,000 mIU/ml
Nonpregnant	<3 mIU/ml
Cortisol	
Serum	
8 AM	5-25 μg/dl
8 PM	<10 μg/dl
Cosyntropin stimulation (30-90 min after 0.25 mg cosyntropin intramuscularly or intravenously)	>10 μg/dl rise over baseline
Overnight suppression (8 AM serum cortisol after 1 mg dexamethasone orally at 11 PM)	≤5 μg/dl
Urine	20-70 μg/24 hr
C peptide, serum	0.28-0.63 pmol/ml
11-Deoxycortisol, serum	
Basal	0-1.4 μg/dl
Metyrapone stimulation (30 mg/kg orally 8 hr prior to level)	>7.5 μg/dl

From Stein: *Internal medicine*, ed 4, St Louis, 1994, Mosby.

Continued

Endocrinologic Normal Values—cont'd

Hormone and Metabolite Normal Values

Epinephrine, plasma	<35 pg/ml	
Estradiol, serum		
Male	20-50 pg/ml	
Female	25-200 pg/ml	
Estrogens, urine (increased during pregnancy; decreased after menopause)	*Male*	*Female*
Total	4-25 µg/24 hr	5-100 µg/24 hr
Estriol	1-11 µg/24 hr	0-65 µg/24 hr
Estradiol	0-6 µg/24 hr	0-14 µg/24 hr
Estrone	3-8 µg/24 hr	4-31 µg/24 hr
Etiocholanolone, serum	<1.2 µg/dl	
Follicle-stimulating hormone, serum		
Male	2-18 mIU/ml	
Female		
Follicular phase	5-20 mIU/ml	
Peak midcycle	30-50 mIU/ml	
Luteal phase	5-15 mIU/ml	
Postmenopausal	>50 mIU/ml	
Free thyroxine index, serum	1-4 ng/dl	
Gastrin, serum (fasting)	30-200 pg/ml	
Growth hormone, serum		
Adult, fasting	<5 ng/ml	
Glucose load (100 g orally)	<5 ng/ml	
Levodopa stimulation (500 mg orally in a fasting state)	>5 ng/ml rise over baseline within 2 hr	
17-Hydroxycorticosteroids, urine		
Male	2-12 mg/24 hr	
Female	2-8 mg/24 hr	
5'-Hydroxyindoleacetic acid (5'-HIAA), urine	2-9 mg/24 hr	
Insulin, plasma		
Fasting	6-20 µU/ml	
Hypoglycemia (serum glucose <50 mg/dl)	<5 µU/ml	
17-Ketosteroids, urine		
Under 8 years old	0-2 mg/24 hr	
Adolescent	0-18 mg/24 hr	
Adult		
Male	8-18 mg/24 hr	
Female	5-15 mg/24 hr	
Luteinizing hormone, serum		
Male adult	2-18 mIU/ml	
Female adult		
Basal	5-22 mIU/ml	
Ovulation	30-250 mIU/ml	
Postmenopausal	>30 mIU/ml	

From Stein: *Internal medicine*, ed 4, St Louis, 1994, Mosby.

Endocrinologic Normal Values—cont'd

Hormone and Metabolite Normal Values

Metanephrines, urine	<1.3 mg/24 hr
Norepinephrine	
Plasma	150-450 pg/ml
Urine	<100 μg/24 hr
Parathyroid hormone, serum	
C-terminal	150-350 pg/ml
N-terminal	230-630 pg/ml
Pregnanediol, urine	
Female	
Follicular phase	<1.5 mg/24 hr
Luteal phase	2.0-4.2 mg/24 hr
Postmenopausal	0.2-1.0 mg/24 hr
Male	<1.5 mg/24 hr
Progesterone, serum	
Female	
Follicular phase	0.02-0.9 ng/ml
Luteal phase	6-30 ng/ml
Male	<2 ng/ml
Prolactin, serum	
Nonpregnant	
Day	5-25 ng/ml
Night	20-40 ng/ml
Pregnant	150-200 ng/ml
Radioactive iodine (^{131}I) uptake (RAIU)	5%-25% at 24 hr (varies with iodine intake)
Renin activity, plasma (mean ± standard deviation)	
Normal diet	
Supine	1.1 ± 0.8 ng/ml/hr
Upright	1.9 ± 1.7 ng/ml/hr
Low-sodium diet	
Supine	2.7 ± 1.8 ng/ml/hr
Upright	6.6 ± 2.5 ng/ml/hr
Diuretics and low-sodium diet	10.0 ± 3.7 ng/ml/hr
Testosterone, total plasma	
Bound	
Adolescent male	<100 ng/dl
Adult male	300-1100 ng/dl
Female	25-90 ng/dl
Unbound	
Adult male	3-24 ng/dl
Female	0.09-1.30 ng/dl
Thyroid-stimulating hormone, serum	<10 μU/ml
Thyroxine (T_4), serum	
Total	4-11 μg/dl
Free	0.8-2.4 ng/dl
Thyroxine-binding globulin capacity, serum	15-25 μg T_4/dl
Thyroxine index, free	1-4 ng/dl
Triiodothyronine (T_3), serum	70-190 ng/dl
T_3 resin uptake	25%-45%
Vanillylmandelic acid (VMA), urine	1-8 mg/24 hr

Endocrine Function Tests

Adrenal Gland

Glucocorticoid suppression: overnight dexamethasone suppression test (8 AM serum cortisol after 1 mg dexamethasone orally at 11 PM)   ≤5 μg/dl

Glucocorticoid stimulation: cosyntropin stimulation test (serum cortisol 30-90 min after 0.25 mg cosyntropin intramuscularly or intravenously)   >10 μg/ml more than baseline serum cortisol

Metyrapone test, single dose (8 AM serum deoxycortisol after 30 mg/kg metyrapone orally at midnight)   >7.5 μg/dl

Aldosterone suppression: sodium depletion test (urine aldosterone collected on day 3 of 200 mEq day/sodium diet)   <20 μg/24 hr

Pancreas

Glucose tolerance test* (serum glucose after 100 g glucose orally)
- 60 min after ingestion   <180 mg/dl
- 90 min after ingestion   <160 mg/dl
- 120 min after ingestion   <125 mg/dl

Pituitary Gland

Adrenocorticotropic hormone (ACTH) stimulation See Adrenal gland, Metyrapone test

Growth hormone stimulation: insulin tolerance test (serum growth hormone after 0.1 U/kg regular insulin intravenously after an overnight fast to induce a 50% fall in serum glucose concentration or symptomatic hypoglycemia)   >5 ng/ml rise over baseline

Levodopa test (serum growth hormone after 0.5 g levodopa orally while fasting)   >5 ng/ml rise over baseline within 2 hr

Growth hormone suppression: glucose tolerance test (serum growth hormone after 100 g glucose orally after 8 hr fast)   <5 ng/ml within 2 hr

Luteinizing hormone (LH) stimulation: gonadotropin-releasing hormone (GnRH) test (serum LH after 100 μg GnRH intravenously or intramuscularly)   4- to 6-fold rise over baseline

Thyroid-stimulating hormone (TSH) stimulation: thyrotropin-releasing hormone (TRH) stimulation test (serum TSH after 400 μg TRH intravenously)   >2-fold rise over baseline within 2 hr

Thyroid Gland

Radioactive iodine uptake (RAIU) suppression test (RAIU on day 7 after 25 μg triiodothyronine orally 4 times daily)   <10% to <50% baseline

Thyrotropin-releasing hormone (TRH) stimulation test. See Pituitary gland, Thyroid-stimulating hormone (TSH) stimulation

---

From Stein: *Internal medicine,* ed 4, St Louis, 1994, Mosby.

*Add 10 mg/dl for each decade over 50 years of age.

Body Mass Index (BMI) Calculator

$$BMI = \frac{Weight\ (kg)}{(Height\ [m])squared} = \frac{Weight\ (lbs)}{(Height\ [m])squared} \times 705$$

Women	Risk Factor*
Less than 19.1	Underweight. The lower the BMI the greater the risk
19.1 to 25.8	Normal, very low risk
25.9 to 27.3	Marginally overweight, some risk
27.4 to 32.2	Overweight, moderate risk
32.3 to 44.8	Severe overweight, high risk
Greater than 44.8	Morbid obesity, very high risk

Modified from the Primary Care Operations Improvement Site prepared by the MGH Laboratory of Computer Science, 2001, The General Hospital Corporation.
*Higher BMI is associated with higher risks of hypertension, diabetes, some cancers and other disorders, and higher overall mortality.

Recommended Dietary Allowances

Food and Nutrition Board, National Academy of Sciences—National Research Council Recommended Dietary Allowances,* Revised 1989 (Designed for the Maintenance of Good Nutrition of Practically All Healthy People in the United States)

							FAT-SOLUBLE VITAMINS			
	CATEGORY						Vitamin A (μg RE)[‡]	Vitamin D (μg)[§]	Vitamin E (mg α-TE)[″]	Vitamin K (μg)
	Age (yr) Condition	Weight[†] (kg)	(lb)	Height[†] (cm)	(in)	Protein (g)				
Women	11-14	46	101	157	62	46	800	10	8	45
	15-18	55	120	163	64	44	800	10	8	55
	19-24	58	128	164	65	46	800	10	8	60
	25-50	63	138	163	64	50	800	5	8	65
	51+	65	143	160	63	50	800	5	8	65
Pregnant						60	800	10	10	65
Lactating	First 6 mo					65	1300	10	12	65
	Second 6 mo					62	1200	10	11	65

Modified from National Academy of Sciences: *Recommended Dietary Allowances*, ed 10. Copyright 1989 by the National Academy of Sciences. Courtesy of the National Academy Press, Washington, DC.

*The allowances, expressed as average daily intakes over time, are intended to provide for individual variations among most normal persons as they live in the United States under usual environmental stresses. Diets should be based on a variety of common foods to provide other nutrients for which human requirements have been less well defined.

[†]Weights and heights of Reference Adults are actual medians for the U.S. population of the designated age, as reported by NHANES II. The median weights and heights of those under 19 years of age were taken from Hamill et al. (1979). The use of these figures does not imply that the height-to-weight ratios are ideal.

[‡]Retinol equivalents. 1 retinol equivalent = 1 μg retinol or 6 μg β-carotene.

[§]As cholecalciferol. 10 μg cholecalciferol = 400 IU of vitamin D.

[″]α-Tocopherol equivalents. 1 mg d-α tocopherol = 1 α-TE.

WATER SOLUBLE VITAMINS							MINERALS						
Vitamin C (mg)	Thiamin (mg)	Ribo-flavin (mg)	Niacin (mg NE)¶	Vitamin B_6 (μg)	Folate (μg)	Vitamin B_{12} (μg)	Calcium (mg)	Phos-phorus (mg)	Mag-nesium (mg)	Iron (mg)	Zinc (mg)	Iodine (μg)	Sele-nium (μg)
50	1.1	1.3	15	1.4	150	2.0	1200	1200	280	15	12	150	45
60	1.1	1.3	15	1.5	180	2.0	1200	1200	300	15	12	150	50
60	1.1	1.3	15	1.6	180	2.0	1200	1200	280	15	12	150	55
60	1.1	1.3	15	1.6	180	2.0	800	800	280	15	12	150	55
60	1.0	1.2	13	1.6	180	2.0	800	800	280	10	12	150	55
70	1.5	1.6	17	2.2	400	2.2	1200	1200	320	30	15	175	65
95	1.6	1.8	20	2.1	280	2.6	1200	1200	355	15	19	200	75
90	1.6	1.7	20	2.1	260	2.6	1200	1200	340	15	16	200	75

¶1 NE (niacin equivalent) is equal to 1 mg of niacin or 60 mg of dietary tryptophan.

The Food Pyramid

THE EASY WAY TO EAT RIGHT!

The Food Guide Pyramid is an outline of what to eat each day based on the Dietary Guidelines. It's not a rigid prescription but a general guide that lets you choose a healthful diet that's right for you.

The Pyramid calls for eating a variety of foods to get the nutrients you need and at the same time the right amount of calories to maintain healthy weight.

Use the Pyramid to help you eat better every day . . . the Dietary Guidelines way. Start with plenty of breads, cereals, rice, pasta, vegetables, and fruits. Add 2 to 3 servings from the milk group and 2 to 3 servings from the meat group. Remember to go easy on fats, oils, and sweets, the foods in the small tip of the Pyramid.

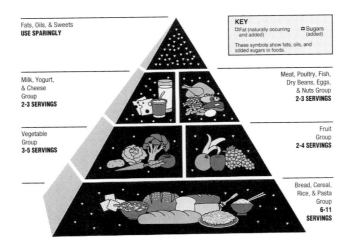

Fats, Oils, & Sweets
USE SPARINGLY

KEY
☐ Fat (naturally occurring and added)   ▨ Sugars (added)
These symbols show fats, oils, and added sugars in foods.

Milk, Yogurt, & Cheese Group
2-3 SERVINGS

Meat, Poultry, Fish, Dry Beans, Eggs, & Nuts Group
2-3 SERVINGS

Vegetable Group
3-5 SERVINGS

Fruit Group
2-4 SERVINGS

Bread, Cereal, Rice, & Pasta Group
6-11 SERVINGS

APPENDIX IX

Calcium

Food Sources of Calcium

	Serving Size	(mg)
Sardines	3 oz	372
Milk, skim	1 cup	300
Milk, whole	1 cup	290
Milk, buttermilk	1 cup	296
Cheese, cheddar	1 oz	210
Cheese, American	1 slice	195
Cheese, mozzarella	1 oz	163
Turnip greens, cooked	⅔ cup	184
Salmon	3 oz	167
Custard	½ cup	161
Tofu	3 oz	128
Ice cream	½ cup	99
Shrimp	3 oz	98
Spinach, cooked	½ cup	88
Broccoli, cooked	½ cup	68
Peanuts, roasted, with husks	⅔ cup	68
Green beans, cooked	½ cup	62
Egg, poached	1 large	51
Beans, cooked	½ cup	50
Cottage cheese	¼ cup	38
Almonds	12 nuts	38
Perrier water	1 cup	32
Cream cheese	1 oz	23
Fish, broiled	4½ oz	20
Bread, enriched white	1 slice	20
Wheat cereal, flakes	1 cup	12

From Cefalo RC, Moos M-K: *Preconceptional health care: a practical guide,* ed 2, St Louis, 1995, Mosby.

Elemental Calcium Available in Some Over-the-Counter Supplements

Brand	Amount of Calcium Carbonate (mg)	Amount of Elemental Calcium (mg)
Os-Cal 500	1250	500
Tums (low sodium)	500	200
Tums (extra strength)	750	300

From Cefalo RC, Moos M-K: *Preconceptional health care: a practical guide*, ed 2, St Louis, 1995, Mosby.

CALCIUM SUPPLEMENTS

Requirements
- Premenopausal women—at least 1000 mg of calcium/day
- Postmenopausal women not on hormonal replacement therapy—1500 mg calcium/day

List of Calcium Supplements and their Prices

Calcium Form	Calcium Per Tablet	Cost for 1 Month Supply*
Calcium Carbonate		
Highly concentrated and best supplement to take with a meal		
Generic 500 mg	500 mg	$
Generic 500 + D	500 mg	$
Generic 600 mg	600 mg	$
Generic 600 + D	600 mg	$
Generic w/Vitamin D and Minerals	600 mg	$
TUMS Regular Strength	400 mg	$$
TUMS Extra Strength	600 mg	$
TUMS Ultra	800 mg	$
Caltrate 600	600 mg	$$$$
Caltrate 600 + D	600 mg	$$
Caltrate w/Vitamin D and Minerals	600 mg	$$
Caltrate 600 + Soy	600 mg	$$$$
Oscal	500 mg	$$
Nature Made 600 + D	600 mg	$
Calcium Citrate		
Absorbed more easily. Less concentrated and therefore more expensive		
Citracal	400 mg	$$$
Citracal + D	500 mg	$$$
Cal Sure	500 mg	$$$$
Calcium Oxide and Hydroxide		
AdvaCal	450 mg	$$$$
Calcium Phosphate		
Posture-D	600 mg	$$

Modified from the Primary Care Operations Improvement Site prepared by the MGH Laboratory of Computer Science, 2001, The General Hospital Corporation.
*Approximate cost for 1 month supply for postmenopausal women taking 1500 mg/day.
$ $7.00-$9.00
$$ $9.50-$12.50
$$$ $13.00-$16.00
$$$$ $20.00 and over

Iron

Food Sources of Iron

	Service Size	Iron (mg)
Calf liver, cooked	3½ oz	14.2
Liverwurst	3 oz	8.7
Chicken livers, cooked	3½ oz	8.5
Prune juice	½ cup	5.2
Ground beef, lean, cooked	3½ oz	3.8
Chickpeas	½ cup	3.0
Steak, cooked	3 oz	2.7
Raisins	½ cup	2.5
Molasses	1 tablespoon	2.3
Prunes, large	4	2.2
Kidney beans	½ cup	2.2
Spinach, cooked	½ cup	2.0
Chicken	¼	1.8
Turkey	3 oz	1.5
Apricots, dried	4 halves	1.3
Avocado	½	1.3
Egg	1	1.1
Blueberries	⅝ cup	1.0
Bread, whole wheat	1 slice	0.8
Bread, enriched white	1 slice	0.6
Dry cereal	Read label; varies widely	

From Cefalo RC, Moos M-K: *Preconceptional health care: a practical guide,* ed 2, St Louis, 1995, Mosby.

Iron Supplements

	Amount of Elemental Iron (%)	Dose Containing 60 mg of Elemental Iron (mg)
Ferrous sulfate	20	300
Ferrous fumarate	32.5	185
Ferrous gluconate	11	545

From Cefalo RC, Moos M-K: *Preconceptional health care: a practical guide,* ed 2, St Louis, 1995, Mosby.

IRON SUPPLEMENTS

Requirements:
- 10-15 milligrams per day

List of Iron Supplements and Their Prices

Iron Supplement	Elemental Iron	Dosing	Cost Per 1 Month Supply ($)
Carbonyl Iron			
Generic Carbonyl Iron-50 mg	50 mg	3 caps a day	$15
Feosol Caplets	45 mg	3 caps a day	$23
Ferrous Fumarate			
Generic iron tablets (150 mg)	50 mg	3 tablets a day	$13
Ferro Sequels Tablets	50 mg	3 tablets a day	$29
Vitron C Tablets	66 mg	3 tablets a day	$19
Ferrous Sulfate			
Generic Ferrous Sulfate	50 mg	3 tablets a day	$21
Slow FE	50 mg	3 tablets a day	$34
Slow FE and Folic Acid	50 mg	3 tablets a day	$34
Ferrous Gluconate			
Fergon	27 mg	4 tablets a day	$11
Polysaccharide Iron Complex*†			
Niferex 150	150 mg	1 tablet a day	$13
Niferex Forte	150 mg	1 tablet a day	$18

Modified from the Primary Care Operations Improvement Site prepared by the MGH Laboratory of Computer Science, 2001, The General Hospital Corporation.

*Fewer side effects.

†Available by prescription only.

APPENDIX **XI**

Soy Supplementation

SOY

The Isoflavone levels in soybean, and, therefore, in any soybean foods, vary. Also many companies cannot say whether their isoflavone numbers include a sugarlike compound that accounts for about 40% of the isoflavone weight.

Drinks and Powders	Isoflavones (mg)	Protein (g)
Solgar Iso-Soy Powder (1 oz)	103	12
Twinlab Isoflavone Powder (1 tsp)	85	34
GeniSoy Natural Protein Powder (1 oz)	74	24
Whole Foods Vanilla Soy Protein Powder (1 oz)	43	24
Edensoy Original drink (8 oz)	41	20
Foods		
White Wave Baked Tofu (3 oz)	52	19
White Wave Tempeh (3 oz)	47	18
GeniSoy Protein Bar (2 oz - 1 bar)	33	14
Ensure, liquid (8 oz)	2	12
Pills		
Nature's Plus Ultra Isoflavone 100 (2)	100	0
Solray Genistein PhytoEstrogen (2)	56	0
Nature's Way Soy Isoflavones (2)	25	0

Company information/ abstracted from Center for Science in the Public Interest Nutrition Action Health Letter: Sept., 1998.

Common Herbal Interventions

Herbal Remedy	Use	Toxicity
Echinacea (Echinacea purpurea and augustifolia)	Stimulates immune system Prophylaxis for common cold	None
Feverfew (Tanacetum parthenium)	Headache treatment Premenstrual syndrome	Withdrawal syndrome: nervousness, headache, insomnia, stiffness, joint pain, and lethargy
Garlic (Allium sativum)	Relief of hemorrhoids Supplemental treatment for hypertension and atherosclerosis	Affects platelet aggregation
Ginkgo (Gingko biloba)	Improving memory and cognition	GI upset and headache Anti-platelet effect
Ginseng (Panax ginseng)	Sexual potency	Hypertension, vomiting, insomnia, headache and epistaxis, and hypoglycemia effect in Type II diabetics
Ma Huang (Ephedra sinica)	Weight loss	Hypertension, seizures, cardiac arrhythmias, death
Saw Palmetto (Serenoa repens)	Diuretic Prostatic hypertrophy	None
St. John's Wort (Hypericum perforatum)	Anxiety Depression Insomnia	Photosensitivity Interacts with tyramine-containing foods
Valerian (Valeriana officinalis)	Tranquilizer Weight control	None

Modified from Tyler VE: *The honest herbal: a sensible guide to the use of herbs and related remedies,* ed 3, Binghamton, New York, 1993, Pharmaceutical Products Press.
Additional information can be downloaded from the Federal Drug Administration (FDA) Website: http://vm.cfsan.fda.gov/-dms/supplmnt.html

Contraception

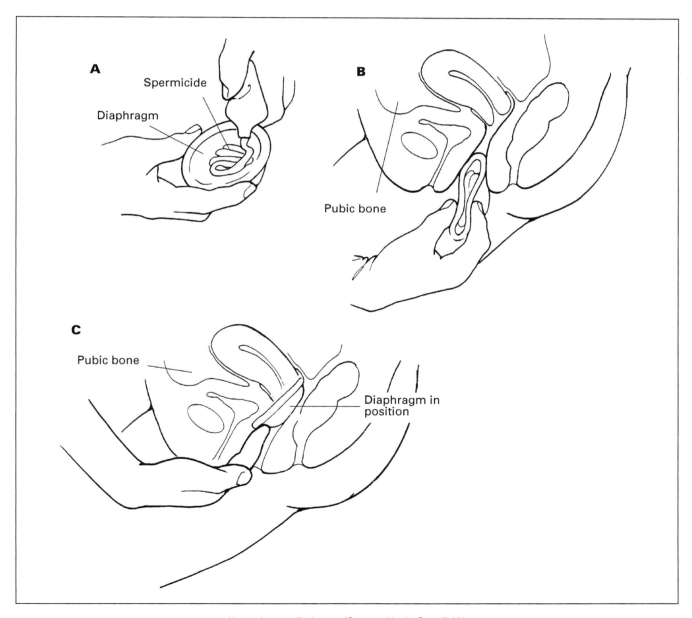

How to insert a diaphragm. (Courtesy Harriet Greenfield.)

Resources

ALCOHOLISM

National Clearinghouse for Alcohol and Drug Information (NCADI), PO Box 2345, Rockville, MD 20852, 1-800-729-6686.

National Council on Alcoholism and Drug Dependence, Inc., 12 West 21st Street, 8th Floor, New York, NY, 10010, 1-800-NCA-CALL.

Materials on alcoholism, fetal alcohol syndrome.

Relapse Prevention Hotline, 1-800-RELAPSE.

Self-Help Groups: AA, Al-Anon, Adult Children of Alcoholics, Narcotics Anonymous, Women for Sobriety.

Listings of meetings can be obtained from headquarter offices with telephone numbers in local directories.

The National Institute on Drug Abuse, Treatment referral hotline 1-800-662-4357.

For drug treatment facilities in local communities.

DEPRESSION

American Association of Suicidology, 2459 South Ave., Denver, CO 80222. For those who have experienced the suicide of someone close.

Depression after delivery, PO Box 1281, Morrisville, PA 19067, (215)295-3994. A resource, not a counselling service. Information request line: 1-800-944-4773.

For women experiencing postpartum depression.

Depression/Awareness, Recognition and Treatment (D/ART), National Institute of Mental Health, Room 15C-05, 5600 Fishers Lane, Rockville, MD 20857.

A federal government/private sector effort to inform primary health care providers, mental health specialists, and the general public about the most up-to-date treatments for depressive illness.

National Depressive and Manic Depression Association, Merchandise Mart, PO Box 3395, Chicago, IL 60654.

For depressed persons and their families.

National Foundation for Depressive Illness, Inc., PO Box 2257, New York, NY 10611, 1-800-248-4344.

Provides referrals to support groups.

PMS Access, PO Box 9326, Madison, WI 53715, 1-800-222-4PMS.

For information on PMS, PMS clinics, support groups.

The National Alliance for the Mentally Ill, 2101 Wilson Blvd., Suite 302, Arlington, VA 22201, (703)524-7600, 1-800-950-6264.

Provides information, emotional support, and advocacy through local and state affiliates for families.

PREGNANCY

American College of Obstetricians and Gynecologists (ACOG), 409 12th Street SW, Washington DC 20024-2188, 1-800-673-8444.

For educational pamphlets on subjects related to women's health.

Healthy Mother, Healthy Babies Coalition (or state chapters) 409 12th Street SW, Room 309, Washington DC 20024, (202)638-5577.

Information and education to improve maternal/infant health.

Local Planned Parenthood Clinic 1-800-230-PLAN(7526).

VIOLENCE

Child Help–Child Abuse Hotline, 1-800-422-4453.

Clearinghouse on Child Abuse and Neglect Information, PO Box 1182, Washington DC 20013, (703)821-2086.

Legal Aid Societies. Numbers are listed in local phone directories.

Local Rape Crisis Center, 1-800-656-HOPE(4673).

National Coalition Against Domestic Violence (NCADV), PO Box 15127, Washington DC 20003-0127, 1-800-333-SAFE.

A national organization of shelters and support service for battered women and their children.

National Organization for Women (NOW), 1000 16th Street NW, Suite 700, Washington DC 20036, (202)331-0066.

Parents United, 232 East Gish Rd., 1st floor, San Jose, CA 95112, (408)453-7616.

For abused children and for adults who were abused as children.

Index

t indicates tables; b indicates boxes; f indicates figures.

H